Basic Neurochemistry

Basic Neurochemistry

THIRD EDITION

EDITED BY

GEORGE J. SIEGEL, M.D.
University of Michigan Medical School,
Ann Arbor

R. WAYNE ALBERS, Ph.D.
National Institute of Neurological
and Communicative Disorders and Stroke,
Bethesda

BERNARD W. AGRANOFF, M.D.
University of Michigan Medical School,
Ann Arbor

ROBERT KATZMAN, M.D.
Albert Einstein College of Medicine
of Yeshiva University, Bronx

Little, Brown and Company   Boston

Library of Congress Catalog Card No. 80-83171

ISBN 0-316-79002-8

Printed in the United States of America

First edition, 1972, edited by R. Wayne Albers, Ph.D., George J. Siegel, M.D., Robert Katzman, M.D., and Bernard W. Agranoff, M.D.

HAL

Jordi Folch-Pi (1911–1979) was a major influence in the growth and development of neurochemistry. His scientific contributions involved studies on the structural components of the brain and the development of methods for their isolation and purification. He elucidated the nature of the cephalin fraction and, without access to the many sophisticated techniques available today, painstakingly determined the structure of phosphatidyl serine and of phosphoinositides. He recognized the importance of adequate methodology as a basis for conceptual progress, and his development of a simple method for the extraction of total brain lipids had a profound and lasting impact on the field of lipid biochemistry. His name is associated as well with studies on gangliosides, sulfatides, and proteolipids. He carried out pioneering studies on lipid-cation interactions and on the chemical maturation of the brain. In recent years, the proteolipids, the hydrophobic membrane proteins which he first described in 1951, became the dominant focus of his work, and he was increasingly occupied with consideration of their membrane-related functions.

In addition to his scientific contributions and international participation in decisions affecting neurochemistry, Folch was active in the formation of both the International and American societies for neurochemistry. His Catalan temperament dominated all his activities, and he pursued his love of life and the outdoors with the same intensity as his dedication to intellectual accomplishment. His colorful personality and incisive wit were loved by all.

In recognition of his wide-ranging contributions to neurochemistry and to neurochemists, the editors dedicate this volume to the memory of Jordi Folch-Pi.

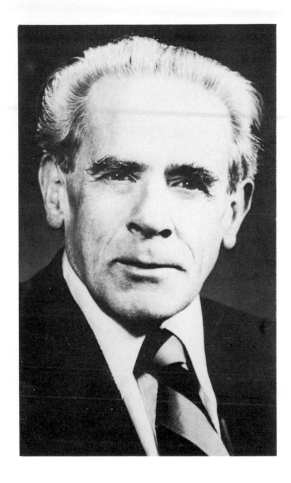

v

Preface

In this edition there are new chapters on the history of neurochemistry (Chap. 1), synaptic transmission (Chap. 8), the opioid peptides and receptors (Chap. 13), neuropeptides (Chap. 14), cytoskeleton proteins (Chap. 20), cell adhesion molecules (Chap. 21), the molecular structure and diseases of the myoneural junction (Chap. 26), and on biochemical hypotheses of mental disorders (Chap. 38). New information and concepts concerning molecular structure and biochemical regulation have been brought into existing chapters. Notable examples include calmodulin, the calcium regulatory protein (Chaps. 3, 6, 15, and 22), the pharmacological classification of aminergic receptors (Chap. 10), amino acid transmitter systems (Chap. 12), thromboxanes (Chap. 16), the molecular composition and growth of nerve terminals and synapses (Chaps. 19, 20, and 23), and, perhaps most exciting today, the use of tracers to produce three-dimensional images of the regional metabolism of intact functioning brain (Chap. 24).

This book is intended to be comprehensive in providing students and instructors with concepts and information pertinent to nervous system and muscle biochemistry. The balance between this objective and size containment is sometimes lost to one side or the other. Many of the chapters can be studied as separate units. Some chapters, combining subjects with a common focus but from widely dispersed literature—for example, ion transport, nucleic acid and protein metabolism, brain growth and regeneration, and muscle biochemistry—are long and are best studied by the beginning reader in sections. Some subjects, such as membrane composition and receptors, myelin, and metabolism of individual classes of brain constituents, are first taken up separately and then iteratively as related

to biochemical regulation, physiology, diseases, and behavior. Cross-references and the index guide the reader along these avenues. We have attempted to curtail bibliographies. Major secondary sources and key articles are marked with asterisks. Some portions of the second edition have been rearranged into other chapters in the third edition.

FROM THE PREFACE TO THE FIRST AND SECOND EDITIONS

In the past half century, neurochemistry has emerged as a distinct, if hybrid, discipline. Its unifying objective is the elucidation of biochemical phenomena that subserve activity of the nervous system or are associated with neurological diseases. For neurochemistry as for all of experimental biology, this unifying objective generates certain subsidiary goals: (1) isolation and identification of components, (2) determination of the functional interactions of the components, and (3) development of integrating hypotheses that account satisfactorily for the activities of the intact organ in terms of molecular events.

A comprehensive description of nervous system function in terms of molecular events presumably would supply intellectually satisfying and socially useful explanations of the neural responses that ultimately mediate mentation and behavior and their pathologies. Advances in neurochemistry already have led to a remarkable increase in our understanding of many of the inherited neurological disorders and to effective diagnostic techniques that may be employed both prenatally and postnatally. In another area, the identification of a deficiency in a specific neurotransmitter associated with Parkinson's disease has led to a useful therapy in this common disorder.

The validity and vitality of neurochemistry are proportionate to the successes of its practitioners in providing biochemical explanations for neural functions. These explanations cannot be derived from chemical analyses alone, and those who wish to contribute to this endeavor must be prepared to pursue various levels of structural and functional organization. The scope of neurochemistry is determined by the junctures that develop between the field of biochemistry and the fields of neurobiology, neurology, and the behavioral sciences. Neurochemists are crucially dependent upon data from these diverse subjects if they are to formulate functionally meaningful molecular hypotheses.

As a result, the student of neurochemistry must become familiar with concepts and information that are widely dispersed in the scientific literature. A number of neurochemistry courses have been organized in medical and graduate schools within recent years, and the organizers have become acutely aware of the difficulties in selecting the most significant material to place within the perspective of neurochemistry. Few existing books are at once comprehensive and sufficiently concise to be practical as texts in these courses.

A conference on neurochemistry curriculum considered these problems in June 1969 and made recommendations for the scope of the subject matter that subsequently was developed into the first edition of *Basic Neurochemistry*. It was anticipated that the experience gained through the construction and use of this text would initiate a continuing reappraisal of the field that could contribute to the evolution of later editions.

ACKNOWLEDGMENT

As with the first two editions, Helene Jordan Waddell, Director of the Rockefeller University Press, has brought to this book her outstanding knowledge of scientific writing, incisive editing, and devotion to scientific education. The editors are grateful for this continued fruitful association.

We thank Marjorie Lees for providing the biography and George Hauser for the photograph of Jordi Folch-Pi.

G.J.S.
R.W.A.
B.W.A.
R.K.

Contents

Part One. General Neurochemistry

Part Two. Medical Neurochemistry

Part Three. Behavioral Neurochemistry

Contributing Authors

Bernard W. Agranoff, M.D.
Professor of Biological Chemistry, Neuroscience Laboratory, Mental Health Research Institute, University of Michigan Medical School, Ann Arbor
Chapter 40

R. Wayne Albers, Ph.D.
Chief, Section on Enzymes, Laboratory of Neurochemistry, National Institute of Neurological and Communicative Disorders and Stroke, Bethesda, Maryland
Chapter 3

Stanley H. Appel, M.D.
Professor and Chairman, Department of Neurology, Baylor College of Medicine, Houston
Chapter 26

Jack D. Barchas, M.D.
Nancy Friend Pritzher Professor of Psychiatry, Stanford University School of Medicine, Stanford, California
Chapter 38

Samuel H. Barondes, M.D.
Professor of Psychiatry, University of California, San Diego, School of Medicine at La Jolla, California
Chapter 21

Joyce A. Benjamins, Ph.D.
Associate Professor of Neurology, Wayne State University School of Medicine, Detroit
Chapter 23

Philip A. Berger, M.D.
Director, Stanford Mental Health Clinical Research Center, Stanford University School of Medicine, Stanford, California
Chapter 38

Murray B. Bornstein, M.D.
Professor of Neurology and Neuroscience, Albert Einstein College of Medicine of Yeshiva University, Bronx, New York
Chapter 32

Roscoe O. Brady, M.D.
Chief, Developmental and Metabolic Neurology Branch, National Institute of Neurological and Communicative Disorders and Stroke, Bethesda, Maryland
Chapter 30

M. J. Brownstein, M.D.
Laboratory of Clinical Science, National Institute of Mental Health, Bethesda, Maryland
Chapters 11 and 14

David O. Carpenter, M.D.
Director, Division of Laboratories and Research, New York State Department of Health, Empire State Plaza, Albany
Chapter 8

Donald D. Clarke, Ph.D.
Professor and Chairman, Department of Chemistry, Fordham University, New York
Chapter 17

Joseph T. Coyle, M.D.
Associate Professor of Pharmacology and Psychiatry, The Johns Hopkins University School of Medicine, Baltimore
Chapter 10

Thomas E. Duffy, Ph.D.
Associate Professor of Biochemistry in the Department of Neurology, Cornell University Medical College, New York
Chapter 35

Pierre M. Dreyfus, M.D.
Professor and Chairman, Department of
Neurology, University of California, Davis,
School of Medicine
Chapter 33

Stanton B. Elias, M.D.
Professor of Neurology, Baylor College of
Medicine, Houston
Chapter 26

Robert A. Fishman, M.D.
Professor and Chairman, Department of
Neurology, University of California, San
Francisco, School of Medicine
Chapter 34

Harold Gainer, Ph.D.
Head, Section on Functional Neurochemistry,
National Institute of Child Health and Human
Development, Bethesda, Maryland
Chapter 14

Stanley E. Geel, Ph.D.
Adjunct Assistant Professor of Neurology,
University of California, Davis, School of Medicine
Chapter 33

John Gergely, M.D., Ph.D.
Director, Department of Muscle Research,
Boston Biomedical Research Institute, Boston
Chapter 27

Paul Greengard, Ph.D.
Professor of Pharmacology, Yale University
School of Medicine, New Haven, Connecticut
Chapter 15

Bertil Hille, Ph.D.
Professor of Physiology and Biophysics, University
of Washington School of Medicine, Seattle
Chapter 5

Jacob M. Hiller, Ph.D.
Research Assistant Professor of Medicine, New
York University School of Medicine, New York
Chapter 13

Y. Edward Hsia, B.M., M.R.C.P., D.C.H.
Professor of Genetics and Pediatrics, University
of Hawaii, Honolulu
Chapter 28

Robert Katzman, M.D.
Professor and Chairman, Department of
Neurology and Professor of Neuroscience, Albert
Einstein College of Medicine of Yeshiva University,
Bronx, New York
Chapter 25

Abel L. Lajtha, Ph.D.
Research Professor of Psychiatry, New York
University School of Medicine, New York
Chapter 17

Raymond J. Lasek, Ph.D.
Professor of Anatomy, Case Western Reserve
University, Cleveland
Chapter 20

F. C. MacIntosh, Ph.D.
Professor of Physiology, McGill University
Faculty of Medicine, Montreal, Quebec, Canada
Chapter 9

Henry R. Mahler, Ph.D.
Research Professor of Chemistry, Indiana
University, Bloomington, Indiana
Chapter 19

Howard S. Maker, M.D.
Associate Professor of Neurology, Mount Sinai
School of Medicine of the City University of New
York, New York
Chapter 17

David B. McDougal, Jr., M.D.
Professor of Pharmacology, Washington
University School of Medicine, St. Louis
Chapter 29

Bruce S. McEwen, Ph.D.
Associate Professor of Neurobiology, Rockefeller
University, New York
Chapter 39

Edith G. McGeer, Ph.D.
Professor and Acting Head, Department of
Neurological Sciences, University of British
Columbia, Vancouver, B.C., Canada
Chapter 12

Patrick L. McGeer, M.D., Ph.D.
Professor and Head, Department of Neurological
Sciences, University of British Columbia,
Vancouver, B.C., Canada
Chapter 12

Guy M. McKhann, M.D.
Kennedy Professor of Neurology and Chairman,
Department of Neurology, The Johns Hopkins
University School of Medicine, Baltimore
Chapter 23

Pierre Morell, Ph.D.
Professor of Biochemistry, University of North
Carolina School of Medicine, Chapel Hill
Chapter 32

James A. Nathanson, M.D., Ph.D.
Assistant Professor of Neurology and Affiliate
in Pharmacology, Harvard Medical School,
Boston
Chapter 15

Elizabeth F. Neufeld, Ph.D.
Chief, Section on Genetics and Biochemistry,
National Institute of Arthritis, Metabolism and
Digestive Diseases, Bethesda, Maryland
Chapter 31

William T. Norton, Ph.D.
Professor of Neurology (Neurochemistry) and
of Neuroscience, Albert Einstein College of
Medicine of Yeshiva University, Bronx, New York
Chapter 4

Sidney Ochs, Ph.D.
Professor of Physiology and Director of Medical
Biophysics Program, University of Indiana School
of Medicine, Indianapolis
Chapter 22

Fred Plum, M.D.
Professor and Chairman, Department of
Neurology, Cornell University Medical College,
New York
Chapter 35

Cedric S. Raine, Ph.D., D.Sc.
Professor of Pathology and Neuroscience, Albert
Einstein College of Medicine of Yeshiva University,
Bronx, New York
Chapters 2 and 32

Thomas S. Reese, M.D.
Head, Section on Functional Neuroanatomy,
National Institute of Neurological and
Communicative Disorders and Stroke, Bethesda,
Maryland
Chapter 8

Fredrick J. Samaha, M.D.
Professor and Chairman, Department of
Neurology, University of Cincinnati Medical
Center, Cincinnati
Chapter 27

Larry J. Shapiro, M.D.
Associate Professor of Pediatrics, University of
California, Los Angeles, School of Medicine
Chapter 31

Hitoshi Shichi, Ph.D.
Research Biochemist, National Institutes of
Health, Bethesda, Maryland
Chapter 7

George J. Siegel, M.D.
Professor of Neurology, University of Michigan
Medical School, Ann Arbor
Chapter 6

Eric J. Simon, Ph.D.
Professor of Medicine and Pharmacology, New
York University School of Medicine, New York
Chapter 13

Solomon H. Snyder, M.D.
Distinguished Service Professor of Pharmacology
and Psychiatry, The Johns Hopkins University
School of Medicine, Baltimore
Chapter 10

Louis Sokoloff, M.D.
Chief, Laboratory of Cerebral Metabolism,
National Institute of Mental Health, Bethesda,
Maryland
Chapter 24

Theodore L. Sourkes, Ph.D.
Professor of Biochemistry in the Department of
Psychiatry, McGill University Faculty of Medicine,
Montreal, Quebec, Canada
Chapters 36 and 37

William L. Stahl, Ph.D.
Professor of Physiology and Biophysics and
Medicine (Neurology), University of Washington
School of Medicine, Seattle
Chapter 6

Kunihiko Suzuki, M.D.
Professor of Neurology and Neuroscience,
Albert Einstein College of Medicine of Yeshiva
University, Bronx, New York
Chapter 18

Phillip D. Swanson, M.D., Ph.D.
Professor and Head, Division of Neurology,
Department of Medicine, University of
Washington School of Medicine, Seattle
Chapter 6

Donald B. Tower, M.D., Ph.D.
Director, National Institute of Neurological
and Communicative Disorders and Stroke,
Bethesda, Maryland
Chapter 1

Barry Wolf, M.D., Ph.D.
Assistant Professor of Human Genetics and
Pediatrics, Medical College of Virginia, Richmond
Chapter 28

Leonhard S. Wolfe, M.D., Ph.D.
Professor of Neurology and Neurosurgery and
Biochemistry, McGill University Faculty of
Medicine, Montreal, Quebec, Canada
Chapter 16

Basic Neurochemistry

Donald B. Tower

Chapter 1. Neurochemistry in Historical Perspective

Neurochemistry is today a mature, established discipline. It has become one of the principal neurosciences, but this is largely a post-World War II phenomenon. In fact, it is only during the last 35 years that the scientific community has come to recognize neurochemistry as a distinct discipline and that the name itself has become generally accepted. Many of us can remember when it was possible to know and keep track of virtually everything going on in the field. As neurochemistry comes to encompass a growing number and diversity of special research areas and subdisciplines, that is no longer possible.

Cornerstones of Neurochemistry

One may consider that there are four "cornerstones" upon which the development of neurochemistry rests. These are knowledge of the chemical composition of the nervous system, recognition of the metabolic bases for neural function, understanding of the chemical foundations for nerve impulse conduction and transmission, and the development of new methodologies.

FROM ALCHEMY TO CHEMISTRY: HENSING TO VAUQUELIN

Despite its relative newness, neurochemistry has its origins in work done in the eighteenth and earlier centuries [1]. The anatomy of the nervous system elucidated by Vesalius and by Willis; the circulation of the blood discovered by Harvey; and the important experiments on the physiology of muscle contraction, digestion, and respiration carried out by others [2-8] mark the beginnings of neurochemistry. The entrenched Aristotelian and Galenical doctrines of "vital" and "animal" spirits and the four "elements," or "humors," proved inadequate to

account for the inherent irritability of animal tissues, for muscle contraction, and for the observations involving isolated muscle and nerve-muscle preparations made by such seventeenth- and eighteenth-century physiologists as Glisson, Swammerdam, Haller, Whytt, Galvani, and Fontana. Other studies demonstrated that digestion of foodstuffs takes place in the absence of mechanical trituration, hence indicating the role of "ferments" in the process, as reported by Sylvius, Haller, Réamur, Stevens, and Spallanzani. A number of physiological and chemical experiments by Boyle, Hooke, Lower, Hales, Priestley, and others culminated in those of Lavoisier, who showed—literally in the midst of the French Revolution—that respiration is clearly analogous to combustion and that bodily oxidations result in the production of heat, carbon dioxide, and water. Others had identified the role of blood circulation through the lungs, but it was Spallanzani who first guessed that the actual site of respiration is at the tissue level. Clearly, these eighteenth-century accomplishments anticipate the emergence of biochemistry and provide important foundations for understanding metabolism in the nervous system.

Although neurosurgeons at the French Academy of Medicine were already deriving accurate knowledge of brain functions from studies of patients with head injuries, much of chemistry still languished in alchemical notions and suffered from inevitable inadequacies in methodology. This is particularly true of the earliest studies on the chemistry of brain and nerves. Like Plato and Aristotle, early seventeenth-century observers, including Bartholin, Burrhus, Lémery, and Leeuwenhoek, speculated on the "temperament" of the brain and its fatty nature, which they compared to spermaceti (a waxlike substance derived from whale oil) [1]. Prominent chemists of the time, such as Lémery, subjected body fluids and tissues, including brain, to the standard alchemical procedures of distillation, digestion, rectification, and calcination to obtain new and better medicinal remedies. However, the first detailed account of chemical analysis of brain tissue and the first report of the isolation of a specific brain substance (phosphorus) are given by the obscure Hessian physician Johann Thomas Hensing (1683–1726) in his monograph *Cerebri examen chemicum ex eodemque phosphorus singularem omnia inflammabilia accendentem*, published at Giessen in 1719 [1].

As one might expect, Hensing's approach was to examine the brain's nature *per ignem* (with fire, which was then the chemist's most powerful tool). According to Hensing, upon heating, beef brain yielded (in order of appearance) a very subtle "water," termed "spirituous"; a volatile, acrid "oil"; a "fixed salt" containing most of the "fixed water," or spirit; and finally, dry "earth" (the *caput mortuum* of the alchemist). He carefully described the isolation and identification of elemental phosphorus from 12 ounces of beef brain and likened it to phosphorus isolated earlier from urine and feces by Brand, Kunckel, and Homberg, and from minerals by Balduin. This was the "*phosphor mirabilis*" examined in detail by Robert Boyle in his 1680 treatise on noctilucence. Hensing, in discussing his own results, suggested that the various substances found in brain were somehow combined and wondered whether the phosphorus could be involved in the functioning of the "animal spirits" that were thought to originate in the brain [1, 9].

Historically, Hensing's work was little more than a curiosity. It had little impact on subsequent studies, although it was cited by Thouret, Sömmering, J. F. John, and Thudichum. During the next century, several inorganic and simple organic substances were isolated from brain, and Hamburger reported that on drying gray and white matter, about 81 percent and 69 percent, respectively, are volatilized. However, it was the analyses of Fourcroy (1793) and of his pupil Vauquelin (1811) that marked the beginnings of modern composi-

tional studies that would culminate in Thudichum's monumental work some fifty years later. Thus, Nicolas-Louis Vauquelin (1763–1829) found human brain to contain 80 percent water; 7 percent "albumen"; about 5 percent fatty materials (clearly distinct from ordinary fats and oils and from the spermaceti and soaps proposed by earlier investigators); "osmazomes" (equivalent to a meat extract); and salts (including phosphates of potash, lime, and magnesia, and common salt and sulfur) accounting for almost 8 percent. The present-day equivalents would be 77.0, 8.05, 11.0, and 3.95 percent, respectively. Except for his lipid analyses, which are low because at that time only alcohol was used as extractant, Vauquelin's data approximate those of Thudichum and present-day investigators [10].

Vauquelin, justifiably one of the leading scientists of his era, succeeded to the chair of chemistry at the Paris Faculté de Médecine in 1809. His teacher Fourcroy, a leading revolutionary, was successor to Lavoisier and a councillor of state under Napoleon. Although not politically involved, Vauquelin served the government in many important capacities. His intimate friends included Lavoisier, Berthollet, De Morveau, Gay-Lussac, Chevreul, and many others. He discovered several chemical elements and a number of organic compounds, including the first amino acid, asparagine. It is not surprising that his "Analyse de la matière cérébrale de l'homme et de quelques animaux" (*Annales de la Muséum d'histoire naturelle*, Vol. 18, pp. 212–239, 1811) had a prompt and widespread impact. The monograph was reprinted in leading French, German, and English scientific periodicals and served as a basis for most subsequent studies on brain chemistry. It is of interest that French chemistry flourished in the social and political turbulence of the Revolution and the First Empire.

FROM COMPOSITION TO METABOLISM:
THUDICHUM TO WINTERSTEIN
During the latter part of the eighteenth century and the beginning of the nineteenth, neurophysiology prospered and came to occupy the central role in studies of the nervous system [2, 4, 5, 8, 11, 12].

The importance of adequate blood supply and oxygen to brain and spinal cord functioning were recognized by Saunders, Monro, Legallois, Cooper, and Brown-Séquard. There were studies by Fontana on the effects of venoms, alcohol, and opium on brain function. These were followed by Davy's observations on the effects of nitrous oxide and the subsequent introduction of other anesthetics. But the great contributions of nineteenth-century neurophysiology concern the functional organization of the nervous system. These included concepts of reflex function put forward by Bell, Hall, and Müller; elucidation of the autonomic nervous system and neural inhibition by the Weber brothers and others; observations on nerve impulse velocity by Helmholtz; and studies of the effects of curare on muscle excitability by Bernard. In the exploration of the central nervous system, the ablation and deafferentation studies by Flourens and by Goltz were especially relevant to subsequent electrophysiological studies that used techniques introduced primarily by DuBois-Reymond. These studies led to the earliest recording of the electroencephalogram by Caton and to the work of Fritsch and Hitzig and Ferrier on stimulation and the electrical excitability of the brain.

During this same period, the development of another major branch of neurology, neuroanatomy, received important impetus from significant improvements in the microscope and from the development of better and more selective histological fixation, sectioning, and staining techniques. The axon, the nerve cell body, dendrites, myelin sheath, glia, and synapse were described by Purkinje, Schwann, Waller, Deiters, Golgi, Nissl, Cajal, and Hortega. Their work provided the structural and cytological bases for the advances being made by the neurophysiologists in the understanding of function.

As the nineteenth century began, organic chemistry burst upon the scene, and a new discipline, biochemistry, emerged [3, 5–7, 13, 14]. From Sweden, there were contributions by Scheele and Berzelius on the concept of organic compounds and methods for their isolation and study. France contributed the discoveries of Berthollet, Fourcroy, and especially Chevreul in lipid chemistry and those of Dumas and Vauquelin on analytical techniques and organic nitrogen-containing compounds. And there were Liebig and Wöhler from Germany, who contributed most importantly to the elucidation of the nature of organic compounds found in plants and animals and to the concept of *Stoffwechsel*, or metabolism—the assimilation, utilization, functional significance, degradation, and excretion of various compounds by living organisms. Liebig served as professor of chemistry at the University of Giessen in Hesse from 1826 to 1852. His was not the first university chemistry laboratory—Lomonosov's in Moscow in 1748 and Thomson's in Glasgow in 1817 preceded his—but Liebig's was the first to offer organized laboratory instruction in chemistry [1, 7]. Moreover, in 1832 he inaugurated the *Justus Liebig's Annalen der Chemie,* one of the earliest media for biochemical communication.

There are several interesting coincidences in the history of neurochemistry. Liebig was appointed professor at Giessen in 1826, the centenary year of the death of Hensing, who had also served as professor of natural and chemical philosophy at the same university. Moreover, one of Liebig's students was Thudichum, who acknowledged his debt to Liebig for the instruction and research inspiration he received as a student and noted that his most prized possession was the analytical combustion train that Liebig gave him and that he used for his analyses of the chemical composition of the brain [15, 16].

With the studies by Liebig and such contemporaries as Wöhler, Kühne and Hoppe-Seyler, organic chemistry and biochemistry rapidly emerged as special branches of chemistry and disciplines in their own right. Progress in organic chemistry continued with the work by Kossel on cytochemistry, proteins, and nucleic acids; Fischer on carbohydrates; Pasteur on stereochemistry; and Faraday, Kekulé, and van't Hoff and Ostwald on gas diffusion, osmotic forces, and dialysis. Biochemistry advanced with the contributions by Bernard, Pasteur, and Büchner on fermentation and enzymes; Pflüger, Hoppe-Seyler and Mac-Munn on respiratory oxidation in tissues; Fick,

Bernard, and Fletcher and Hopkins on the association of carbohydrate utilization and lactic acid production with muscle contraction.

These investigations presaged the surge of research activity early in the present century: the development by Haldane and Barcroft of techniques to analyze blood and tissue gases; the studies by Harden, Neuberg, Embden, and Meyerhof on glycolysis; and the work by Vernon, Batelli and Stern, Winterstein, Wieland, Keilin, Thunberg, Warburg, and many others on tissue oxidation and respiratory pigments. In addition, there were a number of special but significant developments: the discovery of vitamins and their relation to nutritional deficiency states by Eijkman, Goldberg, and Funk; the recognition by Dumas of the role of iodine in goiter; the elucidation by von Mering and Minkowski and Banting and Best of the role of the pancreas and the insulin isolated from it in diabetes; the emergence of the science of genetics and the recognition by Garrod of inborn errors of metabolism and the biochemical basis of genetics; the discovery of x-rays and of radioactive isotopes (by Roentgen and the Curies); the application of radioactive isotopes by Hevesy to biochemical (plant) systems; and the introduction by Tswett of chromatographic techniques [3, 5–7, 13, 17, 18].

All of the foregoing discoveries, as well as many others not mentioned, are important to neurochemistry, but the recognition of this fact did not come rapidly. Much of the problem is referable to the organizational and chemical complexities of the nervous system, which required better investigational techniques than the nineteenth and early twentieth centuries provided. Between the work of Vauquelin in 1811 and that of Thudichum in 1884, there was only modest progress in knowledge of the nervous system's composition [1]. Cholesterol was isolated from brain by Gmelin; lecithin by Gobley and Strecker; phosphatides by Kühne, Couërbe, Frémy, and Gobley; and fatty acids and other simple compounds by most of these workers. J-P. Couërbe (1807–1867) was the first to carry out elementary analyses of the compounds that he isolated (e.g., cholesterol), and he emphasized the importance of phosphorus-containing compounds.

He concluded that phosphorus is the excitation principle of the nervous system. However, it fell to an expatriate German physician in London to put brain chemistry on the scientific "map."

Johann Ludwig Wilhelm Thudichum (1829–1901) was born in Büdingen, Hesse, and graduated with a medical degree from Giessen in 1851. He was forced to emigrate because his political activities made it impossible for him to secure an appointment in Germany [15, 16]. He settled in London in 1853 and established a medical practice in otology and rhinology. Between 1865 and 1882 he devoted much of his time to investigations of brain chemistry, supported by grants of about £2,900 ($15,000) from the Privy Council and the Local Government Board (the predecessor of the British Medical Research Council) to conduct research on the chemical identification of disease. It may seem surprising that Thudichum was supported by the mid-Victorian equivalent of the modern, federally funded research grant, since we tend to view this mechanism as a post–World War II phenomenon. However, it is far from new: Hensing's research in 1719 was supported by grants from the local government in the person of the Landgraf of Hesse-Darmstadt; and in the 1860s, Thudichum was only one of a number of investigators supported by the Local Government Board. Like today's grantees, he did not always stick to the original subject. He never discovered much about brain diseases, but he did a stupendous job in his chemical analyses of the human brain.

The complete studies appeared as a progress report to the Local Government Board for the year 1874 and were published in 1884 as *A Treatise on the Chemical Constitution of the Brain—Based Throughout upon Original Researches* [19]. The monograph was translated into Russian a year later; a second German edition appeared in 1901, the year of the author's death. Thudichum made three major contributions to neurochemistry: he developed important new analytical techniques; he isolated and identified a number of specific chemical constituents of the brain; and he carried out an extraordinarily accurate quantitative analysis of all known constituents of various areas of the human brain. Incidentally, he provided in his publications important historical commentaries on previous studies extending back to Hensing and earlier. Thus, Thudichum isolated and characterized the phosphatides (lecithin and the cephalins), sphingomyelin, the sulfatides and cerebrosides, cholesterol, and most of the trace solutes. He recognized phosphatides as combinations of phosphoglyceric acid with fatty acids (oleic, stearic, and palmitic) and a base (choline, ethanolamine or an unidentified compound); cerebrosides as phosphate-free nitrogen compounds containing galactose; and sphingosine as the basic unit in sphingomyelin. He is responsible for the flowery Greek terminology which has come down to us as the names for most of these constituents. Thudichum believed that he must have complete data on the normal before he could proceed to the study of the abnormal and disease. However, he was convinced that "... it is probable that by the aid of chemistry many derangements of the brain and mind, which are at present obscure, will become accurately definable and amenable to precise treatment, and what is now an object of anxious empiricism will become one for the proud exercise of exact science" [19, pp. 259–260].

Thudichum is one of the neurochemical pioneers whose work forms one of the cornerstones—that of chemical composition and architecture—of today's discipline. In the succeeding half century, only a few investigators carried on similar lines of study, primarily Levine and Waldemar and Mathilde Koch. After Thudichum the emphasis shifted to investigations of the chemical bases of metabolism and function. Today, however, the chemical architecture of the nervous system is again under study.

As part of the general nineteenth-century interest in metabolism, the methods and concepts were inevitably applied to the nervous system. These studies were not numerous; it would be well into the present century before the pace quickened. Nevertheless, the beginnings are discernible toward the end of the nineteenth century [1, 20]. These studies included observations on the blood-brain barrier by Ehrlich; correlation of increased neural activity (induced by electrical stimulation or strychnine)

with increased production of lactic acid, observations quantified on excised samples of spinal cord and brain by Moleschott and Battistini in 1887; and a number of studies on cerebral metabolism in vivo and on frog spinal cord–nerve-muscle preparations in vitro. It is surprising how many early attempts were made to study cerebral metabolism by using simultaneous carotid artery–jugular vein blood level differences in cholesterol, phosphate, sugar, and blood gases. The most ambitious studies on arteriovenous differences in oxygen and carbon dioxide across the cerebral circulation were carried out between 1895 and 1914, principally by Hill and Nabarro, Jensen, and Alexander. Jensen found cerebral blood flow in the dog to be $138 \text{ ml} \cdot 100\text{g}^{-1} \cdot \text{min}^{-1}$, and Alexander and Révész reported the oxygen consumption of "resting" dog brain to be about $600 \, \mu\text{mol} \cdot 100\text{g}^{-1} \cdot \text{min}^{-1}$ (as recalculated by Himwich). These results compare to present-day values for the dog brain of about 60 ml and about $160 \, \mu\text{mol}$, respectively—the discrepancy being the result of measurements by the early workers of what amounted to total head circulation and their overly generous calculation of the cerebral portion.

There were equally impressive in vitro studies, especially those begun in 1907 by Hans Winterstein (1879–1963). He was born in Prague; educated at Prague, Jena, and Göttingen; and served successively as director of the Physiological Institute at Rostock and professor of physiology at Breslau, Istanbul, and Munich. At his death in 1963, Winterstein was the dean of German physiologists [21].

During the period from 1907 to about 1920, he used isolated frog spinal cord–nerve-muscle preparations to investigate the respiration of the spinal cord, its glucose and oxygen utilization and lactate production, and the effects thereon of changes in temperature, osmotic pressure, ionic composition, and of stimulation and narcosis. These studies provided a wealth of data, which Winterstein summarized in his extensive review of central nervous system metabolism published in 1929 [20]. Winterstein is clearly another of the neurochemical pioneers who did much to set in place the metabolic cornerstone of today's discipline. He was followed by a number of others like Batelli and Stern, MacArthur and Jones, Warburg, Szent-Györgyi, Quastel, and many others. Slices or breis of neural tissues were mainly used in their studies. Considerable impetus was given to such work by the introduction of the methods and apparatus for studies of tissue metabolism developed by Otto Warburg. Many graduate students, including myself, began their research on the Warburg apparatus, and manometric studies of brain-slice metabolism continued to be one of the principal experimental approaches.

METABOLISM AND FUNCTION: QUASTEL, PETERS, DALE, LOEWI, AND CANNON

Early studies in the present century were concerned primarily with respiratory and glycolytic metabolism, but the molecular bases for the utilization of oxygen by tissue cells were already being formed [6, 18, 20, 22]. The indophenol oxidase reaction, discovered by Ehrlich, was studied in a variety of tissues, including brain. (This reaction is still used for histochemical purposes.) Warburg believed that these reactions were attributable to an iron-containing respiratory ferment, analogous to hemoglobin—an idea propounded earlier by Spitzer. At the same time, Wieland and Thunberg both found evidence of the existence of hydrogen donors (like glucose) and hydrogen acceptors, concepts confirmed for neural tissues by Winterstein. In 1925, Keilin isolated and identified as cytochromes the "myohaematin" and "histohaematin" described 40 years earlier by MacMunn [18]. Together with Warburg's identification in 1932 of the "yellow enzyme" (various flavoproteins containing flavine-adenine dinucleotide) and cozymase, later designated coenzymes I and II (and still later, the di- and triphosphopyridine nucleotides, DPN and TPN, and now the nicotinamide-adenine dinucleotides, NAD and NADP), these contributions provided the keys to our understanding of the links between glycolysis, the dehydrogenases, and oxygen requirements in tissues [18, 22]. It remained only for the work on the tricarboxylic acid cycle by Szent-Györgyi, Quastel, and Krebs and on the functions of phosphocreatine by Meyerhof to

usher in the modern era of intermediary metabolism [23–25]. Today, neurochemists probably consider the Krebs cycle (tricarboxylic acid or citric acid cycle) mundane, but in medical school less than 40 years ago, these were very new concepts that students and professors were learning together.

The studies of Sir Rudolph Peters, just 50 years ago, on B-vitamin deficiency in pigeons [1, Fig. 10] are especially relevant, because they emphasized the correlation of neural metabolism with neural function and introduced the concept of the "biochemical lesion." When Peters placed pigeons on a polished-rice diet, the birds developed muscular weakness, ataxia, and opisthotonus, correlated with a pronounced accumulation of lactic acid in brain tissues. He conclusively demonstrated that these changes were due to a dietary deficiency of the B-vitamin thiamine and showed that administration of the vitamin in vivo rapidly corrected both symptomatology and biochemical abnormalities and that the latter could be corrected by adding the vitamin in vitro. Peters helped to establish the role of vitamins as coenzymes, put forth the concept of biochemical lesions, and contributed significantly to our understanding of that crucial link between glycolysis and oxidative metabolism, the oxidative decarboxylation of pyruvate [26].

In the 1930s, two of neurochemistry's great pioneers were Peters and fellow Briton Judah H. Quastel, to whom we are indebted for much of what we know today about details of brain metabolism. Quastel's research has been done primarily with brain slices and homogenates in vitro. When I first went to the Montreal Neurological Institute in 1947, Quastel was at work just down the street, and many of my earliest experimental studies utilized the methods and findings that he had published in the *Biochemical Journal* over the previous 15 years. My preceptor was K. A. C. Elliott, who, with Quastel and Irvine H. Page, edited one of the first modern texts on neurochemistry [27]. Elliott [28] has written a warm appreciation of "Q," as Quastel is known to his friends, and points out that "...Q was the first modern biochemist to work extensively in the field [brain chemistry] and he remains one of the leaders in it." Quastel now is busily at work at the University of British Columbia in Vancouver, still pioneering in new neurochemical areas.

CONDUCTION AND TRANSMISSION OF NERVE IMPULSES

Even as these contributions to the metabolic cornerstone of neurochemistry were evolving, the components of the third great cornerstone were being assembled. In the nineteenth century and before, there had been an increasing identification of electricity with the nerve impulse. From studies by Fontana, Galvani, Volta, and many others, the great electrophysiologist DuBois-Reymond had by 1877 accepted the logic of such views, but speculated that these electrical phenomena might well have a chemical basis [11]. Already there were a number of pieces of circumstantial evidence: the effects, demonstrated by Claude Bernard, of curare on blocking nerve stimulation of muscle while the muscle itself remains excitable; the anesthetic properties of nitrous oxide, ether, and chloroform as researched particularly by Snow, and the anticonvulsant properties of bromide, discovered by Locock in 1857, and of phenobarbital, introduced by Hauptmann in 1912 [12]; and the actions of nicotine and pilocarpine on ganglia and muscles, reported by Langley in 1890. In 1904, shortly after Schäfer isolated a pressor principle from the adrenal gland, T. R. Elliott emphasized the parallelism of actions of "adrenalin" and that of sympathetic nerves. In 1906, analogous observations were made by Dixon for muscarine and parasympathetic nerves, and Hunt and Taveau noted the remarkable physiological properties of acetylcholine. Sir Henry Dale [29] in 1914 observed the "muscarinic" and "nicotinic" actions of acetylcholine and its rapid destruction by tissues. In 1921, Otto Loewi [30] published his first paper on the *Vagusstoff*, which was liberated upon stimulation of the frog vagus nerve to the heart and could be detected by its effect in decreasing cardiac contraction when passed in the perfusate to a second heart preparation—an effect that could be blocked by atropine. In that same year, Walter Cannon [31] reported on the liberation from sympathetic nerves of an adrenalin-like substance that he called "sympathin." This was later identified as norepinephrine by von Euler. Subsequent studies on Vagusstoff by Dale showed it to be identical to acetylcholine and led Dale to propose in 1933 the classification of nerves into cholinergic and adrenergic. Further studies by Dale with Feldberg, Gaddum, M. Vogt, and many others, and by Eccles, established acetylcholine as the principal transmitter of nerve impulses at the neuromuscular junction, at preganglionic sympathetic synapses, and at many central synapses. Another significant contribution was made to the field of neurochemistry by David Nachmansohn, who elucidated mechanisms of synthesis and enzymatic inactivation of acetylcholine. Comparable studies on norepinephrine as the first of the catecholamine transmitters were conducted by von Euler, with a great many subsequent contributors, such as Brodie, Udenfriend, and Axelrod [32–38].

To these pioneering investigations of the neurochemical bases of neuronal transmission, we must add the dawning recognition of the role of electrolytes as the basis for action potentials and axonal conduction. Liebig had originally proposed an intracellular locus for potassium and an extracellular locus for sodium. But the membrane studies by Young, Ostwald, Höber, and especially by Nernst and Bernstein at the beginning of the present century anticipated the definitive studies on the squid giant axon, begun in 1939 by Hodgkin and Huxley and continued by Keynes, Cole, and Goldman, among others [39]. There have been many contributors to the elucidation of neuronal conduction and transmission, and no such brief listing can fully do them justice.

METHODOLOGICAL DEVELOPMENT

As World War II began, three of the four cornerstones of neurochemistry had been firmly set in place: the chemical composition and architecture of the nervous system; the metabolic bases for neural function and dysfunction; and the chemical bases for the conduction and transmission of nerve impulses. Why, then, was neurochemistry still not recognized as a distinct discipline by 1941? It was, I think, primarily because many of the essential technical and methodological tools were still lacking. Surely it is largely because of the methodological developments of the 1950s and 1960s that neurochemistry emerged as a discipline and is flourishing today. This factor of methodological developments is what I consider to be the fourth cornerstone of modern neurochemistry. Of course, one must not overlook the impetus provided by the significant postwar increases in research funding, provided mainly, but not exclusively, by the U.S. National Institutes of Health. Other federal and many private research funds, as well as those of medical research councils in other countries, have been important factors. These funding sources made possible the exploitation of methodologies for rapid expansion of our horizons of knowledge. What, then, are some of the key technological developments that comprise this last cornerstone of modern neurochemistry?

Most of us who belong to the post–World War II generations of neurochemists cannot appreciate what research was like in the 1920s and 1930s. Then, relatively few biochemicals were available commercially. One had to devise one's own apparatus, fabricate and repair one's own specialized glassware, prepare one's own enzyme preparations and special reagents like ATP—in fact, almost all the necessities for conducting experiments. One of the most important technological advances since the 1940s has been the commercial availability of complex and unusual biochemical reagents, including enzymes, and growing arrays of analytical equipment and instrumentation, all at affordable prices.

Historically, one of the oldest analytical techniques in biochemistry is chromatography, developed in 1906 by the Russian Mikhail Tswett, who used the technique to separate plant pigments on calcium carbonate columns [6]. However, it was not until the 1940s, when Dent and others introduced paper chromatography, that the versatility of the chromatographic method became appreciated. We have only to recall that its use by Eugene Roberts led to the discovery of γ-aminobutyric acid in brain [40]. Subsequently, thin-layer, column, gas-liquid, and other varieties of chromatography have provided one of the neurochemist's most essential and versatile techniques for preparation, isolation, and analysis. There is also the closely related development of electrophoresis, invented by Tiselius in Sweden and made capable of wide application by the paper techniques developed by Durrum and others. Subsequent derivative procedures have nicely complemented chromatographic methods. In many cases, the use of radioisotopes is an integral part of these and other techniques. Again, the post–World War II growth of the nuclear energy industry was needed to make the biochemical use of radioisotopic techniques generally feasible, but in 1923 Georg Hevesy in Denmark had pioneered the use of radioisotopes in studies on plant metabolism. He showed that thorium B, a radioactive isotope of lead, is handled in an identical manner to stable lead and thus established the basis for the use of isotopes in biochemical research [3, 6].

For cellular and subcellular studies, four other technologies have proved invaluable. The first was the development by Ruska of a practical electron microscope and the adaptation in the 1950s of the electron microscopic fixation and staining techniques developed by Claude and Palade to the special problems posed by neural tissues. For this we are indebted to Fernández-Morán, Wyckoff and Young, Sjöstrand, Hartmann, Luse, Gray, De Robertis, Palay, and many others. Not only has electron microscopy taught us much about the fine structure of the nervous system, it has also greatly enhanced the utility of subcellular fractionation and tissue culture techniques. Subcellular fractionation depended on the development of appropriate ultracentrifugation technology, accomplished primarily by Svedberg, and its adaptation to biological preparations by Claude, Porter, Palade, Siekevitz, and DeDuve, among others [3, 6]. For the nervous system, studies initiated by Palade, Siekevitz, De Robertis, and Whittaker made it possible to investigate such cellular elements as nerve endings (synaptosomes) and synaptic vesicles, mitochondria, and endoplasmic reticulum, and to isolate membrane subfractions, lysosomes, and the like. Several other developments, such as the amino acid sequencing techniques for protein structure worked out by Sanger and the x-ray diffraction studies by Kendrew and Perutz, had important implications for neurochemistry. Tissue culture, originated in the early 1900s by Harrison and Carrel and refined much later by Enders, Eagle, and Gey [41], was not easily applied to the nervous system because of its cellular heterogeneity and complexity. But, again, the work of such pioneers as Margaret Murray, Pomerat, Peterson, Bornstein, Crain, and Hild has permitted unique studies of the neurochemical characteristics of specific glial cell types, investigation of cellular maturation and development of synaptic contacts and myelin sheaths, and studies of the effects of nerve growth factor (discovered by Levi-Montalcini) [42]. Histochemical and microcytochemical techniques have been as valuable as those discussed above in probing the intimate details of cellular architecture and metabolism. These techniques include the fluorescent histochemical procedures developed by Falck and Hillårp and the quantitative cytochemical techniques introduced by Linderstrøm-Lang, Holter, Caspersson, and others. Such neurochemical pioneers as Oliver Lowry, Alfred Pope, and Holger Hydén adapted and elaborated cytochemical methods for the special demands of neural cells and tissues [43].

Other significant methodological contributions were the lipid extraction and analytical techniques designed for the study of neural lipids by Sperry, Klenk, Rossiter, Folch-Pi, and many others; the studies of axoplasmic flow pioneered by Paul A. Weiss, further developed by Ochs, and applied to the retrograde transport of horseradish peroxidase and other proteins by the LaVails; the techniques for measuring cerebral blood flow and metabolism pioneered by Himwich and Gibbs and Lennox in the 1930s and refined in recent years by Kety and Schmidt, Scheinberg, Sokoloff, Ingvar and Lassen, and others; the immunochemical studies on myelin encephalitogenic proteins originated by Rivers and Kabat and Morgan and definitively developed by Kies and Alvord; and the numerous techniques for identifying and studying the various neural transmitters and their receptors. In connection with neural transmitters and receptors, we should not overlook the value of exotic preparations, such as the squid giant axon and the electroplax of the elec-

tric eel, and the value of uniquely specific toxin reagents like fluoroacetate, tetrodotoxin, α-bungarotoxin, and botulinum toxin. In fact, the list is open-ended, but the foregoing examples illustrate the importance of postwar technologies as the last of the cornerstones of neurochemistry.

The Postwar Neurochemical Community

It is difficult to achieve any satisfactory historical perspective for these last three decades. The time span is too short, many developments and trends are still in evolution, and one's own involvement as an active participant tends to blur objectivity. Thus, the end of the story is necessarily incomplete, but some elements can and should be recorded. Surely, one important factor has been the development of a neurochemical "community," first through periodic international symposia, then through the establishment of a journal, and finally through the founding of international and national societies.

In the early 1950s, a group of what must now seem like the "old guard" organized a series of five international neurochemical symposia. The first, on the biochemistry of the developing nervous system, was held in 1954 at Oxford and was organized by Joel Elkes, Louis Flexner, Jordi Folch-Pi, Seymour Kety, and Heinrich Waelsch (United States) and G. W. Harris and Derek Richter (Great Britain) [44]. Others at that meeting included Ansell, Blaschko, Coxon, Feldberg, McIlwain, and Peters (Great Britain); Brante and Hydén (Sweden); Bauer and Klenk (Germany); Palladin and Vladimirov (USSR); and Gerard, Himwich, Lajtha, LeBaron, Lowry, Nachmansohn, Pope, Sperry, and Weil-Malherbe (United States).

In 1956, a second symposium was held at Aarhus, Denmark, on the topic of the metabolism of the nervous system [45]. Most of the same group were present, augmented by, among others, Elliott and Rossiter (Canada); Cumings and Vogt (Great Britain); von Euler and Svennerholm (Sweden); Gjessing (Norway); Lowenthal (Belgium); Magnes (Israel); Mandel (France); and Larrabee, Korey, Schmitt, Sokoloff, and Udenfriend (United States). At the third symposium, held in Strasbourg, France, in 1958 on the subject of the chemical pathology of the nervous system [46], most of the remaining international community became involved. The fourth and fifth symposia followed in 1960 at Varenna on Lake Como, Italy, and in 1962 at St. Wolfgang, Austria, on the subjects, respectively, of regional neurochemistry [47] and comparative neurochemistry [48].

Several other developments deserve mention. One was the Millbank Conference on the Biology of Mental Health and Disease [49] held in New York City in November 1950 with most of the North American investigators in attendance. Two texts were published in 1955, one from North America by Elliott, Page, and Quastel [27] and the other from England by McIlwain [50]; these enjoyed immediate and widespread acceptance. The first of six Soviet conferences on neurochemistry was organized by A. V. Palladin [51] in Kiev in 1953 on the biochemistry of the nervous system [52]. Subsequent conferences were held in Kiev in 1957; in Yerevan, Armenia, in 1962; in Tartu, Estonia, in 1966; in Tbilisi, Georgia, in 1968; and in Leningrad in 1971. These meetings were attended by leading Soviet neurochemists, including V. A. Engelhardt (Moscow); E. M. Kreps, N. N. Demin, M. I. Prokhorova, and I. A. Sytinsky (Leningrad); A. V. Palladin (Kiev); P. A. Kometiani (Tbilisi); and H. Ch. Buniatian (Yerevan).

These symposia focused attention on neurochemistry as an emerging discipline and served to bring together neurochemists from most parts of the world, two processes that were materially assisted by the founding of the *Journal of Neurochemistry* in 1957. It was launched by Pergamon Press (Oxford) as an international journal. Its original editorial board consisted of Engelhardt (Moscow), Engström (Stockholm), Folch-Pi (Waverley), Kety (Bethesda), Klenk (Köln), Pope (Waverley), Richter (London), Rossiter (London, Ontario), M. Vogt (Cambridge), and Waelsch (New York). Volume 1 of the journal contained 376 pages. It has grown to two annual volumes totaling more than 3,500 pages and has engendered a number of "competitors."

By the mid 1960s, neurochemistry had become mature and active enough to form its own professional societies. The International Society for Neurochemistry (ISN) grew out of several preliminary organizational meetings in Göteborg and, notably, in Oxford in 1965, and held its first meeting in Strasbourg, France, in 1967, under the auspices of the original council, composed of Folch-Pi (Secretary), Richter (Treasurer), Hydén, Klenk, McIlwain, Mandel, Palladin, Pope, Rossiter (subsequently appointed Chairman), and Takagaki. There have been subsequent meetings in Milan (1969), Budapest (1971), Tokyo (1973), Barcelona (1975), Copenhagen (1977), Jerusalem (1979), and Nottingham (1981). The ISN has over 600 members from 35 countries. In October 1969, Pergamon Press relinquished ownership of the *Journal of Neurochemistry* to the ISN, which operates it as its official journal.

During the same period, the American neurochemical community established The American Society for Neurochemistry (ASN). The ASN was founded by Folch-Pi, Tower, and Tourtellotte in 1968 and held its first meeting in 1969 in Albuquerque, New Mexico. The original organizing committee comprised Agranoff, Folch-Pi (Secretary), Gál, Kety, Lajtha, LeBaron (subsequently appointed President), Mahler, McKhann, E. Roberts, Tourtellotte, Tower (Treasurer), and Wolfgram. Since then, the ASN has met yearly as follows: Hershey (1971), Seattle (1972), Columbus, Ohio (1973), New Orleans (1974), Mexico City (1975), Vancouver (1976), Denver (1977), Washington (1978), Charleston, SC (1979), Houston (1980), and Richmond (1981). Its membership exceeds 800 from 8 Canadian provinces, 43 states in the United States, 3 Latin American countries, and 12 countries outside the Western Hemisphere. It has sponsored publication of a number of symposium volumes, and accepted sponsorship of the textbook, *Basic Neurochemistry*, of which this volume is the third edition. Other national and regional neurochemical societies have emerged in the Soviet Union, Japan, Great Britain, and Europe. In addition, such relevant groups as the International Brain Research Organization (IBRO) and the Society for Neuroscience in the United States clearly augment these neurochemical efforts.

As one who participated early and actively in almost all of these developments, from the original international symposia, the ISN and the ASN, to a five-year term as chief editor of the *Journal of Neurochemistry*, I can attest personally to their impact in strengthening and maturing neurochemistry as a major neuroscience discipline. I am diffident about trying to appraise the work of the many valued colleagues and friends that these associations have brought me, but I would select three who are now deceased.

Roger Rossiter (1913–1976), Australian by birth, became professor of biochemistry, dean and vice president for health sciences at the University of Western Ontario, and the first chairman of the ISN. Known for his studies of cerebral lipids, he was also a superb teacher and a neurochemical "statesman" [53].

Heinrich Waelsch (1905–1966), born in Brno and educated in Prague, Czechoslovakia, came to the United States in 1938 and at the time of his death was professor of biochemistry at Columbia University and chief of psychiatric research in pharmacology at the New York State Psychiatric Institute, as well as director of the newly created New York State Research Institute for Neurochemistry and Drug Addiction [54]. His research highlighted cerebral amino acid and protein metabolism and cellular metabolic compartmentation. He was active in organizing the international symposia from 1955 to 1964 and in founding the *Journal of Neurochemistry* and the IBRO. With Waelsch's untimely death neurochemistry was deprived of one of its greatest contributors and supporters.

Jordi Folch-Pi (1911–1979), born and educated in Barcelona in Spanish Catalonia, practiced as a physician before coming to the United States to the Rockefeller

Institute in 1935. There he worked with Donald Van Slyke and began his lifelong interest in the chemistry of complex lipids. Folch-Pi left for Harvard in 1944 to take charge of the research laboratories at the McLean Hospital in Belmont, Massachusetts, and in 1956 to become the first professor of neurochemistry at the Harvard Medical School. It was during this period that Folch-Pi reported on his characterization of the cephalins, his discovery of the phosphoinositides, phosphatidyl serine, and proteolipids, and his development of the chloroform-methanol procedure for extraction and initial purification of brain lipids. His procedures revolutionized the lipid chemistry of neural tissues. At this time also Jordi Folch-Pi entered into activities that were to make him one of neurochemistry's most influential leaders and statesmen [55]. He was on the original organizing committee for the International Neurochemical Symposia and on the original editorial board of the *Journal of Neurochemistry*. He was a member of the original council of the International Society for Neurochemistry, its first secretary, and then its chairman for the years 1971–1973. He was one of the organizers of the American Society of Neurochemistry, serving as its first secretary and later as its president for the years 1975–1977. It would be difficult to overstate the contributions that Jordi Folch-Pi made to the phenomenal success of these organizations and to securing formal recognition and establishment of standards of excellence for neurochemistry among the biological sciences.

Current and Future Trends

This account would be incomplete without brief reference to some of the important recent developments in the field [56]. One major area is that concerned with the conduction and transmission of nerve impulses and with muscle contraction. Among many studies are those on the Mg^{2+}-dependent, $(Na^+ + K^+)$-activated adenosinetriphosphatase (ATPase) as the mechanism for transducing cellular energy into the pumping of cations across excitable membranes, as originally proposed by J-C. Skou; on the role of actin, myosin, and calcium ions in muscle contraction, as elucidated by H. E. Huxley; on the details of glycogen storage and breakdown in muscle, including the key function of cyclic AMP discovered by Sutherland; and on the mechanisms of release, reception, and inactivation of transmitters at synapses.

The prototype for studies of the synapse is the neuromuscular junction (NMJ). Earlier investiga-

tions of the NMJ by Nachmansohn and colleagues provided a detailed understanding of the role of acetylcholinesterase, and more recent studies with α-bungarotoxin by Miledi, Potter, Changeux, Patrick and Lindstrom, and others have provided us with purified cholinergic receptor protein. Such research has allowed us to understand the toxic action of the organophosphate cholinesterase inhibitors and the autoimmune nature of myasthenia gravis, thus enabling us to develop methods for treatment of NMJ disorders. At other types of synapses the reception of the transmitter is coupled with the postsynaptic cellular response through the mediation of cyclic AMP, as demonstrated by Greengard. The number and nature of transmitters have proliferated. To acetylcholine and norepinephrine, we may now add γ-aminobutyric acid (GABA) as well as dopamine, serotonin, and probably glycine, glutamic acid, and several types of peptides. The extensive studies by Brodie, Udenfriend, Kaufman, Kopin, and Axelrod have established the metabolic details for most of the catecholamine group of transmitters. Again there are clinical correlates, such as the seizures resulting from vitamin B_6 deficiency, which possibly correlates with impaired GABA metabolism, and the decreases in nigrostriatal dopamine, found by Hornykiewicz to account for the symptomatology in Parkinson's disease. Such correlations lead to therapeutic implications. An important derivative of these developments has been the emergence of neuropharmacology as a very active area of both basic and clinical research. The biochemical circuitry of the central nervous system appears to be among the most promising of current research areas.

The myelin sheath is probably the most thoroughly studied of all biological membranes, with much of the credit going to those successors of Thudichum—Sperry, Rossiter, Klenk, Brante, Folch-Pi, and others—who identified the characteristic myelin lipids. The macromolecular organization of the myelin sheath has been detailed in the physicochemical studies of F. O. Schmitt, Finean and Robertson, and in the electron-microscope observations of Finean, Robertson, and others. In addition, extensive knowledge of the biosynthesis and turnover of myelin lipids has been provided from the metabolic studies of Lynen, Lipmann, Kennedy, Klenk, Svennerholm, Brady, and Suzuki, among many others. The developmental aspects of myelination and the role of the Schwann cell in the peripheral nervous system and the oligodendroglial cell in the central nervous system have been elucidated by Geren, Norton, and many of those already mentioned. Pathological observations have been especially helpful, notably in the studies of Wallerian degeneration by Rossiter, in the use of rodent mutants with a variety of dysmyelinating conditions, and in the autoimmune conditions for which experimental allergic encephalomyelitis (EAE) is a prototype. In the studies of EAE, especially those of Kies and Alvord, Eylar, and Kibler, the discovery of the central role of the myelin basic proteins as the encephalitogens is a major advance toward eventual understanding of that most complicated of neurological disorders, multiple sclerosis. We have also witnessed the identification of myasthenia gravis as an autoimmune disorder of the human nervous system. No doubt there will be others. Neuroimmunology is a very new branch of the neurosciences and has important implications in neurochemistry and clinical neurology.

The blood-brain barrier was discovered by Ehrlich almost a century ago, but it is only today that its nature and operation are finally being understood. Morphological studies with various macromolecules at the electron-microscope level have confirmed the presence of an actual "barrier," primarily attributable to the tight junctions between the endothelial cells lining cerebral capillaries. But it has been the transport studies by Waelsch, Pappenheimer, Lajtha, and others that have revealed the barrier phenomenon as a system of selective transport processes that mediate or facilitate entry into brain of certain solutes and metabolites (such as D-glucose or chloride ions) but prevent the net entry of others (such as L-glutamic acid or penicillin) by actively transporting them out, usually against concentration gradients. A corollary of these observations is that there exists an extraordinary dependence of cerebral metabolism and function on oxygen and glucose supplied by an adequate cerebral blood flow and a very efficient metabolic economy developed by the central nervous system. The aspect of economy was investigated extensively by Heinrich Waelsch with special reference to the mechanisms for supplying carbon skeletons to the Krebs cycle in the absence of glycolytic input or in the presence of α-ketoglutarate withdrawal as glutamic acid and glutamine in ammonia toxicity. Waelsch's studies led to the discovery of carbon dioxide fixation through the pyruvate carboxylase pathway in cerebral neurons and focused on the key roles of glutamate and aspartate in cerebral amino acid and protein metabolism. An important further derivative of these studies has been the recognition of metabolic compartmentation in neural and glial cells. Waelsch pointed out that Hofmeister advanced this concept in 1901 to account for the occurrence of glycogen synthesis, storage, and degradation in the same muscle cell; but Waelsch and Berl have been most persuasive in applying it to the complexities of cerebral metabolism.

Another derivative of such studies has been the recognition of the need for means to study regional and local blood flow and metabolism in the brain in vivo. The classic contributions by Kety and colleagues to the study of total cerebral blood flow and metabolism have already been mentioned. A number of modifications, particularly those of Sokoloff, Lassen, and Ingvar, in which autoradiographic and wash-out techniques were used, have provided experimental approaches to regional and local studies, but none is totally satisfactory. A major step forward has been made possible by Louis Sokoloff's adaptation of 2-deoxy-D-glucose (2-DG) to the problem (see Chap. 24). During the 1950s, the metabolism of this interesting competitor of glucose was investigated by Wick, Woodward, Landau, Ashmore, Sols, Crane, Tower, and other workers. Subsequently, Sokoloff used these data to design experimental animal studies with [14]C- or ^{3}H-labeled 2-DG and autoradiography to delineate the local cerebral uptake of 2-DG as a reflection of regional glucose utilization. A wealth of experimental information has already been obtained as a result of the very extensive application of this technique since its introduction in 1974. Now, with the advent of positron emission transverse tomography, there is the exciting prospect of adapting the principles of the procedure to the examination of the intact living brain in situ, by using ^{18}F- or ^{11}C-labeled 2-DG.

One of the major areas of postwar neurochemical research has been concerned with the biochemical bases of genetically determined disorders of the nervous system. The prototype is, of course, phenylketonuria, originally described in 1934 by Følling in Norway as a metabolic disorder characterized by clinical imbecility and the urinary excretion of abnormal amounts of phenylpyruvic acid. In the post–World War II period, Jervis, Udenfriend, and others followed up on these observations to demonstrate the precise biochemical basis for the disorder and the means for its alleviation. Classically, phenylketonuria results from the genetic deletion or attenuation of hepatic phenylalanine hydroxylase and the consequent block in the metabolism of dietary phenylalanine, which accumulates in the body together with abnormal levels of such minor metabolites as phenylpyruvate and phenyllactate. As a consequence of neonatal screening tests originally developed by Guthrie, and prompt institution of a phenylalanine-free diet, devised by Bickel and others, this disorder need no longer threaten affected infants; but any delay in recognition or dietary treatment results in seizures, dermatitis, and mental retardation. The mental retardation does not reverse when dietary therapy is delayed. The molecular basis of the retardation is not understood, although it may turn out to correlate with the delayed myelination reported by Norman and by Alvord. More recently, Kaufman has uncovered variants of the classic disorder in which the genetically determined biochemical lesions involve the pteridine cofactor for the hydroxylase reaction, the apoenzyme in these variants being entirely normal.

Among the many subsequent examples of neurogenetic lesions, the biochemical nature of the sphingolipid storage diseases, delineated by Brady, Suzuki, O'Brien, and others, has been most instructive. The dozen or more disorders in this group, including Tay-Sachs disease, Gaucher's disease, Niemann-Pick disease, and Fabry's disease are all attributable to genetic deletion or attenuation of a specific enzyme in the respective catabolic pathways, causing abnormal cellular accumulations of the specific sphingolipids. Thus, these are all disorders of lysosomal hydrolases. Brady and colleagues have developed simple diagnostic and screening tests, including testing of amniocentesis specimens to identify fetuses at risk. These developments permit effective genetic counseling and have converted a group of hopeless and usually fatal clinical syndromes of unknown cause into understandable and manageable problems. Brady's group is now examining the possibilities of enzyme replacement therapy as an alternate approach to these problems.

The foregoing examples illustrate some, but by no means all, important areas of recent neurochemical research. Many other discoveries seem to be on the horizon. For example, the whole field of neuroendocrinology is in ferment. One element of this ferment is the discovery and characterization by Guillemin and Schally of the hypothalamic releasing factors for pituitary hormones and the role of such neurotransmitters as dopamine in the process. Another element is the increasing evidence that most hormones, classically regarded as directed to peripheral target organs, are also, and perhaps more importantly, directed to specific areas of the central nervous system. A third element is the discovery of the opioid receptor–enkephalin transmitter modulatory systems in brain. The interactions of neurohormones, neurotransmitters, and neuromodulators seem to provide the types and varieties of biochemical circuitry that would account for the many higher nervous functions involved in learning, memory, plasticity, behavior—in short, all the complexities of central processing.

Perhaps the most essential function of central processing is to deal appropriately and efficiently with the extraordinary variety and volume of incoming sensory stimuli that constantly impinge upon the diversity of peripheral sensory receptors. This input is essential to our orientation in our environment and to appropriate behavioral responses (deafferentation, e.g. deafness, blindness, or leprosy, is usually a disaster) but we still do not understand the sensory transduction processes. Thus, one of the major challenges confronting neuroscience is to determine how photons at the retinal rods and cones, sound waves at the cochlear hair cells, volatile organic chemicals at the olfactory epithelium, or tactile pressure at dermal Meissner's corpuscles are transduced by the various specialized receptors into appropriately encoded nerve signals. One general principle seems to be the modulation by the sensory stimulus of a "dark current," maintained by differential distribution across cell membranes of ions dependent on constantly generated cellular energy. Thus, these are basically neurochemical problems for the future.

Implicit in what I have recounted is the very central and basic role of neurochemistry today in understanding so much of the other neurosciences and of clinical disorders of the nervous system. The historical account outlined here is just an introduction to the neurochemistry of tomorrow. Thudichum believed so nearly a century ago. Today, Seymour Kety writes [57] that the problem that has long challenged philosophers and scientists is the relationship of the mind to the physical universe, and hence the problem of the nature of consciousness and its ultimate reducibility to physicochemical processes. Even a purely mechanistic model of human behavior recognizes it to be the result of two factors: the biological machinery of the brain and the information that it has stored. The language we speak, the values we cherish, our political persuasions, are hardly the results of differences in structure or chemistry of the brain, but quite obviously are dependent on the experiential information it has somehow stored. The synaptic junctions between neurons represent crucial loci for information processing and decision making in the brain and for the activation of the neuronal networks that underlie thought, mood, and behavior.

The recognition that these junctions are mediated by chemical processes provides, for the first time, an appreciation of how a finite number of chemical processes might affect cognition, emotional state, and behavior in definable ways and provides a basis for explaining how genetic deviation, metabolic processes, changes in the chemical milieu, hormones, and drugs might affect psychological processes and could suggest where the biological loci of mental disorders might lie. It is reasonable to think of all neurotransmitters as a biochemical orchestra in the brain, the net output of which depends on the interrelations of a large number of components rather than the expression of a solo instrument. Kety concludes that it is difficult to believe that major mental disorders represent deviations produced in normal biological mechanisms by the psychological experience and information that they store. Despite any role that experience and information may play, we also recognize that there are defects or disturbances in the machinery and that these can be elucidated by research in biological disciplines and corrected by biological means. With Ralph Gerard [49, p. 624] we may conclude: "So the bright area of knowledge ever spreads and, although the dark surface of ignorance is presumably decreasing, the perimeter of contact with the unknown also increases."

References*

1. Tower, D. B. Origins and development of neurochemistry. *Neurology* (Minneap.) 8 (Suppl. 1):3–31, 1958.
2. Fearing, F. *Reflex Action. A Study in the History of Physiological Psychology.* Baltimore: Williams & Wilkins, 1930.
3. Florkin, M. *A History of Biochemistry.* In M. Florkin and E. H. Stotz (eds.), *Comprehensive Biochemistry*, Vol. 30. Amsterdam: Elsevier, 1972.
4. Franklin, K. J. *A Short History of Physiology* (2nd ed.). London: Staples Press, 1949.
5. Garrison, F. H. *An Introduction to the History of Medicine* (4th ed.). Philadelphia: Saunders, 1929.
6. Leicester, H. M. *Development of Biochemical Concepts from Ancient to Modern Times.* Cambridge, Mass.: Harvard University Press, 1974.
7. Moore, F. J. *A History of Chemistry* (3rd ed.). [revised by W. T. Hall]. New York: McGraw-Hill, 1939.
8. Neuberger, M. *Die historische Entwicklung der*

*Most of these references include valuable bibliographical sources.

experimentellen Gehirn- und Rückenmarksphysiologie vor Flourens. Stuttgart: Ferd. Enke, 1897.

9. Tower, D. B. Johann Thomas Hensing (1683–1726). In W. Haymaker and F. Schiller (eds.), *The Founders of Neurology* (2nd ed.). Springfield, Ill.: Thomas, 1970. Pp. 285–289.

10. Tower, D. B. Nicolas-Louis Vauquelin (1763–1829). In W. Haymaker and F. Schiller (eds.), *The Founders of Neurology* (2nd ed.). Springfield, Ill.: Thomas, 1970. Pp. 302–306.

11. Brazier, M. A. B. Rise of neurophysiology in the nineteenth century. *J. Neurophysiol.* 20:212–226, 1957.

12. McIlwain, H. *Chemotherapy and the Central Nervous System.* London: Churchill, 1957.

13. Farber, E. *The Evolution of Chemistry.* New York: Ronald, 1952.

14. Thomson, T. *The Chemistry of Animal Bodies.* Edinburgh: Black, 1834.

15. Drabkin, D. L. *Thudichum: Chemist of the Brain.* Philadelphia: Saunders, 1958.

16. Tower, D. B. Johann Ludwig Wilhelm Thudichum (1829–1901). In W. Haymaker and F. Schiller (eds.), *The Founders of Neurology* (2nd ed.). Springfield, Ill.: Thomas, 1970. Pp. 297–302.

17. Garrod, A. E. *Inborn Errors of Metabolism* (2nd ed.). London: Hodder and Stoughton, 1923.

18. Keilin, D. *The History of Cell Respiration and Cytochrome.* Cambridge: Cambridge University Press, 1966.

19. Thudichum, J. L. W. *A Treatise on the Chemical Constitution of the Brain* [facsimile of the 1884 edition, with introduction by D. L. Drabkin]. Hamden, Conn.: Archon, 1962.

20. Winterstein, H. Der Stoffwechsel des Zentralnervensystems. In A. Bethe, G. v. Bergmann, G. Embden, and A. Ellinger (eds.), *Handbuch der normalen und pathologischen Physiologie.* Berlin: Springer, 1929. Vol. 9, pp. 515–611.

21. Tower, D. B. Hans Winterstein (1879–1963). In W. Haymaker and F. Schiller (eds.), *The Founders of Neurology* (2nd ed.). Springfield, Ill.: Thomas, 1970. Pp. 307–311.

22. Warburg, O. *Heavy Metal Prosthetic Groups and Enzyme Action.* Oxford: Clarendon, 1949.

23. Krebs, H. A. The history of the tricarboxylic acid cycle. *Perspect. Biol. Med.* 14:154–170, 1970.

24. Meyerhof, O. Über die Intermediärvorgänge der enzymatischen Kohlenhydratspaltung. *Ergebn. Physiol.* 39:10–75, 1937.

25. Szent-Györgyi, A. *On Oxidation, Fermentation, Vitamins, Health and Disease.* Baltimore: Williams & Wilkins, 1939.

26. Peters, R. A. *Biochemical Lesions and Lethal Synthesis.* Oxford: Pergamon, 1963.

27. Elliott, K. A. C., Page, I. H., and Quastel, J. H. (eds.). *Neurochemistry. The Chemical Dynamics of Brain and Nerve.* Springfield, Ill.: Thomas, 1955. [A second edition was published in 1962.]

28. Elliott, K. A. C. My colleague Q. *Can. J. Biochem.* 43:vii–ix, 1965.

29. Leake, C. D. Henry Dale (1875–1968). In W. Haymaker and F. Schiller (eds.), *The Founders of Neurology* (2nd ed.). Springfield, Ill.: Thomas, 1970. Pp. 282–285.

30. Browne, J. S. L. Otto Loewi (1873–1961). In W. Haymaker and F. Schiller (eds.), *The Founders of Neurology* (2nd ed.). Springfield, Ill.: Thomas, 1970. Pp. 293–296.

31. Bard, P. Walter Cannon (1871–1945). In W. Haymaker and F. Schiller (eds.), *The Founders of Neurology* (2nd ed.). Springfield, Ill.: Thomas, 1970. Pp. 279–281.

32. Dale, H. H. *Adventures in Physiology.* Oxford: Pergamon Press, 1953.

33. Loewi, O. Aspects of the transmission of the nervous impulse. *J. Mt. Sinai Hosp.* 12:803–816; 851–865, 1945.

34. Cannon, W. B. *Autonomic Neuro-effector Systems.* New York: Macmillan, 1937.

35. Von Euler, U. S. Neurotransmission in the adrenergic nervous system. *Harvey Lect.* 55:43–65, 1959–60.

36. Nachmansohn, D. *Chemical and Molecular Basis of Nerve Activity.* New York: Academic, 1959.

37. Axelrod, J. The metabolism, storage and release of catecholamines. *Recent Prog. Horm. Res.* 21:597–619, 1965.

38. Eccles, J. C. *The Physiology of Nerve Cells.* Baltimore: Johns Hopkins University Press, 1957.

39. Hodgkin, A. L. Ionic movements and electrical activity of the giant axon of the squid. *Proc. R. Soc. London [Biol.]* 148:1–37, 1958.

40. Roberts, E. GABA in Nervous System Function—An Overview. In R. O. Brady and D. B. Tower (eds.), *The Nervous System.* Vol. I: *The Basic Neurosciences.* New York: Raven, 1975. Pp. 541–552.

41. Enders, J. F. Tissue Culture Technics Employed in the Propagation of Viruses and Rickettsia. In T. M. Rivers and F. L. Horsfall, Jr. (eds.), *Viral and Rickettsial Infections of Man* (3rd ed.). Philadelphia: Lippincott, 1959. Pp. 209–229.

42. Nelson, P. G. Nerve and muscle cells in culture. *Physiol. Rev.* 55:1–61, 1975.

43. Lowry, O. H. Quantitative Histochemistry. In R. O. Brady and D. B. Tower (eds.), *The Nervous System.* Vol. 1: *The Basic Neurosciences.* New York: Raven, 1975. Pp. 523–533.

44. Waelsch, H. (ed.). *Biochemistry of the Developing Nervous System.* New York: Academic, 1955.

45. Richter, D. (ed.). *Metabolism of the Nervous System*. London: Pergamon, 1957.

46. Folch-Pi, J. (ed.). *Chemical Pathology of the Nervous System*. Oxford: Pergamon, 1961.

47. Kety, S. S., and Elkes, J. (eds.). *Regional Neurochemistry*. Oxford: Pergamon, 1961.

48. Richter, D. (ed.). *Comparative Neurochemistry*. Oxford: Pergamon, 1964.

49. Millbank Conference. *The Biology of Mental Health and Disease*. New York: Hoeber, 1952.

50. McIlwain, H. *Biochemistry and the Central Nervous System*. London: Churchill, 1955. [Subsequent editions published in 1959, 1966, and 1971.]

51. Kreps, E., and Tower, D. B. Obituary: Aleksandr Vladimirovich Palladin 1885–1972. *J. Neurochem.* 21:723–724, 1973.

52. Tower, D. B. (ed.). *Neurochemistry in the Soviet Union: Report of the Neurochemistry Exchange Mission to the USSR, November 1969*. Washington, D.C.: U.S. Dept. of Health, Education, and Welfare—National Institutes of Health, 1970.

53. McMurray, W. C. Obituary: Roger J. Rossiter. *J. Neurochem.* 27:827–828, 1976.

54. Obituary: Heinrich B. Waelsch. *Internat. J. Neuropharmacol.* 5:i–ii, 1966.

55. Pope, A., Lees, M. B., and Hauser, G. Obituary: Jordi Folch-Pi. *J. Neurochem.* 35:1–3, 1980.

56. Tower, D. B. Neurochemistry—One Hundred Years 1875–1975. *Ann. Neurol.* 1:2–36, 1977.

57. Kety, S. S. The biological substrates of abnormal mental states. *Fed. Proc.* 37:2267–2270, 1978.

Part One. General Neurochemistry

Section I. Morphological Basis of Neurochemistry

Chapter 2. Neurocellular Anatomy

Although our understanding of the functional relationships of the central nervous system (CNS) components is still in its infancy, particularly in the area of neurotransmitters and synaptic modulation, the fine structure of most elements is relatively well worked out [1–7]. The purpose of this chapter is to collate available information and present it in a manner relevant to neurochemistry. The excellent neuroanatomical atlases of Peters [4] and Palay and Chan-Palay [1] should be consulted for a more detailed ultrastructural analysis of specific cell types, particularly of neurons with their diverse forms and connections. This chapter has been compiled to provide a concise description of the major cytoarchitectural features of the nervous system and to provide an entrance into the relevant literature. Although the fine structure of organelles of the CNS and PNS is not peculiar to these tissues, the interrelations of all types, e.g., the synaptic contracts and myelin, are unique. These specializations and those that sequester the CNS from the general circulation, namely, the blood-brain barrier and absence of lymphatics, are major factors in normal and disease processes in the nervous system. For the sake of simplicity, the present section is subdivided first into a section on general organization and then according to major cell types.

General Cellular Organization

Central nervous system parenchyma is made up of nerve cells and their afferent and efferent extensions (dendrites and axons), all closely enveloped by glial cells. Coronal section of the cerebral hemispheres of the brain reveals an outer convoluted rim of gray matter, which overlies white matter (Fig. 2-1). Gray matter also exists as islands within the white matter, contains nerve cell bodies and glia, and lacks significant amounts of myelin, the component responsible for the whiteness of white matter. Further down the neuroaxis in the spinal cord, white matter surrounds the gray matter, which is arranged in a characteristic H formation (Fig. 2-2).

A highly diagrammatic representation of the major CNS elements is shown in Fig. 2-3. The entire central nervous system is bathed both internally and externally by cerebrospinal fluid (CSF), which circulates throughout the ventricular and leptomeningeal spaces. This fluid, a type of plasma ultrafiltrate, plays a significant role in protecting the CNS from mechanical trauma, in the balance of electrolytes and protein, and in the maintenance of ventricular pressure. This subject is reviewed in Chap. 25. The outer surface of the CNS is invested by a triple membrane system, the meninges, composed of flattened fibrous or elastic connective tissue, collagen, and blood vessels. The outermost of the three, the dura mater, is applied tightly to the inner surfaces of the calvaria and has the arachnoid membrane closely applied to its inner surface. The innermost of the meninges, the pia mater, loosely covers the CNS surface. The pia and arachnoid together are called *leptomeninges*. Cerebrospinal fluid occupies the subarachnoid space (between the arachnoid and the pia) and the ventricles. The CNS parenchyma is overlaid by a layer of subpial astrocytes, which, in turn, is covered on its leptomeningeal aspect by a continuous basal lamina material (see Fig. 2-3). On the inner (ventricular) surface, the CNS parenchyma is separated from the CSF by a layer of ciliated ependymal cells, which are thought to facilitate the movement of CSF. In some species, areas of the CNS are lined by nonciliated ependymal cells, for example, the central canal of the human spinal

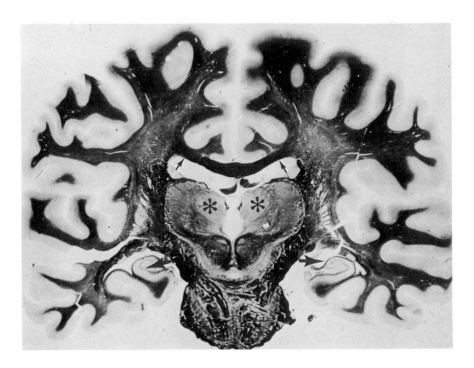

cord. The production and circulation of CSF is maintained by specialized mesodermal elements, which are grapelike collections of vascular tissue and cells that protrude into the ventricles; these elements form the choroid plexus. Resorption of CSF is effected by vascular structures known as *arachnoid villi,* located in the leptomeninges over the surface of the brain.

The ependymal cells abut layers of astrocytes, which, in turn, envelop neurons, neurites, and vascular components. In addition to neurons and glial cells (astrocytes and oligodendrocytes), the CNS parenchyma contains blood vessels, macrophages (pericytes), and microglial cells.

The peripheral and autonomic nervous systems consist of bundles of myelinated and nonmyelinated axons enveloped by Schwann cells—the peripheral nervous system (PNS) counterparts of the oligodendrocytes. The nerve bundles are enclosed by the perineurium and the epineurium—tough, fibrous, elastic sheaths. Between individual nerve fibers are isolated connective tissue (endoneurial) cells and blood vessels. The ganglia (e.g.,

Fig. 2-1. Coronal section of the human brain at the thalamic level stained by the Heidenhain technique for myelin. Gray matter stains faintly; all myelinated regions are black. The thalamus (*) lies beneath the lateral ventricles and is separated at this level by the beginning of the third ventricle. The roof of the lateral ventricles is formed by the corpus callosum (small arrows). The Ammon's horns are shown at the large arrows. Note the outline of gyri and sulci at the surface of the cerebral hemispheres, sectioned here near the junction of the frontal and parietal cortex.

dorsal root and sympathetic ganglia), located peripherally to the CNS, are made up of large neurons, usually unipolar or bipolar, surrounded by satellite cells that are specialized Schwann cells. A dendrite and an axon, both of which can be of great length (up to several feet), arise from each neuron.

The Neuron

FUNCTIONAL FEATURES

From a historical standpoint, no other cell type has attracted as much attention or caused as much

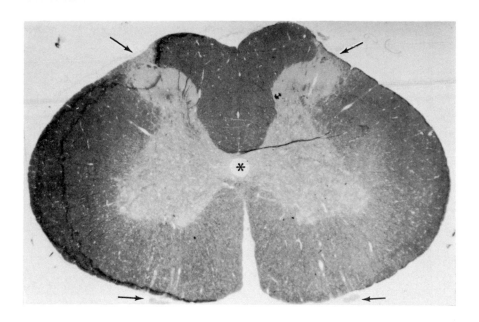

Fig. 2-2. Transverse section of the lumbar spinal cord at L₇ from a normal rabbit. Gray matter is seen as a paler staining area in an H configuration formed by the dorsal and ventral horns with the central canal in the center. The dorsal horns would meet the incoming dorsal spinal nerve roots at the upper arrows. The anterior roots can be seen below (arrows), opposite the ventral horns from which they get their fibers. The white matter occupies a major part of the spinal cord and stains darker. Epon section, 1 μ, stained with toluidine blue.

controversy as the nerve cell. It is impossible in a single chapter to delineate comprehensively the extensive structural, topographical, and functional variation achieved by this cell type. Consequently, despite an enormous literature, the neuron still defies precise understanding, particularly from the functional aspect. It is known that the neuronal population is usually established shortly after birth, that mature neurons do not divide, and that in man there is a daily dropout of neurons amounting to about 20,000 cells. These facts alone make the neuron unique. Development and maturation of neurons are discussed in Chap. 23.

Neurons can be either excitatory, inhibitory, or modulatory in their effect; motor, sensory, or secretory in function. They can be influenced by a large battery of neurotransmitters and hormones (see Chap. 8). Naturally, this enormous repertoire of functions is associated with different developmental influences upon different neurons, largely reflected in the variations of dendritic and axonal outgrowth. Specialization also occurs at axonal terminals, where a variety of junctional complexes (*synapses*) exist. The subtle synaptic modifications are best visualized ultrastructurally, although immunofluorescent staining for light microscopy also permits distinctions among synapses on the basis of the type of transmitter released.

GENERAL STRUCTURAL FEATURES OF NEURONS, DENDRITES, AND AXONS

Although one tends to think of the neuron as a stellate cell with broad dendrites and a fine axon emerging from one pole—an impression gained from the older work of Purkinje, who first described the nerve cell in 1839, and of Deiters, Cajal, and Golgi—this appearance does not hold true for many neurons. The neuron is the most polymorphic cell in the body and defies formal classification on the basis of shape, location, function, fine structure, or

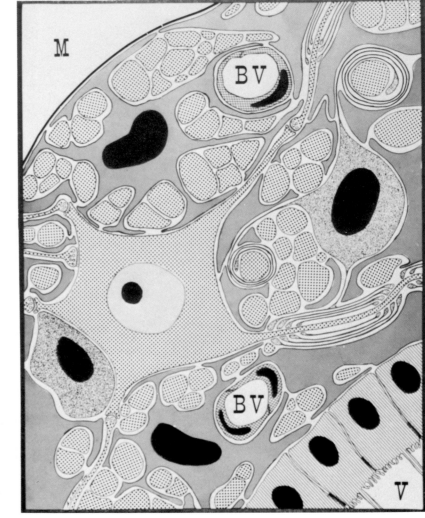

NEURON AND NEURITES

OLIGODENDROGLIA

ENDOTHELIUM

ASTROGLIA

EPENDYMA

NON-NEURONAL NUCLEI

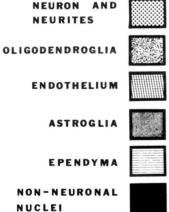

Fig. 2-3. The major components of the CNS and their interrelationships. Microglia are not depicted. In this simplified situation, the CNS extends from its meningeal surface (M), through the basal lamina over the CNS parenchyma (solid black line), subpial astrocytes, parenchyma proper, subependymal astrocytes, to the ciliated ependymal cells lining the ventricular space (V). Note how the astrocyte provides the covering between external factors and CNS parenchyma and also invests blood vessels (BV), neurons, cell processes, etc. One neuron is seen (center) with synaptic contacts on its soma and dendrites. Its axon emerges to the right and is myelinated by an oligodendrocyte (above). Other axons are shown in transverse section, some of which are myelinated. The oligodendrocyte to the lower left of the neuron is of the nonmyelinating, satellite type.

transmitter substance. Early workers described the neuron as a globular mass suspended between nerve fibers, but the teased preparations of Deiters and his contemporaries soon proved this was not the case. Later work, using impregnation staining and culture techniques, elaborated on Deiters' findings. For a long time, before the work of Deiters and Cajal, neurons were believed to form a syncytium, with no intervening membranes—a postulation that also was proposed for neuroglia. Today, of course, we are familiar with the specialized membranes and the enormous variety of neuron shapes and sizes; they range from the small, globular cerebellar granule cells with a perikaryal diameter of about 6 to 8 μ to the pear-shaped Purkinje cells and star-shaped anterior horn cells, both of which may reach diameters of 60 to 80 μ in humans. The perikaryal size, however, is generally a poor index of cell volume. It is a general rule in neuroanatomy that the neurites occupy a greater percentage of the cell surface area than does the soma. For example, the pyramidal cell of the somatosensory cortex has a cell body that accounts for only 4 percent of the total cell surface area, whereas from the dendritic tree, the dendritic spines alone claim 43 percent (Mungai, quoted by Peters et al. [4]). Hydén[2] quotes the work of Scholl (1956), who calculated that the perikaryon of a "cortical cell" represents 10 percent of the neuronal surface area. In the feline reticular formation, certain giant cells possess ratios between soma and dendrites of about 1:5. A single axon is the usual rule, but some cells, for example, the Golgi cells of the cerebellum, are endowed with several axons, some of which may show branching.

The extent of the branching displayed by the dendrites is a useful index of their functional importance. Dendritic trees represent the expression of the receptive fields, and large fields can receive inputs from multiple origins. A cell with less developed dendritic ramification, for example, the cerebellar granule cells, synapses with a more homogeneous population of afferent sources.

The axon emerges from a neuron as a slender thread and frequently does not branch until it nears its target. In contrast to the dendrite and the soma

(with very few exceptions), the axon is frequently myelinated, thus increasing its efficiency as a conducting unit. Myelin, a spirally wrapped membrane (see Chap. 4), is laid down in segments (internodes) by oligodendrocytes in the CNS and in the PNS by Schwann cells. The naked regions of axon between adjacent internodes are known as *nodes of Ranvier*, and it is across these regions of the axon that saltatory conduction (Chap. 5) is effected.

CELLULAR ORGANIZATION OF NEURONS
No unique cytoplasmic features of the neuronal soma serve to characterize this cell as different from any other. Neurons have all the morphological counterparts of other cell types, the structures are similarly distributed, and some of the commonest, for example, the Golgi apparatus and mitochondria, were first described in neurons (Fig. 2-4).

Outer Limiting Membrane
As seen by electron microscopy, the neuron often stands out poorly from the background neuropil, most of which is composed of nonmyelinated neurites (axons and dendrites), synaptic complexes, and glial processes—profiles with similar electron density at low power. Closer inspection shows that, like all cells, the neuron is delineated by a typical triple-layered unit membrane about 75 Å wide, consisting of two dense leaflets about 25 Å thick enclosing a clear space. Some fixation procedures, such as that using glutaraldehyde followed by postosmication, render the inner cytoplasmic leaflet slightly more osmiophilic, giving the unit membrane an asymmetrical appearance.

Nucleus
A large, usually spherical, nucleus containing a prominent nucleolus is typical of many neurons. The nucleochromatin is invariably pale, with little dense heterochromatin. In some neurons, for example, cerebellar granule cells, the karyoplasm may be more differentiated and contain dense heterochromatin. The nucleolus is vesiculated, clearly delineated from the rest of the karyoplasm, and usually contains two textures, the pars fibrosa (fine bundles of filaments) and the pars granulosa, in

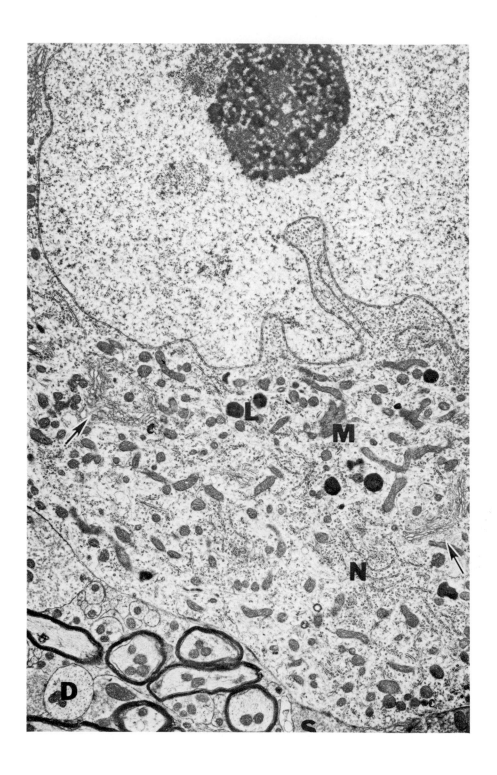

which dense granules predominate. An additional juxtaposed structure, found in neurons of females of some species, is the nucleolar satellite, or sex chromatin, which consists of dense, but loosely-packed, coiled filaments. The nucleus is enclosed by the nuclear envelope, made up on the cytoplasmic side by the inner membrane of the perikaryon (sometimes seen in continuity with the endoplasmic reticulum) and a more regular membrane on the inner, nuclear aspect. Between the two is a clear channel of between 200 and 400 Å. Periodically, the inner and outer membranes of the envelope come together to form a single diaphragm—a nuclear pore (Fig. 2-5). In tangential section, nuclear pores are seen as empty vesicular structures, about 700 Å in diameter. In some neurons, that segment of the nuclear envelope which faces the dendritic pole is deeply invaginated, as in Purkinje cells.

The Perikaryon

The body of the neuron, called the *perikaryon*, is rich in organelles (Fig. 2-4). Among the most prominent features of the cytoplasm is a system of membranous cisternae, divisible into rough endoplasmic reticulum (ER), which forms part of the Nissl substance; smooth (agranular) ER; subsurface cisternae (the hypolemmal system); and the Golgi apparatus. Although these various components are structurally interconnected, and some are even connected to the nuclear envelope, each possesses distinct enzymologic properties. Also present within the cytoplasm are abundant lysosomes, lipofuscin granules (aging pigment), mitochondria, multivesicular bodies, neurotubules, neurofilaments, and ribosomes.

Fig. 2-4. A motor neuron from the spinal cord of an adult rat shows a nucleus containing a nucleolus, clearly divisible into a pars fibrosa and a pars granulosa, and a perikaryon filled with organelles. Among these, Golgi apparatus (arrows), Nissl substance (N), mitochondria (M), and lysosomes (L) can be seen. An axosomatic synapse (S) occurs below and two axodendritic synapses abut a dendrite (D). ×8,000.

NISSL SUBSTANCE. The intracytoplasmic basophilic masses that ramify loosely throughout the cytoplasm and are typical of most neurons are known collectively as *Nissl substance* (Figs. 2-4 and 2-5). The distribution of Nissl substance in certain neurons is characteristic and is used as a criterion for identification. By electron microscopy (EM), this substance is seen to comprise regular arrays or scattered portions of flattened cisterns of rough ER, surrounded by clouds of free polyribosomes (Chap. 19). The membranes of the rough ER are studded with rows of ribosomes. A spacing of 200 to 400 Å is maintained within cisternae. Sometimes, cisternal walls meet at fenestrations. Unlike the rough ER of glandular cells or other protein-secreting cells (e.g., plasma cells), the rough ER of neurons probably produces proteins for its own use, a feature imposed by the extraordinary functional demands placed upon this cell. Nissl substance does not penetrate axons but extends along dendrites.

SMOOTH ER. Most neurons contain at least a few cisternae or tubules of smooth (agranular) ER, which is sometimes difficult to differentiate from rough ER, owing to disorderly arrangement of ribosomes. Ribosomes are not attached to these membranes, and the cisterns usually assume a meandering, branching course throughout the cytoplasm. In some neurons, smooth ER is a quite prominent component, for example, in Purkinje cells. Individual cisterns of smooth ER extend along axons and dendrites. Whether the pockets of smooth ER within axons play a role in the transport or packaging of neurotransmitters or other proteins is uncertain.

SUBSURFACE CISTERNAE. Although not a constant feature of all neurons, a system of smooth, membrane-bound, flattened cisterns can be found in many neurons. These structures, referred to as *hypolemmal cisternae* by Palay and Chan-Palay [1], abut the plasmalemma of the neuron and, in such areas, constitute a secondary membranous boundary within the cell. The distance between these cisternae and the plasmalemma is usually 100 to 120 Å, and on occasion, a mitochondrion may be found in close association with the innermost leaflet (e.g., in Purkinje cells). Similar cisternae have

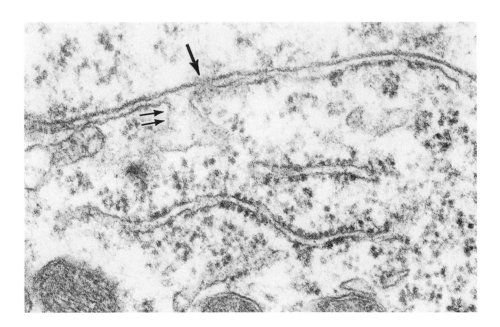

Fig. 2-5. Detail of the nuclear envelope showing a nuclear pore (arrow) and the outer leaflet connected to smooth ER (double arrows). Two cisterns of rough ER with associated ribosomes are also present. ×80,000.

been described as occurring beneath synaptic complexes, but their functional significance is not clearly understood. Some authors have suggested that such a system may play a role in the uptake of metabolites.

GOLGI APPARATUS. Undoubtedly, the most impressive demonstration of the Golgi system, a highly specialized form of agranular reticulum, is achieved by using the metal impregnation techniques of Golgi. Ultrastructurally, the Golgi apparatus consists of aggregates of smooth-walled cisternae and a variety of vesicles, surrounded by a heterogeneous assemblage of organelles, including mitochondria, lysosomes, and multivesicular bodies. In most neurons, the Golgi apparatus encompasses the nucleus, extends into dendrites, but is absent from axons. A three-dimensional analysis of the system reveals that the stacks of cisternae are pierced periodically by fenestrae. Tangential sections of these fenestrations show them to be circular. A multitude of vesicles is associated with each segment of Golgi apparatus, in particular "coated" vesicles, which are proliferated from the lateral margins of flattened cisternae (Fig. 2-6). Such structures have been variously named, but the term

alveolate vesicle seems to be generally accepted. Histochemical staining reveals that these bodies are rich in acid hydrolases, and they are believed to represent primary lysosomes. Acid phosphatase is also found elsewhere in the cisterns but in lesser amounts than in alveolate vesicles.

LYSOSOMES. Lysosomes, the principle organelles responsible for degradation of cellular waste, are common constituents of all cell types of the nervous system and are particularly prominent in neurons, where they can be seen at various stages of development (Fig. 2-4). They range in size from 0.1 to 1 or 2 μ in diameter. The primary lysosome is elaborated from Golgi saccules as a small, vesicular structure (Fig. 2-6). The function of this organelle is to fuse with the membrane of waste-containing vacuoles (*phagosomes*) into which they release hydrolytic enzymes. The sequestered material is degraded within the vacuole. At this stage, the organelle is

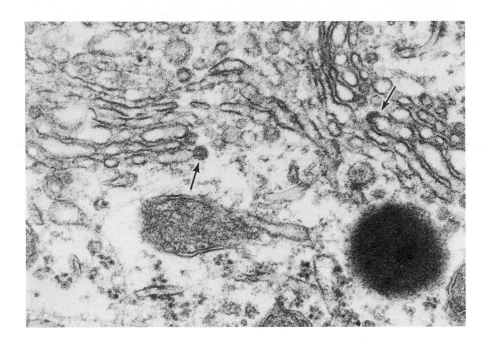

Fig. 2-6. A portion of a Golgi apparatus. The smooth-membraned cisternae appear beaded. The many circular profiles represent tangentially sectioned fenestrae and alveolate vesicles (primary lysosomes). Two of the latter can be seen budding from Golgi saccules (arrows). Mitochondria and a dense body (secondary lysosomes) are also present. ×60,000.

known as a *secondary lysosome* and is usually electron-dense and large. The matrix of this organelle will give a positive reaction when tested histochemically for acid phosphatase. A single limiting membrane is characteristic. Residual bodies containing nondegradable material are considered to be *tertiary lysosomes* and in the neuron are represented by lipofuscin granules (Fig. 2-7). These granules contain brown pigment and lamellar stacks of membrane material and are more common in the aged brain. For a more detailed account of lysosomes, the reader is referred to Novikoff and Holtzman [8].

MULTIVESICULAR BODIES. Multivesicular bodies are usually found in association with the Golgi apparatus and are visualized by EM as small, single membrane-bound sacs about 0.5 μ in diameter. They contain several minute, spherical profiles, sometimes arranged about the periphery. Currently, they are believed to belong in the lysosome series (prior to secondary lysosomes) because they contain acid hydrolases and are apparently derived from primary lysosomes.

NEUROTUBULES. The neurotubule has been the subject of intensive research in recent years. Neurotubules usually are arranged haphazardly throughout the perikaryon of neurons. They are aligned longitudinally in axons and dendrites and, in the latter, form the major filamentous component. Each neurotubule consists of a dense-walled structure enclosing a clear lumen, in the middle of which may be found an electron-dense dot. Sometimes axonal neurotubules display 50 Å filamentous interconnecting side arms. The diameter of neurotubules varies between 220 and 240 Å. High-resolution studies seem to indicate that each neurotubule wall consists of thirteen filamentous subunits arranged helically around the lumen. These structures and the neurofilaments (below) can be seen in the photographs discussed later in connection with astrocytes (see Chaps. 20 and 22).

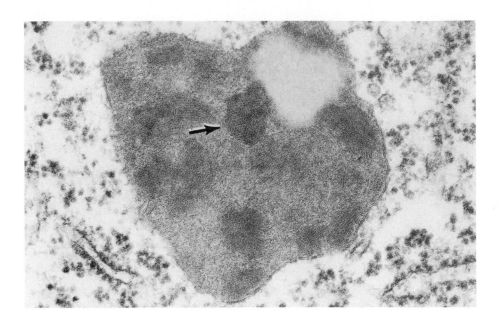

NEUROFILAMENTS. Neurofilaments usually are found in association with neurotubules. The function of the two organelles has been debated for some time, and although it seems reasonable to assume that they play a role in the maintenance of form, their putative role in axoplasmic transport remains to be clarified (see Chap. 22). Neurofilaments have a diameter of about 100 Å, are of indeterminate length, and frequently occur in bundles. They are constant components of axons but are rarer in dendrites. In the axon, individual filaments can be seen to possess a minute lumen and to be interconnected by flocular, proteinaceous side arms, thereby forming a meshwork. Because of these cross-bridges, they do not form tightly packed bundles in a normal axon, in distinction to filaments within glial processes (i.e., astroglia, see Fig. 2-14), which lack cross-bridges. Neurofilaments within neuronal somata do not always display cross-bridges and can be found in tighter bundles. The biochemistry of neurotubules and neurofilaments has been covered by Shelanski and Weisenberg [9]. A form of filamentous structure finer than neurofilaments is seen at the tips of growing neurites, particularly in the growth cones of

Fig. 2-7. A lipofuscin granule from a cortical neuron shows membrane-bound lipid (dense) and a soluble component (gray). The denser component is lamellated. The lamellae appear as paracrystalline arrays of tubular profiles when sectioned transversely (arrow). The granule is surrounded by a single unit membrane. Free ribosomes can also be seen. ×96,000.

developing axons. These 50 Å structures, known as *microfilaments,* facilitate movement and growth, for axonal extension can be arrested pharmacologically by treatment with compounds which depolymerize these structures.

MITOCHONDRIA. Mitochondria are the centers for oxidative phosphorylation. These organelles occur ubiquitously in the neuron and its processes (Figs. 2-4 and 2-6). Their overall shape may change from one type of neuron to another, but their basic morphology is identical to that in other cell types. Mitochondria consist morphologically of double-membraned sacs surrounded by protuberances, or cristae, extending from the inner membrane into the matrix space. The review by Novikoff and Holtzman [9] discusses in more detail the ultra-

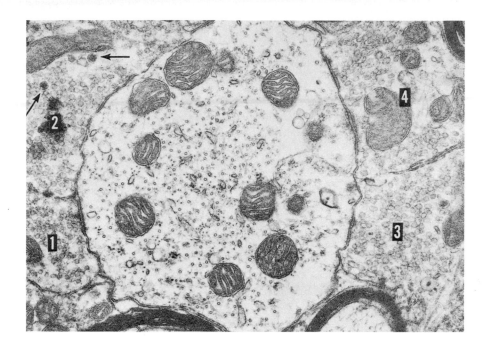

Fig. 2-8. A dendrite emerging from a motor neuron in the anterior horn of a rat spinal cord is contacted by 4 axonal terminals. Terminal 1 contains clear spherical synaptic vesicles, terminals 2 and 3 contain both clear spherical and dense core vesicles (arrows), and terminal 4 contains many clear flattened (inhibitory) synaptic vesicles. Note also the synaptic thickenings and (within the dendrite) the mitochondria, neurofilaments, and neurotubules. ×33,000.

structure and enzymatic properties of mitochondria and the above cellular components.

Axons

As the axon egresses, it is physiologically and structurally divisible into distinct regions—the axon hillock, the initial segment, and the axon proper. These segments are discussed in detail by Peters and coworkers [4]. Basically, the segments differ ultrastructurally in membrane morphology and the content of rough and smooth ER. The axon hillock may contain fragments of Nissl substance, including abundant ribosomes, which diminish as the hillock continues into the initial segment. Here the various axoplasmic components begin to align longitudinally. A few ribosomes and smooth ER still persist, and some axoaxonic synapses occur. More interestingly, however, the axolemma of the initial segment, the region for the generation of the action potential, is underlaid by a dense granular layer similar to that seen at the nodes of Ranvier. Also present in this region are neurotubules, neurofilaments, and mitochondria. The arrangement of the neurotubules in the initial segment, unlike their scattered pattern in the distal axon, is in fascicles; they are interconnected by side arms [4]. Beyond its initial segment, the axon maintains a relatively uniform morphology. It contains an axolemma without any structural modification; microtubules, sometimes cross-linked; neurofilaments interconnected by granular proteinaceous strands; mitochondria; and tubulo-vesicular profiles probably derived from smooth ER. Myelinated axons show granular densifications beneath the axolemma at nodes of Ranvier, and synaptic complexes may also occur in the same regions. The terminal portions of axons arborize and enlarge at their synaptic regions, where they contain synaptic vesicles lying beneath the specialized presynaptic junction.

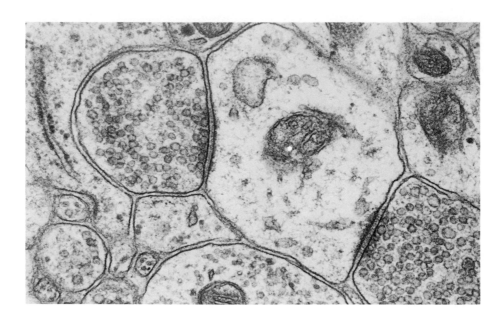

Fig. 2-9. A dendrite (center) is flanked by two axonal terminals packed with clear spherical synaptic vesicles. Details of the synaptic region are clearly shown. ×75,000.

Dendrites

Dendrites, the afferent components of neurons, are frequently arranged around the neuronal soma in a stellate fashion. In some neurons they may arise from a single trunk from which they branch into a dendritic tree. Unlike axons, they are generally lacking in neurofilaments, although they may contain fragments of Nissl substance. Larger branches of dendrites, however, in close proximity to neurons, may contain small bundles of neurofilaments. Some difficulty may be encountered in distinguishing small unmyelinated axons, terminal segments of axons, and small dendrites. In the absence of synaptic evidence, however, they often can be assessed by the content of neurofilaments. The synaptic regions of dendrites occur either along the main stems (Fig. 2-8) or at small protuberances known as *dendritic spines* or *thorns*. Axon terminals abut these structures.

Synapses

The axons and dendrites that emerge from different neurons intercommunicate by means of specialized junctional complexes known as *synapses*, a fact and name first proposed by Sherrington in 1897. Their existence was immediately demonstrable by EM

and today can be recognized in a dynamic fashion by Nomarski optics for light microscopy and by scanning EM. With the development of neurochemical approaches to neurobiology (see Chap. 3 for synaptosomes and Chap. 8 for synaptic transmission), an understanding of synaptic form and function becomes of fundamental importance. As was noted in the first ultrastructural study on synapses (Palade and Palay in 1954, quoted in [5]), synapses display interface specialization and are frequently polarized or asymmetrical. The asymmetry is due to the unequal distribution of electron-dense (osmiophilic) material or thickening applied to the apposing membranes of the junctional complex and the heavier accumulation of organelles within the presynaptic (usually axonal) component. The closely applied membranes constituting the synaptic site are overlaid on the presynaptic and postsynaptic aspects by an osmiophilic material similar to that seen in desmosomes (see Ependymal

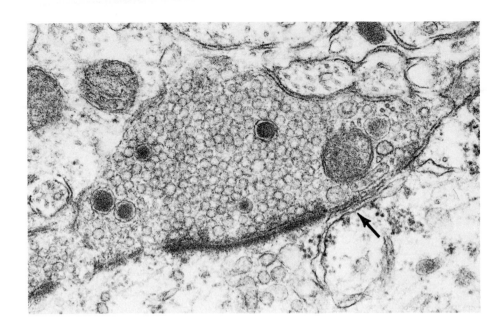

Fig. 2-10. An axonal terminal at the surface of a neuron from the dorsal horn of a rabbit spinal cord contains both dense-core and clear spherical synaptic vesicles lying above the membrane thickenings. A subsurface cisterna (arrow) is also seen. ×68,000.

Cell) and are separated by a gap (cleft) between 150 and 200 Å. The presynaptic component usually contains a collection of clear, 400- to 500-Å synaptic vesicles and various numbers of small mitochondria about 0.2 to 0.5 micron in diameter (Figs. 2-8 to 2-10). Occasional 240 Å microtubules, coated vesicles, and cisternae of smooth ER are not uncommon in this region. On the postsynaptic side is a density, referred to as the *subsynaptic web*; but apart from an infrequent, closely applied packet of smooth ER (subsurface cisterna) belonging to the hypolemmal system, there are no aggregations or organelles in the dendrite.

At the neuromuscular junction, the morphological organization is somewhat different. Here the axon terminal is greatly enlarged and is ensheathed by Schwann cells, and the postsynaptic (sarcolemmal) membrane displays less densification and is deeply infolded.

Before elaborating further on synaptic diversity, it might be helpful to outline briefly other ways in which synapses have been classified in the past. Using the light microscope, Cajal (quoted by Bodian [10]) was able to identify 11 distinct groups of synapses. Nowadays, most neuroanatomists apply a more fundamental classification schema to synapses, depending upon the profiles between which the synapse is formed, that is, axodendritic, axosomatic, axoaxonic, dendrodendritic, somatosomatic, and somatodendritic. Unfortunately, such a list totally disregards the type of transmission (chemical or electrical) and, in the case of chemical synapses, the neurotransmitter involved.

In terms of physiological typing, three groups of synapses are recognized: excitatory, inhibitory, and modulatory. Some neuroanatomical studies (Walberg, 1965, and Uchinozo, 1965, quoted by Bodian [10]) on excitatory and inhibitory synapses have claimed that the excitatory possess spherical synaptic vesicles, whereas inhibitory synapses contain a predominance of flattened vesicles (Fig. 2-8). Other studies, for example, Gray [11], have correlated this synaptic vesicular diversity with physiological data. In his study on cerebellum, Gray showed that neurons with a known predominance of excitatory input on dendrites and an inhibitory input on the cell body possess two corresponding types of synapses. However, although the above interpretation fits well in some loci of the CNS, it does not hold true for all regions. Furthermore, some workers feel that the differences between flat and spherical vesicles may reflect an artifact of aldehyde fixation or a difference in physiological state at the time of sampling. In the light of these criticisms, it is clear that further confirmation as to the correlation between flattened vesicles and inhibitory synapses is required.

Another criterion for the classification of synapses by EM was introduced in 1959 by Gray [11]. Briefly, certain synapses in the cerebral cortex can be grouped into two types, depending upon the length of the contact area between synaptic membranes and the amount of postsynaptic thickening. Relationships have been found between type 1—the membranes of which are closely apposed for long distances and have a large amount of associated postsynaptic thickening—and excitatory axodendritic synapses. Type 2 synapses, on the other hand, are mainly axosomatic, show less close apposition and thickening at the junction, and are believed to be inhibitory. This broad grouping has been confirmed in the cerebral cortex by a number of workers, but it does not hold true for all centers of the CNS.

Most of the data gained from studies on synapses in situ or on synaptosomes (see Chap. 9) have been on cholinergic transmission. Understanding of the vast family of chemical synapses belonging to the autonomic nervous system that utilize biogenic amines (Chap. 10) as neurotransmitter substances is still in its infancy. Morphologically, catecholaminergic synapses are similar but possess, in addition to clear vesicles, dense-core or granular vesicles of variable and slightly larger dimensions (Figs. 2-8 and 2-10). These vesicles were first identified as synaptic vesicles by Grillo and Palay [12], who segregated classes of granular vesicles based on vesicle and core size, but no relationship was made between granular vesicles and transmitter substances. About the same time, EM autoradio-

graphic techniques were being employed, and by using tritiated norepinephrine, Wolfe and co-workers [13] were able to localize the label to granular vesicles within axonal terminals.

Since this work, numerous other labeling techniques for aminergic synapses have been developed. Several of the methods and requirements for detecting such transmitters have been reviewed by Bloom [14]. Catecholaminergic vesicles are generally classified on a size basis, and not all have dense cores.

Another, as yet unclassified, category of synapses may be the so-called silent synapses observed in CNS tissue both in vitro and in vivo. These synapses are morphologically identical to functional synapses but are physiologically dormant.

Finally, with regard to synaptic types, there is the well-characterized electrical synapse [15], in which current can pass from cell to cell across regions of membrane apposition that essentially lack the associated collections of organelles present at the chemical synapse. In the electrical synapse (Fig. 2-11), the unit membranes are closely apposed; the outer leaflets sometimes fuse to form a pentalaminar structure. However, in most places, a gap of about 20 Å exists, producing a so-called gap junction. Not infrequently, such gap junctions are separated by desmosomelike regions [4]. Sometimes electrical synapses exist at terminals that also display typical chemical synapses—in such a case the structure is referred to as a *mixed synapse*. The comparative morphology of electrical and chemical synapses has been reviewed by Pappas and Waxman [16].

The Neuroglia

CLASSIFICATION

Virchow, in 1846, first recognized the existence in the CNS of a fragile, nonnervous, interstitial component made up of stellate or spindle-shaped cells, morphologically distinct from neurons, which he named *neuroglia* ("nerve glue"). It was not until the early part of this century that this interstitial element was classified into distinct cell types [4]. Today, we identify two broad groups of glial cells: (1) the macroglia, embracing astrocytes and oligo-

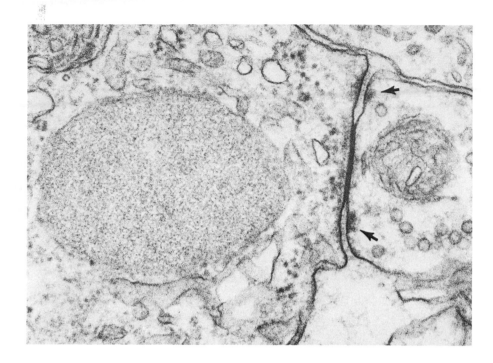

Fig. 2-11. An electrotonic synapse is seen at the surface of a motor neuron from the spinal cord of a toadfish. Between the neuronal soma (left) and the axonal termination (right) a gap junction flanked by desmosomes is visible. Photograph, courtesy of Drs. G. D. Pappas and J. S. Keeter. ×80,000.

dendrocytes, all of ectodermal origin; and (2) the smaller microglia, of mesodermal origin. Macroglial cells develop from a common stem cell, the spongioblast. Microglia invade the CNS at the time of vascularization via the pia mater, the walls of blood vessels, and the tela choroidea.

All glial cells differ from neurons in that they possess no synaptic contacts, and all retain the ability to divide throughout life, particularly in response to injury. The rough schema represented by Fig. 2-1 demonstrates the interrelationships between the macroglia and other CNS components.

MACROGLIAL CELLS

Astrocytes

The complex packing achieved by the processes and cell bodies of astrocytes heralds the potential involvement of this cell type in brain metabolism, because virtually nothing can enter the CNS parenchyma without being confronted by an astrocytic interphase.

Although astrocytes traditionally have been subdivided into protoplasmic and fibrous astrocytes [5], these two forms probably represent the opposite ends of a large spectrum of variation within the same cell type. The morphological components of fibrous and protoplasmic astrocytes are identical; the differences are quantitative. In the early days of electron microscopy, structural differences between the two variants were more apparent, owing to artifactual changes; but with the development of better fixation procedures, it became apparent that the differences were not so great.

Protoplasmic astrocytes range in size from 10 to 40 μ, are frequently located in gray matter in relation to capillaries, and have a clearer cytoplasm than do fibrous astrocytes (Fig. 2-12). Within the perikaryon are scattered 90Å filaments and 240Å microtubules (Fig. 2-13); glycogen granules; lyso-

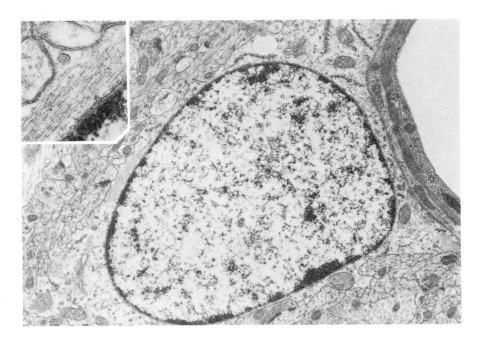

Fig. 2-12. *A protoplasmic astrocyte abuts a blood vessel in rat cerebral cortex. The nucleus shows a rim of denser chromatin, and the cytoplasm contains many organelles, including Golgi and rough ER. ×10,000. Inset: Detail of perinuclear cytoplasm showing filaments. ×44,000.*

somes and lipofuscinlike bodies; isolated cisternae of rough ER; a small Golgi apparatus opposite one pole of the nucleus; and small, elongated mitochondria, often extending together with loose bundles of filaments along cell processes. A centriole is not uncommon. Characteristically, the nucleus is ovoid and the nucleochromatin homogeneous, except for a narrow rim of dense chromatin and one or two poorly defined nucleoli. The fibrous astrocyte occurs in white matter (Fig. 2-13). Its processes are twiglike, being composed of large numbers of glial filaments arranged in tight bundles. The filaments within these cell processes can be distinguished from neurofilaments by their close packing and the absence of cross-bridges (Figs. 2-13 and 2-14). There are often desmosomes between adjacent astrocytic processes.

In addition to protoplasmic and fibrous forms, regional specialization occurs among astrocytes. The outer membranes of astrocytes located in subpial zones and adjacent to blood vessels possess a specialized thickening [17]. Also, desmosomes are common in these regions between astrocytic processes. In the cerebellar cortex, protoplasmic astrocytes can be segregated into three classes—the Golgi epithelial cell, the lamellar or velate astrocyte, and the smooth astrocyte [1], each ultrastructurally distinct.

ASTROCYTE FUNCTION. The functions of astrocytes have long been debated. One of their major roles is related to their connective tissue or skeletal function, since they invest, possibly sustain, and provide a packing for other components. In the case of the astrocytic ensheathment seen around synaptic complexes and the bodies of some neurons, for example, Purkinje cells, it may be speculated that the astrocyte serves to isolate these structures.

One well-known function of the astrocyte is concerned with repair. Subsequent to trauma, astrocytes invariably proliferate, swell, accumulate

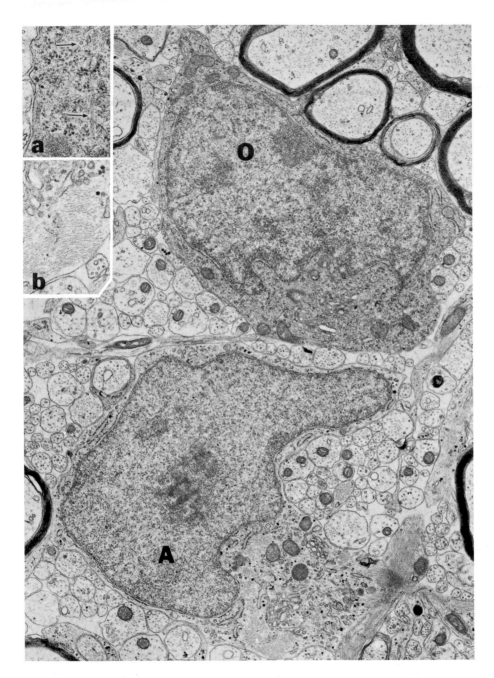

Fig. 2-13. A section from kitten myelinating white matter contains a fibrous astrocyte (A) and an oligodendrocyte (O). The nucleus of the astrocyte has homogeneous chromatin with a denser rim and a central nucleolus. That of the oligodendrocyte is denser and more heterogeneous. Note the denser oligodendrocytic cytoplasm and the prominent filaments within the astrocyte. ×15,000. Inset: (a) Detail of the oligodendrocyte, showing microtubules (arrows) and absence of filaments. ×30,000. (b) Detail of astrocytic cytoplasm showing filaments, glycogen, rough ER, and Golgi apparatus. ×30,000.

glycogen, and undergo fibrosis by the accumulation of filaments. This state of gliosis may be total, in which case all other elements are lost and a glial scar is left; or it may be a generalized response occurring in a background of regenerated or normal CNS parenchyma. Such a phenomenon can occur in both the gray and white matter, thereby indicating common links between protoplasmic and fibrous astrocytes. With age, both fibrous and protoplasmic astrocytes accumulate filaments. In some diseases, astrocytes have been shown to become macrophagous. It is interesting to note that the astrocyte is probably the most disease-resistant component in the CNS, as very few diseases (one of them is alcoholism) can cause depletion or degeneration of astrocytes.

Another putative role of the astrocyte is its involvement in transport mechanisms and in the blood-brain barrier system. It was believed for some time that the transport of water and electrolytes is effected by the astrocyte, a fact never definitively demonstrated and largely inferred from pathological or experimental evidence. It is known, for example, that damage to the brain vasculature, local injury due to heat or cold, and inflammatory changes produce focal swelling of astrocytes, presumably owing to a disturbance in fluid transport. Large molecules can be transferred across the CNS, however, without the involvement of astrocytes. The astrocytic investment of blood vessels might suggest a role in the blood-brain barrier system, but the studies of Reese and Karnovsky [18] and Brightman [19] indicate that the astrocytic endfeet provide little resistance to the movement of molecules and that blockage of passage of material into the brain occurs at the endothelial cell lining blood vessels (see Chap. 25).

Oligodendrocytes

The ultrastructural studies of Schultz and coworkers (1957) and Farquhar and Hartman in 1957, discussed in reference 5, were among the first to contrast the EM features of oligodendrocytes with astrocytes (Fig. 2-12). The study by Mugnaini and Walberg [5] more explicitly laid down morphological criteria for identification of these cells and,

apart from technical improvements apropos quality of preservation, our EM understanding of these cells has changed little since that time. Like the astrocyte, the oligodendrocyte is of ectodermal origin but has fewer cell processes and is spindle shaped.

From a number of EM studies [20], it is apparent that, as with the astrocyte, oligodendrocytes are highly variable, differing in location, morphology, and function, but definable by some morphological criteria. The cell soma ranges from 10 to 20 microns, is roughly globular, and is more dense than that of an astrocyte. The margin of the cell is irregular and compressed against the adjacent neuropil. Few cell processes are seen. Within the cytoplasm, many organelles are found. Parallel cisterns of rough ER and a widely dispersed Golgi apparatus are common. Free ribosomes occur, scattered amidst occasional multivesicular bodies, mitochondria, and coated vesicles. Serving to distinguish the oligodendrocyte from the astrocyte is the apparent absence of glial filaments and the constant presence of 240 Å microtubules (Fig. 2-13), which are most common at the margins of the cell, in the occasional cell process, and in the cytoplasmic loops around myelin sheaths. This absence of filaments, first noticed by Mugnaini and Walberg [5], has been confirmed by several workers. Oligodendrocytic filaments have been observed only in experimental situations. Dense bodies also occur in oligodendrocytes. Most of these are related to lipid droplets, lysosomes, and pigment granules. The nucleus is usually ovoid, but slight lobation is not uncommon. The nucleochromatin stains heavily and contains clumps of denser heterochromatin; the whole structure is sometimes difficult to discern from the background cytoplasm. Desmosomes are known to occur between interfascicular oligodendrocytes.

Ultrastructural studies on the developing nervous system [21, 22] and labeling studies [20] have demonstrated the variability in oligodendrocyte morphology and activity. Mori and Leblond [20] segregated oligodendrocytes into three groups based upon location, stainability, and DNA turnover. Their three classes correspond to satellite,

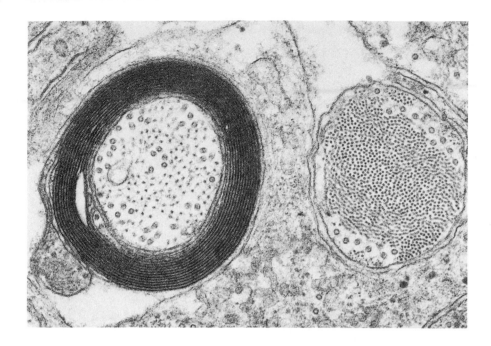

Fig. 2-14. A myelinated axon (left) and the process of a fibrous astrocyte (right) from the spinal cord of an adult dog are sectioned transversely. The axon contains scattered neurotubules and loosely packed neurofilaments interconnected by proteinaceous strands. The astrocytic process contains a bundle of closely packed filaments with no cross-bridges, flanked by several microtubules. Sometimes a lumen can be seen within a filament. ×60,000.

intermediate, and interfascicular (myelinating) oligodendrocytes. Satellite oligodendrocytes are small (about 10 μ), are restricted to the gray matter, and are closely applied to the surface of neurons. They are assumed to play a role in the maintenance of the neuron. Interfascicular oligodendrocytes are large (about 20 μ) during myelination but, in the adult, range from 10 to 15 μ, with the nucleus occupying a large percentage of the volume of the cell soma. Intermediate oligodendrocytes are regarded as potential satellite or myelinating forms. The nucleus in these cells is small, the cytoplasm occupying the greater area of the soma.

OLIGODENDROCYTES AND MYELIN. Myelinating oligodendrocytes have been studied extensively [21, 23, 24]. Examination of the CNS during myelinogenesis (Fig. 2-15) reveals connections between the cell body and the myelin sheath [21]. However, connections between those elements have never been demonstrated in a normal adult animal, unlike the PNS counterpart, the Schwann cell. In contrast to the Schwann cell (see p. 42), the oligodendrocyte is capable of producing many internodes of myelin simultaneously. It is estimated that oligodendrocytes in the optic nerve might produce between 30 and 50 internodes of myelin [23]. In addition to this heavy structural commitment, the oligodendrocyte is known to possess a slow mitotic rate and a poor regenerative capacity. Damage to only a few oligodendrocytes, therefore, can be expected to produce an appreciable area of primary demyelination. Indeed, in most CNS diseases in which myelin is a target, the oligodendrocytes are known to be most vulnerable and among the first CNS elements to degenerate.

Somewhat analogous to the neuron, the relatively small oligodendrocyte cell body produces

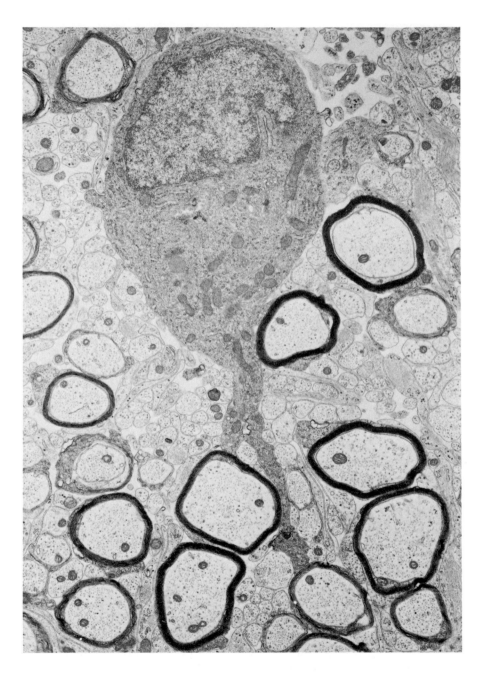

Fig. 2-15. *A myelinating oligodendrocyte from the spinal cord of a two-day-old kitten shows cytoplasmic connections to at least two myelin sheaths. Other myelinated and unmyelinated fibers, as well as glial processes, are seen in the surrounding neuropil.* ×12,750.

and supports many more times its own volume of membrane and cytoplasm. For example, consider an average, 12-μ oligodendrocyte producing 30 internodes of myelin (the lowest number quoted by Peters and Proskauer; see [23]). Each axon has a diameter of 3 μ (small for CNS fibers) and is covered by 6 lamellae of myelin (a conservative estimate), each lamella representing two fused layers of unit membrane. By statistical analysis, taking into account the length of myelin internode (possibly 500 μ) and the length of the membranes of the cell processes connecting the sheaths to the cell body (about 12 μ), the ratio between the surface area of the cell soma and the myelin it sustains is approximately 1:620. The formation of myelin is more completely discussed in Chap. 4.

In some rare instances, oligodendrocytes have been shown to elaborate myelin around structures other than axons. Rosenbluth (1966, discussed in reference 25) was among the first to report the presence of aberrant myelin around neuronal somata and nonaxonal profiles. Since that time, numerous reports have appeared in which myelinated neuronal or oligodendrocytic somata have been described [25].

MICROGLIAL CELLS

Of the few remaining types of CNS cells, the most important, and probably the most enigmatic, is the microglial cell, a cell of mesodermal origin, located in the normal brain in a resting state and purported to become a very mobile, active macrophage in times of need. These cells can be selectively stained and demonstrated by light microscopy using Hortega's silver carbonate method, but no comparable definitive technique exists for their ultrastructural demonstration. The cells have spindle-shaped bodies and a thin rim of densely staining cytoplasm that is difficult to distinguish from the nucleus. The nucleochromatin is homogeneously dense, and the cytoplasm does not contain an abundance of organelles, although representatives of the usual components can be found. During normal wear and tear, some CNS elements degenerate, and microglia can phagocytize the debris (Fig. 2-16). Their identification and numbers (as determined by light

microscopy) differ from species to species. The rabbit CNS is known to be richly endowed. In a number of disease instances, for example, trauma, microglia are known to be stimulated and to migrate to the area of injury where they phagocytize debris. The relatively brief mention of this cell type in EM text books [4], and the conflicting EM descriptions [27, 28], are indicative of the uncertainty attached to their identification. Pericytes, the pericapillary macrophages, are believed to be a resting form of microglial cell.

Ependymal Cells

Ependymal cells are arranged in single-palisade arrays and line the ventricles and central canal. These cells are usually ciliated, their cilia extending from their free (apical) surfaces into the ventricular cavity. Their fine structure has been elucidated by Brightman and Palay [26]. They possess several features that clearly differentiate them from any other CNS cell. The cilia emerge from the apical pole of the cell where they are attached to a blepharoplast, the basal body (Fig. 2-17), which is anchored in the cytoplasm by means of rootlets and a basal foot. The basal foot is the contractile component that apparently determines the direction of the ciliary beat. Like all flagellar structures, the cilium contains the 9 + 2 microtubule arrangement (Fig. 2-17). In the vicinity of the basal body, the arrangement is one of nine triplets; at the tip of each cilium the pattern is one of haphazardly organized single tubules. Also extending from the free surface of the cell are numerous microvilli containing microfilaments (Fig. 2-17). The cytoplasm stains intensely, having an electron density about equal to that of the oligodendrocyte, whereas the nucleus is similar to that of the astrocyte. Microtubules, large whorls of filaments, coated vesicles, rough ER, Golgi apparatus, lysosomes, and abundant small, dense mitochondria are also present. The base of the cell is composed of tortuous processes that interdigitate with the underlying neuropil. The lateral margins of each cell characteristically display long, compound, junctional complexes (Fig. 2-18) made up of desmosomes (*zonulae adhaerentes*) and tight junctions (*zonulae occludentes*).

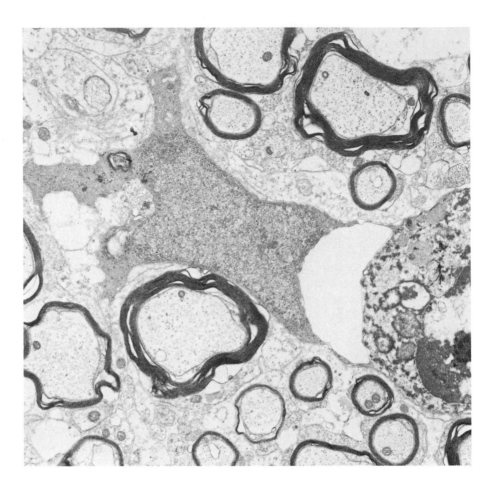

Fig. 2-16. A microglial cell (center) has elaborated two cytoplasmic arms to encompass a degenerating oligodendrocyte (right) in the spinal cord of a three-day-old kitten. The microglial cell nucleus is difficult to distinguish from the narrow rim of densely staining cytoplasm. ×10,000.

The biochemical properties of these structures are well known. Desmosomes display protease sensitivity, divalent cation dependency, and osmotic insensitivity, and the membranes are mainly of the smooth type. In direct contrast to desmosomes, the tight junction (and also gap junctions and synapses) displays no protease sensitivity and no divalent cation dependency, is osmotically sensitive, and morphologically is made up of complex membranes. These facts have been used in the development of techniques to isolate purified preparations of junctional complexes.

Schwann Cells

When axons leave the CNS, they lose their neuroglial interrelationships and traverse a short transi-
tional zone, after which they become invested by Schwann cells. These are the axon-ensheathing cells of the peripheral nervous system, equivalent functionally to the oligodendrocytes of the CNS. Not all PNS fibers are myelinated, but in contrast to nonmyelinated fibers in the CNS, unmyelinated fibers in the PNS are suspended in groups within the Schwann cell cytoplasm, each axon connected to the extracellular space by a short channel, the mes-

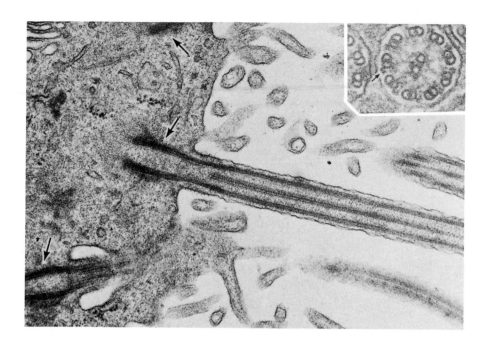

Fig. 2-17. The surface of an ependymal cell contains basal bodies (arrows) connected to the microtubules of cilia, seen here in longitudinal section. Several microvilli are also present. ×37,000. Inset: Ependymal cilia in transverse section possess a central doublet of microtubules surrounded by nine pairs, one of each pair having a characteristic hooklike appendage (arrow). ×100,000.

axon, formed by the invaginated Schwann cell plasmalemma. Myelinated fibers of the PNS, on the other hand, occur singly, are clearly separated, and each internode of myelin is elaborated by one Schwann cell. This ratio of one internode of myelin to one Schwann cell (1:1) is a fundamental distinction between this cell type and its CNS analog, the oligodendrocyte, which is able to proliferate internodes in the ratio of 1:30 or greater. Furthermore, the Schwann cell body always remains in intimate contact with its myelin internode (Fig. 2-19). Periodically, myelin lamellae open up into Schwann cell cytoplasm, producing bands of cytoplasm around the fiber—Schmidt-Lanterman incisures, reputed to be the stretch points along

PNS fibers. These incisures are usually lacking in the CNS. The PNS myelin period is 119 Å in preserved specimens (some 30 percent less than in the fresh state), in contrast to the 106 Å of central myelin. In addition to these structural differences, PNS myelin is known to differ biochemically and antigenically from that of the CNS (Chap. 4).

Ultrastructurally, the Schwann cell is unique and distinct from the oligodendrocyte. Each Schwann cell is surrounded by a basal lamina about 200 to 300 Å thick that does not extend into the mesaxon and is presumably made up of mucopolysaccharide (Fig. 2-19). The basal laminae of adjacent myelinating Schwann cells at nodes of Ranvier are continuous, and the Schwann cell processes interdigitate so that the PNS myelinated axon is never in direct contact with the extracellular space. The Schwann cells of nonmyelinated PNS fibers overlap, and nodes of Ranvier are lacking. The cytoplasm of the Schwann cell is rich in organelles. A Golgi apparatus is located near the nucleus, and cisterns of rough ER occur throughout the cell. Lysosomes, multivesicular bodies, glycogen granules, and lipid granules (*pi granules*)

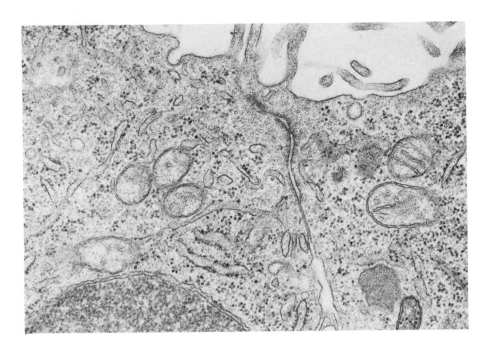

can also be seen. The cell is rich in filaments (in contrast to the oligodendrocyte), and many microtubules are present. The plasmalemma frequently shows pinocytic vesicles. Small, round mitochondria are scattered throughout the soma. The nucleus is flattened, oriented along the nerve fiber, and stains intensely. Aggregates of denser heterochromatin are arranged peripherally. The various features of the Schwann cell are outlined in greater detail by Peters et al. [4].

SCHWANN CELLS DURING DISEASE
In sharp contrast to the oligodendrocyte, the Schwann cell has a vigorous response to most forms of injury. An active phase of mitosis occurs following traumatic insult, and the cells are capable of local migration. Studies on their behavior after primary demyelination have shown that in some cases they are able to phagocytize actively damaged myelin. They possess remarkable mending properties and can begin to lay down new myelin about 1 week after a fiber loses its myelin sheath. Studies on PNS and CNS remyelination by Raine and coworkers [29] have shown that, by 3 months

Fig. 2-18. A typical desmosome and gap junction complex between two ependymal cells. Microvilli and pinocytic vesicles are also seen. ×35,000.

after primary demyelination, PNS fibers are well remyelinated, whereas similarly affected areas in the CNS show relatively little proliferation of new myelin. Under circumstances of severe injury, for example, transection, axons degenerate and the Schwann cells form tubes (*Büngner bands*) containing cell bodies and processes surrounded by a single basal lamina. These structures provide channels along which regenerating axons grow. The presence and integrity of the Schwann cell basal lamina is an essential factor for reinnervation.

Other PNS Elements
The extracellular space between PNS nerve fibers is occupied by bundles of collagen fibrils, blood vessels, and endoneurial cells. The endoneurial cells are elongated, spindle-shaped cells with tenuous processes relatively poor in organelles except for large cisterns of rough ER. There is some evidence

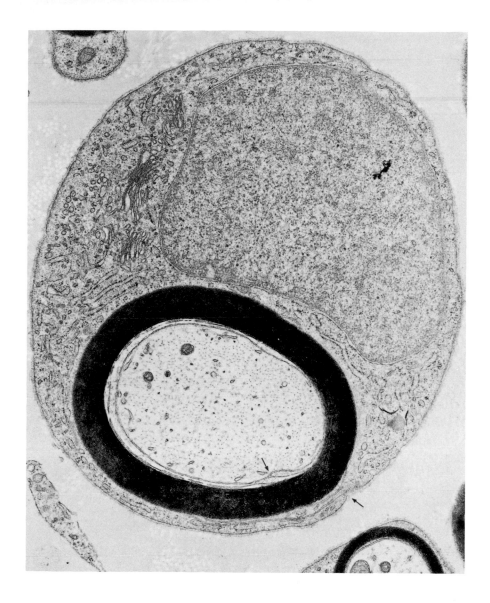

Fig. 2-19. A myelinated PNS axon is surrounded by its Schwann cell. Note the fuzzy basal lamina around the cell, the rich cytoplasm, the inner and outer mesaxon (arrows), the close proximity of the cell to its myelin, and the one-to-one (cell-to-myelin internode) relationship. A process of an endoneurial cell is seen (lower left) and unstained collagen lies in the extracellular space (white dots). ×20,000.

that these cells proliferate collagen fibrils. Sometimes mast cells, the histamine producers of connective tissue, can be seen. Bundles of nerve fibers are arranged in fascicles that are emarginated by flattened connective-tissue cells forming the perineurium, an essential component in the blood-nerve barrier system. Fascicles of nerve fibers are aggregated into nerves and invested by a tough elastic sheath of cells known as the *epineurium*.

Acknowledgments

The author thanks Dr. Robert D. Terry for his helpful discussion. The excellent technical assistance of Everett Swanson, Howard Finch, and Miriam Pakingan is appreciated. I thank Mrs. Mary Palumbo for her secretarial assistance.

The work represented by this chapter was supported in part by grants NS 08952 and NS 03356 from the National Institutes of Health and a grant from the Alfred P. Sloan Foundation.

References

*1. Palay, S. L., and Chan-Palay, V. *Cerebellar Cortex: Cytology and Organization.* New York: Springer, 1974.

*2. Hydén, H. The Neuron. In J. Brachet and A. E. Mirsky (eds.), *The Cell.* New York: Academic, 1960. Vol. 5, pp. 215–323.

*3. Windle, W. F. *Biology of Neuroglia.* Springfield, Ill.: Thomas, 1958.

*4. Peters, A., Palay, S. L., and Webster, H. deF. *The Fine Structure of the Nervous System: The Cells and Their Processes.* New York: Harper & Row, 1970.

*5. Mugnaini, E., and Walberg, F. Ultrastructure of neuroglia. *Ergeb. Anat. Entwicklungsgesch.* 37: 194–236, 1964.

6. Sabatini, D. D., Bensch, K., and Barrnett, R. Cytochemistry and electron microscopic preservation of cellular ultrastructure and enzymatic activity by aldehyde fixation. *J. Cell Biol.* 17:19–56, 1963.

7. Palay, S. L., McGee-Russell, S. M., Gordon, S., Jr., and Grillo, M. A. Fixation of neural tissues for electron microscopy by perfusion with solutions of osmium tetroxide. *J. Cell Biol.* 12:385–410, 1961.

*8. Novikoff, A. B., and Holtzman, E. *Cells and Organelles.* New York: Holt, Rinehart and Winston, 1976.

*Key reference.

*9. Shelanski, M. L., and Weisenberg, R. C. Cytochemical Methods for the Study of Microtubules and Microfilaments. In D. Glick and R. M. Rosenbaum (eds.), *Techniques of Biochemical and Biophysical Cytology.* New York: Wylie, 1972. Vol. 1, pp. 25–50.

*10. Bodian, D. Synaptic Diversity and Characterization by Electron Microscopy. In G. D. Pappas and D. P. Purpura (eds.), *Structure and Function of Synapses.* New York: Raven, 1972. Pp. 45–65.

11. Gray, E. G. Electron microscopy of excitatory and inhibitory synapses: A brief review. *Prog. Brain Res.* 31:141, 1969.

12. Grillo, M. A., and Palay, S. L. Granule-Containing Vesicles in the Autonomic Nervous System. In S. S. Breese (ed.), *Proc. Fifth Int. Cong. Electron Microscopy.* New York: Academic, 1962. P. U-1.

13. Wolfe, D. E., Potter, L. T., Richardson, K. C., and Axelrod, J. Localizing tritiated norepinephrine in sympathetic axons by electron microscopic autoradiography. *Science* 138:440–442, 1962.

*14. Bloom, F. E. Localization of Neurotransmitters by Electron Microscopy. In *Neurotransmitters, Proc. ARNMD.* Baltimore: Williams & Wilkins, 1972. Vol. 50, pp. 25–57.

*15. Bennett, M. V. L. Electrical Versus Chemical Neurotransmission. In *Neurotransmitters, Proc. ARNMD.* Baltimore: Williams & Wilkins, 1972. Vol. 50, pp. 58–90.

*16. Pappas, G. D., and Waxman, S. Synaptic Fine Structure: Morphological Correlates of Chemical and Electrotonic Transmission. In G. D. Pappas and D. P. Purpura (eds.), *Structure and Function of Synapses.* New York: Raven, 1972. Pp. 1–43.

17. Cook, R. D., Raine, C. S., and Wisniewski, H. M. On perivascular astrocytic membrane specializations in monkey optic nerve. *Brain Res.* 57:491–497, 1973.

18. Reese, T. S., and Karnovsky, M. J. Fine structural localization of a blood-brain barrier to exogenous peroxidase. *J. Cell Biol.* 34:207–217, 1967.

19. Brightman, M. The distribution within the brain of ferritin injected into cerebrospinal fluid compartments. II. Parenchymal distribution. *Am. J. Anat.* 117:193–220, 1965.

20. Mori, S., and Leblond, C. P. Electron microscopic identification of three classes of oligodendrocytes and a preliminary study of their proliferative activity in the corpus callosum of young rats. *J. Comp. Neurol.* 139:1–30, 1970.

*21. Bunge, R. P. Glial cells and the central myelin sheath. *Physiol. Rev.* 48:197–248, 1968.

22. Caley, D. W., and Maxwell, D. S. An electron microscope study of the neuroglia during postnatal

development of the rat cerebrum. *J. Comp. Neurol.* 133:45–70, 1968.

*23. Davison, A. N., and Peters, A. *Myelination.* Springfield, Ill.: Thomas, 1970.

24. Hirano, A., and Dembitzer, H. A structural analysis of the myelin sheath in the central nervous system. *J. Cell Biol.* 34:555–567, 1967.

25. Raine, C. S., and Bornstein, M. B. Unusual profiles in organotypic cultures of central nervous tissue. *J. Neurocytol.* 3:313–325, 1974.

26. Brightman, M., and Palay, S. L. The fine structure of ependyma in the brain of the rat. *J. Cell Biol.* 19:415–440, 1963.

27. Mori, S., and Leblond, C. P. Identification of microglia in light and electron microscopy. *J. Comp. Neurol.* 135:57–80, 1969.

28. Blakemore, W. F. Microglial reactions following thermal necrosis of the rat cortex: An electron microscopic study. *Acta Neuropath.* (Berlin) 21:11–22, 1972.

29. Raine, C. S., Wisniewski, H., and Prineas, J. An ultrastructural study of experimental demyelination and remyelination. II. Chronic experimental allergic encephalomyelitis in the peripheral nervous system. *Lab. Invest.* 21:316–327, 1969.

R. Wayne Albers

Chapter 3. Biochemistry of Cell Membranes

The primary functions of neurons include sensing the environment, integrating this input over some range of space and time, and transmitting the resultant signal to other cells. These are functions mediated by cell membranes. From the preceding chapter, it is evident that the principal structural components of cells are membranous. Thus an understanding of the fundamental properties of cell membranes is necessary for exploring the molecular events that underlie neural functions. It is our purpose in this chapter to discuss general principles of membrane biochemistry, to introduce some particular specializations of neural membranes, and to outline some of the important experimental approaches (see also ref. [1]).

The General Structure of Cell Membranes

This is a rapidly advancing area of research. The guiding hypothesis of most current work is the "fluid-mosaic" model of Singer [2]. The structural matrix of cell membranes is a lipid bilayer, predominantly constituted of phospholipids, variable amounts of cholesterol, and glycolipids [3]. Into this matrix are inserted an array of proteins that determine the specific membrane functions that will be discussed in succeeding chapters.

PHYSICAL PROPERTIES OF MEMBRANE LIPIDS
The existence of some form of lipid in natural membranes acting as a barrier to the entrance of small nonelectrolytes was recognized by Overton in 1895 [4]. In 1925, Fricke deduced from electrical impedance measurements that if this barrier was composed of hydrocarbons, it should be about 33 Å thick and suggested that membranes contain a lipid monolayer [5]. In the same year, Gorter and Grendel [6] estimated the surface area of erythrocytes and concluded from their lipid content that there was precisely enough lipid to cover the surface with a bilayer. The existence of bilayers in cell membranes has been established by x-ray diffraction studies [7]. Recent estimates of the thickness of the hydrocarbon part of the bilayer range from 30 to 45 Å.

Early workers felt that certain properties of cell membranes, for example, low surface tension and elasticity, could not be properties of a lipid film. Danielli [8] found that proteins were effective in reducing surface tension at an oil-water interface and proposed that an "unrolled" protein might be adsorbed to the polar surfaces of a lipid bilayer in natural membranes. This model predicts that the ratio of protein to lipid in membranes should be nearly constant and that much of the protein should have an extended (β) secondary structure. Neither of these expectations has been upheld: protein/lipid ratios vary over a wide range from cell to cell and from organelle to organelle [9], and the major component of protein secondary structure in membranes is the α-helical form characteristic of most globular proteins. Moreover, the predominant forces of interaction between membrane proteins and lipids were shown to be hydrophobic rather than polar in nature [2].

Perhaps more forceful than the arguments from physical properties in this regard was the growing appreciation of a wide range of biological functions mediated by membrane proteins that required functional continuity between the inner and outer membrane surfaces, for example, ionic gating (Chap. 5), mediated transport (Chap. 6), and receptor activation of cytoplasmic functions (Chaps. 15 and 16).

The Physical Chemistry of Membranes

The cohesive forces between lipids and between lipids and proteins in membranes are primarily noncovalent bonds that may be classified as ionic, hydrogen, and hydrophobic in character. Such interactions are weak relative to covalent bonds, but a particular complementary orientation among molecules that can maximize the number of these interactions may produce favored stable associations [2].

Molecules are soluble if their interactions with the solvent are stronger than their interactions with other solute molecules. Ionic and polar groups of a molecule will become hydrated, that is, they will interact with the hydrogen or oxygen dipoles of water. If such polar interactions predominate, the molecules of that species will dissolve. Large molecules may have surfaces that lack polar groups, and in aqueous media, such molecules may form aggregates (*micelles*) so organized as to place the nonpolar regions in the interior and the polar groups on the surface. Molecules in which polar and nonpolar groups are segregated are classified as *amphiphilic* and include both the complex lipids and most proteins.

Formation of Lipid Bilayers

The phospholipids can be represented as having a polar "head" composed of a glycerophosphoryl ester moiety and a "tail" composed of two fatty-acid hydrocarbon chains (Chap. 18). Removal of one of the fatty acid moieties produces a lysophosphatide that has marked detergent properties. Aqueous emulsions of lysophosphatides consist of micelles of a few to several hundred molecules, wherein the heads interact with water and the tails are sequestered within. Because of the packing geometry, small, discrete micelles are most readily formed in water from molecules in which the hydrated volume of the polar head group is larger than that of the hydrocarbon tail. In the case of most phospholipids, the packing geometry favors extensive lamellar structures, rather than small micelles. Dispersions of these lamellae form vesicles (*liposomes*). The unit structure is the *bilayer*, an array of phospholipid molecules oriented with polar heads in contact with aqueous media on either side and closely packed hydrocarbon tails inward.

Liposomes are now extensively employed in the study of bilayer properties [10] and in the reconstitution of functional membrane systems (Chap. 6). Single bilayer membranes can be formed from either pure phospholipids or mixtures of amphiphiles by a process of spontaneous thinning, which occurs after a solution in an organic solvent is painted across a small aperture immersed in aqueous medium. The process of thinning can be monitored by the ability of the lipid film to diffract light: the ultimate bilayer membrane thickness is less than the wavelength of visible light and thus appears black after displaying a succession of diffraction colors. The integrity of the membrane can be monitored by its electrical conductance. One of the principal experimental assays for materials that form conductance pathways in membranes (*ionophores*) employs this technique [11].

Physical State of Membrane Lipids

The hydrocarbon region of lipid bilayers can exist in different states of order (phases) that depend upon both temperature and composition. In pure phospholipids, the crystalline (rigid) and liquid-crystalline (fluid in the bilayer plane) states are separated by well-defined transition temperatures. In the lipid mixtures that constitute biological membranes, the situation is more complex: the presence of cholesterol and the heterogeneity of the fatty acid chains cause this transition to occur over a broad temperature range. In the liquid-crystalline state, individual phospholipid molecules have a high degree of mobility within the plane of the membrane, whereas equilibration of phospholipid molecules between the leaflets of a bilayer is relatively slow [12]. Because of the high activation energy required for this "flip-flop," it is possible for asymmetric distributions of phospholipids to persist in bilayers. In fact, biological membranes are highly asymmetrical with respect to the transverse distribution of both lipids and proteins. For example, most plasma membranes contain substantially

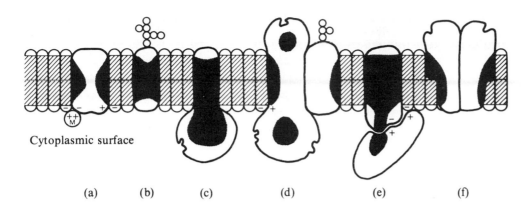

Cytoplasmic surface

(a)   (b)   (c)   (d)   (e)   (f)

Fig. 3-1. Lipid and protein interactions in cell membranes based on some current concepts of structure. Hydrophobic interactions dominate between proteins (shaded areas) and lipids. These are supplemented by electrostatic bonds, including cationic bridges (a). From considerations of protein-folding constraints [16], most intramembrane proteins probably traverse both leaflets of the bilayer. Proteolipids have relatively little interaction with the aqueous environment, but may have internal hydrophilic domains that function as channels (a) and may interact with peripheral proteins (e). Some enzymes are anchored in the membrane but function on only one side (if external, they are termed ecto-enzymes). Others (d) may have functions, such as transport, that require interactions with both sides. Receptors (f) must have stereospecific sites on the external surface and also interact with other membrane proteins.

more phosphatidyl ethanolamine in the cytoplasmic leaflet of the bilayer than in the outer half [13].

Although most of the membrane lipid is in the bilayer configuration, some evidence exists for the occurrence of lipid in other forms. Specific associations with membrane proteins may distort the bilayer structure. Certain cell membrane events, such as fusion, endocytosis, and exocytosis, may also involve transformations from the bilayer structure. The insertion of inverted lipid micelles between bilayer leaflets has been shown to occur in model systems and can produce freeze-fracture images resembling protein particles in electron micrographs [14].

Membrane Proteins

INTRAMEMBRANE PROTEINS

Membrane proteins can be broadly classified as *intramembrane* or *peripheral* (associated), according to whether they interact directly with the hydrophobic region of the bilayer [15].

Intramembrane proteins are found to consist of distinct domains of polar and nonpolar amino acids. In water-soluble proteins, the hydrophobic domains tend to be sequestered in the interior of the folded protein molecules, whereas intramembrane proteins have such regions exposed on their surfaces. The extent of these exposed surfaces has been calculated from measurements of their ability to bind radioactive nonionic detergents. These estimates of nonpolar surface areas range from 20 to 60 percent for different intrinsic membrane proteins [12].

The role of the hydrophobic surfaces must be, in general, to interact with the bilayer lipids (Fig. 3-1). Whether acting as receptors, transport mediators, or enzymes, these specific interactions occur primarily within the aqueous environment, and consequently the functional parts of the protein usually are found in the more hydrophilic domains. In the membrane proteins that function wholly on one side of the membrane, the hydrophobic region may act simply as an anchor. Examples are the microsomal proteins, cytochrome b_5, cytochrome-b_5 reductase, and stearyl coenzyme A (CoA) desaturase [10]. Detergent treatment is required to remove cytochrome b_5 from the microsomal membranes. Subsequent treatment of the protein with trypsin produces a water-soluble cytochrome b_5 which retains catalytic activity but that, in contrast to native protein, cannot be incorporated into liposomes. The trypsin treatment removes a small hydrophobic portion that normally inserts into the lipid bilayer as an anchor.

Bacteriorhodopsin, which functions as a light-driven proton pump in halophilic bacteria, is the best-characterized intrinsic membrane protein [16]. It consists of a single type of polypeptide chain, or subunit, of 247 amino acid residues. Each of these polypeptide chains traverses the lipid bilayer seven times, and each of the seven segments is mostly in α-helical form. Each turn of an α-helix corresponds to 3.6 residues and 5.4 Å displacement along the helix's axis. Using a mean estimate of the thickness of the hydrocarbon bilayer, one may calculate that about 25 residues ($= 3.6 \times [37.5/5.4]$) must be in each segment that traverses the hydrocarbon portion of the bilayer; thus, one concludes that about 70 percent of the total sequence must be contained in these segments.

Several of the enzymes that catalyse active transport (Chap. 6) appear to have hydrophobic domains that extend across the membrane, and globular portions on the cytoplasmic surface that contain the enzyme catalytic sites.

Functional Classes of Intrinsic Membrane Proteins
Membrane receptors (Chaps. 7–16) and ion conductance channels (Chap. 5) are intrinsic membrane proteins of particular importance to neural functions, as are the proteins mediating transport across membranes (Chap. 6). Membrane attachment proteins comprise another functionally defined group. There are specific attachment proteins for actin [17] and spectrin [18]. Tubulin (Chap. 20), in a form similar or identical to that of α-tubulin, occurs as an integral component of synaptic membranes and synaptic vesicle membranes. In the vesicle membranes, α-tubulin appears as a major component [19].

Proteolipids
The proteolipids are a subclass of intrinsic membrane proteins [20, 21]; they are soluble in certain organic solvents, such as chloroform-methanol. Proteolipids were originally identified as constituents of myelin (Chap. 4); later they were also found to be components of the active-transport ATPases [22] and of receptors [23]. In the DCCD-binding protein of the proton-transporting ATPase, the amino acid sequence consists of a short hydrophilic segment flanked by hydrophobic segments of about 25 residues each [24]. In hexameric form, it functions to bind the ATPase to the membrane and probably to form the proton channel.

Glycoproteins
Extensive reviews are available on this subject [25, 26]. External cell surfaces are rich in polysaccharides. These may be extracellular secretions or may be attached covalently to integral membrane components. The latter instance is represented by membrane glycolipids (Chap. 18) and glycoproteins. Members of the largest class of membrane glycoproteins have their polysaccharide moieties linked by N-acetylglucosamine to asparagine residues. Glycoproteins of another class contain carbohydrate linked by N-acetylgalactosamine to serine or threonine residues. Some membrane glycoproteins, such as rhodopsin (Chap. 7), function as receptors and as recognition sites in cellular differentiation processes (Chap. 23). Some are subunits of enzymes, for example, the β subunit of $(Na^+ + K^+)$-stimulated adenosine triphosphatase (see Chap. 6).

Membrane-Associated Proteins
Certain proteins are readily dissociable from membranes by methods that do not disrupt the lipid bilayer, that is, by the use of high or low ionic strength, chaotropic agents, or divalent metal chelators. Acetylcholinesterase is one example of an enzyme that functions extracellularly; it is localized at functionally specialized parts of plasma membranes, such as the end-plate region of skeletal muscle. This enzyme has an attachment segment that resembles collagen in structure and composition [27]. Among the proteins associated with the inner aspect of plasma membranes are a number

that form microfilaments (Chap. 20) and that are structurally related to actin. In several cases, the troponin-C–like calcium-binding protein, cal-modulin, has been associated with such membrane proteins [28] as Ca^{2+}-ATPase [29] and adenylate cyclase [30], where it evidently serves a regulatory function. Calmodulin has been found in high concentration associated with postsynaptic densities [31]. Several guanosine 5'-triphosphate–binding (GTP-binding) proteins are reversibly bound to membranes [32]. One has been shown to mediate the interaction between membrane receptors and adenylate cyclase [41]. Another may represent a tubulin-binding site (Chap. 20 and [33]).

Membrane Dynamics

REGULATION OF MEMBRANE FLUIDITY

The ability of membrane proteins to interact with each other and to undergo the conformational changes necessary to their function often depends on the fluidity of the lipid bilayer [34]. As noted above, this fluidity is determined largely by the nature of the hydrocarbon chains and the cholesterol content. Both of these factors are subject to physiological regulation. For example, hibernating animals change their membrane fatty acid composition during the induction phase of the hibernation process [35]. There is also evidence that neurons increase their membrane fluidity during the process of neurite extension [36].

More rapid fluidity changes may be subject to a different type of regulation: methylation of bilayer phosphatidylethanolamine is catalyzed by intramembrane methyltransferases. The transmethylation of small amounts of phosphatidylethanolamine has been shown to reduce membrane microviscosity. The activity of these methyltransferases is regulated by certain membrane receptors, for example, β-adrenergic; and, in turn, phospholipid methylation has been correlated with changes in receptor properties [37].

Lateral diffusion of membrane proteins appears to be important in many processes, such as receptor activation. For example, several different receptors can activate a given adenylate cyclase molecule. This appears to involve one or more "transducer" proteins, which mediate between the receptor and cyclase proteins. Collision processes by lateral diffusion of membrane proteins would appear necessary to explain these observations. Both lateral and rotary diffusion constants have been measured for membrane proteins. In general, lateral diffusion is slower than free-diffusion theory would predict by one or two orders of magnitude. By contrast, rotary diffusion of membrane proteins appears to be relatively unrestricted. A suggested explanation is that most proteins in cell membranes are hindered in their lateral diffusion by a lattice of proteins that attach to cytoskeletal proteins [38].

Receptor Events in Membranes

Membrane receptor proteins interact stereospecifically with molecules in the extracellular environment to initiate molecular events that alter cell functions. Occupation of the external receptor site by an appropriate agonist results in receptor activation. This activation is only the first of the series of events comprising a cell's response. In some cases, the receptor is closely coupled to the response mechanism. For example, the response to nicotinic cholinergic ligands consists of momentarily opening an ion channel. It is not certain whether the ion channel is integral to the receptor protein, but the rapid response and the interactions of agents acting at the ionophoric site with those acting at the acetylcholine-binding site suggest at least very close apposition of subunits [39] (see also Chap. 9).

In other instances, it is clear that a cascade of protein interactions occurs between the ligand-receptor binding event and the manifest cell response. The ability of membrane proteins to form and disperse in various complexes by diffusing within the bilayer matrix is essential. Members of the class of receptors that can activate adenylate cyclase are prime examples of such diffusion [Chap. 15]. The rate of epinephrine activation of turkey erythrocytes was shown to increase linearly with increases in bilayer fluidity produced by increasing the amount of unsaturated fatty acid in the membranes [40].

The events occurring between receptor activation and modification of adenylate cyclase activity in-

volve, in addition to receptor and enzyme, a GTP-
binding regulatory protein (N-protein). N-proteins
exist in (at least) two forms; these mediate activation and inhibition, respectively. They can be dissociated from the detergent-solubilized adenylate
cyclase. The M_r of one N-protein appears to be of
about 46,000 [41]. A mutant cell line has been
characterized as containing both β-adrenergic
receptors and adenylate cyclase but as not being
capable of cyclase activation by β-adrenergic
agonists. Membranes prepared from these cells can
be induced to cyclase activation by addition of cell
extracts containing N-protein [42].

Data obtained by radiation inactivation suggests
that the receptor, cyclase, and N-proteins exist in
membranes in a variety of different oligomeric complexes corresponding to their states of activation
[43]. The hypothesis advanced by Rodbell [44]
assumes that, in the "resting" state, regulatory and
receptor proteins exist in an oligomeric complex
separated from the cyclase. Agonist activation permits GTP to bind to the N-protein, and this increases the binding affinity between N-protein and
cyclase, so that a ternary complex is formed. Depending upon the nature of the hormone initiating
the process, either inhibition or activation of the
cyclase may result. The activation is turned off by
GTP hydrolysis, although the mechanism for this
has not been established.

In the absence of GTP, the receptor-regulator
complex has an enhanced affinity for agonists, but
agonist binding is incapable of activating the
cyclase. This is a desensitized state of the receptor.
Desensitization is a general consequence of prolonged exposure of receptors to agonists. It is not
well understood, although there have been many
studies of the phenomenon, especially with respect
to the vertebrate neuromuscular junction. A kinetic
model formulated by Katz and Thesleff [45] to
describe cholinergic activation and desensitization
is shown below. The agonist L complexes rapidly
with either the competent receptor R or the desensitized form R'. The activated receptor LR slowly
changes to a more stable, desensitized state, LR';
and the dissociation of LR' is much slower than
that of LR.

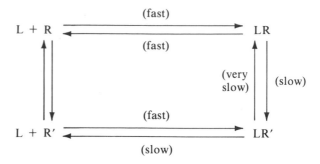

Progressive increases in affinity for cholinergic
ligands have been measured in vitro. The kinetic
form of this transformation corresponds to the
Katz-Thesleff model, except that positive cooperativity has been noted; this suggests that these
receptors may also be oligomeric [46]. In contrast to
the cyclase-activating receptors, no evidence of
metabolic regulation for nicotinic receptors has
been reported. Resensitization of cholinergic receptors has not been accomplished in an in vitro
system; it could involve an energy-requiring step.

MEMBRANE BIOSYNTHESIS

The composite nature of membranes introduces a
number of interdependent questions relating to the
synthesis and assembly of the individual components [47, 48]. How are the newly synthesized lipids
and proteins brought together—as an integrated
supramolecular array of new membrane or as a
result of insertion of new molecules into old membrane? What controls the type of membrane
formed: Is there a genetic control at the supramolecular level or do membranes spontaneously
assemble as determined by the intrinsic characteristics of the individual proteins and lipids? Newly
synthesized phosphatidylethanolamine is initially
inserted into the cytoplasmic leaflet of bacterial cell
membranes; it then rapidly redistributes to the external leaflet. The redistribution has been shown to
be at least 30,000 times faster than the spontaneous
flip-flop rate in synthetic bilayers [49]. It has been
suggested that maintenance of lipid asymmetry,
despite rapid mixing of the newly synthesized pool,
can be explained by selective binding of phospholipids to intramembrane proteins [50].

The site of membrane protein synthesis, in most cases, is the rough endoplasmic reticulum (RER), which consists of an association of endoplasmic reticulum with polyribosomes. As with secretory proteins, the nascent polypeptide precursors of membrane proteins contain one or more hydrophobic signal amino acid sequences that react with RER sites to initiate the transfer of some or all of the nascent polypeptide chain into the lumen of the RER [51]. This signal may be near the N-terminal or within it. The exact function of signal peptides is controversial. One hypothesis is that they interact with specific receptors in the RER. This interaction initiates transport of the nascent polypeptide through the bilayer [47]. An alternative proposal is that signal peptides influence the folding of the growing chain so that the external surface is hydrophobic. The folded chain can then enter the bilayer without the aid of auxiliary proteins [52]. By either model, the signal peptide may subsequently be cleaved by a specific signal protease, which would render the insertion irreversible, or it may remain part of the functional protein. Proteins that traverse the bilayer several times may require multiple signal sequences.

Isolation and Purification of Subcellular Membrane Structures

PRINCIPLES OF FRACTIONATION BY CENTRIFUGATION

A major technical problem in neurochemistry is that of devising methods for obtaining substantial amounts of defined subcellular fractions. In general, the size and density of the subcellular particles are sufficiently different, at least in theory, to define each organelle uniquely. Figure 3-2 shows how one may differentiate the components that might occur in disrupted brain tissue. In practice, however, it is often difficult to separate organelles with small differences in size and density.

The processes of disruption and release of subcellular particles into a suspending medium usually will change particle properties through solvation, osmotic forces, and ion effects. Particles that are permeable to all components of the suspending medium may nevertheless carry a solvation mantle which produces an effective particle-density intermediate between its intrinsic density and that of the medium. In a density gradient within a centrifugal field, however, particles come to equilibrium positions (*isopycnic points*) when the density of the external medium is equal to their intrinsic density. The anhydrous, or intrinsic-particle, densities can be measured in this way. Because vesicular particles usually exhibit some osmotic properties, their effective densities may change with time during centrifugation. Mitochondria and synaptosomes approach the ideal osmometers and, given sufficient time, will equilibrate near their isopycnic point.

Some organelles, such as cell nuclei, respond less readily to fluctuations in osmotic pressure and may exhibit paradoxical volume changes. For example, nuclei swell when transferred from $0.01\ M\ CaCl_2$ to $0.88\ M$ sucrose [53]. Such a response may be related to the high ion exchange capacity of the contents of the nuclei. In this situation, it will be difficult to obtain density gradient separations that are independent of the details of the methods. However, it usually is possible for purposes of fractionation to attain sufficient methodological stability to conduct experiments and ask meaningful questions.

The classic method of differential centrifugation involves only the sedimentation velocity. Particles are dissociated and separated in mediums of relatively low and fixed density, usually isotonic salt or sucrose solutions. Usually, four fractions are obtained by sequential centrifugation steps of increasing rotational velocity and time: a low-speed, short-time nuclear pellet; a medium-speed, medium-time crude mitochondrial fraction; a high-speed, prolonged-time microsomal pellet; and a supernatant fraction containing the soluble cytoplasmic and extracellular components. Although widely used because of its simplicity, this technique has a serious defect—there is an inevitable contamination of the lower-speed fractions with the higher-speed components. As a result, pellets must be washed extensively by repeated centrifugation.

Isopycnic, or buoyant-density, centrifugation aims to order the constituents solely on the basis of intrinsic-particle densities. This is accomplished by

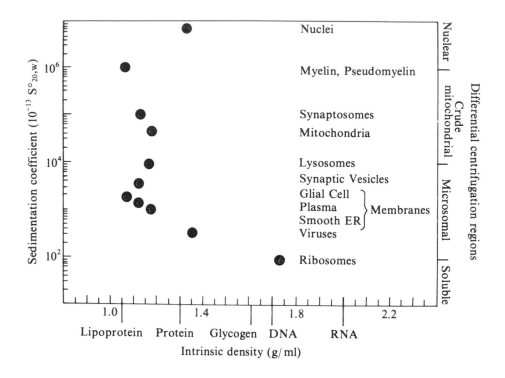

Fig. 3-2. Subcellular particles in a brain homogenate can be separated in a centrifuge on the basis of differential rates of sedimentation (characterized by the sedimentation coefficient, a function of size and intrinsic density) and also on the basis of density gradient centrifugation (characterized by the intrinsic density).

prolonged centrifugation in a medium that contains a density gradient produced by sucrose or by isoosmotic mixtures of sucrose and Ficoll (a sucrose polymer).

Rate-zonal centrifugation is a variant procedure that makes use of the combined velocity-density differences among components. It is based upon the fact that the sedimentation coefficient decreases as the density difference between the particle and medium narrows. Thus, although both dense and light particles move slowly with time, the ratio between their respective sedimentation velocities increases. Thus, the separation of components is improved relative to differential velocity methods, but shorter times are used than are necessary for isopycnic equilibration.

Separation techniques based upon more specific properties of cells and subcellular components are possible. Surface properties may be recognized by specific antibodies, lectins, or other ligands, which in turn, can be attached covalently to chromatographic supports to form so-called affinity columns. Small particles, such as synaptic vesicles, have been purified by size-exclusion chromatography through porous glass columns [54]. There also have been some applications of electronic cell-sorting techniques to subcellular fractionation problems.

CRITERIA OF PURITY

The choice of cell fractionation techniques must be guided by the goals of the particular problem. Accordingly, criteria of purity that are adequate in one problem may not serve in another. For example, cytochrome oxidase is an entirely adequate marker for mitochondrial inner membranes, but the usual cytochrome oxidase assay will not give information about mitochondrial integrity or about the cellular origin of the mitochondria. Lactate dehydrogenase (LDH) is a widely distributed cytoplasmic enzyme, a fact that would seem to make it a poor candidate for a subcellular marker. However, in combination, LDH and cytochrome oxidase assays can be used to assess the content of synaptosomes in a subcellular fraction—synaptosomes are characterized by the presence of both mitochondria and cytoplasmic enzymes encased in a plasma membrane vesicle. These vesicles can be detected by the observation of increased LDH activity after treatment with detergent. However, this assay will not distinguish synaptosomes from vesicles derived from glial or dendritic processes, for example.

Measurements of more specific constituents, such as neurotransmitters, neurotransmitter uptake systems, or specific receptors, are often necessary for adequate assessment of purity. Several proteins have been identified as more or less specific markers for neuronal cell types. The glial fibrillary acidic protein (GFA) is associated with fibrous astrocytes and can be analyzed immunochemically [55]. The acidic protein termed *S-100* appears to be brain-specific but has been reported in both neurons and glia [56]. Another brain-specific protein, originally called *14-3-2*, is found predominantly in neurons and has been shown to be an isozyme of enolase [57]. Myelin contains several specific and well-characterized proteins that can be identified by immunochemical and electrophoretic methods (Chap. 4). Many published reports exist on the purification of subcellular components in brain with the object of characterizing the protein electrophoretic patterns associated with particular organelles and membranes. These are important for comparing the composition and purity of different subcellular fractions.

METHODS FOR ISOLATING SPECIFIC FRACTIONS

Cell Separations

Although it is desirable to begin subcellular fractionation with homogeneous cell populations, homogeneity is particularly difficult to achieve for neural cells, because of the enormous diversity of cell types in the brain. Two general approaches, biological and physical, are possible for selecting bulk quantities of cells of a given type.

Considerable progress has been made in using primary cultures of embryonic brain tissue, usually prepared by dispersing the cells by trypsin treatment [58]. Neurons and glial cells have been separated by virtue of their different tendencies to adhere to glass surfaces under culture conditions. In addition, a variety of neural tumor cell lines have been developed [59]. Differentiated neurons do not divide in culture; this is a serious limitation of the approach. However, various lines of neuroblastoma cells that manifest some of the characteristics of normal neurons have been selected, and because these can be grown in quantity, they are of great value in studying the molecular basis of particular neural functions.

Neural tissue from more mature animals also can be dispersed by mechanical and enzyme treatments in such a way as to leave the component cells relatively intact. Several cell separation methods subject these tissue dispersions to various fractionation procedures to obtain samples relatively rich in neuronal or glial elements. In one such procedure [60], rat brain is minced, incubated with 0.1% trypsin for 90 min, centrifuged at low speed several times in a special medium, and finally passed gently through a nylon screen of 100 to 150 mesh. The filtered dispersion is then layered upon a discontinuous sucrose gradient and centrifuged at 4100 g for 10 min. Neurons are found at the 1.55/2.0 M interface, erythrocytes and endothelial cells at the 1.35/1.55 M interface, and a crude astrocytic fraction at the 0.9/1.35 M interface. Each of these fractions can be further purified by additional gradient separations. Oligodendrocytes can be obtained by an analogous procedure that uses brain white matter as starting material [61]. These isolated cells retain many of their characteristics when examined by electron microscopy, although the number and extent of cell processes are much reduced.

Isolation of Myelin

Myelin consists of the spiral windings of plasma membranes from oligodendrocytes (central nervous system [CNS]) or Schwann cells (peripheral nervous system [PNS]) around axons (Chaps. 2 and

4). Because of the strong interaction between myelin and axolemma, isolates of myelin necessarily include some axonal membranes. Methods for purifying myelin begin with white matter of brain or spinal cord, of which it comprises about 50 percent. Separations are based upon the relatively low density and large size of myelin fragments produced in tissue homogenates. Myelin sediments predominantly with mitochondria in differential centrifugation procedures. It can then be separated from mitochondria by centrifugation through a sucrose density gradient, in which it will form a band at about 0.85 *M*. Another procedure is outlined in Chapter 4.

Myelin-free Axons and Axolemma

One way to obtain purified samples of axons and axolemma is to begin with a tissue rich in unmyelinated axons. Certain peripheral and cranial nerves—particularly the garfish olfactory nerves [62]—cerebellum, and basal ganglia are good starting materials. An alternative method begins with the largely myelinated axons of CNS white matter, isolates the myelin fraction containing the associated axonal fragments, and dissociates the myelin from the axolemma by a prolonged incubation of the fragments in dilute buffer at pH 6. This causes the myelin to swell, form vesicles, and float to the surface during centrifugation, leaving the myelin-free axons as a pellet in the bottom [63].

Nerve-Ending Particles (Synaptosomes)

Homogenization of brain results in shearing of nerve terminals from their axonal terminals. These endings and their contents are relatively resistant to mechanical stress, and their torn surfaces readily reseal to form vesicles called *synaptosomes*. These frequently have an adhering fragment of postsynaptic membrane. Synaptosomes are widely used to study transmitter metabolism and as starting material for the further purification of transmitter-containing vesicles, presynaptic mitochondria, and junctional membranes. Synaptosomes were first purified by de Robertis and coworkers [64] and by Gray and Whittaker [65]. The basic procedure

begins with gentle homogenization of brain tissue in glass or Teflon-and-glass homogenizers with a pestle clearance of about 0.25 mm in a medium of isotonic sucrose. On centrifugation, a pellet forms within 10 min at 1000 *g;* this is discarded. A fraction containing mitochondria, synaptosomes, and some myelin is sedimented at 20,000 *g* within 20 min. Further fractionation by centrifugation of this crude fraction through a discontinuous density gradient is necessary for most purposes. Sucrose gradients were originally used with synaptosomes forming bands in the region of 0.8 to 1.2 *M*. Other procedures use Ficoll-sucrose mixtures to maintain isoosmotic conditions at all densities [66].

SUBFRACTIONATION OF SYNAPTOSOMES. Synaptosomes are readily disrupted by osmotic shock. For some purposes, this step has been applied to the crude fraction obtained by differential centrifugation [67]. Subsequent sucrose density gradient centrifugation produces bands enriched in synaptic vesicles in the 0.4 to 0.6 *M* region, and synaptic membranes at 0.8 to 1.0 *M*. Considerable myelin contamination of the vesicle fraction occurs by this method, and there is a possibility that fragmented mitochondria may not be completely pelleted. A refinement of this technique is to isolate first the synaptosome fraction from a density gradient, lyse the synaptosomes, and employ a second density gradient for the subfractionation [65].

SUBFRACTIONATION OF SYNAPTIC MEMBRANES. The development of techniques for the isolation of the specialized regions of synaptic membrane has presented an opportunity for detailed investigation of their structure and function [68]. Isolation of the so-called synaptic complex was made possible by the demonstration that certain nonionic detergents can release this structure selectively from adjoining pre- and postsynaptic membranes (Chap. 19). A structure associated with the postsynaptic part of this complex can be stained selectively with phosphotungstate [Fig. 3-3]. Treatment of synaptic membranes with other detergents has led to procedures for isolating this postsynaptic density (PSD) and its further purification by density gradient centrifugation (Fig. 3-3).

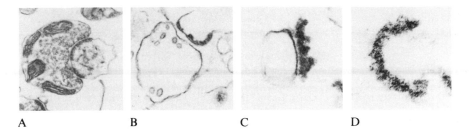

A   B   C   D

Fig. 3-3. Synaptic structures that can be purified from brain. A. Synaptosome with a presynaptic ending containing vesicles and mitochondria. B. Synaptic plasma membranes. C. Synaptic junctions. D. Postsynaptic densities. (Courtesy of Dr. Carl Cotman.)

Isolation of Transmitter-Containing Vesicles

As mentioned above, synaptic vesicles survive the osmotic shock that is sufficient to release the contents of synaptosomes. About 50 percent of the acetylcholine content of synaptosomes can be recovered in association with vesicles of approximately 500 Å diameter that band in densities produced by 0.4 to 0.5 M sucrose. Exposure of the isolated vesicles to distilled water will release the bound acetylcholine. The membranes of these vesicles have a characteristic protein pattern [69]. One of the major proteins is a form of tubulin [19].

Frequently, tissue other than brain is selected for isolation of vesicles containing neurotransmitters. The squid head ganglion is a rich source of acetylcholine vesicles [70]. Catecholamine vesicles are readily isolated from adrenal medullary tissue [71].

Brain Mitochondria

Brain tissue is a rich source of mitochondria and its high rate of glucose and oxygen utilization reflects this fact (Chap. 24). Qualitative and quantitative differences distinguish brain mitochondrial metabolism from that of other organs. There are also differences in the distribution of mitochondrial enzymes throughout the brain that lead one to the conclusion that there are different types of mitochondria within the brain. Mitochondria isolated by differential centrifugation are predominantly found intermixed with synaptosomes. Density gradient procedures can be used to separate free mitochondria from synaptosomes [72]. Another population of mitochondria can be isolated from osmotically lysed synaptosomes. Quantitative differences in the enzyme composition of these two classes have been reported [72]. Some attempts have been made to identify functionally different classes of neuronal mitochondria, but any distinctions that may exist remain to be elucidated.

References

1. Pfenninger, K. H. Organization of neuronal membranes. *Annu. Rev. Neurosci.* 1:445–471, 1978.
2. Singer, S. J. The molecular organization of membranes. *Annu. Rev. Biochem.* 43:805–833, 1974.
3. Tanford, C. The hydrophobic effect and the organization of living membranes. *Science* 200:1012–1018, 1978.
4. Overton, E. Über die osmotischen Eigenschaften der lebenden Pflanzen und Tiergelle. *Vierteljahrsschr. Naturforsch. Ges. Zuer.* 40:159–190, 1895.
5. Fricke, H. A mathematical treatment of the electrical conductivity and capacity of disperse systems. *Phys. Rev.* 26:678–687, 1925.
6. Gorter, E., and Grendel, F. On bimolecular layers of lipoids on the chromocytes of the blood. *J. Exp. Med.* 41:439–443, 1925.
7. Blaurock, A. E. Structure of the nerve myelin membrane. *J. Mol. Biol.* 56:35–52, 1971.
8. Danielli, J. F. Protein films at the oil-water interface. *Cold Spring Harbor Symp. Quant. Biol.* 6:190–195, 1938.
9. Korn, E. D. Structure of biological membranes. *Science* 153:1491–1498, 1966.
10. Bangham, A. D., Hill, M. W., and Miller, N. G. A. Preparation and Use of Liposomes as Models of Biological Membranes. In E. D. Korn (ed.), *Methods in Membrane Biology.* New York: Plenum, 1974. Vol. 1, pp. 1–68.

11. Andreoli, T. E.   Planar Lipid Bilayer Membranes. In S. Fleischer and L. Packer (eds.), *Methods in Enzymology.* New York: Academic, 1974. Vol. 32, pp. 513–539.

12. Rothman, J. E., and Lenard, J.   Membrane asymmetry. *Science* 195:743–753, 1977.

13. Op den Kamp J. A. F.   Lipid asymmetry in membranes. *Annu. Rev. Biochem.* 48:47–71, 1979.

14. Cullis, P. R., and de Kruiff, B.   Lipid polymorphism and the functional roles of lipids in biological membranes. *Biochim. Biophys. Acta* 559:399–420, 1979.

15. Guidotti, G.   The structure of intramembrane proteins. *J. Supramol. Struct.* 7:489–497, 1977.

16. Henderson, R.   The purple membrane from *Halobacterium halobium. Annu. Rev. Biophys. Bioen.* 6:87–109, 1977.

17. Korn, E. D.   Biochemistry of actomyosin-dependent cell motility (a review). *Proc. Natl. Acad. Sci. U.S.A.* 75:588–599, 1978.

18. Tyler, J. M., Hargreaves, W. R., and Branton, D.   Purification of two spectrin-binding proteins. *Proc. Natl. Acad. Sci. U.S.A.* 76:5192–5196, 1979.

19. Zisapel, N., Levi, M., and Gozes, I.   Tubulin: An integral protein of mammalian synaptic vesicle membranes. *J. Neurochem.* 34:26–32, 1980.

20. Folch-Pi, J., and Stoffyn, P. J.   Proteolipids from membrane systems. *Ann. N. Y. Acad. Sci.* 195:86–107, 1972.

21. Lees, M. B., et al.   Structure and function of proteolipids in myelin and non-myelin membranes. *Biochim. Biophys. Acta* 559:209–230, 1979.

22. Hobbs, A. S., and Albers, R. W.   The structure of proteins involved in active membrane transport. *Annu. Rev. Biophys. Bioeng.* 9:259–291, 1980.

23. Taylor, R. F.   Isolation and purification of cholinergic receptor proteolipids from rat gastrocnemius tissue. *J. Neurochem.* 31:1183–1198, 1978.

24. Sebald, W., Graf, T., and Lukins, H. H.   The dicyclohexylcarbodiimide-binding protein of the mitochondrial ATPase complex from *Neurospora crassa* and *Saccharomyces cerevisiae. Eur. J. Biochem.* 93:587–599, 1979.

25. Hughes, R. C.   *Membrane Glycoproteins.* London: Butterworth, 1976.

26. Juliano, R. L.   Techniques for the analysis of membrane. *Curr. Top. Membranes Transp.* 11:107–144, 1978.

27. Lwebuga-Mukasa, G., Lappi, S., and Taylor, P.   Molecular forms of acetylcholinesterase from *Torpedo californica:* Their relationship to synaptic membranes. *Biochemistry* 15:1425–1434, 1976.

28. Cheung, W. Y.   Calmodulin plays a pivotal role in cellular regulation. *Science* 207:19–27, 1980.

29. Niggli, V., Ronner, P., Carafoli, E., and Penniston, J. T.   Effects of calmodulin on the $(Ca^{+2} + Mg^{+2})$-ATPase partially purified from erythrocyte membranes. *Arch. Biochem. Biophys.* 198:124–130, 1979.

30. Toscano, W., et al.   Evidence for a dissociable protein subunit required for calmodulin stimulation of brain adenylate cyclase. *Proc. Natl. Acad. Sci. U.S.A.* 76:5582–5586, 1979.

31. Grab, D., et al.   Presence of calmodulin in postsynaptic densities isolated from canine cerebral cortex. *J. Biol. Chem.* 254:8690–8696, 1979.

32. Pfeuffer, T.   GTP-binding proteins in membranes and the control of adenylate cyclase activity. *J. Biol. Chem.* 252:7224–7234, 1977.

33. Kelly, P. T., and Cotman, C. W.   Synaptic proteins, characterization of tubulin and actin, and identification of a distinct postsynaptic density polypeptide. *J. Cell Biol.* 79:173–183, 1978.

34. Gennis, R. B., and Jonas, A.   Protein-lipid interactions. *Annu. Rev. Biophys. Bioeng.* 6:195–238, 1977.

35. Goldman, S. S.   Cold resistance of brain during hibernation: Evidence of a lipid adaptation. *Am. J. Physiol.* 228:834–838, 1975.

36. de Laat, S. G., et al.   Lateral diffusion of membrane lipids and proteins is increased specifically in neurites of differentiating neuroblastoma cells. *Biochim. Biophys. Acta* 558:247–250, 1979.

37. Hirato, F., et al.   Regulation of β-Adrenergic Receptors by Phospholipid Methylation. In G. Pepeu, M. Kuhar, and S. Enna (eds.), *Receptors for Neurotransmitters and Peptide Hormones.* New York: Raven, 1980. Pp. 91–97.

38. Cherry, R. J.   Rotational and lateral diffusion of membrane proteins. *Biochim. Biophys. Acta* 559:289–327, 1979.

39. Heidemann, T., and Changeux, J.-P.   Structural and functional properties of the acetylcholine receptor protein in its purified and membrane-bound states. *Annu. Rev. Biochem.* 47:317–357, 1978.

40. Hanski, E., Rimon, G., and Levitski, A.   Adenylate cyclase activation by β-adrenergic receptors as a diffusion-controlled process. *Biochemistry* 18:846–853, 1979.

41. Pfeuffer, T.   GTP-binding proteins in membranes and the control of adenylate cyclase activity. *J. Biol. Chem.* 252:7224–7234, 1977.

42. Howlett, A. C., et al.   Reconstitution of catecholamine-sensitive adenylate cyclase. *J. Biol. Chem.* 254:2287–2295, 1979.

43. Schlegel, W., Kempner, E. S., and Rodbell, M.   Activation of adenylate cyclase in hepatic membranes involves interactions of the catalytic unit with multimeric complexes of regulatory proteins. *J. Biol. Chem.* 254:5168–5176, 1979.

44. Rodbell, M.   The role of hormone receptors and

GTP regulatory proteins in membrane transduction. *Nature* 284:17–22, 1980.

45. Katz, B., and Thesleff, S. A study of the "desensitization" produced by acetylcholine at the motor endplate. *J. Physiol. Lond.* 138:63–80, 1957.

46. Sine, S., and Taylor, P. Functional consequences of agonist-mediated state transitions in the cholinergic receptor. *J. Biol. Chem.* 254:3315–3325, 1979.

47. Lodish, H. F., and Rothman, J. E. The assembly of cell membranes. *Sci. Am.* 240:48–63, 1979.

48. Morre, D. J., Kartenbeck, J., and Franke, W. W. Membrane flow and interconversions among membranes. *Biochim. Biophys. Acta* 559:71–152, 1979.

49. Rothman, J. E., and Kennedy, E. P. Rapid transmembrane movement of newly synthesized phospholipids during membrane assembly. *Proc. Natl. Acad. Sci. U.S.A.* 74:1821–1825, 1977.

50. Langley, K. E., and Kennedy, E. P. Energetics of rapid transmembrane movement and of compositional asymmetry of phosphatidylethanolamine in membranes of *Bacillus megaterium*. *Proc. Natl. Acad. Sci. U.S.A.* 76:6245–6249, 1979.

51. Lingappa, V. R., et al. A signal sequence for the insertion of a transmembrane glycoprotein. *J. Biol. Chem.* 253:8667–8670, 1978.

52. Wickner, W. The assembly of proteins into biological membranes: The membrane trigger hypothesis. *Annu. Rev. Biochem.* 48:23–45, 1979.

53. Anderson, N. G., and Wilbur, K. M. Studies on isolated cell components. IV. The effect of various solutions on the isolated rat liver nucleus. *J. Gen. Physiol.* 35:781–796, 1952.

54. Carlson, S. S., Wagner, J. A., and Kelly, R. B. Purification of synaptic vesicles from elasmobranch electric organ and the use of biophysical criteria to demonstrate purity. *Biochemistry* 17:1188–1199, 1978.

55. Bignami, A., and Dahl, D. Astrocyte-specific protein and neuroglial differentiation. *J. Comp. Neurol.* 153:27–37, 1974.

56. Moore, B. W. A soluble protein characteristic of the nervous system. *Biochem. Biophys. Res. Comm.* 19:739–744, 1965.

57. Marangos, P. J., Schmechel, D., Zis, A. P., and Goodwin, F. K. The existence and neurobiological significance of neuronal and glial forms of the glycolytic enzyme, enolase. *Biol. Psychiatry* 14:563–579, 1979.

58. Fischbach, G. D., and Nelson, P. G. Cell Culture in Neurobiology. In E. Kandel (ed.), *Handbook of Physiology, Section 1: The Nervous System, Vol. 1: Cellular Biology of Neurons, Part 2.* Bethesda: Am. Physiol. Soc., 1977. Pp. 719–774.

59. Kimhi, Y. Clonal Systems. In P. G. Nelson and M. Lieberman (eds.), *Excitable Cells in Tissue Culture.* New York: Plenum, 1981. Pp. 173–246.

60. Poduslo, S. E., and Norton, W. T. Neuronal soma and whole neuroglia of rat brain: A new isolation technique. *Science* 167:1143–1145, 1970.

61. Poduslo, S. E., and Norton, W. T. Isolation and some chemical properties of oligodendroglia from calf brain. *J. Neurochem.* 19:727–736, 1972.

62. Chacko, G., Goldman, D., and Pennock, B. Composition and characterization of the lipids of garfish olfactory nerve, a tissue rich in axonal membrane. *Biochim. Biophys. Acta* 280:1–16, 1972.

63. Harford, J. B., Waechter, C. J., Saul, R., and DeVries, G. H. Evidence for the biosynthesis of mannosylphosphoryldolichol and *N*-acetylglucosaminylpyrophosphoryldolichol by an axolemma-enriched membrane preparation from bovine white matter. *J. Neurochem.* 32:91–98, 1979.

64. de Robertis, E., et al. Cholinergic and non-cholinergic nerve endings in rat brain. *J. Neurochem.* 9:23–36, 1962.

65. Gray, E. G., and Whittaker, V. P. The isolation of nerve endings from brain. *J. Anat.* 96:79–88, 1962.

66. Cotman, C. W. Isolation of Synaptosomal and Synaptic Plasma Membrane Fractions. In S. Fleischer and L. Packer (eds.), *Methods in Enzymology* 31, part A. New York: Academic, 1974. Pp. 445–452.

67. Whittaker, V. P., Michaelson, I. A., and Kirkland, R. J. A. The separation of synaptic vesicles from nerve ending particles. *Biochem. J.* 90:293–303, 1964.

68. Cohen, R. S., et al. The structure of postsynaptic densities isolated from dog cerebral cortex. 1. Overall morphology and protein composition. *J. Cell Biol.* 74:181–203, 1977.

69. Wagner, J., and Kelly, R. Topological organization of proteins in an intracellular secretory organelle: The synaptic vesicle. *Proc. Natl. Acad. Sci. U.S.A.* 76:4126–4130, 1979.

70. Dowdall, M. J., and Whittaker, V. P. Comparative studies in synaptosome formation: The preparation of synaptosomes from the head ganglion of the squid, *Loligo pealii. J. Neurochem.* 20:921–935, 1973.

71. Smith, A. D., and Winkler, H. A simple method for the isolation of adrenal chromaffin granules on a large scale. *Biochem. J.* 103:480–482, 1967.

72. Lai, J. C. K., et al. Synaptic and non-synaptic mitochondria from rat brain: Isolation and characterization. *J. Neurochem.* 28:625–631, 1977.

William T. Norton

Chapter 4. Formation, Structure, and Biochemistry of Myelin

This chapter presents a survey of the structure, cellular formation, and biochemistry of the myelin sheath. For a fuller treatment of some subjects, the reader is referred to several books and reviews [1–13], especially the comprehensive volume edited by Morell [7]. An introduction to the histology of oligodendrocytes and myelin is presented in Chap. 2.

The morphological distinction between white matter and gray matter is one that is also useful for the neurochemist. White matter is composed of myelinated axons, glial cells, and capillaries. Gray matter contains, in addition, the nerve cell bodies with their extensive dendritic arborizations, and quite different ratios of the other elements. The predominant element of white matter is the myelin sheath, which comprises about 50 percent of the total dry weight. Myelin is mainly responsible for the gross chemical differences between white and gray matter. It accounts for the glistening white appearance, high lipid content, and relatively low water content of white matter.

The myelin sheath is a greatly extended and presumably modified plasma membrane which is wrapped around the nerve axon in a spiral fashion. The myelin membranes originate from, and are part of, the Schwann cell in the peripheral nervous system (PNS), and the oligodendroglial cells (oligodendrocytes) in the central nervous system (CNS). In the mature myelin sheath, these membranes have condensed into a compact, paracrystalline structure in which each unit membrane is closely apposed to the adjacent one; the protein layers of each unit membrane are fused with, or bound to, the proteins of the unit in apposition. The sheath is not continuous for the whole length of an axon because each myelin-generating cell furnishes myelin

for only a segment of the axon. Between these segments, short portions of the axon are left uncovered. These periodic interruptions, called *nodes of Ranvier,* are critical to the functioning of myelin.

Patterns of Myelination

Myelination does not proceed in all parts of the nervous system at the same time, but follows the order of phylogenetic development [14, 15]. Portions of the PNS myelinate first, then the spinal cord, and the brain last. In all parts of the nervous system there are many small fibers that never myelinate. Even within the brain, different areas myelinate at different rates, the intracortical association areas being the last to do so. It is generally true that pathways in the nervous system become myelinated before they become completely functional. This relationship may be reciprocal, however, and function also appears to stimulate myelination. The relationship of myelination to function is somewhat clouded, because the period of maximum myelination also coincides with many other, less-known, changes in the nervous system. It is not seriously doubted, although somewhat difficult to prove, that much of the loss of function in demyelinating diseases is a result of loss of myelin. (Diseases of myelin are discussed in Chap. 32.)

The importance of myelin to proper performance of the nervous system can be inferred by comparing the different capabilities of newborns of various species. The period at which rapid myelination takes place varies considerably among different species. For instance, the CNS of rats and other nest-building animals myelinates largely postnatally, and the animals are quite helpless at birth. Grazing animals, such as horses, cows, and sheep, have considerably myelin in the CNS at birth and a

63

correspondingly much higher level of complex activity immediately postnatally.

The maximal rate of myelination in humans takes place during the perinatal period. The motor roots begin to myelinate in the fifth fetal month. The brain is almost completely myelinated by the end of the second year of life, although apparently myelination continues in the human neocortex through the end of the second decade, or even longer (see Chap. 23).

Although it is easy to ascertain when myelination begins, it is difficult to determine when the process of accumulation stops. In the rat, myelin is still being deposited in the brain up to 425 days of age and possibly longer [16]. The rat, however, continues to grow in body size and brain weight for many months, and such a prolonged period of myelination may not occur in all species.

Myelin Function

The popular view that myelin acts as an electrical insulator on axons in a manner similar to insulation on a wire is only partly true. Myelin is an insulator, but its function is to facilitate conduction in axons rather than to prevent transfer of signals, or "cross talk," between adjacent fibers. There has been speculation that cross talk, or ephaptic interaction, occurs between neighboring demyelinated axons, but it has not been demonstrated experimentally [17]. The mechanism by which myelin facilitates conduction has no exact analogy in electrical circuitry. In unmyelinated fibers, impulse conduction is propagated by local circuits of current that flow into the active region of the axonal membrane, through the axon, and out through adjacent sections of the membrane (see Fig. 4-1). These local circuits depolarize the adjacent piece of membrane in a continuous sequential fashion. In myelinated axons, the excitable axonal membrane is exposed to the extracellular space only at the nodes of Ranvier. The remainder of the axolemma is covered by the myelin sheath, which has a much higher resistance and much lower capacitance than has the axonal membrane. These passive properties of myelin are probably not peculiar to the myelin membrane but merely reflect the

fact that myelin is composed of many unit membranes stacked on top of each other. Thus, the observed specific resistance and specific capacitance of myelin of a large (15 μm diameter) frog peripheral nerve fiber consisting of 250 unit membranes is roughly equal to that calculated for 250 layers of axonal membrane connected in series [7, pp. 117–159]. When the membrane at the node is excited, the local circuit generated cannot flow through the high-resistance sheath and therefore flows out through and depolarizes the membrane at the next node, which might be 1 mm or farther away (see Fig. 4-1). The low capacitance of the sheath means that little energy is required to depolarize the remaining membrane between the nodes, and this results in an increased speed of local circuit spreading. Active excitation of the axonal membrane jumps from node to node, so this form of impulse propagation is called *saltatory conduction* (Latin *saltare,* "to jump"). It should be emphasized, however, that the action potential moves at a uniform speed down the fiber, but the action currents, which precede the action potential, move discontinuously with time [7, pp. 117–159].

The principal advantages of saltatory conduction are that conduction velocities are greatly increased and energy expenditures reduced relative to conduction in unmyelinated fibers of comparable size. To obtain conduction velocities in unmyelinated fibers equivalent to those in the fastest conducting myelinated fibers, impossibly large unmyelinated fibers and energy expenditures several orders of magnitude greater are required. For example, a myelinated frog nerve of 12 μm diameter conducts at 25 m/sec at 20°C; an unmyelinated nerve (e.g., squid axon) must be 500 μm in diameter to conduct at the same velocity [7, pp. 117–159]. Because only the nodes of Ranvier are excited during conduction in myelinated fibers, sodium flux into the nerve is much less than in unmyelinated fibers, where the entire membrane is involved. It has been shown that, although the 12 μm myelinated nerve conducts at the same speed as the 500 μm squid axon, the squid axon requires 5,000 times as much energy and occupies about 1,500 times as much space [7, pp. 117–159]. Con-

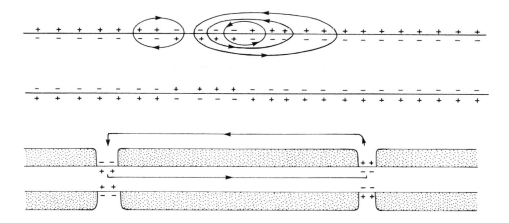

Fig. 4-1. Impulse conduction in unmyelinated (top) and myelinated (bottom) fibers. The arrows show the flow of action currents in local circuits into the active region of the membrane. In unmyelinated fibers the circuits flow through the adjacent piece of membrane, but in myelinated fibers the circuit flow jumps to the next node.

duction velocity in myelinated fibers is proportional to the diameter, while in unmyelinated fibers it is proportional to the square root of the diameter. For this reason, differences in energy and space requirements between the two types of fibers are exaggerated at higher conduction velocities. Velocities of 100 m/sec, which are observed in large mammalian A fibers of 20 μm diameter at 37°C, could only be achieved in unmyelinated fibers with diameters in the order of millimeters. If nerves were not myelinated and equivalent conduction velocities were maintained, the human spinal cord would need to be as large as a good-sized tree trunk. Myelin, then, facilitates conduction while conserving space and energy. Obviously, the evolutionary adaptation of myelin was critical in the development of more highly complex nervous systems.

The calculated ratio of axon diameter to overall myelinated fiber diameter is about 0.6 for optimal conduction velocity. This ratio is close to that observed in myelinated fibers in both PNS and CNS. Myelination does not always confer an advantage; at diameters less than 0.2 μm, unmyelinated fibers will conduct faster than myelinated fibers. At this fiber diameter, the myelin sheath would be only 400 Å (0.04 μm) thick (about four unit membranes) and the axon 0.12 μm in diameter. The core resistance of the axon at these diameters becomes very high and is the limiting factor in conduction speed. In actuality, the minimum diameter of myelinated fibers in the PNS is about 1 μm, whereas it is about 0.3 μm in the CNS, very close to the critical minimum for myelination [18] [see 17–19 for reviews of the function of the myelin sheath in conduction].

Ultrastructure of Myelin

The existence of a sheath surrounding nerve fibers has been known since the early days of light microscopy (Fig. 4-2). Myelin, as well as many of its structural features, such as nodes of Ranvier and Schmidt-Lantermann clefts, can be seen readily in the light microscope. Before the 1930s, sufficient chemical and histological work had been done to indicate that myelin was primarily lipoidal in nature but had a protein component as well. Our current view of myelin as a system of condensed plasma membranes with alternating protein-lipid-protein lamellae is derived mainly from studies by three physical techniques: polarized light, x-ray diffraction, and electron microscopy. The earliest physical studies, in the latter half of the nineteenth century, showed that myelin was birefringent when examined by polarized light. This property indicates a considerable degree of long-range order. As

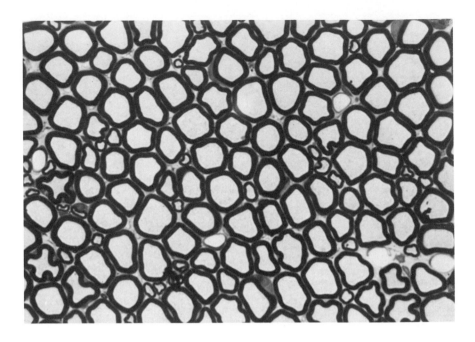

Fig. 4-2. *Light micrograph of a 1 μ Epon section of rabbit peripheral nerve (anterior root), stained with toluidine blue. The myelin sheath appears as a thick black ring around the pale axon. × 600, before 30% reduction. (Courtesy of Dr. Cedric Raine.)*

early as 1913, Göthlin showed that there was both a lipid-dependent and a protein-dependent birefringence and that the lipid-dependent type predominated (see [20] for review). Further work with polarized light by Schmidt and Schmitt and coworkers in the 1930s established that myelin was built up of layers. They also found that the lipid components of these layers were oriented radially to the axis of the nerve fiber, whereas the protein component was oriented tangentially to the nerve. Danielli and Davson had already formulated their concept of the cell membrane as a bimolecular lipid leaflet coated on both sides with protein. So the results of the latter studies were interpreted with the awareness of the possible membrane nature of myelin.

During the same period, in pioneering studies with x-ray diffraction, Schmitt and coworkers [20] found that peripheral nerve myelin had a radial repeating unit of 170 to 180 Å, a distance sufficient to accommodate two bimolecular leaflets of lipid together with the associated protein. In 1939, Schmitt and Bear [21] concluded that the configuration of the lipid and protein in the myelin sheath was as follows: "The proteins occur as thin sheets wrapped concentrically about the axon, with two bimolecular layers of lipoids interspersed between adjacent protein layers," a description nearly consistent with our current view.

The x-ray diffraction studies were extended and elaborated by a series of investigations by Finean and coworkers (reviewed in [22]). Low-angle diffraction studies of peripheral nerve myelin provided an electron density plot of the repeating unit that showed three peaks and two troughs, with a repeat distance of 180 Å. The peaks were attributed to protein plus lipid polar groups and the troughs to lipid hydrocarbon chains. The dimensions and appearance of this repeating unit were consistent with a protein-lipid-protein-lipid-protein structure, in which the lipid portion is a bimolecular leaflet and adjacent protein layers are different in some way.

Similar electron density plots of mammalian

optic nerve showed a repeat distance of 80 Å (Fig. 4-3); that is, adjacent protein layers reacted identically to the x-ray beam. Because 80 Å can accommodate one bimolecular layer of lipid (about 50 Å) and two protein layers (about 15 Å each), this represents the width of one unit membrane; and the main repeating unit of two fused unit membranes is twice this figure, or 160 Å.

The electron density plot reproduced in Fig. 4-3, and similar ones obtained for PNS myelin, were obtained by using the first five diffraction orders. More recent high-resolution studies using more diffraction orders reveal a fine structure in the repeat period that could not be obtained in low-resolution work. These plots have not yet been definitively interpreted in terms of molecular structure [7, pp. 51–90; 23].

The conclusions regarding myelin ultrastructure derived from these two techniques are fully supported by electron microscope studies. Myelin is now routinely seen in electron micrographs as a series of alternating dark and less dark lines separated by unstained zones (Figs. 4-4 through 4-7). The stained or osmiophilic lines are thought to represent the protein layers and the unstained zones the lipid hydrocarbon chains (see Fig. 4-3). The asymmetry in the staining of the protein layers results from the way the myelin sheath is generated from the cell plasma membrane (see following section and Figs. 4-8 through 4-10). The less dark, or intraperiod, line represents the closely apposed outer protein coats of the original cell membrane; the dark, or major period, line is the fused, inner protein coats of the cell membrane.

The x-ray diffraction data and the electron microscope data correlate very well. Myelin in the PNS, when swollen in hypotonic solutions, is found to split only at the intraperiod line, and the electron density plots show that the broadening occurs at the wider of the three peaks in the repeating unit. This combined approach shows the continuity of the membrane junction of the minor period with the extracellular space and proves that the wide electron density peak in peripheral nerve plots corresponds to the intraperiod lines seen in electron micrographs [24]. It also indicates that the

troughs correspond to the light zones between the two dark lines in electron micrographs (see Fig. 4-3). From both x-ray and electron microscope data, it can be seen that the smallest radial subunit that can be called myelin is a five-layered structure of protein-lipid-protein-lipid-protein. This unit, comprising the center-to-center distance between two major period lines, has a spacing in fixed and imbedded preparations of about 120 Å. Because of the considerable shrinkage that takes place after fixation and dehydration, this repeat distance is lower than the 160 to 180 Å period given by x-ray data.

Although a significant difference was found between central and peripheral myelin in the low-angle x-ray diffraction data, the electron micrographs were much the same for both; each showed a major repeat period of about 120 Å with the intermediate, minor period line of low electron density (compare Figs. 4-6 and 4-7). Recently it has been shown that peripheral myelin has an average repeat distance of 119Å and the central myelin of 107Å, confirming the x-ray data for the differences in the size of the period. However, the detailed appearance of electron micrographs is highly dependent on the processing procedures, and some fixation procedures favor retention of the relatively large period seen in x-ray diffraction. Also, with improved methods of perfusion fixation and tissue staining, the intraperiod line is now routinely seen as a double line rather than as a single one (see Figs. 4-6 and 4-7). This ultrastructural appearance indicates that the extracellular sides of the unit membranes are closely apposed but not fused.

So far, only the ultrastructure of the compact, multilamellar portion of the sheath in the internodal region has been discussed. Two adjacent segments of myelin on one axon are separated by a node of Ranvier, and in this region the axon is uncovered. These nodes are present in both central and peripheral axons and apparently have a similar structure. At the paranodal region and the Schmidt-Lanterman clefts, the cytoplasmic surfaces of myelin are not compacted, and Schwann or glial cell cytoplasm is included within the sheath. To visualize these structures one may refer to Figs. 4-8

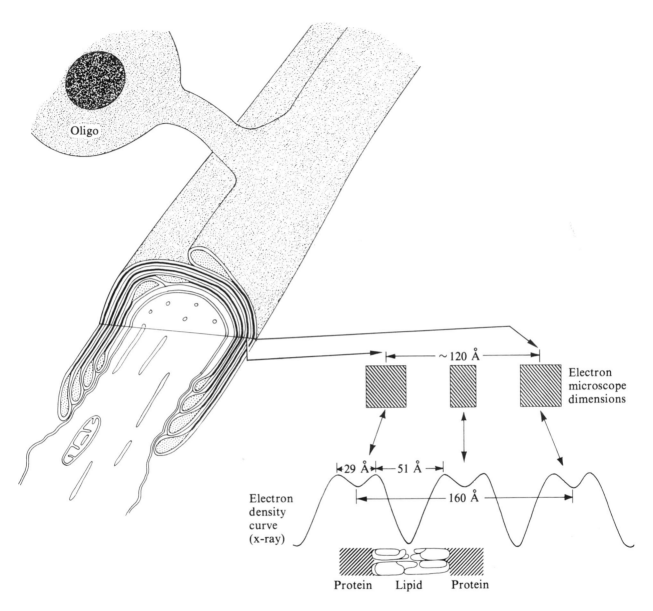

Fig. 4-3. *A composite diagram summarizing some of the ultrastructural data on CNS myelin. At the top an oligodendroglial cell is shown connected to the sheath by a process. The cutaway view of the myelin and axon illustrates the relationship of these two structures at the nodal and paranodal regions. (Only a few myelin layers have been drawn for the sake of clarity.) At the internodal region, the cross section reveals the inner and outer mesaxons and their relationship to the inner cytoplasmic wedges and the outer loop of cytoplasm. Note that in contrast to PNS myelin, there is no full ring of cytoplasm surrounding the outside of the sheath. The lower part of the figure shows roughly the dimensions and appearance of one myelin repeating unit as seen with fixed and embedded preparations in the electron microscope. This is contrasted with the dimensions of the electron density curve of CNS myelin obtained by x-ray diffraction studies in fresh nerve. The components responsible for the peaks and troughs of the curve are sketched below. (Reprinted courtesy of Lea & Febiger, publishers.)*

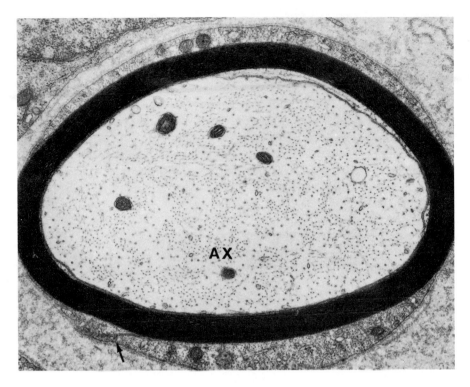

Fig. 4-4. *Electron micrograph of a single peripheral nerve fiber from rabbit. AX, axon. Note that the myelin sheath has a lamellated structure and is surrounded by Schwann cell cytoplasm. The outer mesaxon (arrow) can be seen in lower left. ×18,000. (Courtesy of Dr. Cedric Raine.)*

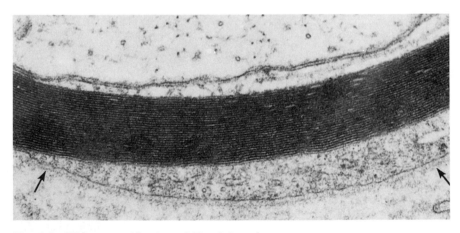

Fig. 4-5. *Higher magnification of Fig. 4-4 to show the Schwann cell cytoplasm covered by basal lamina (arrows). ×50,000.*

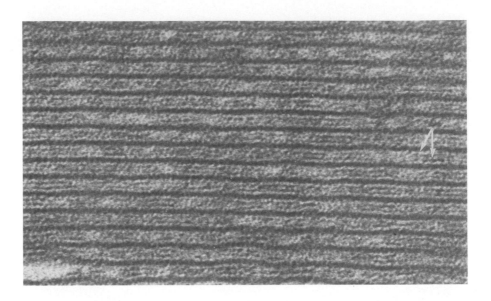

Fig. 4-6. Magnification of the myelin sheath of Figure 4-4. Note that the intraperiod line (arrows) at this high resolution is a double structure. ×350,000. (Courtesy of Dr. Cedric Raine.)

and 4-9, adapted from those of Hirano and Dembitzer [25], which show that if myelin were unrolled from the axon it would be a flat, spade-shaped sheet surrounded by a tube of cytoplasm. This flat sheet may be envisioned as arising from a tubular process full of cytoplasm and enclosed by a membrane. If this process were squeezed in the middle and pressed out toward the edges, the two membrane layers would come together and fuse (with the inside faces forming the major dense line); cytoplasm would be squeezed out toward the periphery of the sheet, forming a thin tube all around the edge. If this sheet were then wrapped around an axon, the regions at the edges of the sheet where the cytoplasmic tubes touch the axon would be the paranodal regions and the regions where the fused membranes wrap up on each other would be the areas of compact myelin (see Figs. 4-2, 4-8, and 4-9). Electron micrographs of longitudinal sections of axon paranodal regions show that the major dense line appears to open up at the edges of the sheet and to loop back upon itself, enclosing cytoplasm within the loop (see Figs. 4-2 and 4-9). These loop-shaped terminations of the sheath at the node are called lateral loops. The loops form membrane complexes with the axolemma called *transverse bands*, whereas myelin in the internodal region is separated from the axon by a gap of extracellular space. The transverse bands are helical structures that seal the myelin to the axolemma but provide, by spaces between them, a tortuous path from the extracellular space to the periaxonal space.

The Schmidt-Lanterman clefts, structures common in peripheral, but rare in central, myelinated axons, appear in the light microscope to be diagonal or funnel-shaped incisures in the internodal sheath. In the electron microscope they are revealed to be regions where the cytoplasmic surfaces of the myelin sheath have not compacted to form the major dense line and therefore contain Schwann or glial cell cytoplasm (Fig. 4-9). These inclusions of cytoplasm are present in each layer of myelin. Therefore, the clefts can be visualized in the unrolled myelin sheet as tubes of cytoplasm similar to the tubes making up the lateral loops but in the middle regions of the sheet, rather than at the edges (Fig. 4-9). [See 7, pp. 1–50, for a more complete description of myelin morphology.]

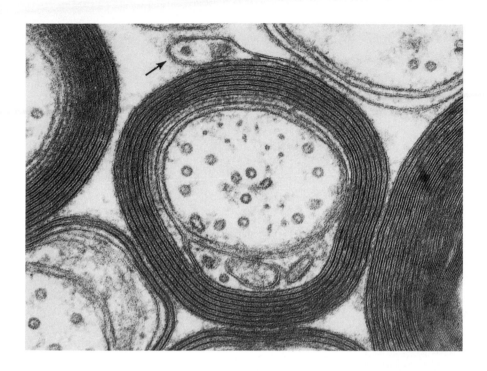

Fig. 4-7. A typical CNS myelinated fiber from the spinal cord of an adult dog. Contrast this figure with the PNS fiber in Figure 4-3. The course of the flattened oligodendrocytic process, beginning at the outer tongue (arrow), can be traced. Note that the fiber lacks investing cell cytoplasm and a basal lamina—as is the case in the PNS. The major dense line and the paler, double intraperiod line of the myelin sheath can be discerned. The axon contains neurotubules and neurofilaments. ×135,000.

Cellular Formation of Myelin

Myelination in the PNS is preceded by invasion of the nerve bundle by Schwann cells, rapid multiplication of these cells, and segregation of the individual axons by Schwann cell processes. Smaller axons (less than 1 μm), which will remain unmyelinated, are segregated; several may be enclosed in one cell, each within its own pocket, similar to the structure shown in Fig. 4-10 A. Large axons (greater than 1 μm) destined for myelination are enclosed singly, one cell per axon per internode. These cells line up along the axons with intervals between them; the intervals become the nodes of Ranvier.

There is evidence that the signal that stimulates the Schwann cell to divide and to begin myelination comes from the axon [26]. All Schwann cells are apparently capable of forming myelin; it is the nature of the axon itself that determines whether it will be myelinated [27, 28].

Geren [29] showed that before myelination the axon lies in an invagination of the Schwann cell (see Fig. 4-10 A). The plasmalemma of the cell then surrounds the axon and joins to form a double membrane structure that communicates with the cell surface. This structure, previously noted in unmyelinated fibers and called the *mesaxon*, then elongates around the axon in a spiral fashion (see Fig. 4-10). Geren postulated that mature myelin is formed in this "jelly-roll" fashion; the mesaxon winds about the axon, and the cytoplasmic surfaces condense into a compact myelin sheath.

In early electron micrographs, cell membranes appeared as single dense lines, the mesaxon as two lines, and myelin as a series of repeating dense lines 120 Å apart. Robertson [24] later reported that the

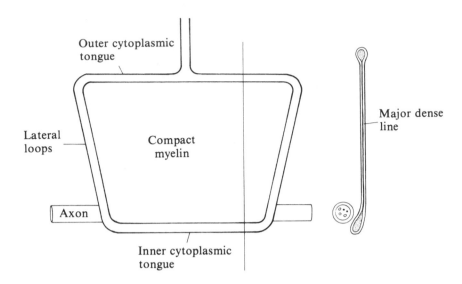

Fig. 4-8. A diagram showing the appearance of CNS myelin if it were unrolled from the axon. One can visualize this structure arising from Fig. 4-3, if the glial cell process were pulled straight up and the myelin layers separated at the intermediate period line. The whole myelin internode forms a spade-shaped sheet surrounded by a continuous tube of oligodendroglial cell cytoplasm. This diagram shows that the lateral loops and inner and outer cytoplasmic tongues are parts of the same cytoplasmic tube. The drawing on the right shows the appearance of this sheet if it were sectioned along the vertical line, indicating that the compact myelin region is formed of two unit membranes fused at the cytoplasmic surfaces. (The drawing is not necessarily to scale.) (Adapted from Hirano, A., and Dembitzer, H. M., J. Cell Biol. 34:555–567, 1967.)

Schwann cell membrane appeared to have a three-layered structure with two dense lines, as illustrated in Fig. 4-10. When the two portions of this membrane come together to form the mesaxon, the two external surfaces appear to join to form a single line that eventually becomes the myelin intra-period line. As a mesaxon spirals into the compact myelin layers, the cytoplasmic surfaces of the mesaxon fuse to form the major dense line. It was thus shown beyond doubt that PNS myelin is morphologically an extension of the Schwann cell membrane. The mesaxon is thus the smallest myelin subunit and has the five-layered structure previously described.

It was reasonable to assume that myelin in the CNS was formed in a similar fashion by the oligodendroglial cell. However, these nerve fibers are not separated by connective tissue, nor are they surrounded by cell cytoplasm; and specific glial nuclei are not obviously associated with particular myelinated fibers. In 1960, it was shown independently by Maturana and by Peters that CNS myelin is a spiral structure similar to PNS myelin; it has an inner mesaxon and an outer mesaxon that ends in a loop, or tongue, of glial cytoplasm (Fig. 4-3; see also [4] for a review of this work).

Unlike peripheral nerve, where the sheath is surrounded by Schwann cell cytoplasm, the cyto-plasmic tongue in the CNS is restricted to a small portion of the sheath. It was assumed that this glial tongue was eventually connected in some way to the glial cell, but confirmation was difficult. Finally, Bunge and colleagues [1] showed that the central myelin sheath is continuous with the plasma membrane of the oligodendroglial cell through slender processes. They also showed that one glial cell apparently can myelinate more than one axon. Peters has calculated that, in the rat optic nerve,

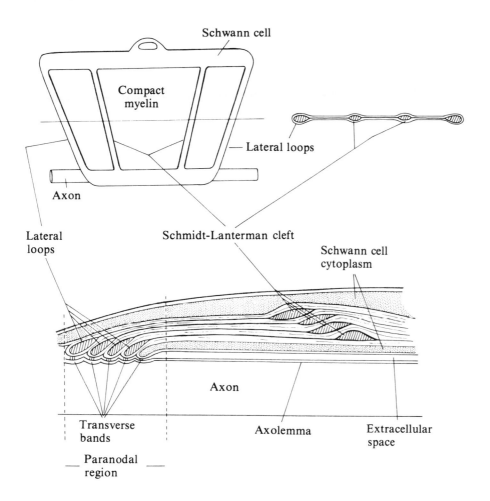

Fig. 4-9. A diagram similar to Fig. 4-8, but showing one Schwann cell and its myelin sheath unrolled from a peripheral axon. The sheet of PNS myelin is, like CNS myelin, surrounded by a tube of cytoplasm and has additional tubes of cytoplasm, which make up the Schmidt-Lanterman clefts, running through the internodal regions. The horizontal section (top right) shows that these additional tubes of cytoplasm arise from regions where the cytoplasmic membrane surfaces have not fused. Diagram (bottom) is an enlarged view of a portion of (top left), with the Schwann cell and its membrane wrapped around the axon. The tube forming the lateral loops seals to the axolemma at the paranodal region, and the cytoplasmic tubes in the internodal region form the Schmidt-Lanterman clefts. (These drawings are not to scale.) (Adapted from Hirano, A., and Dembitzer, H. M., J. Cell Biol. 34:555–567, 1967.)

one oligodendroglial cell myelinates, on the average, 42 separate axons [4].

The actual mechanism of myelin formation is still obscure. In the PNS, a single axon may have up to 100 myelin layers, and it is therefore improbable that myelin is laid down by a simple rotation of the Schwann cell nucleus around the axon. In the CNS, such a postulate is precluded by the fact that one glial cell can myelinate several axons. During myelination, there are increases in the length of the internode, the diameter of the axon, and the number of myelin layers. Myelin is therefore expanding

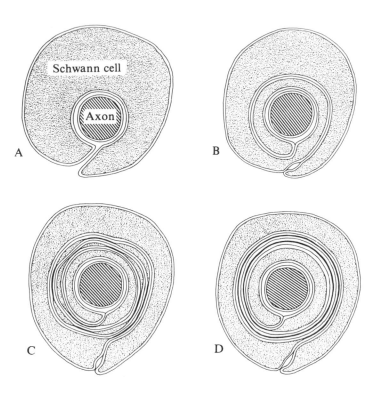

Fig. 4-10. *Myelin formation in the peripheral nervous system. (A) The Schwann cell has surrounded the axon but the external surfaces of the plasma membrane have not yet fused in the mesaxon. (B) The mesaxon has fused into a five-layered structure and spiralled once around the axon. (C) A few layers of myelin have formed but are not completely compacted. Note the cytoplasm trapped in zones where the cytoplasmic membrane surfaces have not yet fused. (D) Compact myelin showing only a few layers for the sake of clarity. Note that Schwann cell cytoplasm forms a ring both inside and outside of the sheath. (Reprinted courtesy of Lea & Febiger, publishers.)*

in all planes at once, and any mechanism to account for this growth must assume the membrane system is flexible. It must be able to expand and contract, and layers probably slip over each other.

Isolation

Myelin is present in all parts of the nervous system but is more concentrated in areas composed mainly of fiber tracts, such as the white matter of brain and spinal cord, and in peripheral nerve trunks, such as sciatic nerve. It is the principal solid component of tissue in these areas. Mammalian brain white matter contains about 50 percent myelin on a dry-weight basis. Even in the whole brain of an adult rat, myelin is about 25 percent of dry weight and accounts for more than 40 percent of the brain lipid [16]. Human brains, which have a higher ratio of white to gray matter than rat brains, have an even higher percentage of myelin. An adult human brain weighing 1,400 g contains 110 g of myelin, 35 percent of the dry weight. Because myelin is a plentiful substance and has singular properties, it can be iso-

lated readily in high yield and purity by conventional methods of subcellular fractionation [7, pp. 161–200; 30].

CNS MYELIN

Myelin is usually isolated by centrifugation of tissue homogenates in sucrose solutions. During homogenization, myelin peels off the axons and reforms in vesicles of the size range of nuclei and mitochondria. (It is important to homogenize the tissue in media of low ionic strength, otherwise much of the myelin remains bound to the axon and the intact myelinated axon fragments present in the homogenate will contaminate the crude myelin preparations.) Because of their high lipid content, these myelin vesicles have the lowest intrinsic density of any membrane fraction of the nervous system. Most isolation methods utilize both of these properties—large vesicle size and low density.

One general class of methods involves the isolation, by differential centrifugation, of a crude mitochondrial fraction that contains mitochondria, synaptosomes, and myelin. This fraction is resuspended in isotonic (0.3 M) sucrose and layered over 0.8 M sucrose. Myelin collects at the interface during centrifugation, whereas mitochondria and synaptosomes sediment through the dense layer. Unless the nuclear fraction is processed similarly, the myelin fragments in that fraction are lost. The advantage of this approach is that most of the smaller microsomal membranes are removed in the differential centrifugation steps. The other general class of methods bypass the initial differential centrifugation step. A homogenate of nervous tissue in isotonic sucrose is layered directly onto 0.85 M sucrose and centrifuged at high speed. A crude myelin layer collects at the interface.

The crude myelin layer obtained by either of these methods is of varying purity, depending on the tissue from which the myelin is isolated. White matter from adult brain yields reasonably pure myelin; myelin from the whole brain of a very young animal might be quite impure. The major impurities are microsomes and axoplasm trapped in the vesicles during the homogenization procedure. Further purification is generally achieved by subjecting the myelin to osmotic shock in distilled water. This opens up the myelin vesicles, releasing trapped material. The larger myelin particles can then be separated from the smaller, membranous material by low-speed centrifugation or by repeating the density gradient centrifugation on continuous or discontinuous gradients, usually of sucrose. On sucrose gradients, myelin forms a band centering at approximately 0.65 M sucrose, equivalent to a density of 1.08g/m. For comparison, mitochondria

have a density of 1.2 (equivalent to about 1.55 M sucrose). These preparations of purified myelin can be further subdivided arbitrarily into fractions of different densities and different compositions by centrifugation on expanded continuous or discontinuous density gradients. The significance of these subfractions will be discussed later (see under Compositional Changes).

Criteria of purity have been difficult to set for myelin preparations because there is no a priori way of knowing what the intrinsic myelin constituents are. The types of criteria for myelin should be the same as for any other subcellular fraction: typical ultrastructure, the absence or minimization of markers characteristic of other particles, and the maximization of markers characteristic of myelin. Most investigators have used the obvious criterion of electron-microscopic appearance. Isolated myelin retains the typical five-layered structure and repeat period of about 120 Å seen in situ. The difficulty of identifying small membrane vesicles of microsomes in a field of myelin membranes and the well-known sampling problems inherent in electron microscopy make this characterization unreliable after a certain purity level has been reached.

The biochemical markers that have been commonly used to assay contamination are succinic dehydrogenase (mitochondria), ($Na^+ + K^+$)-ATPase and 5'-nucleotidase (plasma membranes), NADH—cytochrome-C reductase (microsomes), DNA (nuclei), RNA (nuclei, ribosomes, microsomes), lactate dehydrogenase (cytosol), β-glucosidase (lysosomes), and acetylcholinesterase (neuronal membranes). Although work by various investigators indicates that all of these markers are low in purified myelin, enzyme markers are becoming more suspect as more enzymes are found to be intrinsic to myelin. In particular the classic plasma membrane markers, 5'-nucleotidase and ($Na^+ + K^+$)-ATPase may be normally present in myelin and thus cannot be recommended to detect contaminants (see Enzymes, p. 80).

Markers characteristic of myelin are less useful than negative markers to establish purity, both because they are minimally affected by small amounts of impurities and because they will all be expressed to varying degrees, depending on the developmental stage, by components of oligodendroglial or Schwann cells. Many investigators have used the nearly complete solubility of the final product in chloroform-methanol (2:1, v/v) as an indicator of purity. Although the so-called high molecular weight proteins (including Wolfgram proteins) are insoluble in this mixture, 95 percent of myelin, including the two major proteins (proteolipid protein and basic protein), and all of the lipids are soluble. This test may be unreliable if a new species or very young animals are being examined, or if the proteins have been altered in storage. The myelin-typical marker galactosylceramide (cerebroside) and the myelin-specific enzyme 2′,3′-cyclic nucleotide 3′-phosphohydrolase (CNP) are probably more useful in assaying myelin and oligodendroglial plasma membrane contamination in other fractions than in establishing myelin purity. The myelin protein pattern exhibited in polyacrylamide gel electrophoresis (PAGE) is characteristic and reproducible, but small amounts of contaminating proteins may be difficult to detect and quantitate.

PNS MYELIN
Peripheral nerve myelin can be isolated by similar techniques, but special homogenization conditions are required because of the large amounts of connective tissue and, sometimes, adipose tissue present in the nerve. These more vigorous homogenization conditions also require the use of slightly different gradients to prevent loss of myelin [31]. Because PNS myelin has some proteins different from those in CNS myelin, solubility in chloroform-methanol cannot be used as an indicator of purity. Moreover, the CNP is very much lower in nerve and PNS myelin than in CNS myelin.

Composition
Myelin has a higher lipid-to-protein ratio than have other subcellular fractions. The solids of myelin are 70 to 85% lipid and 15 to 30% protein; the lipids of mammalian CNS myelin are composed of 25 to 28% cholesterol, 27 to 30% galactosphingolipid, and 40 to 45% phospholipid. Early inferences

about myelin composition were made from three types of indirect measurements: comparative analyses of gray and white matter, the measurement of brain constituents during the period of rapid myelination, and studies of brain and nerve composition during experimental demyelination. From such studies it became generally accepted that proteolipid protein, cerebrosides, and sulfatides were exclusively myelin constituents; that sphingomyelin and the plasmalogens were predominantly myelin constituents; that cholesterol and phosphatidylserine were major lipids of myelin as well as of other membranes; and that lecithin was probably not a myelin lipid. These suppositions have now been shown to be only partially correct. Even so, in 1949 Brante [32] calculated that myelin sheath lipids were 25% cholesterol, 29% galactolipids, and 46% phospholipids, figures very close to those obtained by direct analysis of isolated myelin.

No direct determination of water can be made on myelin, although obviously myelin is a relatively dehydrated structure. The low water content of white matter (72%) as opposed to gray matter (82%) is largely due to the high myelin content of white matter. From x-ray diffraction studies on nerve tissue during drying, Finean determined the water content to be about 40% [22]. This is probably a fairly accurate calculation, and all the data on yields of myelin and the composition of myelin and white matter are consistent with about 40% water in the myelin and about 80% water in the nonmyelin portions of white matter, a composition similar to that of the rest of the nervous system.

LIPIDS
Table 4-1 lists the composition of bovine, rat, and human myelin compared to bovine and human white matter, human gray matter, and rat whole brain. (The classification and metabolism of brain lipids are discussed in Chap. 18.) It can be seen that all the lipids found in whole brain are also present in myelin; that is, there are no lipids localized exclusively in some "nonmyelin compartment" except, possibly, cardiolipin. We also know that the reverse is true; that is, there are no myelin lipids

Table 4-1. Composition of CNS Myelin and Brain[a]

Substance[b]	Myelin			White Matter		Gray Matter (Human)	Whole Brain (Rat)
	Human	Bovine	Rat	Human	Bovine		
Protein	30.0	24.7	29.5	39.0	39.5	55.3	56.9
Lipid	70.0	75.3	70.5	54.9	55.0	32.7	37.0
Cholesterol	27.7	28.1	27.3	27.5	23.6	22.0	23.0
Cerebroside	22.7	24.0	23.7	19.8	22.5	5.4	14.6
Sulfatide	3.8	3.6	7.1	5.4	5.0	1.7	4.8
Total galactolipid	27.5	29.3	31.5	26.4	28.6	7.3	21.3
Ethanolamine phosphatides	15.6	17.4	16.7	14.9	13.6	22.7	19.8
Lecithin	11.2	10.9	11.3	12.8	12.9	26.7	22.0
Sphingomyelin	7.9	7.1	3.2	7.7	6.7	6.9	3.8
Phosphatidylserine	4.8	6.5	7.0	7.9	11.4	8.7	7.2
Phosphatidylinositol	0.6	0.8	1.2	0.9	0.9	2.7	2.4
Plasmalogens[c]	12.3	14.1	14.1	11.2	12.2	8.8	11.6
Total phospholipid	43.1	43.0	44.0	45.9	46.3	69.5	57.6

[a]All average figures obtained on adults in the author's laboratory.
[b]Protein and lipid figures in % dry weight; all others in % total lipid weight.
[c]Plasmalogens are primarily ethanolamine phosphatides.

that are not also found in other subcellular fractions of the brain. Even though there are no "myelin-specific" lipids, cerebroside is the most typical of myelin. During development, the concentration of cerebroside in brain is directly proportional to the amount of myelin present [16]. There are only minor differences between the lipid composition of myelin and the corresponding white matter, although myelin lipids tend to have somewhat more cholesterol, cerebrosides, and ethanolamine phosphatides than white matter lipids, and somewhat less sulfatides and lecithin.

Figures expressed in this way give no information about lipid concentrations in either the dry or wet tissue. Thus, although human myelin and white matter lipids have similar galactolipid contents, the total galactolipid is 19.3 percent of the myelin dry weight but 14.5 percent of white matter dry weight. These differences are much greater if a wet-weight reference is used. Then galactolipid is 11.6 percent of myelin but only 4.1 percent of fresh white matter. As another example, total phospho-

lipids are a larger percentage of gray matter lipid than of either myelin or white matter lipids. However, on a total dry-weight basis, phospholipids are 30.2 percent of myelin, 25.2 percent of white matter, and 22.7 percent of gray matter.

Data in Table 4-1 show that many of the suppositions of the earlier deductive work are true. The major lipids of myelin are cholesterol, cerebrosides, and ethanolamine phosphatides in the plasmalogen form. However, lecithin is seen to be a major myelin constituent, and sphingomyelin, a relatively minor one. If the data for lipid composition are expressed in mole percent, most of the preparations analyzed so far contain cholesterol, phospholipid, and galactolipid in molar ratios ranging from 2:2:1 to 4:3:2. Thus, cholesterol constitutes the largest proportion of lipid molecules in myelin, although the galactolipids are usually a greater proportion of the lipid weight.

The composition of brain myelin from all mammalian species studied is very much the same. However, there are some obvious species differences.

For example, rat myelin has less sphingomyelin than does ox or human (Table 4-1).

Besides the lipids listed in the table, there are several others of importance. If myelin is not extracted with acid organic solvents, the polyphosphoinositides remain tightly bound to the myelin protein, and therefore are not included in the lipid analysis. There is good evidence that the portion of brain triphosphoinositide that is stable to postmortem degradation is localized mainly in myelin and may, therefore, have some status as a myelin marker. Triphosphoinositide accounts for between 4 and 6 percent of the total myelin phosphorus, and diphosphoinositide for 1 to 1.5 percent of the myelin phosphorus.

In addition to cerebrosides and sulfatides, there are several minor neutral galactolipids. These include at least three fatty acid esters of cerebroside and two glycerol-based lipids, diacylglycerylgalactoside and monoalkylmonoacylglycerylgalactoside, collectively called *galactosyldiglyceride.*

Although gangliosides, complex sialic acid–containing glycosphingolipids, were once thought to be exclusively situated in neurons, it is now apparent that myelin from mammals contains these lipids at concentrations ranging from 300 μg to greater than 900 μg of sialic acid per gram of myelin, depending on the species and the CNS region; whereas chicken brain and pigeon brain myelin have much higher concentrations, about 2,000 μg sialic acid per gram. Spinal cord myelin has about half the ganglioside content of brain myelin. These levels in mammals are equivalent to about 0.1 to 0.3 percent ganglioside and are 10 to 20 percent of the levels in cerebral gray matter. In mature rat, mouse, ox, cat, and rabbit, the myelin gangliosides have a pattern completely unlike that of whole-brain gangliosides; G_{M1}, the major monosialoganglioside, accounts for about 70 mole percent of the total myelin ganglioside [33–36]. All other membrane fractions have ganglioside patterns that closely resemble those of whole brain and have much higher levels of the polysialo species. Myelin from human, monkey, chimpanzee, and avian CNS contains an additional ganglioside as a major component, sialosylgalactosylceramide (G_{M4} or

G_7) [34, 36]. This ganglioside is derived from cerebroside and has a fatty acid pattern typical of myelin galactolipids, rather than of the other brain gangliosides [34]. Ganglioside G_{M4} is probably specific to myelin and oligodendroglia in certain species.

The long-chain fatty residues of myelin are characterized by a very high proportion of fatty aldehydes. These fatty aldehydes, which are derived primarily from phosphatidalethanolamine and, to a lesser extent, from phosphatidalserine, constitute one-sixth of the total glycerylphosphatide fatty residues and 12 mole percent of the total hydrolyzable fatty chains of the myelin lipids. The phospholipid fatty acids differ considerably from one phospholipid to another but are generally characterized by a high oleic acid content and a low level of polyunsaturated fatty acids. The glycosphingolipids, cerebrosides and sulfatides, have two classes of fatty acids—unsubstituted and α-hydroxy—both of which can be saturated or monounsaturated, whereas sphingomyelin has only unsubstituted fatty acids. The sphingolipid acids are primarily long chain (22 to 26 carbon atoms) with varying amounts of stearic acid. For example, human myelin glycosphingolipids have very little α-hydroxystearic acid but significant amounts of stearic acid, whereas bovine glycosphingolipids have both. These fatty acid patterns are distinctive for myelin and differ considerably from those found for the same lipids in gray matter.

The previous discussion on composition refers primarily to myelin isolated from the brain. Myelin isolated from the spinal cord has a higher lipid/protein ratio than that isolated from the brain of the same species. The differences between myelins isolated from different parts of the CNS are not well documented and deserve further study. We do know, however, that myelin from the PNS has a different composition from myelin of the CNS. Peripheral nerve myelin has not received the same extensive documentation primarily because of the technical difficulty of homogenizing peripheral nerve. The analyses that have been made show that PNS myelin has less cerebroside and sulfatide and considerably more sphingomyelin than CNS myelin. [For general references on myelin lipids, see 3; 4; 6; 7, pp. 161–200; 8, pp. 10–13; 37.]

PROTEINS OF CNS MYELIN

The protein composition of myelin is much simpler than that of other membranes, with two proteins, the proteolipid protein and the basic protein, making up 60 to 80 percent of the total in most species. Mice, rats, and some other rodents have large amounts of an additional smaller basic protein. The remaining proteins include pre-large and pre-small basic proteins, DM-20, several glycoproteins, and the Wolfgram proteins.

With the exception of the basic proteins, myelin proteins are neither easily extractable nor soluble in aqueous media. However, like other membrane proteins, they are soluble in sodium dodecylsulfate (SDS) solutions and can be separated readily by electrophoresis of these solutions in polyacrylamide gels. This technique permits the separation of proteins according to their molecular weight and has made possible the routine analysis of myelin proteins, studies of their synthesis and turnover, and the discovery of new myelin proteins.

Even before myelin had been isolated, the two principal proteins of CNS myelin had been isolated from brain and had been fairly well characterized. In 1951, Folch and Lees discovered that a rather large amount of protein could be extracted from brain white matter with chloroform-methanol mixture. The proteins in this fraction were apparently lipoprotein complexes and were given the generic name *proteolipids,* to distinguish them from water-soluble lipoproteins [38]. Regional and developmental studies made it clear that the proteolipids were primarily myelin constituents. The proteolipid protein fraction isolated from brain by solvent extraction is heterogeneous, although by far the major component is a single protein of 24,000 M_r. This protein has been the subject of much study because of its unusual physical properties; it remains soluble in chloroform even after essentially all of its bound lipids have been removed (for reviews see [2, 7, pp. 201–232; 38]). The major proteolipid protein has about 60% nonpolar amino acids

and 40% polar amino acids. It is very hydrophobic, forms large aggregates in aqueous solution, and is relatively resistant to proteolysis. In spite of these difficulties, sequence studies are now being carried out.

The major basic protein of myelin has been the most extensively studied and characterized [2; 7, pp. 201–232; 39–41] because it is the antigen that, when injected into an animal, elicits a cellular antibody response that produces the CNS autoimmune disease called *experimental allergic encephalomyelitis* (EAE). This disease involves focal areas of inflammation and demyelination that resemble the lesion of multiple sclerosis (see Chap. 32). This disease was first produced many years ago by injections of whole brain or spinal cord homogenates. Extensive studies showed that the responsible antigen was probably a myelin protein. In the late 1950s and early 1960s the pure basic protein was isolated from acid or salt extracts of brain protein from which all lipids had been removed. If isolated myelin is treated with chloroform-methanol (2:1), the basic protein (as well as the proteolipid protein) dissolves; however, it cannot be extracted from whole brain with this solvent. It can be extracted from myelin as well as from brain with either dilute acid or salt solutions; once extracted, it is very soluble in water.

The basic proteins of all species studied are very similar. They are highly basic and highly unfolded, with essentially no tertiary structure in solution. They have molecular weights of around 18,000 and contain approximately 52% polar amino acids and 48% nonpolar amino acids. Cysteine is absent, and there is one mole of tryptophan per mole of protein. This is in contrast to proteolipid protein, which is high in cysteine, methionine, and tryptophan.

The complete amino acid sequence of both the bovine [42] and human [43] basic proteins were published in 1971, and since then the sequences of the proteins of other species have been determined. The bovine protein has 169 residues and differs from the human protein by only 11 residues. If the basic protein is electrophoresed at pH 10, it splits into several bands of different net charge, but of essentially the same molecular weight. This micro-heterogeneity has been shown to be due to a combination of phosphorylation, loss of the C-terminal arginine, and deamidation [44]. There is also heterogeneity in the degree of methylation of an arginine at residue 106. As noted above, mice and rats have a second smaller basic protein of 14,000 M_r. The small basic protein has the same N- and C-terminal sequences as the larger, but differs by a deletion of 40 residues [41, 45].

The other proteins of myelin are conveniently discussed from the viewpoint of SDS-polyacryl-amide gel electrophoresis (SDS-PAGE). The myelin proteins in SDS solutions are usually separated on gels having either a concentration gradient of acrylamide or a fairly high (15%) acrylamide concentration, using a discontinuous buffer system. In the high molecular weight region (M_r greater than 60,000) of the gel, a number of minor uncharacterized bands are found. These vary in amount, depending on species (mouse and rat seem to have the most) and degree of maturity. Some of these may arise from contaminating membranes. In this region is found the major myelin-associated glycoprotein, which has a molecular weight of about 110,000 and amounts to about 1 percent of the total protein. This protein, which can be labeled with fucose, glucosamine, or N-acetylmannosamine, appears to decrease in molecular weight during development [46]. It has now been purified, and its subcellular location is being studied. There are at least two other myelin glycoproteins of lower molecular weight [47].

As one scans down the gel in the direction of decreasing molecular weight, the first prominent bands seen are a doublet in the 50,000 to 60,000 M_r range, the Wolfgram proteins. These were named after their discoverer [48], who realized that proteolipid protein and basic protein could not account for the amino acid analysis of whole myelin proteins and suggested that an acid-soluble proteolipid protein isolated from white matter was a third myelin protein [49]. The Wolfgram proteins plus the minor high molecular weight proteins account for approximately 15 to 20 percent of the total protein.

The next prominent band is proteolipid protein at 24,000 M_r, which constitutes about 40 to 50 percent of the total protein. There are minor bands between proteolipid protein and Wolfgram protein, one of which may be the enzyme CNP (see Enzymes).

Running between proteolipid protein and basic protein (18,000–18,500 M_r) are two minor proteins called variously DM-20 [50] or I proteins. The higher molecular weight protein (about 22,000 M_r) accompanies proteolipid protein during extraction procedures but has not been well-characterized. The lower molecular weight protein in this region stains metachromatically like basic protein and recently has been shown to be the large basic protein with an additional polypeptide sequence of about 3,000 M_r attached to the amino-terminal end of basic protein [51]. It has been called the pre-large basic protein, but there is no evidence that it is a metabolic precursor.

If the myelin being analyzed came from human, bovine, rabbit, guinea pig, cat, monkey, dog, or practically any species except rat and mouse, the large basic protein (18,000 M_r) would be the last protein on the gel and would amount to about 30 to 35 percent of the total. In the rat and mouse, two other basic proteins are found: (1) the protein of 17,000 M_r, which frequently co-migrates with the large basic protein and (2) the small basic protein of 14,000 M_r. The 17,000 M_r protein has been called the pre-small basic protein and bears the same structural relationship to the small basic protein as the pre-large basic protein does to the large basic protein [51]. In mature rats and mice there is more of the small basic protein than the large.

PROTEINS OF PNS MYELIN

PNS myelin proteins are quite different from those of CNS myelin. It has been known since 1951 that peripheral nerves had little or no proteolipid protein. Recent electrophoretic studies show that PNS myelin has four, and possibly five, major proteins, two or three of which are glycoproteins and two of which are basic proteins [2, 52, 53, 56]. The principal protein, P0, is a glycoprotein of 30,000 M_r [54–56] that accounts for more than half of the PNS myelin proteins. There are only a few minor bands of higher molecular weight. Running ahead of P0 on SDS-PAGE are two other glycoproteins: Y (about 25,000 M_r) and X (about 21,000 M_r) [2, 52]. There is now evidence that at least some of the Y protein may be P0 protein with incompletely reduced intramolecular disulfide bonds [57]. The larger of the two basic proteins, P_1, has a molecular weight of 18,000 and appears to be similar or identical to the large basic protein of CNS myelin [58]. However, there is evidence that two proteins are present in this band [53]. The smaller basic protein, P_2, has a molecular weight of 12,000 to 14,000, is unique to the PNS, and is unrelated in sequence to either P_1 or the small CNS myelin basic protein of rodents [56, 59]. It appears that the P_2 protein is the antigen for experimental allergic neuritis, the PNS counterpart of EAE [60]. The total basic protein content is lower in PNS myelin than in CNS myelin, and the ratio of P_1 to P_2 is extremely variable among different species [49, 53]. It is clear that investigations of the structure and composition of PNS myelin proteins are just beginning.[1]

ENZYMES

It was once generally believed that myelin was an inert membrane that did not carry out any biochemical functions. Early studies of selected enzymes that showed little activity in myelin tended to confirm this belief. Recently, however, a large and growing number of enzymes have been discovered in myelin. These findings imply that myelin plays an active metabolic role in synthesis and transport.

These enzymatic activities can be divided into two classes: those believed to be fairly myelin-specific (but probably also present in oligodendroglial membranes); and those known to be present in other subcellular fractions, as well [7, pp. 161–200]. The first group consists of two enzymes: CNP [61–63] and the pH 7.2 cholesterol ester hydrolase [64]. The enzyme CNP is the most extensively studied and has been used as a myelin marker. Isolated myelin contains about 60 percent of total brain activity; the enzyme increases in brain and spinal cord during development in parallel with

myelination, and low levels are present in the myelin-deficient jimpy and quaking mouse mutants. CNP is concentrated more in heavy myelin subfractions than in compact myelin, and is also high in oligodendroglial cells and their plasma membranes. Curiously, it is very low in peripheral nerve and PNS myelin. This enzyme has been recently purified from brain and myelin and found to exist as a dimer of 94,000 to 98,000 M_r, with subunits running on SDS-PAGE with slightly different mobilities at 44,000 to 48,000 M_r [66, 67].[2] The yield of pure enzyme indicates that CNP makes up about 0.3 percent of the total myelin protein. Its physiological function is completely unknown.

The pH 7.2 cholesterol ester hydrolase is one of three such hydrolases in brain that can be distinguished by their pH optima and response to detergents [64, 68]. The relative specific activity of this enzyme in rat brain myelin, compared to whole brain, is 10; a figure two to three times higher than that found for CNP. Isolated myelin accounts for 70 to 80 percent of the total activity. Therefore this enzyme may be more specific to myelin than is CNP. It also fulfills all other criteria for myelin specificity. Since cholesterol esters are not found in normal myelin, the function of this enzyme is obscure.

The enzymes that are not myelin-specific but appear to be intrinsic to myelin and not contaminants are an aminopeptidase [69], nonspecific esterase [70], basic protein kinase [41, 71, 72], phosphoprotein phosphatase [73, 74], a cholesterol esterifying enzyme [75], UDP-galactose:ceramide galactosyltransferase [76], phosphatidylinositol kinase [77], diphosphoinositide kinase [77], CDP-choline:1,2-diradyl-sn-glycerol choline phosphotransferase [78], CDP-ethanolamine:1,2-diradyl-sn-glycerol ethanolamine phosphotransferase [78], carbonic anhydrase [79], 5′-nucleotidase [80], and (Na$^+$ + K$^+$)-ATPase [81]. The functional significance of this heterogeneous collection of enzymes in myelin is not yet clear. The basic protein kinase evidently phosphorylates only a fraction of total myelin basic protein in vivo as well as in vitro. The phosphate group can then be removed by

[1]See page 92.

[2]See page 92.

endogenous phosphatase. Five of these enzymes catalyze steps in the synthesis of major myelin lipids, but whether they play an active role in myelin synthesis is not clear.

Carbonic anhydrase has generally been considered a soluble enzyme and a glial marker, but myelin accounts for a large part of the membrane-bound form in brain. The enzymes 5'-nucleotidase and $(Na^+ + K^+)$-ATPase have long been considered specific markers for plasma membranes. All three of these enzymes play a role in membrane transport; carbonic anhydrase for carbon dioxide, 5'-nucleotidase for adenosine, and $(Na^+ + K^+)$-ATPase for monovalent cations. The presence of these enzymes is evidence that myelin may have an active role in transport of material in and out of the axon. It is likely that other enzyme activities will be discovered as research continues.

Most of the work on myelin enzymes has been done in the CNS. However, the protein kinases [82] and carbonic anhydrase [31] are also present in PNS myelin.

Compositional Changes
DEVELOPING BRAIN
Nervous system development is marked by several overlapping periods, each defined by one major event in brain growth and structural maturation (see Chaps. 19 and 23). These periods can be determined by following the concentration of a specific marker. For example, the period of cellular proliferation can be followed by measuring the amount of DNA per whole brain, and the period of myelination by following a myelin marker such as cerebroside. In the rat, whose CNS undergoes considerable development postnatally, the maximal rate of cellular proliferation occurs at 10 days. The period of rapid myelination overlaps this period of cellular proliferation and is one of the most dramatic in nervous system development. The rat brain begins to form myelin postnatally at about 10 to 12 days. At 15 days of age, about 4 mg of myelin can be isolated from one brain. This amount increases sixfold during the next 15 days, and at 6 months of age, 60 mg of myelin can be isolated from one brain. This represents an increase of about 1,500 percent

over the myelin content of the brains of 15-day-old animals. During the same 5½ month period, the brain weight increases by 50 to 60 percent [16].

It has been convincingly shown by several groups that the myelin that is first deposited has a very different composition from that of the adult. (For reviews, see [4, 9, 16, 83].) As the rat matures, the myelin galactolipids increase by about 50 percent and lecithin decreases by a similar amount. Similar changes are seen in human myelin [84]. The very small amount of desmosterol declines, but the other lipids remain relatively constant. In addition, the polysialogangliosides decrease and the monosialoganglioside, G_{M1}, increases to become the predominant ganglioside. These changes are not complete until the rat is about 2 months old. There is also a change in the composition of the protein portion as well as that of the lipid portion. Both basic protein and proteolipid protein increase in the myelin sheath during development, whereas the amount of higher molecular weight protein decreases [2].

SUBFRACTIONS
The studies summarized above on the composition of myelin from immature brains are consistent with the idea that myelin first laid down by the oligodendroglial cell may represent a transitional form with properties intermediate between those of mature compact myelin and the oligodendroglial cell membrane. As mentioned earlier, in the section on isolation, myelin can be separated into subfractions of different densities. The lighter fractions are enriched in multilamellar myelin, whereas the denser fractions contain a large proportion of single membrane vesicles that resemble microsomes or plasma membrane fragments. Generally speaking, as one goes from light myelin fractions to heavier, the lipid/protein ratio decreases, the amount of basic protein decreases, the amount of unidentified high molecular weight proteins increases, the CNP, carbonic anhydrase, and other enzymes increase, and the amount of proteolipid protein stays relatively constant. Immature animals have a higher proportion of heavier fractions than mature animals; this lends support to the view that

the dense fractions represent transitional forms (see [2; 7, pp. 161–200 and 233–270] and below for further discussions of the significance of this heterogeneity).

DISEASE

Besides the normal changes seen during development, myelin composition is also altered in certain neurological diseases. The myelin abnormalities in human diseases have been found to include both nonspecific and specific changes. The reader is referred to Chap. 32 and [7, pp. 383–414; 85] for full treatment of this subject.

Myelin Metabolism

The principal features of myelin metabolism are its high rate of synthesis during the early stages of myelination and its relative metabolic stability in the adult. Although myelin, once formed, is one of the most stable structures of the body, it is not by any means a completely inert tissue; moreover, there is evidence that its constituents have widely varying metabolic activities.

MYELIN SYNTHESIS

A remarkable amount of synthetic work is done by the oligodendroglial cell during the period of maximum myelination. It has been shown that myelin accumulates in a 20-day-old rat brain at a rate of about 3.5 mg/day [16]. Rough calculations show that there are about 20×10^6 oligodendroglia in such a brain, with each cell body having a dry weight of about 50×10^{-9} mg. Thus, on average, each cell makes about 175×10^{-9} mg of myelin per day, an amount more than three times its own weight. The rates of myelin accumulation increase rapidly prior to this peak and decrease rapidly afterwards. These rates of accumulation depend on three potentially independent biochemical processes: synthesis of separate myelin components, their degradation, and their assembly into myelin. It is not always possible to measure these processes independently. It has been assumed that they are synchronized and that the activities of synthesis and assembly parallel the accumulation

of myelin. This assumption may not be true in all cases.

Myelin synthesis can be measured by studying the activity, in vitro, of enzymes involved in the synthesis of specific myelin components, by measuring incorporation in vivo of labeled precursors into myelin components (with or without isolation of myelin), and by carrying out similar studies in vitro using tissue slices. In a practical sense, the measurement in vitro of specific synthetic enzymes reduces to measurement of the enzymes involved in the synthesis of cerebroside, sulfatide, and galactosyldiglyceride, the only relatively myelin-specific lipids. (Obviously the synthesis of myelin proteins can not be studied by this approach.) For example, the activity of UDP-galactose:ceramide galactosyltransferase (the enzyme that catalyzes the last step of cerebroside synthesis) in mouse brain microsomes increases fourfold from 10 days to a peak activity at 20 days, just preceding the age of maximal rate of myelin accumulation. It then gradually declines, paralleling the declining rate of myelination [86]. The synthesis of glucocerebroside, which is not a myelin lipid, follows a completely different developmental pattern. Many other enzymes involved in lipid synthesis show increases during the period of rapid myelination, even though their products are not myelin specific [7, pp. 233–270]. Most of the lipid synthesis of brain during this period is directed to formation of myelin, independent of whether the lipids are myelin specific, like the galactolipids, or nonspecific, like cholesterol and the phospholipids.

Studies of myelin synthesis in vivo began with the classic studies of Waelsch, Sperry, and Stoyanoff in the 1940s (for a review, see [3]). They found that deuterium from heavy water was incorporated into cholesterol and fatty acid residues of the brains of young myelinating rats quite rapidly, whereas it was incorporated very slowly into adult rat brain — much more slowly than into lipids of other tissues. (This work led to the concept of the metabolic inactivity of myelin in the adult, which will be discussed under Myelin Turnover.) More accurate in vivo studies can be done either by isolating a myelin-specific product from whole brain after the labeling period or by first isolating myelin and then purifying the specific product. Neither procedure may give the component's true rate of synthesis.

In vivo studies using radioactive precursors generally furnish results similar to those of the enzyme assays in vitro. Precursor incorporation increases at the beginning of myelination, peaks during the period of maximum rate of myelination, and then falls off as myelination slows down. For example, in the rat, sulfate incorporation in whole-brain sulfatide increases rapidly between days 10 and 20 and then falls to 5 to 10 percent of the maximum rate by 26 days [87].

Brain and spinal cord slices have been used successfully to study myelin synthesis but are not practical for study of early periods (less than 20 days in the rat) because of the low yields of myelin. Rates of synthesis were highest at the earliest age studied (20 days) and fell to one-tenth of those levels by 60 days of age [88]. The rates of appearance of either labeled lipids or proteins was in the order of spinal cord > brain stem > cerebral cortex, correlating with the myelin content in those areas. These studies showed that in the rat at 30 days, myelin synthesis in the spinal cord accounted for 70 percent of the total lipid synthesis and 15 percent of the total protein synthesis. In the cerebrum, myelin synthesis accounted for a lower percentage of the total; 50 percent of total lipid synthesis and 10 percent of total protein synthesis. It is interesting that, although myelin lipid synthesis decreases greatly with increasing age, so does total lipid synthesis in the nervous system; thus, the proportion devoted to myelin synthesis remains about the same at 60 days. Similar studies in brain slices from young myelinating rats [89] showed that, after incubation with labeled precursor, lecithin and cholesterol had the highest specific activities; these were followed by cerebroside, sphingomyelin, and phosphatidylserine, with phosphatidylethanolamine and sulfatide the lowest. In slices from adult rats, much lower activities were found, but cholesterol had the slowest rate of formation. With different precursors, different relative rates of synthesis of individual lipids are found, but usually the synthesis rates of individual myelin lipids correlate with their long-term turnover rates (see Myelin Turnover).

MYELIN ASSEMBLY

After myelin components have been synthesized in the cell they have to be assembled to form the membrane. The sequence of this process is now being clarified by researchers who are examining the kinetics of entry of components into myelin and its subfractions. It should be kept in mind that assembly of myelin newly formed during development may be a different process from that involved in maintenance and turnover of mature myelin.

The appearance of lipids in myelin relative to other membranes has been studied by many investigators using a variety of labels [7, pp. 233–270]. After short labeling times, microsomal lipids generally have higher specific activities than myelin lipids; but true precursor-product relationships between these membranes have not been proven. At least one lipid, sulfatide, appears to be synthesized in microsomes and then transferred to myelin through a soluble lipoprotein [90], but there is no evidence of such a mechanism with other lipids.

Studies in brain slices of young (17-day-old) rats show that basic protein and Wolfgram proteins appear in myelin with almost no lag after synthesis, but that proteolipid protein enters at a much slower rate for about 45 minutes and then goes in at rates similar to the other proteins [91]. Moreover, if protein synthesis was stopped with cycloheximide, the appearance of basic and Wolfgram proteins into myelin stopped immediately, while proteolipid protein continued to be incorporated into myelin at a normal rate for 30 minutes. This indicates that a pool of proteolipid protein exists that continues to be incorporated into myelin; but it also indicates that there are no such pools of basic and Wolfgram proteins. The myelin glycoproteins acted like proteolipid protein in these experiments, showing a lag in assembly. Investigations of myelin subfraction labeling and of the so-called myelinlike fraction showed that the specific activities of both lipids and proteins of the denser subfractions are higher than the lighter myelin at short labeling times. This suggests, but does not prove, that these fractions may be metabolic precursors of more compact myelin. Double-label studies indicate that the dense subfractions may represent the preexisting pool of proteolipid protein, but that apparently the other proteins enter all fractions simultaneously [92].

If myelin protein synthesis is inhibited in vivo or in vitro with either puromycin or cycloheximide and precursors are then administered, the entry of labeled myelin proteins into newly assembled myelin is halted. However, lipid synthesis continues normally for several hours, and these newly synthesized lipids continue to appear in myelin at a normal rate [93, 94]. Thus, myelin is not assembled synchronously as a unit.

In summing up all of this information on assembly, Benjamins and Morell [2] postulate the following sequence. The high molecular-weight and Wolfgram proteins are present in a lipid-poor precursor membrane. The basic protein and additional Wolfgram protein are added at later stages of transition, but the proteolipid protein and some glycoprotein can enter only at an even later stage. The addition of proteolipid protein would be a rate-limiting or committed step in myelin formation. Lastly, the bulk of the lipids are added and their entry is directed by the proteins already present. This scheme is also based on many developmental studies not covered in this chapter.

It was stated earlier that it is important to distinguish synthesis and assembly as separate processes. Some studies of myelin protein synthesis in the quaking mouse furnish a dramatic example. In this mutant, incorporation of basic and proteolipid proteins into myelin was reduced considerably below normal. However, the synthesis of these proteins in the extra-myelin pool apparently was normal [95], even though the synthesis of myelin lipids is defective in these mutants [7, pp. 489–520]. These data supported a previous assumption that the defect in this mutant was one of assembly.

MYELIN TURNOVER

The sluggish synthesis of myelin components in the adult, first discovered in the earliest experiments

of brain metabolism in which deuterium was used as a label, implies that the turnover of myelin must be slow. Investigations to determine the true turnover rates of myelin are still continuing, and this has proved to be one of the most complex problems in neurochemistry. The concept that myelin, when once formed, is metabolically stable was largely developed by Davison and coworkers [3–5]. Experiments showed that the major myelin constituents—proteolipid protein, cholesterol, sulfatides, and phospholipids—had extraordinarily slow rates of turnover (much slower than components of other tissues). It appeared that all of the myelin lipids had similar turnover rates, and it was concluded that myelin was metabolized as a unit.

Experiments by Smith and colleagues [13] confirmed the relative metabolic stability of myelin but cast doubt on the idea that myelin is metabolized as a unit. Long-term experiments showed that radioactivity is lost from individual myelin lipids at different rates. Phosphatidylinositol, lecithin and phosphatidylserine had half-lives of 5 weeks, 2 months, and 4 months, respectively, whereas ethanolamine phospholipids, cholesterol, sphingomyelin, cerebrosides, and sulfatides had half-lives ranging from 7 months to more than 1 year. By contrast, the half-lives of mitochondrial lipids ranged from 11 to 59 days.

In the wake of these two conflicting viewpoints, a rather large number of turnover studies of myelin lipids was carried out, with little resolution of the confusion. For example, half-lives of lecithin (phosphatidylcholine) in myelin were reported to be as short as 10 days to as long as 167 days. With the more recent work of Jungalwala and coworkers [96, 97], Horrocks and coworkers [98], and Miller and coworkers [99, 100], the picture has now been considerably clarified. It is now known that there are several variables in the experimental design that have considerable influence on these observed (real or apparent) half-lives. These are the precursor used; the time period after injection during which metabolism is studied; and the age of the animal on injection.

Some precursors of synthesis, such as phosphate, acetate, choline, and ethanolamine, are rather extensively reutilized for synthesis after being released by catabolism. Moreover, they are used for resynthesis at different efficiencies, which depend both on the precursor and the product. The more extensively a precursor is reutilized, the longer the apparent half-life will be; thus, for a given lipid the shortest half-life obtained with a series of precursors will be the most accurate one. The precursor of phospholipids that seems to be least reutilized is [2-^{3}H]glycerol [7, pp. 233–270].

When myelin is labeled in a young myelinating animal and the disappearance of label is observed over a period of time, the decay rate follows an exponential curve with more than one rate constant. Rapid decay is seen soon after labeling, and this is followed by increasingly slower decay rates. If short time periods are chosen for decay study, much shorter half-lives will be seen than if decay measurements are pursued over weeks or months. This behavior appears to be real and has been observed with many different precursors and with different lipids and proteins. Usually these decay curves can be approximated as the sum of two processes, a fast and a slow turnover, and indicate that at a minimum there are two metabolic pools in myelin.

Somewhat more confusing are the observations that turnover times are dependent on the age of the animal when labeled. For example, the long-term half-lives of myelin proteins were found to be longer in animals labeled when young than in animals labeled when old [2]. Similar results were found with phosphatidylcholine turnover [100]. Yet, the half-life of the fast component of phosphatidylethanolamine turnover was found to increase with increasing age at injection [98].

The recent experiments of Miller and coworkers [99, 100] on glycerophosphatide turnover illustrate several of the problems discussed above. In the first experiment, rats were injected at 17 days of age with various precursors; turnover was calculated for the first 15-day period after injection (*fast turnover phase*) and for the period of 15 to 80 days after injection (*slow turnover phase*). The turnover times in days for three myelin phospholipids are given in Table 4-2, A.

It can be seen that with all precursors, myelin lipids turned over more slowly than microsomal lipids. [^{3}H]glycerol gives the shortest turnover times and presumably the most accurate. The data in Table 4-2, A, indicate extensive reutilization of the other labels. The ethanolamine lipids (including plasmalogens) seem to reutilize precursors more efficiently than does phosphatidylcholine, giving the appearance of metabolic stability for plasmalogens when glucose or acetate are employed as precursors. These data confirm much of the previous work on turnover with different precursors, but show that the most accurate half-lives in the slow phase are 25 days for phosphatidylcholine and phosphatidylethanolamine, and 34 days for phosphatidalethanolamine, which is the major plasmalogen. To the extent that tritium from glycerol may be reutilized, these can be considered overestimates of the true values.

If animals are labeled at 60 days instead of at 17 days, much faster turnover times are obtained for phosphatidylcholine—very much like the faster phase of turnover seen with young animals. This presumably would also hold true for other lipids (Table 4-2, B).

The turnover times of such other myelin lipids as cholesterol, cerebroside, sulfatide, and sphingomyelin have not been recently reinvestigated with multiple precursors, but it is probable that the earlier results showing slower turnover relative to that of glycerophosphatides are correct and that these lipids are more stable when incorporated into myelin.

Myelin proteins show the same type of biphasic turnover as the lipids. Whereas, in the fast phase, both basic and proteolipid proteins show half-lives of the order of two to three weeks, several studies show that both of these proteins are metabolically stable in the slow phase, showing half-lives too long to be calculated accurately [2, 101]. The Wolfgram proteins and other high molecular weight proteins of myelin do turn over, with half-lives estimated at one to two months in the slow phase. Again, as with the lipids, myelin protein decay curves vary with the precursor used and the age of the animals injected. Shorter half-lives are seen if adult animals are labeled.

In summary, then, Davison's earlier postulate of

Table 4-2. Metabolic Half-Lives of Glycerophosphatides of Myelin and Microsomes of Rat Brain*

Precursor	Phosphatidylcholine		Phosphatidylethanolamine		Phosphatidalethanolamine	
	MY	MIC	MY	MIC	MY	MIC
A. Animals injected at 17 days of age						
[³H]Glycerol	25(10)	13(4)	25(6.5)	14(3)	34(11)	20(4)
[¹⁴C]Choline	39	26	—	—	—	—
[¹⁴C]Ethanolamine	—	—	33	26	58	40
[³²P]Phosphate	30	17	30	29	44	33
[¹⁴C]Glucose	56	35	108	55	stable	54
[¹⁴C]Acetate	54	28	125	65	stable	stable
B. Animals injected at 60 days of age						
[³H]Glycerol	11	6.0				
[¹⁴C]Choline	22	11				
[¹⁴C]Glucose	27	14				

MY, myelin; MIC, microsomes.

*Data in part A from Miller et al. [99], and in part B from Miller and Morell [100]. All times are in days and, except for the numbers in parentheses in line 1, represent half-lives of the slow phase. The numbers in parentheses are half-lives of the rapid phase and are calculated for the first 15 days following injection.

the extreme long-term metabolic stability of most myelin components appears to be confirmed. However, some components do turn over much faster than others, and all components show both a slow and a fast turning-over component. These data indicate that newly formed myelin is catabolized faster than old myelin. It is possible that new membranes are added to regions of the sheath adjacent to cytoplasm, and therefore are also more subject to degradation than components sequestered in compacted layers. However, one study that showed that [³H]cholesterol became evenly distributed throughout PNS myelin in 3 hours does not support this view [102].

MOLECULAR ARCHITECTURE OF MYELIN
The currently accepted view of membrane structure is that of a lipid bilayer with some proteins fully or partially embedded in the bilayer and with others attached to one surface or the other by weaker linkages. Both proteins and lipids are asymmetrically distributed, with the asymmetry of the proteins absolute and that of the lipids partial. Although myelin is an extension of a cell plasma membrane, it probably has a composition quite different

from it. The low protein content and simple protein composition of myelin suggest that in the process of differentiation by which the membrane becomes myelin, it has lost much of its specialized components, producing a skeletal or minimal membrane. Nevertheless, the ultrastructural appearance of myelin suggests it is very much like most membranes, and there is every reason to think that the fluid-mosaic model applies to myelin as well.

In recent years, a number of chemical techniques have been developed to probe the asymmetry of membranes, and some of them have been applied to myelin in an attempt to localize myelin components within the various layers. In addition, antisera specific to myelin components have been raised, and their localization has been studied by immunocytochemical means. The chemical reagents cannot give meaningful information when applied to isolated myelin, because in such fragments both sides of the membrane (cytoplasmic side—*major period line*; external side—*intraperiod line*) are accessible. The technique used is to apply these impermeant reagents to intact portions of the spinal cord. It is postulated that these reagents will react with the external layer of myelin and that this part of the membrane will have a composition identical to that of the intraperiod line. Lactoperoxidase-catalyzed iodination of proteins in such a system resulted in the iodination of proteolipid protein and some high molecular weight proteins, but not in the labeling of basic protein [103], although in isolated myelin fragments, basic protein was labeled.

The interpretation of this experiment is that proteolipid protein is present on the exterior side of myelin, corresponding to the intraperiod line, and that basic protein is on the less-accessible cytoplasmic surface, corresponding to the major dense line. Similar experiments, using pyridoxal phosphate as a probe, after which the complex was reduced with sodium borotritide [104] and using 4,4′-diisothiocyano-2,2′-ditritiostilbene as a probe [105], led to similar conclusions. In an experiment of similar design, treatment with galactose oxidase was followed by reduction with sodium borotritide. In this way, the three major CNS glycoproteins were labeled, indicating that they are on the external surfaces of myelin [106].

Antibodies now exist for Wolfgram proteins, proteolipid protein, basic protein, carbonic anhydrase, cerebroside, CNP, and the major myelin-associated glycoprotein (MAG), among others, but most of the localization studies have been restricted so far to the light microscope level. With the exception of carbonic anhydrase and MAG, the constituents that have been studied appear, at the light microscope level, to be evenly distributed in myelin. MAG appears to be present in areas of myelin adjacent to cytoplasm, but not in compact regions of the sheath [107].

Concanavalin A binds to the intraperiod line of PNS myelin, presumably representing the locus of the P_0 protein [108]. This conclusion has been confirmed by a study showing that in swollen nerves, in which the intraperiod line is opened up, lactoperoxidase can catalyze the iodination of P_0 but not of the basic protein [109].

As yet there are no convincing demonstrations of specific asymmetry of myelin lipids.

Using the results summarized above, several investigators have devised models of how the myelin membrane is constructed at the molecular level (see, for instance [7, pp. 91–116; and 12]). More detailed models of myelin and its structural heterogeneity must await the application of new probes and perfection of ultrastructural immunocytochemical techniques.

Acknowledgment

I wish to thank Dr. Cedric Raine for supplying the elegant photomicrographs that illustrate this chapter.

References

*1. Bunge, R. P. Glial cells and the central myelin sheath. *Physiol. Rev.* 48:197–251, 1968.

*2. Benjamins, J. A., and Morell, P. Proteins of myelin and their metabolism. *Neurochem. Res.* 3: 137–174, 1978.

*3. Davison, A. N., and Dobbing, J. *Applied Neurochemistry.* Philadelphia: Davis, 1978.

*4. Davison, A. N., and Peters, A. *Myelination.* Springfield, Ill.: Thomas, 1970.

*5. Davison, A. N. Biosynthesis of the Myelin Sheath. In *Lipids, Malnutrition, and the Developing Brain* (a Ciba Foundation Symposium). New York: Elsevier, 1972. Pp. 73–90.

*6. Mokrasch, L. C., Bear, R. S., and Schmitt, F. O. Myelin. *Neurosci. Res. Program Bull.* 9:439–598, 1971.

*7. Morell, P. (ed.). *Myelin.* New York: Plenum, 1977.

*8. Norton, W. T. The Myelin Sheath. In E. S. Goldensohn and S. H. Appel (eds.), *Scientific Approaches to Clinical Neurology.* Philadelphia: Lea & Febiger, 1977. Pp. 259–298.

*9. Norton, W. T. Myelin: Structure and Biochemistry. In D. B. Tower (ed.), *The Nervous System.* Vol. I. *The Basic Neurosciences.* New York: Raven, 1975. Pp. 467–481.

*10. O'Brien, J. S. Lipids and Myelination. In H. E. Himwich (ed.), *Developmental Neurobiology.* Springfield, Ill.: Thomas, 1970. Pp. 262–286.

*11. O'Brien, J. S. Chemical Composition of Myelinated Nervous Tissue. In B. Vinken and G. Bruyn (eds.), *Handbook of Neurology.* Amsterdam: North-Holland, 1970. Vol. 7, pp. 40–61.

*12. Rumsby, M. B., and Crang, A. J. The Myelin Sheath—A Structural Examination. In G. Poste and G. L. Nicholson (eds.), *The Synthesis, Assembly, and Turnover of Cell Surface Components.* Amsterdam: North-Holland, 1977. Pp. 247–362.

*13. Smith, M. E. The metabolism of myelin lipids. *Adv. Lipid Res.* 5:241–278, 1967.

*Key reference.

*14. Rorke, L. B., and Riggs, H. E. *Myelination of the Brain in the Newborn*. Philadelphia: Lippincott, 1969.

*15. Yakovlev, P., and Lecours, A. R. The Myelogenetic Cycles of Regional Maturation of the Brain. In A. Minkoski (ed.), *Regional Development of the Brain in Early Life*. Oxford: Blackwell, 1967. Pp. 3–70.

16. Norton, W. T., and Poduslo, S. E. Myelination in rat brain: Changes in myelin composition during brain maturation. *J. Neurochem.* 21:759–773, 1973.

*17. Rasminsky, M. Physiology of Conduction in Demyelinated Axons. In S. G. Waxman (ed.), *Physiology and Pathobiology of Axons*. New York: Raven, 1978. Pp. 361–376.

*18. Waxman, S. G. Variations in Axonal Morphology and Their Functional Significance. In S. G. Waxman (ed.), *Physiology and Pathobiology of Axons*. New York: Raven, 1978. Pp. 169–190.

*19. Hodgkin, A. L. *The Conduction of the Nervous Impulse*. Springfield, Ill.: Thomas, 1964.

20. Schmitt, F. O. Ultrastructure of Nerve Myelin and Its Bearing on Fundamental Concepts of the Structure and Function of Nerve Fibers. In S. R. Korey (ed.), *The Biology of Myelin*. New York: Hoeber-Harper, 1959. Pp. 1–36.

21. Schmitt, F. O., and Bear, R. S. The ultrastructure of the nerve axon sheath. *Biol. Rev.* 14:27–50, 1939.

22. Finean, J. B. Biophysical contributions to membrane structure. *Q. Rev. Biophys.* 2:1–23, 1969.

23. Worthington, C. R. X-Ray Diffraction Studies on Biological Membranes. In D. R. Sanadi and L. Packer (eds.), *Current Topics in Bioenergetics*. New York: Academic, 1973. Vol. 5, pp. 1–39.

24. Robertson, J. D. Design Principles of the Unit Membrane. In G. E. W. Wolstenholme and M. O'Connor (eds.), *Principles of Biomolecular Organization* (a Ciba Foundation Symposium). London: Churchill, 1966. Pp. 357–417.

25. Hirano, A., and Dembitzer, H. M. A structural analysis of the myelin sheath in the central nervous system. *J. Cell Biol.* 34:555–567, 1967.

26. Wood, P. M., and Bunge, R. P. Evidence that sensory axons are mitogenic for Schwann cells. *Nature* 256:662–664, 1975.

27. Weinberg, H. J., and Spencer, P. S. Studies on the control of myelinogenesis II. Evidence for neuronal regulation of myelin production. *Brain Res.* 113: 363–378, 1976.

28. Aguayo, A. J., et al. Multipotentiality of Schwann cells in cross-anastomosed and grafted myelinated and unmyelinated nerves: Quantitative microscopy and radioautography. *Brain Res.* 104:1–20, 1976.

*29. Geren, B. H. The formation from the Schwann cell surface of myelin in the peripheral nerves of chick embryos. *Exp. Cell. Res.* 7:558–562, 1954.

30. Norton, W. T. Isolation of Myelin from Nerve Tissue. In S. Fleischer and L. Packer (eds.), *Methods in Enzymology*. New York: Academic, 1974. Vol. 31, pp. 435–444.

31. Cammer, W. Carbonic anhydrase activity in myelin from sciatic nerves of adult and young rats: Quantitation and inhibitor sensitivity. *J. Neurochem.* 32:651–654, 1979.

32. Brante, G. Studies on lipids in the nervous system with special reference to quantitative chemical determinations and topical distribution. *Acta Physiol. Scand.* 18 (Suppl. 63):1–284, 1949.

33. Suzuki, K., Poduslo, J. F., and Poduslo, S. E. Further evidence for a specific ganglioside fraction closely associated with myelin. *Biochim. Biophys. Acta* 152:576–586, 1968.

34. Ledeen, R. W., Yu, R. K., and Eng, L. F. Gangliosides of human myelin: Sialosylgalactosylceramide (G_7) as a major component. *J. Neurochem.* 21: 829–840, 1973.

35. Ueno, K., Ando, S., and Yu, R. K. Gangliosides of human, cat, and rabbit spinal cords and cord myelin. *J. Lipid Res.* 19:863–871, 1978.

*36. Ledeen, R. W., et al. Gangliosides of the CNS myelin membrane. In P. Mandel and L. Svennerholm (eds.), *Structure and Function of Gangliosides*. New York: Plenum, 1979. Pp. 167–177.

37. Eichberg, J., Hauser, G., and Karnovsky, M. L. Lipids of Nervous Tissue. In G. H. Bourne (ed.), *The Structure and Function of Nervous Tissue*. New York: Academic, 1969. Vol. 3, pp. 185–287.

*38. Folch, J., and Stoffyn, P. Proteolipids from membrane systems. *Ann. N.Y. Acad. Sci.* 195:86–107, 1972.

*39. Eylar, E. H. The structure and immunologic properties of basic proteins of myelin. *Ann. N.Y. Acad. Sci.* 195:481–491, 1972.

*40. Kies, M. W., Martenson, R. E., and Diebler, G. H. Myelin Basic Protein. In A. N. Davison, P. Mandel, and I. G. Morgan (eds.), *Functional and Structural Proteins of the Nervous System*. New York: Plenum, 1972. Pp. 201–214.

*41. Carnegie, P. R., and Dunkley, P. R. Basic Proteins of Central and Peripheral Nervous System Myelin. In B. W. Agranoff and M. H. Aprison (eds.), *Advances in Neurochemistry*. New York: Plenum, 1975. Vol. 1, pp. 95–135.

42. Eylar, E. H., et al. Basic A_1 protein of the myelin membrane, the complete amino acid sequence. *J. Biol. Chem.* 246:5770–5784, 1971.

43. Carnegie, P. R. Amino acid sequence of the encephalitogenic basic protein from human myelin. *Biochem. J.* 123:57–67, 1971.

44. Deibler, G. E., et al. The contribution of phosphorylation and loss of COOH-terminal arginine to the microheterogeneity of myelin basic protein. *J. Biol. Chem.* 250:7931–7938, 1975.

45. Martenson, R. E., et al. Differences between the two myelin basic proteins of the rat central nervous system: A deletion in the smaller protein. *Biochim. Biophys. Acta* 263:193–203, 1972.

46. Matthieu, J.-M., Brady, R. O., and Quarles, R. H. Change in a myelin-associated glycoprotein in rat brain during development: Metabolic aspects. *Brain Res.* 86:55–65, 1975.

47. Poduslo, J. F., Everly, J. L., and Quarles, R. H. A low molecular weight glycoprotein associated with isolated myelin: Distinction from myelin proteolipid protein. *J. Neurochem.* 28:977–986, 1977.

48. Wolfgram, F., and Kotorii, K. The composition of the myelin proteins of the central nervous system. *J. Neurochem.* 15:1281–1290, 1968.

49. Wolfgram, F. A new proteolipid fraction of the nervous system. I. Isolation and amino acid analyses. *J. Neurochem.* 13:461–470, 1966.

50. Agrawal, H. C., et al. Partial characterization of a new myelin protein component. *J. Neurochem.* 19:2083–2090, 1972.

51. Barbarese, E., Braun, P. E., and Carson, J. H. Identification of pre-large and pre-small basic protein in mouse myelin and their structural relationship to large and small basic protein. *Proc. Natl. Acad. Sci. U.S.A.* 74:3360–3364, 1977.

52. Greenfield, S., et al. Protein composition of myelin of the peripheral nervous system. *J. Neurochem.* 20:1207–1216, 1973.

53. Singh, H., Silberlicht, I., and Singh, I. J. A comparative study of the polypeptides of mammalian peripheral nerve myelin. *Brain Res.* 144:303–312, 1978.

54. Everly, J. L., Brady, R. O., and Quarles, R. H. Evidence that the major protein in rat sciatic nerve myelin is a glycoprotein. *J. Neurochem.* 21:329–334, 1973.

55. Wood, J. G., and Dawson, R. M. C. A major myelin glycoprotein of sciatic nerve. *J. Neurochem.* 21:717–719, 1973.

56. Brostoff, S. W., et al. Isolation and partial characterization of the major proteins of rabbit sciatic nerve myelin. *Brain Res.* 86:449–458, 1975.

57. Cammer, W., Sirota, S., and Norton, W. T. The effect of reducing agents on the apparent molecular weight of the myelin P_0 protein and the possible identity of the P_0 and "Y" proteins. *J. Neurochem.*, in press, 1980.

58. Brostoff, S. W., and Eylar, E. H. The proposed amino acid sequence of the P_1 protein of rabbit sciatic nerve myelin. *Arch. Biochem. Biophys.* 153:590–598, 1972.

59. Brostoff, S. W., Sacks, H., and DiPaola, C. The P_2 protein of bovine root myelin: Partial chemical characterization. *J. Neurochem.* 24:289–294, 1975.

60. Kadlubowski, M., and Hughes, R. A. C. Identification of the neuritogen for experimental allergic neuritis. *Nature* 277:140–141, 1979.

61. Kurihara, T., and Tsukada, Y. The regional and subcellular distribution of 2',3'-cyclic nucleotide 3'-phosphohydrolase in the central nervous system. *J. Neurochem.* 14:1167–1174, 1967.

62. Olafson, R. W., Drummond, G. I., and Lee, J. F. Studies on 2',3'-cyclic nucleotide 3'-phosphohydrolase from brain. *Can. J. Biochem.* 47:961–966, 1969.

*63. Sims, N. R., and Carnegie, P. R. 2'-3'-Cyclic nucleotide 3'-phosphodiesterase. In B. W. Agranoff and M. H. Aprison (eds.), *Advances in Neurochemistry*. New York: Plenum, 1978. Vol. 3, pp. 1–41.

64. Eto, Y., and Suzuki, K. Cholesterol ester metabolism in rat brain. A cholesterol ester hydrolase specifically localized in the myelin sheath. *J. Biol. Chem.* 248:1986–1991, 1973.

65. Yamaguchi, S., and Suzuki, K. A novel magnesium-independent neutral sphingomyelinase associated with rat central nervous system. *J. Biol. Chem.* 253:4090–4092, 1978.

66. Drummond, R. J. Purification of 2',3'-cyclic nucleotide 3'-phosphohydrolase from bovine brain by immunoaffinity chromatography: Further biochemical characterization of the protein. *J. Neurochem.* In press.

67. Sprinkle, T. J., Grimes, M. J., and Eller, A. G. Isolation of 2',3'-cyclic nucleotide 3'-phosphodiesterase from human brain. *J. Neurochem.* 34:880–887, 1980.

68. Igarashi, M., and Suzuki, K. Solubilization and characterization of the rat brain cholesterol ester hydrolase localized in the myelin sheath. *J. Neurochem.* 28:729–738, 1977.

*69. Marks, N. Myelin enzymes and protein metabolism. *Adv. Exp. Med. Biol.* 32:263–273, 1972.

70. Rumsby, M. G., Getliffe, H. M., and Riekkinen, P. J. On the association of nonspecific esterase activity with central nerve myelin preparations. *J. Neurochem.* 21:959–968, 1973.

71. Steck, A. J., and Appel, S. H. Phosphorylation of myelin basic protein. *J. Biol. Chem.* 249:5416–5420, 1974.

72. Miyamoto, E. Phosphorylation of endogenous proteins in myelin of rat brain. *J. Neurochem.* 26:573–577, 1976.

73. Miyamoto, E., and Kakiuchi, S. Phosphoprotein phosphatases for myelin basic protein in myelin and

cytosol fractions of rat brain. *Biochim. Biophys. Acta* 384:459–465, 1975.

74. McNamara, J. O., and Appel, S. H. Myelin basic protein phosphatase activity in rat brain. *J. Neurochem.* 29:27–36, 1977.

75. Choi, M.-U., and Suzuki, K. A cholesterol-esterifying enzyme in rat central nervous system myelin. *J. Neurochem.* 31:879–886, 1978.

76. Costantino-Ceccarini, E., and Suzuki, K. Evidence for presence of UDP-galactose:ceramide galactosyltransferase in rat myelin. *Brain Res.* 93:358–362, 1975.

77. Deshmukh, D. S., Bear, W. D., and Brockerhoff, H. Polyphosphoinositide biosynthesis in three subfractions of rat brain myelin. *J. Neurochem.* 30:1191–1193, 1978.

78. Ledeen, R. W., and Wu, P. S. Evidence for presence of CDP-choline:1,2-diradyl-*sn*-glycerol choline phosphotransferase and CDP-ethanolamine:1,2,-diradyl-*sn*-glycerol ethanolamine phosphotransferase in rat CNS myelin. Seventh Meeting of International Society for Neurochemistry, 1979. Abstract, p. 117.

79. Cammer, W., et al. Brain carbonic anhydrase: Activity in isolated myelin and the effect of hexachlorophene. *J. Neurochem.* 27:165–171, 1976.

80. Cammer, W., et al. 5′-Nucleotidase in rat brain myelin. *J. Neurochem.* 35:367–373, 1980.

81. Reiss, D. S., Lees, M. B., and Sapirstein, V. S. Is Na$^+$,K$^+$-ATPase a myelin-associated enzyme? Seventh International Meeting of International Society for Neurochemistry, 1979. Abstract, p. 118.

82. Singh, H., and Spritz, N. Protein kinases associated with peripheral nerve myelin. I. Phosphorylation of endogenous myelin proteins and exogenous substrates. *Biochim. Biophys. Acta* 448:325–337, 1976.

83. Horrocks, L. A. Composition and metabolism of myelin phosphoglycerides during maturation and aging. *Prog. Brain Res.* 40:383–395, 1973.

84. Svennerholm, L., Vanier, M.-T., and Jungbjer, B. Changes in fatty acid composition of human brain myelin lipids during maturation. *J. Neurochem.* 30:1383–1390, 1978.

*85. Suzuki, K. Biochemistry of Myelin Disorders. In S. G. Waxman (ed.), *Physiology and Pathobiology of Axons.* New York: Raven, 1978. Pp. 337–348.

86. Costantino-Ceccarini, E., and Morell, P. Biosynthesis of brain sphingolipids and myelin accumulation in the mouse. *Lipids* 7:656–659, 1972.

87. McKhann, G. M. and Ho, W. The in vivo and in vitro synthesis of sulfatides during development. *J. Neurochem.* 14:717–724, 1967.

88. Smith, M. E. A regional survey of myelin development: Some compositional and metabolic aspects. *J. Lipid Res.* 14:541–551, 1973.

89. Rawlins, F. A., and Smith, M. E. Myelin synthesis in vitro: A comparative study of central and peripheral nervous tissue. *J. Neurochem.* 18:1861–1870, 1971.

90. Benjamins, J. A., Miller, K., and McKhann, G. M. Myelin subfractions in developing rat brain: Characterization and sulfatide labeling. *J. Neurochem.* 20:1589–1603, 1973.

91. Benjamins, J. A., Iwata, R., and Hazlett, J. Kinetics of entry of proteins into the myelin membrane. *J. Neurochem.* 31:1077–1085, 1978.

92. Benjamins, J. A., Gray, M., and Morell, P. Metabolic relationships between myelin subfractions: Entry of proteins. *J. Neurochem.* 27:571–575, 1976.

93. Benjamins, J. A., et al. The effects of inhibitors of protein synthesis on incorporation of lipids into myelin. *J. Neurochem.* 18:729–738, 1971.

94. Smith, M. E., and Hasinoff, C. M. Biosynthesis of myelin proteins in vitro. *J. Neurochem.* 18:739–747, 1971.

95. Greenfield, S., Brostoff, S. W., and Hogan, E. Evidence for defective incorporation of proteins in myelin of the quaking mutant mouse. *Brain Res.* 120:1507–1515, 1977.

96. Jungalwala, F. B., and Dawson, R. M. The turnover of myelin phospholipids in the adult and developing rat brain. *Biochem. J.* 123:683–693, 1972.

97. Jungalwala, F. B. Synthesis and turnover of cerebroside sulfate of myelin in adult and developing rat brain. *J. Lipid Res.* 15:114–123, 1974.

*98. Horrocks, L. A., et al. Synthesis and Turnover of Brain Phosphoglycerides—Results, Method of Calculation, and Interpretation. In G. Porcellati, L. Amaducci, and C. Galli (eds.), *Function and Metabolism of Phospholipids in the Central and Peripheral Nervous Systems.* New York: Plenum, 1976. Pp. 37–54.

99. Miller, S. L., Benjamins, J. A., and Morell, P. Metabolism of glycophospholipids of myelin and microsomes in rat brain. *J. Biol. Chem.* 252:4025–4037, 1977.

100. Miller, S. L., and Morell, P. Turnover of phosphatidylcholine in microsomes and myelin in brains of young and adult rats. *J. Neurochem.* 31:771–777, 1978.

101. Sabri, M. I., Bone, A. H., and Davison, A. N. Turnover of myelin and other structural proteins in the developing rat brain. *Biochem. J.* 142:499–507, 1974.

102. Rawlins, F. A. A time-sequence autoradiographic study of the in vivo incorporation of

[1,2-^{3}H]cholesterol into peripheral nerve myelin. *J. Cell Biol.* 58:42–53, 1973.

103. Poduslo, J. F., and Braun, P. E.   Topographical arrangement of membrane proteins in the intact myelin sheath. *J. Biol. Chem.* 250:1099–1105, 1975.

104. Golds, E. E., and Braun, P. E.   Organization of membrane proteins in the intact myelin sheath. *J. Biol. Chem.* 251:4729–4735, 1976.

105. Wood, D. D., Epand, R. M., and Moscarello, M. A.   Localization of the basic protein and lipophilin in the myelin membrane with a nonpenetrating reagent. *Biochim. Biophys. Acta* 467:120–129, 1977.

106. Poduslo, J. F., Quarles, R. H., and Brady, R. O.   External labeling of galactose in surface membrane glycoproteins of the intact myelin sheath. *J. Biol. Chem.* 251:153–158, 1976.

107. Sternberger, N. H., et al.   Immunochemical demonstration of myelin-associated glycoprotein. *Trans. Am. Soc. Neurochem.* 10:86, 1979.

108. Wood, J. G., and McLaughlin, B. J.   The visualization of concanavalin A binding sites in the interperiod line of rat sciatic nerve myelin. *J. Neurochem.* 24:233–235, 1975.

109. Peterson, R. G., and Gruener, R. W.   Morphological localization of PNS myelin proteins. *Brain Res.* 152:17–30, 1978.

110. Greenfield, S., Brostoff, S. W., and Hogan, E. L.   Characterization of the basic proteins from rodent peripheral nervous system myelin. *J. Neurochem.* 34:453–455, 1980.

111. Drummond, R. S., and Dean, G.   Comparison of 2′,3′-cyclic nucleotide 3′-phosphodiesterase and the major component of Wolfgram protein W1. *J. Neurochem.* 35:1155–1165, 1980.

112. Sprinkle, T. J., Wells, M. R., Garver, F. A., and Smith, D. B.   Studies on the Wolfgram high molecular weight CNS myelin proteins: Relationship to 2′,3′-cyclic nucleotide 3′-phosphodiesterase. *J. Neurochem.* 35:1200–1208, 1980.

[1] Rat and mouse myelins have a basic protein of molecular weight similar to P_2, and it had been assumed that it was the same as P_2 from other species. It has now been shown that these rodents have only small amounts of P_2. The major protein in the 14,000 to 15,000 M_r range in rats and mice has a slightly higher M_r than P_2. It has been named P_r and seems to be immunologically related to P_1 but not to P_2 [110].

[2] Two studies show that the Wolfgram protein doublet at 42,000 to 50,000 M_r corresponds in molecular weight, amino acid composition, and immunologic properties with CNP [111, 112].

Section II. Function of Neural Membranes

Bertil Hille

Chapter 5. Excitability and Ionic Channels

The nervous systems of higher animals enable the organisms to receive and act upon internal and external stimuli with speed and in a coordinated manner. The activity of the nervous system is reflected in a variety of electrical and chemical signals that arise in the receptor organs, the nerve cells, and the effector organs, including muscles and secretory glands. Consider, for example, a simple reflex arc mediating reflex withdrawal of the hand from a hot surface. Four cell types are involved in a network shown diagrammatically in Fig. 5-1. The message travels from skin receptors through the network as a volley of electrical disturbances, terminating in contraction of some muscles. This chapter concerns the physical basis of the electrical potentials in such excitable cells. As we shall see, the electrical potentials are generated by the passive movements of ions such as Na^+, K^+, Ca^{2+}, and Cl^- through highly selective molecular pores in the cell surface membrane called *ionic channels*. Ionic channels play a role in membrane excitation as central as the role of enzymes in metabolism. Opening and closing of specific pores shapes the potential changes and gives rise to characteristic electrical messages. The subject of this chapter has been treated in more detail in other books and reviews [1–6].

Electrical Phenomena in Excitable Cells

All excitable cells have a resting potential; the entire cytoplasm is electrically more negative than the external bathing fluid by 30 to 100 mV. All of this potential drop appears across the extremely thin external cell membrane, as may be ascertained by recording with an electrolyte-filled glass pipette microelectrode. When such an electrode is used to probe potentials around an excitable cell, a sudden negative drop appears at the moment the thin tip of the pipette penetrates the cell surface. By convention, the membrane potential is always reported in terms of "inside" minus "outside," so the resting potential is a negative number, for example, −70 mV in a myelinated nerve fiber. Signals that make the cytoplasm more positive are said to *depolarize* the membrane, and those making it more negative are said to *hyperpolarize* the membrane.

The electrical signals recorded from cells are basically of two types: the highly stereotyped *action potential*, characteristic of each cell type, and a variety of *slow potentials* [4]. The action potential of axons is a brief, spikelike depolarization that propagates regeneratively as an electrical wave without decrement and at a high, constant velocity from one end of the axon to the other. It is used for all rapid signaling over a distance. For example, in the reflex arc of Fig. 5-1, action potentials in motor axons might carry the message from spinal cord to arm, telling the muscle fibers of the biceps to contract. In large mammalian axons at body temperature, the action potential at any one patch of membrane may last only 0.4 msec as it propagates at a speed of 100 meters per second. The action potential is normally elicited when the cell membrane is depolarized by some type of stimulus to beyond a threshold level; and it is said to be produced in an *all-or-nothing* manner because a subthreshold stimulus gives no propagated response, whereas every suprathreshold stimulus elicits the stereotyped propagating wave. Action potentials are also frequently referred to as *spikes*, or *impulses*. Most nerve cell and muscle cell membranes can make action potentials and are said to be *electrically excitable*, but a few cannot.

By contrast, slow potentials are localized membrane depolarizations and hyperpolarizations, with time courses ranging from several milliseconds to minutes. They are associated with a variety of transduction mechanisms. For example, slow potentials arise at the membrane site of action of neurotransmitter molecules and of some hormones, and also in sensory endings of chemosensors, mechanosensors, and other receptor cells. These electrical signals in sensory endings are frequently called *generator,* or *receptor, potentials,* and the signals arising postsynaptically at chemical synapses are called *postsynaptic* potentials. Slow potentials are graded in relation to their stimulus and sum with each other both spatially and temporally while decaying passively over a distance of no more than a few millimeters from their site of generation. The natural stimulus for the initiation of action potentials is a depolarizing slow potential exceeding the firing threshold. Thus, impulses in a wide variety of presynaptic cells often give rise to a barrage of excitatory (depolarizing) and inhibitory (hyperpolarizing) postsynaptic potentials in the dendrites of a postsynaptic neuron, and these potentials sum in the cell body to provide the drive stimulating (or suppressing) the initiation of action potentials in the axon. In each of the four cell populations involved in the reflex arc in Fig. 5-1, depolarizing slow potentials give rise to propagating action potentials as the message moves forward.

The Ionic Hypothesis and the Membrane Theory

In the late nineteenth century, such scientific giants as Kohlrausch, Arrhenius, Ostwald, Nernst, and Planck elucidated the nature of ionic dissociation and movement in aqueous solution, and physiologists realized that the currents and potentials in excitable cells might be due to the diffusion of ions. This view was put in a clear and quite modern form as early as 1902 by Julius Bernstein [7, 8] in his "membrane theory." He postulated that (1) electrical potentials arise across a semipermeable plasma membrane that completely envelops each cell; (2) the potential arises because of concentration gradients of ions such as K^+ across the membrane and because the membrane is not equally

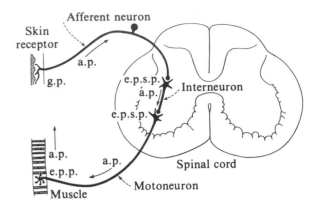

Fig. 5-1. Path of excitation in a simplified spinal reflex that mediates withdrawal of the arm from a painful stimulus. In each of the three neurons and in the muscle cell, excitation starts with a localized slow potential and is propagated via an action potential (a.p.). The slow potentials are: generator potential (g.p.) at the skin; excitatory postsynaptic potentials (e.p.s.p.) at the interneuron and the motoneuron; and end-plate potential (e.p.p.) at the neuromuscular junction. Each neuron makes additional connections to other pathways that are not shown.

permeable to all ions; and (3) the potentials change when some chemical alteration in the membrane changes the ionic permeability [7]. Although 50 more years of electrophysiological work was required to complete the proof, the membrane theory is now fully tested and no longer needs to be considered a hypothesis. However, before we can discuss its consequences in further detail, we must review the physical chemistry of electrodiffusion.

Rules of Ionic Electricity

To see how membrane potentials arise, consider the electrolyte system represented in Fig. 5-2 (left) where a porous membrane separates aqueous solutions of unequal concentrations of a fictitious salt, KA. Two electrodes permit the potential difference between the two solutions to be measured. Now, assume that the membrane pores are permeable exclusively to K^+ and that K^+ begins to diffuse across the membrane but A^- does not. For simple statistical reasons, the movement of K^+ from the concentrated side to the dilute side will initially exceed the movement in the reverse

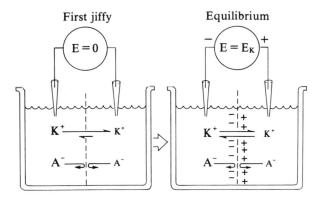

First jiffy   Equilibrium

Fig. 5-2. Origin of the membrane potential in a purely K^+-permeable membrane. The porous membrane separates unequal concentrations of the dissociated salt $K^+ A^-$. In the first "jiffy," the membrane potential, E, recorded by the electrodes above, is zero, and K^+ diffuses to the right down the concentration gradient. The anion A^- cannot cross the membrane, so a net positive charge builds up on the right side and a negative charge on the left. At equilibrium, the membrane potential, caused by the charge separation, has built up to the Nernst potential E_K, and the fluxes of K become equal in the two directions.

direction, and we speak of a *net flux* of K^+ down the concentration gradient. However, this process does not continue very long, as K^+ carries a positive charge from one compartment to the other, leaving a net negative charge behind. The charge separation creates an electrical potential difference, called *membrane potential,* between the two solutions, with a positive sign on the dilute side; it thereby sets up an electrical force tending to oppose further net movement of K^+.

EQUILIBRIUM POTENTIAL

The membrane potential reached in a system with only one permeant ion and no perturbing forces is called the *equilibrium,* or *Nernst, potential* for that ion, that is, the final membrane potential for the system in Fig. 5-2 is the potassium equilibrium potential, symbolized E_K. At that potential, there is no further *net* movement of K^+, and unless otherwise disturbed, the membrane potential and ionic gradient will remain stable indefinitely. The value of the Nernst potential is readily derived

from thermodynamics by recognizing that the change of electrochemical potential ($\Delta\mu_j$) for moving the permeant ion j^{+z} across the membrane must be zero at equilibrium:

$$\Delta\mu_j = 0 = RT \ln \frac{[j]_o}{[j]_i} - zFE \tag{5-1}$$

where R = the gas constant (8.31 joules/degree/ mole)

     T = absolute temperature in °K (°C + 273.2)

     F = Faraday's constant (96,500 coulombs/ mole)

Using terms appropriate to biology, $[j]_i$ represents activities of ion j^{+z} outside and inside a cell, z is the ionic valence, and E the membrane potential defined as "inside-minus-outside." Solving for E and calling it E_j to denote the ion at equilibrium gives the Nernst equation:

$$E_j = \frac{RT}{zF} \ln \frac{[j]_o}{[j]_i} \tag{5-2}$$

For practical use at 20°C, the Nernst equation can be rewritten

$$E_j = \frac{58 \text{ mV}}{z} \log \frac{[j]_o}{[j]_i} \tag{5-3}$$

showing that for a 10:1 transmembrane gradient, a monovalent ion can give 58 mV of membrane potential. Table 5-1 gives approximate intracellular and extracellular concentrations of the four electrically most important ions in a mammalian skeletal muscle cell and the Nernst potentials calculated from these numbers at 37°C (neglecting possible activity coefficient corrections). Experimentally, it is found that the resting muscle membrane is primarily permeable to K^+ and Cl^-, and therefore the resting potential in muscle is -90 mV, close to the equilibrium potentials E_K and E_{Cl}. During a propagated action potential, pores permeable to Na^+ are opened, some Na^+ enters the fiber, and the membrane potential swings transiently toward E_{Na}. When these pores close again, the membrane potential returns to near E_K and E_{Cl} again.

Table 5-1. Approximate Free Ion Concentrations in Mammalian Skeletal Muscle

Ion	Extracellular Concentration (mM)	Intracellular Concentration (mM)	$\dfrac{[\text{Ion}]_o}{[\text{Ion}]_i}$	Nernst Potential[a] (mV)
Na^+	145	12	12	$+66$
K^+	4	155	0.026	-97
Ca^{2+}	1.5	$<10^{-3}$	>1500	$>+97$
Cl^-	120	4^b	30^b	-90^b

[a]Equilibrium potentials calculated at 37°C from the Nernst equation.
[b]Calculated assuming a -90 mV resting potential for the muscle membrane and assuming that chloride ions are at equilibrium at rest.

FLUXES AND NONEQUILIBRIUM POTENTIALS

Although the concept of equilibrium potentials is essential for understanding and predicting the membrane potentials generated by ionic permeability, real cells are actually never at equilibrium, both because different ionic channels open and close during excitation and because, even at rest, several types of channels are open simultaneously. Under these circumstances, the ionic gradients are being dissipated constantly, albeit slowly, and ionic pumps are always needed in the long run to maintain a steady state (see Chap. 6). The net passive flux, M_j, of each ion is proportional to the permeability, P_j, for that ion and is often given, at least approximately, by an empirical formula called the *Goldman-Hodgkin-Katz flux equation* [5, 9, 10]:

$$M_j = P_j z_j \frac{EF}{RT} \frac{[j]_o - [j]_i \exp(z_j\, EF/RT)}{1 - \exp(z_j\, EF/RT)} \quad (5\text{-}4)$$

Experimentally, these fluxes may be measured as an electric current, or by using radioactive tracer techniques, or with sensitive indicator substances responding to the ion in question by fluorescence or other optical changes. In many cases, the fluxes are too small to detect by the less-sensitive, classical method of chemical analysis for total amount of an ion.

When the membrane is permeable to several ions, the steady state potential is given by the sum of contributions of the permeant ions, weighted according to their relative permeabilities [5, 9, 10]:

$$E = \frac{RT}{F} \ln \frac{P_{Na}[Na^+]_o + P_K[K^+]_o + P_{Cl}[Cl^-]_i}{P_{Na}[Na^+]_i + P_K[K^+]_i + P_{Cl}[Cl^-]_o} \quad (5\text{-}5)$$

This Goldman-Hodgkin-Katz voltage equation is often used to determine the relative permeabilities to ions from experiments where the bathing ion concentrations are varied and changes in the membrane potential are recorded. It has the same form as the equation usually used to describe the responses of ion-selective electrodes in analytical work in the laboratory.

During excitation, ionic channels open or close, ions move, and the membrane potential changes. The extra ionic fluxes during activity act as an extra load on the Na^+-K^+ pump that stimulates an extra burst of respiration until the original gradients are restored [11]. How large are these fluxes? The physical minimum, calculated from the rules of electricity, is a very small number. Only 10^{-12} equivalents of charge need be moved to polarize 1 sq cm of membrane by 100 mV, meaning that ideally the movement of 1 picomole per square centimeter of monovalent ion would be enough to depolarize the membrane more than fully. This quantity, related to the electrical capacitance of the membrane, is a constant throughout the animal and plant kingdoms, as would be the case if the effective thickness and dielectric constant of the insulating (hydrophobic) part of all cell plasma membranes are similar. In practice, unmyelinated axons gain about 4 to 8 pmoles of Na^+ and lose about the same amount of K^+ per square centimeter for one action potential [12, 13]. The figure is higher than the physical ideal because the oppositely directed fluxes of Na^+ and K^+ overlap considerably in time, working against each other. With this kind of Na^+ gain, a squid giant axon of 1 mm diameter could be stimulated 10^5 times, and a mammalian unmyelinated fiber of 0.2 μm diameter only 10 to 15 times before the internal Na^+ concentration would be doubled—assuming that the Na^+-K^+ pump, which normally exports Na^+ and imports K^+ (see Chap. 6), has been blocked. In myelinated nerve, the Na^+ gain in one impulse is very small, amounting to only 2×10^{-10} moles per gram of nerve or 2×10^{-17} moles per centimeter of single fiber length [14]. These values are very low because of the special low-capacitance properties of myelin. In other tissues where the fluxes have not been measured, using a value several times the physical minimum of 1 pmol/sq cm for 100 mV might be a reasonable first estimate. To use such a number requires knowledge of the area of surface membrane and invaginations of the cells in question.

The equations just discussed are those for passive electrodiffusion in ionic channels where the only motive forces on ions are thermal and electrical, and they do indeed explain almost all the potentials of excitable cells. However, there is one more type of electric current source in cells that can generate potentials: the ion pumps and other membrane devices that couple ion movements to the movements of other molecules. In excitable cells, the most prominent of these current-generating membrane functions is the Na^+-K^+ pump, which gives a net export of positive charge and hence tends to hyperpolarize the cell-surface membrane in proportion to the rate of pumping [15, 16]. But hyperpolarization is typically only a modest few millivolts. By contrast, mitochondria have very powerful current sources in their proton transport systems. The membrane potentials of such organelles are at times dominated by this crucial bioenergetic transformation system and would then not be describable in terms of diffusion in simple passive channels.

Electrically Excitable Cells

PERMEABILITY CHANGES OF THE ACTION POTENTIAL

Given the rules of ionic electricity, the major biological problem in understanding action potentials is to describe and explain the ionic permeability mechanisms in the membrane. Physiologists have regarded the opening and closing of ionic channels in the membrane as purely passive conformational changes that require no direct input of metabolic energy, a view that has been dramatically confirmed in studies with internally perfused or dialysed cells. For example, the great majority of the axoplasm may be squeezed out of one cut end of a squid giant axon, and then the axon may be reinflated with a continuously flowing column of salt solution that enters at one end and leaves at the other, and still excitability can be preserved [17]. A giant axon perfused with isotonic potassium sulfate can continue to fire several hundred thousand impulses. As a further extreme, much of the remaining axoplasm can be removed by a short perfusion with papain or other proteolytic enzymes, and even potassium fluoride is an excellent internal perfusion medium. Analogous experiments that used dialysis techniques or diffusion of ions through holes cut in cells have been done with other axons, skeletal muscle, and invertebrate and vertebrate neuronal cell bodies. These experiments prove that ATP and other intracellular, small molecules of metabolism are quite unnecessary, either for many cycles of opening and closing of ionic channels or for the depolarizing and repolarizing ionic current flows. Of course, in the long term, ATP and other molecules are needed to fuel the Na^+-K^+ pump and to maintain the biochemical structure and integrity of the membrane and its channels.

In a classic series of experiments, Hodgkin, Huxley, and Katz [1, 2, 4, 5, 18] measured the kinetics of ionic permeability changes in squid giant-axon membranes by a direct electrical method called the *voltage clamp*. As the name implies, the method controls the membrane voltage electrically (often to follow step changes of potential), while ionic movements are recorded directly as electric current flowing across the membrane. The recorded current may be resolved into individual ionic components by changing the ions in the solutions that bathe the membrane. In modern use, this technique has achieved such sensitivity that the flux of amounts as small as 10^{-18} mole of ion in less than a millisecond can be described. The voltage clamp may be regarded as a rapid and sensitive assay for studying the opening and closing of ionic channels.

By using the voltage clamp, Hodgkin and Huxley [18] discovered that the processes underlying *gating* (the opening and closing conformational changes) of channels are controlled by the membrane potential and therefore derive their energy from the work done by the electric field on charges or dipolar groups associated with the channel macromolecule. Hodgkin and Huxley identified currents from two types of ion-selective channels, *Na+ channels* and *K+ channels,* which account for almost all of the current in squid axon membranes, and they made a kinetic model of the opening and closing steps, which may be simplified as follows:

Na+ Channels

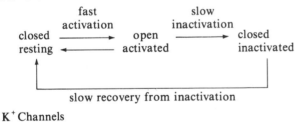

K+ Channels

Depolarization of the membrane is sensed by the channels and causes the reactions to proceed to the right. Repolarization or hyperpolarization causes them to proceed to the left. We can understand the action potential in these terms. The action potential, caused by a depolarizing stimulus, involves a transient opening of Na+ channels that allows Na+ to enter the fiber and depolarize the membrane fully, followed by a transient opening of K+ channels that allows K+ to leave and repolarize the membrane. Figure 5-3 shows a calculation of the temporal relation between channel opening and membrane-potential changes in an axon at 18.5°C, using the model of Hodgkin and Huxley [18].

If there are no chemical or mechanical signals for electrically excitable channels to open, how does the action potential propagate smoothly down an axon, bringing new ionic channels into play ahead of it? Any electrical depolarization or hyperpolarization of a cell membrane spreads a small distance in either direction from its source by a purely passive process often called *cable,* or *electrotonic, spread.* The spread occurs because the intracellular and extracellular media are much better conductors than is the membrane, so any charges injected at one point across the membrane repel each other and disperse over the membrane surface. Electrophysiologists usually describe this process in terms of current flow in an electrical equivalent circuit, with resistors and capacitors representing the geometry of the cell and its membranes. One of the common resulting equations is called the *cable equation,* in analogy to the similar description of how signals spread in electrical cables. The lower part of Fig. 5-3 shows diagrammatically the so-called local circuit currents that spread the depolarization forward. In this way, the excited depolarized membrane area smoothly depolarizes unexcited regions ahead of the action potential, bringing them above firing threshold, opening their Na+ channels, and advancing the wave of excitation. The action potential in the upper part of the figure is calculated by combining the known "cable properties" of the squid giant axon with the rules of ionic electricity and the kinetic equations (Hodgkin-Huxley equations) for the voltage-dependent gating of Na+ and K+ channels. The complete success of the calculation means that the factors described are all those needed to understand action-potential propagation.

A wide variety of cells has now been studied by voltage clamp methods, and quantitative descriptions of their permeability changes are available. All axons, whether vertebrate or invertebrate, operate on the same principles; they have a small background permeability, primarily to K+, which sets the resting potential, and display brief,

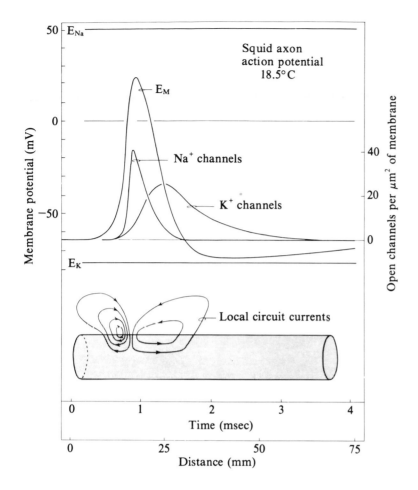

Fig. 5-3. Events of the propagated action potential calculated from the Hodgkin-Huxley [18] kinetic model. Because the action potential is a nondecrementing wave, the diagram shows equivalently the time-course of events at one point in the axon or the spatial distribution of events at one time as the excitation propagates to the left. Upper: Action potential (E_M) and the opening and closing of Na^+ and K^+ channels. Lower: Local circuit currents. The intense loop on the left spreads the depolarization to the left into the unexcited membrane.

dramatic openings of Na^+ and K^+ channels in sequence to shape the action potentials. Chapter 4 describes myelin, a special adaptation of larger (1 to 20 μm diameter) vertebrate nerve fibers for higher conduction speed. In myelinated nerves, like unmyelinated ones, the depolarization spreads from one excitable membrane patch to another by local circuit currents; but because of the insulating properties of the coating myelin, the excitable patches of axon membrane (the nodes of Ranvier)

may be more than a millimeter apart, and the rate of progression of the impulse is faster. The wavelength of an action potential is such that 20 to 40 nodes of Ranvier are active at one time, and every 15 to 20 μsec a new node in front begins to depolarize and an old one behind finishes repolarizing. Nodes of Ranvier have the same Na^+ and K^+ channels as other axon membranes, but they have at least 10 times as many per unit area to depolarize the long, passive, internodal myelin. The Na^+-K^+

pump may be distributed similarly (Chap. 6). The internodal axon membrane has K^+ channels but not Na^+ channels. However, hidden underneath the myelin, these K^+ channels are not in a position to contribute to action potentials. In some cases, after experimental demyelination by diphtheria toxin (a process taking several days), Na^+ channels and excitability can develop in a formerly internodal section of axon [19].

To look for diversity in types of channels, one need not look to evolution, for channels seem to be conservative and quite similar among animals with nervous systems. Rather, diversity is found in the different cell types in any one organism, where the repertoire of functioning channels is adapted to the special role each cell plays in the body. All axons have only to transmit brief action potentials that code a message by their frequency, so their channels are similar. However, the action potential of a variety of muscles and secretory cells may serve instead to time the duration or fix the intensity of a contraction or a secretory response, and their action potentials are never as brief and rarely as invariant as those of axons. Usually, neuron cell bodies also have longer action potentials than does the axon coming from them. In all of these cell types, it is not uncommon to find Ca^{2+} channels that open with depolarization, supplementing the depolarizing effect of Na^+ channels by adding a slower, depolarizing Ca^{2+} influx or sometimes even acting alone to depolarize the membrane without Na^+ channels [20, 21]. Ca^{2+} channels have a special importance, because often the entering Ca^{2+} plays the role of a chemical messenger to activate exocytosis (secretion), contraction, a ciliary reorientation, metabolic pathway, etc. Indeed, whenever an electrical message activates any nonelectrical event, a change of the intracellular free Ca^{2+} concentration acts as an intermediary. In addition, muscles, secretory cells, and neuron cell bodies usually have several types of K^+ channels, some opened by depolarization, as in axons, some opened by raised intracellular free Ca^{2+}, and some turned *off* by depolarization. The electric eel electroplax has a high density of conventional Na^+ channels to generate the strong currents of the electric dis-

charge and resting K^+ channels that turn off with depolarization to avoid opposing the effect of the Na^+ channels [22].

Properties of Voltage-Dependent Channels
Most of what we know about ionic channels comes from functional studies with voltage clamp methods on channels still imbedded in the cell membrane, rather than from attempts to isolate or analyze them chemically [3, 5, 6, 23]. Figure 5-4A summarizes the major functional properties in terms of a fanciful cartoon. Ionic channels are macromolecules or macromolecular complexes that form aqueous pores in the lipid membrane. The pore is narrow enough in one place, the ionic selectivity filter, to "feel" each ion and to distinguish among Na^+, K^+, Ca^{2+}, and Cl^-. The channel also contains charged or dipolar components that sense the electric field in the membrane and drive conformational changes that, in effect, open and close gates controlling the permeability of the pore. In Na^+ and K^+ channels, the gates seem to close the axoplasmic mouth of the pore and the selectivity filter seems to be near the outer end of the pore. This type of information is not yet available for Ca^{2+} channels.

The Na^+ channel is so essential to successful body function that it has become the target in evolution of several potent poisons. The pharmacology of such agents has provided important insights in further defining functional regions of the channel [3, 5, 6, 24]. Figure 5-4B shows the supposed sites of action of the four most prominent classes of Na^+ channel agents. At the outer end of the channel is a site where the puffer-fish poison, tetrodotoxin (TTX), a small, lipid-insoluble, charged molecule, binds with a K_i of 1 to 10 nM and blocks Na^+ permeability. An analogous substance, saxitoxin (STX), also called *paralytic shellfish poison,* has the same action. Both of these molecules have been tritiated and are widely used to count the number of sodium channels in a tissue, as diagnostic tools in physiological experiments, and as markers for chemical isolation of channels. For example, there are 200 to 500 toxin-binding sites per square micrometer of membrane in squid giant

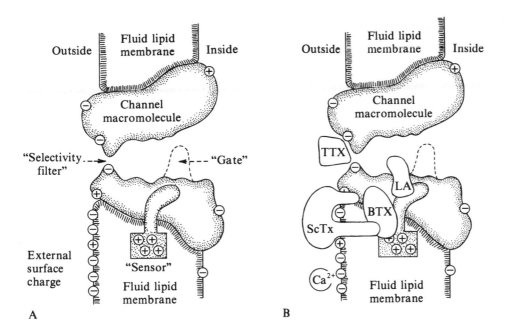

Fig. 5-4. Diagram of the functional units of an ionic channel (A) and the hypothesized binding sites for several drugs and toxins affecting Na^+ channels (B). The drawing is fanciful and the dimension and shapes of the parts are not known. Drug receptors: TTX, tetrodotoxin and saxitoxin; ScTx, scorpion toxins and anemone toxins; BTX, batrachotoxin and aconitine (perhaps also veratridine and gray-anotoxin); LA, local anesthetics; Ca^{2+}, divalent ions screening and associating with surface negative charge.

axons and in frog skeletal muscle. A second important class of Na^+ channel blockers includes such clinically useful local anesthetics as lidocaine and procaine. They are lipid-soluble amines with a hydrophobic end and a polar end, and they bind to a hydrophobic site within the channel where they also interact with the inactivation gating machinery. The relevant clinical actions of local anesthetics are fully explained in their mode of blocking Na^+ channels. Two other classes of toxins either open Na^+ channels spontaneously or prevent them from closing normally once they have opened. These are lipid-soluble steroids, such as the arrow poison, batrachotoxin (BTX), the plant alkaloids aconitine and veratridine, both acting within the membrane, and peptide toxins from scorpion and

anemone venoms, which act only from the outer surface of the membrane. Most scorpion and anemone toxins block the inactivation gating step specifically. All of these reagents are expected to play an important role in future studies of the molecular properties of Na^+ channels.

Far fewer specific agents are known that affect K^+ channels or Ca^{2+} channels. K^+ channels can be blocked by tetraethylammonium ion, Cs^+ and Ba^{2+}, and 4-aminopyridine. Except for 4-aminopyridine, there is good evidence that these ions become lodged within the channel at a narrow place from which they may be dislodged by K^+ coming from the other side [3]. Ca^+ channels can be blocked by verapamil and the related substance D-600, by many divalent ions applied externally, including particularly Mn^{2+}, Co^{2+}, Cd^{2+}, and Ni^{2+}, and by F^- in the internal medium.

How do we know that a channel is a pore? By far the most convincing evidence is the large ionic flux a single channel can handle. Combining estimates of channel density, from counts with radioactively labeled tetrodotoxin or saxitoxin, with measurements of Na^+ current density from voltage clamp studies shows that a single open Na^+ channel can easily pass 4000 Na^+ per millisecond, even near 0°C. The flux of K^+ in a single open K^+ channel is comparable. A turnover number of 4×10^6/sec is several orders of magnitude faster than known enzymatic carrier mechanisms and agrees well with the theoretical properties of a pore of atomic dimensions. Similar fluxes have been observed with pore-forming antibiotic peptides in model systems. These substances, including gramicidin A, alamethicin, and monazomycin, spontaneously form pores permeable to water and small ions in lipid bilayer membranes, as well as in biological membranes [25]. Their antibiotic effect can be attributed to the collapsing of ionic gradients across membranes. They are small enough to be synthesized in many variants in the laboratory and are an excellent model system for elucidating structure-function relations in ionic pores. Several of the antibiotic substances even have very steeply voltage-dependent gating. However, none of the pore-forming agents characterized so far can discriminate between small cations to the degree that Na^+ channels or K^+ channels can.

It was once stated in the biological literature that ions bind water molecules to form a hydrated ion with a defined radius and a specific hydration number. This fictional particle had then to fit through the pore to pass across the membrane. It is correct that a small ion like Na^+ is strongly attracted to the oxygen end of the H_2O dipole, as it is also attracted to oxygen dipoles of alcohols, carbonyls, and, to some extent, ethers. However, the permanence of this interaction should not be exaggerated in comparison with the already strong interaction of H_2O with H_2O. Now we know that water molecules break and make hydrogen bonds with other waters 10^{11} and 10^{12} times per second, and that alkali ions exchange water molecules or other oxygen ligands at least 10^9 times per second [26]. In these terms, the progress of an ion across the membrane is not the movement of a fixed hydrated complex, but rather a continual exchange of oxygen ligands as the ion dances through the sea of free water molecules and of polar groups that form the wall of the pore. It is generally assumed that polar groups and even charged groups are in the pore to provide stabilization energy to the permeating ion. This would compensate for the water molecules

that must be left behind as the ion enters into the pore. Evidence for important negative charges at the mouth or in the selectivity filter of Na^+ and K^+ channels comes from a block of their permeability as the pH of the external medium is lowered below pH 5.5 [27].

The minimum size of ionic channels has been determined from the van der Waals dimensions of ions that will go through them [27]. For example, Na^+ channels will pass at least ten ions other than Na^+, most of them organic ions. The largest is aminoguanidinium, which requires an orifice of somewhat more than 3×5 Å in the selectivity filter of the channel. A sodium ion (ionic diameter 1.90 Å) crossing such a narrow region would have to be partly, but not fully, dehydrated. It might still be in contact with three water molecules (diameter 2.80 Å) at the moment of maximum dehydration.

Because channels are narrow and neither geometrically nor chemically uniform along their length, ionic fluxes cannot be perfectly described by the equations of free diffusion already discussed, and theories capable of describing temporary binding to attractive sites and jumps over barriers are now being explored. Formally, the kinetics of flux through channels are construed similarly to enzyme kinetics. It is assumed that the channel passes through a sequence of "channel-ion complexes" as it catalyzes the progression of an ion across the membrane. The enzyme kinetic theories also can describe other properties of ionic channels such as selectivity, saturation, competition, and block by permeant ions.

The molecular basis of gating is unknown both in biological systems and in antibiotic models, although in the latter, the molecules are at least defined. Several useful indirect methods of study exist. There are the pharmacological agents already discussed, which permit selective blocking of steps in gating. There are more specific chemical agents, such as the enzyme(s) pronase, and the amino-acid modifying reagents that attack arginine and lysine. When perfused inside an axon, these agents irreversibly eliminate the inactivation process in Na^+ channels [28]. There are traditional kinetic studies of channel opening and closing, in which the goals are to define better the number of conformational steps involved. Finally, there is the new "gating current" method, in which sensitive recording methods applied to membranes with all ionic currents blocked detect tiny currents caused by the movements of the charged and dipolar components of the channel macromolecule itself [3].

Sensitive as the traditional approaches may be, these need augmentation by the direct chemical methods of isolation, structure determination, and reconstitution. Of the electrically excitable channels, only the Na^+ channel has been pursued vigorously by biochemists. A high molecular weight, tetrodotoxin-binding component has been solubilized and purified from electric organs and other excitable tissues [24, 29]. Whether the whole Na^+ channel is recovered in a "functional" state is not known. The future for such work is excellent.

OTHER CHANNELS

The channels used in the action potential contrast with those generating slow potentials at synapses and sensory receptors by having strongly voltage-dependent gating. The other channels have gates controlled by chemical transmitters, hormones, or other molecules (as in taste or smell) or by other energies, such as mechanical deformations in touch and hearing. In general, less is known about these channels than about Na^+ and K^+ channels of action potentials, with the exception of the acetylcholine-sensitive channel of the neuromuscular junction (see Chaps. 8, 9, and 26). The ionic mechanisms of these channels include a very broad, monovalent, anion permeability at inhibitory synapses, a cation permeability (about equal for Na^+ and K^+) at several excitatory synapses, at the neuromuscular junction, and at many sensory transducers, and other more selective K^+ and Na^+ permeabilities in other synapses. The acetylcholine receptor of the neuromuscular junction has been solubilized and chemically purified (see Chap. 26).

Acknowledgment

The preparation of this chapter was supported by grant NS 08174 from the National Institutes of Health.

References

*1. Hodgkin, A. L. *The Conduction of the Nervous Impulse.* Springfield, Ill.: Thomas, 1964.

*2. Katz, B. *Nerve, Muscle and Synapse.* New York: McGraw-Hill, 1966.

*3. Armstrong, C. M. Ionic pores, gates, and gating currents. *Q. Rev. Biophys.* 7:179–210, 1975.

*4. Kuffler, S. W., and Nicholls, J. G. *From Neuron to Brain.* Sunderland, Mass.: Sinauer, 1976.

*5. Hille, B. Ionic Basis of Resting and Action Potentials. In J. M. Brookhart et al. (eds.), *Handbook of Physiology,* Vol. 1. Washington, D.C.: American Physiological Society, 1977.

*6. Ulbricht, W. Ionic channels and gating currents in excitable membranes. *Annu. Rev. Biophys. Bioen.* 6:7–31, 1977.

7. Bernstein, J. Untersuchungen zur Thermodynamik der Bioelektrischen Ströme, Part I. *Pfleugers Arch.* 92:521–562, 1902.

8. Bernstein, J. *Electrobiologie.* Braunschweig: Wieweg, 1912.

9. Goldman, D. E. Potential, impedance, and rectification in membranes. *J. Gen. Physiol.* 27:37–60, 1943.

*10. Hodgkin, A. L., and Katz, B. The effect of sodium ions on the electrical activity of the giant axon of the squid. *J. Physiol.* (London) 108:37–77, 1949.

11. Connelly, C. M. Recovery processes and metabolism of nerve. *Rev. Mod. Phys.* 31:475–484, 1959.

12. Keynes, R. D. The ionic movements during nervous activity. *J. Physiol.* (London) 114:119–150, 1951.

13. Cohen, L. B., and De Weer, P. Structural and metabolic processes directly related to action potential propagation. In J. M. Brookhart et al. (eds.), *Handbook of Physiology.* Washington, D.C.: American Physiological Society, 1977. Vol. 1, pp. 137–159.

14. Asano, T., and Hurlbut, W. P. Effects of potassium, sodium, and azide on the ionic movements that accompany activity in frog nerves. *J. Gen. Physiol.* 41:1187–1203, 1958.

*15. Ritchie, J. M. Energetic aspects of nerve conduction: the relationships between heat production, electrical activity and metabolism. *Prog. Biophys. Mol. Biol.* 26:147–187, 1973.

*16. Thomas, R. C. Electrogenic sodium pump in nerve and muscle cells. *Physiol. Rev.* 52:563–594, 1972.

17. Baker, P. F., Hodgkin, A. L., and Shaw, T. I. Replacement of the axoplasm of giant nerve fibres with artificial solutions. *J. Physiol.* (London) 164:330–354, 1962.

*18. Hodgkin, A. L., and Huxley, A. F. A quantitative description of membrane current and its applica-

*Key reference.

tion to conduction and excitation in nerve. *J. Physiol.* (London) 117:500–544, 1952.

19. Bostock, H., and Sears, T. A. The internodal axon membrane: electrical excitability and continuous conduction in segmental demyelination. *J. Physiol.* (London) 280:273–301, 1978.

*20. Hagiwara, S., and Byerly, L. Calcium channel. *Ann. Rev. Neurosci.* 4:69–125, 1981.

*21. Reuter, H. Divalent cations as charge carriers in excitable membranes. *Prog. Biophys. Mol. Biol.* 26:1–43, 1973.

22. Nakamura, Y., Nakajima, S., and Grundfest, H. Analysis of spike electrogenesis and depolarizing K inactivation in electroplaques of *Electrophorus electricus,* L. *J. Gen. Physiol.* 49:321–349, 1965.

*23. Hille, B. Ionic channels in excitable membranes. Current problems and biophysical approaches. *Biophys. J.* 22:283–306, 1978.

*24. Catterall, W. A. Neurotoxins acting on sodium channels. *Annu. Rev. Pharmacol. Toxicol.* 20: 15–43, 1980.

*25. McLaughlin, S., and Eisenberg, M. Antibiotics and membrane biology. *Annu. Rev. Biophys. Bioeng.* 4:335–366, 1975.

26. Diebler, H., Eigen, M., Ilgenfritz, G., Maass, G., and Winkler, R. Kinetics and mechanisms of reactions of main group metal ions with biological carriers. *Pure Appl. Chem.* 20:93–115, 1969.

*27. Hille, B. Ionic Selectivity of Na and K Channels of Nerve Membranes. In G. Eisenman (ed.), *Membranes—A Series of Advances,* Vol. 3. New York: Marcel, 1975.

28. Eaton, D. C., et al. Arginine-specific reagents removed sodium channel inactivation. *Nature* 271: 473–476, 1978.

29. Agnew, W. S., et al. Purification of the tetrodotoxin binding component associated with the voltage-sensitive sodium channel from *Electrophorus electricus* electroplax membranes. *Proc. Natl. Acad. Sci. U.S.A.* 75:2606–2610, 1978.

Addendum

Another useful review of Na^+ channels has appeared [30]. The absence of Na^+ channels and presence of K^+ channels in the region of axon covered by myelin has now been demonstrated directly [31]. A new biophysical technique, the patch clamp, has made it practical to record clear square steps of ionic current as a *single* ionic channel opens and closes in a small patch of membrane [32, 33].

*30. Cahalan, M. Molecular properties of sodium channels in excitable membranes. In C. W. Cotman et al. (eds.), *The Cell Surface and Neuronal Function.* Amsterdam, The Netherlands: Elsevier/North Holland Biomedical Press, 1980. Pp. 1–47.

*31. Chiu, S. Y., and Ritchie, J. M. Evidence for the presence of potassium channels in the internodal region of acutely demyelinated mammalian single nerve fibres. *J. Physiol.* (London) 315: (in press), 1981.

*32. Conti, F., and Neher, E. Single channel recordings of K^+ currents in squid axons. *Nature* 285:140–143, 1980.

*33. Neher, E. Unit conductance studies in biological membranes. In P. F. Baker (ed.), *Techniques in Cellular Physiology.* Amsterdam, The Netherlands: Elsevier/North Holland Biomedical Press, 1981. Pp. 116–131.

George J. Siegel
William L. Stahl
Phillip D. Swanson

Chapter 6. Ion Transport

General Considerations

Different cellular and subcellular compartments of the body are separated from each other and from the external environment by a series of membranes. To maintain the compartmental concentrations of essential nutrients and ions at levels necessary for normal cellular activity, membrane transport processes are essential. Each compartment has a reasonably characteristic composition. Steep chemical and electrical gradients often exist across the membranes. These are often important links in cellular function. For example, sodium and potassium ions are involved in the generation and propagation of the action potential in nerve and muscle tissues.

Movement of molecules through membranes can, in some instances, be described in terms of simple forces that are sufficient to bring about movement without the addition of metabolic energy. In these passive transport processes, a net flux of material arises due to dissipation of the total free energy of the system. The energy of the system decreases until thermodynamic equilibrium is reached and all net fluxes are zero. In other instances, movements of molecules across membranes require expenditure of energy (active transport).

The rate of passage of a molecule through a membrane depends on the magnitude of forces responsible for the movement (concentration or electrical potential gradients) and the relative ease with which the molecule passes through the membrane, expressed in terms of membrane permeability. Mechanisms of movement remain largely unproved but may involve direct movement through the membrane, passage through membrane pores, and pinocytosis.

Stein [1] has carefully examined data on the permeation of a large number of substances through membranes. *Passive diffusion* involves movement of a solute across a membrane as a result of random molecular motion. Membrane charge may alter the rate of diffusion. The model of a simple bimolecular leaflet with substances directly diffusing through the hydrophobic lipid phase accounts for much of the assembled permeability data for nonelectrolytes as based on considerations of the permeant's size, the number of potential hydrogen-bonding groups, and, in some cases, the number of bare methylene groups in relation to the oil-water partition coefficient. However, this model does not account for the anomalous permeability of water, urea, and ions in most natural membrane systems. Alternatively, a model that postulates movement of the permeant within channels penetrating through the hydrophobic environment of the membrane predicts that diffusion might be determined exclusively by the size of the penetrating species. This view is not wholly adequate because no single value for the pore radius can account completely for the available data. Penetration of many molecules may occur through nonrigid lattice spaces between the lipoprotein chains of the membrane matrix. There is probably a range of such pore sizes in any given membrane.

It is well known that a number of molecules—glucose and glycerol, for example—pass through cell membranes faster than is predicted on the basis of the above considerations. This mediated transport of specific molecules imparts great functional flexibility to the membrane. Systems controlling the rate at which specific molecules enter the cell down a preexisting concentration gradient have been termed *facilitated diffusion* systems.

107

These systems do not require metabolic energy. The kinetics of such systems have been interpreted successfully in terms of membrane *carriers*. Reversible binding of a permeating substance *P* with a membrane component *C*, designated as the carrier, is postulated (Fig. 6-1). The complex then traverses the membrane and dissociates, thereby releasing the permeant into the cell. The carrier then returns to the opposite face of the membrane to complete the cycle. Assuming the presence of carriers enables one to explain many of the known kinetic characteristics of membrane transport processes, including saturation, specificity, and competition. Coupling of the inward movement of one substance with the outward movement of another can also be encompassed in such models. Although the mechanism shown in Fig. 6-1 indicates movement of the carrier through the membrane, the carrier molecule could be viewed as rotating or changing in conformation to permit movement of the permeant through the membrane.

Cells are able to maintain steady state concentrations of many substances far from equilibrium by supplying energy derived from metabolic processes. Therefore, *active transport* of a substance is transport against its electrochemical or osmotic gradient, requiring a source of energy to bring about vectorial movement of particles through a membrane. Energy might be supplied at one or more of the steps shown in Fig. 6-1 in such a way that transfer of permeant is more effective in one direction than in the other. A useful example is the movement of sodium ions (Na^+). During the initial phase of a nerve action potential, Na^+ moves rapidly into the cell by passive diffusion, due to forces that result from its concentration and electrical potential gradients. During the recovery phase, however, Na^+ moves out of the cell against these gradients. Thus, the transport during the recovery phase is an "active" process requiring energy for the transport.

Active transport of Na^+ out of the cell is important for maintenance and restoration of ion gradients that are necessary for initiation of an action potential, as well as for regulation of intracellular cation concentrations and for maintenance

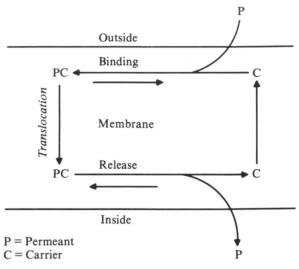

P = Permeant
C = Carrier

Fig. 6-1. Carrier-mediated transport.

of a constant cell volume. The concentrations of Na^+ and K^+ within the cell undoubtedly influence the rates of a variety of enzyme reactions. Complex systems, such as mitochondrial oxidative phosphorylation, are inhibited by high Na^+ or low K^+ concentrations.

The necessity of active transport for cell volume stabilization has been discussed in theoretical terms by Stein [1] and by Post and Jolly [2]. Animal cells are surrounded by water-permeable, nonrigid membranes that vary in volume if placed in media of varying tonicity. The steady state volume will change if a cell is prevented from metabolizing appropriate substrates. The membrane is permeable to some solutes (e.g., inorganic ions) and not to others (e.g., certain proteins). If there were no active transport, the permeable constituents would become distributed in equilibrium with equal internal and external concentrations or, in the case of ions, distributed according to a Donnan equilibrium ratio (see Chap. 5). Because of the presence of impermeable substances within the cell, water would move into the cell, thus increasing the volume. As developed by Post and Jolly [2], the three factors that control the volume of a cell without a rigid cell wall are (1) the amount of fixed intracellular material; (2) the concentration of external permeable material; and (3) the ratio of the rate constants of the "leak" to the "pump." Increasing leakiness or decreasing pump rates will bring about an increased cell volume.

Na$^+$ and K$^+$ Transport

The maintenance of ionic gradients between the inside of the cell and the extracellular fluid is characteristic of almost all mammalian cells. The approximate intracellular and extracellular concentrations of major ions are listed in Table 6-1. This chapter deals primarily with Na$^+$, K$^+$, and Ca^{2+} because these ions are transported by active processes. Cl$^-$ is probably distributed passively according to the electrochemical gradient. Free hydrogen ions are present in similar concentrations on both sides of the plasma membrane, and the bicarbonate (HCO$_3^-$) concentration depends on concentrations of H$^+$ and CO$_2$. Though much lower than the total content, the free intracellular Mg^{2+} concentration is similar to that in the extracellular fluid [3].

The prevalence of low sodium and high potassium intracellular concentrations was interpreted by Boyle and Conway [4] to suggest that cell membranes are impermeable to Na$^+$ but permeable to K$^+$. Later, numerous observations with radiolabeled sodium showed that cell membranes are in fact permeable to Na$^+$. The hypothesis was then introduced by Dean in 1941 that an active sodium pump extrudes Na$^+$, which continuously diffuses into the cells. Where K$^+$ gradients are removed from equilibrium, this premise was extended to the inward pumping of K$^+$ as well [5]. The next phase of investigation involved cation flux studies with red-cell ghosts and giant axons, the intracellular and extracellular milieus of which could be controlled conveniently in the laboratory. Experiments showed that Na$^+$ extrusion is simultaneous with K$^+$ influx and that this coupled flux depends on the availability of ATP as the immediate and sufficient source of energy [5–7]. The third critical phase was initiated with the discovery by Skou in 1957 of the enzyme (Na$^+$ + K$^+$)-stimulated adenosine-triphosphatase in crab nerve membranes. Skou postulated that this enzyme is the molecular machinery for the sodium-potassium pump in the membrane [8].

The principal facts establishing this relationship are listed in Table 6-2. The usual criterion of Na$^+$-K$^+$ pump activity is sensitivity to such cardioactive steroids as ouabain, since no other specific transport system or enzyme is known to be directly inhibited by these substances. This relationship is operationally useful although it is not proof of identity. That (Na$^+$ + K$^+$)-ATPase and the "pump" are identical has been established conclusively by experimental reconstitution of pump activity in artificial vesicles composed only of lipids and the purified protein components of the enzyme [9, 10]. A conference proceedings [10] and several recent reviews on this enzyme have been published [11–15].

Na$^+$-K$^+$ Pump

SOLUTE MOVEMENTS: PHYSICS AND PHYSIOLOGY

Unequal concentrations of Na$^+$ and K$^+$ across a membrane (*concentration gradients*) are produced

Table 6-1. Approximate Concentrations of Ions in Brain

Ion	Extracellular Conc. (mEq/liter)	Intracellular Conc. (mEq/liter)	Ratio Ion$_e$/Ion$_i$
Na$^+$	145	12	12.1
K$^+$	3	155	0.019
Cl$^-$	120	4	30
HCO$_3^-$	27	8	3.4
Ca^{2+}	2.3	10^{-4}	2.3×10^4
Mg^{2+}	2.4	1.2–2.6	≈ 1

Table 6-2. Properties of Na^+ and K^+ Transport and of the $(Na^+ + K^+)$-ATPase that Demonstrate Its Role in Active Na^+ and K^+ Transport

1. It is located in the cell membrane.
2. Its cation requirements are similar to those of the active transport system: there is a higher affinity for Na^+ than K^+ on the intracellular side of cell membrane and opposite affinity on the outside of cell membrane.
3. Substrate requirements are similar to those of the active transport system: ATP is utilized as the energy source for movement of cations.
4. The enzyme system hydrolyzes ATP at a rate dependent on the concentrations of Na^+ inside and K^+ outside the cell.
5. The system is found in all cells that have active, linked transport of Na^+ and K^+.
6. The system is inhibited by cardiac glycosides.
7. There is good correlation between enzyme activity and rates of cation flux in different tissues.
8. The purified reconstituted enzyme catalyzes coupled Na^+ and K^+ transport and the stoichiometry of Na^+-K^+–pumped/ATP hydrolyzed is 3:2:1, as observed in red cells and nerve.

by energy-utilizing processes (active transport) in the face of continuous dissipation of the gradients through passive diffusion. This section shows how to calculate the amount of work performed by the cell to produce Na^+ and K^+ concentration gradients. The kinetics of solute movements across the cell membranes and the resulting concentration gradients will be analyzed in terms of two components. One component is passive diffusion (leak) and the other is active transport (energy dependent).

The rate of diffusion (dn/dt) is given by Fick's law

$$\frac{dn}{dt} = DA\,\frac{dc}{dx} \qquad (6\text{-}1)$$

where n = number of molecules, D = diffusion coefficient, A = area, c = concentration, and x = distance. If we are interested only in the rate of movement from one compartment to another across a biological membrane and not in the rate per unit distance, then

$$\frac{dn}{dt} = -PA\,[c_1 - c_2] \qquad (6\text{-}2)$$

for a membrane of given permeability properties and thickness, P.

It is seen from equation 6-2 that the rate of diffusion is proportional to the difference in concentrations and to the membrane area. In addition, changes in membrane permeability properties or thickness can regulate the rate of diffusion. Through conformational changes, membrane components may reorient chemical groups, which changes the resistance to the passage of ions by virtue of binding, steric, or electrostatic properties. Such reorientations are viewed as the opening or closing of "gates" to channels through which the solute diffuses down its concentration or electrochemical gradient. (These are discussed in Chaps. 3, 5, and 8.)

The Gibbs free energy ($\triangle G$) involved in diffusion for each molecule of solute is calculated from the equation

$$\triangle G = RT \ln c_2/c_1 \qquad (6\text{-}3)$$

Also, work is expressed as $\triangle G \times n$ and power as $\triangle G \times dn/dt$ where n is the number of molecules of solute, t is the time, R equals 1.99 cal/mol/deg, and T is the temperature in degrees Kelvin. In diffusion, when $c_1 > c_2$, $\triangle G$ is negative and the process is exergonic. The released energy can serve to drive some endergonic process. The energy released in equalizing c_1 and c_2 is equal to that needed to restore the same concentration gradient if only concentrative work were involved. The work of establishing the gradient is proportional to the logarithm of the ratio of concentrations, but unlike the rate of movement, it is not proportional to the concentration difference. Thus, for a given total number of molecules diffused, the work to remove these molecules depends on the fractional change in concentration, and not on the number of molecules.

Cell membranes separate electrical charge, and in tissues, therefore, translocation of charged solutes involves electrical potential as well as chemical concentration gradients (see Chap. 5 for a detailed discussion). For our purpose here, the energy related to electrical potential is given by

$$\triangle G = ZF\Psi \qquad (6\text{-}4)$$

where Z is the valence, F is the Faraday constant (23,500 cal/volt/mol), and Ψ represents the transmembrane potential difference. The minimal amount of total free energy change related to movement of one molecule of a solute with respect to the combined electrochemical gradient is the addition of equations 3 and 4:

$$\triangle G = RT \ln c_2/c_1 + ZF\Psi \qquad (6\text{-}5)$$

If the chemical and electrical components are not equal and opposite, then $\triangle G$ is not equal to zero and work is performed by some other exergonic process to maintain a steady state. The amount of work needed per unit time (*power*) will be proportional to the rate of passive leak down the electrochemical gradient.

The work performed in cells to maintain a steady state electrochemical gradient for Na^+ and K^+ can be calculated as follows:
The sum of $\triangle G$ for both Na^+ and K^+ gradients is

$$\triangle G_{total} = RT(\ln[Na^+_e]/[Na^+_i] + ZF\Psi + \ln[K^+_i]/[K^+_e]$$
$$- ZF\Psi)$$

$$\triangle G_{total} = RT(\ln[Na^+_e]/[Na^+_i] + \ln[K^+_i]/[K^+_e]) \qquad (6\text{-}6)$$

Assuming some typical values (see Table 6-1),

$$\triangle G \text{ total} = (1.99 \text{ cal/mol/deg}) (300 \text{ deg}) (\ln 12.1 + \ln 51.6)$$

$$\triangle G \text{ total} = 3.84 \text{ kcal/mol of } Na^+ \text{ exchanged for } K^+.$$

The hydrolysis of ATP yields about 12 kcal/mol, thus permitting the exchange of about 3 moles of cation per mole of ATP hydrolyzed to ADP plus P_i. It can be seen that the total $\triangle G$ produces a larger gradient for K^+ than for Na^+, that is, less energy input is needed for each mole of K^+ than for Na^+. This follows since the K^+ influx is in the direction of the membrane electrical potential, whereas Na^+ efflux is against this potential. We shall see later that the coupled Na^+ and K^+ transport seems crucial for the performance of concentrative work for both cations, even though the larger portion of chemical energy seems directed to the Na^+ efflux (see Operation of the Na^+-K^+ Pump).

CONTROL OF CATION GRADIENTS BY $(Na, + K^+)$-ATPase
Gradients for a number of ions discussed are shown in Table 6-1. Energy for the work of producing the

gradients for Na^+ and K^+ is provided by the hydrolysis of ATP. Where other ions are found in concentrations removed from their electrochemical equilibria, similar ATP-dependent pumps are sought.

Table 6-3 shows the Na^+-K^+ flux and $(Na^+ + K^+)$-ATPase activities in a number of tissues. If the concentration gradients during the flux measurements are in a steady state, these flux values represent the average passive diffusion leaks and an equal, but oppositely directed, active transport. Despite an enormous range in absolute values, the constant ratio of flux to enzyme activity among these tissues permits us to presume that most of the measured flux is due to gradients produced by $(Na^+ + K^+)$-ATPase.

The free energy of hydrolysis of ATP is transduced by $(Na^+ + K^+)$-ATPase into driving Na^+ and K^+ against their electrochemical gradients by the enzyme embedded in the membrane. In the steady state, the rate of ATP hydrolysis is proportional to the rate of leak and is regulated by the concentrations of Na^+ and K^+ accessible to critical sites on the enzyme. The *set point* of the concentration gradient is that combination of concentrations that, under a given set of conditions, is always restored by the enzyme through increases or decreases in its pumping rate after a perturbation. The gradient set point is determined by the sensitivity of the enzyme to small changes in concentrations of Na^+ and K^+. The enzyme properties that influence this regulation may include its sensitivity to other ligands, such as Mg^{2+}, ATP, ADP, and P_i. These ligands modify the reactivity of the enzyme with Na^+ and K^+ in ways that are not entirely understood. The capacity of the enzyme pump to keep pace with leaks and the rate at which it can respond to perturbations in the gradient are determined by the maximal enzyme velocity and the concentration of active molecules. With this introduction, we can discuss the relationships among the Na^+-K^+ pump, membrane potentials, and energy requirements for active transport in neural tissue.

RELATIONSHIP OF Na^+-K^+ PUMP TO MEMBRANE POTENTIALS
In many resting neural membranes, permeability

Table 6-3. $(Na^+ + K^+)$-ATPase Activity and Cation Flux in Tissues

Tissue	Temp. (°C)	A Cation Flux (10^{-14} mol/ sq cm/sec)	B $(Na^+ + K^+)$-ATPase* (10^{-14} mol/ sq cm/sec)	(A)/(B)
Human erythrocytes	37	3.87	1.38 ± 0.36	2.80
Frog toe muscle	17	985	530 ± 94	1.86
Squid giant axon	19	1,200	400 ± 79	3.00
Frog skin	20	19,700	$6,640 \pm 1,100$	2.97
Toad bladder	27	43,700	$17,600 \pm 1,640$	2.48
Electric eel, noninnervated membranes of Sachs' organ	23	86,100	$38,800 \pm 4,160$	2.22
Average	. . . .	. . . .	. . . .	2.56 ± 0.19

*ATPase activities were determined by standard methods on portions of lyophilized and reconstituted tissue homogenates or micro-dissected samples of frozen-dried tissue.
Data from Bonting and Caravaggio, *Arch. Biochem. Biophys.* 101:37, 1963.

to K^+ is about 50 times greater than to Na^+. This feature allows the resting membrane potential to respond mainly to changes in the concentration gradient for K^+ (see Chap. 5). The larger the K^+ gradient, the larger the membrane potential. The Na^+-K^+ pump rate, therefore, is a major factor in determining the resting membrane potential. During the action potential, channels with very high Na^+ conductance (500-fold increase) and others with high K^+ conductance open briefly in sequence, allowing high rates of diffusion down the electrochemical gradients. When the Na^+ conductance channel is open, the membrane potential is responsive to the Na^+ concentration gradient and almost reaches the Na^+ equilibrium potential. Thus, by regulating the steady state Na^+ gradient, the pump rate also is a major factor in determining the height of the action potential. Similarly, during postsynaptic excitatory or inhibitory potentials, changes in specific permeability to Na^+, K^+, or other ions allow these ions to move down their electrochemical gradients and allow the membrane potential to approach the equilibrium potential for the ion(s) whose channel was specifically altered.

To summarize, mediation of the Na^+-K^+ pump provides the immediate energy reservoir for these special properties of excitable tissue: the resting cell membrane potential, the conducted action potential, and postsynaptic potentials that involve Na^+ and K^+. In addition, a small proportion of the membrane potential under certain conditions is due to the inequality of the Na^+-K^+ exchange. This electrogenic component of the Na^+-K^+ pump is discussed later.

ENERGY REQUIREMENTS OF NEURAL TISSUE FOR ACTIVE TRANSPORT
Cation flux during action potentials is two to three orders of magnitude greater than in the resting state (see Chap. 5). The Na^+ entry and K^+ efflux from a squid giant axon during a single action potential (duration is about 1 msec) is about 3×10^{-12} mol/ sq cm membrane [16]. The resting membrane flux in this tissue is 12×10^{-12} mol/sq cm/sec (Table 6-3). It may take the pump about one second to discharge the flux of one spike. Based on these estimates, at conduction frequencies ranging from 10 to 100 impulses/sec, the Na^+-K^+ pump rate would have to respond through a range of one to two orders of magnitude in order to maintain a steady state when the neuron is conducting. Postsynaptic membrane excitatory or inhibitory potentials

(about 10 mV) produce ion flux probably about one-tenth of that produced during an action potential but these may last 10 to 1,000 times longer than action potentials and may occupy larger membrane areas.

The geometry of the cellular elements is another factor in considering energetics of cation flux. The ratio of surface area (S) to volume (V) for a cylinder of a given radius, r, equals $2/r$, and for a sphere this ratio is about $3/r$. For either a sphere or a cylinder, the ratio of S/V varies inversely with the radius. In addition, the S/V ratio is larger for a sphere than for a cylinder of a given radius if the cylinder ends, which are not bounded by membrane, are ignored. The proportionate effect of cation exchange on the intracellular cation concentration increases as the radius of the fiber decreases. This is because the ratio of membrane area to volume increases as the radius decreases, whereas the flux varies with membrane area (eq. 6-2). Thus, in a smaller tube an impulse produces a larger fractional change in the intracellular concentration (see Chap. 5). Since $\triangle G$ is proportional to the logarithm of the fractional change in concentration (eq. 6-3), the energy expenditure for reestablishing the gradient is relatively larger for smaller axons. The same relationship holds for cation flux in the resting membrane. Changing the shape of the cellular unit also affects the energetics, as spheres have a larger ratio of membrane area to volume than do cylinders of the same radius. Finally, from the same considerations, the larger the number of separate membrane-bounded units contained within the volume the more the energy that will be required by a given volume of tissue for maintaining steady state concentration gradients.

Myelination is a third factor. Only the axolemma underlying the node of Ranvier is completely depolarized by action potentials, so a myelinated fiber will have lower total flux per unit length than an unmyelinated fiber of the same radius (see Chaps. 4 and 5).

In summary, the energy utilized to maintain cation gradients in a volume of heterogeneous nerve tissue—cortex for example—will be determined by (1) the distribution of cellular elements with differing shapes, diameters, and extent of myelination, and (2) the superimposed distribution of differing action potential frequencies and postsynaptic potentials.

COUPLING OF NEURONAL METABOLISM AND FUNCTION

The hypothesis now widely held for the coupling of neuronal metabolism and neuronal function states that the changes in metabolic rate that accompany neuronal potential changes are caused by increased ATP hydrolysis, which, in turn, is caused by active cation transport (see also Chap. 24). To test this hypothesis, we can pose the question: What are the magnitudes and time courses of changes in cation flux and in metabolic rate that accompany neuronal activity? Eventually, we wish to know what portion of the cation flux is dependent on ATP utilization and what portion of the available ATP is used only for cation transport.

In considering the coupling of whole brain metabolism and function, three additional problems are introduced that are not solvable by examining individual cells. One is that the metabolic contribution of glial cells when responding in an environment together with neurons may differ from that of isolated glial cells. The second lies in the heterogeneity of neuronal elements. The third is that responses of a multicellular system may involve reorganization of activity among the separate units, as well as net quantitative changes in the whole system, and an energy cost for redistribution of activity.

With these reservations in mind, we are interested in seeing what the brain's caloric expenditure for transport might be. One strategy is to study how extracellular K^+ is regulated. Under physiological conditions, the brain extracellular K^+ concentration, $[K^+_e]$, is very closely maintained at 2.8 to 3 mM. Measurements of $[K^+_e]$ are made either with K^+-specific, ion-exchanger microelectrodes or by measuring the membrane potential response of cortical glial cells. The glial cells are electrically inexcitable, and their membrane potentials respond linearly to the logarithm of $[K^+_e]$ with a slope of 34 to 38 mV per tenfold change in $[K^+_e]$. They behave as if they are K^+-specific electrodes [17]. It is also possible to measure $[K^+_e]$ along with the intracortical concentration of NADH by reflectance spectrophotometry in the intact exposed cerebral cortex [18].

Studies have shown that cortical potentials evoked by electrical stimulation may be accompanied by an increase in $[K^+_e]$ from 3 to 12 mM and that a direct relation exists between NADH oxidation and the logarithm of the $[K^+_e]$ increase. Although a plateau is eventually reached for $[K^+_e]$, oxidation continues to increase [18]. Stimulating cortex with epileptogenic drugs or stimulation of nerves afferent to the cortex also usually produces rises in $[K^+_e]$ to a maximum of about 10 to 12 mM [17, 19]. Superfusion of a higher $[K^+_e]$ produces sustained depolarization, very large K^+ efflux, greatly increased metabolic rate, and depressed electrocerebral activity with an isoelectric encephalogram [17]. These effects spread across the cortex and are subsumed under the expression "spreading depression."

Various interpretations of these results are possible. At the least, these results indicate (1) that depolarization or increased firing frequency is accompanied by increased K^+ efflux and increased oxidative metabolism, (2) that there is regulation of $[K^+_e]$ (at a level of about 10 mM under these conditions), and (3) that this regulation may require increasing energy expenditure. It seems that $[K^+_e]$ higher than 10 to 20 mM completely overloads the regulatory capacity and produces massive depolarization. That $[K^+_e]$ is allowed to rise during these experimental stimulations from the usual plateau of 3 mM to a new plateau of 10 mM suggests a mechanism for changing the set point of regulation. This could involve either the coming into play of different biochemical mechanisms or the switching of the sensitivity of a single biochemical mechanism.

Extracellular K^+ might be removed by diffusion through the extracellular fluid (ECF), by active transport from ECF through capillary endothelial cells into blood, by active transport into neurons and glia, by passive transport into blood or glia, or by a combination of these processes (see K^+ Redistribution by Glia, below). Rates of $[K^+_e]$ clearance

in cortex after electrical pulsation vary with the duration and frequency of stimulation. As measured by glial membrane potentials from different cortical cells in awake cat, average clearance rates ranged from 0.57 to 1.06 mM/sec after 10 sec and from 0.93 to 1.88 mM/sec after 40 sec of 30 Hz pulsation, but many values clustered about 1 mM/sec [19].

A clearance rate of 1 mM/sec, assuming 15% ECF, represents 0.15 μmol/g brain/sec. If all of the $[K^+_e]$ clearance were energy dependent, which is not known, and 2 moles of K^+ were transported per mole of ATP, then the maximum rate of ATP utilization for this rate of K^+ removal would be 0.075 μmol ATP/g/sec. It is estimated that cortex normally synthesizes 0.25 to 0.5 μmol ATP/g/sec. Thus, the K^+ clearance under these conditions would require 15 to 30 percent of the cortex ATP utilization [17].

To estimate the proportion of metabolic rate that may subserve cation transport, brain slices have been either electrically pulsed or incubated in various media, with and without ouabain, while their oxygen consumption was measured. About 25 to 40 percent of metabolic rate may be dependent on cation flux [20, 21]. Similarly, in preparations of isolated nerves, inhibition of active transport may reduce oxygen consumption by 20 to 50 percent, whereas nerve stimulation produces increases in oxygen consumption that are largely blocked by ouabain [22, 23]. Seizures in animals produce several-fold increases in brain ATP utilization that are believed to result from the greatly increased cation flux (see Chaps. 24 and 36).

Although whole-brain and single nerve fibers utilize similar proportions of the energy metabolism for cation transport, they are not alike in their metabolic expenditure per gram of tissue. Estimates of cortex metabolic rate obtained from data related to spike activity in single fibers are about one-tenth or less of the metabolic rate actually measured in brain [24]. It has been pointed out that these discrepancies suggest much larger energy demands of small-diameter nerve terminals, dendrites, and synaptic processes in cortex than can be anticipated from studies of single fibers in which only action potential spikes are measured [24]. It can be calculated that biosynthetic activity, including resynthesis of the whole brain content of acetylcholine, catecholamines, and indoleamines [25] and turnover of proteins and lipids, would account for less than 10 percent of total brain ATP metabolic rate. The contribution or function of various Mg^{2+}- and Ca^{2+}-dependent ATPases found in brain has not been established. These might be involved in vesicle storage of transmitters [26], synaptosomal Ca^{2+} transport [27], and axoplasmic transport systems critical for cortical function (see Chap. 22).

REGULATION BY CATIONS OF CATION FLUX
Most of the information concerning ion movements has been obtained from studies of erythrocytes because their internal and external milieus can be controlled conveniently in laboratory experiments. Under physiological conditions, most results indicate outward movement of 3 Na^+ and inward movement of 2 K^+ for each molecule of ATP hydrolyzed to $ADP + P_i$. Similar ratios have been found for nerve, muscle, and other tissues. Some evidence suggests that the coupling ratio may vary at different membrane potentials or internal Na^+ concentrations, but Na^+ extrusion is almost always larger than K^+ entry. It is this inequality in exchange that directly produces a potential difference (inside negative) of a few millivolts [11, 13].

The regulation of sodium-potassium exchange by the compositions of internal and external media is very complicated. When in physiologically low concentrations in these compartments, intracellular Na^+ and extracellular K^+ stimulate normal Na^+-K^+ exchange (Na^+ efflux and K^+ influx). When in physiologically high concentrations, intracellular K^+ and extracellular Na^+ inhibit normal Na^+-K^+ exchange but may stimulate a reverse exchange. Under physiological conditions in high-K^+ cells, the principal rate-limiting ligand concentration is that of intracellular Na^+ [11, 13].

Kinetic analysis of flux activation with erythrocytes can be interpreted in different ways. The general picture suggests the existence of three extracellular Na^+ sites of relatively low affinity ($K_d \approx 30$ mM) and three intracellular Na^+ sites of high affinity ($K_d \approx 0.2$ mM). Sites for K^+ show the opposite asymmetry. Data are consistent with two different extracellular K^+ sites of relatively high affinity (K_d less than 0.5 mM). The range of K_d for the intracellular K^+ sites is 10 mM and higher [13].

The sensitivity of the pump to Na^+ and K^+ may vary under different conditions or in different tissues. As stated earlier, this sensitivity is one of the enzyme properties that determines the gradient set point. For example, in goat red cells, which are low in potassium, the ratio of affinities for Na^+ and K^+ at internal activation sites is much lower than is the ratio in human erythrocytes, which contain high intracellular K^+. The lower sensitivity to activation by internal Na^+ could account for internal K^+ concentration in the goat cells being lower than in the human cells [11].

OPERATION OF THE Na^+-K^+ PUMP
Extensive studies by Glynn and colleagues [11] have shown that the ouabain-sensitive, Na^+-K^+ pump in erythrocytes can be made to operate in five different modes depending on the compositions of the intracellular and extracellular media (Table 6-4). In this context, channel refers to carrier-mediated ion translocation.

1. *Forward Na^+-K^+ exchange in normal direction.* This depends on the usual physiological gradients for Na^+ and K^+. Intracellular ATP is hydrolyzed while Na^+ leaves and K^+ enters the cell with a ratio of 3:2:1 for Na^+/K^+/ATP. This is the only mode in which concentrative work is performed by the pump. Requirements are ATP and Na^+ at the internal surface, and K^+ at the external surface. It has been shown that cytoplasmic Na^+ stimulates phosphorylation of membrane-bound enzyme by ATP [28].

2. *Uncoupled Na^+ efflux.* Erythrocytes incubated in media without Na^+ or K^+ show an efflux of sodium, which does not appear to exchange for any other cation. This efflux is dependent on the presence of intracellular ATP and is accompanied by Na^+-stimulated ATP hydrolysis at a ratio of about 3 Na^+ extruded per mole of ATP. The Na^+ extrusion is not against, but rather down, its concentration gradient. The free energy of hydrolysis presumably is lost. In fact, external Na^+ of about 5 mM inhibits the uncoupled efflux, whereas higher $[Na^+_e]$ produces

Table 6-4. Transport Modes in Erythrocytes and Their Presumed Underlying Reactions

Pump Mode	Pump Requirements	Pump Activation Sites		Enzyme Reaction	Reaction Requirements
		Internal	External		
Normal Na^+-K^+ exchange (concentrative work)	In: Na^+, Mg^{2+}, ATP Out: K^+	High affinity Na^+	High affinity K^+	Net: $H_2O + ATP \rightarrow ADP + P_i$	Na^+, K^+, Mg^{2+}, ATP
Na^+ efflux	In: Na^+, Mg^{2+}, ATP	High affinity Na^+		$E + ATP \rightarrow ADP + EP$ $EP + H_2O \rightarrow E + P_i$ Net: $ATP + H_2O \rightarrow ADP + P_i$	Na^+, Mg^{2+}, ATP
Na^+-Na^+ exchange	In: Na^+, Mg^{2+}, ATP, ADP Out: Na^+	High affinity Na^+ (? also K^+)	Low affinity Na^+	$E + ATP \rightarrow ADP + E{\sim}P$ $E{\sim}P + [^{14}C]ADP \rightarrow E + [^{14}C]ATP$ Net: $[^{14}C]ADP + ATP \leftrightarrow [^{14}C]ATP + ADP$	Na^+, low Mg^{2+}, ATP, ADP
K^+-K^+ exchange	In: K^+, Mg^{2+}, ATP, P_i Out: K^+	Low affinity K^+	High affinity K^+	$E + P_i \rightarrow EP$ $EP + [^{18}O]H_2O \rightarrow E + [^{18}O]P_i$ Net: $[^{18}O]H_2O + P_i \leftrightarrow [^{18}O]P_i + H_2O$	K^+, Mg^{2+}, P_i
Reversed Na^+-K^+ exchange (ATP synthesis)	In: high K^+, Mg^{2+}, high $[ADP][P_i]/[ATP]$ Out: high Na^+	Low affinity K^+	Low affinity Na^+	Net: $ADP + P_i \rightarrow ATP + H_2O$	Two steps: ADP + high $[Na^+]$ added to P_i + low $[Na^+]$

Na^+-Na^+ exchange. The effect of increasing the external Na^+ concentration may be due to the decreased gradient, to a regulatory effect on the pump, or both. Since, in the presence of even high concentrations of $[Na^+_e]$, the addition of low $[K^+_e]$ would actually increase the Na^+ efflux (forward Na^+-K^+ exchange), $[K^+_e]$ probably is critical to the coupling of the energy of ATP hydrolysis to the enzyme in such a way as to produce concentrative work for Na^+. This energy-translocation coupling effect seems distinct from the reaction permitting Na^+ translocation that is not dependent on K^+. The same may be true of K^+ translocation, because no concentrative work for K^+ is observed without the same for Na^+.

3. *Na^+-Na^+ exchange.* When the extracellular medium is high in Na^+ and contains no K^+, an exchange between internal and external Na^+ is observed without net change in concentration.

Intracellular ADP and ATP are needed for the exchange. However, ATP is not hydrolyzed and the critical reaction for opening Na^+ channels may instead be ATP-ADP transphosphorylation. Low $[Na^+_i]$ and high $[Na^+_e]$ stimulate the Na^+-Na^+ exchange.

4. *K^+-K^+ exchange.* When erythrocytes contain K^+ but little or no Na^+, the K^+-K^+ exchange is 1:1 and is dependent on the presence of intracellular ATP and P_i. However, no ATP is hydrolyzed. The reaction for opening K^+ channels might involve reversible phosphorylation of the pump by P_i, and this reaction may be allosterically modified by ATP. The K^+-K^+ exchange rate is stimulated by internal and external K^+ with asymmetrical sensitivities opposite to the relationship for Na^+-Na^+ exchange.

5. *Reversed Na^+-K^+ exchange.* When the concentration gradients for Na^+ and K^+ are greater than normal and the intracellular ratio of [ATP]/

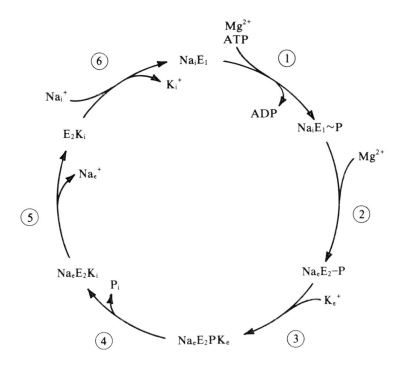

Fig. 6-2. Reaction model for $(Na^+ + K^+)$-ATPase. Stoichiometry and number of monomers are not specified. Uncoupled reactions and translocations may be accommodated by assuming side paths that are less favored under physiological conditions: $Na_iE_1 \sim P \cdot ADP \leftrightarrow Na^+_e + E_1 \sim P \cdot ADP$; Na_eE_2-$P + H_2O \to Na^+_e + E_2 + P_i$; $K^+_e + E_2 \xrightarrow{Mg^{2+},ATP,P_i} K^+_i + E_2 \leftrightarrow E_1$. There is controversy, however, about the exact reactions. From Siegel in [10] pp. 287–299. Reprinted with permission from Academic Press.

[ADP] [P_i] is lower than normal, Na^+ moves into and K^+ out of the cell, while ATP is synthesized. Extracellular K^+ inhibits the synthesis of ATP and this reversed Na^+-K^+ exchange.

Biochemistry of $(Na^+ + K^+)$-ATPase

REACTIONS CATALYZED

In contrast to cation flux, most of the information concerning the chemical reactions catalyzed by the enzyme has been obtained by using fragmented membranes or purified enzyme in suspension. In these enzymatic assays, all of the various ligand sites are exposed to the same medium. Under

various conditions $(Na^+ + K^+)$-ATPase is able to catalyze a number of reactions that may be viewed as portions of a cycle leading to ATP hydrolysis [29] (Fig. 6-2). The reader is referred to the review articles [11–13].

$(Na^+ + K^+)$-Activated ATPase

ATP is hydrolyzed in the presence of Mg^{2+}, Na^+, and K^+. This reaction accompanies the forward Na^+-K^+ exchange. The apparent affinity for Na^+ depends on the concentration of K^+, and vice versa. Sensitivity to activation by either cation is reduced by increasing the concentration of the other. Either cation also produces inhibition; sensitivity to inhibition also is reduced by increasing the other cation. Maximal activity is usually obtained in the presence of 1 to 3 mM $MgCl_2$ and ATP, 80 to 100 mM NaCl, and 10 to 20 mM KCl. K^+ can be replaced by its congeners, NH_4^+, Rb^+, Cs^+, Tl^+, but Na^+ cannot be replaced. Li^+, while a poor substitute for Na^+ or K^+, actually may share certain properties with both. Kinetic data suggest two activating sites or effects for K^+; one might be essential for catalysis and the other for regulation. The optimal Mg^{2+} concentration depends on the ATP concentration, and Mg^{2+} appears to act on the enzyme as a regulator at Mg^{2+} sites, as well as being part of the substrate, $MgATP^{2-}$. There appear to be two sites for $MgATP^{2-}$, one with affinity of less than 10 μM and one of 200 to 600 μM. For optimal hydrolysis activity, both sites are saturated. However, the high-affinity site alone appears sufficient to account for enzyme phosphorylation. Therefore, the low-affinity site may have a regulatory role. Nucleotides other than ATP can be hydrolyzed, but affinities for them are much lower.

Na$^+$-Dependent Phosphorylation
Enzyme phosphorylation is stimulated by Na^+ in the presence of Mg^{2+} and ATP, but without K^+. A slow rate of Na^+-dependent ATP hydrolysis can then be measured. This reaction accompanies uncoupled Na^+ efflux in red cells. The addition of K^+ produces acceleration in the rate of dephosphorylation. In addition, K^+ reduces both the apparent affinity for Na^+ and the maximum steady state level of phosphoenzyme (EP). The inhibition of EP formation is an effect of K^+ separate from that of acceleration of hydrolysis rates. When the ATP concentration is in the micromolar range, or if it is replaced by a nucleotide with very low affinity, such as UTP, then the addition of K^+ inhibits nucleotide hydrolysis, as well as the formation of EP. K^+ also inhibits binding of ATP to the enzyme.

Na$^+$-Dependent ADP-ATP Transphosphorylation
When Na^+ is added to 0.1 to 0.5 mM $MgCl_2$, ADP-^{14}C, and ATP, it stimulates phosphate transfer from phosphorylated enzyme to ADP. This is a reversal of enzyme phosphorylation and provides evidence for a high-energy phosphorylated intermediate (E~P) state of the enzyme. The transphosphorylation may underlie Na^+-Na^+ exchange in red cells: phosphorylation by ATP opens an efflux channel, and transfer of phosphate back to ADP permits Na^+ influx.

K$^+$-Dependent Phosphorylation by P$_i$
In the presence of Mg^{2+} and K^+ without Na^+, the enzyme incorporates $^{32}P_i$ onto the same acceptor site as that phosphorylated by ATP in the Na^+-dependent reaction. This reaction can also be shown by the exchange, stimulated by K^+, of ^{18}O between medium P_i and H_2O. It represents reversibility of the K^+-dependent enzyme dephosphorylation. These K^+-dependent reactions are supposed to accompany the K^+-K^+ exchange observed in red cells, although the K^+ translocation depends also on ATP binding.

ATP Synthesis
Some EP, formed from P_i in the presence of Mg^{2+} and low Na^+, without K^+, transfers the phosphate to ADP when the EP is incubated in a separate step with ADP and a high concentration of Na^+. This complete sequence of reversals corresponds to the synthesis of ATP from P_i observed in red cells under conditions of reversed Na^+-K^+ exchange.

K$^+$-Dependent Phosphatase (K$^+$-pNPPase)
Several nonphysiological phosphoric acid anhydrides can be hydrolyzed in the presence of Mg^{2+} and K^+ without Na^+. The most often used is p-nitrophenylphosphate. It is supposed that the supplied anhydride is a substitute for the enzyme acyl phosphate, and that it is acted upon by a phosphatase catalytic site. No cation flux, such as uncoupled K^+ influx, has been found linked to this reaction.

Coupling of Na$^+$ and K$^+$
Recently, some evidence has been adduced for an enzyme reaction stimulated simultaneously by Na^+ and K^+. Pb^{2+} inhibits hydrolysis activity but stimulates enzyme phosphorylation by ATP in the absence of Na^+. Utilizing Pb^{2+}-dependent phosphorylation as a probe, it was found that Na^+ is synergistic with K^+ in reducing steady state EP levels under certain conditions. The reduction in Pb · EP is specific for Na^+, but K^+ can be replaced by its congeners. The affinities for Na^+ and K^+ in this reaction are most consistent with those of externally oriented sites—low affinity for Na^+ and high affinity for K^+ [29]. Studies on phosphorylation by acetylphosphate also suggest that, in addition to stimulating phosphorylation, Na^+ acts synergistically with K^+ on EP [30]. Another line of evidence

is that Na^+ plus K^+ exert synergistic effects on the rate of enzyme alkylation by a sulfhydryl-reactive probe [31]. Further work is needed to elucidate the multiple interactions.

SIDEDNESS OF THE $(Na^+ + K^+)$-ATPase REACTIONS

In the intact cell or in reconstituted vesicles, the enzyme catalytic protein spans the membrane and has active sites exposed to both surfaces. Ouabain binds almost irreversibly to the enzyme and inhibits all the transport and catalytic reactions but stimulates incorporation of P_i onto the same phosphoryl-acceptor site as that phosphorylated by ATP. Ouabain binds only from the extracellular surface; tritiated ouabain is a marker for counting and localizing enzyme sites in tissues [11, 13]. ATP phosphorylates only from the cytoplasmic surface. Both the phosphoryl-acceptor site and the major binding site for derivatives of ouabain are on the large (α) polypeptide. ATP at the cytoplasmic surface increases ouabain-binding rates; K^+ at the extracellular surface decreases these rates. Conformational effects on the catalytic polypeptide produced by ATP are transmitted through the membrane, either through phosphorylation or through binding of ATP itself [32]. Recent evidence for an endogenous ouabainlike substance in mammalian brain suggests the possibility of a physiological role for the ouabain-binding site [33].

Na^+ at the cytoplasmic surface stimulates phosphorylation [28] while K^+ at either extracellular or cytoplasmic surfaces inhibits Na^+-dependent phosphorylation. The intracellular, but not extracellular, K^+ inhibition of red-cell membrane phosphorylation at $37°C$ is overcome by intracellular Na^+.

Vanadate, analogous in structure to phosphate, is taken up by red cells and inhibits $(Na^+ + K^+)$-ATPase activity from the cytoplasmic surface. K^+ at the extracellular surface potentiates vanadate inhibition. Vanadate is of possible physiological significance, as it is inhibitory in the nanomolar concentrations found in tissues, and injections of vanadate cause diuresis and sodium excretion (see [34] for references).

CONFORMATION STATES OF THE ENZYME

It has been proposed that the Na^+-dependent EP can exist in two states—$E_1 \sim P$ and $E_2 - P$, distinguished by their energy levels and reactivity with ADP or H_2O. This is based on the fact that Na^+-dependent ADP-ATP exchange is seen at low Mg^{2+} concentrations or in the presence of sulfhydryl alkylating reagents, N-ethylmaleimide (NEM), oligomycin, and BAL-arsenite. These conditions inhibit ATP hydrolysis but do not change the steady state levels of total EP. Partial digests of phosphoenzyme derived under various conditions from ATP or from P_i show that high-energy and low-energy EP have the same labeled phosphopeptides. It is further assumed that an equilibrium exists between two nonphosphorylated enzyme species such that E_1 has a higher affinity for Na^+ and reactivity with ATP for phosphorylation, and E_2 has a higher affinity for K^+ and is not phosphorylated by ATP. The enzyme conformational transitions are represented as follows [35–38]:

$$\text{I. } E_1 + MgATP^{2-} \xrightarrow{\quad Na^+ \quad} E_1 \sim P + ADP$$

$$\text{II. } E_1 \sim P \xrightarrow{\quad Mg^{2+} \quad} E_2 - P + \text{large } \triangle G$$

$$\text{III. } E_2 - P + H_2O \xrightarrow{\quad K^+ \quad} E_2 + P_i$$

$$\text{IV. } E_2 \xrightarrow{\quad\quad} E_1$$

Many kinetic experiments have supported the basic assumptions of two phosphorylated and two dephosphorylated enzyme species [see 11 to 13 for references].

ENZYMATIC REACTIONS AND Na^+-K^+ TRANSLOCATION

The demonstrated modes of transport in red cells (Table 6-4) indicate that reactions facilitating nonconcentrative cation translocation through the pump carriers, or channels, can be independent for Na^+ and K^+. However, the coupling of ATP chemical energy to concentrative work seems to be achieved only when channels for both Na^+ and K^+ are conducting in specific directions. Under this condition, not only are the channels open, but energy is supplied for propulsion through both. This implies that a biochemical link is made between the channels and that this linkage is requisite to performance of work. Both topological factors and chemical reactivity presumably determine the nature of this linkage.

The simplest model that accounts for independent reactions and that also incorporates a coupling reaction is shown in Fig. 6-2. The cycle proceeds through both consecutive and simultaneous reactions with Na^+ and K^+. The enzyme is asymmetrical, with Na^+-K^+ antagonism at E_1 and synergism at E_2-P sites. Translocations of Na^+ and K^+ are consecutive within each cycle, despite the coupling reaction [29]. The precise nature of the coupling reaction, however, is open to question in the absence of sufficient physical or topological information to restrict possibilities.

TRANSPORT MODELS

The enzyme reaction model can be applied to physical models for transport if certain postulates are adopted:

1. The enzyme conformational changes produced by the binding of ligands permit translocations of cations through ionophoric domains of the transport enzyme complex.
2. Conformational changes associated with concentrative work produce a force gradient within the ionophoric domain. The gradient may relate to accessibility to, affinity for, or propulsive effects on the cation. Recognition of cation and direction of movement, and an ability to separate charges, conceivably, are factors.
3. The vector for the series of enzyme conformational transitions and, hence, of the concentrative work, is imposed by the large free-energy change in transition of phosphoenzyme from a species with high ADP reactivity to one with high K^+ affinity and H_2O reactivity and insensitivity to ADP.
4. There is a biochemical linkage between Na^+ and K^+ ionophores and the catalytic domain, such that concentrative work for the two cations is coupled.

The first three postulates are applicable, generally, to any active transporting enzyme complex; for example, the SR-ATPase involved in muscle relax-

ation. This is the Ca^{2+}-stimulated ATPase of sarcoplasmic reticulum (SR) that transports Ca^{2+} out of the sarcoplasm into SR vesicles. Ca^{2+} stimulates phosphorylation on an aspartyl residue of SR-ATPase; Ca^{2+} also stimulates ADP-ATP transphosphorylation, as well as ATP hydrolysis catalyzed by this enzyme. The SR-ATPase is an integral membrane polypeptide of about 115,000 molecular weight. The phosphorylation site is at the sarcoplasmic surface. ATP hydrolysis leads to 2 Ca^{2+} transported into SR vesicles per mole ATP. The reversal of Ca^{2+} transport leads to ATP formation. The ionophoric function can be dissociated from catalytic activity and the Ca^{2+} translocation site is separate from the $CaATP^{2-}$ binding site. Ca^{2+} accelerates EP formation. The metal ion complexed to the substrate can be replaced by Mg^{2+}, Mn^{2+}, or Co^{2+}, but the translocation site is specific for Ca^{2+}. Recent evidence is consistent with transition of EP from a species sensitive to ADP and Ca^{2+}, to EP insensitive to ADP and with reduced Ca^{2+} affinity, to another EP, also insensitive to ADP, but whose hydrolysis is accelerated by Mg^{2+} and K^+. A counter port ion has not been demonstrated. (See [39] for references.) It can be assumed that the EP undergoes a conformational change during the translocation of Ca^{2+}.

The fourth postulate is necessary for an exchange pump, in which the concentrative work is coupled in both directions across the membrane.

A useful scheme for coupling both Na^+ and K^+ channels with energy transfer, assuming that EP is an intermediate in transport, is provided by the reciprocating flip-flop model [31]. This model is based on the half-sites reactivity principle. In this view, two catalytically competent enzyme monomers operate 180 degrees out of phase so that the $E_1 \rightarrow E_2$-P transition in one is linked to the $E_2 \rightarrow E_1$ transition in the other monomer. The complete active transport unit is thus a dimer. The catalytic sites exert negative cooperativity between the monomers, so that one site has high affinity for ATP and is phosphorylated while the other binds ATP with low affinity. Na^+ binding to one unit leads through phosphorylation of one monomer to conformational changes in the other. The units are interconvertible. The essential features are coexistence of two equivalent and interconvertible catalytic centers that are negatively cooperative and coexistence of separate Na^+ and K^+ ionophoric centers [31].

Difficulties with these models are the uncertainties regarding the ratios of subunits and phosphorylation per active oligomer (see *Functional Groups*), and the fact that all the enzyme can be either in the Na^+ or K^+ form (see *Trypsin Cleavage*). Satisfactory models will have to account for independent as well as coupled Na^+ and K^+ reactions and translocations. [See reviews 11 to 13 for references.]

PURIFICATION

The isolation of an enzyme in pure form and with high activity has been very difficult, in part because the $(Na^+ + K^+)$-ATPase is an integral membrane protein. The protein must either be solubilized and then fractionated by use of standard biochemical techniques, or impurities must be extracted selectively while leaving the enzyme in a particulate state. Recent successful procedures have utilized electric organ [40], shark rectal gland [41], and dog and sheep kidney [42–44]. The brain enzyme remains only partially purified [45]. Purification techniques generally involve treating membranes with sodium iodide to remove impurities, solubilizing with detergents, column chromatography, density gradient centrifugation, and/or precipitating with glycerol or salts. In one case, sonic irradiation without detergents has been used successfully with the electric eel enzyme.

COMPOSITION AND STRUCTURE

Ultrastructure

The purified enzyme is particulate and contains lipid and carbohydrate. Where preparations have been examined by electron microscopy, they appear as membrane fragments or vesicles [46].

FREEZE-FRACTURE AND NEGATIVE-STAINING STUDIES. Purified $(Na^+ + K^+)$-ATPase preparations have been studied by negative-staining and freeze-fracture techniques to ascertain the morphology, distribution, and size of the enzyme and its subunits. These studies show that purified enzyme preparations contain membranelike fragments and vesicles with a substructure of globular particles exposed on each face of the membrane (Fig. 6-3A). After negative staining, the preparations contain granules about 30 to 50 Å in diameter; these appear at about the same density on both sides of the membrane. The granules, assumed to be protein particles, often have a stalklike appearance on the side generally thought to be the "cytoplasmic" surface. The portion of the particle extending to the "external" surface is less defined and often has a fine granular appearance.

When membranes are freeze-fractured, they split within the lipid bilayer so that exposed surfaces belong either to the original cytoplasmic or to the external half of the membrane, and embedded particles may often be visualized (Fig. 6-3B and C). Generally, one fracture face (Fig. 6-3B), probably originally facing the cytoplasmic side, has a two- to fourfold higher density of particles than does the external face. Despite the density difference, particles on either face tend to have diameters of about 100 Å [47], that is, nearly twice the size of those observed after negative staining. The density of particles within the freeze-fractured membrane is about one-fourth that found in negatively stained preparations [47, 48], suggesting that application of the latter technique may cause disaggregation of membrane particles.

The freeze-fracture technique is more likely to preserve the enzyme in its physiological state than would negative staining, because the latter method is relatively harsh and involves drying specimens in the presence of phosphotungstic acid, ammonium molybdate, or uranyl salts, all of which greatly diminish enzyme activity.

Freeze-fracture followed by rotary shadowing exposes particles with an apparent oligomeric structure (Fig. 6-3D). Some of these have a quadripartite structure and may be composed of smaller subunits. One interpretation, suggested by Haase and Koepsell [47], is that those quadripartite particles with a diameter of about 100 Å may be complexes of the units with diameters of 30 to 50 angstroms seen in negatively stained preparations. These workers have estimated a molecular weight of 170,000 for the negatively stained particle. The molecular weight of the oligomer seen in freeze-

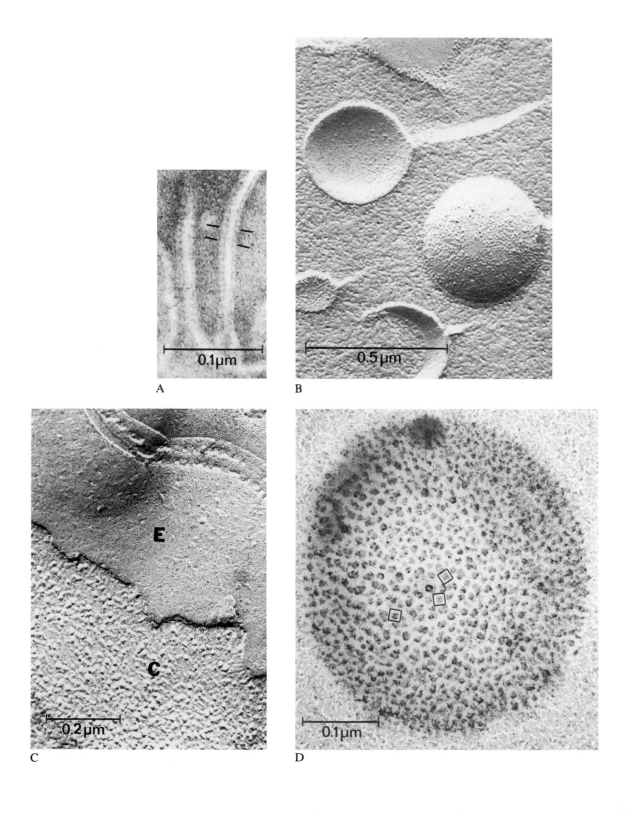

A

B

C

D

fractured preparations would likely be greater than 500,000, which is in the range of molecular weights suggested in several studies in which radiation inactivation and column chromatographic techniques were used. However, it is probably too early to calculate confidently the weight of the oligomers.

Subunits
Purified $(Na^+ + K^+)$-ATPase preparations have been examined by polyacrylamide gel electrophoresis in the presence of sodium dodecyl sulfate (SDS-PAGE) and generally are judged to be at least 70 to 90 percent pure [46, 49]. Although two major polypeptides are found, several minor components are also evident. Nearly all purified preparations of the $(Na^+ + K^+)$-ATPase contain the larger polypeptide, often called the α *subunit*, $M_r = 85,000$ to $120,000$, and a small glycopeptide, the β *subunit*, $M_r = 42,000$ to $60,000$. However, recent studies [50] show that the larger polypeptide also contains carbohydrate, albeit at a much lower level than the smaller peptide (Table 6-5). In addition to the α and

Fig. 6-3. Ultrastructure of the $(Na^+ + K^+)$-ATPase [see 47]. A. Micrograph of negatively stained $(Na^+ + K^+)$-ATPase. Distinct particles are located on both sides of the membrane. Note stalklike appearance of particles. Each particle seems to be coordinated with a particle on the opposite face of the membrane. B. Micrograph of freeze-fractured $(Na^+ + K^+)$-ATPase preparation isolated from rat kidney. (Specific activity: approximately 200 μmoles of ATP are split per milligram of protein per hour.) Two different fracture faces can be distinguished: convex faces appear with a high particle density; faces with a low particle density are generally concave. C. Freeze-fracture from intact cells of the thick ascending limb of Henle's loop. The fracture face with high particle density (C) is thought to be the cytoplasmic half of the membrane, whereas the half with low density (E) is likely the extracellular face. ×41,000. D. Rotary-shadowed membrane-bound $(Na^+ + K^+)$-ATPase. Rat kidney enzyme (B. above) was freeze-fractured and rotary-shadowed [47]. The fracture face has a high particle density, and many particles show a quadrapartite substructure (squares) and have a diameter of about 100 A. (Micrographs courtesy of Hermann Koepsell.)

β peptides, a third peptide has been implicated as a component of the $(Na^+ + K^+)$-ATPase. Forbush and coworkers [51] found that exposure of the purified $(Na^+ + K^+)$-ATPase to ultraviolet light in the presence of a radioactive photoaffinity derivative of ouabain led to covalent attachment of the derivative and irreversible inhibition of the enzyme. SDS-PAGE analyses showed that both the α polypeptide and a smaller polypeptide of about $12,000$ M_r were appreciably labeled. The small peptide, an acidic proteolipid, is present in low concentrations in the enzyme preparation but seems to be closely associated with the $(Na^+ + K^+)$-ATPase, although its function, like that of the glycopeptide, remains unknown.

Most studies have used SDS-PAGE and calibration with protein markers to estimate the molecular weight of the α and β peptides. From these studies, subunit stoichiometries of $\alpha_2\beta$, $\alpha_2\beta_3$, $\alpha_2\beta_2$, and $\alpha_4\beta_2$ have been suggested (see [12]). Only recently has equilibrium ultracentrifugation been used to establish protein and peptide molecular weights with detergent-solubilized enzyme [52]. In this study, purified shark rectal gland $(Na^+ + K^+)$-ATPase (specific activity $1,300-1,500$ μmol P_i/mg protein/hr) was solubilized with the detergent Lubrol WX. The smallest enzymatically active detergent-lipid-protein complex contains two α polypeptides of molecular weight $106,000 \pm 3,000$ each, and four β peptides of molecular weight $36,600 \pm 1,500$ each. The molecular weight of the small peptide is $51,700$ when corrected for carbohydrate. The active enzyme complex contains approximately 9% lipid, 13% carbohydrate, and 78% protein. Hastings and Reynolds [52] find a molecular weight of $380,000$ for the protein components of the enzymatically active complex and a ratio of $\alpha_2\beta_4$. In contrast, Peters and colleagues find a ratio of $\alpha_2\beta_2$ and a protein molecular weight of $326,800$ for kidney enzyme in the absence of detergent. The ratio of phosphorylation per mole of α unit is almost one [53].

The α chain contains the site for phosphorylation [43] and the main ouabain-binding site [51]. The role of the β peptide is unknown. Cross-linking experiments using suberimidate suggest that the two peptides are in close contact [54], and conformational changes in the larger polypeptide affect the susceptibility of the glycopeptide to proteolysis. Antibodies obtained against the glyco-

Table 6-5. Composition of Purified $(Na^+ + K^+)$-ATPase[a]

Substance	Amount
Cholesterol	0.3–0.6 μmol/mg protein
Phospholipid	0.92–1.1 μmol/mg protein
Phosphatidylcholine	36–50%
Sphingomyelin	6–18%
Phosphatidylserine	8–15%
Phosphatidylethanolamine	28–43%
Phosphatidylinositol	1–6%
Carbohydrate	moles/100 moles amino acids
Glycopeptide	
Total carbohydrate	22–26
Total neutral sugars	16 (1.3)[b]
Sialic acid	1–4 (0.09)
Amino sugars	2–8 (0.30)

[a] Data from purified preparations from shark rectal gland, electric organ, rabbit and lamb kidney.
[b] Values in parentheses show carbohydrate content of the α polypeptide of the $(Na^+ + K^+)$-ATPase [50].
Source: Perone et al., *J. Biol. Chem.* 250:1035–1040, 1975; DePont et al., *Biochim. Biophys. Acta* 508:464–477, 1978; and unpublished data of Stahl.

peptide inhibit $(Na^+ + K^+)$-ATPase in the native enzyme [55].

The polypeptides have only been separated by preparative chromatography or electrophoresis in the presence of SDS [see, for instance, 44, 56, 57]. The high concentrations of SDS required in this approach lead to denaturation and loss of enzymatic activity. Attempts to reconstitute an enzymatically active enzyme after separation of subunits have not been successful. Nonetheless, compositional analyses of the individual subunits have been done, and antibodies have also been obtained.

The α peptides obtained from various sources have similar amino acid compositions [58]. This is also true of the β peptides as a class; however, the β subunits clearly have a composition different from that of the α subunit. There is a striking difference in peptide tyrosine content, which is two times higher in the β than in the α peptide. The α peptide has low carbohydrate content (Table 6-5), but the β contains appreciable amounts of amino sugars, sialic acid, fucose, mannose, galactose, and, perhaps, glucose [57, 58]. Carbohydrate composition varies markedly in β peptides isolated from dif-

ferent sources, but removal of all of the carbohydrate from the purified electric organ holoenzyme has no effect on enzymatic activity [58]. However, the presence of carbohydrate on the β peptide is responsible for microheterogeneity of this subunit. Marshall and Hokin [59] have found that isoelectric focusing on a polyacrylamide gel leads to separation of the β peptide into about nine individual components. Neuraminidase treatment of the initial β peptide removes all of the sialic acid, and subsequent isoelectric focusing shows a reduction from nine to four bands. Microheterogeneity must therefore be due in part to the charge imparted to the β peptide by the attached sialic acid groups. Amino sugars may also contribute to this microheterogeneity.

Functional Groups

The β-carboxyl group of one of the *aspartic acid* residues of the α peptide has been established as the group phosphorylated by ATP to form an acid-stable acyl phosphate [58]. It is not yet certain whether half or all of the phosphorylation sites can be occupied at once [53, 57]. It also has been reported that tyrosine [40] and arginine [60] are within the active site of the enzyme, although the positions of these residues remain unknown and must await peptide sequencing and studies with conformational probes.

The enzyme contains about 36 sulfhydryl groups per molecule (based on an assumed M_r of 250,000) [61]. Two of these are absolutely necessary for ATP hydrolysis and for transport to occur. Work by Albers and coworkers [62] with the *Electrophorus electricus* electric-organ enzyme has shown that sulfhydryl-specific reagents like NEM inhibit the net $(Na^+ + K^+)$-ATPase but stimulate the ADP-ATP exchange reaction. Different thiol groups of the $(Na^+ + K^+)$-ATPase are labeled by thiol-blocking reagents like NEM in the presence of ligands known to promote different states of the enzyme, for example, E_1, E_2, $E_1{\sim}P$, and $E_2{-}P$ [63, 64]. This indicates that the thiols are selectively exposed or shielded from alkylating reagents in these states and provides good evidence that the phosphorylated species represent different conformations of the enzyme. In addition, fluorescent thiol-blocking reagents have been used to modify the native enzyme. The fluorescent reporter group is sensitive to changes from nonphosphorylated to phosphory-lated states of the enzyme, as shown by dramatic increases in fluorescence, again providing evidence that phosphorylation of the enzyme causes conformational changes [65, 66].

Trypsin Cleavage

Another approach that provides structural evidence for the existence of different conformations of the $(Na^+ + K^+)$-ATPase has come from Jørgensen's work with tryptic digestion [67]. He found that trypsin cleaves at only a few points on the α peptide, and these cleavages are sensitive to the presence of Na^+ and K^+. In the presence of ligands promoting E_2 or $E_2{-}P$, trypsin cleaves the α peptide into fragments of 41,000 and 58,000 M_r (K^+ form, Fig. 6-4). Formation of the E_1 state (Na^+ form, Fig. 6-4) of the enzyme gives a different pattern of fragments. The time course of proteolysis is more complex than that for the K^+ form, but the final product has a molecular weight of 77,000. Further work by Castro and Farley (Fig. 6-4) on the sites of proteolytic cleavage has shown that chymotrypsin cleaves the Na^+ form at the same site as does trypsin but that ouabain modifies the conformation of the $(Na^+ + K^+)$-ATPase so that an additional site becomes available for attack by chymotrypsin. The structural studies described in this section, as well as the kinetic experiments (described under Conformational States of the Enzyme, above) provide overwhelming evidence that ligands modifying

Fig. 6-4. Proteolytic cleavage sites of the large subunit of the $(Na^+ + K^+)$-ATPase. Arrows indicate sites of cleavage by chymotrypsin (CHY), trypsin in the presence of Na^+ (TRY,Na), trypsin in the presence of potassium (TRY,K), and chymotrypsin in the presence of ouabain (CHY,oua). From ref. 154, and reprinted by permission of the authors.

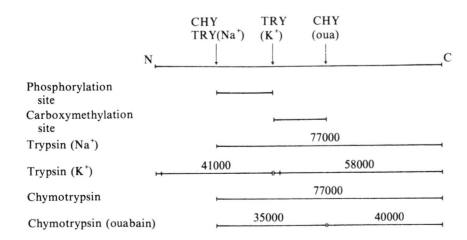

$(Na^+ + K^+)$-ATPase activity also modulate conformational changes within the enzyme.

Lipids

The lipid composition of the enzymatically active, purified enzyme has been of interest in view of the divergence of opinion regarding whether specific lipids are required for the enzyme to function (see [68, 69]). Several studies, utilizing membranes that contain the $(Na^+ + K^+)$-ATPase, apparently showed that exogenous phosphatidylserine or acidic phospholipids are specifically required for activation of the enzyme after the native phospholipids have been removed or altered with detergents or phospholipases. More recent work does not support this idea but indicates instead that there is no absolute requirement that the phospholipid have a specific polar head group. De Pont and coworkers [70, 71] convincingly proved this point by incubating the $(Na^+ + K^+)$-ATPase with phosphatidylserine decarboxylase, which converted phosphatidylserine to phosphatidylethanolamine without loss of $(Na^+ + K^+)$-ATPase activity.

However, there is little doubt that a general phospholipid requirement exists for $(Na^+ + K^+)$-ATPase activity to be demonstrated. For example, when the apoenzyme is solubilized with detergents and separated from phospholipids by gel filtration, 98 to 99 percent of the $(Na^+ + K^+)$-ATPase and K^+-$pNPPase$ activities are lost. These activities may be regained completely by adding heat-treated tissue (containing a mixture of phospholipids) or may be partially reactivated by adding phosphatidylcholine or phosphatidylethanolamine [72]. The phospholipid composition of purified enzyme preparations varies considerably in the enzyme isolated from different sources but closely resembles the composition of the parent membrane from which it was derived. It may be that certain preferential lipid-phospholipid interactions do, in fact, take place in such membrane-associated enzymes as $(Na^+ + K^+)$-ATPase

Generally, 100 to 300 molecules of phospholipid are present per molecule (defined as one molecular unit containing one ouabain-binding site or phosphorylation site) of the isolated $(Na^+ + K^+)$-ATPase. Less than 90

molecules of phospholipid seem to be required for full enzymatic activity [71]. Ottolenghi [72] has studied the process of relipidation of the detergent-treated, enzymatically inactive form of the $(Na^+ + K^+)$-ATPase and found that gradual reappearance of enzymatic activity was accompanied by addition of clumps of 18 to 25 molecules of phospholipid in the presence of mixed detergents. In these studies, the K^+-$pNPPase$ was first reactivated, and this was followed by restoration of $(Na^+ + K^+)$-ATPase activity.

Cholesterol has also been implicated in modifying the activity of $(Na^+ + K^+)$-ATPase [73, 74], and at present a reasonable explanation of such effects may be through modifications in membrane fluidity. The importance of lipids in modulating activity of membrane-associated enzymes is well established [75]. An excellent correlation between the activation energy of $(Na^+ + K^+)$-ATPase and fluidity of the associated lipids has been demonstrated. Generally, the enzyme undergoes a large decrease in activation energy (from about 33 to 15 kcal/mole) as temperature is increased above 20 to 22°C, a point that corresponds approximately to the "melting" of the fatty acyl chains of the phospholipids [76, 77]. The fluidity of the lipids is affected by chain length and degree of unsaturation of the fatty acyl group and by cholesterol content. This sort of effect suggests that the observed transition is a fundamental property related primarily to the lipid composition of the particular membrane system under study. Temperature-dependent transitions may also reflect cooperative interactions between membrane lipids and proteins (in this case, the $(Na^+ + K^+)$-ATPase), but the primary effect is probably due to changes in fluidity of the boundary lipids near the active site of the enzyme.

Reconstitution of the Pump

A primary goal has been to purify the $(Na^+ + K^+)$-ATPase and to reconstitute it into an ATP-dependent system that actively pumps sodium and potassium ions. This has now been achieved and provides the final proof that the enzyme and pump are the same entity [9]. For reconstitution, the enzyme had to be inserted into phospholipid vesicles. This was done by (1) solubilizing the enzyme in the presence of excess phospholipid, and the detergent sodium cholate, followed by extensive dialysis to form closed vesicles that contain the enzyme in the bilayer; or (2) by sonication of the enzyme in the presence of phospholipid, a process that also produces vesicles that incorporate enzyme. Using these techniques, reconstitution of the pump is relatively low (<15%), and it appears that, in about half of the vesicles, the $(Na^+ + K^+)$-ATPase is oriented inside out and the remaining vesicles contain right-side-out enzyme. Only the ATP hydrolyzing sites on the inside-out $(Na^+ + K^+)$-ATPase vesicles are accessible to ATP in the medium, and sodium uptake into these vesicles could be investigated. The vesicles were loaded previously with potassium, and it was found that the stoichiometry of Na^+/K^+-pumped ATP hydrolyzed is 3:2:1; this is consistent with the coupling ratios observed in erythrocytes and nerve. In addition to ATP-dependent Na^+ transport, other reactions characteristic of the enzyme, including K^+–K^+ exchange, Na^+–Na^+ exchange, and Na^+-coupled K^+ transport, have been demonstrated in the reconstituted system. Enzyme has been reconstituted into vesicles of pure phosphatidylcholine and into vesicles containing phosphatidylethanolamine–phosphatidylcholine mixtures [78]. Reconstituted systems of defined composition will be valuable for study of the transport mechanism.

Are There Two Brain $(Na^+ + K^+)$-ATPases?
Several lines of evidence have suggested that more than one functional $(Na^+ + K^+)$-ATPase may exist in brain. Inhibition of the brain enzyme by cardiotonic steroids shows a complex inhibition curve [79, 80], suggesting two inhibition sites. On the other hand, only one inhibition site is implicated in nonnervous tissue. In another study [81], the potassium affinities of the $(Na^+ + K^+)$-ATPase were found to differ in isolated neuronal and glial preparations. However, the clearest evidence for two molecular forms comes from Sweadner's recent work [80], in which $(Na^+ + K^+)$-ATPase preparations of nervous and nonnervous tissue organs were examined. The enzyme was identified on low density polyacrylamide gels after SDS-PAGE by using Na^+-dependent, K^+-sensitive phosphorylation by ATP. Two forms of the phosphorylated catalytic subunit from brain were separated on these gels. The two bands, probably representing isozymes, differed in their molecular weight by only a few thousand, and structural analysis showed that they are closely related. The two forms (α and $\alpha+$) were found in nervous tissue, but only the lower molecular weight form (α) was found in such nonneuronal tissues as skeletal muscle, cardiac muscle, kidney, and pigment epithelium of the retina. Interestingly, the higher molecular weight form was absent from astrocytes prepared from primary cultures; this suggests a different cellular localization for these two forms of the $(Na^+ + K^+)$-ATPase. This work may help to resolve questions regarding $(Na^+ + K^+)$-ATPase reactivities and function in neurons and glia.

ANTIGENICITY
A number of different $(Na^+ + K^+)$-ATPase holoenzyme and subunit preparations have been used to generate antisera in rabbits [see 82 for review]. Even a highly purified polypeptide produces a population of antibody molecules that appear to be specific for different regions of the polypeptide chain. Use of less purified antigenic material could therefore lead to very complex mixtures of antibodies. In early experiments, partially purified rat brain was used to obtain antisera. These antisera caused complete inhibition of $(Na^+ + K^+)$-ATPase activity when mixed with rat brain microsomes but had little effect on K^+-pNPPase activity [83]. These experiments suggested that the sodium-dependent phosphorylation was inhibited, whereas the potassium-dependent dephosphorylation was unaffected, by antisera. The two activities therefore may have antigenically distinct regions on the catalytic subunit of the enzyme. Further, antisera to the purified rabbit kidney $(Na^+ + K^+)$-ATPase only inhibits the sodium pump in red blood cells when available to the inner surface of the cell membrane; this suggests that antibodies to the catalytic subunit were produced in this case [84]. On the other hand, antibodies raised against the canine kidney holoenzyme probably react with antigenic determinants on either side of the plasma membrane [85]. Recently, pure catalytic unit from goldfish brain has been obtained. Antiserum to this subunit reacts with the axolemma membrane (see Cellular Localization). The protein purity, lipid content, and method of immunization would likely affect the characteristics of the antisera produced.

Studies in Schwartz's laboratory [85] clearly demonstrated antigenic differences among $(Na^+ + K^+)$-ATPases isolated from various organs and species. For example, antiserum against the canine kidney enzyme inhibited the enzyme from the same source by approximately 90 percent, but this same antiserum inhibited enzyme activity in rat and pig kidney by only 50 percent. In dog, rat, and cow, antiserum against canine kidney enzyme inhibited brain microsomal $(Na^+ + K^+)$-ATPase by about 25 percent. These studies suggest at least partial homology among $(Na^+ + K^+)$-ATPases from different sources, but probably there are unique antigenic species and organ differences. These differences have been brought into focus by Sweadner [80], who found that the larger subunit of the brain $(Na^+ + K^+)$-ATPase may have two isozymic forms, whereas the kidney enzyme has only one isozymic large polypeptide.

DISTRIBUTION

The enzyme is found in very high activity in electrically excitable tissues (Table 6-3) such as electric organ of eel, brain, nerve, and muscle of other species. In brain, cortex has the highest activity. High activity is present in secretory organs, including kidney, choroid plexus, and the ciliary body.

Subcellular Fractions

In every tissue that has been examined, $(Na^+ + K^+)$-ATPase activity has been found in subcellular fractions that contain particulate material derived from cell membranes. In mammalian brain dispersions prepared in isotonic sucrose, the higher specific activity is found in the primary microsomal fraction, which consists morphologically of membrane fragments, and in the synaptosomal fraction that is prepared by centrifuging the primary "mitochondrial" fraction on a sucrose density gradient [86]. Lowest specific activities are found in the supernatant and purified mitochondrial fractions. When synaptosomes are disrupted by dispersion in water, $(Na^+ + K^+)$-ATPase activity is absent from the synaptic vesicle subfraction and is concentrated in fractions that contain membrane fragments derived

from external synaptosomal membranes. Localization of the enzyme in membranes, especially plasma membranes, is consistent with the enzyme's role in active Na^+ and K^+ transport. The high activity in brain cortex and synaptosomes parallels metabolic demands in these tissues.

Cellular Localization

Introduction of new techniques has greatly stimulated research into the sites of the sodium pump in many tissues. Three methods have emerged [see 87]. These involve (1) a cytochemical procedure for localizing K^+-pNPPase (see section on Enzyme Reactions), which uses p-nitrophenylphosphate as substrate and strontium to capture the precipitated phosphate; (2) autoradiography of [^{3}H]ouabain bound to the pump; and (3) immunocytochemical methods involving binding and visualization of specific antibodies raised to the purified $(Na^+ + K^+)$-ATPase. The cytochemical and immunohistochemical techniques may be used at the electron-microscope level and have high sensitivity. The autoradiographic method of Stirling is useful in physiological studies and is more amenable for quantitative analyses of the number of pump sites in a tissue. However, the level of resolution is not high, and electron microscopy generally is not useful with this latter technique.

$(Na^+ + K^+)$-ATPase is preferentially located on the basolateral or inward-facing membranes of transporting epithelia regardless of the direction of net transport or the tonicity of the absorbates or secretions (Fig. 6-5). As an example of reabsorptive epithelia, Shaver and Stirling [88] studied [^{3}H]-ouabain in renal tubules and found almost exclusive basolateral localization of medullary $(Na^+ + K^+)$-ATPase in the thick ascending limb (Fig. 6-5B); these findings were in agreement with biochemical studies of microdissected rat nephrons (Fig. 6-5A). Little enzyme was found in thin limbs by using either technique. This corroborates the K^+-pNPPase histochemical data of Ernst [89] and the immunocytochemical approach [90]. The localization has been important in considering the role of different portions of the nephron in active Na^+ transport. Relatively high concentrations of

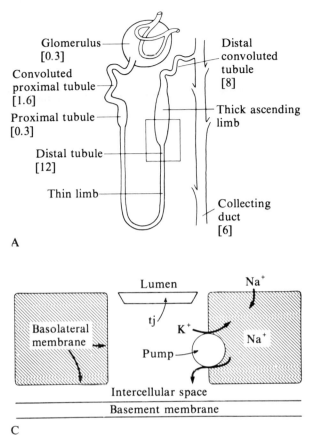

A

C

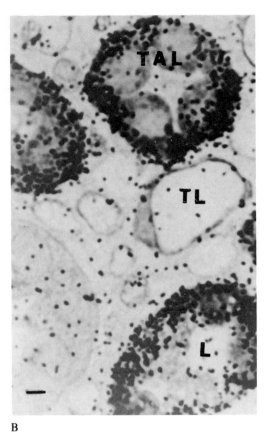

B

Fig. 6-5. (Na+ + K+)-ATPase of reabsorptive epithelia.
A. Diagram of juxtamedullary rat nephron with
relative (Na+ + K+)-ATPase values in brackets derived
from direct biochemical assay [155]. B. Binding sites of
[³H]-ouabain primarily associated with basolateral
membranes of thick ascending limbs (TAL) of rabbit
kidney [88]; this study was carried out on specimens
obtained from the general area enclosed by the
rectangle in A. Little activity is associated with the
thin limbs (TL). Bar, 2 μm. Reprinted by permission
of the authors [88] and by Journal of Cell Biology. C.
Diagram of epithelial tubule cells showing basolateral
localization of the (Na+ + K+)-ATPase. TJ, tight
junction; L, lumen.

$(Na^+ + K^+)$-ATPase are present in the distal tubule, so that major sodium reabsorption takes place in that portion of the nephron. The plasma membranes of the epithelial cells have high $(Na^+ + K^+)$-ATPase activity on the basolateral surfaces and low activity on the luminal side, suggesting that the sodium pump drives net reabsorption of Na^+ across the distal tubule (Fig. 6-5C). Na^+ may flow into the cell at the luminal surface down a concentration gradient and then be actively transported out of the cell basolaterally [see 90].

Clearly, knowledge of the cellular localization of the $(Na^+ + K^+)$-ATPase has helped in the development of theories of sodium transport in nonnervous tissue. However, the detailed cellular localization of $(Na^+ + K^+)$-ATPase activity in nervous tissue remains unresolved. Its presence in neurons was established from early work with crab nerve [8] and squid axon [6], but its relative levels in mammalian neurons and glia are still unknown [see 91, 92]. In general, studies with neurons and glia isolated from brain have shown either similar levels of activity in neuronal and glial cell bodies or somewhat higher levels in glial cell bodies (Table 6-6). Studies by Kimelberg and coworkers [93] suggest that cultured astrocytes have much lower activity than do glial cells isolated from rat cerebral cortex; however, incubation of astrocytes with dibutyryl cyclic AMP led to increased $(Na^+ + K^+)$-ATPase, possibly associated with process extension by these cells. Other studies that relied on histochemical [91, 92] or immunocytochemical [94] demonstrations of $(Na^+ + K^+)$-ATPase activity have suggested that neuronal and glial cell bodies (in contrast to their extensions) have similar levels of activity. However, the cytochemical work shows very high activity associated with large dendritic processes in mammalian cerebral cortex (see [95] and Fig. 6-6A and B). One concern about the cellular fractionation studies is that the glial fractions isolated from rat brain are perhaps contaminated by these dendritic membranes and that this leads to an erroneous assumption of high $(Na^+ + K^+)$-ATPase activity in the glia. Also, the biochemical data on relative activities of $(Na^+ + K^+)$-ATPase in neurons and glia may be misleading in that neuronal perikarya constitute only 2 to 5 percent of the cortical volume.

Despite the problems outlined above, progress is being made in localizing the $(Na^+ + K^+)$-ATPase, especially in less complex nervous systems [94, 96]. Fig. 6-6C is an electron micrograph of the goldfish optic nerve showing localization of $(Na^+ + K^+)$-ATPase antigenic sites at a node of Ranvier. This localization is consistent with the need for active Na^+ and K^+ pumping at this site, because resting and active potentials are generated only at the nodes in myelinated nerves. Retinal ganglion neurites growing in explants, however, show a continuous distribution of sites [96]. Intensive study will be required to obtain a more complete picture of cellular maturation and localization of the $(Na^+ + K^+)$-ATPase in nervous tissue.

SOME FUNCTIONAL IMPLICATIONS IN BRAIN

Electrogenic Pumping
It was pointed out that the ratio of Na^+ to K^+ exchanged is greater than 1. In nerve and muscle tissues, various ratios—from 2:1 to 4:3 to 5:1—have

been estimated. If the excess Na^+ extruded is not balanced by an equal number of other positive charges entering, or negative charges leaving, the cell interior, the pump produces hyperpolarization directly and is not entirely electroneutral. It has been shown that after nerve fibers are loaded with Na^+, as by immersion at low temperatures or in zero K^+ media or with transiently increased Na^+ conductance produced by acetylcholine, activation of the pump produces hyperpolarization. The potential transiently drops below the K^+ equilibrium potential. The extent of hyperpolarization is expected to depend on the actual coupling ratio and the rate of the pump activity under the given conditions, on the membrane electrical resistance, and on the extent to which anions such as Cl^- may comigrate with Na^+. Under steady state conditions, the electrogenic component of the pump appears to

Table 6-6. $(Na^+ + K^+)$-ATPase in Selected Preparations

Preparation	$(Na^+ + K^+)$-ATPase Activity (μmoles P_i formed/mg protein/hr)
Rat brain	13.9
Rat cerebral cortex, layers 1–3	14.2
Rat astrocytes nodules	0.68
Rat glioma C-6	0.61
Rat glioma C-6	1.05
Mouse neuroblastoma 2A (1300)	0.44
Rat cerebral cortex	4.91
Rat "neuronal" fraction	3.28
Rat "glial" fraction	21.69
Beef brain "neuronal" fraction	3.90
Beef brain "glial" fraction	3.72
Rat "neuronal" fraction	6.3
Rat "glial" fraction	18.9
Rat astrocytes (primary cultures)	1.06
Rat astrocytes treated with dibutyryl cyclic AMP	2.7

Source: Stahl and Broderson [91] and Kimelberg et al. [93] for detailed references.

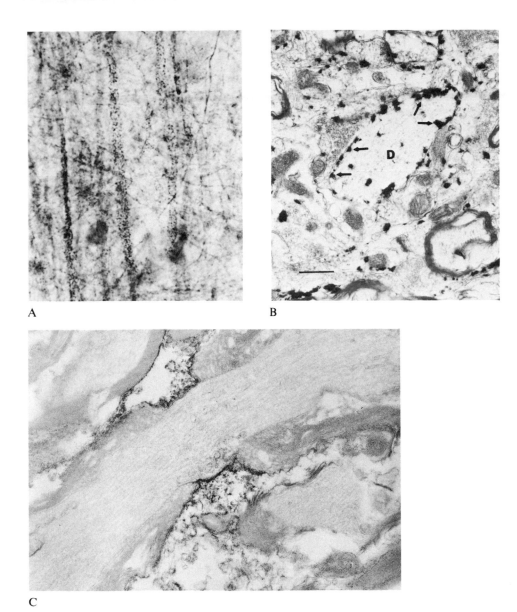

A

B

C

Fig. 6-6. Localization of (Na⁺ + K⁺)-ATPase in nervous tissue. A. Association of K⁺-pNPPase activity with large (dendritic) processes in layer 4 of the somatosensory cortex demonstrated using the cytochemical method [91]. Note the reticular nature of the reaction product. A complex meshwork of smaller reactive processes are also demonstrated. ×1600, before 34% reduction. B. EM localization of K⁺-pNPPase activity in dendritic (D) process of somatosensory cortex of the rat [95]. Reaction product (arrows) is mainly associated with cytoplasmic aspect of the dendritic plasmalemma. Bar, 0.5 μm. C. Immu-nocytochemical localization of (Na⁺ + K⁺)-ATPase in goldfish optic nerve. Rabbit antibodies to the goldfish brain catalytic subunit of the (Na⁺ + K⁺)-ATPase were used and the enzyme was localized using the immunocytochemical peroxidase-antiperoxidase method. Reaction product (dark precipitate) is found at the axolemma only at the nodes of Ranvier and apparently at the outer lamellae of myelin. ×41,000, before 30% reduction. The later micrograph was provided through the courtesy of Schwartz, Agranoff, Ernst, and Siegel [see 96].

be negligible, or up to 10 millivolts in some tissues. The effect is more noticeable after perturbations such as the action potential and may account for the negative afterpotential. Some postsynaptic inhibitory potentials may be due to the electrogenic component. The electrogenic effect also may be seen in nerves that depolarize quickly when the Na^+-K^+ pump is inhibited by metabolic factors or poisons.

The effects of membrane potential on the Na^+/K^+ coupling ratio are not established, but it is expected that a significant effect would modify the interdependence of metabolic rate, membrane potential, and cation gradients. The inequality of Na^+-K^+ exchange also has implications for transient cation regulation of resting membrane potential. Transient reductions in $[K_e^+]$, which tend to hyperpolarize the membrane, would also reduce the pump rate and, hence, Na^+ extrusion, with a rapid resultant decrease in potential. Depending on the coupling ratio and the relative sensitivities, these two effects may cancel, thus resisting transient fluctuations in membrane potential [97–100].

Potassium Redistribution by Glia

Neuronal discharge may normally lead to increased levels of extracellular K^+ of about 1 to 3 mM; however, during epileptogenesis, levels may be 3 or 4 times higher. Elevated $[K_e^+]$ may increase neuronal excitability [see 101], so control of $[K_e^+]$ in the CNS is of critical importance. The present question is whether glia contribute to K^+ reuptake and, if so, what mechanism is involved.

It would seem that neurons reaccumulate K^+ almost exclusively by the Na^+-K^+ pump, that is, through active transport [102]. The exact role of glia in regulating K^+ uptake is still in question; however, both active and passive transport processes may be involved. Although $[K_i^+]$ in glia is much higher than in extracellular fluid (ECF), the K^+ permeability is also very high, and the electrochemical gradient across the glial membrane is so close to equilibrium for K^+ that passive transport of K^+ into the glial cell is possible. The K^+ could then be released to the extracellular fluid from a glial process at some distance from the original source. The

K^+ released at a distance may be reassimilated by neurons via the active $(Na^+ + K^+)$-transport system. This proposed mechanism of passive K^+ transport in glia is called *spatial buffering* [see 102] and is favored by many neurophysiologists. Evidence exists for such a functional syncytium of glia in nervous systems of mammals as well as nonmammals [see 101].

The role of active K^+ transport by glia is more difficult to assess. Clearly, glia must possess a $(Na^+ + K^+)$-ATPase to maintain the gradient, and as pointed out earlier, the set point of the Na^+-K^+-pump will determine the resting membrane potential. An important question is whether the Na^+-K^+ pump in glia is appreciably influenced by the extracellular load. Studies in vitro with bulk-isolated glia and glial cell lines suggest that this may be the case. For example, Franck and coworkers [103] found that the maximum velocity of the $(Na^+ + K^+)$-ATPase in bulk-isolated glia was observed with 20 mM K^+, whereas the maximum activity for isolated neurons was observed in 5 mM K^+.

One might predict especially high levels of $(Na^+ + K^+)$-ATPase activity in glia if active transport of K^+ were an especially important function of these cells. As discussed above under Cellular Localization, the levels of $(Na^+ + K^+)$-ATPase in native functional glia remain in question.

In summary, both active and passive transport processes are probably important in regulating extracellular K^+ levels. However, the relative importance of these processes, as well as the specific contributions of neurons versus glia to K^+ homeostatis, remains uncertain.

Effects of Neurotransmitters

It is known that transmitter release from nerve terminals is dependent on free cytoplasmic Ca^{2+} (see Chaps. 8 to 12). The relationship between intracellular Na^+ and Ca^{2+} is such that increases in the intracellular Na^+ lead to increases in free cytoplasmic Ca^{2+}, presumably because Ca^{2+} is released from bound stores in cellular organelles (see Neurotransmitter Release, below). Thus, it can be shown that the introduction of Na^+-laden or Ca^{2+}-laden liposomes into cells of adrenal gland slices leads to increased catecholamine release. Liposomes loaded with Na^+ plus EGTA or with K^+ do not promote release [104]. Therefore, conditions that reduce Na^+ intracellular levels may reduce transmitter release and vice versa. It has been found that norepinephrine, epinephrine, and dopamine stimulate $(Na^+ + K^+)$-ATPase and reduce catecholamine or acetylcholine release in a number of tissues. Conversely, ouabain has been found to increase transmitter release [105, 106]. It is believed that one mechanism for feedback inhibition of endogenous amine release may involve amine stimulation of $(Na^+ + K^+)$-ATPase in presynaptic terminals. While there is evidence that specific aminergic receptors may be involved in the stimulation of the enzyme, it has also been suggested that the amines can abolish enzyme inhibition caused by vanadate by chelating the vanadate [107–109].

Stimulation of $(Na^+ + K^+)$-ATPase by neurotransmitters can affect the membrane potential directly. For example, it has been found that in frog heart muscle epinephrine augments the portion of Na^+ current attributable to the electrogenic pump [110] and that ouabain antagonizes amine depression of cortical neurons [111]. In these cases, the amines produce hyperpolarization, which, it is thought, could be due to stimulation of the electrogenic pump as for inhibitory postsynaptic potentials mentioned above (Electrogenic Pumping).

Na^+-Dependent Cotransport of Organic Solutes

Na^+ gradients established by the Na^+-K^+ pump are critical for transport of sugars, amines, and certain amino acids into many types of cells, including brain. In these cases, it is presumed that there is a saturable carrier in the membrane. Na^+ binds first to the carrier and increases the affinity of externally oriented carrier sites specific for the transported ligand. The Na^+-carrier-ligand complex with filled external sites is in equilibrium with the binding sites oriented toward the interior of the cell (Fig. 6-1). Because of the Na^+ gradient, association is favored at extracellular sites, and dissociation is favored at intracellular sites. This leads to transport of both Na^+ and the organic solute [112, 113]. Ouabain inhibits this transport.

Such Na^+-dependent transport systems with high affinity for transmitter amines and amino acids believed to act as transmitters (GABA, glutamate, glycine, aspartate, proline) are found in synaptosomal fractions from specific neurocellular locations. These carrier systems function in the presynaptic reuptake of the specific substance from the synaptic cleft (see Chaps. 10 and 12).

Na^+-dependent inhibition of opiate binding to neural receptors is another membrane function related to the ionic milieu. In this case, presumably, the binding of ligand does not lead to its transport but to effects of the receptor-ligand complex on the synaptic membrane (see Fig. 13-1).

It is evident that CNS effects due to inhibition of $(Na^+ + K^+)$-ATPase, such as ouabain-induced seizures, might arise from many factors [114]. Various changes in nervous system function may ensue from effects on $(Na^+ + K^+)$-ATPase, depending on the precise cellular location of the effect.

Hormone Effects on $(Na^+ + K^+)$-ATPase

The most-characterized hormonal influence is that of thyroxine. It is known that thyroid hormone increases metabolic rate of tissues, excluding mature brain. In tissues taken from thyroidectomized rats treated for several days with thyroid hormones to produce a hyperthyroid state, the ouabain-sensitive oxygen utilization rate and $(Na^+ + K^+)$-ATPase activity increase. Mature brain, however, is not affected. Thyroid hormones injected into rats produce increased numbers of ouabain-binding sites and phosphoenzyme per milligram of protein in various tissues, excluding brain. The effect of thyroid hormone in rats appears to be the induction of increased synthesis of $(Na^+ + K^+)$-ATPase molecules. It is believed that the resulting increased cation flux in target tissues contributes to the thermogenic responses to thyroid hormone [115]. The effect of thyroid function on $(Na^+ + K^+)$-ATPase in immature brain would be of interest.

Adrenal hormones, both glucocorticoid and mineralocorticoid, can alter $(Na^+ + K^+)$-ATPase activity levels in a number of tissues, including kidney, intestine, and other osmoregulatory tissues, such as fish gills [116]. These hormones serve adaptive functions related to salt and water balance. The inductive effect of adrenal hormones on $(Na^+ + K^+)$-ATPase may be even more prominent in the developing animal. Maternal adrenalectomy and administration of Metopirone (metyrapone) almost completely prevents the normal rise in kidney enzyme activity in the fetus [117]. Significant stimulation of immature kitten and rat cerebral $(Na^+ + K^+)$-ATPase (but not that of adult brain) has been produced by administration of cortisol, methylprednisolone, or ACTH to the intact animals [118].

Little information is available concerning ovarian steroids, but an effect of estrogen on anterior pituitary $(Na^+ + K^+)$-ATPase activity in ovariectomized rats has been reported [119]. Some potentially useful synthetic derivatives of progesterone [120] and of prednisolone [121] are interesting in that they inhibit $(Na^+ + K^+)$-ATPase, produce myocardial inotropic effects, and inhibit ouabain binding.

Insulin has the effect of reducing extracellular K^+ and intracellular Na^+ in muscle. This effect is not completely understood, but there is evidence that insulin in vitro stimulates $(Na^+ + K^+)$-ATPase activity in some muscle preparations [122] under conditions of less than maximal enzyme activation. Insulin stimulation of Na^+ efflux from muscle seems to involve both ouabain-sensitive and -insensitive components [123]. Insulin appears to have a direct effect on the transport system; its action is rapid as contrasted to the inductive effects of the thyroid and adrenal hormones.

Development and Differentiation
The activity of rat brain $(Na^+ + K^+)$-ATPase expressed as units per milligram of microsomal protein increases about 10 times from fetal to adult stages [124]. This increased activity is proportional to increased amounts of enzyme in the recovered microsomal fractions. This suggests a critical time for the developmental regulation of the type of proteins being synthesized for or inserted into the membranes disposed in the microsomal fraction. The stage of most rapid increase in $(Na^+ + K^+)$-ATPase is prior to myelination; it corresponds to the time of glial cell proliferation and the intricate elaboration

of neuronal and glial processes. This stage is one in which membranes maturely specialized for cation transport are built up; it is possible that cation conductance channels also are built up at this point. Membranes expected to have particularly high densities of transport sites are those destined to underlie nodes of Ranvier in myelinated nerves (see Fig. 6-5C), fine nerve processes, and possibly, glial membranes crucial for clearing K^+ from synaptic cleft regions [95, 96]. Effects of hormones on this critical development stage are not yet known.

$(Na^+ + K^+)$-ATPase in the choroid plexus and brain capillaries may be involved in CSF production and regulation of CSF and ECF. This is discussed in Chap. 25.

Calcium Transport
The concentration of Ca^{2+} within cells has been estimated to be between 10^{-8} and 10^{-7} M, whereas a 1 M concentration would be expected if this cation were distributed according to a Donnan ratio. Regulation of intracellular calcium concentration is increasingly recognized as vital for function of all cells [125]. Calcium ions function as ligands in a variety of intracellular reactions. Certain enzymes, such as the $(Na^+ + K^+)$-ATPase and some glycolytic enzymes, are inhibited; others are stimulated either directly or indirectly through mediation of calmodulin. Of particular note in nervous tissue are actions on (1) calmodulin, a soluble protein that plays a role in the control of number of Ca^{2+}-dependent enzymes [126], and (2) the process of neurotransmitter release.

CALMODULIN
A calcium-dependent modulator protein with a molecular weight of about 15,000 has been detected in a variety of tissues including brain (Chap. 3). This protein was first discovered in the late 1960s by Cheung and coworkers (see [127] for review) who were studying enzymes involved with cyclic AMP metabolism in brain. During the purification process, the phosphodiesterase enzyme lost activity after it was passed through an anion exchange column. This inactivation was due to removal of a protein, now termed *calmodulin,* during purifica-

tion. Since its discovery, calmodulin has been found to increase the activities of a number of other Ca^{2+}-dependent enzyme systems. These are listed in Table 6-7. See also Axoplasmic Transport.

Calmodulin binds 4 Ca^{2+} per mole, with dissociation constants ranging from 4 to 8 μM [128]. The binding is accompanied by conformational changes that convert the protein to an active form.

Calmodulin has been found localized within cells by immunofluorescence techniques. In mouse basal ganglia, antibody to calmodulin is detected in postsynaptic densities and dendritic microtubules. Isolated postsynaptic densities from dog cerebral cortex contain calmodulin [129]. The function of this protein in the postsynaptic density is not yet certain, but the suggestion has been made that it activates membrane-bound enzymes in the dendrites or regulates the rate of receptor desensitization of the postsynaptic membrane.

It is also of interest that in the presence of Ca^{2+}, calmodulin binds tightly to the phenothiazine drug trifluoperazine and thereby becomes biologically inactive.

There are other Ca^{2+}-binding proteins in muscle and other cells. None is as widely distributed as calmodulin. Since the primary structure is very similar in calmodulin isolated from widely divergent species, it is suggested that this protein is the most ancient in the family of calcium-binding proteins and has a pivotal role in mediating the function of Ca^{2+} [126, 127].

NEUROTRANSMITTER RELEASE
It is known that release of neurotransmitters at neuromuscular junctions or from synaptosomes will not take place unless calcium ions are present in the bathing media. It is assumed that an increase in calcium conductance occurs in nerve endings in response to depolarization, then calcium ions diffuse down their electrochemical gradient into the presynaptic terminals. In a poorly understood fashion, synaptic vesicles are triggered to release neurotransmitter (Chap. 9). As emphasized by Blaustein and coworkers [130, 131], this process lasts only 1 to 2 msec and the terminal must again be ready to respond within a few more milliseconds. Internal application of calcium ions at the squid giant synapse terminal augments the background rate of transmitter release [132]; this supports the assumption that the internal Ca^{2+} concentration is important.

At very low extracellular concentrations, a reversed electrochemical gradient for calcium can be produced at the frog neuromuscular synapse [133, 134]. Stimulation of such nerves at a rate of 0.09 to 2 Hz reduces the frequency of miniature end-plate potentials (MEPP). However, on high-frequency stimulation (10–100 Hz), a small increase in MEPP

Table 6-7. Some Calmodulin-Regulated Reactions

Enzyme	Action
Phosphodiesterase	Hydrolysis of cyclic AMP and cyclic GMP
Adenylate kinase	Synthesis of cyclic AMP
Phospholipase A_2	Deacylation of phosphoglycerides
Plasma membrane Ca^{2+}-ATPase	Extrusion of Ca^{2+} from cell
Myosin light-chain kinase	Phosphorylation of a myosin light-chain protein activating actomyosin ATPase and contraction of smooth muscle or nonmuscle myosin
Phosphorylase kinase	Degradation of glycogen
Protein kinases	Phosphorylation of membrane components
NAD kinase	Conversion of NAD to NADP in plant and sea urchin eggs
Guanylate cyclase	Synthesis of GMP in a protozoan

was observed, which suggested that release of Ca^{2+} from intracellular stores could take place under appropriate conditions.

TECHNIQUES FOR STUDYING CALCIUM MOVEMENTS

Calcium ions are readily bound by a number of proteins and phospholipids. Study of calcium movements is therefore difficult, and in many studies estimation of calcium concentration has been very approximate. Measurement of calcium *content* of tissues is readily accomplished by extracting tissue with acid and by measuring the extract's calcium content with an atomic absorption spectrophotometer. The isotope ^{45}Ca has been effectively used to examine calcium ion movements [135, 136]. Measuring free calcium ion *concentrations* has been much more difficult, but great progress has been made in recent years. Calcium-sensitive indicators have been used to measure free Ca^{2+} concentrations. These include the metallochromic indicator dyes murexide and arsenazo III and the calcium-binding proteins aequorin and obelin. These proteins are extracted from certain jellyfish. When exposed to low concentrations of calcium, the proteins emit light, which can be measured with a photomultiplier tube. Light output usually is proportional to the square of ionized calcium concentration. The newest techniques for measuring ionized calcium use Ca^{2+}-sensitive electrodes [137]. Electrodes contain membranes prepared with ion-selective ligands and a neutral carrier, such as polyvinyl chloride. The EMF is directly proportional to the log of the calcium activity within limits that also depend on the presence of other ions. Some electrodes are sensitive to as little as 10^{-8} M calcium ion.

CONTROL OF INTRACELLULAR FREE CALCIUM IONS

Several processes are available to cells for controlling intracellular calcium ion concentrations (Fig. 6-7).

Regulation at Plasma Membrane

An ATP-dependent outward-directed Ca^{2+} pump has been demonstrated in erythrocytes and squid axons. These preparations also contain a Ca^{2+}-activated ATPase, and it seems likely that both activities represent the same process. As in erythrocytes, ATP-driven Ca^{2+} pumping and Ca^{2+}-ATPase activity can be stimulated several-fold by addition of exogenous calmodulin [138]. Presumably under physiological conditions, elevation of calcium levels to the low micromolar range (for example, by depolarization of a nerve cell) leads to formation of an activated Ca^{2+}-ATPase complex containing calmodulin, so that calcium can be pumped out of the cell at an increased rate by a mechanism that is insensitive to sodium ion.

A Na^+-Ca^{2+} exchange mechanism for extruding calcium also exists at the outer membrane (Fig. 6-7). In this system, energy for Ca^{2+} extrusion may be provided by inward movement of Na^+, although the mechanism for coupling these processes remains unclear. Studies (see [139] for references) with squid axon, brain slices, and synaptosomes have shown that the efflux of $^{45}Ca^{2+}$ is reduced when external Na^+ is replaced by Li^+, choline, or dextrose. Metabolic inhibitors—or ouabain, which specifically inhibits Na^+ and K^+ transport—increase net Ca^{2+} uptake. At present, the relative contribution of the Ca^{2+}-ATPase and Na^+-Ca^{2+} exchange to overall Ca^{2+} homeostasis remains unknown. Recent studies have demonstrated that vesicles prepared from brain microsomal or synaptosomal membranes are capable of sequestering calcium ions by both a Na^+-Ca^{2+} exchange process and an ATP-dependent process. Presumably these vesicles are "inside-out", so that accumulation really represents the extrusion process at the external membrane [140, 141].

Regulation by Mitochondria and Other Cellular Organelles

MITOCHONDRIA. An extensive literature exists on calcium uptake by mitochondria [142]. Mitochondria from all sources exhibit energy-dependent calcium uptake mechanisms. Calcium uptake can be supported either by ATP hydrolysis or by oxidation of respiratory substrates such as succinate. Uptake is inhibited by Ruthenium Red. The driving force for Ca^{2+} movement across the mitochondrial membrane may be the nonphosphorylated high-

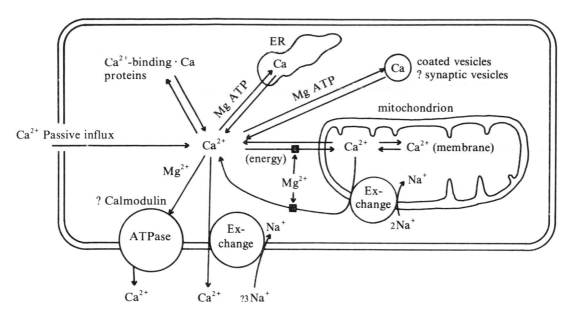

Fig. 6-7. Calcium transport processes. Uptake of calcium by cells is a passive process through Ca²⁺-selective channels. A small portion is bound to Ca²⁺-binding proteins. Intracellular concentration may be regulated by Ca²⁺-Na⁺ exchange or by a calmodulin regulated (Mg²⁺ + Ca²⁺)-ATPase at the plasma membrane; by active transport into mitochondria and Ca²⁺-Na⁺ exchange by mitochondria; and by MgATP-dependent binding by endoplasmic reticulum and possibly other vesicular structures. Mitochondrial uptake is inhibited by Mg²⁺, as is Na⁺-stimulated efflux. Outer membrane Ca²⁺-Na⁺ exchange is energy-dependent because the (Na⁺ + K⁺)-ATPase maintains the sodium gradient across the plasma membrane [P. D. Swanson, G. D. Schellenberg, A. F. Clark, and I. J. Roman. Calcium buffering systems in brain, in R. Rodnight, H. Bachelard, and W. Stahl (eds.), Chemisms of Brain, London: Churchill Livingstone, 1981. Reproduced with permission.].

energy intermediate thought to be involved in oxidative phosphorylation, or the force may involve the membrane potential. In the latter case, the driving force is viewed as being the electrical component of the proton electrochemical gradient across the inner mitochondrial membrane [142]. Still, other mechanisms seem to be involved in Ca²⁺ release from mitochondria. These are insensitive to Ruthenium Red. The efflux system seems to be regulated by the oxidation-reduction state of the mitochondrial carriers. The other system of special interest to neurochemists is mediated by a Na⁺-Ca²⁺ exchange mechanism. Na⁺ has been shown to inhibit mitochondrial calcium *uptake* [143] and to stimulate mitochondrial calcium release under conditions in which further uptake is inhibited by Ruthenium Red [144]. Similar effects of Na⁺ on calcium release are present in mitochondria from heart, parotid gland, adrenal cortex, and skeletal muscle, but cannot be shown in mitochondria from kidney, liver, lung, or smooth muscle. It is tempting to suggest that modulation of mitochondrial calcium transport by Na⁺ could have physiological significance. Half-maximal velocity of Ca²⁺ efflux was achieved at a Na⁺ concentration of 7 to 12 mEq/liter, a concentration that could occur under physiological conditions. The mitochondria may take up or release Ca²⁺ in response to Na⁺ shifts secondary to membrane depolarization (Fig. 6-7). Whether shifts of significant magnitude occur under ordinary conditions is not known. In certain pathological states, such as epilepsy, greater Na⁺ shifts might release additional Ca²⁺ ions and hence trigger excess release of neurotransmitter. The existence of Na⁺-Ca²⁺ exchange in mitochondria and the lack of specific inhibitors of the process make it difficult to characterize or distinguish the mechanism of Na⁺-Ca²⁺ exchange at the plasma membrane from the mitochondrial process.

NONMITOCHONDRIAL UPTAKE. Although mitochondria are the most obvious intracellular source of Ca^{2+}, endoplasmic reticulum has also been suggested as a calcium-sequestering site in neurons (Fig. 6-7). In squid axon, at low Ca^{2+} concentrations (30 nM), calcium ion uptake by mitochondria is slower than uptake by nonmitochondrial organelles [145]. Blaustein and coworkers [131], using synaptosomes from rat brain, have demonstrated a nonmitochondrial ATP-dependent sequestration of Ca^{2+}. This system is also more sensitive to low concentrations of Ca^{2+} (1 μM) than are the mitochondria, where K_m for Ca^{2+} uptake under physiological conditions is about 20 to 40 μM. This uptake may be nonmitochondrial because Ca^{2+} sequestration occurred in the presence of such metabolic inhibitors as DNP, oligomycin, and azide.

Several investigators have demonstrated both Ca^{2+}-stimulated ATPase activity and $(Mg^{2+}+ATP)$-dependent Ca^{2+} uptake associated with "vesicles" isolated from osmotically shocked synaptosomes [146], coated vesicles isolated from brain homogenates [147], and brain microsomal preparations [148, 149]. The vesicles studied should not be assumed to be synaptic vesicles, because purified synaptic vesicles do not appear to accumulate calcium actively [149]. The vesicles may be derived from endoplasmic reticulum, but plasma membrane fragments may also be present in such preparations. The Ca^{2+} transport activity in these preparations is thought to be evidence for the existence of Ca^{2+}-sequestering vesicles or reticulum-type structures that function intraneuronally to regulate Ca^{2+} levels. Initial attempts at identifying specific proteins involved in nonmitochondrial Ca^{2+} fluxes in brain focused on searching for Ca^{2+}-stimulated ATPase activity. Ca^{2+}-stimulated ATPase activity has been found by numerous laboratories in membranous fractions, including synaptic vesicles and microsomes [149–153]; and when reconstituted, such preparations do catalyze ATP-dependent Ca^{2+} uptake [27, 153]. Much remains to be learned about the relative roles of membrane extrusion processes, mitochondrial and nonmitochondrial sequestration, and release mechanisms in the control of intracellular Ca^{2+} concentration.

Acknowledgments

Portions of the work reported in this chapter were supported in part by NSF grant 7805174, NIH grant NS 05424, and by the Medical Research Service of the Veterans Administration.

References

1. Stein, W. D. *The Movement of Molecules Across Cell Membranes.* New York: Academic, 1967.
2. Post, R. L., and Jolly, P. C. The linkage of sodium, potassium, and ammonium active transport across the human erythrocyte membrane. *Biochim. Biophys. Acta* 25:118–128, 1957.
3. Veloso, D., et al. The concentrations of free and bound magnesium in rat tissues: Relative constancy of free Mg^{2+} concentrations. *J. Biol. Chem.* 248:4811–4819, 1973.
4. Boyle, P. J., and Conway, E. J. Potassium accumulation in muscle and associated changes. *J. Physiol.* (London) 100:1–63, 1941.
5. Wilbrandt, W. Some recent developments in the field of alkali cation transport. *Int. Rev. Cytol.* 13:203–220, 1962.
6. Caldwell, P. C., et al. The effects of injecting energy-rich phosphate compounds on the active transport of ions in the giant axons of *Loligo. J. Physiol.* (London) 152:561–590, 1960.
7. Hoffman, J. The link between metabolism and the active transport of Na^+ in human red cell ghosts. *Fed. Proc.* 19:127, 1960.
8. Skou, J. C. The influence of some cations on an adenosine triphosphatase from peripheral nerve. *Biochim. Biophys. Acta* 23:394–401, 1957.
9. Goldin, S. M. Active transport of sodium and potassium ions by sodium and potassium ion-activated adenosine triphosphatase from renal medulla—reconstitution of purified enzyme into a well-defined in vitro transport system. *J. Biol. Chem.* 252:5630–5642, 1977.
10. Skou, J. C., and Nørby, J. G. (eds.). *Na, K-ATPase Structure and Kinetics.* New York: Academic, 1979.
11. Glynn, I. M., and Karlish, S. J. D. The sodium pump. *Annu. Rev. Physiol.* 37:13–55, 1975.
12. Hobbs, A. S., and Albers, R. W. The structure of proteins involved in active membrane transport. *Annu. Rev. Biophys. Bioeng.* 9:259–291, 1980.
13. Robinson, J. D., and Flashner, M. S. The $(Na^+ + K^+)$-activated ATPase. Enzymatic and transport properties. *Biochim. Biophys. Acta* 549:145–176, 1979.
14. Skou, J. C. Enzymatic basis for active transport of Na^+ and K^+ across cell membrane. *Physiol. Rev.* 45:596–617, 1965.

15. Wallick, E. T., Lane, L. K., and Schwartz, A. Biochemical mechanism of the sodium pump. *Annu. Rev. Physiol.* 41:397–411, 1979.

16. Hodgkin, A. L., and Keynes, R. D. Active transport of cations in giant axons from *Sepia* and *Loligo. J. Physiol.* (London) 128:28–60, 1955.

17. Katzman, R., and Grossman, R. Neuronal activity and potassium movement. In D. H. Ingvar and H. Lassen (eds.), *Brain Work: The Coupling of Function, Metabolism and Blood Flow in Brain.* Copenhagen: Mukegaard, 1975. Pp. 149–156.

18. Jobsis, R., et al. Metabolic activity in epileptic seizures. In D. H. Ingvar and H. Lassen, cited in [17], pp. 185–196.

19. Ransom, B. R., and Goldring, S. Slow hyperpolarization in cells presumed to be glia in cerebral cortex of cat. *J. Neurophysiol.* 36:879–892, 1973.

20. Bachelard, H. S., Campbell, W. J., and McIlwain, H. The sodium and other ions of mammalian cerebral tissues, maintained and electrically stimulated in vitro. *Biochem. J.* 84:225–232, 1962.

21. Keesey, J. C., and Walgren, H. Movements of radioactive sodium in cerebral cortex slices in response to electrical stimulation. *Biochem. J.* 95:301–310, 1965.

22. Baker, P. F., and Connelly, C. M. Some properties of the external activation site of the sodium pump in crab nerve. *J. Physiol.* (London) 185:270–297, 1966.

23. Rang, H. P., and Ritchie, J. M. The dependence on external cations of the oxygen consumption of mammalian nonmyelinated nerve fibers at rest and during activity. *J. Physiol.* (London) 196:163–181, 1968.

24. Creutzfeldt, O. D. Neurophysiological correlates of different functional states of the brain. In D. H. Ingvar and H. Lassen, cited in [17], pp. 21–46.

25. Bachelard, H. S. Energy utilized by neurotransmitters. In D. H. Ingvar and H. Lassen, cited in [17], pp. 79–81.

26. Toll, L., and Howard, B. D. Role of Mg^{2+}-ATPase and a pH gradient in storage of catecholamines in synaptic vesicles. *Biochemistry* 17:2517–2523, 1978.

27. Papazian, D., Rahamimoff, H., and Goldin, S. M. Reconstitution and purification by "transport specificity fractionation" of an ATP-dependent calcium transport component from synaptosome-derived vesicles. *Proc. Natl. Acad. Sci. U.S.A.* 76:3708–3712, 1979.

28. Blostein, R. Side specific effects of sodium on (Na,K)-ATPase. Studies with inside-out red-cell membrane vesicles. *J. Biol. Chem.* 254:6673–6677, 1979.

29. Siegel, G. J., Iyengar, S., and Fogt, S. K. *Electrophorus electricus* $(Na^+ + K^+)$-ATPase: Evidence for simultaneous Na^+ and K^+ binding in the presence of Pb^{2+}. *J. Biol. Chem.* 255:3935–3943, 1980.

30. Swann, A. C., and Albers, R. W. (Na^+,K^+)-ATPase of mammalian brain: Differential effects on cation affinities of phosphorylation by ATP and acetylphosphate. *Arch. Biochem. Biophys.* 203:422–427, 1980.

31. Grosse, R., et al. Analysis of function-related interactions of ATP, sodium and potassium ions with Na^+- and K^+-transporting ATPase studied with a thiol reagent as tool. *Acta Biol. Med. Germ.* 37:83–96, 1978.

32. Siegel, G. J., and Fogt, S. K. Effects of Pb^{2+} and other divalent cations on ouabain binding to *E. electricus* electroplax $(Na^+ + K^+)$-adenosinetriphosphatase. *Mol. Pharmacol.* 15:43–48, 1979.

33. Haupert, G. T., Jr., and Sancho, J. M. Sodium transport inhibitor from bovine hypothalamus. *Proc. Natl. Acad. Sci. U.S.A.* 76:4658–4660, 1979.

34. Grantham, J. J., and Glynn, I. M. Renal Na,K-ATPase: Determinants of inhibition by vanadium. *Am. J. Physiol.* 236:F530–F535, 1979.

35. Post, R., Hegyvary, C., and Kume, S. Activation by adenosine triphosphate in the phosphorylation kinetics of Na^+ and K^+ transport adenosine triphosphatase. *J. Biol. Chem.* 247:6530–6540, 1972.

36. Albers, R. W., Koval, G. J., and Siegel, G. J. Studies on the interaction of ouabain and other cardioactive steroids with sodium-potassium–activated adenosine triphosphatase. *Mol. Pharmacol.* 4:324–336, 1968.

37. Fahn, S., Koval, G. J., and Albers, R. W. Sodium-potassium–activated adenosinetriphosphatase of *Electrophorus* electric organ. I. An associated sodium-activated transphosphorylation. *J. Biol. Chem.* 241:1882–1889, 1966.

38. Siegel, G. J., and Goodwin, B. Sodium-potassium activated adenosine triphosphatase: Potassium regulation of enzyme phosphorylation. *J. Biol. Chem.* 247:3630–3637, 1972.

39. Yamada, S., and Ikemoto, N. Reaction mechanism of calcium-ATPase of sarcoplasmic reticulum. *J. Biol. Chem.* 255:3108–3119, 1980.

40. Cantley, L. C. Jr., Gelles, J., and Josephson, L. Reaction of (Na + K)-ATPase with 7-chloro-4-nitrobenzo-2-oxa-1,3-diazole: Evidence for an essential tyrosine at the active site. *Biochemistry* 17:418–425, 1978.

41. Dixon, J. F., and Hokin, L. E. A simple procedure for the preparation of highly purified (Na + K)-ATPase from the rectal salt gland of *Squalus acanthias* and the electric organ of *Electrophorus electricus. Anal. Biochem.* 86:378–385, 1978.

42. Jørgensen, P. L. Purification and characterization of Na,K-ATPase. III. Purification from outer

medulla of mammalian kidney after selective removal of membrane components by sodium dodecyl sulfate. *Biochim. Biophys. Acta* 356:36–52, 1974.

43. Kyte, J. Purification of the sodium- and potassium-dependent adenosine triphosphatase from canine renal medulla. *J. Biol. Chem.* 246:4157–4165, 1971.

44. Lane, L. K., Potter, J. D., and Collins, J. H. Large scale purification of Na,K-ATPase and its subunits from lamb kidney medulla. *Prep. Biochem.* 9:157–170, 1979.

45. Sweadner, K. J. Purification from brain of an intrinsic membrane protein fraction enriched in $(Na^+ + K^+)$ATPase. *Biochim. Biophys. Acta* 508:486–499, 1978.

46. Jørgensen, P. L. Purification of $(Na^+ + K^+)$-ATPase: Active site determination and criteria of purity. *Ann. N.Y. Acad. Sci.* 242:36–52, 1974.

47. Haase, W., and Koepsell, H. Substructure of membrane-bound Na,K-ATPase protein. *Pflug. Arch.* 381:127–135, 1979.

48. Vogel, F., et al. Electron microscopic visualization of the arrangement of the two protein components of (Na + K)-ATPase. *Biochim. Biophys. Acta* 470:497–502, 1977.

49. Jørgensen, P. L. Purification and characterization of $(Na^+ + K^+)$-ATPase. IV. Estimation of the purity and of the molecular weight and polypeptide content per enzyme unit in preparations from the outer medulla of rabbit kidney. *Biochim. Biophys. Acta* 356:53–67, 1974.

50. Churchill, L., Peterson, G. L., and Hokin, L. E. The large subunit of (Na + K)-activated ATPase from electroplax of *Electrophorus electricus* is a glycoprotein. *Biochem. Biophys. Res. Commun.* 90:488–490, 1979.

51. Forbush, B., III, Kaplan, J. H., and Hoffman, J. F. Characterization of a new photoaffinity derivative of ouabain: Labelling of the large polypeptide and of a proteolipid component of the Na,K-ATPase. *Biochemistry* 17:3667–3676, 1978.

52. Hastings, D. F., and Reynolds, J. A. Molecular weight of $(Na^+ + K^+)$-ATPase from shark rectal gland. *Biochemistry* 18:817–821, 1979.

53. Peters, W. H. M., et al. $(Na^+ + K^+)$ATPase has one functioning phosphorylation site per α subunit. *Nature* 290:338–339, 1981.

54. Kyte, J. Properties of the two polypeptides of Na- and K-dependent ATPase. *J. Biol. Chem.* 247:7642–7649, 1972.

55. Rhee, H. M., and Hokin, L. E. Inhibition of the purified Na-K–activated ATPase from rectal gland of *Squalus acanthias* by antibody against the glycoprotein subunit. *Biochem. Biophys. Res. Commun.* 63:1139–1145, 1975.

56. Jean, D. H., Albers, R. W., and Koval, G. J. Sodium-potassium–activated ATPase of *Electrophorus* electric organ. X. Immunochemical properties of the Lubrol-solubilized enzyme and its constituent polypeptides. *J. Biol. Chem.* 250:1035–1040, 1975.

57. Perrone, J. R., et al. Molecular properties of purified (Na + K)-activated ATPases and their subunits from rectal gland of *Squalus acanthias* and the electric organ of *E. electricus*. *J. Biol. Chem.* 250:4178–4184, 1975.

58. Hokin, L. E. Purification and properties of the (Na + K)-activated ATPase and reconstitution of sodium transport. *Ann. N.Y. Acad. Sci.* 242:12–23, 1974.

59. Marshall, P. J., and Hokin, L. E. Microheterogeneity of the glycoprotein subunit of the (Na + K)-activated ATPase from the electroplax of *Electrophorus electricus*. *Biochem. Biophys. Res. Commun.* 87:476–482, 1979.

60. DePont, J. J. H. H. M., et al. An essential arginine residue in the ATP-binding centre of $(Na^+ + K^+)$-ATPase. *Biochim. Biophys. Acta* 482:213–227, 1977.

61. Schoot, B. M., DePont, J. J. H. H. M., and Bonting, S. L. Studies on the $(Na^+ + K^+)$-activated ATPase. XLII. Evidence for two classes of essential sulfhydryl groups. *Biochim. Biophys. Acta* 522:602–613, 1978.

62. Albers, R. W., Fahn, S., and Koval, G. J. The role of Na^+ in the activation of *Electrophorus* electric organ ATPase. *Proc. Natl. Acad. Sci. U.S.A.* 50:474–481, 1963.

63. Hart, W. M., Jr., and Titus, E. O. Isolation of a protein component of Na-K transport ATPase containing ligand-protected sulfhydryl groups. *J. Biol. Chem.* 248:1365–1371, 1973.

64. Hart, W. H., Jr., and Titus, E. O. Sulfhydryl groups of sodium-potassium transport ATPase. *J. Biol. Chem.* 248:4674–4681, 1973.

65. Harris, W. E., and Stahl, W. L. Conformational changes of purified $(Na^+ + K^+)$-ATPase detected by a sulfhydryl fluorescence probe. *Biochim. Biophys. Acta* 485:203–214, 1977.

66. Stahl, W. L., and Harris, W. E. A fluorescent sulfhydryl probe for studying conformational changes of the Na^+,K^+-ATPase. In J. C. Skou and J. G. Nørby, cited in [10], pp. 157–167.

67. Jørgensen, P. L. Purification and characterization of (Na, K)-ATPase. V. Conformational changes in the enzyme. Transitions between the Na-form and K-form studied with tryptic digestion as a tool. *Biochim. Biophys. Acta* 401:399–415, 1975.

68. Roelofsen, B., and Van Deenen, L. L. M. Lipid requirement of membrane-bound ATPase. Studies

on human erythrocyte ghosts. *Eur. J. Biochem.* 40: 245–257, 1973.

69. Stahl, W. L.   Role of phospholipids in the Na$^+$, K$^+$-stimulated ATPase system of brain microsomes. *Arch. Biochem. Biophys.* 154:56–67, 1973.

70. DePont, J. J. H. H. M., Van Prooijen-Van Eeden, A., and Bonting, S. L.   Studies on the (Na$^+$-K$^+$)-activated ATPase. XXXIV. Phosphatidylserine not essential for (Na$^+$ + K$^+$)-ATPase activity. *Biochim. Biophys. Acta* 323:487–494, 1973.

71. DePont, J. J. H. H. M., Van Prooijen-Van Eeden, A., and Bonting, L.   Role of negatively charged phospholipids in highly purified (Na + K)-ATPase from rabbit kidney outer medulla. Studies on (Na$^+$ + K$^+$)-activated ATPase. XXXIX. *Biochim. Biophys. Acta* 508:464–477, 1978.

72. Ottolenghi, P.   The relipidation of delipidated Na,K-ATPase. *Eur. J. Biochem.* 99:113–131, 1979.

73. Järnefelt, J.   Lipid requirements of functional membrane structures as indicated by the reversible inactivation of (Na$^+$ + K$^+$)-ATPase. *Biochim. Biophys. Acta* 266:91–96, 1972.

74. Kimelberg, H. K.   Alterations in phospholipid-dependent (Na$^+$ + K$^+$)-ATPase activity due to lipid fluidity. Effects of cholesterol and Mg^{2+}. *Biochim. Biophys. Acta* 413:143–156, 1975.

75. Sandermann, H.   Regulation of membrane enzymes by lipids. *Biochim. Biophys. Acta* 515:209–237, 1978.

76. Charnock, J. S., and Bashford, C. L.   A fluorescent probe study of the lipid mobility of membranes containing Na,K-dependent ATPase. *Mol. Pharmacol.* 11:766–774, 1975.

77. Swanson, P. D.   Temperature dependence of sodium ion activation of the cerebral microsomal ATPase. *J. Neurochem.* 13:229–236, 1966.

78. Racker, E., and Fisher, L. W.   Reconstitution of an ATP-dependent Na pump with an ATPase from electric eel and pure phospholipids. *Biochem. Biophys. Res. Commun.* 67:1144–1150, 1975.

79. Marks, M. J., and Seeds, N. W.   A heterogeneous ouabain-ATPase interaction in mouse brain. *Life Sci.* 23:2735–2744, 1978.

80. Sweadner, K. J.   Two molecular forms of (Na$^+$ + K$^+$)-ATPase in brain. *J. Biol. Chem.* 254: 6060–6067, 1979.

81. Grisar, T., Franck, G., and Schoffeniels, E.   K$^+$-activation mechanism of the (Na,K)-ATPase of bulk isolated glia and neurons. In E. Schoffeniels, G. Franck, D. B. Tower and L. Hertz (eds.), *Dynamic Properties of Glia Cells*. New York: Academic, 1978. Pp. 359–369.

82. Schwartz, A., Lindenmayer, G. E., and Allen, J. C.   The Na,K-Adenosine triphosphatase: Pharma-cological, physiological and biochemical aspects. *Physiol. Rev.* 27:3–134, 1975.

83. Askari, A., and Rao, S. N.   (Na$^+$-K$^+$)-ATPase complex: Effects of anticomplex antibody on the partial reactions catalyzed by the complex. *Biochem. Biophys. Res. Commun.* 49:1323–1328, 1972.

84. Jørgensen, P. L., et al.   Antibodies to pig kidney (Na$^+$ + K$^+$)-ATPase inhibits the Na$^+$ pump in human red cells provided they have access to the inner surface of the cell membrane. *Biochim. Biophys. Acta* 291:795–800, 1973.

85. McCans, J. L., et al.   Antigenic differences in (Na + K)-ATPase preparations isolated from various organs and species. *J. Biol. Chem.* 250: 7257–7265, 1975.

86. Hosie, R. J. A.   The localization of adenosine-triphosphatase in morphologically characterized subcellular fractions of guinea pig brain. *Biochem. J.* 96:404–412, 1965.

87. DiBona, D. R., and Mills, J. W.   Distribution of Na$^+$-pump sites in transporting epithelia. *Fed. Proc.* 38:134–143, 1979.

88. Shaver, J. L. F., and Stirling, C.   Ouabain binding to renal tubules of the rabbit. *J. Cell Biol.* 76:278–292, 1978.

89. Ernst, S. A.   Transport ATPase cytochemistry: Ultrastructural localization of potassium-dependent and potassium-independent phosphatase activities in rat kidney cortex. *J. Cell Biol.* 66:586–608, 1975.

90. Kyte, J.   Immunoferritin determination of the distribution of (Na$^+$ + K$^+$)-ATPase over the plasma membranes of renal convoluted tubules. I. Distal segment. *J. Cell Biol.* 68:287–303, 1976.

91. Stahl, W. L., and Broderson, S. H.   Localization of Na,K-ATPase in brain. *Fed. Proc.* 35:1260–1265, 1976.

92. Stahl, W. L., et al.   Studies on cellular localization of (Na$^+$-K$^+$)-ATPase activity in nervous tissue. In E. Schoffeniels et al., cited in [81], pp. 371–381.

93. Kimelberg, H. K., et al.   (Na$^+$ + K$^+$)-ATPase, ^{86}Rb$^+$ transport and carbonic anhydrase activity in isolated brain cells and cultured astrocytes. In E. Schoffeniels et al., cited in [81], pp. 347–357.

94. Wood, J. G., et al.   Immunocytochemical localization of sodium, potassium–activated ATPase in knifefish brain. *J. Neurocytol.* 6:571–581, 1977.

95. Broderson, S. H., Patton, D. L., and Stahl, W. L.   Fine structural localization of K$^+$-stimulated p-nitrophenylphosphatase activity in dendrites. *J. Cell Biol.* 77:R13–R17, 1978.

96. Schwartz, M., et al.   Goldfish brain (Na$^+$,K$^+$)-ATPase: Purification of catalytic polypeptide and production of specific antibodies. *J. Neurochem.* 34:1745–1752, 1980.

97. Akasu, T., Omura, H., and Koketsu, K. Roles of electrogenic Na$^+$ pump and K$^+$ conductance in the slow inhibitory postsynaptic potential of bullfrog sympathetic ganglion cells. *Life Sci.* 23:2405–2410, 1978.

98. Gorman, A. L. F., and Marmor, M. F. Steady-state contribution of the sodium pump to the resting potential of a molluscan neuron. *J. Physiol.* (London) 242:35–48, 1974.

99. Johnson, E. A., et al. Some electrophysiological consequences of electrogenic sodium and potassium transport in cardiac muscle. *J. Theor. Biol.* 87:737–756, 1980.

100. Thomas, R. C. Electrogenic sodium pump in nerve and muscle cells. *Physiol. Rev.* 42:563–594, 1972.

101. Prince, D. A., Pedley, T. A., and Ranson, B. R. Fluctuations in ion concentrations during excitation and seizures. In E. Schoffeniels et al., cited in [81], pp. 281–303.

102. Somjen, G. Electrophysiology of neuroglia. *Annu. Rev. Physiol.* 37:163–190, 1975.

103. Franck, G., et al. Potassium transport in mammalian astroglia. In E. Schoffeniels et al., cited in [81], pp. 315–325.

104. Gutman, Y., et al. Increased catecholamine release from adrenal medulla by liposomes loaded with sodium or calcium ions. *Biochem. Pharmacol.* 28:1209–1211, 1979.

105. Vizi, E. S. Na$^+$-K$^+$–activated adenosinetriphosphatase as a trigger in transmitter release. *Neuroscience* 3:376–384, 1978.

106. Wu, P. H., and Phillis, J. W. Effects of alpha-adrenergic and beta-adrenergic blocking-agents on biogenic-amine–stimulated (Na$^+$ + K$^+$)-ATPase of rat cerebral cortical synaptosomal membrane. *Gen. Pharmacol.* 9:421–424, 1978.

107. Meyer, E., and Cooper, J. Correlations between Na$^+$-K$^+$-ATPase activity and acetylcholine release in rat cortical synaptosomes. *J. Neurochem.* 36:467–475, 1981.

108. Hudgins, P. M., and Bond, G. H. Reversal of vanadate inhibition of Na,K-ATPase by catecholamines. *Res. Commun. Chem. Pathol. Pharmacol.* 23:313–326, 1979.

109. Wu, P. H., and Phillis, J. W. Effects of vanadate on brain (Na$^+$ + K$^+$)-ATPase and para-nitrophenylphosphatase: Interactions with monovalent and divalent ions and with noradrenaline. *Int. J. Biochem.* 10:629–635, 1979.

110. Akasu, T., Ohta, Y., and Koketsu, K. Effect of adrenaline on electrogenic Na$^+$ pump in cardiac muscle cells. *Experientia* 34:488–490, 1978.

111. Sastry, B. S. R., and Phillis, J. W. Antagonism of biogenic-amine–induced depression of cerebral cortical neurones by (Na$^+$ + K$^+$)-ATPase inhibitors. *Can. J. Physiol. Pharmacol.* 55:170–179, 1977.

112. Christensen, H. N. Developments in amino acid transport, illustrated for the blood-brain barrier. *Biochem. Pharmacol.* 28:1989–1992, 1979.

113. Wheeler, D. D. A kinetic analysis of sodium-dependent glutamic acid transport in peripheral nerve. *J. Neurochem.* 26:239–246, 1976.

114. Davidson, D. L., Tsukada, Y., and Barbeau, A. Ouabain-induced seizures—site of production and response to anticonvulsants. *Can. J. Neurol. Sci.* 5:405–411, 1978.

115. Smith, T. J., and Edelman, I. S. Role of sodium transport in thyroid thermogenesis. *Fed. Proc.* 38:2150–2153, 1979.

116. Charney, A. N., and Donowitz, M. Prevention and reversal of cholera enterotoxin–induced intestinal secretion by methylprednisolone induction of (Na$^+$ + K$^+$)-ATPase. *J. Clin. Invest.* 57:1590–1599, 1976.

117. Geloso, J., and Basset, J. Role of adrenal glands in development of fetal rat kidney (Na$^+$ + K$^+$)-ATPase. *Pfluegers Arch.* 348:105–113, 1974.

118. Huttenlocher, P. R., and Amemiya, I. M. Effects of adrenocortical steroids and of adrenocorticotropic hormone on (Na$^+$ + K$^+$)-ATPase in immature cerebral cortex. *Pediatr. Res.* 12:104–107, 1978.

119. Knudsen, J. F. Estrogen (EB) and EB + progesterone (P) induced changes in pituitary sodium, potassium adenosine-triphosphatase activity (ATPase). *Endocr. Res. Commun.* 3:281–295, 1976.

120. LaBella, F. S., Bihler, I., and Kim, R. S. Progesterone derivative binds to cardiac ouabain receptor and shows dissociation between sodium pump inhibition and increased contractile force. *Nature* 278:571–573, 1979.

121. Yamamoto, S. Prednisolone-3, 20-bisguanylhydrazone: Mode of interaction with rat brain sodium and potassium-activated adenosine triphosphatase. *Eur. J. Pharmacol.* 50:409–418, 1978.

122. Gavryck, W. A., Moore, R. D., and Thompson, R. C. Effect of insulin upon membrane-bound (Na$^+$ + K$^+$)-ATPase extracted from frog skeletal muscle. *J. Physiol.* (London) 252:43–58, 1975.

123. Clausen, T., and Kohn, P. G. Effect of insulin on transport of sodium and potassium in rat soleus muscle. *J. Physiol.* (London) 265:19–42, 1977.

124. Bertoni, J. M., and Siegel, G. J. Development of (Na$^+$ + K$^+$)-ATPase in rat cerebrum: Correlation with Na$^+$-dependent phosphorylation and K$^+$-paranitrophenylphosphatase. *J. Neurochem.* 31:1501–1511, 1978.

125. Scarpa, A., and Carafoli, E. (eds.). *Calcium Transport and Cell Function. Ann. N.Y. Acad. Sci.* Vol. 307, 1978.

126. Bartfai, T. Cyclic nucleotides in the central nervous system. *Trends Biochem. Sci.* 10:121–124, 1978.

127. Cheung, W. Y. Calmodulin plays a pivotal role in cellular regulation. *Science* 207:19–27, 1980.

128. Lin, Y. M., Liu, Y. P., and Cheung, W. Y. Cyclic 3′:5′-nucleotide phosphodiesterase. Purification, characterization, and active form of the protein activator from bovine brain. *J. Biol. Chem.* 249: 4943–4954, 1974.

129. Grab, D. J., et al. Presence of calmodulin in post-synaptic densities isolated from canine cerebral cortex. *J. Biol. Chem.* 254:8690–8696, 1979.

130. Blaustein, M. P., Ratzlaff, R. W., and Kendrick, N. K. The regulation of intracellular calcium in the presynaptic nerve terminals. *Ann. N.Y. Acad. Sci.* 307:195–211, 1978.

131. Blaustein, M. P., et al. Calcium buffering in pre-synaptic nerve terminals. I. Evidence for involvement of a nonmitochondrial ATP-dependent sequestration mechanism. *J. Gen. Physiol.* 72:15–42, 1978.

132. Miledi, R. Transmitter release induced by injection of calcium ions into nerve terminals. *Proc. R. Soc. Lond.* [Biol.], Series B 183:421–425, 1973.

133. Erulkar, S. D., and Rahamimoff, R. The role of calcium ions in tetanic and post-tetanic increase of miniature end-plate potential frequency. *J. Physiol.* (London) 278:501–511, 1978.

134. Erulkar, S. D., Rahamimoff, R., and Rotshenker, S. Quelling of spontaneous transmitter release by nerve impulses in low extracellular calcium solutions. *J. Physiol.* (London) 278:491–500, 1978.

135. Stahl, W. L., and Swanson, P. D. Movements of Ca and other cations in isolated cerebral tissues. *J. Neurochem.* 18:415–427, 1971.

136. Stahl, W. L., and Swanson, P. D. Calcium movements in brain slices in low Na or Ca media. *J. Neurochem.* 19:2395–2407, 1972.

137. Simon, W., et al. Calcium-selective electrodes. In A. Scarpa and E. Carafoli, cited in [125], pp. 52–69.

138. Kuo, C-H., et al. Regulation of ATP-dependent Ca uptake of synaptic plasma membranes by Ca-dependent modulator protein. *Life Sci.* 25:235–240, 1979.

139. Swanson, P. D., Anderson, L., and Stahl, W. L. Uptake of Ca ions by synaptosomes from rat brain. *Biochim. Biophys. Acta* 356:174–183, 1974.

140. Gill, D. I., Grollman, E. F., and Kohn, L. D. Calcium transport mechanisms in membrane vesicles from guinea pig brain synaptosomes. *J. Biol. Chem.* 256:184–192, 1981.

141. Schellenberg, G. D., and Swanson, P. D. Sodium-dependent and calcium-dependent calcium transport by rat brain microsomes. *Biochim. Biophys. Acta* (in press).

142. Bygrave, F. L. Mitochondria and the control of intracellular calcium. *Biol. Rev.* 53:43–79, 1978.

143. Swanson, P. D., and Stahl, W. L. Effects of sodium on calcium uptake by brain mitochondria. Fifth Meeting of International Society for Neurochemistry, 1975. Abstract, p. 191.

144. Crompton, M., et al. The interrelations between the transport of sodium and calcium in mitochondria of various mammalian tissues. *Eur. J. Biochem.* 82:25–31, 1978.

145. Henkart, M. P., Reese, T. S., and Brinley, F. J. Endoplasmic reticulum sequesters calcium in the squid giant axon. *Science* 202:1300–1303, 1978.

146. Rahamimoff, H., and Abramovitz, E. Ca transport and ATPase activity of synaptosomal vesicles from rat brain. *FEBS Lett.* 92:163–167, 1978.

147. Blitz, A. L., Fine, R. E., and Toselli, P. A. Evidence that coated vesicles isolated from brain are calcium-sequestering organelles resembling sarcoplasmic reticulum. *J. Cell Biol.* 75:135–147, 1977.

148. Nakamuru, Y., and Konishi, K. Mechanism of adenosine triphosphate–dependent Ca^{++} uptake of brain microsomes. *J. Biochem.* 75:1129–1133, 1974.

149. Tsudzuki, T. Adenosine triphosphatase-dependent calcium uptake of synaptic vesicle fraction is largely due to contaminating microsomes. *J. Biochem.* 86:777–782, 1979.

150. Ichida, S., et al. Effects of La^{2+}, Mn^{2+}, and ruthenium red on Mg-Ca–ATPase activity and ATP-dependent Ca binding of the synaptic plasma membrane. *J. Pharmacol.* 26:39–43, 1976.

151. Nakamuru, Y., and Schwartz, A. ATP-dependent calcium-binding vesicles, magnesium, calcium ATP and sodium, potassium ATPase distribution in dog brain. *Arch. Biochem. Biophys.* 144:16–29, 1971.

152. Robinson, J. D. (Ca + Mg)-stimulated ATPase activity of a rat brain microsomal preparation. *Arch. Biochem. Biophys.* 176:366–374, 1976.

153. Saermark, T., and Vilhardt, H. Isolation and partial characterization of magnesium ion– and calcium ion–dependent adenosine triphosphatase activity from bovine brain microsomal fraction. *Biochem. J.* 181:321–330, 1979.

154. Castro, J., and Farley, R. A. Proteolytic fragmentation of the catalytic subunit of the Na and K–ATPase. Alignment of tryptic and chymotryptic fragments and location of sites labeled with ATP and iodoacetate. *J. Biol. Chem.* 254:2221–2228, 1979.

155. Schmidt, U., and Dubach, U. C. Activity of (Na^+,K^+)-stimulated–ATPase in the rat nephron. *Pfluegers Arch.* 306:219–226, 1969.

156. Bonting, S. L., and Caravaggio, L. L. Studies on Na-K–activated ATPase. V. Correlation of enzyme activity with cation flux in six tissues. *Arch. Biochem. Biophys.* 101:37–46, 1963.

Hitoshi Shichi

Chapter 7. Molecular Biology of the Visual Process

Physiological Background

The eye detects light and transmits its signal to the brain, so we expect the presence of light-absorbing pigments within the organ. In the vertebrate eye, such pigments are indeed found in the visual (photoreceptor) cells of the retina. Each visual cell is composed of two principal parts, the metabolically more active inner segment, which contains nucleus, mitochondria, and other subcellular organelles, and the outer segment, in which the visual pigment is localized exclusively (see Fig. 7-1). The inner segments of the visual cells have terminals that synapse with horizontal cells and bipolar cells. The bipolar cells, in turn, form junctions with ganglion and amacrine cells, as illustrated in Fig. 7-1.

The visual cells are classified into two types, based on their morphology: *rod cells* have elongated outer segments and contain rhodopsin, the visual pigment responsible for dim-light (black-and-white, or scotopic) vision; *cone cells,* which possess cone-shaped outer segments, are photoreceptors for daylight (color, or photopic) vision. Microspectroscopic techniques have revealed the presence of three (morphologically indistinguishable) types of cone cells in the human retina. Each cell contains one of three pigments, with absorption maxima at 445, 535, and 570 nm, respectively. The number of pigments and their absorption maxima vary in different species. One estimate is that the human eye contains 120 million rod cells in the peripheral region of the retina and 6.5 million cone cells concentrated mainly in the central (foveal) region.

Na^+ entering through the outer-segment membrane is pumped out by the sodium pump believed to be located mainly in the inner-segment plasma membrane. The Na^+ permeability of the outer segment is higher in the dark than in the light. Thus, the plasma membrane of the vertebrate rod cell is depolarized (i.e., excited) during the dark adaptation. Light reduces the Na^+ permeability of the outer segment and hyperpolarizes, or de-excites, the membrane. Therefore, "visual excitation" in the vertebrate photoreceptor means that the depolarized visual-cell plasma membrane is inhibited by light. The release of chemical transmitter at the synaptic terminal of the visual cell in the dark also is inhibited by light. The presence of α-aminobutyric acid, glycine, acetylcholine, dopamine, and taurine has been reported in the retinal neurons [1, 2]. If these compounds are the retinal chemical transmitters, it remains to be determined which transmitters are associated with the individual cell types.

Absorption of light by a single pigment molecule in rod cells triggers a series of events that results in a particular pattern of excitation of retinal neurons and, eventually, of cerebral neurons. In rod vision, the magnitude of neural excitation is directly related to perception of the brightness of light. To discriminate color, absorption of light by at least two cone pigments with different absorption maxima is essential. The ratio of magnitudes of excitation thus induced determines the type of color perceived. The arrays of visual signals generated by the photoreceptor cells and programmed by retinal neurons, principally bipolar cells, are transmitted to the lateral geniculate bodies via ganglion cell axons, which make up the optic nerves and tracts. Impulses are conveyed by the geniculocalcarine radiations to the visual cortex of the brain, where the signals representing light intensity and wavelength are presumed to be decoded separately by

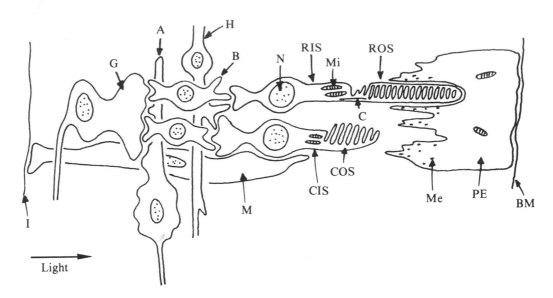

Fig. 7-1. The vertebrate retina: (A) amacrine cell; (B) bipolar cell; (BM) Bruch's membrane; (C) cilium; (CIS) cone inner segment; (COS) cone outer segment; (G) ganglion cell; (H) horizontal cell; (I) inner limiting membrane; (M) Müller cell; (Me) melanin granule; (Mi) mitochondrion; (N) nucleus; (PE) pigment epithelium; (RIS) rod inner segment; (ROS) rod outer segment.

different neurons. The visual process related to the coding and decoding of visual signals is an important area of electrophysiology, but is not covered here. This chapter deals primarily with the structural and functional aspects of photoreceptors and molecular events that take place after photon absorption by the visual cells. General references are found in [3–6].

Photoreceptor Membranes

PROPERTIES OF ROD MEMBRANES

Photoreceptor membranes are made of a continuous bilayer of phospholipids and rhodopsin, which is the major membrane protein. Other attached membrane proteins are probably mostly enzymes. The phospholipids contain high concentrations of polyunsaturated fatty acids. The outer segment of a rod visual cell is comprised of a stack of several hundreds of discs encased in a sack of the plasma membrane (Fig. 7-1). In 1963, Droz showed by means of autoradiography that in vertebrate animals injected with radioactive amino acids, labeled proteins migrate as a distinct band from the base toward the apex of a rod outer segment. Young [7] subsequently showed that radioactive amino acids injected into animals are first incorporated into the proteins synthesized on ribosomes in the rod inner segment. A part of the synthesized protein, pre-

sumably including opsin, moves to the Golgi apparatus and then to the junction between the inner and outer segments. The protein that reaches the outer segment through a narrow passage of the cilium is finally incorporated into the plasma membrane of the rod (Fig. 7-2). Incorporation of opsin into the membrane occurs as a part of disc formation, which is initiated by invagination of the plasma membrane in the basal region of the rod outer segment. The membranous infoldings thus formed become detached from the plasma membrane as they are displaced by the formation of newer discs. The discs that eventually reach the apical region of the rod outer segment are shed from the tip of the segment and are phagocytized by the pigment epithelial cell. Disc shedding is minimal in the dark and follows a circadian rhythm; a burst of shedding occurs soon after the onset of light [8, 9]. In this manner, the rod undergoes constant turn-

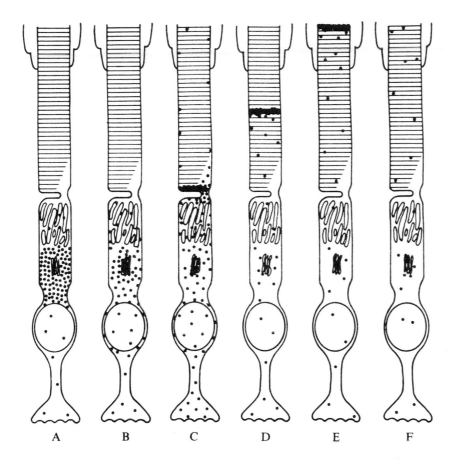

A   B   C   D   E   F

Fig. 7-2. Protein renewal in rod visual cells. Radioactive amino acids are first incorporated into proteins on the ribosomes and in the Golgi of the inner segment (A and B). Part of the newly synthesized protein moves to the cilium region, then to the base of the outer segment (C). The proteins incorporated into discs (D) are displaced by repeated formation of newer discs and reach the apical region of the outer segment (E), from which they are shed in small packets (F).

over at rates ranging from a few days to months, depending upon the species.

This is a remarkably active membrane synthetic system. For example, the turnover rate of a frog rod is 8.5 weeks. Assuming that a frog has 3 million rods (1,800 discs per rod) per eye, and noting that a disc is 6×10^{-6} meter (m) in diameter, one can calculate that a frog eye synthesizes 2.5 sq cm of disc membrane every hour. Disc membranes are not capable of synthesizing membrane components. Thus, such individual membrane components as protein, carbohydrate, and lipid must all be synthesized in the inner segment and then transported to the outer segment, where membrane assembly occurs. The incorporation of phospholipids, fatty acids, and vitamin A into the rod membranes also occurs independently of membrane assembly. These components are exchangeable with their respective counterparts in the old discs, and therefore are redistributed continuously through the outer segment.

In contrast to rod outer segments, the cone outer segments of animals injected with radioactive amino acids do not show a distinct radioactive band of newly synthesized protein. The cone discs generally remain continuous with the plasma membrane (see Fig. 7-1). A rapid randomization of radioactive protein may explain the absence of a distinct band of radioactivity in the membrane system.

Studies of animal models of retinal dystrophy are important both for clinical implications (e.g., remedies for retinitis pigmentosa) and for understanding the regulatory mechanism of disc-membrane turnover. In rats with inherited retinal dystrophy, rod outer segments grow abnormally long and accumulate as lamellar bundles in the extracellular space between the visual cell and the pigment epithelium. This overproduction is the result of a failure of the rod membranes to be phagocytized by the pigment epithelium. In another type of hereditary retinal dystrophy, found in mice, the rod outer segments fail to develop to full maturation, probably owing to a genetic defect in the disc assembly mechanism.

Rod outer segment membranes ($>$95 percent disc membranes, $<$5 percent plasma membrane) consist of 60 percent protein and 40 percent phospholipid. In vertebrate photoreceptors, about 80 percent of the phospholipid is accounted for by phosphatidylethanolamine and phosphatidylcholine. The most abundant polyunsaturated fatty acid is docosahexaenoic acid (22 carbons and 6 unsaturated bonds), linked exclusively to the middle carbon of the glycerol moiety of phospholipids.

Important to the function of photoreceptor membranes is the degree of freedom of movement of rhodopsin molecules within the membrane. Owing to the high content of polyunsaturated fatty acids, rod membranes are highly fluid at physiological temperature and demonstrate various properties predicted by the fluid-mosaic model of biomembranes [10]. These properties include spinning motion (rotational freedom) of rhodopsin, with the

rotational axis perpendicular to the longer axis of the disc, and diffusion (translational freedom) of the molecule in a direction parallel to the longer axis of the disc. In disc membranes, the retinal chromophore of rhodopsin is oriented in a plane parallel to the longer axis of the disc. If the chromophores do not rotate in the plane, the rods will demonstrate dichroic properties because one of the linearly polarized light components that propagates parallel to the longer axis is preferentially absorbed. By means of rapid-recording spectroscopy, however, a transient dichroism (lifetime = 20 μsec) was detected in fresh frog rods. If rhodopsin protein in the tissue is fixed with glutaraldehyde, the chromophore is also fixed, and a permanent dichroism is observed [11]. These results indicate that rhodopsin has rotational as well as translational freedom in the disc membrane. Rhodopsin is a glycoprotein with its carbohydrate moiety protruding from the inner surface of the disc membrane. The carbohydrate moiety is attached to an asparagine residue and has the structure [12, 47]:

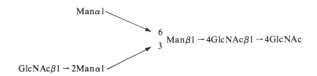

It is not thermally feasible for the carbohydrate moiety to go through the hydrophilic and hydrophobic layers of membrane. Therefore, the pigment molecule may not tumble from one side of the membrane to the other.

Translational freedom of the rhodopsin molecule was also demonstrated in another way. When one side of the rod is bleached by light, the absorbance at 530 nm of the irradiated side is decreased. When the rod remains in the dark for a few seconds, the absorbance of the irradiated side rises, with a concomitant decrease in the absorbance of the unirradiated side (see Fig. 7-3). The rate of equilibration becomes greater as the temperature is raised. Glutaraldehyde fixation of the tissue inhibits the equilibration process. From these results, Poo and

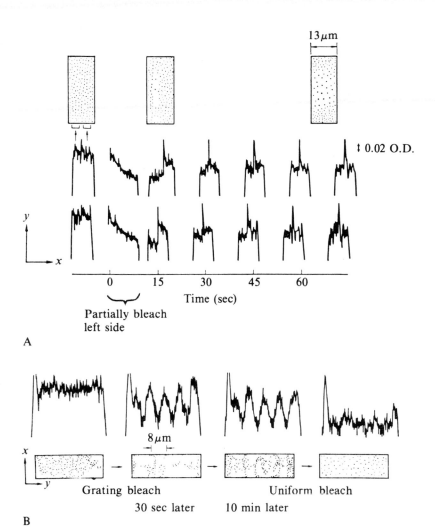

A

B

Fig. 7-3. Lateral diffusion of rhodopsin in the disc membrane. A. Rhodopsin diffusion after partial bleaching of the left-hand side of the rod. B. Absence of rhodopsin diffusion along the rod axis [see 13].

Cone [13] concluded that the rhodopsin molecule can translate freely in the disc membrane. From the rate of rhodopsin diffusion, the viscosity of the disc membrane was estimated to be about 2 poise (approximately equal to the fluidity of olive oil). The highly fluid nature of rod membranes may be important for irradiated rhodopsin to move around in the membranes and activate cyclic nucleotide phosphodiesterase and GTPase, as described in a

later section (see Biochemical Model). If the rod is bleached with a grating pattern, lines of which are at right angles to the long axis of the outer segment, the absorbance of the bleached region remains unchanged during the subsequent dark incubation. This result indicates that rhodopsin cannot migrate from one disc to another.

STRUCTURE OF DISC MEMBRANES

Although the regular stacking of the discs in outer segments of vertebrate rods had been known for some time, the double-membrane architecture of the disc was not recognized until 1960. Electron-microscope studies indicated that the disc mem-

brane is symmetrical in cross section, with the
hydrocarbon region of the lipids in the center zone
of the membrane, and that dense particles, presumably rhodopsin, are present in the membrane.
Freeze-etched rod membranes show an asymmetric distribution of the dense particles. Low-angle
X-ray diffraction studies on outer segments in frog
eyes showed that discs are stacked up with an inter-
discal distance of 300 Å and contain a regular array
of particles 40 Å in diameter. Fourier synthesis of
X-ray diffraction patterns of rod disc membrane
and lipid bilayers are shown in Fig. 7-4A. High
electron density peaks indicate phospholipid head
groups, and low-density troughs correspond to lipid
hydrocarbon regions. That the electron density is
greater in both the hydrocarbon and head group
regions of disc membrane than in lipid bilayers may
be attributed to the presence of rhodopsin. Thus,
rhodopsin is considered to span the membrane, as
shown in Fig. 7-4B [14]. The model is also supported by neutron diffraction data and chemical
labeling experiments. The size of the pigment
molecule determined by energy-transfer measurements between fluorescent probes is at least 75 Å
in length [15]. The N-terminus of opsin is exposed
on the inner (intradiscal) surface. The C-terminal
peptide is found on the outer (extradiscal) surface
of membrane and is accessible to proteolytic
enzymes.

Photochemistry of Visual Pigments

GENERAL STRUCTURAL AND SPECTRAL PROPERTIES

Rod pigments and cone pigments are both composed of protein (opsin), and retinal. Retinal$_1$,
which has one unsaturated bond in the cyclohexene
ring, is the chromophore of visual pigments of ter-
restrial vertebrates. On the other hand, the
chromophore of visual pigments in the marine
vertebrate is retinal$_2$, which has two double bonds
in the ionone ring. Whether a pigment has retinal$_1$
or retinal$_2$ for its chromophore is correlated with
the wavelength of the sunlight that reaches the
environment in which the animal lives. For example, the major visual pigment of the tadpole is
porphyropsin ($\lambda_{max} = 520$ nm), which contains

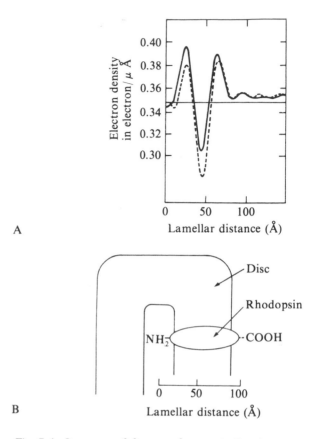

Fig. 7-4. Structure of disc membrane. A. Fourier
series representations. Disc membrane (———); disc lipid
bilayers (– – –). B. Localization of rhodopsin.

retinal$_2$; this is appropriate because the blue, but
not the red, component of sunlight is largely absorbed by water before it reaches the eye. After
metamorphosis of the tadpole, the visual pigment
of frog rhodopsin ($\lambda_{max} = 502$ nm) contains
retinal$_1$.

In rhodopsin, the aldehyde group of retinal is
linked to the ϵ-amino group of a lysine residue of
opsin through Schiff base formation. Protonated
Schiff base complexes between retinal and any of a
variety of amino acids show absorption maxima
around 440 nm. Therefore, an additional shift
toward the longer wavelength side that occurs in the
visual pigments is probably caused by interaction

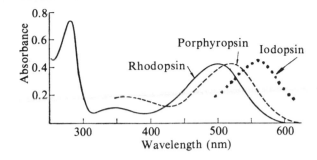

Fig. 7-5. *Absorption spectra of visual pigments.*

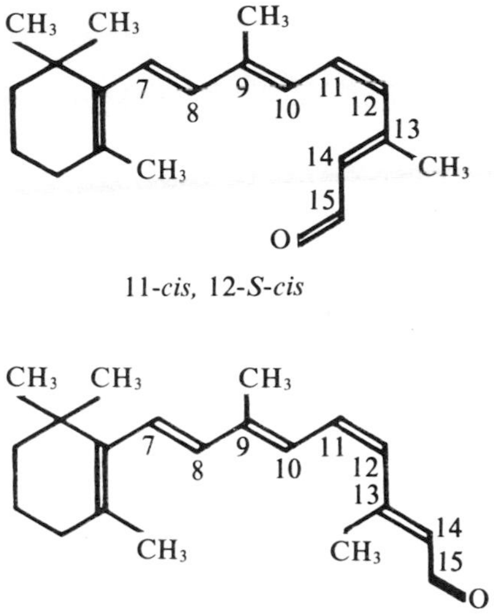

11-*cis*, 12-S-*cis*

11-*cis*, 12-S-*trans*

Fig. 7-6. *Formulas of the 11-cis, 12-S-cis and 11-cis, 12-S-trans conformers of retinal.*

of the chromophore with the opsin conformation.

As shown in Fig. 7-5, rhodopsin has maximum absorption bands at 498 nm (α band, $\epsilon_M = 41,000$) and 340 nm (β band, $\epsilon_M = 10,000$) at room temperature. The α and β bands of porphyropsin are found at 523 nm and 360 nm. The chromophore of visual pigments is 11-*cis* retinal. Two stereoisomers of 11-*cis* retinal are possible with respect to the orientation of the 13-14 double bond. If the 13-14 double bond and the 11-12 double bond are in trans configuration, the isomer is called 11-*cis*, 12-S-*trans* retinal (Fig. 7-6). If they are in cis configuration, the isomer is called 11-*cis*, 12-S-*cis* retinal. X-ray crystallography reveals that crystalline 11-*cis* retinal is in the 11-*cis*, 12-S-*cis* form. The retinal in visual pigments is believed to be in the 11-*cis*, 12-S-*trans* configuration. Supporting evidence for this conclusion comes from studies on visual pigment analogs. For example, 11-*cis*, 14-methylretinal exists only in the 12-S-*trans* configuration because of steric hindrance between the methyl group at carbon 14 and the hydrogen atom at carbon 10. Nevertheless, a light-bleachable visual pigment analog can be synthesized when opsin is mixed with the chemically synthesized 11-*cis*, 14-methylretinal in the 12-S-*trans* form [16]. Both rhodopsin and porphyropsin show positive circular dichroic bands in wavelength regions corresponding to the α and β absorption maxima. The circular dichroism is due to the optical asymmetry of the chromophore, induced by an interaction between opsin protein and optically inactive 11-*cis* retinal.

PHOTON ABSORPTION

Early studies established that photon absorption by rhodopsin results in the photic isomerization of the chromophore to the all-*trans* form (Fig. 7-7). This reaction occurs before lumirhodopsin is formed.

During the thermal process that follows the photochemical reaction, rhodopsin undergoes a series of spectrally distinct changes (Fig. 7-8) that can be identified by ordinary spectroscopy at different temperatures [6]. As examples, if rhodopsin is irradiated at −195°C with light of 437 nm, bathorhodopsin (previously called *prelumirhodopsin*) is formed; irradiation at −268°C instead gives rise to hypsorhodopsin, which, in turn, is converted to bathorhodopsin. By using a high-resolution flash photolysis apparatus, the rates of formation of bathorhodopsin and of metarhodopsin II from metarhodopsin I were recently determined at physiological temperatures [17, 18]. Decay of metarhodopsin I (lifetime $\simeq 3 \times 10^{-4}$ sec) is believed to be related to the photocurrent generation (latency $\simeq 10^{-4}$ sec) by the rod.

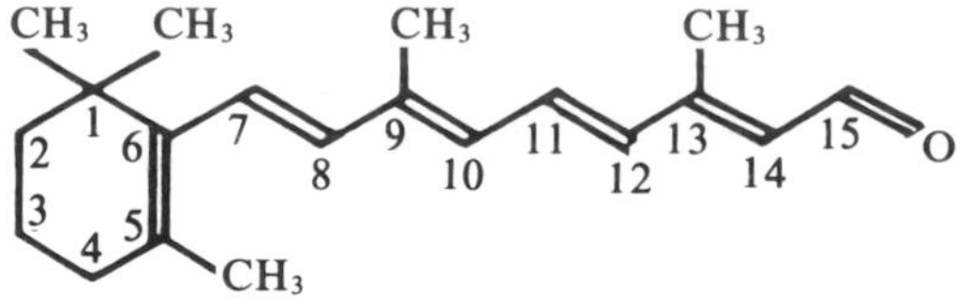

Fig. 7-7. Formula for all-trans retinal.

Studies on detergent-extracted rhodopsin indicate that the conversion of metarhodopsin I to metarhodopsin II is accompanied by the appearance of SH groups and proton uptake. The equilibrium between metarhodopsin I and metarhodopsin II can be shifted toward metarhodopsin II under high pressures (1068 atm). Although these results suggest a conformational change of opsin protein during the conversion of metarhodopsin I to metarhodopsin II, circular dichroism and ^{13}C nuclear magnetic resonance measurements of membrane-associated rhodopsin in the far ultraviolet region show little change in opsin conformation produced by photic bleaching. Any change of opsin conformation must be very small, therefore, and should not involve extensive unfolding or reordering of the peptide chain.

A birefringence loss was observed in outer segments of frog rod exposed to light [19]. The change in birefringence is related directly to the conversion of metarhodopsin I to metarhodopsin II and is attributed to reorientation of one phospholipid molecule per mole of rhodopsin. The chromophore of rhodopsin is optically active. This property is retained to the level of metarhodopsin II.

Metarhodopsin III is optically inactive. This suggests that, in going from metarhodopsin II to metarhodopsin III, retinal may be transferred from its original binding site either to a different site or to a different molecule. Studies involving chromophore fixation with borohydride at different bleaching stages support this possibility [20].

COLOR VISION

In contrast to what we know about rod pigments, very little is known about the chemistry of cone pigments. In 1937, Wald extracted a cone pigment named *iodopsin* (see Fig. 7-5) from the retinas of domestic fowl. After photic bleaching of iodopsin ($\lambda_{max} = 562$ nm), the following intermediates can be identified spectrally: bathoiodopsin ($\lambda_{max} = 640$ nm), lumiiodopsin ($\lambda_{max} = 518$ nm), metaiodopsin I ($\lambda_{max} = 495$ nm), and metaiodopsin II ($\lambda_{max} = 380$ nm). Microspectroscopic measurements of single cones of isolated human retinas reveal the presence of three pigments with absorption maxima at 445 nm, 535 nm, and 570 nm, respectively. Examination of color-blind subjects by ophthalmoscopic densitometry has demonstrated that red blindness and green blindness are related to a deficiency of the 570 nm pigment and the 535 nm pigment, respectively [21].

Regeneration of Visual Pigments

To maintain unimpaired vision, the visual pigments bleached by absorption of light must be regenerated. Regeneration of visual pigments takes place by two different mechanisms: (1) as a part of de novo synthesis of disc membrane; (2) reisomerization of all-*trans* retinal to 11-*cis* retinal and combination with opsin; this combination is much faster with iodopsin than with rhodopsin. As already described, opsin protein is synthesized in the inner segment and incorporated into the plasma membrane of the outer segment. Thus, there is little doubt that the first mechanism contributes to regeneration of rhodopsin.

Pigment regeneration by the second mechanism was first reported a century ago. Boll observed in 1876 that retinas excised from light-adapted animals were colorless, whereas the purple color was restored in retinas of animals that had been exposed to light and subsequently kept in the dark. Wald and associates established that the biochemical basis of pigment regeneration is a combination of opsin with a specific retinal isomer, 11-*cis* retinal [22].

How, then, is 11-*cis* retinal formed from all-*trans* retinal? A number of mechanisms have been considered. Because rhodopsin regeneration takes place in the dark, the isomerization of retinal was first believed to be an enzymatic process, and many attempts were made to identify "retinal isomerase." However, attempts have failed to demonstrate that

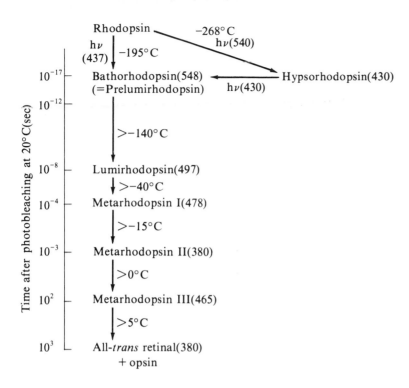

Time after photobleaching at 20°C(sec)

Rhodopsin
hν
(437) │ −195°C
−268°C
hν(540)

10^{-17} Bathorhodopsin(548) ← Hypsorhodopsin(430)
(=Prelumirhodopsin) hν(430)

10^{-12}

>−140°C

10^{-8} Lumirhodopsin(497)
>−40°C
10^{-4} Metarhodopsin I(478)

>−15°C

10^{-3} Metarhodopsin II(380)

>0°C

10^{2} Metarhodopsin III(465)

>5°C

10^{3} All-*trans* retinal(380)
+ opsin

Fig. 7-8. Intermediates detected spectrally after photic bleaching of vertebrate rhodopsin. The numbers in parentheses are wavelengths of light in nanometers used for irradiation or absorbed maximally by the individual intermediates.

11-*cis* retinal is formed by incubating, in the dark, all-*trans* retinal with excised retinas or rod outer segments. On the other hand, all-*trans* retinal is photochemically isomerized to 11-*cis* retinal in the presence of rod outer segments [23]. This activity is not due to an enzyme, because it is not destroyed by protein-denaturing agents. It can be accounted for by a mechanism of phosphatidylethanolamine catalysis [24]. Phosphatidylethanolamine forms a protonated Schiff base with retinal and, upon irradiation, effectively isomerizes all-*trans* retinal to the 11-*cis* form (Fig. 7-9). Rhodopsin in vitro is regenerated to opsin by transfer of the 11-*cis* isomer as a phospholipid complex. The transfer reaction occurs both in the light and in the dark and can explain rhodopsin regeneration during dark adaptation.

Photic isomerization of free retinal was long considered to be of little physiological importance, because 380 nm light, which would be absorbed by free retinal is found in the rod. These objections before it reaches the retina and because little or no free retinal is found in the rod. These objectives can be met, however, if in vivo isomerization of retinal occurs by absorption of the 460 nm light that the Schiff base complex absorbs maximally and if the retinal that is released from bleached pigment immediately forms a complex with phosphatidylethanolamine.

Another proposed mechanism involves the pigment epithelium. Dowling [25] irradiated albino rats with intense light (1000 foot-candles) and showed that the all-*trans* retinal released is reduced to retinol in the retina and stored in the pigment epithelium. He showed also that the stored retinol is sent back to the retina for pigment regeneration in the dark. From these results, a visual cycle involving a shuttle of retinol between the retina and the pigment epithelium was proposed (Fig. 7-10). It is

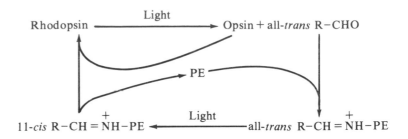

Fig. 7-9. The in situ visual cycle in the rod outer segment of the vertebrate retina. PE and R stand for phosphatidylethanolamine and $C_{19}H_{27}$, respectively.

not known if retinal is isomerized to the 11-*cis* form in the pigment epithelium or in the retina.

This mechanism may be operative under intense light, which is known to cause disintegration of rod membranes. When this happens, retinal is reduced to retinol and removed from the rod by the scavenger action of the pigment epithelium. However, this cannot be the only mechanism for regeneration of visual pigment. For example, rhodopsin regeneration in albino rats takes place efficiently without the pigment epithelium if the retina is incubated in a small, sealed chamber [26]. In addition, if retinol is shuttled between the retina and the pigment epithelium during adaptation cycles, the specific radioactivity of rhodopsin of animals that are labeled with radioactive retinol would increase with repetitions of the adaptation cycles. In both albino rats [27] and frogs [28], the specific radioactivity of the visual pigment was not increased by alternate adaptations to moderate lighting and darkness. These results suggest that, unless the rods are extensively bleached by intense light, the retinol released from bleached pigment may not migrate to the pigment epithelium. Under mild bleaching conditions, rhodopsin regeneration might also occur by a retinal utilization mechanism in situ in the rod outer segment (Fig. 7-9).

A third mechanism for regeneration would not depend on prior release of the all-*trans* retinal. For example, in squid rhodopsin, all-*trans* retinal is not released from bleached pigment, and pigment regeneration occurs by photic reisomerization of retinal at pH 10 and subsequent dark incubation [29]. When cone pigments are bleached by light, pigments can be regenerated by absorption of a second photon. This occurs by photic reisomerization of all-*trans* retinal still attached to opsin. These

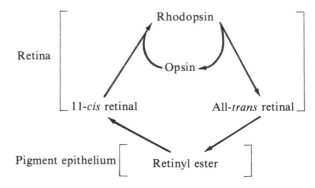

Fig. 7-10. The visual cycle in the vertebrate eye, in which both the retina and the pigment epithelium are involved.

mechanisms have yet to be confirmed by in vivo observations, and there may be other means for visual regeneration in vivo.

Visual Excitation

BIOPHYSICAL MODEL

The outer-segment membranes of vertebrate rods and cones show a resting potential of -30 to -40 mV, inside negative. Vertebrate cells are hyperpolarized by photobleaching of the visual pigment, whereas invertebrate cells (e.g., in *Limulus*) are depolarized by light. In view of the highly ordered structure of photoreceptors that resemble macromolecular crystals, a mechanism involving electron or hole conduction was proposed for light-dependent

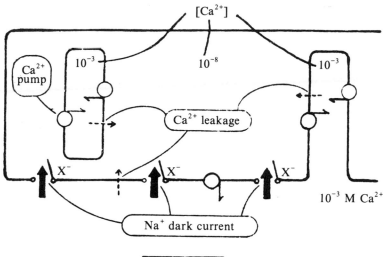

A. Dark

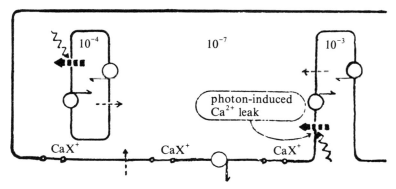

B. Light

Fig. 7-11. Modulation of Na⁺ current by Ca²⁺ for visual excitation in vertebrate rods and cones [32].

modulation of the membrane potential [30]. Accumulated evidence [31], however, is overwhelmingly in favor of the ionic mechanism and gives little support to the semiconduction mechanism.

According to the ionic mechanism, the steady potentials of vertebrate photoreceptor membranes in the dark result from the entry of Na^+ into outer segments and the pumping out of Na^+ across the plasma membrane of the inner segment. Light blocks the entry of Na^+ without affecting the sodium pump. A decrease in intracellular Na^+ con-

centration results in hyperpolarization of the membrane. This mechanism is supported by the observations that the transmembrane potentials are reduced by lowering Na^+ concentrations in the medium and are inhibited by ouabain, the inhibitor of (Na^+-K^+)-ATPase. The extent of light-induced hyperpolarization of vertebrate photoreceptors (or of depolarization, in the case of invertebrate photoreceptors) depends on the wavelength and intensity of irradiating light.

Bleaching of the visual pigment occurs in disc membranes, but it is the plasma membrane that is hyperpolarized. How can a signal generated by photon absorption in the disc membrane be transmitted to the plasma membrane? Hagins [32] has

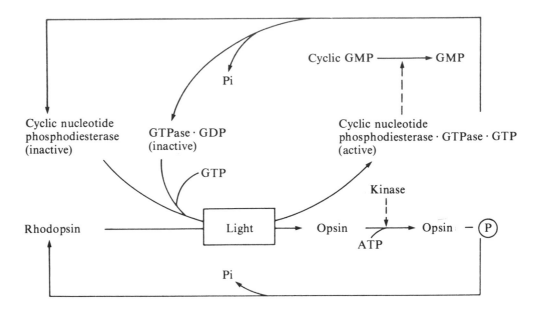

Fig. 7-12. Light-elicited biochemical reactions.

proposed a model in which visual excitation of vertebrate rod and cone photoreceptors is modulated by Ca^{2+}. According to this model (Fig. 7-11), the outer-segment membrane shows high Na^+ permeability in the dark. As soon as rhodopsin molecules in the disc membrane are bleached by light, Ca^{2+} sequestered inside the disc is released and closes the Na^+ entry channels in the plasma membrane. Since the Na^+ pump is not affected by light, pumping Na^+ out of the cell continues in the light. The decreased intracellular Na^+ concentration results in hyperpolarization of the plasma membrane. The number of Na^+ entry channels in the outer-segment plasma membrane of a rod cell is calculated at about 1,000. Closing off a few percent of the channels should suffice to induce the hyperpolarization actually measured. Cone discs are continuous with the plasma membrane, and Ca^{2+} inside the disc and in the outside medium are not separated. The model suggests, therefore, that photobleaching of visual pigments in cone photoreceptors is coupled with rapid movement of external Ca^{2+} into the cytoplasm. For the model to function continuously, there must be a mechanism by which Ca^{2+} is accumulated within the discs in the dark. Firm experimental evidence for the Ca^{2+} hypothesis has yet to be presented.

In addition to an inflow of Na^+, formation of a proton gradient across the photoreceptor membrane may also contribute to generation of the transmembrane potential. For example, the amplitude of electroretinograms evoked by a high-intensity light increases with a rise in the pH and decreases at lowered pH [33]. The pH of the medium in which retinas are bathed rises rapidly upon illumination [34]. Light-induced proton uptake in bovine outer segments accompanies changes in disc volumes [35]. In this connection, an interesting observation was made on bacteriorhodopsin, a rhodopsinlike pigment present in the purple membrane of halobacteria [36]. When the membrane is irradiated by light, a proton gradient is formed across the membrane and a transmembrane potential as high as 50 mV is generated [37].

BIOCHEMICAL MODEL
Biochemical reactions that occur immediately after photobleaching of visual pigments are summarized in Fig. 7-12.

The light-dependent phosphorylation of rhodopsin [38–40] is too slow to be involved in visual transduction. The protein kinase involved is specific for rhodopsin and is not stimulated by cyclic nucleotide [41]. Two other enzymes, cyclic nucleotide phosphodiesterase [42] and GTPase [43–44], in the rod are activated by light. Phosphodiesterase requires GTP for activation, and its hydrolysis to GDP by light-activated GTPase for inactivation. Thus, phosphodiesterase activation by light occurs as a transient phenomenon. The activated form of phosphodiesterase is probably a complex of the enzyme with GTPase and GTP. If the phosphodiesterase activation occurs within a few milliseconds after light absorption and a large number of cyclic GMP molecules are hydrolyzed per photon absorbed, the regulation of cyclic nucleotide phosphodiesterase can serve as a biochemical amplification mechanism. In attempts to link biochemical findings to electrophysiology, the effect of cyclic GMP on rod membrane potentials was studied. Cyclic GMP caused effects similar to those of lowered extracellular Ca^{2+} concentrations and depolarized rod membranes [45]. Intracellular injection of cyclic GMP resulted in an increase in the latency of the membrane to be hyperpolarized by light [46]. The biochemical mechanism underlying the effect of cyclic GMP on rod membranes remains unidentified.

References

*1. Graham, L. T.   Comparative Physiology. In H. Dawson and L. T. Graham (eds.), *The Eye,* Vol. 6. New York: Academic, 1974.

*2. Bonting, S. L. (ed.).   *Transmitters in the Visual Process.* Oxford: Pergamon, 1976.

*3. Jung, R. (ed.).   *Handbook of Sensory Physiology.* Vol. 7/3. Part A, *Central Processing of Visual Information;* Part B, *Visual Centers in the Brain.* Heidelberg: Springer-Verlag, 1973.

*4. Zeki, S.   Functional specialization in the visual cortex of the rhesus monkey. *Nature* 274:423–428, 1978.

*5. Fuortes, M. G. F. (ed.).   *Physiology of Photoreceptor Organs. Handbook of Sensory Physiology,* Vol. 7/2. Heidelberg: Springer-Verlag, 1972.

*6. Knowles, A., and Dartnall, H. J. A.   The Photobiology of Vision. In H. Dawson (ed.), *The Eye,* Vol. 2B. New York: Academic Press, 1977.

*7. Young, R. W.   Visual cells and the concept of renewal. *Invest. Opthalmol.* 15:700–725, 1976.

8. LaVail, M. M.   Rod outer segment disk shedding in rat retina: Relationships to cyclic lighting. *Science* 194:1071–1074, 1976.

9. Basinger, S., Hoffman, R., and Matthes, M.   Photoreceptor shedding is initiated by light in the frog retina. *Science* 194:1074–1076, 1976.

10. Singer, S. J., and Nicolson, G. L.   The fluid model of the structure of cell membranes. *Science* 175:720–731, 1972.

11. Brown, P. K.   Rhodopsin rotates in the visual receptor membrane. *Nat. New Biol.* 236:35–38, 1972.

12. Liang, C-J., et al.   Structure of the carbohydrate moieties of bovine rhodopsin. *J. Biol. Chem.* 254:6414–6418, 1979.

13. Poo, M., and Cone, R. A.   Lateral diffusion of rhodopsin in the photoreceptor membrane. *Nature* 247:438–441, 1974.

14. Chabre, M.   X-ray diffraction studies of retinal rods. I. Structure of the disc membrane, effect of illumination. *Biochim. Biophys. Acta* 382:322–335, 1975.

15. Wu, C. W., and Stryer, L.   Proximity relationship in rhodopsin. *Proc. Natl. Acad. Sci. U.S.A.* 69:1104–1108, 1972.

16. Chan, W. K., et al.   Properties of 14-methylretinal, 13-desmethyl-14-methylretinal, and visual pigments formed therefrom. *J. Am. Chem. Soc.* 96:3642–3644, 1974.

17. Busch, G. E., et al.   Formation and decay of prelumirhodopsin at room temperatures. *Proc. Natl. Acad. Sci. U.S.A.* 69:2802–2806, 1972.

18. Applebury, M. L., et al.   Rhodopsin. Purification and recombination with phospholipids assayed by the metarhodopsin I–metarhodopsin II transition. *Biochemistry* 13:3448–3458, 1974.

19. Liebman, P. A., et al.   Membrane structure changes in rod outer segments associated with rhodopsin bleaching. *Nature* 251:31–36, 1974.

20. Rotmans, J. P., Daemen, F. J. M., and Bonting, S. L.   Biochemical aspects of the visual process. XXVI. Binding site and migration of retinaldehyde during rhodopsin photolysis. *Biochim. Biophys. Acta* 357:151–158, 1974.

21. Rushton, W. A. H.   A cone pigment in the protanope. *J. Physiol.* (London) 168:345–359, 1963; A foveal pigment in the deuteranope. *J. Physiol.* (London) 176:24–37, 1965.

22. Wald, G., and Brown, P. K.   Synthesis and bleaching of rhodopsin. *Nature* 177:174–176, 1956.

23. Hubbard, R.   Retinene isomerase. *J. Gen. Physiol.* 39:935–962, 1955.

24. Shichi, H., and Somers, R. L.   Possible involvement of retinylidene phospholipid in photoisomeri-

*Key reference.

zation of all-*trans* to 11-*cis* retinal. *J. Biol. Chem.* 249:6570–6577, 1974.

25. Dowling, J. E.   Chemistry of visual adaptation in the rat. *Nature* 188:114–118, 1960.

26. Cone, R. A., and Brown, P. K.   Spontaneous regeneration of rhodopsin in the isolated rat retina. *Nature* 221:818–820, 1969.

27. Bridges, C. D. B., and Yoshikami, A.   Uptake of tritiated retinaldehyde by the visual pigment of dark-adapted rats. *Nature* 221:275–276, 1969.

28. Hall, M. O., and Bok, D.   Incorporation of [^{3}H] vitamin A into rhodopsin in light- and dark-adapted frogs. *Exp. Eye Res.* 18:105–117, 1974.

29. Suzuki, T., Sugahara, M., and Kito, Y.   An intermediate in the photoregeneration of squid rhodopsin. *Biochim. Biophys. Acta* 275:260–270, 1972.

30. Rosenberg, B.   A physical approach to the visual receptor process. *Adv. Radiat. Biol.* 2:193–241, 1966.

*31. Tomita, T.   Electrical activity of vertebrate photoreceptors. *Q. Rev. Biophys.* 3:179–222, 1970.

*32. Hagins, W. A.   The visual process: Excitatory mechanisms in the primary receptor cells. *Annu. Rev. Biophys. Bioeng.* 1:131–158, 1972.

33. Winkler, B. S.   The electroretinogram of the isolated rat retina. *Vision Res.* 12:1183–1198, 1972.

34. Ostroy, S. E.   Hydrogen ion changes of rhodopsin. pK changes and the thermal decay of metarhodopsin II$_{380}$. *Arch. Biochem. Biophys.* 164:275–284, 1974.

35. McConnel, D. G.   Relationship of the light-induced proton uptake in bovine retinal outer segment fragments to Triton-induced membrane disruption and to volume changes. *J. Biol. Chem.* 250: 1898–1906, 1975.

36. Oesterhelt, D., and Stoeckenius, W.   Rhodopsin-like protein from the purple membrane of *Halobacterium halobium. Nat. New Biol.* 233:149–152, 1971.

37. Drachev, L. A., et al.   Electrogenesis by bacteriorhodopsin incorporated in a planar phospholipid membrane. *FEBS Lett.* 39:43–45, 1974.

38. Kuhn, H., Cook, J. H., and Dreyer, W. J.   Phosphorylation of rhodopsin in bovine photoreceptor membranes. A dark reaction after illumination. *Biochemistry* 12:2495–2501, 1973.

39. Bownds, D., et al.   Phosphorylation of frog photoreceptor membranes induced by light. *Nat. New Biol.* 237:125–127, 1972.

40. Frank, R. N., Cavanaugh, H. D., and Kenyon, K. R.   Light-stimulated phosphorylation of bovine visual pigments by adenosine triphosphate. *J. Biol. Chem.* 248:596–609, 1973.

41. Shichi, H., and Somers, R. L.   Light-dependent phosphorylation of rhodopsin. Purification and properties of rhodopsin kinase. *J. Biol. Chem.* 253: 7040–7046, 1978.

42. Miki, N., et al.   Purification and properties of the light-activated cyclic nucleotide phosphodiesterase of rod outer segments. *J. Biol. Chem.* 250:6320–6327, 1975.

43. Robinson, W. E., and Hagins, W. A.   A light-activated GTPase in retinal rod outer segments. *Biophys. J.* 17:196a, 1977.

44. Wheeler, G. L., and Bitensky, M. W.   A light-activated GTPase in vertebrate photoreceptors: Regulation of light-activated cyclic GMP phosphodiesterase. *Proc. Natl. Acad. Sci. U.S.A.* 74:4238–4242, 1977.

45. Lipton, S. A., Rasmussen, H., and Dowling, J. E.   Electrical and adaptive properties of rod photoreceptors in *Bufo marinus*. II. Effects of cyclic nucleotides and prostaglandins. *J. Gen. Physiol.* 70:771–791, 1977.

46. Nicol, G. D., and Miller, W. H.   Cyclic GMP injected into retinal rod outer segments increases latency and amplitude of response to illumination. *Proc. Natl. Acad. Sci. U.S.A.* 75:5217–5220, 1978.

47. Fukuda, M. N., et al.   Rhodopsin carbohydrate. Structure of small oligosaccharides attached at two sites near the NH$_2$ terminus. *J. Biol. Chem.* 254: 8201–8207, 1979.

Section III. Synaptic Function

David O. Carpenter
Thomas S. Reese

Chapter 8. Chemistry and Physiology of Synaptic Transmission

In 1921, Loewi [1] reported the first of a series of studies that showed that the inhibitory nerves to the heart exert their effect through release of a chemical neurotransmitter, acetylcholine. Chemical transmission is now accepted as the principal means of communication between a neuron and its target, whether that be another neuron, a muscle, or a gland. The process of synaptic transmission involves synthesis and storage of a transmitter substance in the presynaptic terminal, release of that substance into extracellular space, and interaction of the transmitter with specific receptors on the postsynaptic membrane that trigger either electrical or biochemical alteration in the postsynaptic cell.

Synaptic Transmission

Much of the detailed knowledge of the process of synaptic transmission has come from study of the vertebrate neuromuscular junction, which uses acetylcholine as an excitatory neurotransmitter. At this synapse, and at many others, there is a close approximation of the nerve terminal and the postsynaptic cell, with transmission occurring at discrete sites characterized by specializations of presynaptic and postsynaptic membranes. It has been customary to distinguish a "neurotransmitter," released where there is intimate association between presynaptic and postsynaptic elements, from a "neurohormone," which is released into the circulation to travel some distance before reaching its receptor. That is, however, a description of only two extremes of chemical transmission and is not a very useful distinction.

In some tissues, such as intestine, nerve terminals are without close association to specific smooth muscle cells and release transmitter into extra-cellular space, where it diffuses locally to influence a number of cells. A particular transmitter may act locally at some synapses but may be released from a different store to act at distant receptors. For example, norepinephrine neurons in the central nervous system form contacts with close association to the postsynaptic cell; chromaffin cells of the adrenal medulla release norepinephrine into the circulation, from which it is carried to smooth muscle throughout the body. Moreover, the effects of a particular transmitter may be quite different on different tissues and at different sites. The recent demonstrations of neurotransmitter roles for substances previously known only as digestive system hormones are consistent with the broad generalization that nature may use a substance for very different, but specific, functions at different locations, depending upon which effector mechanism is coupled to the receptor.

The mechanisms of synthesis, storage, and release of neurotransmitters are, in general, not different from those in nonnervous cells that secrete very different products, such as enzymes and hormones. With the possible exception of some lipophilic molecules, such as steroids, the secretory product is stored in granules or vesicles and is released by the process of exocytosis, where the membrane-bound vesicle fuses with the plasma membrane and releases its contents into the extracellular medium. The most critical event for release is Ca^{2+} entry. In all systems where exocytosis is known to occur, it is Ca^{2+} dependent [2].

Most neurons are electrically excitable, and the function of the action potential is both to carry information rapidly over long distances and to trigger Ca^{2+} entry into the terminal to induce transmitter release. Electrical excitability is not an exclusive property of neurons, however, as other secretory cells, such as the β cells of the pancreas, chromaffin cells of the adrenal medulla, and endocrine cells of the pituitary pars distalis and intermedia also generate action potentials [3, 4]. On the other hand, not all neurons convey action potentials. Many neurons in retina (receptor, horizontal, and bipolar cells) and some neurons in olfactory bulb function without generation of action potentials [5] and release transmitter in a graded manner, which presumably is regulated by a graded, voltage-dependent Ca^{2+} permeability. Although these considerations make it difficult to define which cells are neurons and which are not, it seems certain that release of neurotransmitters occurs by Ca^{2+}-dependent exocytosis, whether or not the entry of Ca^{2+} is triggered by an action potential.

Putative Neurotransmitters

The number of substances endogenous to nerve cells that may act as transmitters has increased considerably in the past few years. In addition to acetylcholine (Chap. 9), the catecholamines (dopamine, norepinephrine, and epinephrine) have been shown convincingly to be neurotransmitters in both peripheral and central nervous systems. For dopamine, norepinephrine, and the indoleamine 5-hydroxytryptamine (serotonin), identification of neurons containing the transmitter has been facilitated by the development of fluorescent histochemical techniques (see Chaps. 10 and 11). Other primary amines (histamine, octopamine, phenylethylamine, and phenylethanolamine) and polyamines (putrecine, spermine, and spermidine) may also be transmitters. A number of amino acids also have well-documented effects on neurons. These include glutamic and aspartic acids, glycine, β-alanine, γ-aminobutyric acid (GABA), taurine, and possibly proline (Chap. 12). An evaluation of the physiological function of these substances is complicated by their ubiquitous distribution in cells. Other relatively small molecules have at times been suggested as neurotransmitters; these include calcium ion, adenosine, adenosine triphosphate (ATP), cyclic adenosine monophosphate (cyclic AMP), guanosine triphosphate (GTP), cyclic

guanosine monophosphate (cyclic GMP), cytosine triphosphate (CTP), estrogen, testosterone, corticosterone, and various prostaglandins.

A major development within the past few years has been the appreciation of the role of small peptides as neurotransmitters. Substance P, an 11–amino-acid peptide, was described as an active agent as early as 1931 by von Euler and Gaddum [6], but it was only with the work of Leeman and associates, who determined the sequence and developed radioimmunoassay methods for identification, that this peptide has been widely recognized as an important neurotransmitter [see 7]. A variety of peptides are present and distributed asymmetrically in nervous tissue. These range in size from carnosine and thyrotropin-releasing hormone (TRH) (2 and 3 amino acids, respectively) to neurotensin and somatostatin (13 and 14 amino acids, respectively). Other putative peptide neurotransmitters include the enkephalins and endorphins, which may be the brain's natural morphine; agents that have hormone actions elsewhere, such as insulin, angiotensin I and II, vasoactive intestinal polypeptide, cholecystokinin, prolactin, vasopressin, and oxytocin; and releasing factors, such as luteinizing hormone–releasing hormone (LH-RH), melanocyte-stimulating hormone release inhibiting hormone (MIF-1), and somatostatin release-inhibiting hormone. A number of other active peptides have been described in both invertebrates and vertebrates, but with less knowledge of structure and action (see Chaps. 13 and 14).

The number of substances that must be considered putative neurotransmitters is at present at least 50, and is growing rapidly. However, there has been a rigorous proof of transmitter function for only a very few. With the realization that small peptides can be neurotransmitters, the possibilities for active agents becomes mind-boggling and the difficulties in chemical and physiological identification become enormous.

CRITERIA FOR IDENTIFICATION OF NEUROTRANSMITTERS

A number of criteria must be met to consider a substance a proven neurotransmitter. None of these criteria is adequate by itself, but it is also unlikely that all can be clearly established for each substance. The criteria fall into the following categories:

1. The neurotransmitter is present in nerve terminals. The content may be demonstrated by chemical measurement, histofluorescence, or immunological markers. Autoradiographical localization after administration of a labeled transmitter or precurser is suggestive of a transmitter role but must not be considered proof, because uptake systems may not be specific. Demonstration of lack of content in a cell body does not disprove the possibility that the substance is a transmitter, because synthesis may occur only in the terminals. In peripheral organs, the transmitter stores should disappear subsequent to denervation and reappear on innervation. This criterion applies only to tissues in which the nerve terminals degenerate and are not supported by glia after being severed from the cell body. Although this is a helpful criterion in peripheral tissues, it is often difficult to achieve selective and total denervation in the central nervous system. Furthermore, multiple inputs to a single area of brain may use the same transmitter, complicating interpretation of the results of denervation.

2. A transmitter is released upon nerve stimulation. However, not every substance released need be considered a neurotransmitter. For instance, adrenal medullary cells release adenine, ATP, ADP, AMP, and dopamine β-hydroxylase, together with catecholamines [8]. The postsynaptic response is due principally or solely to norepinephrine, and the other substances presumably are released only because they are stored in the same granules.

3. The effects of the putative neurotransmitter, when applied to the postsynaptic membrane, are the same as those caused by stimulation of the presynaptic nerve and occur in concentrations within the range of transmitter concentrations released from the nerve terminal.

4. The dose-response curve of the applied putative neurotransmitter is altered by drugs in the same direction and magnitude as are the natural synaptic potentials.

5. A mechanism exists locally to inactivate the neurotransmitter. A variety of mechanisms are possible. Acetylcholine is degraded by acetylcholinesterase; amino acids are probably inactivated principally by transport into either nerve terminals or glial cells. Catecholamines are either transported into nerve terminals or degraded, and peptides are probably degraded by peptidases. This criterion is important in identification of transmitters at discrete synapses, but it is also important not to have too rapid removal of substances which must reach their target tissue through the blood or by diffusion over considerable distances. Thus, diffusion and dilution may also be mechanisms of inactivation.

Dale's Principle

In 1933, Sir Henry Dale [9] proposed that the term *cholinergic* be used for neurons that release acetylcholine, and the term *adrenergic* be applied to neurons that release norepinephrine (adrenalin). Later [10] he noted that, upon regeneration of specific neurons, the original transmitter was restored. In 1957, Eccles [11] proposed a generalization that he called *Dale's principle*. Spinal motoneurons of mammals have two axons: a large one to muscle; and a small one (the *recurrent collateral*), which excites an interneuron (the *Renshaw cell*) that inhibits the motoneuron. Eccles and his colleagues demonstrated that the excitatory neurotransmitter at the synapse between the recurrent collateral of spinal motoneurons and Renshaw cells in the spinal cord was acetylcholine, as it is at the neuromuscular junction [12]. On the basis of these studies and Dale's observations, Eccles proposed [11]: (1) a given neuron contains and releases only one neurotransmitter, and (2) a neuron is either excitatory or inhibitory, but it cannot exert different functional effects at different termination sites. This principle has been widely accepted by a generation of neurobiologists and has been a valuable generalization.

However, while it is clear that many or most neurons use primarily one transmitter, there is now sufficient evidence contrary to both tenets of Dale's principle to indicate that it should be abandoned. Kandel and coworkers [13] definitively disproved the second premise by demonstrating that a single interneuron (cell L_{10}) in the abdominal ganglion of the marine mollusk *Aplysia* released acetylcholine, which caused a monosynaptic, Na^+-dependent excitation of one neuron (cell R_{15}) and a monosynaptic Cl^--dependent inhibition of another (cell L_3). The response depends on the postsynaptic membrane, as well as on the transmitter. It now has been shown that individual sympathetic neurons maintained in tissue culture may contain and release either acetylcholine, norepinephrine, or both [14]. Although these results could be questioned on the basis of being obtained from cultured cells, which may not be normally differentiated, there is also biochemical evidence that many large, single invertebrate neurons contain [15], and possibly release [16], more than one neurotransmitter; and there is morphological evidence that mammalian neurons contain peptides and nonpeptides in the same terminal [17–19]. Evidence for the presence of two putative transmitters is not proof that both are released or that there are postsynaptic receptors for both, but it appears very likely that these terminals do use more than one transmitter and that the substances may have quite different postsynaptic effects. As discussed under Synaptic Modulation below, peptides in particular frequently have been found to modulate the postsynaptic responses to other transmitters; and the presence of two transmitters in one terminal may signify an ability to modulate synaptic efficiency at that synapse.

Mechanisms of Transmitter Release

Many of the fundamental discoveries concerning release of transmitter from synapses were made on isolated frog nerve-muscle preparations. The preparations have the advantage that recordings are readily made from the muscle near neuromuscular junctions. Such recordings led to one of the most important and well-known discoveries in neurobiology—that the transmitter is released in quanta, or packets, each containing approximately 10,000 molecules of acetylcholine [20]. Even in the absence of neural activity, quanta are released con-

tinuously, at a rate that approaches 1 per second. When an action potential in the nerve invades the nerve terminals on the muscle, this rate is increased more than four orders of magnitude, so a few hundred quanta are released in just a few milliseconds. Quantal release is now known to take place at a variety of other types of synapses. Furthermore, the morphology of the apparatus for the release of quanta (see Presynaptic Active Zone, below) seems to be a universal feature of synapses [21, 22], so there is no reason to reject the notion that release of quanta is the usual means of releasing neurotransmitters from synapses in both the brain and in the peripheral nervous system. Acetylcholine also leaks directly across the membranes of nerve terminals, but it remains to be seen whether it influences the muscle [23].

The electron microscope was used to examine synapses only after the quantal nature of transmitter release had been discovered. It was learned that the motor nerve terminal contains about a half-million vesicles filled with acetylcholine. Opening a vesicle could result in releasing many acetylcholine molecules, perhaps the 10,000 that constitute the physiological quantum [24]. This notion, that one synaptic vesicle contains and releases one quantum, came to be known as the "vesicle hypothesis." Because vesicles are definitive of synapses in the peripheral and central nervous systems of both vertebrates and invertebrates, it became important to know whether the vesicle hypothesis is true (Fig. 8-1). As time passed, that hypothesis has seemed more and more correct, although some conflicting evidence has appeared [25]. Other views are discussed also in Chap. 9.

One of the most striking pieces of evidence for the vesicle hypothesis is that isolated synaptic vesicles contain transmitters (see Chaps. 9–11). We have already mentioned that release of quanta requires calcium. In this respect, the process resembles the release of hormones and other secretory substances from gland and blood cells by the process of exocytosis [26]. The question, then, is whether transmitter is released from nerve terminals by exocytosis, and whether each exocytosis results in the release of one quantum.

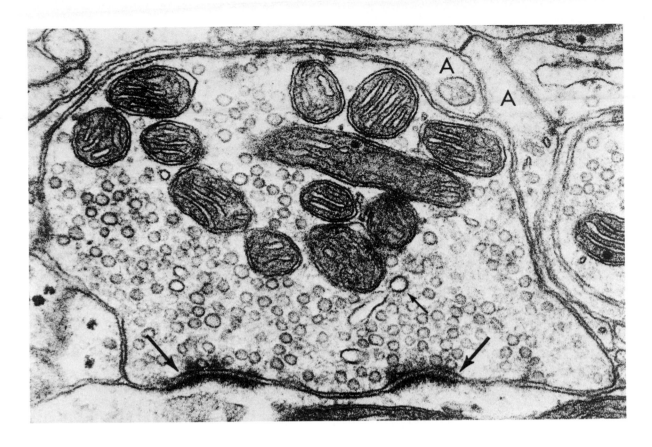

Fig. 8-1. Synapse from brain stem showing two active zones (large arrows). Typical contents are synaptic and coated (small arrow) vesicles, mitochondria, and variously shaped cisterns of endoplasmic reticulum. Vesicles cluster near active zones and nestle between the patches of dense fuzz on its cytoplasmic surface. Synapse is surrounded by astrocytic processes (A). From [21] with permission. ×60,000

Another piece of evidence for the vesicle hypothesis comes from examination of nerve-muscle or nerve-nerve synapses after intense activity induced by nerve stimulation. Transmitter release results in the depletion of synaptic vesicles, concomitant with an increase in presynaptic membrane surface area. This finding could be explained neatly if synaptic vesicles add their membrane to the surface membrane during activity [27, 28]. Other evidence emerged from stimulating adrenergic nerve-muscle synapses. Here it was shown that a protein, dopamine β-hydroxylase, is released concomitantly with the catecholamine transmitter; it is difficult to point to any mechanism other than exocytosis that could account for this stoichiometric release of a protein along with a transmitter [29].

Nevertheless, it proved difficult to visualize exocytosis directly in conventional electron micrographs, perhaps because the exocytotic opening is smaller than the thickness of typical sections. The freeze-fracture technique seemed more promising for this purpose, because when tissue is fixed, frozen, and broken open, the fracture tends to split membranes and therefore to follow their hydrophobic interiors. While still frozen, this fractured surface can be replicated with platinum and examined with a resolution of approximately 2 nm, which is fine enough to see where intrinsic membrane proteins cross the lipid bilayer. With this approach, the stomata of synaptic vesicles in the act of exocytosis were seen consistently in synapses fixed during quantal release, and any agent that blocked release blocked the exocytosis [30]. Furthermore, exocytosis did not depend on action potentials in the nerve, because it occurred when such agents as spider venom acted directly on nerve terminals to release transmitter [31].

The Presynaptic Active Zone

The striking finding that emerged from freeze-fracture studies of synapses is that exocytosis is limited to certain regions of the synapse or nerve terminal, and therefore uses only a small percentage of the synaptic membrane surface [30, 32]. This confirmed Couteaux's prescient suggestion that a nerve has "active zones" for transmitter release [33]. Recognition of active zones led to the interesting concept that the majority of *individual* active zones fail to release a quantum after a nerve impulse. For instance, there are approximately 500 active zones in the frog nerve-muscle synapse, yet less than half this number of quanta are released after a nerve stimulation (Fig. 8-2) [20]. At nerve-nerve synapses, a single nerve may form huge calyces or branch to form multiple boutons, each with one or a few active zones on the same or multiple target cells [34]. Where boutons from a single nerve are deployed on many different target cells, the patterns of synaptic connectivity could vary considerably from impulse to impulse if the number of quanta were close to or less than the number of boutons (Fig. 8-1).

The morphology of active zones also suggests important questions for further investigation. Large intramembrane particles are present near the active zone, and consideration of their universal deployment and numbers at presynaptic active zones leads to the suggestion that they are the channels that admit the calcium that initiates transmitter release (Fig. 8-3) [30]. The cytoplasm of nerve terminals near active zones always contains a fuzzy material that makes contact with the releasable active-zone vesicles. It is important to know the role of this material in inserting a new vesicle back into the active zone after it undergoes

exocytosis, or for initiating the membrane interactions that lead to exocytosis (Figs. 8-1 and 8-2). Finally, it remains to be determined whether all chemical synaptic transmission is at active zones [21].

At the same time that evidence was accumulating that quantal release depends on exocytosis [35], other evidence suggested that the relationship might not be one quantum to one vesicle. Indeed, freeze-fracture micrographs taken through active synapses revealed many more vesicle openings than would be expected if the chemical fixatives were capturing only one or a few cycles of release [30]. Also, unit potentials that were only a fraction of the size of the quantum potential were found at frog nerve-muscle synapses; a quantum seemed to be made up of several concomitant smaller release events [36]. Finally, a glimpse at the statistical properties of quantal release from individual active zones was made possible by extracellular recordings from short segments of nerve terminal. The variability from release cycle to release cycle turned out to be very high, suggesting that the active zones themselves were the basic statistical unit of release. If the 10,000 or more vesicles at the active zones were the pool from which the several quanta were drawn, the variability between release cycles should have been a Poisson rather than the observed binomial distribution [37]. These dis-

Fig. 8-2. Longitudinal thin section through a nerve terminal on a frog muscle fiber. This view represents approximately 1/100 the length of the several terminals which comprise a neuromuscular junction. Active zones at asterisks should be compared with those in the nerve-nerve synapse in Fig. 8-1: they appear smaller because they are bar-shaped and the bar has been cross-sectioned. The postsynaptic component of the active zone, represented by the thicker membrane at the tops of the folds in the muscle surface, is much more extensive. Finally, there are many more active zones, though it must be noted that an axon in the brain may give rise to many synapses containing active zones such as those shown in Fig. 8-1. Nerve terminal is surrounded by flat processes of Schwann cells (S) which periodically interdigitate between the terminal and the muscle. From [21] with permission. ×40,000

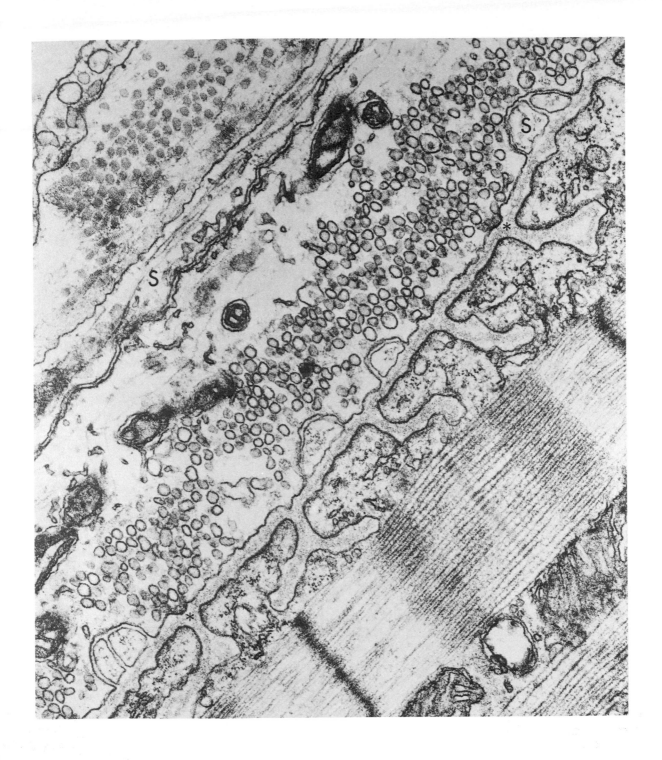

parate observations could be given a unified explanation if each exocytotic event released only part of a quantum, a "microquantum," which then would somehow be synchronized with several other microquanta. One could imagine that the necessary synchrony between exocytotic events could most easily be accomplished if all the release constituting a quantum were at the same active zone, which would then be regarded as the basic structural unit of transmitter release.

A choice between this concept of synaptic transmission and a one-to-one vesicle hypothesis (which would leave the morphological basis of microquanta [38] unexplained!) could only be made by techniques that could show morphological events in real time, that is, by freezing the synapse directly by a process requiring only a few milliseconds, rather than the many seconds that are required for chemical fixation [21]. By this means, the number of quanta released at a frog nerve-muscle synapse could be compared to the number of exocytotic events that result from a single nerve stimulation (Fig. 8-3). It turned out that, over a wide range of transmitter release (augmented by potassium-blocking agents such as 4-aminopyridine), one quantum accompanies one exocytotic event, implying that in this preparation the vesicle hypothesis is correct [35].

The fate of the synaptic vesicle membrane inserted into the nerve terminal membrane during exocytosis must now be considered. It was mentioned that nerve terminals and synapses increase in circumference during activity. This was interpreted to mean that synaptic-vesicle membrane is at least transiently added to their surfaces. When the freezing technique was applied to stimulated nerve terminals, it was possible to add the observation that a particulate component of the synaptic vesicle membrane was added at the active zone and diffused out, to be collected and internalized several seconds later by endocytosis of coated vesicles [39]. This interpretation, however, is currently under debate [40]. The process has been followed less directly with tracer proteins, such as horseradish peroxidase, which are taken up in coated vesicles and end up in synaptic vesicles. A scheme for "recycling" synaptic vesicle membrane locally at the frog nerve-muscle synapse summarizes these observations, but exactly how synaptic vesicle membranes are sorted out and made into new synaptic vesicles remains to be seen (Fig. 8-4) [41].

Other important questions in synaptic structure are where transmitter is inserted into new synaptic vesicles, how and the extent to which local recycling is supplemented by axoplasmic transport, and the extent to which noncholinergic, central nervous system synapses depend on local recycling [42].

Little is known about the final stages in the development of the presynaptic active zone, but the remarkable cytoplasmic reorganization that occurs when an axonal growth cone moving over a substrate in a culture meets an appropriate neuronal target may be representative of the earlier stages in the process [43]. This transformation may be triggered by small junctions, which form almost immediately after contact, or by undefined soluble factors, but the inducing factor produces the striking result that the growth cone flattens against the target cell and no longer emits microspikes [44]. Inside, the extensive tubular and vesicular systems, and the filamentous matrix and lysosomal systems characteristic of a motile growth cone, are replaced by the filamentous microtubular synaptic core and the synaptic vesicle domains associated with active zones.

Structure of the Postsynaptic Active Zone

Postsynaptic active zones also have been recognized where synaptic terminals make contact with nerves or muscles [21]. The position, but not necessarily the size, of the postsynaptic active zone matches that of the presynaptic active zone (Figs. 8-1 and 8-2). The internal membrane structure of postsynaptic active zones varies with the type of transmitter used, but it would not be surprising if the secretory mechanism were the same for different transmitters, which, however, require different ion channel–receptor complexes [45]. Nevertheless, certain generalities apply to the structure of the postsynaptic active zone.

At most types of postsynaptic active zones, intramembrane particles are more concentrated

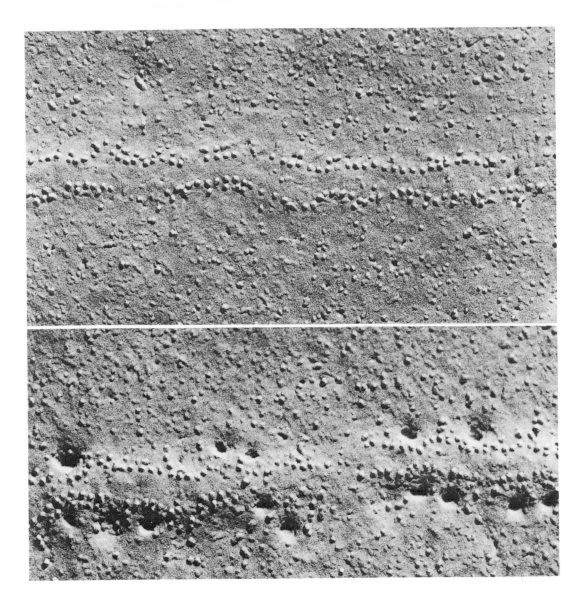

Fig. 8-3. Freeze-fractured active zones from frog resting and stimulated neuromuscular junction. The active zone is the region of presynaptic membrane surrounding double rows of intramembrane particles, which may be channels for the calcium entry that initiates transmitter release. Holes that appear in active zones during transmitter release (lower picture) are openings of synaptic vesicles engaged in exocytosis. This muscle was prepared by quick-freezing, and transmitter release was augmented with 4-amino-pyridine, so the morphological events (opening of synaptic vesicles) could be examined at the exact moment of transmitter release evoked by a single nerve shock. From [39] with permission. ×120,000

than over the rest of the membrane (Fig. 8-5). This concentration varies up to 10,000 per sq μm in cholinergic systems (a 100 to 1 increase over that on the remaining membrane [30]) and down to aggregates barely discernible from those in the rest of the membrane at certain central nervous system synapses [46, 47]. The organization within the aggregate can also vary from linear arrays to dispersed types of spacings where distances between particles are relatively constant.

For cholinergic nerve-muscle synapses, there is good evidence that these particles are the sites of ion channel–receptor complexes, and that the heads of these particles protrude beyond the outer surface of the postsynaptic active zone into the synaptic cleft. The synaptic cleft contains a basement membrane, or a similar, fuzzy material, concentrated in the center of the cleft at nerve-nerve synapses, and side-arms periodically arise from the central skein of cleft material to make contact with the surface of the postsynaptic active zone [47]. At nerve-muscle synapses, the cytoplasmic side of this membrane is also "thickened" by a coat of fuzzy material 5 to 10 nm wide, and similar coats of material seem to be a general feature of postsynaptic active zones, regardless of the chemical type of the synapse (Fig. 8-2).

Structural variability between the active zones of different chemical types of synapses is mainly in the concentration, size, and fracturing characteristics of the intramembrane components, and in the extent to which this component, or perhaps additional components, extend into the cytoplasm. The postsynaptic active zone, therefore, is a membrane complex that involves both the cytoplasmic and external surfaces of the postsynaptic membrane [21]. Its edges are very sharp, and the sharpness persists even at the edges of large postsynaptic active zones, where groups containing several hundred receptors separate into patches. These membrane complexes are more stable than the rest of the membrane. Turnover of cholinergic receptors at the active zone has a time course of days, and active zones in general maintain their organization in the face of metabolic or mechanical damages that alter the rest of the surface membrane [48].

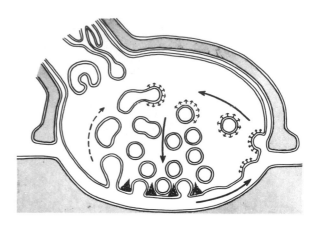

Fig. 8-4. *Current scheme for re-formation of synaptic vesicles by recycling their membranes. After a vesicle opens, it collapses into the surface membrane of the nerve terminal. Membrane is recovered by endocytosis of coated vesicles (on right) or by direct invagination of the extra surface membrane (on left). Whether direct invagination is used during normal synaptic function and exactly how new synaptic vesicles are formed from the internalized surface membrane are not known.*

Development of the postsynaptic active zones requires the laying down of synaptic cleft material and the proper deployment of receptors and the submembranous components of the active zone. Unfortunately, the exact sequences of the different structural changes are not known, although it is known that the postsynaptic active zone in muscle regenerates at its former position, provided the cleft material, a basement membrane in this instance, is left intact [49]. Alternatively, brains of mutant mice show instances in which the postsynaptic active zone is completed in the absence of presynaptic nerve terminals or a cleft [50].

In cultured muscle, receptors exchange rapidly between the insides of cells and the surface membrane and are spread out over the entire muscle surface [51]. The intramembrane components of receptors seem to enter or leave the surface membrane in small groups [52]. This finding suggests that the transmitter-sensitive regions of the muscle fibers could be assembled from small, prefabricated arrays of receptor membrane. Studies on the de-

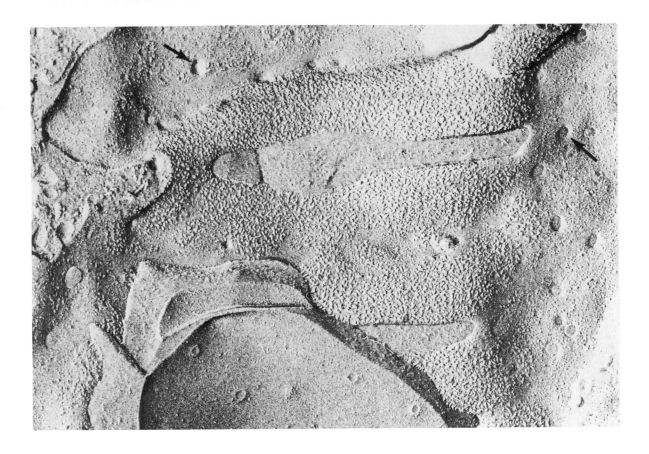

Fig. 8-5. In this freeze-fracture view the nerve terminal (below) has been ripped away, exposing the surface of muscle under it. The postsynaptic active zones clearly differ from the rest of the muscle membrane, which is marked by the caveolae characteristic of muscle cells (arrow). More important are the numerous intramembrane particles at the active zones on the tops of the folds; these are thought to be acetylcholine receptors. The vesicle openings on the outer leaflet of the nerve terminal below are formation sites of coated pits, like those diagrammed in Fig. 8-4. These occur following transmitter release, but outside of the active zones. From [21] with permission. ×75,000

velopment of intracellular junctions in other systems suggest that an anlage, manifested by shape changes within the membrane, may be established prior to the deployment of intramembrane components. The intramembrane components at the presynaptic active zone also seem to be assembled in patches suggestive of prefabricated arrays, although a temporal difference between the deployment of intramembrane and extramembrane components has not been resolved as yet.

In a number of instances, the postsynaptic active zones are deployed on special folds or protrusions of the postsynaptic cell. At many types of nerve-muscle synapse, the surface of the muscle is a series of folds (in vertebrates) (Fig. 8-2), cylindrical invaginations (electric organ), or cylindrical protrusions (insects). The postsynaptic active zones typically are found at the apices of these protrusions, although the purpose of this arrangement is not yet clear. At frog neuromuscular junctions, the folds themselves are supported by a core of intermediate-sized filaments and microtubules that run parallel to the axis of the fold [53] (Fig. 8-2). A fine network of neurofilaments, in turn, connects this core with the fuzz on the cytoplasmic side of the active zone.

In brain cortex, cylindrical protrusions called *dendritic spines* are also sites of postsynaptic active zones; a single cortical neuron has on the order of 50,000 such spines. Although the special detail afforded by current freezing and staining techniques is not yet available for brain, older work has shown that spines are characterized by their content of fine filamentous material [22]. Active zones isolated from the cerebral cortex show further details of the relationship between the postsynaptic membrane and the cytoskeleton. The cytoplasmic side of the active zone shows a prominent band of fuzz, which, in turn, is in contact with a meshwork of microfilaments [54]. The similarity of central nervous system spines with the folds at the neuromuscular junction lies in this contact between the active zone and the cytomatrix; the difference lies in the lack of a microtubule-filament complex in the core of the spine. Cortical spines are of particular interest, because there is evidence that size and shape of the spines may affect the input from their active zones to the cell body [55]. Furthermore, spines change shape under certain experimental conditions. This suggests that they may act similarly in life; they are in a strategic position for these shape changes to result in changes in information processing [56].

In this section, we have considered individual active zones in their most organized form, such as that found at neuromuscular junctions or at many of the interneuronal connections in the brain. Not all types of synapses are so highly organized, and it is not clear whether their transmission mechanisms are organized into active zones. Alternatively, differences between different types of synapses could be merely a question of the shapes and sizes of the active zones; some organized in the discrete patches discussed above, and others with the same components more spread out in small units not readily recognized by current methods of analysis [46]. The varicosities of the adrenergic terminals in peripheral end-organs and inhibitory synapses in certain regions of the central nervous system may

be examples of the spread-out type of organization [46].

Responses of the Postsynaptic Cell to Neurotransmitters

Neurotransmitters can alter the excitability of a postsynaptic cell in two principal ways: by changing membrane potential and by changing membrane resistance. Although many common synaptic responses result in a change of both potential and resistance, this is not always the case. Furthermore, the effects of changing potential may either add to or oppose the effects of changing resistance.

In a typical electrically excitable neuron that has an axon projecting to some distant point, there is an integration of synaptic inputs from dendrites and soma at the axon hillock. At this site, the action potential is initiated that will trigger transmitter release at the axon terminals [11]. The level of depolarization that must be reached at the axon hillock for spike initiation is relatively constant, and thus the effect of potential is simple, in that depolarization brings the cell closer to firing threshold, whereas hyperpolarization brings the cell further from threshold. Although some neurons may show varying degrees of accommodation to a maintained depolarization, in general a neuron will fire repetitively if depolarized beyond the critical firing threshold.

The best-understood mechanism of transmitter action involves binding to a specific receptor; this causes a change in the transmembrane permeabilities to one or more ions. The effect on potential depends upon which ionic permeabilities are changed. Because the ions in tissue usually are not in equal concentration on both sides of the cell membrane, there is a driving force, determined by the concentration gradient, for each ionic species (see Chap. 6). The asymmetrical ionic concentrations are maintained by the relative membrane impermeability to some ions and the activity of the Na^+-K^+ pump. By the Nernst equation (see Chap. 5), we can define an equilibrium potential for any ion (E_X). The equilibrium potential is the one at which the electrical gradient is exactly equal to the chemical concentration gradient for that ion.

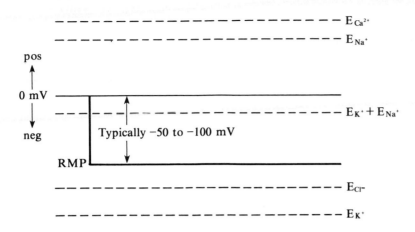

$$E_{Ca^{2+}}$$

$$E_{Na^+}$$

pos

↑

0 mV

↓

neg

Typically −50 to −100 mV

$$E_{K^+} + E_{Na^+}$$

RMP

$$E_{Cl^-}$$

$$E_{K^+}$$

Fig. 8-6. Typical ionic equilibrium potentials in excitable tissues. Resting membrane potential (RMP) is usually between −50 and −100 mV. The equilibrium potentials (E) for various ions are indicated. At the equilibrium potential, the electrical gradient for that ion is exactly equal to the concentration gradient, so that as many ions enter as leave the cell.

Figure 8-6 shows in diagrammatic form the equilibrium potentials for the major ionic species involved in determining potential shifts in neurons. To a first approximation, resting membrane potential (RMP) can be described by the Goldman-Hodgkin-Katz equation [57], which considers the contributions of Na$^+$, K$^+$, and Cl$^-$ (see Chap. 5). Since the interior of cells is high in K$^+$ and low in Na$^+$ and Cl$^-$, RMP is determined by the balance of the electrical and chemical driving forces on all of these ions. Under resting conditions, K$^+$ permeability predominates and RMP is relatively near to E_{K^+}. The degree to which RMP deviates from E_{K^+} reflects active transport and the relative permeabilities to and the concentration gradients of the other ions. Ca^{2+} is not in electrochemical equilibrium, but its resting permeability is low enough so that the Ca^{2+} gradient does not contribute significantly to RMP.

When a transmitter increases permeability to a single ion, the membrane potential will move in the direction of the equilibrium potential for that ion. If a transmitter causes a specific decrease in the permeability to one ionic species, the membrane potential will move away from the equilibrium potential for that ion and toward that of the ion with the dominant permeability. Table 8-1 lists the variety of known responses to neurotransmitters. The best-studied responses are the result of increased permeabilities to one or two ionic species.

Because E_{K^+} is more negative than RMP, an increase in K$^+$ permeability will hyperpolarize, whereas an increase in Na$^+$ permeability will depolarize, the cell. In most neurons, E_{Cl^-} is more negative than RMP, and consequently most specific Cl$^-$ permeability increases are hyperpolarizing. However, in some neurons, such as dorsal root ganglion cells, E_{Cl^-} is less negative than RMP, and an increase in Cl$^-$ permeability results in a depolarization. At the vertebrate neuromuscular junction, and probably at most receptors mediating fast excitation in vertebrates, the transmitter acts to open a channel that allows movement of both Na$^+$ and K$^+$ [58]. This is a quite different channel from those specific for Na$^+$ and K$^+$, which are turned on sequentially to generate action potentials (see Chap. 5); it is, however, probably homologous to the transmitter-activated fast Na$^+$ channel of invertebrates. The equilibrium potential for the response at the neuromuscular junction is about −15 mV, that is, approximately midway between E_{K^+} and E_{Na^+}. In invertebrates, several transmitters have been found that activate a slower and pharmacologically distinguishable Na$^+$-permeability increase [59] and a specific Ca^{2+} permeability [60].

Table 8-1. How Neurotransmitters Act

Change in Permeability (P)	Effect on Postsynaptic Cell
A. Directly alter membrane permeability	
1. Simultaneous fast ↑ P_{Na+} + ↑ P_{K+}	(Excit)
2. Fast ↑ P_{Na+}	(Excit)
3. Slow ↑ P_{Na+}	(Excit)
4. ↑ P_{K+}	(Inhib)
5. ↑ P_{Cl-}	(Inhib)
6. ↑ P_{Ca2+}	(Excit)
7. ↓ P_{Na+}	(Inhib)
8. ↓ P_{K+}	(Excit)
9. ↓ P_{Ca2+}	(Inhib)
B. Biochemical mechanisms	
1. Stimulate adenylate cyclase	
2. Stimulate guanylate cyclase	
3. ? Stimulate $(Na^+ + K^+)$-ATPase	
4. ? Alter prostaglandin levels	

Excit, excitation (depolarization); Inhib, inhibition (hyperpolarization).

Because Ca^{2+} has so many regulatory influences on a variety of neuronal functions, transmitter control of Ca^{2+} permeability may have significant influences beyond the immediate voltage changes. Permeability increase responses can easily be detected by measuring transmembrane resistance. Permeability has an inverse relation to resistance, so the resistance falls during a response associated with an increased permeability to any ion. Resistance usually is measured by passing small pulses of current across the membrane and measuring the resulting voltage deflection. If current is kept constant, the voltage produced will reflect the changes in resistance according to Ohm's law.

Permeability increase responses are fast and require no energy beyond that necessary to maintain concentration gradients, but many responses to neurotransmitters are not associated with a decreased resistance. In both vertebrates and invertebrates, responses associated with either a clear increase in resistance or, in some cases, no measurable resistance change have been obtained with several different transmitters. These responses may be either hyperpolarizing (presumably the result of a specific decrease of Na^+ permeability) or depolarizing (a decreased K^+ permeability), and they tend to be slower in time course. The mechanisms that generate the potentials are unknown, but they are probably energy requiring and may involve a second messenger. Although cyclic AMP and cyclic GMP have been suggested as being involved in several of these slow responses and although synthesis of both substances may be stimulated by neurotransmitters, it is not possible at present to rigorously correlate these biochemical changes with electrical changes (see Chap. 15). Some responses not accompanied by a clear conductance change have been ascribed to a transmitter activation of an electrogenic Na^+-K^+ pump (see Chap. 6), but this conclusion also is controversial. An elucidation of the mechanisms involved in responses not caused by permeability increases is one of the obvious challenges in neurobiology today.

For at least two types of neurotransmitter actions, the effects on membrane resistance are probably of considerably greater importance than is potential change. In some neurons, E_{Cl-} is very near to RMP. If a transmitter increases permeability to Cl^-, and E_{Cl-} is equal to RMP, there would be no change in potential. Even so, any other input would be reduced in effectiveness. This is most easily understood by viewing the action of the second input as a current which, by Ohm's law, will produce less voltage when resistance has fallen. Since E_{Cl-} is never very far from RMP, the short-circuiting effect of increasing Cl^- permeability may be very significant. An example is presynaptic inhibition, a process that has best been studied in the spinal cord, where it results from a synaptic ending on the presynaptic terminal of primary afferent fibers. The effect of activating this pathway onto the presynaptic terminal is to release GABA, which causes increased Cl^- permeability and a Cl^--dependent depolarization in the presynaptic terminal (in these fibers E_{Cl-} is less negative than is RMP). In a manner not totally understood, there is a reduction in the amount of transmitter released from the presynaptic terminal when the afferent fiber discharges. The mechanism may be a short-circuiting of the terminal, due to increased Cl^- permeability, with blockade of impulse invasion into the terminal branches where transmitter release occurs. In contrast, the effects of neurotransmitters associated with a decrease in permeability may increase the responsiveness of neurons to other synaptic inputs. The permeability decrease responses are often associated with only modest voltage shifts, and the alteration of membrane resistance may be the most significant result of this type of synaptic action.

Fig. 8-7. Presynaptic and postsynaptic neurotransmitter receptors. The squares, circles, and triangles represent three different transmitter substances, and the receptors for each are represented by the blocks with the matching hole. Although many patterns probably exist in the nervous system, in this schematic drawing the afferent terminal is shown to contain two transmitters, one of which acts on both presynaptic and postsynaptic membranes, whereas the other acts only on the presynaptic membrane. At the synapse between another neuron and the afferent terminal, a different transmitter has receptors on both membranes.

Synaptic Modulation

Modulation is a term that encompasses a variety of mechanisms whereby one neurotransmitter affects the response to or release of a second transmitter. There are two major levels of modulation: (1) modulation of transmitter release through presynaptic receptors and (2) modulation of postsynaptic receptors and responses. Although a number of examples of each are known, we are, unfortunately, only beginning to understand the variety of mechanisms involved.

Presynaptic inhibition and facilitation have been known for 20 years from studies in cat spinal cord, but only recently has it become apparent that there are receptors on presynaptic terminals for a great variety of substances [61]. Figure 8-7 shows how these receptors might be organized in a typical synapse. Many terminals appear to have receptors for their own transmitter (autoreceptors) that would be activated every time release occurs (see also Chap. 10). The action site of peptides present in terminals that contain principally nonpeptide transmitter may be presynaptic. At many terminals, there is a presynaptic innervation from other nerve cells. This presynaptic synapse may use a different

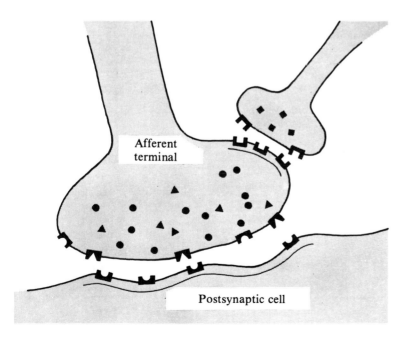

Afferent terminal

Postsynaptic cell

transmitter and may act through any of a variety of mechanisms to inhibit or facilitate the efficacy of the synapse. Because the terminal is so small as to be inaccessible to direct electrophysiological investigation, we do not know many of the mechanisms of presynaptic inhibition or facilitation.

One mechanism of presynaptic inhibition may be a short-circuiting of the terminal by the increase of Cl^- permeability, as already discussed, but it is also likely that neurotransmitters may directly increase [60] or decrease [62] Ca^{2+} permeability. Because Ca^{2+} is so critical for transmitter release, such a mechanism would be very efficient.

Modulation of postsynaptic responsiveness may result through several different mechanisms. Any transmitter that induces a prolonged increase in resistance will increase the responsiveness to all other input in a nonselective fashion. In some systems, aspartate selectively potentiates the responsiveness to glutamate by blocking glutamate uptake [63]. Any mechanism that retards transmitter removal will potentiate the response. Other systems have specific modulatory interactions between two transmitters. One example is given in Fig. 8-8, which shows a recording from a pyramidal tract neuron in cat cortex. This neuron showed very little response to either acetylcholine or TRH, but when application of acetylcholine was paired with a single application of TRH, a prolonged potentiation of the response to acetylcholine took place. This modulation has been reported to be specific for acetylcholine receptors [64], but the mechanism is unknown.

The Organization of Neurotransmitter Receptor Complexes

Only a few years ago, it was generally accepted that excitation in the central nervous system is mediated primarily by receptors for glutamate, whereas inhibition is caused by GABA and glycine, with minor roles taken by catecholamines and indoleamines. We now have a large number of likely neurotransmitters and at least a dozen possible ionic or biochemical changes that may be elicited by them. Furthermore, any one transmitter may activate quite different ionic responses on different

cells, depending on the postsynaptic membrane. For example, in different cells of the relatively simple nervous system of *Aplysia,* serotonin causes increased permeability to Cl^-, K^+, or Ca^{2+}, fast or slow increases in Na^+ permeability, depolarizing or hyperpolarizing responses with decreased permeability, stimulation of cyclic AMP synthesis, and modulation of the actions of another neurotransmitter [59, 60, 65, 66]. In vertebrates, acetylcholine causes a simultaneous Na^+-K^+ excitation at the neuromuscular junction, a fast inhibition (probably Cl^--dependent) at some central neurons, a K^+-dependent inhibition in the heart, a slow depolarizing resistance-increase response on pyramidal tract neurons ([67] Fig. 8-8), and a stimulation of cyclic GMP in several areas [68].

Figure 8-9 shows a model of the organization of neurotransmitter receptors [69] that is consistent with most available information and helps to explain the great variety of responses that may be elicited by a single transmitter. The model assumes that the transmitter binding site (the *receptor*) is a molecule separate and distinct from the *ionophore* (the membrane structure that causes the change in membrane permeability). In the functional unit, called the *receptor complex,* the receptor and ionophore are intimately associated in such a way that binding of the transmitter to the receptor induces a conformation change, first in the receptor and secondarily in the ionophore, resulting in an opening of a gate that allows ions to flow through the ionophore. The ionic species that moves is determined by a selectivity filter (see Chap. 5). This is the narrowest portion of the channel that is opened in the ionophore by withdrawal of the gate, and it screens, by both size and charge, the ions that may pass on. The model proposes that different transmitter-specific receptors may be associated with the same ionophore. Thus, as illustrated, an ionophore that passes only Cl^- ions may be coupled to an acetylcholine receptor in one cell and to a dopamine receptor in another. Furthermore, the model allows for a single receptor to be coupled at different sites to different ion-specific ionophores. Enzymes and regulatory proteins may be linked to the receptor complex (see Chap. 3).

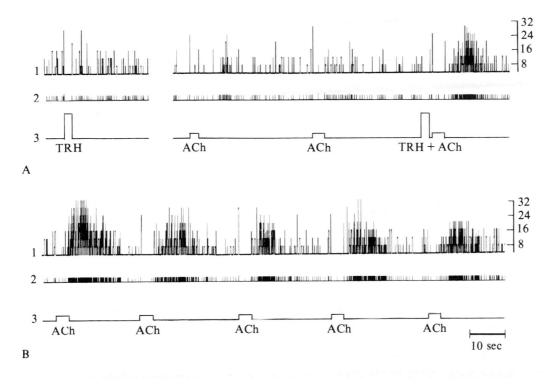

Fig. 8-8. Modulation of a response to acetylcholine (ACh) by thyrotropin-releasing hormone (TRH). Recordings were made from a pyramidal tract neuron from sensorimotor cortex of a chloralose-anesthetized cat and identified by antidromic activation by a stimulating electrode in the medullary pyramid. Trace 1 shows a histogram of frequency of discharge in spikes per second. Trace 2 shows a single pulse for each action potential. Trace 3 shows the period of application of ACh and TRH. A. Application of TRH alone caused no response; ACh alone was essentially ineffective. B. After a single pairing of TRH and ACh (end of A), the response to ACh was brisk and remained so for over two minutes. (Courtesy of C. Auker, D. Braitman, and D. Carpenter.)

Several observations support this model of receptor complex organization:

1. In some cells, where a β-adrenergic receptor activates adenylate cyclase, it has been possible to separate the receptor and the cyclase molecules and even to develop cell clones in which both molecules are present, but are uncoupled [70].

2. In *Aplysia* neurons, every combination of nine different receptors and three different ionic responses have been found [71].

3. In *Aplysia*, when different receptors activate the same ionic response, the time course, temperature sensitivities, and ionic selectivities are identical [69, 72].

4. In the central nervous system, most transmitters (including peptides) excite some neurons, inhibit others, and do not affect·the remainder. The model predicts that no substance is either exclusively excitatory or inhibitory. Consistent with this view are demonstrations that glutamate, previously believed to be only excitatory, causes inhibitory effects on cerebellar granule cells [73], whereas GABA, previously thought to be inhibitory only in vertebrates, causes an inhibitory response on some dendrites of hippocampal pyramidal neurons but excitatory responses on others [74].

The model also provides an important framework for the analysis of transmitter antagonist

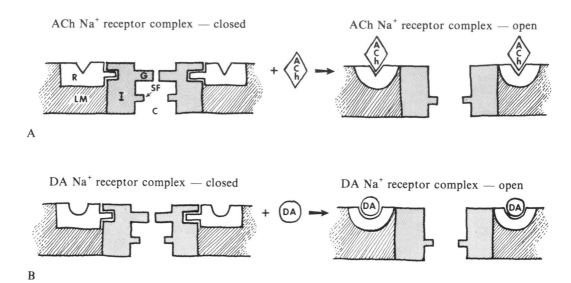

ACh Na⁺ receptor complex — closed   ACh Na⁺ receptor complex — open

A

DA Na⁺ receptor complex — closed   DA Na⁺ receptor complex — open

B

action. Drugs might act (1) on the receptor, in which case they should block all responses to a given transmitter; (2) at the ionophore, in which case they block all similar ionic responses, regardless of which transmitter elicits them; or (3) only on a specific combination of receptor and ionophore. Examples of mechanism (1) for each transmitter are discussed in detail in the chapter dealing with the specific transmitter. Several examples consistent with the second mechanism, an antagonist blocking an ionophore, have been reported. Penicillin, bicuculline, and picrotoxin block Cl⁻ responses to a variety of different transmitters [72, 75]. Curare blocks Na⁺ and Cl⁻ responses of invertebrates and Na⁺-K⁺ and Cl⁻ responses of vertebrates to several transmitters [71].

In spite of the complexity of the mammalian central nervous system, several generalizations on the mechanisms of synaptic transmission may be made with moderate confidence:

1. Transmitter release results from a Ca^{2+}-dependent exocytosis.
2. Any single transmitter substance may produce different responses at different locations.
3. A particular ionic or biochemical response can be elicited by different transmitters at different locations.

Fig. 8-9. Model of organization of neurotransmitter receptor complexes in nerve membranes. The receptor complex is embedded in a lipid membrane (LM). The receptor (R) and ionophore (I) portions are shown to be distinct entities. A receptor in B, for dopamine (DA), may couple with the same ionophore as shown coupled to an acetylcholine (ACh) receptor in A. After attachment of the transmitter to its binding site, a conformational change is induced in the receptor that causes a conformational change in the ionophore so as to open the gate (G), which prevented ions from flowing in the resting state. When the gate is opened, ions flow through the channel (C). The species that passes through the channel is determined by selectivity filter (SF), which screens ions by size, charge, and free energies of hydration. The model assumes that several different ionophores may be associated with any particular receptor, and that those ionophores differ principally in their ionic selectivities.

4. Although many details of synaptic transmission are still unknown, the basic principles of the process which have been elucidated from study of invertebrate neurons and of the neuromuscular junction are applicable to the central nervous system.

References

1. Loewi, O. Über humorole Übertragborkeit der Herznervenwirkung. I. Mitteilung. *Pflüegers Arch.* 189:239–242, 1921.

2. Rubin, R. P. The role of calcium in the release of neurotransmitter substances and hormones. *Pharmacol. Rev.* 22:389–428, 1970.

3. Douglas, W. W., and Taraskevich, P. S. Action potentials in gland cells of rat pituitary pars intermedia: Inhibition by dopamine, an inhibitor of MSH secretion. *J. Physiol.* (London) 285:171–184, 1978.

4. Matthews, E. K., and O'Connor, M. D. L. Dynamic oscillations in the membrane potential of pancreatic islet cells. *J. Exp. Biol.* 81:75–91, 1979.

5. Shepherd, G. M. *The Synaptic Organization of the Brain: An Introduction.* New York: Oxford University Press, 1974.

6. von Euler, U.S., and Gaddum, J. H. An unidentified depressor substance in certain tissue extracts. *J. Physiol.* (London) 72:74–87, 1931.

7. Leeman, S. E., and Mroz, E. A. Substance P. *Life Sci.* 15:2033–2044, 1975.

8. Douglas, W. W., and Poisner, A. M. Evidence that the secreting adrenal chromaffin cell releases catecholamines directly from ATP-rich granules. *J. Physiol.* (London) 183:236–248, 1966.

9. Dale, H. H. Nomenclature of fibres in the autononomic system and their effects. *J. Physiol.* (London) 80:10–11P, 1933.

10. Dale, H. H. Pharmacology and nerve endings. *Proc. Roy. Soc. Med.* 28:319–332, 1935.

11. Eccles, J. C. *The Physiology of Nerve Cells.* Baltimore: Johns Hopkins Press, 1957.

12. Eccles, J. C., Fatt, P., and Koketsu, K. Cholinergic and inhibitory synapses in a pathway from motor-axon collaterals to motoneurones. *J. Physiol.* (London) 126:524–526, 1954.

13. Kandel, E. R., et al. Direct and common connections among the identified neurons in the abdominal ganglion of *Aplysia. J. Neurophysiol.* 30:1352–1376, 1967.

14. Furshpan, E. J., et al. Chemical transmission between rat sympathetic neurons and cardiac myocytes developing in microcultures: Evidence for cholinergic, adrenergic and dual-function neurons. *Proc. Natl. Acad. Sci. U.S.A.* 73:4225–4229, 1976.

15. Brownstein, M. J., et al. Coexistence of several putative neurotransmitters in single identified neurons of *Aplysia. Proc. Natl. Acad. Sci. U.S.A.* 71:4662–4665, 1974.

16. Cottrell, G. A. Does the giant cerebral neurone of *Helix* release two transmitters: ACh and serotonin? *J. Physiol.* (London) 259:44–45P, 1976.

17. Chan-Palay, V., Jonsson, G., and Palay, S. L. Serotonin and substance P coexist in neurons of the rat's central nervous system. *Proc. Natl. Acad. Sci. U.S.A.* 75:1582–1586, 1978.

18. Hökfelt, T., et al. Occurrence of somatostatin-like immunoreactivity in some peripheral sympathetic noradrenergic neurons. *Proc. Natl. Acad. Sci. U.S.A.* 74:3587–3591, 1977.

19. Pickel, V. M., Reis, D. J., and Leeman, S. E. Ultrastructural localization of substance P in neurons of rat spinal cord. *Brain Res.* 122:534–540, 1977.

20. Katz, B. *The Release of Neural Transmitter Substance.* Liverpool: Liverpool University Press, 1969.

21. Heuser, J. E., and Reese, T. S. Structure of Synapse. In E. Kandell (ed.), *The Handbook of Physiology, The Nervous System I.* Bethesda: American Physiological Society, 1977. Pp. 261–294.

22. Peters, A., Palay, S. L., and Webster, H. de F. *The Fine Structure of the Nervous System.* Philadelphia: Saunders, 1976.

23. Katz, B., and Miledi, R. Transmitter leakage from motor nerve endings. *Proc. R. Soc. Lond. [Biol.]* 196:59–72, 1977.

24. Del Castillo, J., and Katz, B. Biochemical aspects of neuromuscular transmission. *Prog. Biophys. Mol. Biol.* 6:121–170, 1956.

25. Marchbanks, R. N. The vesicular hypothesis questioned. *Trends Neurosci.* 1:83–84, 1978.

26. Llinas, R., and Heuser, J. E. Depolarization-release coupling. *Neurosci. Res. Bull.* 15:555–687, 1977.

27. Heuser, J. E., and Reese, T. S. Morphology of Synaptic Vesicle Discharge and Reformation at the Frog Neuromuscular Junction. In M. V. L. Bennett (ed.), *Synaptic Transmission and Neuronal Interaction.* New York: Raven Press, 1974. Pp. 59–77.

28. Pysh, J. J., and Wiley, R. G. Synaptic vesicle depletion and recovery in cat sympathetic ganglion electrically stimulated in vivo. Evidence for transmitter secretion by exocytosis. *J. Cell Biol.* 60:363–374, 1974.

29. Weinshilbaum, R. M., et al. Proportional release of norepinephrine and dopamine β-hydroxylase from sympathetic nerves. *Science* 174:1349–1351, 1972.

30. Heuser, J. E., Reese, T. S., and Landis, D. M. D. Functional changes in frog neuromuscular junctions studied with freeze-fracture. *J. Neurocytol.* 3:109–131, 1974.

31. Pumplin, D. W., and Reese, T. S. Membrane ultrastructure of the giant synapse of the squid *Loligo pealei. Neuroscience* 3:685–696, 1978.

32. Sandri, C., Van Buren, J. M., and Akert, K. (eds.). Membrane Morphology of the Vertebrate Nervous System. *Prog. Brain Res.* Vol. 46, 1977.

33. Couteaux, R., and Pecot-Dechavassine, M. Vesicules synaptiques et poches au niveau des "zones actives" de la junction neuromusculaire. *C. R. Acad. Sci. Ser. C. Sci. Chem.* 271:2346–2349, 1970.

34. Gulley, R. L., Landis, D. M. D., and Reese, T. S. Internal organization of membranes at end bulbs of Held in the anteroventral cochlear nucleus. *J. Comp. Neurol.* 180:707–742, 1978.

35. Heuser, J. E., et al. Synaptic vesicle exocytosis captured by quick freezing and correlated with quantal transmitter release. *J. Cell Biol.* 81:275–300, 1979.

36. Kriebel, M. E., Llados, R., and Matteson, D. R. Spontaneous subminiature end-plate potentials in mouse diaphragm muscle: Evidence for synchronous release. *J. Physiol.* (London) 262:553–581, 1976.

37. Wernig, A., and Striner, H. Quantum amplitude distribution points to functional unity of the synaptic "active zone." *Nature* 289:820–822, 1977.

38. Kriebel, M. E., Llados, F., and Matteson, D. R. Multimodal distribution of frog miniature end-plate potentials in adult, denervated, and tadpole leg muscle. *J. Gen. Physiol.* 192:407–436, 1976.

39. Heuser, J. E., and Reese, T. S. Synaptic Vesicle Exocytosis Captured by Quick Freezing. In F. O. Schmitt and F. G. Worden (eds.), *The Neurosciences Fourth Intensive Study Program.* Cambridge, Mass.: M.I.T. Press, 1979. Pp. 573–600.

40. Ceccarelli, B., Grohovaz, F., and Hurlbub, W. P. Freeze-fracture studies of frog neuromuscular junctions during intense release of transmitter. *J. Cell Biol.* 81:163–192, 1979.

41. Heuser, J. E., and Reese, T. S. Evidence for recycling of synaptic vesicle membrane during transmitter release at the frog neuromuscular junction. *J. Cell Biol.* 57:315–344, 1973.

42. Basbaum, C., and Heuser, J. E. Morphological studies of stimulated adrenergic nerve varicosities in the mouse vas deferens. *J. Cell Biol.* 80:310–325, 1979.

43. Rees, R. P., Bunge, M. B., and Bunge, R. P. Morphological changes in the neuritic growth cone and target neuron during synaptic development in culture. *J. Cell Biol.* 68:240–263, 1976.

44. Rees, R. P. Structure of cell coats during initial stages of synapse formation on isolated cultured sympathetic neurons. *J. Neurocytol.* 7:679–691, 1978.

45. Landis, D. M. D., Reese, T. S., and Raviola, E. Differences in membrane structure between excitatory and inhibitory components of the reciprocal synapse in the olfactory bulb. *J. Comp. Neurol.* 155:67–92, 1974.

46. Landis, D. M. D., and Reese, T. S. Differences in membrane structure between excitatory and inhibitory synapses in the cerebellar cortex. *J. Comp. Neurol.* 155:93–126, 1974.

47. Heuser, J. E., and Salpeter, M. Organization of acetylcholine receptors in quick-frozen, deep-etched, and rotary-shadowed *Torpedo* postsynaptic membrane. *J. Cell Biol.* 82:150–173, 1979.

48. Heuser, J. E., Reese, T. S., and Landis, D. M. D. Preservation of synaptic structure by rapid freezing.

Cold Spring Harbor Symp. Quant. Biol. 15:17–24, 1976.

49. Sanes, J. E., Marshall, L. M., and McMahon, U. J. Reinnervation of muscle fiber basal lamina after removal of myofibers. *J. Cell Biol.* 78:176–198, 1978.

50. Landis, D. M. D., and Reese, T. S. Structure of the Purkinje cell membrane in staggerer and weaver mutant mice. *J. Comp. Neurol.* 171:247–260, 1977.

51. Fambrough, D. Development of Cholinergic Innervation of Skeletal, Cardiac, and Smooth Muscle. In A. M. Goldberg and I. Hamin (eds.), *Biology of Cholinergic Function.* New York: Raven Press, 1976. Pp. 101–160.

52. Cohen, S. A., and Pumplin, D. W. Clusters of intramembrane particles associated with binding sites for α-bungarotoxin in cultured chick myotubes. *J. Cell Biol.* 82:494–516, 1979.

53. Couteaux, R., and Pecot-Dechavassine, M. Particulantes structurales du sarcoplasme sous-mural. *C. R. Acad. Sci. Ser. D (Paris)* 266:8–10, 1968.

54. Cohen, R. S., et al. The structure of postsynaptic densities isolated from dog cerebral cortex. I. Overall morphology and protein composition. *J. Cell Biol.* 74:181–203, 1977.

55. Rall, W., and Rinzel, J. Dendritic spines and synaptic potency explored theoretically. *Int. Cong. Physiol. Sci. Proc.* 9:1384, 1971.

56. Fifkova, E., and Van Harreveld, A. Long-lasting morphological changes in dendritic spines of dentate granular cells following stimulation of entorhinal area. *J. Neurocytol.* 6:211–230, 1977.

57. Hodgkin, A. L., and Katz, B. The effect of sodium ions on the electrical activity of the giant axon of the squid. *J. Physiol.* (London) 108:37–77, 1949.

58. Dionne, V. E., and Ruff, R. L. End-plate current fluctuations reveal only one channel type at frog neuromuscular junction. *Nature* 266:263–265, 1977.

59. Gerschenfeld, H. M., and Paupadin-Tritsch, D. Ionic mechanisms underlying the responses of molluscan neurones to 5-hydroxytryptamine. *J. Physiol.* (London) 243:427–456, 1974.

60. Pellmar, T. C., and Carpenter, D. O. Voltage-dependent calcium current induced by serotonin. *Nature* 277:483–484, 1979.

61. Starke, K., Taube, H. D., and Borowski, E. Presynaptic receptor systems in catecholaminergic transmission. *Biochem. Pharmacol.* 26:259–268, 1977.

62. Dunlap, K., and Fischbach, G. D. Neurotransmitters decrease the calcium component of sensory neurone action potentials. *Nature* 276:837–839, 1978.

63. Crawford, A. C., and McBurney, R. N. The synergistic action of L-glutamate and L-aspartate at crus-

tacean neuromuscular junction. *J. Physiol.* (London) 268:697–709, 1977.

64. Yarbrough, G. G. TRH potentiates excitatory actions of acetylcholine on cerebral cortical neurones. *Nature* 263:523–524, 1976.

65. Cedar, H., and Schwartz, J. H. Cyclic adenosine monophosphate in the nervous system of *Aplysia californica*. II. Effects of serotonin and dopamine. *J. Gen. Physiol.* 60:570–587, 1972.

66. Weiss, K. R., Cohen, J., and Kupfermann, I. Potentiation of muscle contraction: A possible modulatory function of an identified serotonergic cell in *Aplysia*. *Brain Res.* 99:381–386, 1975.

67. Krnjević, K. Chemical nature of synaptic transmission in vertebrate. *Physiol. Rev.* 54:418–540, 1974.

68. Kebabian, J. W., Steiner, A. L., and Greengard, P. Muscarinic cholinergic regulation of cyclic guanosine 3′,5′-monophosphate in autonomic ganglia: Possible role in synaptic transmission. *J. Pharmacol. Exp. Ther.* 193:474–488, 1975.

69. Swann, J. W., and Carpenter, D. O. The organization of receptors for neurotransmitters on *Aplysia* neurons. *Nature* 258:751–754, 1975.

70. Haga, T., et al. Adenylate cyclase permanently uncoupled from hormone receptors is a novel variant of S49 mouse lymphoma cells. *Proc. Natl. Acad. Sci. U.S. A.* 74:2016–2020, 1977.

71. Carpenter, D. O., Swann, J. W., and Yarowsky, P. J. Effects of curare on responses to different putative neurotransmitters in *Aplysia* neurons. *J. Neurobiol.* 8:119–132, 1977.

72. Yarowsky, P. J., and Carpenter, D. O. A comparison of similar ionic responses to gamma-aminobutyric acid and acetylcholine. *J. Neurophysiol.* 41:531–541, 1978.

73. Yamamoto, C., Yamashita, H., and Chujo, T. Inhibitory action of glutamic acid on cerebellar interneurones. *Nature* 262:786–787, 1976.

74. Anderson, P., et al. Two Mechanisms for Effects of GABA on Hippocampal Pyramidal Cells. In R. W. Ryall and J. S. Kelly (eds.), *Iontophoresis and Transmitter Mechanisms in the Mammalian Central Nervous System*. Amsterdam: Elsevier, 1978. Pp. 179–181.

75. Pellmar, T. C., and Wilson, W. A. Penicillin effects on iontophoretic responses in *Aplysia californica*. *Brain Res.* 136:89–101, 1977.

Acetylcholine (ACh) is a compound of considerable antiquity. We can be fairly sure that it arrived on the evolutionary scene before nervous systems did, proved itself to be a versatile performer, and was tried out in a variety of parts before being assigned its major role as a synaptic transmitter in the higher animals. The evidence for this is that there are still many bacteria, fungi, protozoa, and plants that manufacture acetylcholine and store it. Even in mammals, it can be found in high concentration at sites where it has no known function. The best-known mammalian examples are the cornea, some ciliated epithelia, the spleen in certain ungulates, and the human placenta. As we have little information about the functional significance of ACh in any of these tissues, the rest of this chapter will be concerned with ACh in its role as a synaptic transmitter. In this role, ACh has a great variety of actions, but all of them depend on its ability to combine with specific protein receptors imbedded in cell membranes. By so doing, it changes the configuration of the receptors; and this often, perhaps always, leads to the opening of cation-selective channels, with consequences that depend both on the ionic species that can traverse the channels and on the nature of the ion-sensitive mechanisms inside the cell. If ACh ever acts by combining directly with intracellular receptors, that action has so far been overlooked.

Chemistry of Acetylcholine

The structure of ACh was deduced from crystallographic analyses by Pauling and coauthors [1]. They pointed out that, though either end of the ACh ion (C2 — N — C4 — C5 or C5 — O1 — C6 — C7) has all four atoms coplanar, rotation can occur around the bonds C4 — C5 and C5 — O1.

$$\begin{matrix} & (2) & & & & (1) \\ & O & & & & CH_3 \\ & \parallel & & & & | \\ H_3C & — C & — O — CH_2 — CH_2 & — N & — CH_3 \\ (7) & (6) & (1) \quad (5) \qquad (4) & | & \\ & & & & CH_3 & (3) \end{matrix}$$

Acetylcholine

Because of this double hinge, the two planes are twisted somewhat away from each other, so that O2 tends to approach C1, and further displacement can occur when the ion interacts with a protein receptor. As noted later, under Cholinergic Receptors, there are two kinds of ACh receptors, nicotinic and muscarinic, mediating quick and slow responses respectively. Pauling's group analyzed the structures of molecules that elicit or block one type of response; this analysis included a number of molecules more rigid than those of ACh. They concluded that the ACh ion attached to a receptor site has about the same conformation in each case but has a different orientation: the *methyl side* of the ion has a high affinity for muscarinic receptors, and the *carbonyl side* has a high affinity for nicotinic receptors. Naturally, it is somewhat risky to suppose that the ACh ion in solution or close to a receptor takes the same shape that it has in a crystal of an ACh salt; but the results of quantum chemical analyses [2] seem to agree reasonably well with the work on crystals. There is no doubt that the onium head of ACh, with its positive charge spread over the methyl cluster, is an important structural feature for both muscarinic and nicotinic action, whereas the negatively charged carbonyl O atom and the distance between it and the N atom are significant features on the nicotinic side.

Under ordinary laboratory conditions, or in vivo, the only part of the ACh molecule susceptible to chemical attack is the ester linkage. The hydrolysis of ACh at this site is accelerated by hydroxyl ions and to a much smaller degree, by hydrions, as obtains with aliphatic esters generally. ACh is stable in solution at pH 4, and at pH 7.4 and 37°C its half-life is many hours unless an esterase is present; but at pH 12 or higher it is destroyed within seconds. This fact provides the basis of a useful test to determine whether a tissue extract owes its biological activity to ACh.

Both ACh and choline form salts of low water solubility with a number of inorganic and organic anions and may be separated in this way from other materials in tissue extracts. Chloroaurate, reineckate, dipicrylamate, and tetraphenylborate salts have been used for this purpose. Separation of ACh from choline can be achieved on the basis of the differential solubility of some of these salts in suitable organic solvents, or by means of chromatography.

Cholinergic Neurons

SPECIFIC CONSTITUENTS OF CHOLINERGIC NEURONS

Cholinergic neurons synthesize, store, and release ACh. Such neurons also synthesize choline acetyltransferase (ChAT), the enzyme that catalyzes the formation of ACh (reaction 1), and acetylcholinesterase (AChE), the most important of the enzymes that catalyze the hydrolysis of ACh (reaction 2):

$$\text{Choline} + \text{acetyl-CoA} \rightarrow \text{ACh} + \text{CoA} \qquad (9\text{-}1)$$

$$\text{ACh} + H_2O \rightarrow \text{choline} + \text{acetic acid} \qquad (9\text{-}2)$$

ChAT and AChE are made in the neuronal soma and are transported (see Chap. 22) down the axon to the synapses, where they are put to work. According to the current majority view, the presence of ACh in the axon is a by-product of the transport of ChAT: acetylcholine functions only as a synaptic transmitter, and does not have a role in the conduction of impulses along the axon.

Choline acetyltransferase and ACh itself are present throughout the whole length of every cholinergic neuron. Their highest concentrations, however, are in the axon's terminal swellings, commonly referred to as *nerve endings*. (This term will be retained, although it is a misnomer in many cases. Usually the swellings are spaced out along the axon's distal course like beads on a string, but at some junctions, for example, those between motor axons and the end-plates of skeletal muscle fibers, all the presynaptic elements do have a terminal location.) Cell fractionation studies show that much of the ACh of the nerve endings is contained in the synaptic vesicles, but some of it is free in the cytosol. Most of the ChAT is also free in the cytosol, but some of it may adhere to the outside of the vesicles [3].

AChE has a somewhat wider distribution in the nervous system than ACh or ChAT. Besides being a regular constituent of cholinergic neurons, it is made by some neurons, for example, afferent neurons in vertebrates, that do not appear to be cholinergic. Whereas the presence of ChAT and ACh in a neuron is reliable evidence that the neuron is cholinergic, the presence of AChE is not, unless its concentration is very high. It has proved to be a useful marker, however, because it is much easier to detect histochemically than are ChAT or ACh. Except for such histochemical tests, there is no way of distinguishing cholinergic from noncholinergic neurons by their appearance. AChE is also made extraneuronally to a much greater extent than is ChAT. It is a constituent of erythrocyte membranes, and at some cholinergic synapses, notably the motor end-plate, most of the AChE is attached to the postsynaptic cell. As these examples indicate, AChE is characteristically a membrane-bound enzyme. At synapses, most of its active sites face outward, enabling the enzyme to hydrolyze newly released ACh; but cholinergic axons and nerve endings outside the central nervous system apparently contain some inward-facing AChE as well.

ChAT and AChE have been studied intensively for decades. AChE has had special attention because a number of drugs, insecticides, and "nerve gases" act by inhibiting it. Neurochemical studies since 1970 have added two further items to the list of substances that seem to be specifically associated with cholinergic nerve endings: (1) a membrane carrier, presumed to be a protein but not yet isolated, that mediates the *high-affinity uptake of choline* for ACh synthesis [4]; and (2) vesiculin [5], an incompletely defined mucopolysaccharidelike

Table 9-1. Cholinergic Pathways in the Peripheral Nervous System

Pathway	Neuronal Cell Bodies in:	Axonal Endings on:[a]	Receptors[f]	Action[g]
Somatic motor	CNS	Skeletal muscle fibers	N	
Preganglionic	CNS	Neurons in autonomic ganglia	N,M	E
		Interneurons in ganglia	M	E
		Adrenomedullary cells	N,M	E
		Neurons in gut plexuses	N	E
Postganglionic	Parasympathetic ganglia	Smooth muscle[b]	M	E
		Smooth muscle[c]	M	I
		Heart muscle fibers	M	I
		Gland cells[d]	M	E
Postganglionic	Sympathetic ganglia	Smooth muscle[e]	M	I
		Sweat gland cells	M	E
Gut wall, instrinsic	Gut plexuses	Gut smooth muscle	M	E

[a]Endings that supply smooth muscle are often distant from cells.
[b]Includes smooth muscle of iris (constrictor of pupil), ciliary body, bronchioles, bladder, etc.
[c]Includes vascular smooth muscle in brain, exocrine glands, genitalia, etc.
[d]Includes lachrymal, nasal, salivary, gastric glands, exocrine pancreas; also endocrine cells producing gastrin, insulin.
[e]Includes vascular smooth muscle in microcirculation of muscles in some animals.
[f]M, muscarinic; N, nicotinic; where both are listed, the first is more prominent.
[g]E, excitatory; I, inhibitory. (Cholinergic inhibition of smooth muscle is sometimes indirect: a third kind of cell is involved.)

material that is present in the interior of the synaptic vesicles and may have a role in ACh storage.

DISTRIBUTION OF CHOLINERGIC NEURONS
Details of the distribution and functional significance of peripheral cholinergic pathways in mammals can be found in textbooks of physiology or pharmacology. Table 9-1 gives a summary and also indicates the nature of the postsynaptic receptors in each case. The cholinergic pathways in other vertebrates have about the same distribution as in mammals. The electric organ, present in some species of fish, is excellent material for neurochemical studies because of the density of its cholinergic innervation.

It is not yet possible to present a table of central cholinergic pathways, but the data for it are gradually accumulating [6]. A number of well-documented examples may be cited:

1. The axons of motoneurons send excitatory branches within the spinal cord to nearby neurons (*Renshaw cells*) whose discharge inhibits the same and other motoneurons. (Because these axon collaterals arise from cholinergic neurons, they are cholinergic themselves, but the Renshaw cells are not.)
2. A well-defined cholinergic tract from the septal region synapses with neurons in the hippocampus.
3. Another compact tract, descending from the habenular nuclei to the midbrain interpeduncular nucleus, accounts for the latter's extraordinarily high content of ACh.
4. The major striatal nuclei, especially the caudate and putamen, are also very rich in ACh, most of which seems to be in short intrastriatal neurons.
5. Although few, if any, sensory axons are cholinergic, some involvement of ACh in sensory function is made likely by its presence in the efferent olivocochlear bundle and in some layers of the retina.
6. Ascending fibers account for most of the ACh in cortex, but their suspected relationship to the "arousal" projections from the mesencephalic reticular system is now in doubt; instead, they are thought to arise from

several nuclei deeper in the forebrain. It seems that few, if any, of the wholly intracortical neurons are cholinergic.

At present, the mapping of central cholinergic neurons has to rely on the use of a combination of techniques, none of which is wholly reliable by itself. Unfortunately, there are no generally accepted methods as yet for the histochemical detection of ACh, ChAT, or the high-affinity choline carrier, the three truly specific components of the cholinergic neuron. Such methods, however, are likely to be available soon, and should then provide anatomical information of quality comparable to that now available for aminergic neurons.

Assay of Acetylcholine and Choline

Until the 1960s, to measure the ACh stored in or released from a tissue, one had to choose one of the bioassay methods [for references, see 7]. Among the favorite test objects were the frog rectus abdominis muscle, leech body wall, cat or rat blood pressure, guinea pig ileum, toad lung, and clam heart. These methods are tricky and tedious, but sensitive (down to 1–10 pmole), and with practice they can be made to give results that are reliable within error limits of 10 percent or less. They are still being used to some extent, but during the last 10 years a number of investigators have accepted the challenge of devising chemical assay methods of comparable sensitivity, and as a result a dozen or more acceptable procedures are now available [8]. Several of these procedures allow free choline to be determined in parallel with ACh, an obvious advantage for studies of ACh metabolism. A promising new approach is the development of a radioimmunoassay.

In studying the ACh metabolism of intact brain, the experimenter must be aware that excising the tissue or severing the animal's neck can alter ACh and choline levels within seconds. The worker can minimize these artifacts by working with anesthetized animals, or with very small ones like mice whose brain enzymes can be inactivated by such drastic measures as putting the animals' heads into liquid air or into a focused microwave beam.

Cholinergic Receptors

Cells that respond to injected ACh or to ACh released at nerve endings are termed *cholinoceptive*.

Generally, their responses can be assigned to one or the other of the two broad classes identified by Dale in 1914: (1) *nicotinic responses* are typically quick, lasting for milliseconds; they are always excitatory, at least initially; they can be evoked by nicotine as well as by ACh; and they can be blocked by drugs of the curare type or by an excess of either nicotine or ACh itself; (2) *muscarinic responses* are typically slow, lasting for seconds; they may be either excitatory or inhibitory; they can be evoked by muscarine, a mushroom alkaloid, as well as by ACh; they can be blocked by atropine or scopolamine. These two kinds of responses both result from the temporary combination of ACh with *muscarinic* or *nicotinic receptors*. One or the other kind of receptor—occasionally both—is present on the surface of every vertebrate cholinoceptive cell.

The existence of these receptors had been a convenient postulate for decades before they were characterized chemically [9]. It is now well established that they are integral membrane proteins, deeply imbedded in the membrane's lipid matrix. After cell disruption, they are often found in membrane fragments along with AChE but are harder to detach: detergents are generally used, but their separation from the receptor protein during the later stages of its purification may be awkward.

Solubilized nicotinic and muscarinic receptors retain much of their pharmacological specificity, combining selectively and reversibly with ACh and with the numerous basic drugs that mimic or oppose its action in vivo. In addition, agents have been found that combine specifically, and more or less irreversibly, with one or the other receptor type. Such an agent can be given a radioactive or fluorescent label and used as a receptor probe. In this way, tissue receptors can be visualized, and the number of receptors per unit area can be estimated. The purification of solubilized receptor material is thus facilitated. The most useful ligands are of two kinds, acetylcholine analogs or protein toxins: (1) either nicotinic or muscarinic receptors can be labeled with basic alkylating agents that are chemically related to ACh; (2) nicotinic receptors can be labeled with protein neurotoxins isolated from the venoms of several genera of snakes, especially α-bungarotoxin from the krait and α-toxin from the cobra. The discovery of these selective agents in the 1960s was a powerful stimulus to research on cholinergic receptors. With electric organ (by far the richest source) as starting material, the nicotinic receptor has been harvested in excellent yield and fair purity, and a good deal has been learned about its chemistry. There is no comparably rich source of the muscarinic receptor, but in recent years substantial progress has been made toward its isolation and chemical characterization.

In spite of these remarkable advances we are still, as the following paragraphs will illustrate, a long way from understanding either nicotinic or muscarinic action at the molecular level. Most of what we have learned about these processes has come from studying intact tissues.

THE NICOTINIC RECEPTOR

As harvested from electric organ, the receptor is a glycoprotein of rather conventional amino acid composition [10]. Current estimates of its molecular weight are in the vicinity of 250,000. Within this receptor unit are four types of subunit, the smallest of which (about 40,000 daltons) is duplicated and appears to contain the major ACh-binding sites. The electron micrographic evidence [10, 11] suggests a hollow cylindrical structure, 7 to 9 nm in diameter, which protrudes from the outer, and perhaps also from the inner, face of the postsynaptic membrane. The idea of a central pore that ACh can convert into a cation channel [12] is attractive but not yet proven.

Little is known about the structure of the ACh-binding sites. Presumably at least one anionic group is present, since nicotinic agonists and antagonists typically possess at least one strongly electropositive group, usually centered on a quaternary N atom. A disulfide bond may be nearby, for the responses to some agonists are reversibly suppressed by the reducing agent dithiothreitol, which opens such bonds.

All nicotinic receptors do not behave alike. For example, tetraethylammonium and hexamethonium are classic competitive antagonists of ACh at ganglionic synapses, but they have little ability to block its action at neuromuscular synapses; gallamine has just the opposite

$$(CH_3)_3\overset{+}{N} - (CH_2)_6 - \overset{+}{N}(CH_3)_3$$
Hexamethonium

Gallamine

$$(CH_3)_3\overset{+}{N} - (CH_2)_{10} - \overset{+}{N}(CH_3)_3$$
Decamethonium

Tubocurarine

specificity; decamethonium has a strong ACh-like action on muscle end-plates, but little action on ganglion cells. Such findings suggest that the spacing of the anionic sites may be regular, but different, in the two kinds of location. (Tubocurarine, the classic neuromuscular blocking agent, blocks ganglionic synapses nearly as well.)

In solution, the purified receptors retain their high affinity for ACh. But when they have been inserted into artificial membranes and then treated with ACh, they have usually displayed little of their original ability to increase the membranes' cation conductance—a rather disappointing result in view of the success achieved in comparable experiments with the purified Ca^{2+}-transport protein. The latest efforts at reconstitution [13] seem, however, to have been more successful, and suggest that the receptor subunits themselves are the only materials needed to create the ionophore.

Nicotinic Action

The nicotinic action of ACh [14] is basically the same wherever it occurs: it opens membrane channels for cations. Both G_{Na} and G_K (Na^+ and K^+ conductances) are increased; G_{Na}, which in the absence of ACh is only a small fraction of G_K, rises to exceed it. The opening of these ionic channels short-circuits the membrane potential, causing a local depolarization (*end-plate potential* or *excitatory postsynaptic potential*), which if it reaches a critical level, will generate a conducted impulse (*action potential* or *spike*). Anion conductance is unaffected by nicotinic action, so it seems likely that the channels are aqueous pores lined with fixed negative charges, which reject anions. One can imagine that the channels, once opened, might become plugged if a base of matching molecular dimensions is present in the environment; and, in fact, it has been shown recently that some of the best-known nicotinic blocking drugs do act mainly in that way, rather than by preventing the attachment of ACh to the receptor sites.

Analysis of "end-plate noise" [15] has shown that in frog muscle exposed to ACh each channel opens for about a millisecond at a time, allowing the passage of at least 10^4 Na ions. Sophisticated biophysical studies [for review, see 16 and 17] reveal that the duration of this elemental event is affected by changes in temperature and transmembrane voltage and varies with the nicotinic agonist involved. It is also clear that there is some sort of interaction (cooperativity) between the ACh-binding subunits in a single receptor. As yet, however, it is not possible to give a simple account of either the kinetics of agonist-receptor interaction or of the relationship between receptor occupancy and channel opening.

Nicotinic responses are often brief, even when the agonist is kept in contact with the receptors. This may happen for either, or both, of two reasons: (1) The local depolarization, though initially sharply focused, gradually spreads beyond the receptor area, because the adjacent membrane voltage is discharged by current flowing through the opened channels; as a result, action potentials are no longer generated (*depolarizing block*). (2) Persistent contact with the nicotinic agent leads to *receptor desensitization*, a rather mysterious phenomenon that may represent a configuration of the receptor-ionophore complex that is different from either its resting or its active state.

THE MUSCARINIC RECEPTOR

Muscarinic receptors in vivo can be identified and labeled with the aid of specific reversible (or slowly reversible) antagonists such as benzilylcholine mustard [9] and its derivatives and 3-quinuclidinyl benzilate [18]. Receptors of this kind are less closely packed on cholinoceptive cell surfaces than are nicotinic receptors on end-plate and electroplaque membranes. In longitudinal gut muscle, for example, there are about 200 receptor sites per sq μm; but muscarinic sites are often scattered over a large part of the cell's surface, whereas nicotinic sites usually have a more restricted distribution. In brain, most of the cholinergic synapses are muscarinic, and the relative abundance of muscarinic receptors in different parts of the brain agrees rather well with the concentration of ChAT.

Although in vivo labeling of muscarinic and nicotinic receptors began at about the same time, progress toward the isolation and purification of the muscarinic variety has been comparatively slow. It appears that most of the procedures involving solubilization with detergents that work well with the nicotinic receptor either damage the muscarinic receptor or fail to detach it. However, some success has been obtained recently [19, 20], and it has been reported that the specific binding of muscarinic ligands in tissues from several species is associated with a single protein whose molecular weight is about 80,000.

The kinetic data obtained with antagonists applied to intact tissues also indicate that the sites are uniform everywhere: binding is in accordance with mass action, and the calculated affinity constants for a series of antagonists agree very well with their relative pharmacological potency. The binding of agonists, however, does not conform to this simple scheme. The same population of receptors is indeed involved; but to account for the kinetic data it is necessary to postulate that the binding sites form two major subpopulations and that the affinity of an agonist for one kind of site can be up to 300 times its affinity for the other kind [20a]. Surprisingly, it is the low-affinity site that is believed to be the functionally active one, perhaps because it is constrained through being coupled to an ionophore or a cyclase; the GTP level may be influential here. A further surprise is that choline is a potent muscarinic agonist in the brain [20b], though not in the periphery. The significance of this finding is still obscure.

Muscarinic Action

The consequences of muscarinic receptor activation differ from tissue to tissue [9] and cannot be stated simply. In many cases, the opening or closing of ionophores is a prominent, and perhaps the primary, event. If G_{Na} is increased or G_K is decreased, the response will be excitatory; if G_{Na} is decreased or G_K is increased, the response will be inhibitory. Each of these conductance changes can be observed in one or another type of cell; in central neurons, changes in G_K are mainly responsible for both excitation and inhibition [14]. Another frequent concomitant of muscarinic responses is the activation of guanylate cyclase [21]. This may appear early and may even be the primary event in some cases, but nothing is known about the nature of the coupling between receptor and cyclase. As in other systems, the respective roles of intracellular free Ca^{2+} and cyclic GMP are not easily sorted out [22]: a rise in the level of either might be responsible for some of the conductance changes mentioned earlier (see Chap. 15).

In comparison with nicotinic responses, observable muscarinic responses always develop and fade slowly; seconds are required, even in brain. Their minimum latency (at least 100 msec) seems too long for a conformational change to occur in an ionophore that is attached to the ACh-binding protein. It is easier to suppose that some kind of second messenger is involved, and that the delay represents the time required for an enzyme-mediated mechanism to operate, or for Ca^{2+} to be translocated as a result of the primary receptor perturbation.

PRESYNAPTIC RECEPTORS

Not all cholinergic receptors are postsynaptic. It is now well established that many of them have a presynaptic location, which may be close enough to transmitter release sites for the receptors to be involved in feedback control. Most commonly, the receptors involved are muscarinic, and the feedback is negative [23]; but presynaptic nicotinic receptors

play a minor role at mammalian neuromuscular junctions [24] and presumably elsewhere as well.

To make matters still more complicated, there are also muscarinic and nicotinic receptors on some adrenergic terminals and adrenergic (usually α) receptors on some cholinergic terminals (see Chap. 10), as well as presynaptic receptors for adenosine derivatives, prostaglandins, and a number of endogenous neuropeptides. It seems remarkable that they can all be accommodated in the space available. It is risky to generalize from a great number of scattered instances, but perhaps two comments can be offered in this context: (1) transmitter release during high-frequency synaptic activation is often limited by feedback mechanisms operating via presynaptic receptors; and (2) presynaptic inhibition at axoaxonal synapses, including those close to cholinergic junctions, sometimes depends on muscarinic or α-adrenergic action. As a cautionary note, it should be added that there are synapses where presynaptic receptor action seems to be negligible and others where the effects that have been ascribed to such action may really have been due to local changes in extracellular K^+ or Ca^{2+} resulting from the postsynaptic responses.

Synthesis of Acetylcholine

CHOLINE ACETYLTRANSFERASE

Location

Choline acetyltransferase was recognized as a distinct enzyme by Nachmansohn and Machado in 1943; its second substrate, acetyl-CoA, was not isolated until a few years later. As already noted, its distribution is like that of ACh; both are present throughout the length of cholinergic neurons and are concentrated in the axonal endings. It is now agreed that most of the ChAT in brain synaptosomes is free in the cytoplasm, and this is probably true for all cholinergic nerve endings in situ. But it is recognized that ChAT, especially in some species, tends to adhere to membranes, and it has been suggested that part of the nerve-ending ChAT is attached during life to the outer surface of the synaptic vesicles. It is further proposed that ACh newly synthesized by ChAT in that location might be placed favorably for transport into the interior of the vesicles, a point that will be discussed later.

Properties

ChAT [25, 26], extracted from the nervous tissue of different species and partially purified, is a stable, relatively basic, globular protein of about 68,000 M_r. The positive charge on the molecule varies with the species, and it is thought that several isoenzymes with different isoelectric points may be present in a single tissue [3]. These variations probably determine the proportion of enzyme that becomes bound to vesicles, and that proportion, in turn, may influence the relative turnover rates of vesicular and extravesicular ACh.

Not much has been learned about the composition of ChAT except that basic amino acids predominate. There may be a "dinucleotide fold" at the active site: this structure is thought to be characteristic of enzymes that depend on nucleotide-based coenzymes. A plausible candidate for participation at that site is the imidazole ring of histidine. In fact, free imidazole can catalyze the transfer of acetyl groups from CoA to choline in the absence of any enzyme. ChAT is readily inhibited by thiol reagents, but the critical thiol groups are probably not at the active site.

The substrate specificity of ChAT is by no means extreme, especially when it is in its natural environment. It can acetylate many alcoholic bases besides choline, and it can accept acyl groups other than acetyl from CoA as donor. But normally its only product, at least in vertebrate nervous tissue, is ACh, because normally the only substrates that are presented to it are choline and acetyl-CoA. (Whittaker [7] has reviewed the occurrence of other choline esters in nonnervous tissue and in invertebrates.)

Kinetics

All investigators agree that the reaction catalyzed by ChAT is reversible, and that acetyl-CoA has a higher affinity for the enzyme than does choline. Estimated Michaelis constants are of the order of $1\ mM$ for choline and $10\ \mu M$ for acetyl-CoA. Kinetic analyses [25, 26] on the brain enzyme (the placental enzyme behaves differently) are consistent with an ordered mechanism of the Theorell-Chance type, with the sequence of events shown in Fig. 9-1; ACh is thought to leave very soon after choline attaches.

In life, ChAT seldom, if ever, acetylates choline at anything like the rate it can achieve when it is in solution with an optimal supply of its substrates.

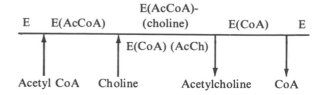

Fig. 9-1. Reaction mechanism of choline acetyltransferase.

ACh synthesis is slow in the absence of nerve impulses, but it accelerates greatly along with ACh release when synaptic traffic becomes brisk. In brain, in vivo synthesis can attain 25 percent of the in vitro rate [27]; in peripheral tissues, the percentage is always lower. Experimentally, the synthesis can, of course, be slowed by interfering with the supply of either substrate. But the question of how synthesis is controlled under physiological conditions of neural rest and activity is embarrassingly difficult to answer; some of the possible mechanisms are discussed on page 199.

SOURCE OF CHOLINE

Neurons, unlike liver cells, cannot synthesize choline de novo. The ultimate source of choline for ACh synthesis is, therefore, the free choline of the plasma. This is homeostatically maintained at a rather constant level, 10 to 20 μM, by renal and other mechanisms. In vivo, the small pool of extracellular free choline undergoes constant turnover, exchanging with both intracellular free choline (probably 8 to 40 nmol/g in brain [28]) and the much larger pool of choline covalently bound in tissue phospholipid. In vitro, phospholipid catabolism is likely to be dominant, and the free choline that diffuses out of a tissue placed in an initially choline-free artificial medium may soon attain a concentration adequate to support net ACh synthesis at an optimal rate. This fact has sometimes been ignored by neurochemists who apply radioactive choline to isolated tissues to study choline uptake or ACh turnover. No convincing evidence exists as yet that nerve endings can make direct use of phospholipid as a source of choline for ACh synthesis. It has been shown that lysophosphatidylcholine (and perhaps other choline esters) in the circulation can provide choline to make ACh in brain [29], but probably the bound choline becomes available for uptake only after it has been split off extraneurally.

Concentrative uptake of radioactive choline has been demonstrated for a number of tissues. Many other quaternary bases, including ACh, are taken up by the same mechanism, though usually more slowly; the hemicholiniums (HC-3 is the compound generally used) are the most potent of many bases that block uptake. In the first studies of this kind, the Michaelis constants (K_m) for the uptake of choline appeared to be in the range of 10 to 100 μM for most tissues, including brain. It seemed odd that the ChAT of nervous tissue should have to depend for its supply of substrate on a carrier that could not be efficiently loaded at a level of 10 μM, which is the plasma concentration of free choline, especially as experiments on perfused ganglia [30] had shown this level to be adequate to maintain ACh synthesis, even during maximal demand. In fact, according to the same experiments, active nerve endings have an extraordinary capacity for converting plasma choline into ACh: some 20 percent of the choline in the plasma can be trapped in this way, even though the plasma leaves the ganglion only a second or so after it enters.

This apparent paradox was resolved by the discovery in 1973 of a transport system in brain synaptosomes that has a much higher affinity for choline, with K_m values close to 1 μM. There is now convincing evidence [4] that this high-affinity system is located exclusively in cholinergic nerve endings and that most of the choline it transports is converted into ACh. Noncholinergic cells and terminals posses only the low-affinity mechanism discovered earlier. The high-affinity mechanism is carrier mediated, and Na^+- and Cl^--dependent; it is inhibited by low concentrations of HC-3 (K_i values below 0.1 μM have been reported); it does not significantly mediate the uptake of ACh, but it can transport a number of bases that are close chemical relatives of choline. The chemistry and the precise location of the high-affinity carrier, and the manner in which it is related (as it seems to be) to both ACh release and ACh synthesis, are problems for future research. There is no evidence that the high-affinity transport is directly coupled to an energy transducer such as an ATPase, but the process seems to be more complex than facilitated diffusion across the nerve-terminal plasma membrane. It may turn out that the carrier is somehow activated or made accessible to choline by vesicular exocytosis or, more likely, by some other event associated with the arrival of the nerve impulse [31, 32].

There is now much evidence [33] that cholinergic nerve endings recapture and reuse up to 60 percent of the choline formed by hydrolysis of the ACh they release. They do not recapture ACh, the transmitter itself; in this they differ from their adrenergic cousins, and probably from most other kinds of chemically transmitting nerve endings. Much of the uptake of choline during activity is accounted for by the reuptake, so it seems likely that the high-affinity uptake mechanism is particularly active for a few milliseconds after the arrival of each nerve impulse. After any longer period, the choline just formed from released ACh would have diffused away from the synapses and could not compete for uptake with the choline supplied by the circulation.

Choline diffuses readily across the capillary wall in most tissues, but it can penetrate the blood-brain barrier only by way of a low-affinity ($K_m = 220$ μM) transport system [34]. Consequently, most of the ACh that is being made in brain at any moment comes from choline that has been recycled locally through ACh or phospholipid; only a few percent come from choline that has just left the circulation [29]. The level of choline in the interstitial fluid of brain may be nearer to the level in the cerebrospinal fluid, which is only 1 to 5 μM [29], than to the plasma level. Thus, it has been suggested that ACh synthesis in brain may be limited by the supply of choline, especially when synaptic activity is accelerated; this is much less likely to occur in peripheral tissues.

SOURCE OF ACETYL-CoA
Experiments with labeled precursors leave little doubt that, in mammalian brain, the acetyl moiety of ACh is derived almost wholly from pyruvate

generated from glucose via the Embden-Meyerhof pathway [28, 35]. Curiously, acetate is a relatively poor source of acetyl-CoA for ACh synthesis in mammalian brain, although it is a good source of acetyl-CoA for lipid synthesis in that tissue and for ACh synthesis in *Torpedo* electroplaques, rabbit cornea, and lobster nerve. In all tissues studied, acetyl-CoA is primarily a product of the mito-chondrial inner compartment and is supposed not to leak out, so the problem of how mitochondrion-generated acetyl-CoA can give rise to cytoplasmic acetyl-CoA has been a continuing puzzle. Several ingenious explanations based on known metabolic pathways have been suggested, but at present none of them seems very likely [28]. It may be that in these nerve endings acetyl-CoA can, after all, leave the mitochondria [28] or can be made in the cyto-plasm with the aid of an enzyme, such as pyruvic dehydrogenase [36].

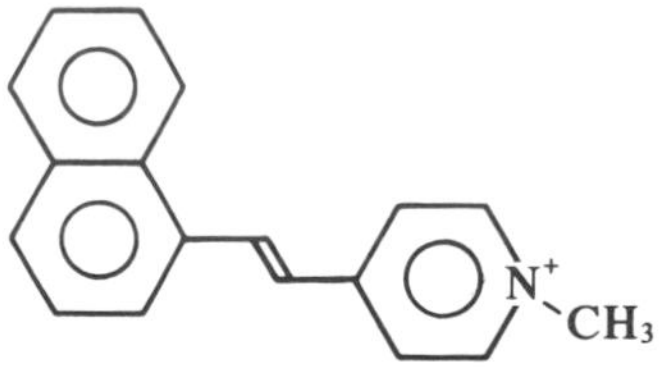

INHIBITORS OF ACETYLCHOLINE SYNTHESIS
A number of reversible and irreversible inhibi-tors of ChAT have been synthesized and studied [25, 37]. The most potent are a series of styryl-pyridines and some alkyl disulfides of CoA. Un-fortunately, these compounds, though active in vitro, have little effect on ChAT in its natural setting within the nerve ending, probably because they do not reach the enzyme in sufficient concen-tration. At present, the only reliable inhibitors of ACh synthesis in vivo are the compounds that com-pete with choline for the high-affinity carrier. They are all quaternary bases [38]. The best-known, and perhaps still the most potent, is HC-3, but some of the other hemicholiniums are little, if any, less active. (The hemicholiniums are characterized by the presence of a choline moiety cyclized through hemiacetal formation into a 6-membered ring.) Another inhibitor of interest is the triethyl analog of choline, known as *triethylcholine* (TEC). In vivo, these bases are delayed-action poisons and are effective in low dosage. In such dosage, they have no obvious effect on cholinergic transmission until the synapses have been activated long enough, or at high enough frequency, to deplete stored ACh below a critical level. Because the site of the high-

4 - (1 - naphthylvinyl) - 1 - methylpyridinium

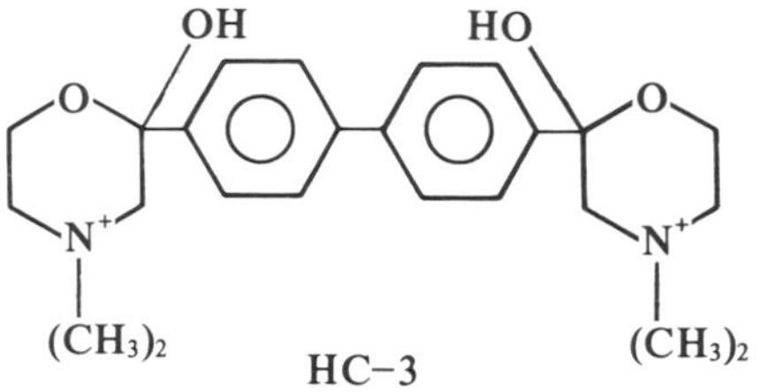

HC-3

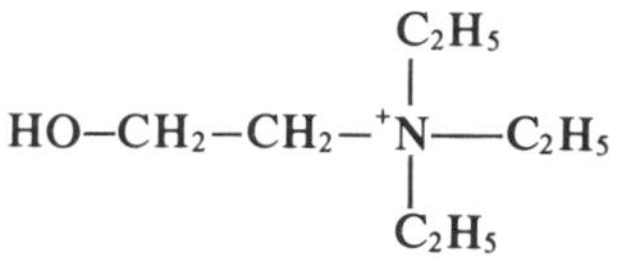

TEC

affinity transport system is still uncertain, the site at which its inhibitors act is also uncertain. TEC acts partly by generating a false transmitter (p. 199) and thus usurping ACh storage capacity in vesicles. HC-3 does not act in this way, but it is still unproved that the drug's only significant effect is to prevent the entry of choline into the presynaptic cytosol. Inhibition by the drug (or its acetyl ester) of ACh transfer from cytosol to vesicles remains a distinct possibility.

ACETYLCHOLINE UPTAKE BY BRAIN TISSUE
Though peripheral cholinergic endings trap choline efficiently, they cannot capture ACh [39]. Brain tissue can do so, however, apparently by the same mechanism that mediates the low-affinity uptake of choline. This uptake of ACh can be observed only when an organophosphate AChE inhibitor is used to protect the ACh; the uptake is blocked by physostigmine as well as by HC-3. The ACh that enters the tissue does not gain access to synaptic vesicles, and it is not released by stimulation. The

phenomenon is thus an artifact, the principal significance of which is that it can mislead the neurochemical experimenter.

Storage of Acetylcholine

COMPARTMENTATION OF NEURONAL ACETYLCHOLINE

ACh is presumed to be present with ChAT in the cell bodies and dendrites of vertebrate cholinergic neurons, but its concentration and location are not known. Axonal ACh appears to be free in the axoplasm, because when a nerve trunk is homogenized in an anticholinesterase-containing medium, nearly all of its ACh is found in the supernatant. The concentration of ACh in the axoplasm has been estimated as 0.3 mM. About 20 percent of the preformed ACh of brain tissue is released by simple homogenization: no doubt much of this free ACh, as it is called, originates from cell bodies and axons.

ACh in nerve endings behaves differently [40]. Osmotic or mechanical lysis of synaptosomes releases no more than half of this ACh (*labile-bound ACh*). The rest of it remains sedimentable (*stable-bound ACh*): much of this can be recovered in a well-defined fraction of very small particles, which, when examined with the electron microscope, cannot be distinguished from synaptic vesicles. The remainder is in vesicle-containing debris. It seems reasonable to conclude that stable-bound ACh represents ACh that was in the vesicles during life. But it is probably less safe to conclude that labile-bound ACh represents ACh that was in the terminal cytosol during life: some of the vesicular ACh might have become free during the manipulations.

Reliable information about ACh levels in the presynaptic cytosol and vesicles of brain neurons would be of great interest. The information we have is not very reliable, unfortunately, partly because of the just-mentioned uncertainty about leakage, but even more because we do not know what proportion of the harvested synaptosomes are cholinergic. Whittaker's guess, 10 to 15 percent, seems as good as any. On that basis, he calculated [see 41] that there would be some 2,000 ACh molecules in a vesicle; this would make the ACh concentration in the vesicle core about 0.2 M if all the ACh is in the form of free ions. Whittaker's estimate agrees well with one based on data for vesicles harvested from sympathetic ganglia, in which most of the synapses can be assumed to be cholinergic. After correcting for various biasing factors, Wilson and coworkers [42] arrived at a figure of 1,630 molecules per vesicle. Taken at face value, these estimates for mammalian vesicles suggest that the vesicular fluid is approximately isotonic with its surroundings and that ACh is its principal cation.

The data for cholinergic vesicles from the *Torpedo* electric organ [41] are firmer than those for vesicles from mammalian brain, and support the same conclusion. As *Torpedo* vesicles are much larger and are situated in a medium of higher osmolarity, they hold much more ACh, up to 300,000 molecules per vesicle. *Torpedo* vesicles are smaller when depleted of their ACh by exhaustive stimulation; there is some evidence that mammalian vesicles behave similarly.

BINDING OF VESICULAR ACETYLCHOLINE

Torpedo vesicles contain ATP. The molar ratio of ACh to ATP is about 16, which is similar to the ratio found for vesicles from the electric tissues of other fish species and also to the amine-ATP ratios reported for several kinds of amine storage particle [43]. Also present in the vesicle core is vesiculin [5], now characterized as a glycosaminoglycan, which contains sulfate, binds free amino acids strongly, and may exist in vivo as part of a proteoglycan. It is natural to suppose that ATP and a vesiculin complex are counterions for ACh and help to keep it inside the vesicles, but this has not yet been demonstrated.

In life, the vesicles must take up and retain ACh against a fairly steep concentration gradient; this suggests that there might be some sort of pump in the vesicular membrane. Its action could be to exchange Na^+ or choline for ACh, or to create an electrical gradient favoring ACh accumulation, or simply to move ACh uphill; but none of these mechanisms has been detected, nor is it known whether there is an electrical gradient across the membrane. Indeed, isolated vesicles placed in an ACh-containing medium have shown little capacity for either net uptake or exchange of ACh.

There is evidence from *Torpedo* that ATP and ACh are released by stimulation [43] and that ATP replenishment is assisted by a high-affinity uptake system for adenosine [44]. The fate of vesiculin lost during synaptic activity is uncertain.

SURPLUS ACETYLCHOLINE

When a peripheral tissue supplied by cholinergic axons is treated with a suitable anticholinesterase, its ACh content rises during an hour or so to about twice its initial value, even in the absence of nerve impulses [for references, see 28]. The ACh formed under these conditions has been called *surplus ACh*. It is clearly intracellular, and there are several reasons for thinking that it is presynaptic: the postsynaptic elements have little capacity for making ACh or for taking it up from outside; a tissue deprived of its cholinergic supply loses its ability to form surplus ACh; and cholinergic axons whose AChE is inactivated also accumulate additional ACh [45]. These findings, and others, suggest that some of the presynaptic AChE in peripheral tissues is inward-facing, and that when it is inhibited the level of ACh in the nerve endings rises as a result of continuing synthesis to a higher than normal level. There is now conclusive evidence [46] that surplus ACh in ganglia and muscles cannot be released by nerve impulses (although it can slowly exchange with releasable ACh in muscles). It can, however, be released by K^+ and by nicotinic agonists, including ACh itself; these agents release no ACh from the normal synaptic store. Surplus ACh must therefore be held in some compartment other than the one that holds most of the normal store, which is 80 to 90 percent releasable. Certainly, the simplest interpretation is to suppose that surplus ACh is in the presynaptic cytosol outside the vesicles; but other interpretations have been preferred [28], and decisive evidence is lacking. Surplus ACh is an experimental artifact, but one of considerable significance. Its rate of formation is a measure of intracellular ACh turnover at rest. If the location just suggested for it can be proved, the evidence that nerve impulses release ACh by vesicular exocytosis—a hypothesis that is still often challenged—will be greatly strengthened.

Surplus ACh formation, as just discussed, is a phenomenon that has been described for peripheral synapses. The evidence that it occurs at central cholinergic synapses is less satisfactory [28]. Perhaps only peripheral cholinergic endings possess inward-facing AChE and, therefore, normally have little ACh outside the vesicles.

Release of Acetylcholine

QUANTAL TRANSMISSION

Much of our information about ACh release has come from electrophysiological experiments. These show that ACh is released in multimolecular packets or quanta [47] at some, and probably all, cholinergic synapses. When the nerve ending is at rest, the quanta are released singly and with nearly random timing. When the nerve ending is partly depolarized, for example, by applying K^+ or a cathodal current, the quanta are released more often: the greater the depolarization, the higher the frequency. When the nerve ending is invaded by an impulse and therefore fully depolarized (there is actually a reversal of its membrane potential), the frequency of release is greatly increased for a brief instant. In the special case of the neuromuscular junction, a few hundred quanta may be released almost synchronously from numerous sites on the motor axon's terminal expanse. At more typical nerve endings, an impulse probably releases no more than one or two quanta from any one varicosity.

The probability that an ACh quantum will emerge from a given release site at any selected instant depends, as has just been seen, on the presynaptic transmembrane potential at that site. It also depends on a second major factor, the concentration of Ca^{2+} in the extracellular medium, or—more accurately—at some critical site or sites in the nerve ending itself. As the nerve ending becomes depolarized, Ca^{2+} enters (along with Na^+) and forms a temporary complex with some nerve ending constituent. The amount of complex formed determines the probability of quantal release. This probability is small in the absence of external Ca^{2+}, and also if the external Mg^{2+} concentration is high;

Mg^{2+} competes with Ca^{2+}, preventing formation of the complex.

The material with which Ca^{2+} combines has not been identified. Either the binding of Ca^{2+}, or some later step in the release process, shows cooperativity, for as external Ca^{2+} is gradually raised from zero there is a more than proportionate increase in the number of quanta released by an impulse. One mathematical analysis of the biophysical data has suggested that four calcium ions must attach in order to activate a single release site [48].

An intriguing finding, the significance of which has not yet been evaluated, is the presence of a discrete Ca^{2+}-binding site on each synaptic vesicle [49]. It is tempting to theorize that the divalent calcium ion is able to attach itself simultaneously to presynaptic membrane and vesicles, and thus to promote vesicular exocytosis, but this notion is certainly an oversimplification [50]. It does seem safe to conclude, however, that the Ca^{2+} complex has only a brief existence and that thereafter the Ca^{2+} that has entered is trapped by other nerve ending constituents, as well as by the mitochondria, before eventually being extruded. It is also probable that intracellular Na^+, here as in other kinds of cells, can displace trapped intracellular Ca^{2+} and so make it available for promoting release. During repetitive excitation both Na^+ and Ca^{2+} will accumulate, so each impulse may release more quanta even when the total stock of ACh is being depleted. Metabolic poisons also potentiate release temporarily in many cases; they can do so by interfering with both Na^+ and Ca^{2+} extrusion.

Quantum Size

All the influences discussed above act to determine the number of quanta released, not the size of the individual quanta. Quantum size, that is, the amount of ACh per quantum, is generally rather uniform, at least at the neuromuscular junction. It can be increased, however, by various treatments (e.g., high concentrations of Ca^{2+}, or vinblastine) that cause vesicles to coalesce, and it can be decreased by repetitive stimulation when ACh synthesis is blocked by HC-3 [51]. Even in the absence of such drugs, some quanta of substandard size are released, and these may predominate in junctions that have been subjected to prolonged stimulation or poisoned with botulinum toxin [52], an agent that somehow interferes with the action of

Ca^{2+} [53]. It has been argued [52] that each normal-sized quantum is made up of a number, up to 10 to 15, of these smaller quanta. An extension of the argument would be that the smaller, rather than the larger, quantum represents the ACh in a single vesicle.

There are numerous estimates of the number of ACh molecules in a mammalian quantum, but the smallest recent estimate, 6,250 molecules [54], is larger than the estimates quoted for mammalian vesicles. The best estimates for snake and frog quanta [55, 56] are also larger than those for vesicles.

Are Quanta Preformed?

The observations just mentioned have offered a challenge to the vesicle hypothesis of transmitter release, at least in its original form, which equates the quantum to the ACh contained in a vesicle. A more radical attack on the hypothesis is the assertion that quanta are not normally released by vesicular exocytosis but by some quite different mechanism, which is usually conceived to be the transient opening of membrane channels, through which ACh escapes from the cytosol, or from a small compartment that refills from the cytosol [57–61]. On this basis, the vesicular ACh would be regarded as a reservoir, serving only to replenish the releasable store during synaptic activity: there is, in fact, no doubt that vesicular ACh turns over rapidly in such circumstances. The original hypothesis has been amplified and warmly defended, especially by Heuser, Whittaker, Zimmermann and their coworkers [41, 50, 62, 63], and is probably still favored by the majority of workers in the field (see Chap. 8), although it is agreed that the details of the interaction between vesicular and presynaptic membranes are not understood. Those who wish to sample the flavor of this important controversy, which, even if unsettled, has stimulated research of lasting value, may consult the papers above; there are also some less committed reviews [e.g., 64–66].

Stimulation of adrenergic pathways releases the soluble proteins and ATP of the vesicles along with the norepinephrine. From this result it is naturally inferred that the release depends upon exocytosis. Similar experiments on cholinergic pathways have been attempted but so far have not provided convincing evidence for exocytosis [65].

SOME SUGGESTED RELEASE MECHANISMS
A role for *cyclic nucleotides* in ACh release has been postulated to account for the finding that both caffeine and dibutyryl cyclic AMP increase nerve-evoked ACh discharge at the neuromuscular junction. The numerous examples of mutual feedback between Ca^{2+} transport and nucleotide-cyclase systems make such a mechanism plausible enough in principle, but there have been some negative findings [65], and a convincing case has not yet been made. This is further discussed in Chap. 15.

One of the prostaglandins, PGE_1, is known to be involved in the negative-feedback control of norepinephrine release (see Chap. 16), but it seems to have no significant action on ACh release [65]. The prostaglandins are more likely to be involved in ACh mobilization, the process by which ACh in the depots is made more readily available for release.

The evidence that contractile proteins are involved in some way in ACh release is provocative but still incomplete [67]. Possible roles for such proteins would include the movement of vesicles toward the presynaptic membrane, the supposed exocytotic process itself, and the subsequent recycling of vesicular membrane components. The *active zones* of transmitter release, especially at the neuromuscular junction, have been brilliantly visualized by both thin-section and freeze-fracture electron microscopy [50, 61]. These zones form parallel ridges on the outer face of the presynaptic membrane, facing the postsynaptic folds; each ridge is adorned with a double array of fine particles and, under conditions of intense transmitter release, is bordered by images that look like exocytotic (or endocytotic) figures. Filamentous or microtubular material adherent to the vesicles at these zones must at least be concerned with the nonrandom distribution of vesicles within the presynaptic axoplasm. What further roles all these particles and granules may play will be hard to decide until they are better characterized chemically.

Removal of Acetylcholine
CHOLINESTERASES
Acetylcholinesterase is one of a number of cholinesterases. It is the one that splits ACh most rapidly and is the only one, so far as we know, that is functionally important at cholinergic synapses. The other cholinesterases are collectively referred to as *acylcholinesterases*, or sometimes as *pseudocholinesterases*. The best known of these is a plasma enzyme, the preferred substrate of which is butyrylcholine; its physiological role is ill defined.

ACETYLCHOLINESTERASE
Location
AChE is manufactured in cholinergic cell bodies, and its intracellular location there has been verified by histochemistry at the ultrastructural level. It is delivered to the synapses by axonal transport (see Chaps. 20 and 22). Koelle and coauthors [68] noted that only part of the AChE of brain behaves as if it were accessible to quaternary substrates and inhibitors. They supposed that this fraction of the enzyme (*functional AChE*) is outward facing, and the remainder (*reserve AChE*) is inward facing and in transit. The ability of peripheral cholinergically innervated tissues to form surplus ACh [46] in the presence of an anticholinesterase suggests that at least a small part of the enzyme transported by peripheral axons is still in the reserve orientation as it nears the synapses; cerebral cortex, which seems to have less of that ability, may possess only functional AChE.

As has already been noted, much of the body's AChE does not originate in neurons. In skeletal muscle, even the junctional AChE is largely postsynaptic and is synthesized by muscle rather than by nerve cells.

Properties and Kinetics
Most tissues contain several forms of AChE [79, 80, 87]. These are catalytically identical glycoproteins, but they differ in molecular weight, ease of extraction, and physical properties. In order of increasing size they are: a monomer of about 65,000 daltons, the likely precursor of the other forms; a dimer and

a tetramer, which are partly in solution and partly membrane-bound; and several asymmetric species that have a cluster of monomers attached to a collagen tail. In neurons the enzyme is transported along the axon and eventually externalized; when this happens, part remains attached to the neurilemma, but part is secreted into the extracellular space [96]. At nicotinic junctions the collagen-tailed variants predominate; they are not membrane-bound, but reside in the synaptic cleft.

The active center of each subunit has been described as incorporating *anionic* and *esteratic* sites, which fit respectively the cationic trimethyl cluster and the ester carbonyl of ACh, but binding at the anionic site depends more on hydrophobic than on coulombic interactions. The esteratic site incorporates a serine side chain, as do many hydrolytic enzymes; a histidine imidazole is also present. The enzyme's substrates and inhibitors are varied chemically, but all of them combine with it in precisely the same way. The irreversible (or very slowly reversible) organophosphorus inhibitors, including the awesomely toxic nerve gases, inactivate the enzyme by phosphorylating the serine hydroxyl; most of the other well-known inhibitors, including physostigmine (eserine) and neostigmine, are carbamates and carbamylate the same group, but reversibly. Kinetic studies of the enzyme indicate a three-step reaction with ACh (Fig. 9-2). The final deacetylation is probably the rate-controlling step. AChE is one of the fastest enzymes, with a turnover number higher than 10^{-4} sec^{-1}; but its velocity falls off at high substrate concentrations, because of the increased probability that two ACh molecules might attach at a single active center and thus prevent each other's hydrolysis (substrate inhibition).

Physiological Significance

The role of AChE at synapses can be studied by applying a drug such as physostigmine, the principal action of which is to inhibit the enzyme. The lifetime of synaptically released ACh is then prolonged. Ongoing muscarinic actions are intensified. Ongoing nicotinic actions are also intensified initially, but nicotinic blockade may follow if the frequency of synaptic activation is high. The reason

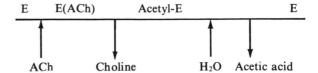

Fig. 9-2. *Reaction mechanism of acetylcholinesterase.*

that blockade is not seen at lower activation frequencies is that simple diffusion can remove released ACh from the synaptic area within milliseconds. As was pointed out earlier, ACh, unlike norepinephrine and probably unlike most other transmitters, is not recaptured to any extent by the nerve endings that have released it; only the choline derived from its breakdown can be taken up and reused. So AChE has a double function: on the postsynaptic side, it prevents released ACh from acting longer than is necessary; and on the presynaptic side, it helps to ensure an adequate supply of choline for ACh synthesis.

Anticholinesterase poisoning, if not too severe, can be relieved by treatment with atropine, supplemented by a suitable oxime ($R \cdot CH \cdot NOH$), if the poisoning is the result of a long-acting organophosphorus inhibitor. The oxime combines chemically with the phosphorus atom of inhibitor and so reactivates the enzyme. The outstanding example is pralidoxime (*N*-methylpyridinium-2-aldoxime chloride). Pharmacology texts give further information.

Turnover of Acetylcholine

MEASUREMENT OF TURNOVER

In vivo, choline is ACh's only precursor and also its only breakdown product, except for the acetyl moiety. In theory, therefore, one should be able to determine the turnover of tissue ACh under steady state conditions by measuring either (1) the rate at which choline is being turned into ACh, or (2) the rate at which ACh is being turned into choline. In practice, neither of these approaches is easy.

As an index of (1), one can observe the rate at which labeled plasma choline enters the ACh store; but this will result in underestimation of turnover, because endogenous choline is always being recycled through ACh, and there is no way of finding the specific activity of only that choline that is being presented to the tissue's ChAT. As an index of (2), one can measure the rate at which ACh is released when its destruction is prevented by an anticholinesterase; but that is often technically difficult, and even when it is possible, it is hard to be sure how the drug may have affected the intraterminal compartmentation and metabolism of ACh. Rather similar objections can be raised to all the other methods that have been suggested for quantitating ACh turnover in vivo [71], including those methods based on labeling the acetyl group. Nevertheless, such turnover studies are still a useful approach to the assessment of cholinergic function in the intact brain [27, 72, 73]. Alterations of turnover can generally be detected, even if the absolute values remain somewhat uncertain. Mere measurement of changes in ACh content gives less reliable information.

The problems of measuring ACh turnover in isolated cell and tissue preparations are usually less severe, although the use of drugs to block ACh synthesis or breakdown always introduces some uncertainties.

RESTING TURNOVER
Two kinds of observation show that synaptic ACh is being synthesized and destroyed even in the absence of nerve impulses. The ACh store increases in size (surplus ACh formation) when the extracellular medium contains a penetrating anticholinesterase, and the store becomes labeled when the medium contains radioactive choline. Reported ACh turnover rates, measured in either of these ways, are 0.5 to 1.5 percent per minute in ganglia, muscles, and salivary glands [65]. Most of this resting turnover is intracellular, at least in ganglia; no more than 10 to 20 percent of it can be accounted for by the ACh that escapes into the medium. ACh turnover at central synapses during rest appears to be faster than at these peripheral synapses. Rates of about 5 percent per minute can be calculated from labeling measurements on anesthetized whole brain in situ [27] and on cortical slices treated with tetrodotoxin to eliminate nerve impulses. In brain,

however, the ACh that is released probably accounts for most of the turnover, for brain tissue is less able to form surplus ACh than are peripheral tissues. Relatively high rates of resting ACh release and turnover also have been reported for neuroeffector synapses in intestine [65].

TURNOVER DURING ACTIVITY
The experimental data from ganglia [30] and skeletal muscles [74] are in good agreement. In these tissues, synaptic activity accelerates both synthesis and release of ACh, and the increase in both is frequency-dependent up to a maximum, which is reached at about 16 Hz in the case of plasma-perfused ganglia subjected to prolonged stimulation. When driven at this frequency, either set of synapses can maintain an ACh turnover rate of 7 to 10 percent per minute, whereas their stored ACh remains at about the resting level.

These rates are impressive, but those for mammalian brain in situ are an order of magnitude higher. Several laboratories [72, 73] have now reported mean turnover times of only 1 to 2 minutes for part or all of the brain ACh. The fastest of these turnover rates is about 25 percent of the rate at which the ChAT present could synthesize ACh under optimal conditions. There is some reason to think that an even higher rate might be reached in animals subjected to stress. The effects of anesthetics and other drugs suggest that ACh turnover in brain, as in peripheral tissues, depends on the frequency of synaptic activation, but no quantitative relationship has been established.

POOLS, COMPARTMENTS, AND MOBILIZATION
The preceding paragraphs have dealt with synaptic ACh turnover under steady state conditions, but often such conditions do not exist. The commonest reason for departure from steady state conditions is a change in the frequency of synaptic activation. When this occurs, the amounts of ACh released by successive nerve impulses are determined by the interaction of several processes that are poorly understood at present. Some of these processes increase, and some decrease the release. According to the quantum hypothesis, which assumes that

there is a store of preformed quanta in the nerve ending, all the processes influence one or both of two parameters: (1) the number of quanta that at a given moment are available for release, because they are in a particular state or location, and (2) the probability that any of these quanta will be released by the next impulse.

As to (1), many neurochemical and neurophysiological analyses support the idea that all the nerve ending ACh is not equally releasable but is distributed between two or more *pools*. In the simplest model [30], there is a smaller *readily available* pool and a large *reserve* pool. The process by which the first pool is replenished from the second has been called *mobilization,* and there is no doubt that it is often rate-limiting for release. In an effort to accommodate all the experimental data, subdivisions of the two pools have sometimes been postulated. One further modification is certainly required: experiments on several tissues whose ACh stores were partly replaced by radioactive ACh showed clearly that newly synthesized ACh is preferentially released [65]; apparently the readily available pool is replenished largely by new synthesis, not just by mobilization of old ACh from the reserve pool.

As to (2), studies of peripheral synapses have shown that the major factor determining the probability of release is undoubtedly the level of Ca^{2+} in the nerve ending [75]. This Ca^{2+} includes both the Ca^{2+} that enters during a given impulse and the Ca^{2+} that entered previously and became trapped reversibly. The exact locations of the active and the trapped Ca^{2+} are unknown, as was stated earlier.

It would be a forward step if the notion of *pools* could be discarded and, if instead, ACh metabolism could be described in terms of morphologically identifiable *compartments*. At present, however, this would be a step into the dark or, at best, into an area of dimly lit pitfalls. The *readily available* pool has been plausibly conceived as representing the ACh in those vesicles that are close to the presynaptic release sites or perhaps actually adherent to them. There is some morphological support for this concept [50], and although it is not yet overpowering, there is a good deal of evidence, especially from *Torpedo* [63], that there are two vesicle populations differing in their lability or their degree of filling. An earlier proposal [76] was that there are two kinds of vesicular ACh, *internal* and *surface-bound*. Reference has already been made to the competing hypothesis that the immediate source of released ACh is the cytosol rather than the vesicles: on that basis, the vesicular ACh would constitute the reserve pool.

FALSE TRANSMITTERS

A number of bases related to choline that are not normally present in the body can enter cholinergic nerve endings by the high-affinity mechanism and be acetylated there [77]. When this happens, the acetyl base enters the normal transmitter store. It can be released by nerve impulses if Ca^{2+} is present, and it will then exert a postsynaptic action, although a weaker one than that of ACh. It thus qualifies as a *false transmitter*. Research on this phenomenon has brought a number of significant facts to light, of which two may be mentioned: (1) some choline homologs are efficiently acetylated by ChAT in nerve endings, though hardly at all by ChAT in solution; (2) when both ACh and a false transmitter are present, they behave very similarly—they both enter vesicles, they contribute to the same quanta [78], and they are equally available for release. These last findings show that releasable ACh behaves as if it were in a fairly well-stirred compartment, but they do not identify the compartment morphologically.

RATE-LIMITING FACTORS

ACh synthesis in nerve endings depends on the availability of choline, glucose (or lactate or pyruvate), and O_2 from the extracellular medium [28, 65]. Extracellular Na^+ is also a requisite, because it supports both choline uptake and ACh storage. In vivo, the plasma levels of all these factors are normally well maintained by efficient homeostatic mechanisms; and so far as peripheral nerve endings are concerned, there is no convincing evidence that the extracellular level of any of them is limiting for ACh synthesis, unless a disease process or a poison (e.g., HC-3) is present.

The situation in brain may be different. At cortical synapses, as already noted, ACh turnover is much faster; the extrasynaptic space is limited; and one of the extracellular factors, free choline, can enter that space only by a low-affinity carrier. Thus, it would not be surprising if ACh synthesis in brain were limited by the availability of choline, at least in some circumstances. In support of that notion, it has been demonstrated that brain ACh levels rise significantly when plasma choline is increased [79, 80], and it has also been shown that certain neurological abnormalities thought to be caused by central cholinergic hypofunction are relieved by prolonged administration of choline or lecithin in amount sufficient to produce hypercholinemia. In these cases, however, the evidence is incomplete that choline is acting primarily as an ACh precursor to accelerate ACh synthesis; it is possible that it may be acting mainly as a muscarinic agonist. (Muscarinic agonists are known to raise brain ACh, mainly because they act on presynaptic receptors to reduce ACh release; and choline is a fairly potent muscarinic agonist in cortex.) But whatever the role of choline may be, it is clear in any case that the synthesis of ACh in brain is less closely coupled to its release than it is in peripheral tissues [28, 65]. Ganglia and muscles, for example, can maintain their ACh stores almost undiminished even during intense synaptic activity, whereas in cortex the stores are always in a state of partial depletion, except perhaps during deep sleep or anesthesia: the greater the synaptic activity, the more severe the depletion.

Because the action of ChAT is reversible, its equilibrium position with respect to its substrates and products must determine both the net rate of ACh synthesis and the level of free ACh in the cytosol [81]. This statement implies that the ratio of CoA to acetyl-CoA in the vicinity of the enzyme may be at least as important as the ratio of ACh to choline. Unfortunately, we have no reliable information about either ratio in any set of nerve endings during life. There has been much speculation about how synthesis is regulated and linked to release, and most of the conceivable rate-controlling factors have been suggested at one time or another. Some of these (which may not be entirely independent of one another) are activation of the choline uptake system by depolarization or by ion movements resulting from depolarization; inactivation of that system by accumulating ACh; inhibition of ChAT by ACh; allosteric suppression of that inhibition by Cl^- entering the cytosol during depolarization; translocation of newly synthesized ACh into the vesicular compartment or of CoA into mitochondria; transport of acetyl-CoA out of mitochondria or the reacetylation of CoA by a cytoplasmic enzyme system. These factors are evaluated in a number of reviews [28; see also 4, 26, 59, 65, 69, 79, 82].

ACh mobilization is the limiting process for ACh release at peripheral synapses that are being activated at high frequency. Under these conditions, ACh output per unit of time cannot be maintained at its initial maximum but declines to a steady level that is independent of the frequency [30]. The decline is not the result of failure of ACh synthesis, because there is little change in the level of stored ACh and there is no reason to suppose that release has become less efficient. By exclusion, release must be determined by the rate of mobilization, and neurochemical studies have revealed only that in ganglia it is promoted by an unidentified factor present in normal plasma [30]. Little is known about ACh mobilization at central synapses.

ACh release at physiological rates of activation is controlled by Ca^{2+} influx, as has been stressed. Some secondary factors that promote release may be mentioned: CO_2, which may increase intracellular calcium ionization; intraterminal Na^+, which competes with Ca^{2+} for binding sites; presynaptic hyperpolarization, which results from repetitive activation and augments the nerve ending spike; and numerous drugs, acting by a variety of mechanisms [65]. As yet, there is no biochemical explanation for the extraordinary ability of botulinum toxin (and, to a lesser degree, certain other toxic proteins made by bacteria and animal venom glands) to block ACh release irreversibly, while doing nothing to interfere with the functioning of noncholinergic synapses.

As indicated earlier, the major problem in constructing models for ACh turnover in cholinergic endings has been that of deciding how to set the biochemical information in its morphological context. That problem remains perplexing, even though it seems to have been largely solved for the analogous case of adrenergic endings, and even though there is a wealth of clearly relevant data from both biochemical and morphological studies. As soon as the nerve ending compartment from which ACh quanta emerge has been conclusively identified, all these data, and also the biophysical data, will contribute precision to an integrated scheme. Readers who cannot wait for this to happen can examine the facts and arguments presented in the references cited here [58–61, 63–66] and try to make up their own minds.

Other Aspects of Cholinergic Function

Neurotransmitter systems are influenced by development, by aging, and by use and disuse. These aspects of cholinergic function have been considered in a number of reviews [28, 65, 83–86].

References

*1. Pauling, P. The Shapes of Cholinergic Molecules. In P. G. Waser (ed.), *Cholinergic Mechanisms.* New York: Raven, 1974. Pp. 241–249.

*2. Green, J. P., Johnson, C. L., and Kang, S. Application of quantum chemistry to drugs and their interactions. *Annu. Rev. Pharmacol.* 14:319–342, 1974.

*3. Fonnum, F. Molecular Aspects of Compartmentation of Choline Acetyltransferase. In R. Balazs and J. E. Cremer (eds.), *Metabolic Compartmentation in the Brain.* New York: Wiley, 1972. Pp. 35–45.

4. Kuhar, M. J., and Murrin, L. C. Sodium-dependent, high affinity choline uptake. *J. Neurochem.* 30:15–21, 1978.

5. Stadler, H., and Whittaker, V. P. Identification of vesiculin as a glycosaminoglycan. *Brain Res.* 153: 408–413, 1978.

*6. Kuhar, M. J., and Atweh, S. F. Distribution of some suspected neurotransmitters in the central nervous system. *Rev. Neurosci.* 3:35–76, 1978.

*7. Whittaker, V. P. Identification of Acetylcholine and Related Choline Esters of Biological Origin. In G. B. Koelle (ed.), *Handbuch der experimentellen Pharmakologie: Cholinesterases and Anticholinesterase Agents.* Berlin: Springer-Verlag, 1963. Suppl. 15, pp. 1–39.

*8. Hanin, I. (ed.). *Choline and Acetylcholine: Hand-*

book of Chemical Assay Methods. New York: Raven, 1974.

*9. Rang, H. P. Acetylcholine receptors. *Q. Rev. Biophys.* 7:283–399, 1974.

*10. Briley, M. S., and Changeux, J-P. Isolation and purification of the nicotinic receptor and its functional reconstitution into a membrane environment. *Int. Rev. Neurobiol.* 20:31–63, 1977.

11. Potter, L. T., and Smith, D. S. Postsynaptic membranes in the electric tissue of *Narcine.* I. Organization and innervation of electric cells. Fine structure of nicotinic receptor-channel molecules revealed by transmission microscopy. *Tissue Cell* 9:585–594, 1977.

*12. Potter, L. T. Acetylcholine Receptor-Channel Molecules. In G. S. Levey (ed.), *Hormone Receptor Interaction: Molecular Aspects.* New York: Dekker, 1976. Pp. 401–431.

*13. Wu, W. C.-S., and Raftery, M. A. Reconstitution of acetylcholine receptor function using purified receptor protein. *Biochemistry* 20:694–701, 1981.

*14. Krnjević, K. Chemical nature of synaptic transmission in vertebrates. *Physiol. Rev.* 54:418–540, 1974.

*15. Katz, B., and Miledi, R. The Analysis of Endplate Noise—A New Approach to the Study of Acetylcholine/Receptor Interaction. In S. Thesleff (ed.), *Motor Innervation of Muscle.* New York: Academic, 1976. Pp. 31–50.

*16. Colquhoun, D. Mechanisms of drug action at the voluntary muscle end-plate. *Annu. Rev. Pharmacol.* 15:307–325, 1975.

17. Stevens, C. F. Synaptic actions of acetylcholine: Problems for future research. *Fed. Proc.* 37:2651–2653, 1978.

18. Yamamura, H. I., Kuhar, M. J., and Snyder, S. H. In vivo identification of muscarinic cholinergic receptor binding in brain. *Brain Res.* 80:170–176, 1974.

19. Aronstam, R. S., Schuessler, D. C., Jr., and Eldefrawi, M. E. Solubilization of muscarinic acetylcholine receptors of bovine brain. *Life Sci.* 23: 1377–1382, 1978.

20. Hulme, E. C., Birdsall, N. J. M., and Burgen, A. S. V. A study of the muscarinic receptor by gel electrophoresis. *Br. J. Pharmacol.* 66:337–342, 1979;

20a. Hulme, E. C., Birdsall, N. J. M., and Burgen, A. S. V. The binding of agonists to brain muscarinic receptors. *Mol. Pharmacol.* 14:723–736, 1978.

20b. Krnjević, K., and Reinhardt, W. Choline excites cortical neurons. *Science* 206:1321–1323, 1979.

21. Greengard, P. Possible role for cyclic nucleotides and phosphorylated membrane proteins in postsynaptic actions of neurotransmitters. *Nature* 260: 101–108, 1976.

*Key reference.

*22. Krnjević, K.   Acetylcholine and Cyclic GMP. In D. J. Jenden (ed.), *Cholinergic Mechanisms and Psychopharmacology*. New York: Plenum, 1978. Pp. 261–266.

*23. Szerb, J. C.   Characterization of Presynaptic Muscarinic Receptors in Central Cholinergic Neurons. In D. J. Jenden (ed.), *Cholinergic Mechanisms and Psychopharmacology*. New York: Plenum, 1978. Pp. 49–60.

*24. Miyamoto, M. D.   The actions of cholinergic drugs on motor terminals. *Pharmacol. Rev.* 29: 221–247, 1977.

*25. Mautner, H. G.   Choline acetyltransferase. *CRC Crit. Rev. Biochem.* 4:341–370, 1977.

*26. Rossier, J.   Choline acetyltransferase: A review with special reference to its cellular and subcellular location. *Int. Rev. Neurobiol.* 20:283–337, 1977.

*27. Sparf, B.   On the turnover of acetylcholine in brain. *Acta Physiol. Scand.* (Suppl. 397):7–47, 1973.

*28. Tuček, S.   *Acetylcholine Synthesis in Neurons.* London: Chapman and Hall, 1978.

29. Freeman, J. J., and Jenden, D. J.   The source of choline for acetylcholine synthesis in brain. *Life Sci.* 19:949–962, 1976.

30. Birks, R., and MacIntosh, F. C.   Acetylcholine metabolism of a sympathetic ganglion. *Can. J. Biochem. Physiol.* 39:787–827.

31. Collier, B., and MacIntosh, F. C.   The source of choline for acetylcholine synthesis in a sympathetic ganglion. *Can. J. Physiol. Pharmacol.* 47:127–135, 1969.

32. Collier, B., and Ilson, D.   The effect of preganglionic nerve stimulation on the accumulation of certain analogues of choline by a sympathetic ganglion. *J. Physiol.* (London) 264:489–509, 1977.

33. Collier, B., and Katz, H. S.   Acetylcholine synthesis from recaptured choline by a sympathetic ganglion. *J. Physiol.* (London) 238:639–655, 1974.

34. Pardridge, W. M., and Oldendorf, W. H.   Transport of metabolic substrates through the blood-brain barrier. *J. Neurochem.* 28:5–12, 1977.

*35. Blass, J. P., and Gibson, G. E.   Cholinergic Systems and Disorders of Carbohydrate Metabolism. In D. J. Jenden (ed.), *Cholinergic Mechanisms and Psychopharmacology*. New York: Plenum, 1978. Pp. 791–803.

36. Lefresne, P., Beaujouin, J. C., and Glowinski, J.   Origin of the acetyl moiety of acetylcholine synthesized in rat striatal synaptosomes: A specific pyruvic dehydrogenase involved in ACh synthesis? *Biochimie* 60:479–487, 1978.

*37. Haubrich, D. R.   Choline Acetyltransferase and Its Inhibitors. In A. M. Goldberg and I. Hanin (eds.), *Biology of Cholinergic Function*. New York: Raven, 1976. Pp. 239–268.

*38. Bowman, W. C., and Marshall, I. G.   Inhibitors of Acetylcholine Synthesis. In J. Cheymol (ed.), *International Encyclopedia of Pharmacology and Therapeutics, Section 14, Vol. 1. Neuromuscular Blocking and Stimulating Agents*. Oxford: Pergamon, 1972. Pp. 357–390.

39. Katz, H. S., Salehmoghaddam, S., and Collier, B.   The accumulation of radioactive acetylcholine by a sympathetic ganglion and by brain: Failure to label endogenous stores. *J. Neurochem.* 20:569–579, 1973.

40. Dowdall, M. J.   Synthesis and Storage of Acetylcholine in Cholinergic Nerve Terminals. In S. Berl, D. D. Clarke, and D. Schneider (eds.), *Metabolic Compartmentation and Neurotransmission*. New York: Plenum, 1975. Pp. 585–607.

*41. Whittaker, V. P.   The Electromotor System of Torpedo as a Model Cholinergic System. In D. J. Jenden (ed.), *Cholinergic Mechanisms and Psychopharmacology*. New York: Plenum, 1978. Pp. 323–345.

42. Wilson, W. S., Schulz, R. A., and Cooper, J. R.   The isolation of cholinergic synaptic vesicles from bovine superior cervical ganglion and estimation of their acetylcholine content. *J. Neurochem.* 20: 659–667, 1973.

43. Zimmermann, H.   Turnover of adenine nucleotides in cholinergic synaptic vesicles of the *Torpedo* electric organ. *Neuroscience* 3:827–836, 1978.

44. Meunier, F. M., and Morel, N.   Adenosine uptake by cholinergic synapses from *Torpedo* electric organ. *J. Neurochem.* 31:845–851, 1978.

45. Evans, C. A. L., and Saunders, N. R.   An outflow of acetylcholine from normal and regenerating ventral roots of the cat. *J. Physiol.* (London) 240:15–32, 1974.

46. Collier, B., and Katz, H. S.   The synthesis, turnover and release of surplus acetylcholine in a sympathetic ganglion. *J. Physiol.* (London) 214:537–552, 1971.

*47. Katz, B.   *Nerve, Muscle and Synapse.* New York: McGraw-Hill, 1966.

*48. Rahamimoff, R.   The Role of Calcium in Transmitter Release at the Neuromuscular Junction. In S. Thesleff (ed.), *Motor Innervation of Muscle*. New York: Academic, 1976. Pp. 117–149.

49. Politoff, A. L., Rose, S., and Pappas, G. D.   The calcium-binding sites of synaptic vesicles of the frog neuromuscular junction. *J. Cell Biol.* 61:818–823, 1974.

*50. Heuser, J. E., Reese, T. S., Dennis, M. J., Jan, Y., Jan, L., and Evans, L.   Synaptic vesicle exocytosis captured by quick freezing and correlated with quantal transmitter release. *J. Cell Biol.* 81:275–300, 1979.

51. Elmqvist, D., and Quastel, D. M. J. Presynaptic action of hemicholinium at the neuromuscular junction. *J. Physiol.* (London) 177:463–482, 1965.

52. Kriebel, M. E., Llados, F., and Matteson, D. R. Spontaneous subminiature end-plate potentials in mouse diaphragm muscle: Evidence for synchronous release. *J. Physiol.* (London) 262:553–581, 1976.

53. Cull-Candy, S. G., Lundh, H., and Thesleff, S. Effects of botulinum toxin on neuromuscular transmission in the rat. *J. Physiol.* (London) 260:117–203, 1976.

54. Fletcher, P., and Forrester, T. The effect of curare on the release of acetylcholine from mammalian motor nerve terminals and an estimate of quantum content. *J. Physiol.* (London) 251:131–144, 1975.

55. Kuffler, S. W., and Yoshikami, D. The number of transmitter molecules in a quantum: An estimate from iontophoretic application of acetylcholine at the neuromuscular junction. *J. Physiol.* (London) 251:465–482, 1975.

56. Miledi, R., Molenaar, P. C., and Polak, R. L. An analysis of acetylcholine in frog muscle by mass fragmentography. *Proc. R. Soc. Lond. [Biol.]* 197:285–297, 1977.

57. Birks, R. I. The relationship of transmitter release and storage to fine structure in a sympathetic ganglion. *J. Neurocytol.* 3:133–160, 1974.

58. Israël, M., Dunant, Y., and Manaranche, R. The present status of the vesicular hypothesis. *Progr. Neurobiol.* 13:237–275, 1979.

59. Marchbanks, R. M. Role of Storage Vesicles in Synaptic Transmission. In C. R. Hopkins and C. J. Duncan (eds.), *Society for Experimental Symposium XXXIII, Secretory Mechanisms.* Cambridge, England: Cambridge University Press, 1979. Pp. 251–276.

*60. Tauc, L. Transmitter Release at Cholinergic Synapses. In G. A. Cottrell and P. N. R. Usherwood (eds.), *Synapses.* Glasgow: Blackie, 1977. Pp. 64–78.

*61. Gray, E. G. Presynaptic Microtubules, Agranular Reticulum and Synaptic Vesicles. In G. A. Cottrell and P. N. R. Usherwood (eds.), *Synapses.* Glasgow: Blackie, 1977. Pp. 6–18.

62. Giompres, P., Zimmermann, H., and Whittaker, V. P. New Evidence in Favour of the Vesicle Theory of Transmitter Release. In J. Taxi (ed.), *INSERM Symposium no. 13, Ontogenesis and Functional Mechanism of Peripheral Synapses.* Amsterdam: Elsevier, 1980. Pp. 91–98.

*63. Zimmermann, H. Commentary: Vesicle cycling and transmitter release. *Neuroscience* 4:1773–1803, 1979.

*64. Osborne, M. P. Role of Vesicles with Some Ob-

servations on Vertebrate Sensory Cells. In G. A. Cottrell and P. N. R. Usherwood (eds.), *Synapses.* Glasgow: Blackie, 1977. Pp. 40–63.

*65. MacIntosh, F. C., and Collier, B. The Neurochemistry of Cholinergic Terminals. In E. Zaimis (ed.), *Handbook of Experimental Pharmacology: Organization, Function and Pharmacology of the Neuromuscular Junction.* Berlin: Springer-Verlag, 1976. Pp. 99–228.

*66. MacIntosh, F. C. The Present Status of the Vesicle Hypothesis. In D. J. Jenden (ed.), *Cholinergic Mechanisms and Psychopharmacology.* New York: Plenum, 1978. Pp. 297–322.

67. Trifaró, J. M. Contractile proteins in tissues originating in the neural crest. *Neuroscience* 3:1–24, 1978.

*68. Koelle, G. B. Cytological Distributions and Physiological Functions of Cholinesterases. In G. B. Koelle (ed.), *Handbuch der experimentellen Pharmakologie: Cholinesterases and Anticholinesterase Agents.* Berlin: Springer-Verlag, 1963. Suppl. 15, pp. 187–298.

*69. Rosenberry, T. L. Acetylcholinesterase. *Adv. Enzymol.* 43:103–218, 1975.

70. Trevor, A. J., et al. Acetylcholinesterases. *Life Sci.* 23:1209–1220, 1978.

*71. Jenden, D. J. Estimation of Acetylcholine and the Dynamics of its Metabolism. In D. J. Jenden (ed.), *Cholinergic Mechanisms and Psychopharmacology.* New York: Plenum, 1978. Pp. 139–162.

*72. Cheney, D. L., and Costa, E. Pharmacological implications of brain acetylcholine turnover measurements in rat brain nuclei. *Annu. Rev. Pharmacol. Toxicol.* 17:369–386, 1977.

*73. Nordberg, A. Apparent regional turnover of acetylcholine in mouse brain: Methodological and functional aspects. *Acta Physiol. Scand.* (Suppl. 445):1–51, 1977.

74. Potter, L. T. Synthesis, storage and release of ^{14}C acetylcholine in isolated rat diaphragm muscles. *J. Physiol.* (London) 206:145–166, 1970.

*75. Hubbard, J. I. Neuromuscular Transmission: Presynaptic Factors. In J. I. Hubbard (ed.), *The Peripheral Nervous System.* New York: Plenum, 1974. Pp. 151–180.

76. Marchbanks, R. M., and Israël, M. The heterogeneity of bound acetylcholine and synaptic vesicles. *Biochem. J.* 129:1049–1061, 1972.

77. Collier, B., Boksa, P., and Lovat, S. False cholinergic transmitters. *Prog. Brain Res.* 49:107–121, 1979.

78. Large, W. A., and Rang, H. P. Factors affecting the rate of incorporation of a false transmitter into mammalian motor nerve terminals. *J. Physiol.* (London) 285:1–24, 1978.

79. Haubrich, D. R., and Chippendale, T. J. Regula-

tion of acetylcholine synthesis. *Life Sci.* 20:1465–1478, 1977.

80. Ulus, I. H., et al. Effect of Choline on Cholinergic Function. In D. J. Jenden (ed.), *Cholinergic Mechanisms and Psychopharmacology.* New York: Plenum, 1978. Pp. 525–538.

81. Potter, L. T. Synthesis, Storage and Release of Acetylcholine from Nerve Terminals. In G. H. Bourne (ed.), *The Structure and Function of Nervous Tissue.* New York: Academic, 1972. Vol. 4, pp. 105–128.

*82. Jenden, D. J. An Overview of Choline and Acetylcholine Metabolism in Relation to the Therapeutic Uses of Choline. In A. Barbeau, J. H. Growdon, and R. J. Wurtman (eds.), *Nutrition and the Brain,* Vol. 5, *Choline and Lecithin in Brain Disorders.* New York: Raven, 1979, Pp. 13–24.

*83. Black, I. B. Regulation of autonomic development. *Annu. Rev. Neurosci.* 1:183–214, 1978.

*84. Varon, S. S., and Bunge, R. P. Trophic mechanisms in the peripheral nervous system. *Annu. Rev. Neurosci.* 1:327–361, 1978.

*85. Fambrough, D. M. Control of acetylcholine receptors in skeletal muscle. *Physiol. Rev.* 59:165–227, 1979.

86. Landmesser, L., and Pilar, G. Interaction between neurons and their targets during synaptogenesis. *Fed. Proc.* 37:2016–2022, 1978.

Note added in proof

1. Evidence is growing [88] that some cholinergic neurons may store and release active *peptides* along with ACh (see Chap. 8).

2. ACh uptake by isolated vesicle preparations has been demonstrated [88, 89, 91].

3. On the question of vesicle-quantum equivalence [92, 93], the minority view that vesicular exocytosis is no more than a minor mode of ACh discharge is still maintained [58, 59], with the further proposal that the principal function of exocytosis is to extrude intraterminal Ca [94, 95]. On the majority side, the molecular aspects of impulse-evoked exocytosis have been examined in detail [92]. It seems increasingly likely that there are two processes for vesicle-membrane recycling: a rapid one, in which exocytosis is immediately followed by endocytosis at the same site; and a slower one, in which the retrieved membrane is incorporated into coated vesicles and cisternae before becoming available for a second exocytosis.

4. It has been suggested [cf. 92] that nonquantal synaptic leakage of ACh is comparable in amount to quantal release and therefore large enough to compromise the interpretation of neurochemical (vs. neurophysiological) studies of ACh release. The suggestion is based on experiments with isolated skeletal muscles. In these preparations the nonquantal release can indeed be embarrassingly large, but it has been argued [93] that the leakage is mostly an artefact of the particular experimental situation.

87. Bon, S., Vigny, M., and Massoulié, J. Asymmetric and globular forms of acetylcholinesterases in mammals and birds. *Proc. Natl. Acad. Sci. U.S.A.* 76:2546–2550, 1979.

88. Hökfelt, T., Johansson, D., Ljungdahl, A., Lundberg, J. M., and Schultzberg, M. Peptidergic neurons. *Nature* 284:515–521, 1980.

89. Giompres, P., and Luqmani, Y. A. Cholinergic synaptic vesicles isolated from *Torpedo marmorata:* Demonstration of acetylcholine and choline uptake in an isolated system. *Neuroscience* 5:1041–1052, 1980.

90. Diebler, M.-F., and Morot-Gaudry, Y. Incorporation of Acetylcholine into Torpedo Synaptic Vesicles In Vitro. In M. Brzin, D. Sket, and H. Bachelard (eds.), *Synaptic Constituents in Health and Disease.* Oxford: Pergamon Press, 1980. Pp. 111–112.

91. Parsons, S. M., and Koenigsberger, R. Specific stimulated uptake of acetylcholine by *Torpedo* electric organ synaptic vesicles. *Proc. Natl. Acad. Sci. U.S.A.* 77:6234–6238, 1980.

*92. Kelly, R. B., Deutsch, J. W., Carlson, S. S., and Wagner, J. A. Biochemistry of neurotransmitter release. *Annu. Rev. Neurosci.* 2:399–466, 1979.

93. MacIntosh, F. C. The Role of Vesicles in Cholinergic Systems. In M. Brzin, D. Sket, and H. Bachelard (eds.), *Synaptic Constituents in Health and Disease.* Oxford: Pergamon Press, 1980. Pp. 11–50.

94. Dunant, Y., Babel-Guérin, E., and Droz, B. Calcium metabolism and acetylcholine release at the nerve-electroplaque junction. *J. Physiol.* (Paris) 76:471–478, 1980.

95. Israël, M., Manaranche, R., Marsal, J., Meunier, F.-M., Morel, N., Frachon, P., and Lesbats, B. Calcium uptake by cholinergic synaptic vesicles. *J. Physiol.* (Paris) 76:479–485, 1980.

96. Skau, K. A., and Brimijoin, S. Release of acetylcholinesterase from rat hemidiaphragm preparation stimulated through the phrenic nerve. *Nature* 275:224–226, 1978.

Joseph T. Coyle
Solomon H. Snyder

Chapter 10. Catecholamines

The catecholamines—dopamine, norepinephrine, and epinephrine—are neurotransmitters in a number of brain areas subserving functions relating to emotion, attention, and visceral regulation. Although dopamine serves as the precursor for norepinephrine, and norepinephrine may be N-methylated to form epinephrine, the three catecholamines also have separate localizations in distinct neuronal pathways. One major theme of recent research is that of identifying specific behavioral and physiological roles served by individual catecholamine neuronal pathways. Other major research concerns are biochemical specification of catecholamine receptors, the identification of multiple receptors for each catecholamine, and dynamic changes in receptors that parallel altered synaptic functioning.

Biosynthesis of Catecholamines

Of the synthetic pathways for neurotransmitters, the enzymatic processes involved in the formation of catecholamines have been most completely characterized. All the component enzymes in the synthesis pathway have been purified to homogeneity, which has allowed for detailed analysis of their kinetics of interaction with substrates, cofactors, activators, and inhibitors (Fig. 10-1). Furthermore, with specific antibodies raised against the purified enzymes, precise localization of the enzymes has been made possible through immunocytochemical techniques.

Tyrosine hydroxylase (TH), an enzyme located uniquely in tissues that synthesize catecholamines, is the initial and rate-limiting enzyme in their biosynthetic pathway [15]. TH uses molecular oxygen and tyroxine as its substrates and biopterin as its cofactor; it catalyzes the addition of a hydroxyl group to the meta position of tyrosine, thus forming L-dopa (3,4-dihydroxy-L-phenylalanine). TH can also hydroxylate phenylalanine to tyrosine, which is then converted to L-dopa; this alternative synthetic route may be of significance in patients affected with phenylketonuria, in which phenylalanine hydroxylase activity is depressed. TH has a K_m for L-tyrosine in the micromolar range; as a result, it is virtually saturated by the high tissue concentrations of endogenous L-tyrosine. Although L-tyrosine does not ordinarily limit the rate of amine synthesis, recent evidence indicates that the cofactor, biopterin, is at subsaturating concentrations within the catecholaminergic neurons and thus may play an important regulatory role in the velocity of this reaction. TH is primarily a soluble enzyme, localized in the cytosol of catecholaminergic neuronal processes; however, interactions with such membrane constituents as phosphatidylserine have been shown to alter its kinetic characteristics.

Dopa decarboxylase (DDC) is a pyridoxine-dependent enzyme that catalyzes the removal of the carboxyl group from dopa to form dopamine [2]. The enzyme has a low K_m and high velocity with respect to L-dopa; thus, endogenous L-dopa is efficiently converted to dopamine, and negligible amounts of L-dopa occur in catecholaminergic tissue. DDC also decarboxylates 5-hydroxytryptophan, the precursor to serotonin, as well as other aromatic amino acids; accordingly, it has also been called *aromatic amino acid decarboxylase*. DDC has widespread distribution in the body, where it is found both in catecholaminergic and serotonergic neurons and in nonneuronal tissues, such as kidney and vascular pericytes. For the dopaminergic neurons, this is the final step in the synthesis pathway for their neurotransmitter.

205

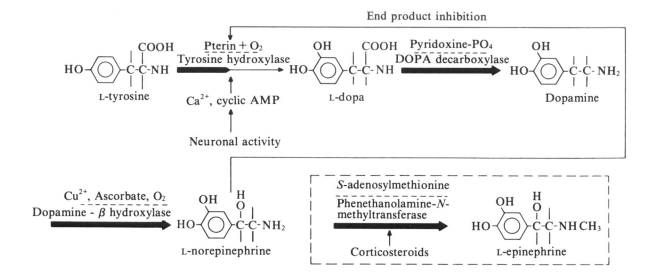

Fig. 10-1. *Biosynthetic pathway for catecholamines.*
See text for details of the enzymatic processes and
regulatory mechanisms.

For neurons that use epinephrine or norepinephrine for their neurotransmitters, dopamine β-hydroxylase (DBH) is the next step in the biosynthetic pathway[7]. Like tyrosine hydroxylase, DBH is a mixed-function oxidase that uses molecular oxygen to form the hydroxyl group added to the β carbon on the side chain of dopamine. The enzyme contains cupric ions that are involved in electron transfer in reaction; accordingly, copper chelators, such as diethyldithiocarbamate, act as potent inhibitors of the enzyme. DBH is concentrated within the vesicles that store catecholamines; most of the enzyme is bound to the inner vesicular membrane but some is free within the vesicles.

For a small group of neurons in the brain stem that utilize epinephrine as their neurotransmitter and for the adrenal medullary cells for which epinephrine is the primary neurohormone, the final enzyme in the synthesis pathway is phenylethanolamine N-methyltransferase (PNMT). This enzyme transfers a methyl group from S-adenosylmethionine to the amine terminus of norepinephrine [3]. Curiously, the PNMT exists in a soluble state in the cytosol outside the catecholamine storage vesicles. The level of PNMT in adrenergic tissue is regulated by the corticosteroids; and high activity of PNMT in the adrenal medulla reflects the high concentrations of corticosteroids released

into the venous sinuses that drain the adrenal cortex. Conditions such as hypophysectomy, that reduce corticosteroid levels, result in marked reductions in the amount of this enzyme in adrenergic tissue; conversely, administration of large amounts of corticosteroids, particularly during the neonatal period, results in the synthesis of PNMT in sympathetic neurons that do not ordinarily contain the enzyme.

Storage and Release of Catecholamines

Catecholamines are concentrated within storage vesicles that are present in high density within the nerve terminals; ordinarily, low concentrations of the catecholamines remain free and unprotected in the cytosol. Thus, conversion of tyrosine to L-dopa and L-dopa to dopamine occurs in the cytosol; dopamine then is taken up within the storage vesicles; for the noradrenergic neurons, the final hydroxylation occurs within the vesicles. The mechanism that concentrates the catecholamines within the vesicles is an ATP-dependent process linked to a proton pump[8]. The intravesicular concentration of catecholamines, which exist in a complex with adenosine triphosphate (ATP), acidic proteins known as *chromagranins,* and soluble DBH, is approximately 0.5 *M.* The vesicular uptake process has broad substrate specificity and can transport a variety of biogenic amines, including tryptamine, tyramine, and amphetamines; these amines compete with endogenous catecholamines for the vesicular storage capacity. Reserpine is a specific, potent, and irreversible inhibitor of the vesicular amine pump that terminates the ability of the vesicles to concentrate the amines. Treatment with reserpine causes a profound depletion of endogenous catecholamines in neurons.

The vesicles play a dual role: they maintain a ready supply of catecholamines at the terminal, and they mediate the process of their release. When an action potential reaches the nerve terminal, calcium (Ca^{2+}) channels open, allowing an influx of the cation into the terminal; increased intracellular Ca^{2+} promotes the fusion of vesicles near the synaptic specialization with the neuronal membrane. The vesicles then discharge their soluble contents, including norepinephrine, ATP, and DBH, into the extraneuronal space [20]. The demonstration that the large enzyme (300,000 M_r) DBH is released concurrently and proportionately with norepinephrine established that release occurs by the process of exocytosis. Exocytotic release from sympathetic neurons may be the source of some of the DBH that circulates free in the blood plasma. Indirectly acting sympathomimetics, like tyramine and amphetamine, release the catecholamines by a different mechanism, one that is neither dependent upon calcium nor associated with release of DBH. These drugs displace catecholamines from storage vesicles, resulting in neurotransmitter leakage from the nerve terminals.

Regulation of Catecholamine Biosynthesis

In spite of marked fluctuations in the activity of catecholaminergic neurons, the levels of catecholamines within the nerve terminals remain relatively constant. Hence, efficient regulatory mechanisms must operate to modulate the rate of synthesis of catecholamines, depending upon need.

A long-term process affecting the rate of catecholamine synthesis involves alterations in the amount of enzyme molecules in the synthetic pathway that is available at the nerve terminals. When catecholaminergic neuronal firing remains high for prolonged periods, the rates of synthesis of TH and DBH are increased in the neuronal perikarya; notably, DDC does not appear to be modulated by this process. The supranormal number of enzyme molecules are then transported down the axon to the nerve terminals.

Whereas alterations in the rate of synthesis of biosynthetic enzyme molecules provides a gradual and delayed method of control, two servomechanisms operative at the level of the nerve terminal play an important role in the short-term modulation of catecholamine synthesis and are responsive to momentary changes in neuronal activity. First, TH, as the rate-limiting enzyme in the synthesis pathway, is modulated by end-product inhibition. Thus, when adequate intraneuronal stores of catecholamines have been achieved, excess catecholamines inhibit the further activity of this enzyme by competing at the site that binds the pteridine cofactor; conversely, as catecholamines are released, the free levels fall, resulting in disinhibition of the enzyme. Second, with depolarization of the catecholaminergic terminals, TH undergoes activation; the kinetic characteristics of the enzyme change so that it has a higher affinity for its pteridine cofactor and becomes less sensitive to end product inhibition. Recent evidence suggests that this transient modification of the molecule may occur as a result of reversible phosphorylation or influx of Ca^{2+}. Thus, through such mechanisms as end-product inhibition, transient activation, and enzyme induction, the neuron can accommodate to alterations in utilization of catecholamine neurotransmitters [9].

Catabolism of Catecholamines

Two enzymes are primarily responsible for the catabolic inactivation of catecholamines: monoamine oxidase (MAO) and catechol-*O*-methyltransferase (COMT) (Fig. 10-2). Dopamine metabolites are discussed in Chap. 36. These enzymes

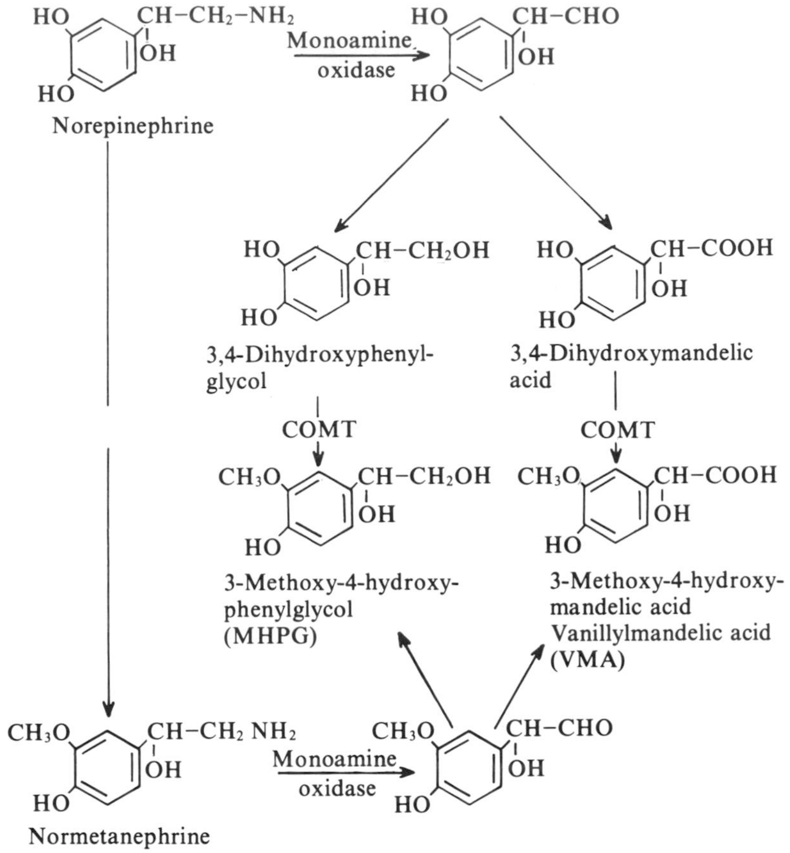

Fig. 10-2. Pathways of norepinephrine degradation.

have a fairly ubiquitous distribution throughout the body. MAO is a flavin-containing enzyme located on the outer membrane of the mitochondria [4]. This enzyme oxidatively deaminates catecholamines to their corresponding aldehydes; in turn, these can be converted by aldehyde dehydrogenase to analogous acids. Because of its intracellular localization, MAO plays a strategic role in inactivating catecholamines that are free within the nerve terminal and not protected by storage vesicles. Accordingly, drugs that interfere with vesicular storage, like reserpine, or indirectly acting sympathomimetics, such as amphetamines, cause a marked increase in deaminated metabolites. Isozymes of MAO have been characterized with differential substrate specificites; MAO-A preferentially deaminates norepinephrine and serotonin, whereas MAO-B acts on a broad spectrum of phenylethylamines. MAO plays an important pro-

tective role in the gut and the liver by preventing access to the general circulation of ingested, indirectly acting amines, such as tyramine and phenylethylamine, that are contained in food; however, patients treated with MAO-inhibitor antidepressants are not afforded this protection and can suffer severe hypertensive crises after ingesting foods that contain high amounts of tyramine. A methyl substituent on the α carbon of the phenylethylamine side chain protects against deamination by MAO; the prolonged action of amphetamine and related indirectly acting stimulants is caused by this α-methyl group, which prevents their inactivation by MAO.

COMT is located primarily on the outer plasma membrane of nearly all cells, including erythrocytes

[14]; thus, COMT acts on extraneuronal catecholamines. The enzyme, which requires Mg^{2+}, transfers a methyl group from the cosubstrate, S-adenosylmethionine, to the 3-hydroxy group on the catecholamine ring. COMT has broad substrate specificity, methylating virtually any catechol compound, regardless of the side-chain constituents; for this reason, there has been little success in the development of potent competitive inhibitors of the enzyme that are of pharmacological significance.

Measurement of catecholamine metabolites can provide insight into the rate of release or turnover of catecholamines in brain. In clinical studies, the catecholamine metabolites are generally assayed in the cerebrospinal fluid (CSF), because the large quantities derived from the peripheral sympathomedullary system obscure the small central contribution from brain to urinary levels. However, the acid metabolites are actively excreted from CSF; more reliable estimates of turnover in brain are obtained when this transport process is blocked by pretreatment with the drug probenecid.

4-Hydroxy-3-methoxy-phenylacetic acid, more commonly known as *homovanillic* acid (HVA), is a major metabolite of brain dopamine. Spinal fluid HVA levels provide insight into the turnover of dopamine in the striatum (they are depressed, for example, in Parkinson's disease). A metabolite of norepinephrine formed relatively selectively in the brain is 3-methoxy-4-hydroxyphenylglycol (MHPG). Because this is a minor metabolite for the much larger amounts of norepinephrine metabolized in the periphery, it is estimated that between 30 and 50 percent of the MHPG excreted in urine is derived exclusively from brain. This metabolite has been measured in CSF and in urine to provide an index of norepinephrine turnover in the brain and has been found to be decreased in certain forms of psychiatric depression.

Reuptake Inactivation of Synaptically Released Catecholamines

The action of catecholamines released at the synapse is terminated primarily by reuptake into the nerve terminals that release the neurotransmitters. Catecholamines that have not been effectively removed from the synaptic cleft by the transport process diffuse into the extracellular space, where they are catabolized by MAO and COMT. The catecholamine reuptake process was discovered by Axelrod and coworkers [1]. They found that when radioactive norepinephrine was injected intravenously, it accumulated in tissues in direct proportion to the density of the tissues' sympathetic innervation. The amine taken up into the tissues was protected from catabolic degradation, and subcellular studies revealed its localization in synaptic vesicles. Ablation of the sympathetic input to organs abolished their ability to accumulate and store the radioactive norepinephrine. Subsequent studies demonstrated that this uptake process is a characteristic feature of catecholamine neurons in both the periphery and the brain; the transport process has been extensively studied in sheared-off nerve terminals or synaptosomes isolated from brain.

The uptake process is mediated by a carrier located on the outer membrane of the catecholaminergic neurons. It is saturable and obeys a Michaelis-Menten type of kinetics. A transport process selective for norepinephrine is found only on noradrenergic neurons, whereas a carrier with different specificity is found on dopaminergic neurons [5]. The uptake process is energy-dependent, since it can be inhibited by incubation at a low temperature or by a metabolic inhibitor. The energy requirements reflect a coupling of the uptake process with the sodium gradient across the neuronal membrane; drugs, such as ouabain, that inhibit the $(Na^+ + K^+)$-ATPase, or drugs such as veratridine that open sodium channels, inhibit the uptake process noncompetitively. The linkage of uptake to the sodium gradient may be of physiological significance, since transport temporarily ceases at the time of depolarization-release of catecholamines. Because of the differential specificity of the transport processes for dopaminergic and for noradrenergic neurons, they can be inhibited selectively by drugs, including tricyclic antidepressants and cocaine. In addition, a variety of phenylethylamines, such as amphetamine, bind to the carrier; thus, they can be concentrated within catecholaminergic neurons as well as compete with the catecholamines for transport. Active uptake is the mechanism whereby the catecholamine neurotoxin, 6-hydroxydopamine, is accumulated selectively to high concentrations within catecholaminergic neurons and destroys them through the auto-oxidative liberation of hydrogen peroxide.

Distribution of Catecholaminergic Neurons and Their Processes in the Brain

The understanding of catecholamine neuronal function in brain has been greatly aided by the development of neuroanatomical methods to visualize these neurons in the central nervous system and in the periphery [12]. Nearly two decades ago, Falck and Hillarp took advantage of the fact that, in the presence of formaldehyde, catecholamines cyclize to form intensely fluorescent products. With a fluorescence microscope, the neurons containing the catecholamines could be visualized in thin sections obtained from tissue previously exposed to formaldehyde vapor. Investigators have used this technique to map the distribution of the catecholamine-containing cell bodies and axonal pathways in the brain. A recent modification of the method uses glyoxylic acid and has resulted in enhanced sensitivity and a more stable fluorophor for even better visualization of the fine axons and terminals.

By purifying the enzymes that synthesize catecholamines, it is possible to make potent antiserum against each enzyme. Thin sections of tissue are incubated with antibody against a particular enzyme (e.g., rabbit anti-DBH). The section is then incubated with a second antibody against the first. The second antibody is linked to a marker, such as fluorescein (e.g., fluorescein-labeled, goat anti-rabbit IgG) or horseradish peroxidase. The neurons containing these enzymes are thus stained specifically. By this technique, the PNMT-containing neurons that synthesize epinephrine can be distinguished from noradrenergic neurons that are devoid of PNMT; similarly, noradrenergic neurons that contain DBH can be separated from the dopaminergic neurons that do not possess this enzyme.

Finally, advantage has been taken of the highly selective uptake process for catecholaminergic neurons. Thus, after incubation with radioactive norepinephrine, noradrenergic axons can be demonstrated at the ultrastructural level by autoradiographic techniques. Alternatively, after administration of the congener, 5-hydroxydopamine, which is taken up actively and stored within the vesicles, the catecholaminergic terminals can be distinguished by the presence of dense precipitates of 5-hydroxydopamine within their vesicles. Notably, all these techniques for visualizing the catecholaminergic neurons take advantage of their specific biochemical characteristics.

NOREPINEPHRINE

The cell bodies of the noradrenergic neurons cluster in the medulla oblongata, pons, and midbrain and are considered to be anatomically part of the reticular formation (Fig. 10-3). On the basis of their major axonal projections, they can be divided roughly into two major pathways, the dorsal and ventral bundles. The cell bodies of origin for the dorsal bundle are contained in a dense nucleus known as the *locus coeruleus,* located in the lateral aspect of the fourth ventricle. The locus sends noradrenergic axons that innervate the spinal cord and cerebellum and course anteriorly through the medial forebrain bundle to innervate the entire cerebral cortex and hippocampus. This highly divergent projection nevertheless exhibits patterns of fiber distribution unique to each of the regions innervated. The ventrally located cell bodies send fibers that innervate the brainstem and hypothalamus at particular nuclei that may receive markedly different degrees of innervation. As demonstrated by immunocytochemical techniques, there are scattered in the ventral portion of the pons and medulla a small number of neurons that contain PNMT; the axons of these epinephrine-utilizing neurons terminate primarily in the brain stem and hypothalamus.

DOPAMINERGIC NEURONS

The cell bodies of the dopaminergic neurons are located primarily in the midbrain. These can be

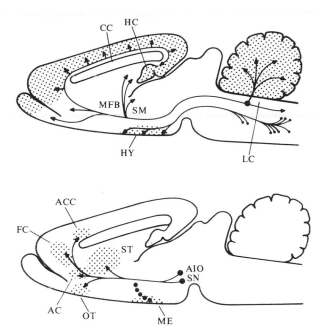

Fig. 10-3. Catecholaminergic neuronal pathways in the rat brain. Upper: noradrenergic neuronal pathways. Lower: dopaminergic neuronal pathways. AC, nucleus accumbens; ACC, anterior cingulate cortex; CC, corpus callosum; FC, frontal cortex; HC, hippocampus; HY, hypothalamus; LC, locus coeruleus; ME, median eminence; MFB, median forebrain bundle; OT, olfactory tubercle; SM, stria medullaris; SN, substantia nigra; ST, striatum.

divided into three main groups: nigrostriatal, meso-cortical, and tuberohypophysial. The major dopaminergic tract in brain originates in the zona compacta of the substantia nigra and sends axons that provide a dense innervation to the caudate nucleus and putamen of the corpus striatum; nearly 80 percent of all the brain's dopamine is found in the corpus striatum. In Parkinson's disease, the nigrostriatal dopaminergic tract degenerates—this accounts for the symptoms in the disorder.

Dopaminergic cell bodies that lie medial to the substantia nigra provide a diffuse, but more modest, innervation to the forebrain, including the frontal and cingulate cortex, the septum, nucleus accumbens, and olfactory tubercle. It has been hypothesized that antipsychotic neuroleptic drugs exert their therapeutic action through blockade of the effects of dopamine released by this system.

Dopaminergic cell bodies situated in the arcuate and periventricular nuclei of the hypothalamus send axons that innervate the intermediate lobe of the pituitary and the median eminence. These neurons play an important role in regulating the release of pituitary hormones, especially prolactin. In addition to these major dopaminergic pathways, dopaminergic interneurons have been demonstrated in the olfactory bulb and in the neural retina.

Catecholaminergic Receptors

The brain contains three catecholamine neurotransmitters—dopamine, norepinephrine, and epinephrine. However, there seem to be multiple types of receptors for each catecholamine (Table 10-1). Postsynaptic receptors for dopamine and norepinephrine are distinct. It is not yet known whether receptors for epinephrine-containing neurons differ in their properties from receptors postsynaptic to norepinephrine neurons, because the limited distribution of epinephrine neurons in the brain has precluded any characterization of their receptors.

AUTORECEPTORS

One important distinction separates postsynaptic receptors from autoreceptors. The postsynaptic receptors on any given neuron receive information from transmitters released by another neuron. Typically, the postsynaptic receptor is located on the dendrite or cell body of the neuron, but it also may occur on axons or nerve terminals; in the latter case, an axoaxonic synaptic relationship effects "presynaptic" inhibition or excitation. In contrast, autoreceptors are situated on a given neuron and respond to transmitter molecules released by the same neuron. Autoreceptors may be distributed over the entire surface of the neuron. At the nerve terminal, they respond to transmitter molecules discharged into the synaptic cleft; on the cell body, they may respond to transmitter molecules released by dendrites. Functionally, auto-

Table 10-1. Distinguishing Features of Multiple Postsynaptic Catecholamine Receptors

Dopamine Receptors
    Dopamine-1 (D-1) Receptors
        Linked to adenylate cyclase
        Ergot alkaloids (e.g., bromocryptine) are antagonists
        Flupenthixol, dopamine, and apomorphine are partially (about 65%) selective ligands
        Butyrophenone neuroleptics are weak antagonists
        Largely absent in pituitary
        Present in corpus striatum on intrinsic neurons sensitive to kainic acid
    Dopamine-2 (D-2) Receptors
        Not linked to adenylate cyclase
        Ergot alkaloids are agonists
        Butyrophenones are partially (about 70%) selective ligands
        Butyrophenone neuroleptics are potent antagonists
        Present in pituitary
        Present in corpus striatum largely on axons and terminals of corticostriate pathway

Norepinephrine β Receptors
    β_1 Receptors
        Linked to adenylate cyclase
        Epinephrine and norepinephrine are equally potent agonists
        Practalol is a selective antagonist
        Marked regional variations in brain
        No selective ligands

    β_2 Receptors
        Linked to adenylate cyclase
        Epinephrine is more potent than norepinephrine
        Terbutaline and salbutamol are selective agonists
        Uniformly distributed in brain
        No selective ligands

Norepinephrine α Receptors
    α_1 Receptors
        Prazosin, indoramin, and WB-4101 (2-([2′,6′-dimethoxy]-phenoxyethylaminol methylbenzodioxane) are
            selective antagonists on receptors localized in heart and vas deferens
        WB-4101 is a selective ligand and antagonist
    α_2 Receptors
        Piperoxan and yohimbine are relatively selective antagonists
        Clonidine and other imidazolines are selective agonists
        Localized in pancreas and rabbit duodenum
        Clonidine, epinephrine, and norepinephrine are selective ligands

α_1 and α_2 Receptors are blocked to a similar extent by ergots and phentolamine. Both receptors are present throughout the brain, though regional variations in rat are greater for α_2 receptors

receptors appear to regulate transmitter release in such a way that the released transmitter, acting upon the autoreceptors, inhibits further release. Autoreceptors have been identified for norepinephrine-, dopamine-, serotonin-, and GABA-containing neurons. However, the most detailed information is available about norepinephrine neurons. The major type of autoreceptor described in both the peripheral sympathetic nervous system and the brain has pharmacological properties resembling those of the α_2 receptor, the properties of which will be detailed below [11, 17, 18]. In general, the drug specificity of the dopamine autoreceptors appears similar to that of the postsynaptic dopamine receptors.

In the peripheral sympathetic nervous system, autoreceptors of the β-adrenergic type have also been described. These differ markedly from all other autoreceptors reported, since norepinephrine acting upon these β-autoreceptors facilitates transmitter release and thus amplifies the effects of neuronal firing. This effect contrasts with the inhibitory action of α-adrenergic and dopamine autoreceptors, which exert a negative feedback upon transmitter release.

POSTSYNAPTIC RECEPTORS

The most extensive biochemical data regarding catecholamine receptors deal with the postsynaptic receptors, which can be labeled readily in binding studies. In contrast, autoreceptors have not been directly labeled. One can study a neurotransmitter receptor biochemically either indirectly by measuring a related enzyme, such as adenylate cyclase, or directly by use of binding procedures that employ radioactive neurotransmitters or related drugs.

Dopamine Receptors

The dopamine receptor has been studied through both receptor-linked adenylate cyclase activity and binding techniques in which are used tritiated ligands. The first biochemical studies of dopamine receptors involved demonstration of a dopamine-sensitive adenylate cyclase, which will be discussed

in detail in Chapter 15. Dopamine receptors have been labeled in binding studies through the use of dopamine itself or ligands such as apomorphine or ADTN (2-amino-6,7-dihydroxy-1,2,3,4-tetrahydronaphthalene), agonist agents that bind to receptors and mimic the effects of the natural transmitter. Dopamine receptors can also be labeled by such drugs (also ligands) as the antischizophrenic butyrophenones, spiroperidol and haloperidol, which block dopamine receptors. In typical binding experiments, tritiated forms of the ligands are incubated with brain membranes under conditions in which the majority of the radioactivity bound to the membranes is associated with dopamine receptors [6]. Drugs and transmitters can be grouped by their relative potencies in displacing or inhibiting the binding of any other given tritiated ligands.

Binding studies have revealed multiple classes of dopamine receptors. The pattern of ligand displacement shows that such agonists as dopamine, apomorphine, and ADTN and such antagonists as haloperidol and spiroperidol all label physiological dopamine receptors. However, agonists are more potent in competing with agonists than with antagonists, whereas antagonists are more potent in competing with antagonists than with agonists for binding sites. These differences have been interpreted to mean that the dopamine receptor, like the opiate receptor, can exist in distinct, interconvertible states that favor binding of agonists or antagonists respectively. Additional differences in drug potencies, however, which do not fully parallel the agonist-antagonist continuum suggest that, in part, the agonists and antagonists may label physically distinct dopamine receptors.

The relative potencies of drugs in competing with agonists for binding sites resemble fairly closely their potencies in affecting the dopamine-sensitive adenylate cyclase, so it is likely that the dopamine receptors labeled predominantly by agonists represent those that are linked to the dopamine-sensitive adenylate cyclase. Brain lesion studies support this view. Kainic acid injection in the corpus striatum selectively destroys intrinsic neurons and essentially abolishes the dopamine-sensitive adenylate cyclase, but it reduces antagonist binding to dopamine receptors by only about 50 percent. The remaining dopamine receptors labeled by tritiated antagonists are removed by lesions of the major neuronal projection from the cerebral cortex to the corpus striatum. This suggests that receptors labeled by antagonists include those dopamine receptors localized on intrinsic neurons in the corpus striatum that are linked to adenylate cyclase and dopamine receptors situated on axons and nerve terminals of the corticostriate projection that are not associated with adenylate cyclase (Fig. 10-4).

Differences between the pituitary and the brain also indicate distinctions of dopamine receptors. Ergot drugs, such as bromocriptine, act like agonists at pituitary dopamine receptors, because they reduce the pituitary secretion of prolactin that is markedly enhanced by classical dopamine antagonists. In contrast, the same ergots behave as dopamine antagonists on the adenylate cyclase of corpus striatum homogenates. The pituitary gland lacks a dopamine-sensitive adenylate cyclase.

In summary, dopamine receptors in the pituitary and on the corticostriate path in the corpus striatum are not linked to adenylate cyclase; these are referred to as *dopamine-2 receptors*. Receptors related to the dopamine-sensitive adenylate cyclase are referred to as *dopamine-1 receptors* [10].

What are the functions of the two types of dopamine receptors? The antischizophrenic actions of dopamine-antagonist neuroleptic drugs are believed mediated by blockade of dopamine-2 receptors, since butyrophenone neuroleptics—the most potent known antischizophrenic agents—are extremely potent in blocking dopamine-2 receptors but are weak in blocking dopamine-1 receptors. The fact that such ergots as bromocriptine act as dopamine agonists in relieving the symptoms of Parkinson's disease, although they are antagonists at dopamine-1 receptors, indicates that these drugs also exert their therapeutic actions through dopamine-2 receptors. In the pituitary gland, dopamine antagonists enhance prolactin activity with potencies that parallel their actions at dopamine-2,

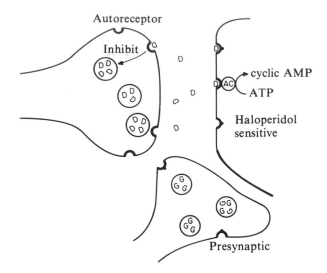

Fig. 10-4. *Dopamine receptor heterogeneity. A postsynaptic receptor (D-1) is linked to adenylate cyclase (AC). A second dopamine receptor (D-2), which exhibits high affinity for butyrophenones like haloperidol, is found on postsynaptic neurons as well as on the terminals of striatal glutaminergic (G) afferents. The third dopamine receptor (autoreceptor) is localized on dopaminergic terminals (D) and regulates the release of dopamine.*

rather than dopamine-1, receptors. Moreover, bromocriptine acts as an agonist in inhibiting prolactin secretion in the pituitary. Thus, the pituitary dopamine receptors involved in the hormonal actions of various drugs are also dopamine-2 receptors. The pharmacological or physiological role of dopamine receptors associated with adenylate cyclase are as yet unclear since no major therapeutic drugs have been shown to exert their effects via these receptors.

Alpha- and Beta-Adrenergic Receptors
The distinctions between α-adrenergic and β-adrenergic receptors for norepinephrine in the peripheral sympathetic nervous system have been known since the late 1940s. Norepinephrine and epinephrine act at both α and β receptors, but isoproterenol, the agonist catecholamine, acts only at β receptors. Numerous adrenergic antagonists

also differentiate α and β receptors. The classical β-blocking drug propranolol is essentially inactive at α receptors; the α-blocker phentolamine is very weak at β receptors.

Physically distinct subtypes of β and α receptors exist and have important pharmacological consequences. Of the β receptors, those known as β_1 receptors predominate in the heart; β_2 receptors are largely confined to the lung. A major side effect of such catecholamines as isoproterenol, which is used to treat asthma, is cardiac acceleration. Relatively selective β_2-agonist drugs relieve asthmatic symptoms by dilating the bronchi at doses which do not markedly affect the heart.

The brain contains both β_1 and β_2 receptors, which cannot, however, be so differentiated by physiological functions. Moreover, radioactive drugs which bind exclusively to one or the other type of β receptors are not yet available. However, one can label all β receptors with a tritiated drug and selectively block the binding to one of the subtypes of β receptors with β_1- or β_2-selective agents. The density of β_1 receptors varies more markedly in different brain areas than does that of β_2 receptors [13].

Distinct subtypes of postsynaptic α-adrenergic receptors have also been described. As with the dopamine receptor, tritiated α antagonists and α agonists can be used to label α receptors in both the brain and the peripheral tissues. As with β receptors, the binding properties of α receptors are essentially the same in brain and periphery. Drug specificities for α receptors labeled by either agonists or antagonists differ in a fashion similar to the differences in dopamine receptors. In general, agonists are more potent in competing with and inhibiting the binding of agonists than antagonists, whereas antagonists are more potent in competing with antagonists than agonists. Interestingly, this pattern is not apparent for β receptors, for which drug specificities and potencies are identical whether competition with agonists or antagonists is assayed.

The binding properties of α-adrenergic receptors do differ from those of dopamine receptors, as there is no evidence for interconvertibility of sites

labeled by α agonists and α antagonists. Instead they appear to label completely distinct receptors [19]. The α receptors labeled by agonists are referred to as α_2 *receptors;* those labeled by antagonists are referred to as α_1 *receptors.* Some tissues possess only postsynaptic α_1, others postsynaptic α_2, and some organs have a mixture of both. The proportion of α_1 and α_2 receptors also varies in different brain regions. Some areas possess exclusively α_1, others exclusively α_2, and a third area has mixtures of the two. The physiological consequences of the two types of α receptors in the brain are unclear at the present time. Strikingly, the drug specificity of postsynaptic α_2 receptors closely resembles that of adrenergic autoreceptors, which are, therefore, also referred to as α_2 *receptors.* In peripheral tissues, pharmacological effects of drugs in contracting smooth muscle of various organs differ, and these differences in relative potencies parallel differences in binding properties of α receptors in the various organs.

DYNAMICS OF CATECHOLAMINE RECEPTORS
Neurotransmitter receptors are not static entities. In rats, changes in the numbers of receptors appear to be associated with altered synaptic activity. In both the peripheral sympathetic nervous system and the brain, destruction of catecholamine-containing nerves is associated with functional supersensitivity of postsynaptic sites [16]. Destruction of the dopamine-containing nigrostriatal pathway has well-observed behavioral consequences. Because this pathway is uncrossed, a unilateral nigrostriatal lesion causes asymmetry in dopamine innervation between the two cerebral hemispheres. Behavioral studies demonstrate that the dopamine receptors in the denervated corpus striatum are supersensitive, because apomorphine, a dopamine agonist that stimulates dopamine receptors selectively, causes rotational behavior in the treated rats. The extent of receptor supersensitivity can be quantified by measuring the amount of rotational behavior.

After selective nigrostriatal lesions have been produced in rats by injections of 6-hydroxydopamine in the substantia nigra, the number of dopamine receptors in the ipsilateral corpus striatum increases markedly, and the extent of augmentation of binding in individual animals correlates with the extent of behavioral supersensitivity as monitored by rotational behavior [6]. Thus, the increase in receptor density appears to play a role in the behavioral supersensitivity of these animals.

Changes in the numbers of dopamine receptors may also be involved in pharmacological actions of neuroleptic drugs. One of the most serious side effects of the neuroleptic drugs is *tardive dyskinesia,* a disfiguring, excessive, motor activity of the tongue, face, arms, and legs in patients treated chronically with large doses of the drugs. Paradoxically, reduction of the dosage worsens the symptoms, whereas increasing the dosage alleviates the symptoms, so clinicians have speculated that tardive dyskinesia reflects supersensitivity of dopamine receptors that have been chronically blocked. This hypothesis gains support from direct demonstrations that chronic treatment with neuroleptic drugs produces an increase in the number of dopamine receptors in the corpus striatum [6]. Moreover, the ability of neuroleptics to elicit this increase correlates with their ability to block dopamine receptors.

α-Adrenergic and β-adrenergic receptors also demonstrate supersensitivity in binding studies. The numbers of α_1 and α_2 receptors increase after the noradrenergic neurons in the brain have been destroyed by 6-hydroxydopamine injections. Interestingly, after this induced destruction of norepinephrine-containing neurons, the number of β_1 receptors increases markedly, but no changes occur in the number of β_2 receptors [13].

In contrast to the success in linking dopamine receptors to adenylate cyclase in brain homogenates, results with α and β receptors have been equivocal. It is well established that β-adrenergic stimulation increases adenylate cyclase activity in many peripheral tissues. Such effects can be demonstrated with high concentrations of catecholamines in brain slices. However, in brain homogenates, β-receptor effects on cyclic AMP levels are not observed reproducibly. In peripheral tissues such as platelets, α-receptor stimulation is associated with decreases in cyclic AMP levels and adenylate cyclase activity. These effects are not observed in brain homogenates. Exposure of brain slices to norepinephrine can elicit an increase in the formation of cyclic AMP, which is partially affected by the relationship to α receptor–active drugs. Adrenergic mechanisms and cyclic nucleotides will be discussed in detail in Chap. 15.

References

*1. Axelrod, J. Noradrenaline: Fate and control of its biosynthesis. *Science* 173:598–606, 1971.

2. Christenson, J. G., Dairman, W., and Udenfriend, S. Preparation and properties of homogenous aromatic L-amino acid decarboxylase from hog kidney. *Arch. Biochem. Biophys.* 141:356–367, 1970.

3. Connett, R. J., and Kirshner, N. Purification and properties of bovine phenylethanolamine-*N*-methyltransferase. *J. Biol. Chem.* 245:329–334, 1970.

*4. Costa, E., and Sandler, M. *Monoamine Oxidase: New Vistas.* New York: Raven, 1972.

5. Coyle, J. T., and Snyder, S. H. Catecholamine uptake by synaptosomes in homogenates of rat brain: Stereospecificity of different areas. *J. Pharmacol. Exp. Ther.* 170:221–231, 1969.

*6. Creese, I., Burt, D. R., and Snyder, S. H. Biochemical actions of neuroleptic drugs: Focus on the dopamine receptor. In L. L. Iversen, S. D. Iversen and S. H. Snyder (eds.), *Handbook of Psychopharmacology.* New York: Plenum, 1978. Vol. 10, pp. 37–90.

7. Craine, J. E., Daniels, G., and Kaufman, S. Dopamine-β-hydroxylase: The subunit structure and anion activation of the bovine adrenal enzyme. *J. Biol. Chem.* 248:7838–7844, 1973.

8. Holz, R. W. Evidence that catecholamine transport into chromaffin vesicles is coupled to vesicle membrane potential. *Proc. Natl. Acad. Sci. U.S.A.* 75:5190–5194, 1978.

9. Joh, T. H., Park, D. H., and Reis, D. J. Direct phosphorylation of brain tyrosine hydroxylase by cyclic AMP–dependent protein kinase: Mechanism of enzyme activation. *Proc. Natl. Acad. Sci. U.S.A.* 75:4744–4748, 1978.

10. Kebabian, J. W., and Calne, D. B. Multiple receptors for dopamine. *Nature* 277:93–96, 1979.

11. Langer, S. Z. Presynaptic regulation of catecholamine release. *Biochem. Pharmacol.* 23:1793–1800, 1974.

*Key reference.

*12. Lindvall, O., and Bjorklund, A. Organization of catecholamine neurons in the rat central nervous system. In L. L. Iversen, S. D. Iversen and S. H. Snyder (eds.), *Handbook of Psychopharmacology.* New York: Plenum, 1978. Vol. 9, pp. 139–231.

13. Minneman, K. P., et al. β-1 and β-2-Adrenergic receptors in rat cerebral cortex. *Science* 204:866–868, 1979.

14. Nikodejevic, B., Sinoh, S., Daly, J. W., and Creveling, C. R. Catechol-O-methyltransferase II: A new class of inhibitors of catechol-O-methyltransferase; 3,5 dihydroxy-4-methoxy benzoic acid and related compounds. *J. Pharmacol. Exp. Ther.* 174:83–93, 1970.

15. Shiman, R., Akino, M., and Kaufman, S. Solubilization and partial purification of tyrosine hydroxylase from bovine adrenal medulla. *J. Biol. Chem.* 246:1330–1340, 1971.

*16. Snyder, S. H. Receptors, neurotransmitters, and drug responses. *N. Engl. J. Med.* 300:465–472, 1979.

*17. Starke, K. Regulation of noradrenaline release by presynaptic receptor systems. *Rev. Physiol. Biochem. Pharmacol.* 77:1–124, 1977.

*18. Stjarne, L. Basic mechanisms and local feedback control of secretion of adrenergic and cholinergic neurotransmitters. In L. L. Iversen, S. D. Iversen and S. H. Snyder (eds.), *Handbook of Psychopharmacology.* New York: Plenum, 1975. Vol. 6, pp. 179–233.

19. U'Prichard, D. C., and Snyder, S. H. Distinct α-noradrenergic receptors differentiated by binding and physiological relationships. *Life Sci.* 24:79–88, 1979.

20. Weinshilboum, R. M., et al. Proportional release of norepinephrine and dopamine β-hydroxylase from sympathetic nerves. *Science* 174:1349–1351, 1971.

Michael J. Brownstein

Chapter 11. Serotonin, Histamine, and the Purines

Serotonin

In the middle of the last century, a vasoactive substance was discovered in serum. It was not until the late 1940s, however, that this vasoconstrictor was isolated in a complex crystalline form and characterized as *5-hydroxytryptamine* (5HT). Before its characterization by Page and his collaborators, the material was called *serotonin,* a name that has been retained.

At the same time that serotonin was being purified from serum, Erspamer and his coworkers were studying the substance in enterochromaffin cells of the gut that gives these cells their unique histochemical appearance. They called this substance *enteramine* and demonstrated its existence in a number of mammalian tissues. Shortly after 5-hydroxytryptamine in blood was described, they showed that enteramine and serotonin were identical. Thus, by the time serotonin had been identified as 5HT, it was known to be a normal constituent of several mammalian tissues.

Serotonin is not unique to mammals; it is widely distributed among plants and animals [1–3]. It occurs in coelenterates, arthropods, mollusks, tunicates, and vertebrates. It is also found in such fruits as bananas, pineapples, plums, in nuts, and in various venoms.

Like acetylcholine and the catecholamines, serotonin acts on many organs of the body either directly or by a neuronal reflex. Its actions on the cardiovascular, respiratory, and gastrointestinal systems are especially prominent.

SEROTONIN IN THE MAMMALIAN CENTRAL NERVOUS SYSTEM

The central nervous system contains a relatively small part (about 1 percent) of the serotonin in the body. The distribution of serotonin in the brain is uneven. The hypothalamus, midbrain, and brain stem have high concentrations; the cerebral cortex, hippocampus, and striatum have moderate concentrations; and the cerebellum has a low concentration [4] (Table 11-1). The anatomy of serotonin-producing neurons was first studied by determining the effect of lesions in one part of the brain on amine levels elsewhere [5, 6]. The crude outlines of the serotoninergic system were drawn in this way, but the details began to emerge only after the introduction of the histochemical method of Falck and Hilarp [7]. With this method, serotonin-containing neurons could be visualized directly, the serotonin in them having been converted into a fluorophore by exposure to formaldehyde [8–10]. Unfortunately, the fluorophore derived from serotonin is not produced as efficiently as are fluorophores derived from catecholamines. Furthermore, the serotonin fluorescence bleaches rapidly in ultraviolet light. Therefore, the fluorescence histochemical method has not proved to be quite as valuable for serotonin as it has for catecholamines. It has been augmented, however, by newer techniques: immunocytochemical localization of tryptophan hydroxylase, orthograde transport of labeled amino acids, retrograde transport of horseradish peroxidase, and autoradiographic localization of tritiated serotonin. All these methods have contributed to our picture of the central serotoninergic system.

A family of neurons in the pons and mesencephalon is the primary source of serotonin in the brain (Fig. 11-1). These neurons are found in or near the midline, or raphe, in clusters. The more rostrally placed cells send processes to the telencephalon and diencephalon; the more caudally placed cells project to the medulla and spinal cord. Neurons in the median raphe nucleus innervate limbic struc-

219

Table 11-1. Regional Distribution of
Serotonin in Rat Brain

Tissue	μg/g Wet Wt
Whole brain	0.62
Cerebral cortex	0.57
Hippocampus	0.53
Striatum	0.57
Midbrain	0.97
Hypothalamus	0.98
Brain stem (pons and medulla oblongata)	0.83
Cerebellum	0.07
Pineal gland	73.00
Pituitary gland	0.56

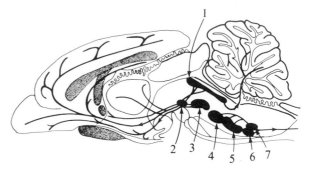

Fig. 11-1. Serotonin in the central nervous system. Most of the serotonin in the brain is made by neurons in the raphe nuclei: (1) nucleus raphe dorsalis, (2) nucleus linearis, (3) nucleus centralis superior, (4) nucleus raphe pontis, (5) nucleus raphe magnus, (6) nucleus raphe pallidus, (7) nucleus raphe obscurus. Raphe neurons send ascending and descending projections to the remainder of the brain and spinal cord.

tures preferentially; neurons in the dorsal raphe nucleus project primarily to the neostriatum, cerebral cortex, thalamus, and cerebellum.

There is evidence that some serotonin-producing cells in the brain reside outside the raphe complex [11]. Complete isolation (*deafferentation*) of the medial basal hypothalamus, for example, depletes this area of 70 percent of its serotonin; presumably, the remainder is made locally. Some of the serotonin intrinsic to the hypothalamus is likely to be present in mast cells, some has been said to be in *tanycytes,* specialized ependymal cells that line the third ventricle, and some may be in neurons [12]. Similarly, cells in the pineal gland—a gland that originates as an evagination of the diencephalon—manufacture serotonin. The pineal organ is extraordinarily rich in serotonin (Table 11-1), and its cells are unique in the way that they metabolize this monoamine (see Role of Serotonin in the Pineal Gland).

Serotonin is stored in synaptic vesicles in nerve endings. It appears to be synthesized outside the vesicles and then taken into them [13]. Finally, it is released by an exocytotic process (see Chap. 8).

SYNTHESIS AND METABOLISM

The biosynthesis and degradation of serotonin are depicted in Fig. 11-2. The first step in the biosynthesis of serotonin is the active uptake of trypto-

phan into serotoninergic neurons. The tryptophan is derived primarily from the diet.

After tryptophan enters the cell, it is hydroxylated by tryptophan hydroxylase [14], the activity of which limits the rate of serotonin synthesis. This mixed-function oxidase requires elementary oxygen and a pteridine cofactor, tetrahydrobiopterin. When tetrahydrobiopterin is provided, the K_m of tryptophan hydroxylase for tryptophan is 5×10^{-5} M. Apparently the enzyme is not normally saturated with tryptophan in vivo. Thus, giving animals excess tryptophan increases serotonin levels; depriving them of tryptophan or giving them a great deal of phenylalanine, an amino acid that competes with tryptophan for uptake into cells, has the opposite effect [15]. Whether the changes in the serotonin content of the brain that accompany alterations in the availability of tryptophan are of physiological import is a matter of debate [16]. Similarly, the increase in serotonin synthesis when animals are given 100% oxygen to breath may or may not be physiologically significant. It remains to be seen whether the tryptophan- or oxygen-induced modifications of serotonin levels are reflected in increases in serotonin release at specific synapses.

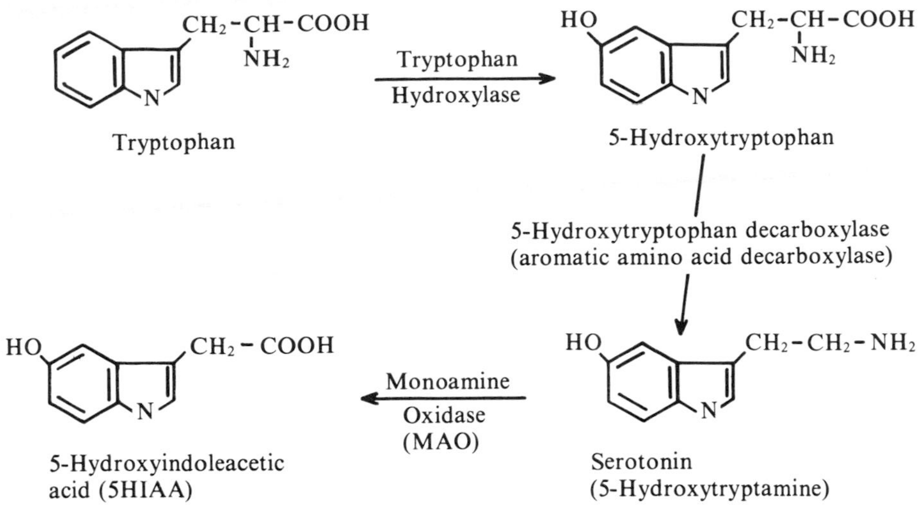

Fig. 11-2. Metabolism of serotonin.

Feedback inhibition of tryptophan hydroxylase by serotonin or its principal metabolite has not been demonstrated in vivo. Drugs that cause 5-hydroxyindoleacetic acid to accumulate by blocking its elimination from the brain do not affect the apparent rate of serotonin production. Thus, at present, little can be said about processes that modulate the rate of tryptophan hydroxylation in the brain.

It should be noted, however, that the activity of indoleamine 2,3-dioxygenase may be important in controlling free tryptophan levels and, by implication, the rate of serotonin synthesis. This enzyme catalyzes the oxidative cleavage of tryptophan to yield kynurenine and is ubiquitously present in the brain. Thus, much of the tryptophan in the brain may be metabolized by ring cleavage [17].

After tryptophan is hydroxylated to yield 5-hydroxytryptophan (5HTP), the latter is decarboxylated to form serotonin (5-hydroxytryptamine). The 5HTP decarboxylase is present in vast excess; inhibition of its activity by more than 80 percent hardly alters serotonin levels. Inhibition of tryptophan hydroxylase by the same amount causes a substantial drop in the serotonin content of the brain.

Whether 5HTP decarboxylase is a different enzyme from dopa decarboxylase is moot. They seem to be immunologically indistinguishable.

The most important enzyme in catabolizing serotonin is monoamine oxidase A, which oxidizes the amino group of serotonin to form an aldehyde, 5-hydroxyindoleacctaldehyde. The aldehyde is usually rapidly oxidized further to yield 5-hydroxyindoleacetic acid, but it also can be reduced to form an alcohol, 5-hydroxytryptophol.

A serotonin sulfotransferase is present in the brain, and its product, serotonin-O-sulfate, has been detected in brain extracts. Sulfatation of serotonin is an especially important route of metabolism in the periphery; 33 percent of the urinary metabolites of serotonin are O-sulfates [18].

N-methylated (bufotenin) and N-formylated (tryptoline) derivates of serotonin have received a great deal of attention because they produce behavioral abnormalities. These so-called psychotogens seem to be present in brain in tiny amounts, but more work is needed before it can be concluded that they are generated there enzymatically and are not artifacts [19].

On the other hand, N-acetylated derivatives of serotonin are made in the body, especially in the pineal gland [20]. In the pineal, serotonin is first N-acetylated and then O-methylated [21]. The product of these reactions, melatonin [22], is an antigonadotropic substance that is secreted into the systemic circulation.

REUPTAKE

Enzymatic degradation of serotonin by monoamine oxidase (MAO) helps to limit its biological actions; so does reuptake into nerve terminals. Both serotonergic endings and other monoaminergic endings can take up serotonin. The uptake process can be blocked by several drugs (Table 11-2). Other agents interfere with the biosynthesis, storage, and metabolism of serotonin. Still other drugs mimic or antagonize serotonin's action on postsynaptic receptors.

ROLE OF SEROTONIN IN THE PINEAL GLAND

The synthesis of melatonin in the pineal gland [23] has been mentioned earlier. The rate-limiting enzyme in the pathway leading to melatonin is serotonin N-acetyltransferase (Fig. 11-3). The levels of this enzyme and its products are high during the night and low during the day. Conversely, serotonin in the pineal falls at night, when much of it undergoes N-acetylation, and increases again during the day.

The N-acetyltransferase activity increases at night because then more norepinephrine is released from sympathetic nerves innervating the pineal. During the day administration of β-adrenergic agonists (e.g., isoproterenol) induces the N-acetyltransferase. Induction of the enzyme and maintenance of elevated enzyme activity seems to depend on an intracellular increase in cyclic AMP.

The "sensitivity" of pineal cells to β-adrenergic agonists (i.e., the concentration of agonist required for half maximal induction of N-acetyltransferase, the maximum activity attained, and the lag period that precedes the induction of the enzyme) is related to their previous exposure to the agonist. When the cells are deprived of β-adrenergic stimulation, they become supersensitive. They exhibit a shift to the left in the dose-response curve for isoproterenol, an increase in the maximum enzyme activity that can be induced by the drug, and an increase in the time required for induction of the enzyme. Protracted exposure to β-adrenergic agonists leaves

Table 11-2. Drug Action at Serotonergic Synapses

Drug	Action/Site
p-Chlorophenylalanine, α-propyldopacetamide	Inhibit TH, decrease 5HT
Iproniazid, clorgyline	Inhibit MAO, increase 5HT
Probenecid	Inhibits removal of 5HIAA from the brain
Reserpine, tetrabenazine	Deplete 5HT from granules
Tricyclic antidepressants, tryptolines (imipramine, chlorimipramine, amitryptyline)	Inhibit reuptake by 5HT endings
5,6-Dihydroxytryptamine	Destroys 5HT endings
Methysergide, cinaserin	5HT receptor antagonists
LSD	5HT receptor agonist

5HIAA, 5-hydroxyindoleacetic acid; 5HT, 5-hydroxytryptamine; MAO, monoamine oxidase; TH, tyrosine hydroxylase.

the cells subsensitive. These alterations in sensitivity reflect several changes in the ecology of the pinealocytes. There are changes in the number of β-adrenergic receptors on the surface of the cells, in the coupling of the receptors to adenylate cyclase, in the activity of phosphodiesterase, and in the responsiveness to cyclic AMP of the biochemical machinery responsible for de novo synthesis and maintenance of N-acetyltransferase.

One wonders whether the biosynthesis of serotonin or other neurotransmitters in central neurons is regulated in as complex a manner as is the biosynthesis of melatonin.

RELEASE OF SEROTONIN

In mollusks, serotonin serves as a mediator of cardiac acceleration. There is good evidence that it is released from nerve endings in clam hearts. In the central and peripheral nervous systems of other animals, serotonin release has not been shown to occur at specific synapses as clearly as it has in the clam. It is evident, however, that serotonin can be released from brain slices and synaptosomes in response to depolarizing stimuli and that it can be released into the cerebrospinal fluid when raphe neurons are electrically excited.

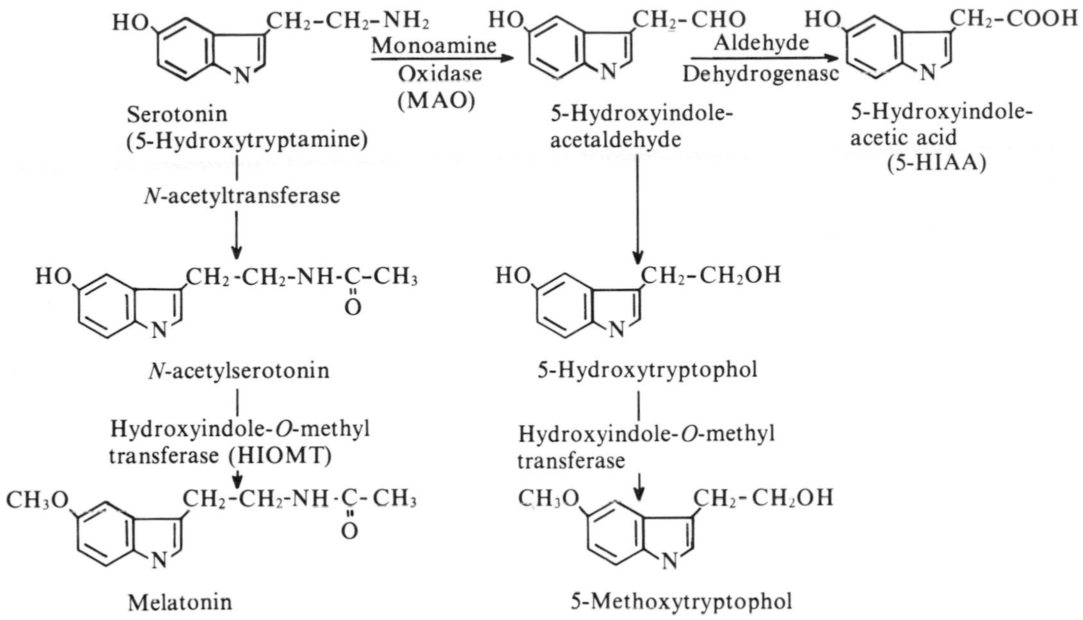

Fig. 11-3. Pathways of serotonin metabolism in the pineal gland.

SEROTONIN RECEPTORS

Microiontophoretic studies have revealed that both serotonergic and nonserotonergic neurons have serotonin receptors [24]. Occupation of presynaptic 5HT "autoreceptors" on serotonin-containing neurons reduces the neurons' rate of spontaneous firing. This provides a mechanism for feedback inhibition of neuronal activity that is coupled to release of transmitter. The predominant action of 5HT receptors on nonserotonergic cells seems to be inhibition of firing, although some excitatory serotonin receptors have been described.

In general, serotonin analogs (e.g., LSD, psilocin, dimethyltryptamine) are more potent on presynaptic than on postsynaptic receptors. Peripheral serotonin antagonists (e.g., cinaserin, cyproheptadine, metergoline, methiothepin, methysergide) work poorly at central inhibitory synapses; but, interestingly, they do inhibit the effect of the amine at central excitatory synapses.

Two ligands have been used to study serotonin binding sites in mammalian brain: d-LSD-^3H and 5HT-^3H [25]. These two ligands bind saturably, reversibly, and with high affinity. The D stereoisomer of LSD binds with a much greater affinity than does the L stereoisomer. Binding to presynaptic serotonergic elements has not been detected with either ligand; that is, lesioning central serotonergic neurons does not depress binding in the remainder of the brain. Both ligands appear to bind chiefly to neurons, but it seems unlikely that D-LSD and 5HT bind to identical macromolecular elements. Peripheral serotonergic antagonists displace LSD-^3H from its binding sites more effectively than they do 5HT-^3H. Tryptamines with 5-hydroxy substituents are more effective in competing for "5-HT-^3H receptors" than "LSD-^3H receptors." Whether there is a single serotonin receptor in the brain with antagonist- and agonist-preferring states, or two separate receptors, remains to be determined.

ROLE OF SEROTONIN IN THE BRAIN

Serotonin has been implicated in numerous central processes, including regulation of the anterior pituitary, sleep, appreciation of pain, thermoregulation, control of blood pressure, appetitive behavior, drinking, respiration, heart rate, rhythmic behavior, and memory.

Histamine

Histamine was synthesized in 1907 by Windaus and Vogt and subsequently was found in body tissues. At first, histamine was suspected to be a product of putrefaction and not a natural body constituent. Dale and Laidlaw, however, demonstrated that animals sensitized to otherwise inert proteins developed symptoms that resembled those of histamine poisoning (anaphylactic shock) when these proteins were administered. Best, Dale, and Dudley then showed that histamine could be extracted from fresh samples of lung and liver. Therefore, Dale concluded in the late 1920s that histamine was likely to mediate diverse phenomena, including some of the body's reactions to injury and foreign agents. Histamine's presence in a number of different tissues (Greek, *histos,* "tissue") supported Dale's thesis.

Histamine is found in bacteria and in a variety of plants and animals. It is present, moreover, in many venoms and noxious secretions. Almost all mammalian tissues contain some histamine. The skin, intestinal mucosa, and lungs are especially rich in this amine; the brain, on the other hand, has a low concentration of histamine, but turns it over very quickly. Thus, it should not be inferred from the relatively low steady state level of histamine in the brain (1×10^{-10} to 3×10^{-10} moles per gram of brain tissue) that the amine is unimportant there.

Histamine and histidine decarboxylase, the enzyme responsible for its biosynthesis, are unevenly distributed among different regions of the central nervous system [26–28] (Table 11-3). Highest concentrations are found in the hypothalamus, especially in the medial and ventral nuclei [29]. The midbrain, thalamus, and basal ganglia are moderately rich in histamine; the cerebral cortex has a modest amount of histamine; and the cerebellum, medulla, and spinal cord have a small amount.

Students of histamine have been hampered by the lack of a sensitive and specific histochemical technique for its localization. As a result, it has not

been possible to visualize histamine-containing elements in the brain or to estimate what fraction of the histamine is in neurons and what fraction is in nonneuronal cells, such as mast cells. Peritoneal mast cells each contain about 13 pg of histamine, so fewer than 10,000 such cells could provide the brain with all of its histamine. Mast cells have been seen in the central nervous system. They are especially numerous in the meninges, the pituitary, and the median eminence, but they have also been detected in parenchymal areas. Their parenchymal distribution roughly parallels that of histamine in the central nervous system.

There is evidence, however, that not all the histamine in the brain is in mast cells. Histamine and histidine decarboxylase are found in *synaptosomes* (a preparation of pinched-off nerve endings) from cortical tissue [30–31]. More important, the levels of histamine and histidine decarboxylase decrease in the hippocampus and other cortical regions after ascending pathways are destroyed [32–33]. In fact, after total deafferentation of specific cortical areas, histidine decarboxylase disappears almost entirely, but a small amount of histamine remains [34]. This residual histamine may be in mast cells, which, as has been mentioned, have a large amount of histamine but a very low histidine decarboxylase activity. The locations of the cell bodies that provide the cerebral cortex with its presumed histaminergic input remain to be discovered.

HISTAMINE SYNTHESIS AND METABOLISM

Histamine is formed by decarboxylation of histidine (Fig. 11-4). Two enzymes can catalyze this reaction: L-aromatic aminoacid decarboxylase and the "specific" L-histidine decarboxylase. The first of these is found in catecholaminergic and serotonergic neurons, in which it decarboxylates dopa and 5HTP, respectively. Although the affinity of the L-aromatic amino acid decarboxylase for histidine is relatively low, catecholaminergic and serotonergic neurons could, in theory, produce some or all of the brain's histamine. There is evidence, however, that cerebral histamine biosynthesis takes place in another population of neurons, which resist destruction by 6-hydroxydopamine

Table 11-3. Histamine and Histidine Decarboxylase in the Nervous System

| Tissue | Histamine (ng/g net wt) | | Histidine Decarboxylase (nmole/g tissue/hr) Rat |
	Mouse (enzymatic assay)	Rat (fluorometric assay)	
Whole brain	48	48	—
Brain stem	61	30	0.42
Cerebellum	26	25	0.08
Midbrain	—	54	1.53
Striatum	58	61	1.44
Cerebral cortex	35	42	1.17
Hippocampus	34	48	1.18
Hypothalamus	104	197	6.06
Spinal cord	—	—	0.11

and 5,7-dihydroxytryptamine [35–36], and which contain the specific histidine decarboxylase. This enzyme in brain homogenates behaves in much the same way as the enzyme isolated from stomach [28], for example. Its optimum pH is inversely related to substrate concentrations, and its affinity for histidine is fairly high (K_m about 4×10^{-4} M). The enzyme does not appear to be saturated with substrate in vivo. Histidine loading causes an increase in brain histamine levels, and availability of histidine may be important in regulating the rate of histidine biosynthesis. The activity of the specific decarboxylase is inhibited by α-hydrazinohistidine and brocresine (as are other pyridoxal phosphate–

dependent enzymes), but it is not inhibited by α-methyldopa, as L-aromatic aminoacid decarboxylase is.

The effects of decarboxylase inhibitors on histamine formation in vivo are consistent with the view that most of the histamine synthesis in the brain is catalyzed by the specific enzyme. Methyldopa does not affect histamine formation from histidine in doses that block serotonin formation from 5-hydroxytryptophan. On the other hand, α-hydrazinohistidine and brocresine do depress histamine synthesis in the brain markedly.

The key enzyme in the metabolism of histamine is histamine N-methyltransferase, which transfers a methyl group from S-adenosylmethionine to an imidazole-ring nitrogen, yielding methylhistamine

Fig. 11-4. Synthesis and metabolism of histamine.

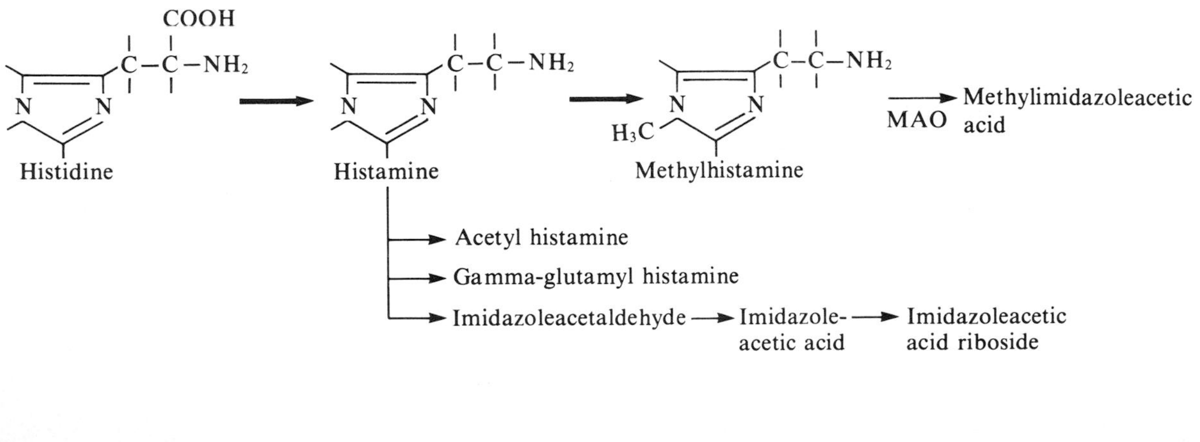

[37]. Subsequently, some of the methylhistamine is oxidized, and finally 1,4-methylimidazoleacetic acid is produced. A small amount of histamine in the brain seems to be converted into γ-glutamylhistamine. The role of this and of such other amides as γ-glutamylserotonin and γ-glutamyldopamine is unknown. In the periphery, part of the histamine is oxidized by histaminase, and part is acetylated. These modes of metabolism do not seem particularly important in the brain. Furthermore, reuptake of histamine does not appear to play a major part in terminating its action.

HISTAMINE RELEASE
Because there is no evidence that exogenous histamine mixes uniformly in the brain with the endogenous pool, histamine-^3H cannot be used as have labeled serotonin and catecholamines to study release in vivo or in vitro. The efflux of histamine from brain slices has been studied, however. Histamine release in vitro follows potassium depolarization and is calcium dependent. Thus, it seems to occur by means of exocytosis.

The turnover of histamine has been studied in vivo by blocking its synthesis (with α-hydrazinohistidine, for example) and determining its rate of decay [26]. The drug-induced depletion of histamine is very rapid, although only partial. The half-life of the pool of histamine that is depleted (30 to 40 percent of the total) is less than 1 minute.

HISTAMINE RECEPTORS
In the periphery, two types of histamine receptors are recognized: H_1 and H_2. H_1 agonists, such as 2-methylhistamine and 2-pyridylethylamine, cause contraction of smooth muscle in a variety of organs, among them the gut and bronchi [38]. H_2 agonists, the most specific of which is 4-methylhistamine, stimulate acid secretion by the stomach, increase the heart rate, and inhibit rat uterine contractions [39]. H_2 receptor agonists are specifically antagonized by metiamide and by cimetidine. Mepyramine is a potent H_1 antagonist, but it is not perfectly specific; it partially antagonizes 4-methylhistamine, as well as norepinephrine and serotonin.

Many neurons in the central nervous system respond to the iontophoretic application of histamine [40]. In the hypothalamus, the majority of cells appear to be excited by histamine. In the cerebral cortex, on the other hand, the predominant response to histamine is inhibition. This histamine-induced depression of neurons seems to involve activation of both H_1 and H_2 receptors.

Histamine is a very potent stimulator of adenylate cyclase activity in brain slices, and some of the effects of histamine [41] on central neurons may be mediated by intracellular increases in cyclic AMP levels. The histamine-induced stimulation of cyclic AMP accumulation seems to result partly from occupation of H_1 receptors and partly from occupation of H_2 receptors [42].

HISTAMINE FUNCTION IN THE NERVOUS SYSTEM
Histamine has been implicated in the central regulation of a number of physiological processes, among them water intake, vasopressin release, emesis, arousal, thermoregulation, anterior pituitary function, and cardiovascular function.

Purines
The case for purinergic transmission is considerably weaker than that for serotonergic transmission. Nevertheless, the evidence obtained to date has persuaded a number of workers that purines are involved in communication among cells.

DISTRIBUTION AND RELEASE OF PURINES
The purine nucleotides are essential constituents of all cells; therefore, it is not surprising that they are found in nervous tissue (see Chap. 19). Adenosinetriphosphate (ATP) is found in synaptic vesicles along with catecholamines and acetylcholine. It is released with the other contents of the vesicles when the nerve endings are depolarized. It may be degraded to adenosine and recaptured by cells, with or without acting on receptors.

The purines are synthesized in the form of 5′-mononucleotides (Fig. 11-5). The first step in the biosynthesis of purines is the conversion of α-D-ribose-5-phosphate into 5-phospho-α-D-ribose-1-pyrophosphate (PRPP) (Fig. 11-5). PRPP is used in making both purines and pyrimidines, and is

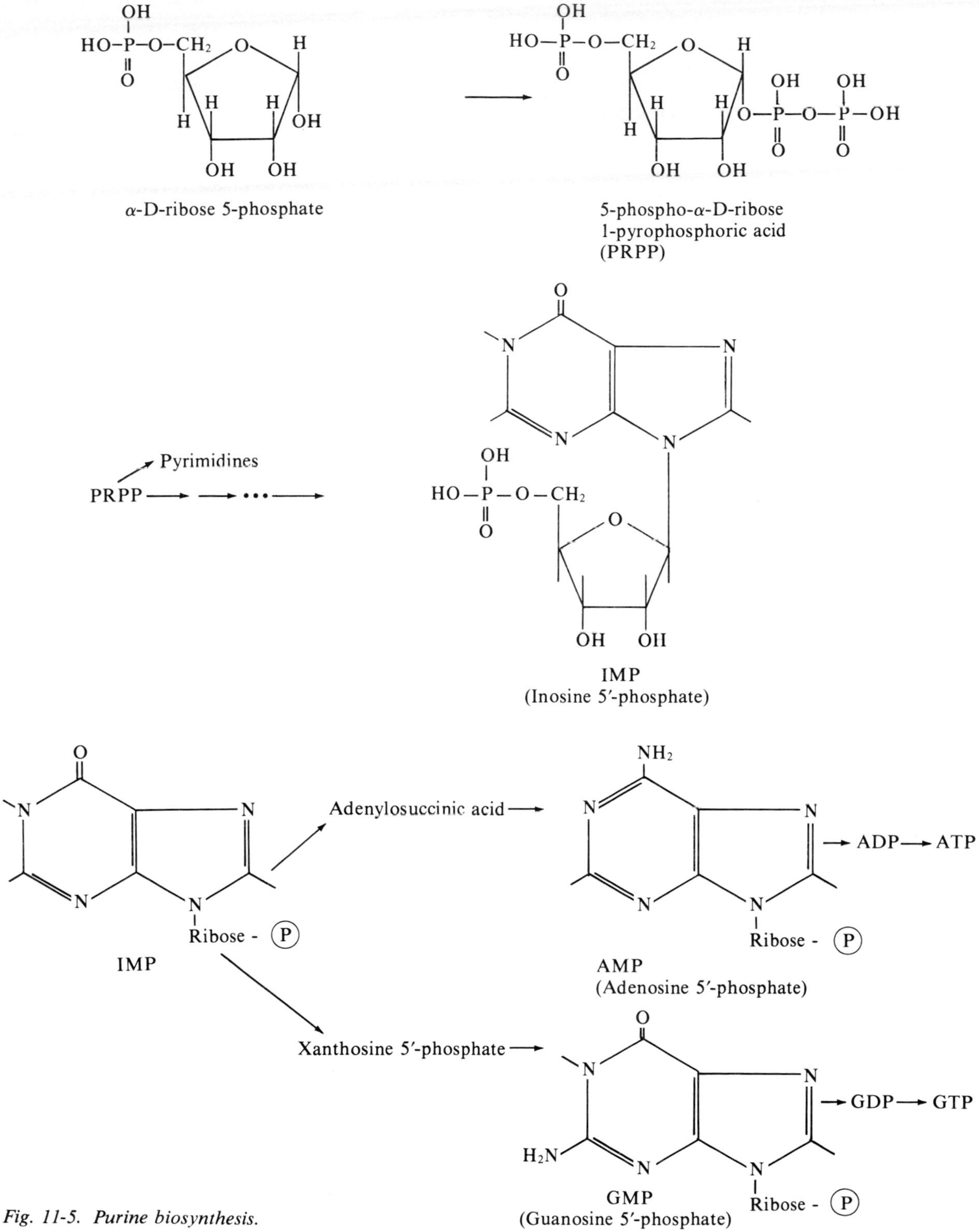

α-D-ribose 5-phosphate

5-phospho-α-D-ribose
1-pyrophosphoric acid
(PRPP)

Pyrimidines

PRPP ⟶ ⟶ ⋯ ⟶

IMP
(Inosine 5′-phosphate)

Adenylosuccinic acid ⟶

Xanthosine 5′-phosphate ⟶

IMP

AMP
(Adenosine 5′-phosphate)

ADP ⟶ ATP

GMP
(Guanosine 5′-phosphate)

GDP ⟶ GTP

Fig. 11-5. Purine biosynthesis.

important for the salvage of purines as well (see below and Chap. 19). The synthesis of purines from PRPP is complex; the purine ring is built step by step onto PRPP by successive additions of carbons and nitrogens from glycine, $N^5,10^{10}$-methenyltetrahydrofolate, glutamine, CO_2, aspartate, and N^{10}-formyltetrahydrofolate. The first product in the biosynthetic pathway to have a complete purine ring is inosinic acid (IMP). The production of IMP is expensive; six high-energy phosphates from ATP are used in converting α-D-ribose-5-phosphate into IMP.

IMP serves as a precursor for adenosine 5'-phosphate (AMP) and guanosine 5'-phosphate (GMP), which can be converted into their respective diphosphates (ADP, GDP) and triphosphates (ATP, GTP). These nucleotides are ubiquitously present in cells that use them in the transfer of chemical energy and in the production of RNA. The nucleosides and free bases, on the other hand, are found in only trace amounts in healthy tissue and seem to be by-products of the enzymatic hydrolysis of nucleic acids and nucleotides. Whether there are neurons that make and release purines, purine nucleosides, or purine nucleotides exclusively is not known.

Purine nucleosides and purines are ultimately degraded to uric acid (Fig. 11-6). Most of the free purines formed daily are not broken down, however. Instead, they seem to be salvaged by a variety of cells, including neurons (Fig. 11-7). (The salvage pathway is discussed in Chap. 19.) Exogenously administered adenosine, for example, is concentrated by nervous tissue. Presumably, adenosine released from nerve endings (or ATP released and metabolized to adenosine) is taken up by the nerves and recycled. It may be that the uptake mechanism serves to inactivate purine neurotransmitters in addition to conserving them.

A deficiency in one of the enzymes involved in purine salvage—guanine (hypoxanthine) phosphoribosyltransferase—is responsible for the Lesch-Nyhan syndrome. This enzyme allows guanine and hypoxanthine to accept a phosphate group from PRPP to form GMP and IMP, respectively. In the absence of the enzyme, guanine and

hypoxanthine are metabolized to uric acid instead of being saved, and there is a marked compensatory increase in purine synthesis. The uric acid builds up in the kidneys, resulting in renal failure. In addition, patients with Lesch-Nyhan syndrome suffer from mental retardation, spastic cerebral palsy, choreoathetosis, seizures, and self-mutilation [43]. Since hyperuricemia alone is not associated with the neurological and behavioral abnormalities seen in Lesch-Nyhan syndrome, it has been suggested that these abnormalities are a consequence either of the deleterious effects of excess xanthine and hypoxanthine or of a decrease in the availability of IMP and GMP. Parenteral administration of caffeine or theophylline (both methylxanthines) to rats and rabbits causes the animals to mutilate their limbs. This finding supports the notion that toxic purine metabolites are responsible for the Lesch-Nyhan syndrome. Adenine has been given to people with Lesch-Nyhan disease in the hope that it would serve as a substrate for IMP and GMP production and, at the same time, reverse the body's compensatory overproduction of xanthine and hypoxanthine. Unfortunately, adenine partly corrected the biochemical deficits in the patients without affecting the course of their disease [44].

PURINE RECEPTORS

Indisputably, purines have significant actions on excitable tissues. Iontophoresis of adenine derivatives onto cortical neurons, for example, results in a decrease in their firing rate [45]. Agents that block the neuronal uptake of adenosine (dipyridamole, hexabendin) and that should prolong its availability to extracellular receptors potentiate its actions. Drugs like caffeine and aminophylline, on the other hand, block the depressant effect of adenosine and are thought to be receptor antagonists.

Similar results are obtained when purines are applied to brain slices in vitro and the accumulation of cyclic AMP is measured [4]. Adenosine elicits a marked increase in cyclic AMP production, as do ATP, ADP, and AMP. However, the activity of these nucleotides appears to be dependent on a prior hydrolysis to adenosine. Most alterations in the ribose or purine portion of adenosine cause

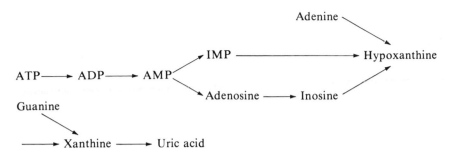

Fig. 11-6. Degradation of purines.

$$Adenine + PRPP \longrightarrow AMP + PP_i$$

$$Guanine + PRPP \longrightarrow GMP + PP_i$$

$$Purine + ribose\ 1\text{-}phosphate \longrightarrow purine\ nucleoside + P_i$$

$$Adenosine + ATP \longrightarrow AMP + ADP$$

Fig. 11-7. Purine salvage mechanisms.

a loss of stimulatory activity. In fact, 5′-deoxy-adenosine, theophylline, caffeine, and 3-isobutyl-1-methylxanthine have been found to antagonize adenosine.

Combinations of adenosine and norepinephrine, histamine, or serotonin have much greater than additive effects on the accumulation of cyclic AMP in cerebral cortical slices [46]. Compounds that block adenosine uptake into cells potentiate low concentrations of adenosine.

Recently, inosine and hypoxanthine have been shown to displace diazepam-^3H from stereospecific, high-affinity binding sites on brain membrane preparations [47]. These two purines were isolated from brain extracts in the course of a search for an endogenous diazepamlike ligand. High concentrations of inosine [48] and adenosine [49] act as anticonvulsants, and hypoxanthine and inosine elicit a rapidly desensitizing excitatory response and a nondesensitizing inhibitory response when they are applied to cultured spinal neurons [50]. Flurazepam blocks the inhibitory and mimics the excitatory response.

On the basis of the experiments summarized in the last four paragraphs, it is evident that there may be a number of purine receptors in the central nervous system, including separate receptors for adenosine and for inosine-hypoxanthine. Some of these receptors may be coupled to adenylate cyclase, and in occupying their receptors, the purines may function either as neurotransmitters or as agents that modulate the effects of other neurotransmitters. Whether the purine receptors are physiologically important or pharmacological curiosities remains to be seen.

References

*1. Collier, H. O. J. The Occurrence of 5-Hydroxytryptamine (5HT) in Nature. In G. P. Lewis (ed.), *5-Hydroxytryptamine*. New York: Pergamon, 1958. Pp. 5–19.

*2. Garattini, S., and Valzelli, L. *Serotonin*. New York: Elsevier, 1965.

*3. Page, I. H. *Serotonin*. Chicago: Year Book, 1968.

4. Saavedra, J. M., Brownstein, M., and Axelrod, J. A specific and sensitive enzymatic-isotopic microassay for serotonin in tissues. *J. Pharmacol. Exp. Ther.* 186:508–515, 1973.

*Key reference.

5. Heller, A., Harvey, J. A., and Moore, R. Y. A demonstration of a fall in brain serotonin following central nervous system lesions in the rat. *Biochem. Pharmacol.* 11:859–866, 1962.

6. Heller, A., and Moore, R. Y. Effect of central nervous system lesions on brain monoamines in the rat. *J. Pharmacol. Exp. Ther.* 150:1–9, 1965.

*7. Falck, B., et al. Fluorescence of catecholamines and related compounds condensed with formaldehyde. *J. Histochem. Cytochem.* 10:348–354, 1962.

*8. Ungerstedt, U. Stereotaxic mapping of the monoamine pathways in the rat brain. *Acta Physiol. Scand.* 82 (Suppl. 367):1–48, 1971.

*9. Dahlström, A., and Fuxe, K. Evidence for the existence of monoamine-containing neurons in the central nervous system. I. Demonstration of monoamines in the cell bodies of brain stem neurons. *Acta Physiol. Scand.* 62 (Suppl. 232):1–55, 1964.

*10. Dahlström, A., and Fuxe, K. Evidence for the existence of monoamine neurons in the central nervous system. II. Experimentally induced changes in the intraneuronal amine levels of bulbospinal neuron systems. *Acta Physiol. Scand.* 64 (Suppl. 247):1–36, 1965.

11. Brownstein, M. J., Palkovits, M., and Kizer, J. S. Effect of surgical isolation of the hypothalamus on its neurotransmitter content. *Brain Res.* 117:287–295, 1976.

12. Smith, A. R., and Ariëns Kappers, J. Effect of pinealectomy, gonadectomy, pCPA, and pineal extracts on the rat parvocellular neurosecretory hypothalamic system: A fluorescence histochemical investigation. *Brain Res.* 86:353–371, 1975.

13. Joh, T. H., et al. Brain tryptophan hydroxylase: Purification of, production of antibodies to, and cellular and ultrastructural localization in serotonergic neurons of rat midbrain. *Proc. Natl. Acad. Sci. U.S.A.* 72:3575–3580, 1975.

14. Tong, J. H., and Kaufman, S. Tryptophan hydroxylase. Purification and some properties of the enzyme from rabbit hindbrain. *J. Biol. Chem.* 250:4152–4158, 1975.

15. Wurtman, R. J., and Fernstrom, J. D. Control of brain monoamine synthesis by diet and plasma amino acids. *Am. J. Clin. Nutr.* 28:638–647, 1975.

16. Gallager, D. W., and Aghajanian, G. K. Inhibition of firing of raphe neurons by tryptophan and 5-hydroxytryptophan: Blockade by inhibiting serotonin synthesis with RO-4-4602. *Neuropharmacology* 15:149–156, 1976.

17. Fujiwara, M., et al. Indoleamine 2,3-dioxygenase. *J. Biol. Chem.* 253:6081–6085, 1978.

18. Hidaka, H., Nagatsu, T., and Yagi, K. Occurrence of a serotonin sulphotransferase in the brain. *J. Neurochem.* 16:783–785, 1969.

*19. Koslow, S. Biosignificance of *N*- and *O*-methylated indoles to psychiatric disorders. In E. Usdin, D. A. Hamburg, and J. D. Barchas (eds.), *Neuroregulators and Psychiatric Disorders.* New York: Oxford, 1977. Pp. 210–219.

20. Weissbach, H., Redfield, B. G., and Axelrod, J. Biosynthesis of melatonin: Enzymatic conversion of serotonin to *N*-acetylserotonin. *Biochim. Biophys. Acta* 43:352–353, 1960.

21. Axelrod, J., and Weissbach, H. Purification and properties of hydroxyindole-*O*-methyltransferase. *J. Biol. Chem.* 236:211–213, 1961.

22. Lerner, A. B., et al. Isolation of melatonin, the pineal gland factor that lightens melanocytes. *J. Am. Chem. Soc.* 80:2587–2591, 1958.

*23. Nir, I., Reiter, R. J., and Wurtman, R. J. *The Pineal Gland, J. Neural. Transm.* (Suppl. 13), 1978.

24. Haigler, H. J., and Aghajanian, G. K. Serotonin receptors in the brain. *Fed. Proc.* 36:2159–2164, 1977.

*25. Bennett, J. P., Jr., and Snyder, S. H. Serotonin synaptic receptors in the mammalian central nervous system. *Fed. Proc.* 37:137–138, 1978.

26. Taylor, K. M., and Snyder, S. H. Dynamics of the regulation of histamine levels in mouse brain. *J. Neurochem.* 19:341–354, 1972.

27. Ronnberg, A. L., and Schwartz, J. C. Répartition régionale de l'histamine dans le cerveau de rat. *C. R. Acad. Sci.* (Paris) 268:2376–2379, 1969.

28. Schwartz, J. C., Lampart, C., and Rose, C. Properties and regional distribution of histidine decarboxylase in rat brain. *J. Neurochem.* 17:1527–1534, 1970.

29. Brownstein, M. J., et al. Histamine content of hypothalamic nuclei of the rat. *Brain Res.* 77:151–156, 1974.

30. Carlini, E. A., and Green, J. P. The subcellular distribution of histamine, slow-reacting substance, and 5-hydroxytryptamine in the brain of the rat. *Br. J. Pharmacol.* 20:264–277, 1963.

31. Baudry, M., Matres, M.-P., and Schwartz, J.-C. The subcellular localization of histidine decarboxylase in various regions of the brain. *J. Neurochem.* 21:13–21, 1973.

32. Garbarg, M., et al. Histaminergic pathway in rat brain evidenced by lesions of the medial forebrain bundle. *Science* 186:833–835, 1974.

33. Barbin, G., et al. Histamine synthesizing afferents in the hippocampal region. *J. Neurochem.* 26:259–263, 1976.

34. Barbin, G., et al. Decrease in histamine content and decarboxylase activities in an isolated area of cerebral cortex of the cat. *Brain Res.* 92:170–174, 1975.

35. Garbarg, M., et al. Evidence for a specific decarboxylase involved in histamine synthesis in an ascending pathway in rat brain. *Agents Actions* 4:181–182, 1974.

36. Schwartz, J.-C. Histamine as a transmitter in brain. *Life Sci.* 17:503–518, 1975.

37. Brown, D. D., Tomchick, R., and Axelrod, J. Distribution and properties of a histamine-methylating enzyme. *J. Biol. Chem.* 234:2948–2950, 1959.

38. Ash, A. S. F., and Schild, H. O. Receptors mediating some actions of histamine. *Br. J. Pharmacol. Chemother.* 27:427–439, 1966.

39. Black, J. W., et al. Definition and antagonism of histamine H_2-receptors. *Nature* 236:385–390, 1972.

40. Sastry, B. S. R., and Phillis, J. W. Depression of rat cerebral cortical neurons by H_1 and H_2 histamine receptor agonists. *Eur. J. Pharmacol.* 38:269–273, 1976.

41. Kakiuchi, S., and Rall, T. W. Studies on adenosine 3′, 5′-phosphate in the rabbit cerebral cortex. *Mol. Pharmacol.* 4:379–388, 1968.

42. Baudry, M., Matres, M.-P., and Schwartz, J.-C. H_1 and H_2 receptors on the histamine induced accumulation of cyclic AMP in guinea-pig brain slices. *Nature* 253:362–364, 1975.

*43. Nyhan, W. L. Purine metabolism and abnormal behavior in children. *Adv. Behav. Biol.* 1:281–301, 1971.

*44. Nyhan, W. L. The Lesch-Nyhan syndrome. *Annu. Rev. Med.* 24:41–60, 1973.

45. Phillis, J. W., Kostopoulos, G. K., and Limacher, J. L. A potent depressant action of adenine derivatives on cerebral cortical neurones. *Eur. J. Pharmacol.* 30:125–129, 1975.

*46. Daly, J. Role of cyclic nucleotides in the nervous system. In L. L. Iverson, S. D. Iverson, and S. H. Snyder (eds.), *Handbook of Psychopharmacology. V. Synaptic Modulators.* New York: Plenum, 1975. Pp. 47–130.

47. Skolnick, P., et al. Inosine, an endogenous ligand of the brain benzodiazepine receptor, antagonizes pentylenetetrazole-evoked seizures. *Proc. Natl. Acad. Sci. U.S.A.* 76:1515–1518, 1979.

48. Skolnick, P., et al. Identification of inosine and hypoxanthine as endogenous inhibitors of ^3H-diazepam binding in the central nervous system. *Life Sci.* 23:1473–1480, 1978.

49. Maitre, M., et al. Protective effect of adenosine and nicotinamide against audiogenic seizure. *Biochem. Pharmacol.* 23:2807 2816, 1974.

50. MacDonald, J. F., et al. Purines may be endogenous ligands for benzodiazepine receptors on cultured spinal neurons. *Science* 205:715–717, 1979.

P. L. McGeer
E. G. McGeer

Chapter 12. Amino Acid Neurotransmitters

In this chapter we discuss amino acids for which a role as a neurotransmitter either has been proven or is considered possible. If there is doubt, the amino acid is described as a *putative neurotransmitter*. In cases where only suggestive evidence exists, the amino acid is described as a *neurotransmitter candidate*.

So far, it may be said that γ-aminobutyric acid (GABA) and glycine are proven neurotransmitters; glutamate and aspartate are putative neurotransmitters; and taurine, proline, serine, and *N*-acetyl-aspartate are neurotransmitter candidates.

Specific Amino Acids

GABA

GABA is the most thoroughly documented of all neurotransmitter compounds. It has been the object of intensive study, with many elegant chemical and physiological techniques being applied to an elucidation of its role.

Eugene Roberts [1] and Jorge Awapara [2] independently discovered the presence of GABA in brain tissue in 1950. In 1953, Florey discovered in mammalian brain a mysterious "factor I" that inhibited the crayfish stretch-receptor neuron. Bazemore, Elliott, and Florey [3] identified this as GABA, the year before Kuffler and Edwards [4] showed that it duplicated the transmitter action at certain crayfish cord synapses. Obata and Takeda [5] first showed its release in mammalian systems, demonstrating its presence in the fourth ventricle after Purkinje cells were stimulated. Fonnum and coworkers [6] then demonstrated that cutting Purkinje axons resulted in a disappearance of glutamic acid decarboxylase (GAD), the synthesizing enzyme, from the terminals. Elegant final proof of GABA's role in Purkinje cells was developed by the Roberts team; they purified glutamic acid decarboxylase, developed antibodies against it, and showed by the immunohistochemical method that it was localized to Purkinje cell terminals [7].

Chemistry of GABA

Glucose, the main energy source of the brain, is a particularly efficient precursor of GABA and is probably the principal in vivo source. Pyruvate and several other amino acids can also serve as precursors. They feed into the so-called GABA shunt (Fig. 12-1). The shunt is actually a closed loop that acts to conserve the supply of GABA. The first step is the transamination of α-ketoglutarate, an intermediate in the Krebs cycle, to glutamic acid. Glutamic acid is then decarboxylated by GAD to form GABA. GABA is transaminated by GABA α-oxoglutarate transaminase (GABA-T) to form succinic semialdehyde, but the transamination can only take place if α-ketoglutarate is the acceptor of the amine group. This transforms α-ketoglutarate into the GABA precursor, glutamate, thereby guaranteeing a continuity of supply. Thus, a molecule of GABA can be destroyed metabolically only if a molecule of precursor is formed to take its place. The succinic semialdehyde formed from GABA is rapidly oxidized to succinic acid by succinic semialdehyde dehydrogenase (SSADH) to reenter the Krebs cycle. Ancillary to the GABA shunt is a *glutamine loop:* released GABA can be picked up by glial cells, where a similar transamination by GABA-T can take place. The glutamate formed cannot, however, be converted to GABA in the glia, since they lack GAD. Instead, it is transformed by glutamine synthetase (Glu Synth) into glutamine, after which it can be returned to the nerve ending. In the nerve ending, the enzyme glutaminase converts

233

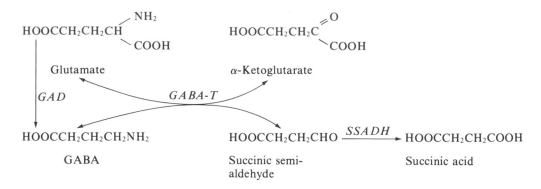

Glutamate

α-Ketoglutarate

GAD

GABA-T

HOOCCH₂CH₂CH₂NH₂

GABA

Succinic semi-
aldehyde

Succinic acid

the glutamine back to glutamate, thus completing the loop and conserving the supply of GABA precursor.

Figure 12-2 is a schematic diagram showing the intracellular localization of the components of the GABA shunt and glutamine loop in the region of the synapse. As shown in the figure, GABA-T and SSADH are attached to mitochondria. Glutaminase, GAD, and Glu Synth are cytoplasmic enzymes, with GAD occurring only in neurons, Glu Synth only in glia, and glutaminase in both. An internal segment of the shunt operates entirely within the nerve ending, but the glutaminase loop comes into play when GABA is released from the nerve ending.

Viewed in terms of energy, the GABA shunt yields three ATP molecules. It is therefore less efficient than the portion of the Krebs cycle that converts α-ketoglutarate to succinic acid through the usual pathway. This direct route, used principally by brain, as well as exclusively by all other tissues, yields three molecules of ATP and one of GTP.

It is still not certain to what extent glucose, the principal fuel for the brain, is diverted through the shunt rather than being stripped through the standard Krebs cycle. Figures based on in vivo turnover rates of GABA as compared with Krebs cycle intermediates suggest 10 percent [8]. Since the amount of GABA actually utilized for neurotransmitter function is not known, it is impossible to determine whether any of that produced is designed primarily as a contribution to the energy pool. It may be that GABA is being continuously formed in nerve endings at a rate well in excess of that re-

Fig. 12-1. Schematic diagram showing the reactions of the GABA shunt.

quired for neurotransmission, with the surplus being metabolized presynaptically and winding up as a supplemental energy source.

GAD, the key enzyme in the formation of GABA, has been purified from mouse brain by Wu [9] and his collaborators. It has a molecular weight of 85,000 and requires pyridoxal phosphate as a cofactor. The K_m is 0.7 mM for glutamate and 0.05 mM for pyridoxal phosphate—in each case well below the in vivo tissue level. Consequently, the enzyme should normally be fully saturated with its substrate and its cofactor. Antibodies to the purified enzyme have been produced in rabbits, and localization to nerve endings has been confirmed submicroscopically by the immunocytochemical technique (Fig. 12-3).

GABA-T has also been purified to homogeneity from mouse brain and antibodies to it have been prepared [9]. It has a molecular weight of 109,000 and, like GAD, requires pyridoxal phosphate as cofactor. The K_m for GABA is 1.1 mM. The availability of α-ketoglutarate may play an important role in the destruction of GABA. This is particularly true when respiration ceases: since the Krebs cycle depends on aerobic metabolism, the level of α-ketoglutarate rapidly declines. GABA cannot then be destroyed, although it can still be formed from glutamate, because GAD is an anaerobic enzyme. There is, therefore, a rapid increase in brain GABA levels post mortem, accompanied by a rapid decline in glutamate.

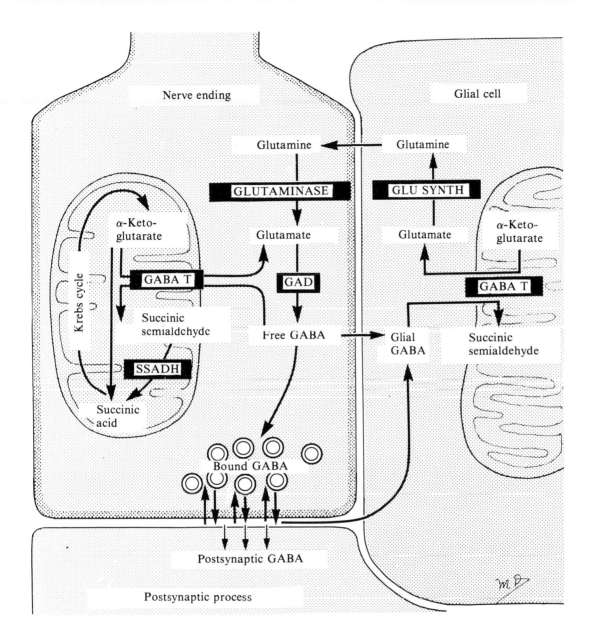

Fig. 12-2. Schematic diagram showing relationship of GABA nerve ending, a postsynaptic process, and a glial cell. Enzymes are shown in black rectangles and endogenous intermediates in white.

The mitochondria containing GABA-T are in several locations. They are in GABA-containing synaptosomes and glial cells, and may be in postsynaptic neuronal processes. In the first location they participate in maintaining appropriate presynaptic concentrations of GABA, whereas in the latter two they participate in its destruction after release (Fig. 12-2). The final enzyme in the GABA shunt, SSADH, is closely coupled to GABA-T and is similarly distributed in brain. The high tissue content required to saturate the enzyme relative to that for GABA-T probably explains why succinic semialdehyde has never been detected as an endogenous metabolite in neural tissue. That which is formed from GABA is very rapidly converted to succinic acid, which then enters the Krebs cycle.

Other routes have been described for GABA in brain. It can be formed from putrescine or from γ-hydroxybutyrate. It may be a precursor of other significant brain metabolites, such as homocarnosine (the dipeptide derivative of GABA and histidine), γ-hydroxybutyrate, γ-aminobutyrylcholine, γ-butyrylbetaine, γ-guanidinobutyric acid, and several others. None of these alternate routes, however, has been established as being of major importance either metabolically or physiologically [8].

Considerable biochemical work in recent years has been concentrated on GABA receptors. It is believed that high-affinity binding to postsynaptic neurotransmitter receptor sites can generally be distinguished from binding to presynaptic uptake sites on the basis of the role played by Na^+. Presynaptic uptake is Na^+-dependent, whereas postsynaptic binding is not. Na^+-independent, high-affinity binding of radioactive GABA, muscimol, or N-methylbicuculline to synaptic membrane preparations has the regional distribution expected for postsynaptic GABA receptors and is inhibited by GABA agonists and antagonists; it is not affected by presynaptic uptake inhibitors [10, 11]. Both physiological and binding studies indicate the existence of more than one type of GABA receptor. Some, but not all, are coupled to a benzodiazepine recognition site, which allows modulatory interactions between GABA and benzodiazepines (and

Fig. 12-3. Localization of GAD by immunohistochemistry. A. A neuron (N) from a deep cerebellar nucleus treated with anti-GAD serum is surrounded by profiles of dense, punctate, GAD-positive Purkinje cell axon terminals (long arrows). Numerous GAD-positive terminals are demonstrated on the surface of one of the grazed neuronal processes (short arrows). Bar represents 10 μm. (From Barber et al., Brain Res. 141:355, 1978). B. The inset shows a semithin (1 μm) section of the pars reticulata with obliquely and transversely sectioned dendrites encircled by punctate structures containing GAD-positive reaction product (arrows). The electron micrograph shows an obliquely sectioned dendrite in the substantia nigra surrounded by many axon terminals filled with GAD-positive reaction product that are equivalent to the puncta observed in the inset. Some of these terminals form symmetric synapses (arrows), whereas the unstained terminal contains round synaptic vesicles and forms an asymmetric synapse (arrowhead) with this dendritic shaft. Each marker indicates 1 μm. A multivesicular body (MVB) is identified. (From Ribak et al., Brain Res. 116:287, 1977). C. Immunocytochemical localization of GAD in laminae II–III of rat lumbar spinal cord 24 hr after ipsilateral dorsal root lesions. A dense, degenerating primary afferent terminal (T_{PA}) is surrounded by GAD-positive axon terminals (T_G) and by dendritic profiles (d). One of the GAD-positive axon terminals (T_{G1}) invaginates into the primary afferent terminal from a tissue level not included in this sectioning plane. Two of the GAD-positive terminals appear to be presynaptic (double arrows) to the degenerating primary afferent terminal. These axoaxonal synaptic relationships are consistent with the evidence that implicates GABA as one of the neurotransmitters which mediate presynaptic inhibition in the dorsal spinal cord. In addition to being postsynaptic to GAD-positive terminals, the primary afferent terminal is also presynaptic (single arrows) to some of the surrounding dendritic profiles. Magnification ×79,000. (Electron micrography courtesy of James E. Vaughn, City of Hope National Medical Center, Duarte, California). (Barber et al., Brain Res. 141:35, 1978).

presumably, the so far unidentified endogenous ligand for the benzodiazepine receptor) [12]. GABA binding is greatly enhanced by freezing and detergent treatment of the tissue and is apparently inhibited by an endogenous protein which masks some of the receptor sites in freshly prepared homogenates.

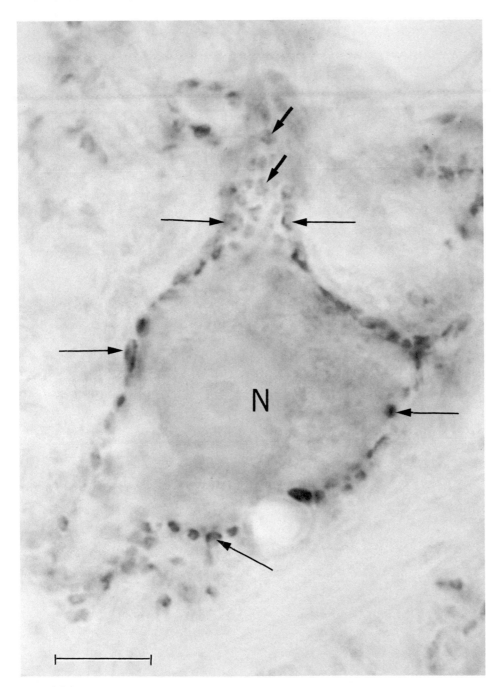

Fig. 12-3A

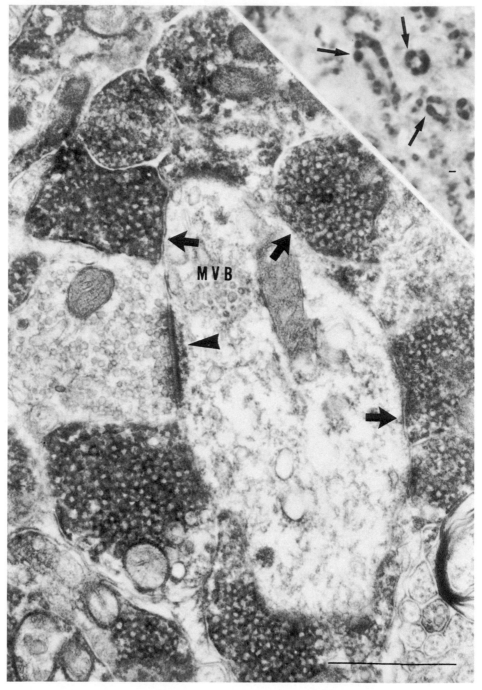

Fig. 12-3B

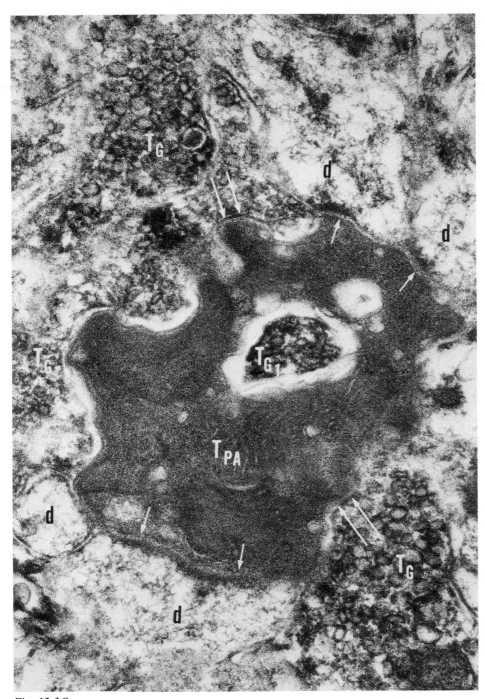

Fig. 12-3C

Physiology and Pharmacology of GABA

For technical reasons, some of the most convincing tests of neurotransmitter action cannot be performed on the CNS, but must be carried out on isolated nerves that can be obtained only in the periphery. In the case of GABA, such tests must be carried out on invertebrates, as in most vertebrates, particularly mammalians, GABA is almost exclusively limited to CNS. Lobster nerves are an ideal model. Otsuka and coworkers [12] first showed that stimulation of single inhibitory, but not excitatory, nerves of lobster nerve-muscle preparations resulted in markedly increased GABA release. This release was reduced by lowering calcium levels in the extracellular medium, as is the case for the release of all neurotransmitters. Furthermore, GABA mimicked the action of the endogenous transmitter when applied iontophoretically. It increased conductance of the postsynaptic membrane by selectively enhancing permeability to Cl^-. Both the natural transmitter and GABA proved ineffective in solutions where Cl^- was replaced by anions too large to penetrate the postsynaptic membrane.

The physiological actions of GABA as an inhibitory neurotransmitter of mammalian synapses can be summarized by considering the classical evidence obtained for its action in the cerebellar Purkinje cell. It is the following:

1. Stimulation of Purkinje cells results in hyperpolarization of postsynaptic cells in the deep cerebellar nuclei and Deiters' nucleus. This hyperpolarization becomes a depolarization when the resting membrane potential of the postsynaptic cell is artificially increased beyond the equilibrium potential for the inhibitory postsynaptic potential (IPSP).
2. The postsynaptic membrane is permeable to chloride and other anions of comparably small size during transmitter action.
3. Picrotoxin and bicuculline, which are classical GABA antagonists, block the effects of stimulation; strychnine, which is not a GABA blocker, is ineffective.
4. Stimulation of Purkinje cells results in the re-

lease of detectable amounts of GABA into the perfusion fluid of the fourth ventricle or into the output field of a push-pull cannula inserted into the area of the deep cerebellar nuclei.

Detailed accounts of the ionic actions of GABA can be obtained by reference to a number of excellent review articles [13].

Pharmacological agents exist that are capable of interacting with GABA in all of the classic areas for manipulation of neurotransmitters. These are sites of synthesis, storage, extraneuronal release, presynaptic reuptake, postsynaptic destruction, and postsynaptic action.

Some of the better-known agents are listed in Table 12-1. So far, few of them have found their way into clinical medicine. Many of them interact prominently with other systems, so their specificity is limited. Moreover, inconsistencies appear in a number of cases between the presumed mechanism of action and the overall physiological effects. In general, however, drugs that diminish GABA activity cause convulsions; those that enhance it cause sedation. Such global effects would be anticipated in a general inhibitory transmitter.

GABA levels can be lowered by a variety of agents that inhibit GAD synthesis. 3-Mercaptopropionic acid, for example, inhibits GAD almost totally at a concentration of 10^{-3} M. After this agent is administered to rats, convulsions commence in about 7 minutes, at a time when GABA levels are reduced by about one-third. Allylglycine has a similar effect. High-pressure oxygen, which also inhibits GAD activity and reduces GABA levels, produces the same results. Most of the known GAD inhibitors, however, belong to the group of so-called carbonyl trapping agents, which act against the cofactor pyridoxal phosphate and therefore affect both GAD and GABA-T. The drawback of such compounds is that GABA levels may not necessarily be decreased. For example, some agents, such as isonicotinylhydrazide, will both raise and lower GABA levels, depending upon the time after administration of the drug and the dose. Those carbonyl trapping agents that appear to inhibit GAD more specifically than GABA-T

Table 12-1. Some Drugs That Affect GABA Action[a]

Drug	Presumed Action Mechanism	Physiological Effect
Synthesis		
Allylglycine	GAD inhibitor	Convulsant
3-Mercaptopropionic acid	GAD inhibitor	Convulsant
High-pressure oxygen	GAD inhibitor	Convulsant
Isonicotinylhydrazide	B_6 antagonist	Convulsant in high doses
Thiosemicarbazide	B_6 antagonist	Convulsant in high doses
Release		
Tetanus toxin	Inhibitor of GABA and glycine release	Convulsant
Pump		
cis-3-Aminocyclohexanecarboxylic acid[b]	GABA neuronal pump inhibitor	
Nipecotic acid	GABA neuronal pump inhibitor	
β-Alanine	GABA glial pump inhibitor	
Haloperidol	Monoamine blocker and weak GABA neuronal pump inhibitor	Antipsychotic
Chlorpromazine	Monoamine blocker and weak GABA neuronal pump inhibitor	Antipsychotic
Imipramine	Monoamine and GABA pump inhibitor	Antidepressant
Destruction		
Aminoxyacetic acid	B_6 antagonist for GABA-T	Sedative
n-Dipropylacetate	GABA-T inhibitor[c]	Anticonvulsant
Hydrazinopropionic acid	GABA T inhibitor	Sedative
Gabaculine	GABA-T inhibitor	Anticonvulsant
γ-Acetylenic GABA	GABA-T inhibitor	
γ-VinylGABA	GABA-T inhibitor	
Antagonist		
Bicuculline	GABA antagonist	Convulsant
Picrotoxin	GABA antagonist	Convulsant
Agonist		
Muscimol	GABA agonist	Psychotomimetic
Imidazoleacetic acid	Weak GABA agonist	Weak sedative
Homotaurine	GABA agonist	
Baclofen	Possible GABA agonist[d]	Muscle relaxant
γ-Hydroxybutyrate	Possible GABA agonist	Weak sedative

[a]For most references see McGeer et al. [24], pages 220–225. [b]Neal et al. *Brain Res.* 176:285, 1979. [c]Blume et al. *Brain Res.* 171:182, 1979. [d]Hill and Bowery. *Nature* 290:149, 1981.

have a greater tendency to decrease GABA; they therefore produce seizures in animals. Classical examples are isoniazide, semicarbazide, and thiosemicarbazide. They inhibit GAD in concentrations of 10^{-4} to 10^{-3} M in vitro and in vivo. However, other carbonyl trapping agents, such as aminooxyacetic acid, hydroxylamine, and hydrazinopropionic acid, which have a greater effect on GABA-T than on GAD, tend to raise GABA levels and thus have a sedative effect. Unfortunately, these agents reverse their effects at higher doses, producing convulsions. They are therefore not used in humans. Many MAO inhibitors are weak carbonyl trapping agents that preferentially reduce GABA-T activity and raise GABA levels in animals. This always occurs at doses beyond those used clinically, and therefore the antidepressant action is probably unrelated to changing GABA levels.

The most useful GABA-T inhibitor so far developed is sodium *n*-dipropylacetate, which may, however, also interact with excitatory amino acid systems. Clinically, it has proved effective in treating certain forms of epilepsy. Other GABA-T inhibitors are γ-acetylenic GABA, γ-vinyl GABA, and GABAculine (5-amino–1,3-cyclohexadiene-carboxylic acid), all of which have a long-lasting effect in vivo but are not completely specific.

One action of tetanus toxin, a convulsant peptide, is to inhibit the presynaptic release of the inhibitory transmitters GABA and glycine. For example, when injected directly into the cerebellum, the toxin suppresses basket cell inhibition of cerebellar Purkinje cells but does not influence the postsynaptic inhibitory effect of GABA administered microelectrophoretically; this indicates that it has no effect on receptor sites.

Uptake pump inhibitors enhance and prolong the inhibitory action of GABA, but the physiological effects of the compounds so far investigated vary according to their action on other systems. GABA pump inhibitors include such GABA analogs as 2-hydroxy-2-chloroGABA and 4-methylGABA, as well as those agents with major effects on aromatic amine systems such as chlorpromazine, imipramine, and haloperidol.

One of the confusing aspects is that a GABA pump system exists for glia as well as synaptosomes. The two processes are not identical because they are affected by different inhibitors. β-Alanine, for example, inhibits glial uptake 200 times more powerfully than it does neuronal uptake. *cis*-3-Aminocyclohexanecarboxylic acid is the most specific neuronal uptake inhibitor so far identified.

Picrotoxin and bicuculline are potent blockers of GABA whether it is endogenously released from synaptic terminals or applied iontophoretically. Accordingly, these two agents are regarded as classic GABA antagonists. Both produce convulsions. Bicuculline has a mild anticholinesterase action but nevertheless is regarded as being highly specific.

Strychnine, another convulsant, blocks glycine inhibitory receptors but not GABA receptors. Thus, strychnine and bicuculline are an important combination for the study of inhibitory mechanisms. Strychnine-sensitive, bicuculline-insensitive inhibitory synapses are usually glycinergic, whereas strychnine-insensitive, bicuculline-sensitive ones are GABAnergic.

Muscimol, a psychotomimetic isoxazole isolated from the mushroom *Amanita muscaria,* is a potent agonist of the bicuculline-sensitive, strychnine-insensitive receptors of spinal cord characteristic of GABA inhibitory sites. The reason for its seemingly unrelated psychotomimetic pharmacological action is unknown. Binding of labeled muscimol has been employed as a method for mapping GABA receptor sites [10, 11]. Several other compounds, including two aminocyclopentanecarboxylic acids and homotaurine, have been shown through screening procedures to have actions similar to those of GABA at receptor sites. Imidazoleacetic acid, a naturally occurring metabolite of histamine, acts like GABA on the stretch-receptor neuron of the crayfish, and inhibits GABA "receptor binding." Pharmacologically, it resembles a minor tranquilizer with sedative, muscle-relaxing, and hypothermic properties. β-(*p*-Chlorophenyl)GABA, also termed *baclofen* (Lioresal), is a GABA derivative used clinically as a muscle relaxant, but the extent to which it is a GABA agonist is undetermined. It does not activate GABA receptors on cortical neurons and does not affect GABA transport. More recent evidence suggests it may act by inhibiting the release of excitatory amino acids. γ-Hydroxybutyric acid (γ-OH) is another GABA-like agent in clinical use as a basal anesthetic, or at lower doses, as a mild sedative. Whether it acts directly as an agonist or is converted to GABA in vivo remains undetermined.

Anatomical Distribution of GABA Pathways in Brain

The brain content of GABA is 200 to 1,000 times greater than that of such neurotransmitters as dopamine, noradrenaline, acetylcholine, and serotonin. It is widely distributed, as might be anticipated for a transmitter suspected of serving the inhibitory interneurons found in almost all areas of brain.

Table 12-2 lists neuronal systems currently considered to be GABA-containing, along with the techniques that have been used to establish their identity. It is based upon only partially adequate methodology and is obviously far from complete. One expects that there will be many additions, and possibly some deletions, in future years.

The most convincing evidence for specific GABA neurons comes from immunohistochemical studies of GAD. Figure 12-3 shows the localization of GAD in some typical areas, including cerebellar Purkinje cells and other cerebellar cells at the light level, and substantia nigra and spinal interneuron terminals at the electron microscope level. However, in none of the systems described in Table 12-2 did immunohistochemistry provide the first significant evidence. Inhibitory activity of specific neurons and of GABA itself applied iontophoretically near their terminals, the effects of lesions on GABA and GAD levels, and the uptake

Table 12-2. Some Proposed Neuronal Pathways Involving GABA

Pathway	Evidence*
Purkinje cells	Inhibitory action, pharmacological, release, lesions, axoplasmic flow, immunohistochemistry
Cerebellar Golgi, stellate and basket cells	Uptake, inhibitory action, immunohistochemistry
Hippocampal basket cells	Uptake, inhibitory action, lesions, immunohistochemistry[a]
Nigrotectal/thalamic	Lesions[d], inhibitory action[e]
Pallidonigral	Uptake, lesions, axoplasmic flow, release[f]
Pallidothalamic	Lesions[g]
Pallidohabenular	Lesions[h], inhibitory action[h]
Striatopallidal	Inhibitory action[b], lesions[i]
Accumbopallidal	Lesions[j]
Accumbens to supraoptic n.	Lesions[u]
Neostriatal interneurons	Uptake, lesions
Spinal cord interneurons	Uptake, inhibitory action, localization, immunohistochemistry[a]
Cochlear interneurons	Lesions[k]
Cortical interneurons	Lesions[l], uptake, inhibitory action
Olfactory bulb interneurons	Immunohistochemistry[m], inhibitory action, uptake[n]
N. accumbens interneurons	Lesions[o]
Retinal amacrine and/or horizontal cells	Uptake, localization[p], immunohistochemistry[q]
Amygdala to bed nucleus of stria terminalis	Lesions[r]
Amygdala interneurons	Lesions[r]
Raphe interneurons	Lesions[s,t], uptake[t]

*Where no reference is given, the literature is cited and discussed in McGeer et al. [24], pages 204–214. The term *lesions* used here generally refers to changes in GAD activity after selection lesions.
[a]C. E. Ribak et al., *Brain Res.* 140:315, 1978; [b]K. Obata and M. Yoshida, *Brain Res.* 64:455, 1973; [c]J. A. M. van der Heyden, *J. Neurochem.* 32:469, 1979; [d]S. R. Vincent et al., *Brain Res.* 151:159, 1978; [e]J. M. Deniau et al., *Exp. Brain Res.* 32:409, 1978; [f]Y. Kondo and K. Iwatsubo, *Brain Res.* 154:395, 1978; [g]J. B. Penney, Jr. and A. B. Young, *Brain Res.* 207:195, 1981; [h]Z. Gottesfeld and D. M. Jacobowitz, *Brain Res.* 152:609, 1978. D. L. Jones and G. J. Mogansen, *Brain Res.* 188:93, 1980; [i]F. Fonnum et al., *Brain Res.* 143:125, 1978; [j]A. Dray and N. R. Oakley, *Experientia* 34:68, 1978; [k]R. J. Wenthold, *Brain Res.* 162:338, 1979; [l]M. V. Johnston and J. T. Coyle, *Brain Res.* 170:133, 1979; G. G. S. Collins, *Brain Res.* 171:552, 1979; [m]R. P. Barber et al., *Brain Res.* 141:35, 1978; C. E. Ribak et al., *Brain Res.* 126:1, 1977; [o]I. Walaas and F. Fonnum, *Neuroscience* 4:209, 1979; [p]S. J. Berger et al., *J. Neurochem.* 28: 159, 1977; [q]D. M. K. Lam et al., *Nature* 278:565, 1979; [r]G. Le Gal La Salle et al., *Brain Res.* 155:397, 1978; [s]E. G. McGeer et al., *Brain Res.* 168:375, 1979; [t]M. F. Belin et al., *Brain Res.* 170:279, 1979; [u]D. K. Mayer et al., *Brain Res.* 200:165, 1980.

of labeled GABA followed by autoradiography have been of great initial importance. Where a number of techniques agree—as in the case of Purkinje cells and cerebellar basket cells—the assignment seems reasonably certain. In many cases, however, where GABA is proposed as the neurotransmitter on the basis of only lesion or uptake studies or both (Table 12-2), the assignment must be regarded as highly tentative.

GLYCINE

Glycine is the simplest of the amino acids in structure and is involved in a multitude of metabolic pathways. As a consequence, it was not seriously considered as a neurotransmitter candidate at the time its inhibitory neurophysiological properties were first noted by Purpura and coworkers [14] and Curtis and coworkers [15], who considered it only a weakly active agent. However, a study of its distribution in spinal cord by Aprison and Werman [16] showed that glycine had the predicted distribution of the postsynaptic inhibitory transmitter. This study was quickly followed by one which showed that after temporary aortic occlusion there was a significant loss of glycine and aspartate, but not of GABA or glutamate, in the gray matter of the spinal cord. Moreover, the loss of glycine and aspartate correlated with the amount of interneuronal disruption seen in histological sections [17].

A rigorous neurophysiological comparison showed that glycine iontophoresed onto motor neurons duplicated the action of the inhibitory transmitter released on stimulation of these spinal interneurons [18].

Further confirmatory chemical evidence came when it was shown that there was a high-affinity uptake system for glycine in slices and homogenates of cat or rat spinal cord [19] and that glycine was preferentially localized to synaptosomes on subcellular fractionation studies. On the basis of these findings in spinal cord, it can be said that glycine is a proven neurotransmitter.

Chemistry of Glycine

In mammals, glycine is a nonessential amino acid that makes up 1 to 5 percent of typical dietary proteins. It crosses the blood-brain barrier with ease and thus may be transported to brain and spinal cord from blood. It is incorporated into peptides, proteins, nucleotides, and nucleic acids; and its fragments participate in other metabolic sequences. It can be synthesized from glucose and other substrates. Thus, it is one of the more versatile compounds in brain.

The immediate precursor of glycine is serine. Studies using radioactive precursors suggest that some of the glycine in brain is derived from de novo synthesis from glucose through serine (Fig. 12-4) and not from transport. The enzyme serine hydroxymethyltransferase (SHMT) is responsible for converting serine to glycine. It requires tetrahydrofolic acid, pyridoxal phosphate, and manganese ions, and is strongly inhibited by such antipyridoxal compounds as aminooxyacetic acid. Unfortunately, the activity of SHMT cannot be used as an index of the presence of glycinergic neurons. The rate of formation from serine appears constant from area to area, and there is no distinct correlation with the presumed presence of glycinergic cell bodies or nerve endings.

The metabolic disposal of glycine is unclear. It has been shown in vitro that glycine can be converted to glutathione, guanidinoacetic acid, glyoxylate, or even back to serine through a cleavage mechanism (Fig. 12-4). Again, however, there is no correspondence between the activity of this cleavage system or other disposal mechanisms and the probable occurrence of glycine neurons.

Sodium-dependent synaptosomal uptake of radioactive glycine has been demonstrated in spinal cord and certain areas of brain (Fig. 12-5). It is easily distinguished from the low-affinity uptake system, which is shared by other small amino acids, is present in all CNS areas, and presumably is concerned with other aspects of glycine metabolism.

Glycine and strychnine bind to synaptosomal membrane fragments by a high-affinity Na^+-independent system characteristic of specific receptor sites. The parallelism between regional strychnine-^3H binding and glycine uptake (Fig. 12-5) and the correlation between the neurophysiological actions of glycinelike amino acids and their ability to inhibit strychnine-^3H binding have been

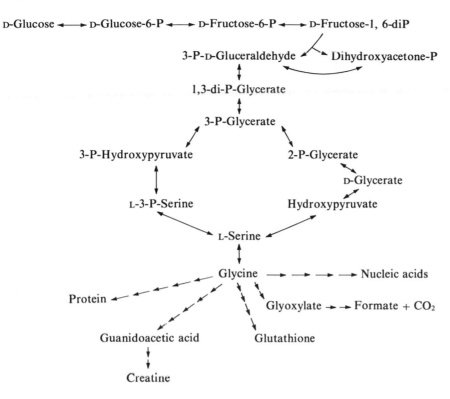

Fig. 12-4. *Probable synthetic pathway and possible metabolic routes for glycine in nervous tissue.*

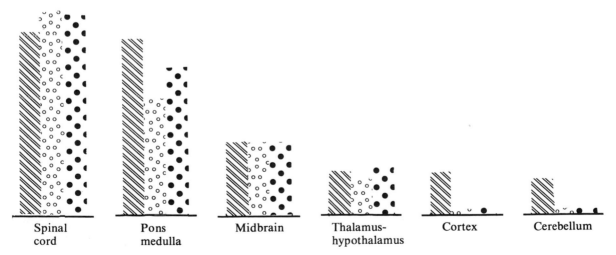

Fig. 12-5. *Glycine levels (\\\\\\ ), glycine uptake (○ ○ ○ ○ ○ ○) and strychnine binding (• • •) in various regions of rat brain relative to values in midbrain.*

taken to mean that specific strychnine-^3H binding involves synaptic receptor sites for glycine [20].

Obviously, much still remains to be discovered about the chemical reactions important for glycine synthesis and disposal, the control of glycine levels, and the chemistry of the glycinergic receptor.

Physiology and Pharmacology of Glycine

Glycine fulfills the physiological criteria expected of the transmitter released by inhibitory interneurons in the spinal cord. Its iontophoretic action duplicates the effects of synaptic activation. It hyperpolarizes the membrane, brings about a large fall in membrane resistance, and increases Cl⁻ permeability. Although these actions are also produced by GABA, glycine is blocked by strychnine, and GABA by bicuculline. The action of spinal inhibitory interneurons is prevented by strychnine, but not by bicuculline, confirming that glycine is the true transmitter [18].

There are several other substances besides strychnine that block the action of glycine, but not of GABA, on spinal neurons. Examples are brucine, thebaine, and 4-phenyl-4-formyl-N-methylpiperidine.

Anatomical Distribution of Glycine

As a dietary amino acid, glycine is found in all tissues. The discovery of unusually high levels in the spinal cord was fundamental in indicating a neurotransmitter role. Similarly, high glycine levels and specific uptake in particular regions of the retina suggested a similar function in some retinal interplexiform and amacrine cells [21]. The demonstration in retina of K⁺-stimulated, Ca²⁺-dependent release of glycine, and of lesion-induced decreases in synaptosomal glycine uptake provide supporting evidence [22]. Regional distribution data suggest the presence of glycine nerve endings in the pons, medulla, midbrain, and possibly the diencephalon (Fig. 12-5). There have been suggestions that glycine may be a transmitter in the corticohypothalamic projection and for some inhibitory fibers that descend in the cord, particularly from the medullary reticular formation. Further exploration is clearly needed.

GLUTAMATE AND ASPARTATE

Although the transmitter is unknown for the vast majority of excitatory cells in the CNS, glutamate and aspartate are extremely promising candidates. Glutamate has been recognized for some time as the probable neurotransmitter in certain invertebrate synapses, such as the crayfish neuromuscular junction [28]. These two amino acids are present in high concentration in brain tissue and possess many of the requisite physiological and chemical properties for neurotransmitters. They can thus be described as putative neurotransmitters, although they obviously have other roles in the CNS. For example, glutamate is incorporated into proteins and peptides, is involved in fatty acid synthesis, contributes (along with glutamine) to the regulation of ammonia levels and the control of osmotic or anionic balance, serves as precursor for GABA and for various Krebs cycle intermediates, and is a constituent of at least two important cofactors (glutathione and folic acid). It is not surprising that it should be the most plentiful amino acid in the adult CNS, having a concentration 3 to 4 times as high as taurine, glutamine, or aspartate, the three amino acids that are next most abundant (Table 12-3).

Two lines of biochemical evidence have proven critical in separating out neurotransmitter glutamate and aspartate from that portion concerned with other metabolic functions. The first was the demonstrations of a high-affinity uptake [23] and K⁺-induced, Ca²⁺-dependent release. The second was the demonstration of decreases in both uptake

Table 12-3. Content of Some Amino Acids in Whole Rat Brain (in μmol/g wet wt)

Glutamate	13.6 ± 0.4
Taurine	4.8 ± 0.3
Glutamine	4.4 ± 0.2
Aspartate	3.7 ± 0.2
GABA	2.3 ± 0.1
Glycine	1.7 ± 0.1
Serine	1.4 ± 0.1
Alanine	1.1 ± 0.1
Lysine	0.4 ± 0.0

and release following lesions to specific neuronal tracts (Table 12-4).

Chemistry of Glutamate and Aspartate

Both glutamic and aspartic acids are nonessential amino acids synthesized from glucose and other precursors by means of the tricarboxylic acid cycle (Fig. 12-6).

There are other possible sources. As we have already noted, glial cells have a very active enzyme (glutamine synthetase) for converting glutamate into glutamine (Eq. 12-1). The glutamine formed by this process can be transferred to neurons and reconverted in neurons or glia to glutamate by the enzyme glutaminase (Eq. 12-2).

This may be a significant source of glutamate in glutamate neurons, just as it appears to be a major source of glutamate in GABA nerve endings (see Fig. 12-2). Unfortunately, lesion experiments have so far failed to demonstrate localization of glutaminase in presumed glutamate tracts in either the hippocampus or striatum [25].

Aspartate is apparently synthesized by the transamination route, with glutamate as an indirect precursor.

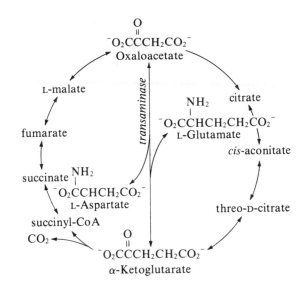

Fig. 12-6. Intermediates of the Krebs cycle, showing the formation of L-glutamate and L-aspartate by transamination reactions.

It is not known if there are specific metabolic routes for neuronally released aspartate and glutamate. Much of the aspartate and glutamate released is apparently taken back into the nerve endings, for

$$\underset{\substack{| \\ \text{glutamate}}}{\overset{NH_2}{HOOCCH_2CH_2CHCOOH}} + NH_3 + ATP \xrightarrow[\text{synthetase}]{\text{glutamine}} \underset{\substack{| \\ NH_2 \\ \text{glutamine}}}{H_2NOCCH_2CH_2CHCOOH} + ADP + P_i \qquad (12\text{-}1)$$

$$\underset{\substack{| \\ NH_2 \\ \text{glutamine}}}{H_2NOCCH_2CH_2CHCOOH} + H_2O \xrightarrow{\text{glutaminase}} \underset{\substack{| \\ NH_2 \\ \text{glutamate}}}{HOOCCH_2CH_2CHCOOH} + NH_3 \qquad (12\text{-}2)$$

high-affinity synaptosomal uptake has been demonstrated. Uptake also occurs into glial cells. No pharmacological method has been found to distinguish between the uptake systems of glial and synaptosomal transport. As in the case of GABA, Na^+-dependent binding seems to be to presynaptic transport sites, while at least some of the Na^+-independent binding seems to be to postsynaptic receptors.

Physiology and Pharmacology of Glutamate and Aspartate

Important evidence that L-glutamate and L-aspartate are neurotransmitters comes from their iontophoretic actions. Both these dicarboxylic amino acids powerfully excite virtually all neurons with which they come in contact. The characteristics of glutamate excitation are its extraordinary sensitivity (under optimal conditions cells can be excited with as little as 10^{-15} mole), its instantaneous onset, and the rapid termination of its action. This is accompanied by a marked fall in membrane resistance and an increase in sodium and other ion permeability comparable to that observed when acetylcholine is applied near the muscle end-plate [24]. The action is not prevented by tetrodotoxin, so it cannot be mediated by the sodium channels responsible for the propagation of the action potential and must represent specific excitation of receptor sites. In most respects, L-aspartate has an iontophoretic action comparable to that of glutamate, although it is generally less potent.

There may be many excitatory transmitters discovered in the future, but according to our present understanding of brain mechanisms there need not be a large variety: glutamate and aspartate could suffice. Thus, they could be the "workhorses" of excitatory action, just as GABA and glycine appear to be the workhorses of inhibitory action.

The identification of either glutamate or aspartate as the transmitter of a specific pathway would be greatly facilitated by the discovery of specific antagonists of synaptic and amino acid-induced excitation. Of the antagonists so far suggested, D-α-aminoadipate, D-α-aminosuberate, 2-amino-5-phosphonovalerate, 2-amino-4-phosphonobutyrate, cis-2,3-piperidinedicarboxylate, γ-D-glutamyl-glycine, and diethyl glutarate are probably the most specific for excitatory amino acids vis-a-vis other neurotransmitters such as acetylcholine and substance P. The problem is complicated by the growing evidence that there are probably several different types of receptors at which glutamate and aspartate can act. Three have been distinguished, for example, at which N-methyl-D-aspartate (NMDA), quisqualate (QA) and kainate (KA) are selective agonists; the antagonists 2-amino-5-phosphonovalerate and D-α-aminoadipate appear to act preferentially at the NMDA receptor, diethyl glutarate at the QA receptor and γ-D-glutamyl-glycine at the KA receptor. Glutamate and aspartate as agonists, and cis-2,3-piperidinedicarboxylate as antagonist, seem to act at all three types of receptors but glutamate is more active than aspartate at the QA receptor (and probably at the KA receptor) while the converse is true at the NMDA receptor [27]. The structure of these agonists is given in Fig. 12-7.

Conflicting data exist on the relative agonist and antagonist actions of many of the compounds, perhaps because of the particular preparation and experimental conditions chosen.

An important feature of excitatory analogs of glutamate and aspartate is that they possess neurotoxic activity. Systemically administered L-glutamate or L-aspartate themselves, in addition to excitatory analogs, produces degeneration of cells in the retina and the hypothalamus in immature animals if given in high enough doses. Seizures may also occur, and the same result is produced in mature animals with intraventricular administration. Microinjections of excitatory amino acids into various brain areas produce an acute reaction that selectively destroys certain neurons in the area. These observations have both theoretical and practical applications since these amino acids serve as useful chemical lesioning agents. The order of toxicity generally parallels their excitatory potency, with kainic acid (KA) being the most active. Others include N-methyl-D-aspartate, ibotenate, and β-N-oxalyl-L-α, β-diaminopropionate (OLDP) [28]. OLDP is a potent neurotoxin which has been implicated in the etiology of human neurolathyrism caused by eating the seeds of Lathyrus satidus.

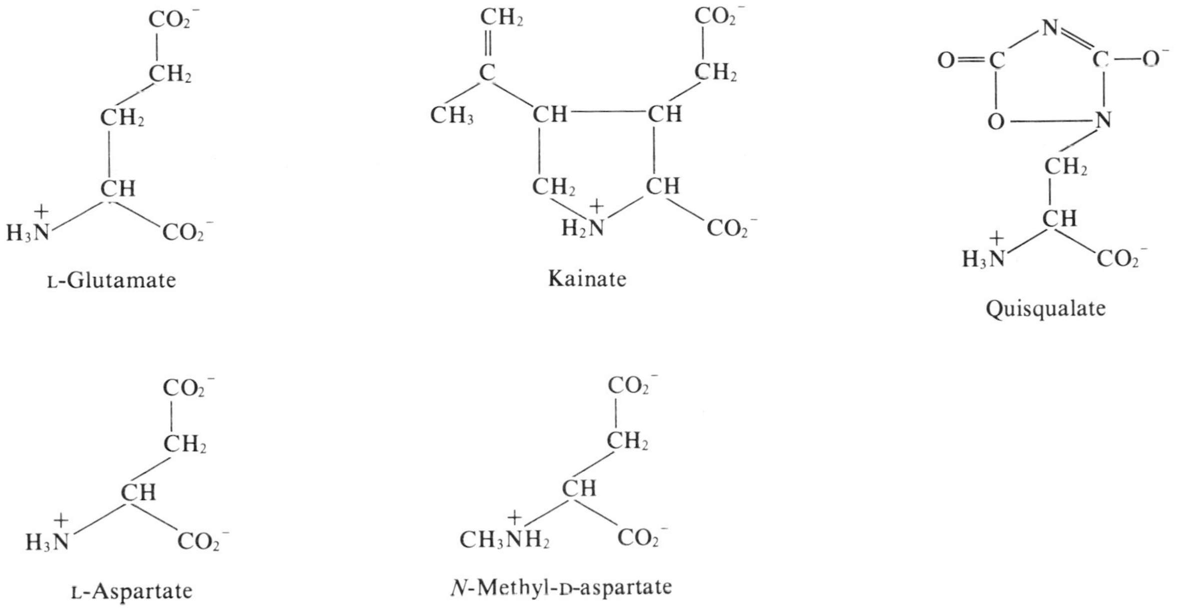

Fig. 12-7. Structural formulas for L-glutamate, kainate, quisqualate, L-aspartate, and N-methyl-D-aspartate.

Studies of the toxic effects also suggest a number of different kinds of receptors for the various amino acids. The toxicity of KA, for example, apparently depends largely upon an intact glutamate input to the affected neurons, whereas the toxicity of ibotenate and glutamate seem to be independent of such an input. It has been proposed, therefore, that glutamate and ibotenate may exert their neurotoxic effects by direct action at excitatory postsynaptic glutamate receptors; the action site of KA may be at some other, subsidiary or modulatory, receptor.

It might be anticipated from these data that high doses of glutamate and aspartate would be toxic in humans, but there are no firm data to support this supposition. No reports of neurotoxicity have appeared, but some individuals experience strange sensations after eating in Chinese restaurants. This "Chinese restaurant syndrome" involves the production of burning sensations, facial pressure, and chest pains in sensitive individuals. The effects are probably at least partially peripheral. Caution should be exercised with infants, however, where the blood-brain barrier might not be fully developed.

Anatomy of Glutamate and Aspartate

Some proposed pathways for glutamate and aspartate are listed in Table 12-4. They are highly tentative, of course, but they serve as a base upon which future data may be built. The most firmly based assignments for glutamate are the corticostriate, entorhinal-hippocampal, and cerebellar granule cells; and for aspartate, the hippocampal commissural path. It must be iterated that the present techniques for identifying glutamate and/or aspartate paths have major weaknesses. Physiological methods are technically difficult and suffer from lack of selective antagonists. Biochemical approaches involve measuring changes in release, uptake, or levels in a given area after various lesions. Release measurements have technical difficulties, uptake measurements do not distinguish between aspartate and glutamate, and levels tend to be an insensitive index of the neuronal pools (Fig. 12-8). The development of better biochemical or histochemical technique would represent a major advance.

OTHER AMINO ACIDS

A number of other amino acids occur in brain and possess some physiological activity. These include taurine, serine, proline, N-acetylaspartic acid, α- and β-alanine, and L-cysteinesulfinic acid. Of these, only the first four deserve further mention as possible neurotransmitters.

Taurine

A decade after the discovery of high concentrations of taurine in brain by Awapara [2] and Roberts [1], Curtis and Watkins [29] demonstrated that it had a strong inhibitory action on spinal neurons. Jasper and Koyama [30] added further interest by demonstrating its increased release from the cerebral

Table 12-4. Some Proposed Glutamate and/or Aspartate Pathways

Pathway	Evidence*
Corticostriate	Physiological, uptake, levels, release[a,b]
Perforant path	Uptake, release, levels, physiological*[c-e]
Hippocampal commissural	Uptake, release, levels, physiological*[d,f]
Hippocampal/subiculoseptal/mammillary	Levels, uptake[g,h]
Subiculum to accumbens	Uptake[i]
Cerebellar granule cells	Uptake, levels, release, localization, physiological*[j-m]
Primary auditory fibers to cochlear	Levels, release, physiological[o-q]
Lateral olfactory tract	Release, levels, uptake*[r,s]
Retinotectal	Uptake of radioactive*
Visual corticotectal	Uptake, levels*
Visual corticogeniculate	Uptake, levels*[t]
Cortical pyramidal layer 6 → layer 4	Uptake of radioactive[t]
Corticothalamic	Uptake,* levels[u]
Other corticofugal to red nucleus, basis pontis, and spinal cord	Uptake[u]
Retinal photoreceptors	Localization, physiological[v,w]
Stria medullary afferents to habenula	Uptake[x]
Primary afferent fibers	Uptake, levels[y]
Baroreceptor afferents	Uptake, physiological[z]

*Literature not cited here may be found in McGeer et al. [28], pages 184–190. Uptake and levels refer here generally to changes in uptake or levels following lesions.
[a]Kim et al., *Brain Res.* 132:370, 1977. [b]Reubi et al., *Brain Res.* 176:185, 1979; Godukhin, *Fiziol. Zh. SSSR* 65:1544, 1979. [c]Hamberger et al., *Brain Res.* 168:513, 1979. [d]White et al., *Nature* 270:356, 1977, *Brain Res.* 164:177, 1979; Wheal and Miller, *Brain Res.* 182:145, 1980; Hicks and McLennan, *Can. J. Physiol. Pharmacol.* 57:973, 1979. [e]Lauro et al., *Brain Res.* 207:476, 1981. [f]Nitsch et al., *ASN* 3/80, p. 108; Nitsch and Okada, *J. Neurosci. Res.* 4:161, 1979. [g]Nitsch et al., *Neurosci. Lett.* 11:295, 1979; Walaas and Fonnum, *Neuroscience* 5:1691, 1980. [h]Storm-Mathisen and Woxen Opsahl, *Neurosci. Lett.* 11:295, 1978; Zaczek et al., *Exp. Neurol.* 65:145, 1979. [i]Walaas and Fonnum, *Neuroscience* 4:209, 1979. [j]Tran and Snyder, *Brain Res.* 167:345, 1979; Rohde et al., *J. Neurochem.* 32:1431, 1979; Campbell and Shank, *Brain Res.* 153:618, 1978. [k]Roffler-Tarlov and Sidman, *Brain Res.* 142:269, 1978. [l]Sandoval and Cotman, *Neuroscience* 3:199, 1978. [m]Mikoshiba and Changeux, *Brain Res.* 142:487, 1978. [n]Stone, *Br. J. Pharmacol.* 66:291, 1979; Messer, *Adv. Cell Neurobiol.* 1:179, 1980. [o]Wenthold and Gulley, *Brain Res.* 158:295, 1978; Wenthold, *Brain Res.* 143:544, 1978. [p]Wenthold, *Brain Res.* 162:338, 1979; Canzek and Reubi, *Exp. Brain Res.* 38:437, 1980. [q]Martin and Adams, *Neuroscience* 4:1097, 1979. [r]Matsui and Yamamoto, *J. Neurochem.* 24:245, 1975; Yamamoto and Matsui, *J. Neurochem.* 26:487, 1976; Bradford and Richards, *Brain Res.* 105:168, 1976; White et al., *Nature* 270:356, 1977. [s]Collins, *J. Physiol. Lond.* 291:51, 1979; *Brain Res.* 171:552, 1979; Collins and Probett, *Brain Res.* 209:231, 1981. [t]Baughman and Gilbert, *Nature* 287:848, 1980. [u]Young et al., *J. Neurosci.* 3:241, 1981. [v]Voaden et al., *Neurochem. Int.* 1:151, 1980. [w]Slaughter and Miller, *Science* 211:182, 1981. [x]Gottesfeld and Jacobowitz, *Brain Res.* 152:609, 1978. [y]Roberts and Hill, *J. Neurochem.* 31:1549, 1978. [z]Talman et al., *Science* 209:213, 1980.

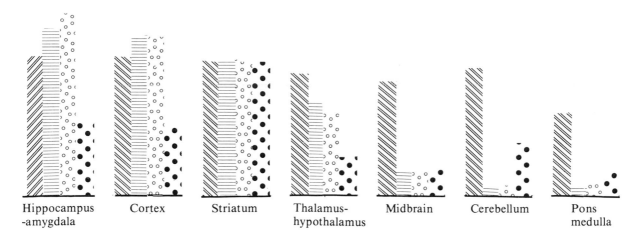

Hippocampus   Cortex   Striatum   Thalamus-   Midbrain   Cerebellum   Pons
-amygdala   hypothalamus   medulla

Fig. 12-8. Glutamate levels (//////), glutamate uptake (═══), aspartate uptake (°₀°₀°₀°) and kainate binding (● ● ●) in various regions of rat brain as percent of values in striatum. Note very close parallelism between aspartate and glutamate uptakes and the relatively slight regional variation in glutamate levels.

cortex of cats during arousal. Since these initial reports, there has been a continuing controversy as to whether taurine might play a neurotransmitter role in brain. An alternative hypothesis suggests that taurine is a generalized stabilizer of membrane excitability.

Taurine is believed to be formed in brain by a route starting from cysteine. This is converted to cysteinesulfinic acid, hypotaurine, and finally taurine. The key enzyme is believed to be the decarboxylase that converts cysteinesulfinic acid to hypotaurine. Some taurine may also be taken up from the periphery, particularly in newborn animals. Alternative routes through cysteic acid or cysteamine are generally considered less probable.

Taurine is mostly excreted unchanged, or conjugated with bile acids. Turnover of total brain taurine is far slower than for any of the established neurotransmitters (9–16 hr for fast decay, and 40–238 hr for slow decay). In view of this, as well as the postnatal decrease in total taurine levels and the rather even regional distribution of taurine, it is generally accepted that much of the taurine in brain is present in nonneurotransmitter pools. This

is also true, however, of established or putative amino acid neurotransmitters, such as glycine, glutamate, and aspartate.

Although the regional distribution of taurine is rather even, higher than average levels are found in the pituitary and pineal glands, the retina, cerebellum, olfactory bulb, and striatum. Particular taurine systems proposed, therefore, include cerebellar stellate cells, retinotectal neurons, and interneurons of the retina, olfactory bulb, and striatum. In no case is the evidence of a neurotransmitter role completely convincing.

Positive evidence cited in favor of a neurotransmitter role for taurine are its physiological activity; the existence of a high-affinity uptake system; release of taurine from brain slices or retina on electrical stimulation, and from the retina by light; and apparent synaptosomal localization of cysteinesulfinic acid decarboxylase (CSAD) activity [31].

All are controversial. Thus, antagonistic studies with strychnine and bicuculline have suggested that taurine may be acting in various regions at glycine or GABA receptors, and the high-affinity uptake system into synaptosomes has been reported to be of low efficacy, and easily confused with that into glia. Although K^+-stimulated release of taurine in the neostriatum and olfactory bulb has been reported by some authors, others were unable to demonstrate such release from the retina, striatum, cerebellum, or various other areas under conditions in which GABA or glycine release was easily shown. Finally, work on CSAD is suspect because purified GAD has been reported to accept cysteinesulfinic acid as a substrate, and regional distribution and lesion-induced changes in CSAD parallel those seen in GAD; hence the relatively low apparent CSAD activities measured in brain homogenates or fractions may be due to GAD.

Although a neurotransmitter role in the retina has not been proven for taurine, it seems to be clearly involved in maintaining the structural integrity, and a defect in taurine transport or storage, or both, may be related to retinitis pigmentosa, a degenerative disease in humans. An association of taurine deficiency with epilepsy has also been suggested, and a mild anticonvulsant activity of taurine has been reported in humans and in some, but not all, experimental models of epilepsy [31].

Serine

The chief interest in serine is that it is interconvertible with glycine in the CNS. It also has a weak glycinelike action in iontophoretic studies. Serine does not influence the high-affinity uptake system of glycine, and so far, it has been associated only with low-affinity uptake in brain tissue from adult animals. Thus, evidence for neurotransmitter action is very weak.

Proline

Although proline is present at relatively low concentrations in mammalian brain, very high concentrations have been reported in the nervous systems of both crabs and lobsters. Significantly higher concentrations occur in dorsal than in ventral roots in the spinal cord. It has a weak glycinelike action on cat spinal neurons and appears to be taken up into synaptosomes by a high-affinity sodium-dependent system. Some believe, however, that it may be taken up as a precursor for peptides such as TRH. Again, evidence for neurotransmitter action is weak.

N-Acetylaspartic Acid

N-Acetylaspartic acid is reported to have a distribution restricted to the brains of vertebrate species

and has a concentration about twice that of GABA (5–6 μmol/g). Some evidence of a regional disparity in concentration and of an association with synaptosomes has been reported as indicative of a possible neurotransmitter role. Little physiological information is available.

Summary

There is excellent evidence that four amino acids are the major ionotropic neurotransmitters in brain with GABA and, to a lesser extent, glycine being inhibitory and glutamate and aspartate excitatory. There is little convincing evidence that any other amino acid serves as a neurotransmitter in mammalian brain. GABAergic and glycinergic systems can be distinguished both chemically and physiologically, but good methods are not yet available for a clear distinction between aspartate and glutamate neurons. Both physiological and binding studies suggest that there are several different types of receptors for GABA [32, 33, 34] and for glutamate/aspartate [35]. Considerable attention is being given to defining the characteristics and functions of these various types of receptors and, particularly, that type of GABA receptor which is coupled with a benzodiazepine recognition site into a unit which allows interaction between GABA and the benzodiazepines [33, 34, 36, 37].

References

1. Roberts, E., and Frankel, S. γ-Aminobutyric acid in brain: Its formation from glutamic acid. *J. Biol. Chem.* 187:55–63, 1950.
2. Awapara, J., et al.   Free γ-aminobutyric acid in brain. *J. Biol. Chem.* 187:35–39, 1950.
3. Bazemore, A. W., Elliott, K. A. C., and Florey, E. Isolation of factor I. *J. Neurochem.* 1:334–339, 1957.
4. Kuffler, S. W., and Edwards, C.   Mechanism of gamma-aminobutyric acid (GABA) and its relation to synaptic inhibition. *J. Neurophysiol.* 21:589–610, 1958.
5. Obata, K., and Takeda, K.   Release of GABA into the fourth ventricle induced by stimulation of the cat cerebellum. *J. Neurochem.* 16:1043–1047, 1969.
6. Fonnum, F., Storm-Mathisen, J., and Walberg, F. Glutamate decarboxylase in inhibitory neurons. A study of the enzyme in Purkinje cell axons and boutons in the cat. *Brain Res.* 20:259–275, 1970.

7. Saito, K., et al. Immunohistochemical localization of glutamate decarboxylase in rat cerebellum. *Proc. Natl. Acad. Sci. U.S.A.* 71:269–277, 1974.

8. Baxter, C. F. Some Recent Advances in Studies of GABA Metabolism and Compartmentation. In E. Roberts, T. N. Chase, and D. B. Tower (eds.), *GABA in Nervous System Function.* New York: Raven Press, 1976. Pp. 61–87.

9. Wu, J. Y. Purification, Characterization and Kinetic Studies of GAD and GABA-T from Mouse Brain. In E. Roberts, T. N. Chase, and D. B. Tower (eds.), *GABA in Nervous System Function.* New York: Raven Press, 1976. Pp. 7–60.

10. Lester, B. R., and Peck, E. J. Kinetic and pharmacologic characterization of gamma-aminobutyric acid receptive sites from mammalian brain. *Brain Res.* 161:79–97, 1979.

11. DeFeudis, F. V. Vertebrate GABA receptors. *Neurochem. Res.* 3:263–280, 1978.

12. Costa, E., and Guidotti, A. Molecular mechanisms in the receptor action of benzodiazepines. *Ann. Rev. Pharmacol. Toxicol.* 19:531–545, 1979.

13. Roberts, E., Chase, T. N., and Tower, D. B. (eds.). *GABA in Nervous System Function.* New York: Raven Press, 1976.

14. Purpura, D. P., et al. Structure-activity determinants of pharmacological effects of amino acids and related compounds on central synapses. *J. Neurochem.* 3:238–266, 1959.

15. Curtis, D. R., Phillis, J. W., and Watkins, J. C. Actions of amino acids on the isolated hemisected spinal cord of the toad. *Br. J. Pharmacol.* 16:262–283, 1961.

16. Aprison, M. H., and Werman, R. The distribution of glycine in cat spinal cord and roots. *Life Sci.* 4:2075–2083, 1965.

17. Davidoff, R. A., et al. Changes in amino acid concentrations associated with loss of spinal interneurons. *J. Neurochem.* 14:1025–1031, 1967.

18. Werman, R., Davidoff, R. A., and Aprison, M. H. Inhibitory effect of glycine in spinal neurons in the cat. *J. Neurophysiol.* 31:81–95, 1968.

19. Logan, W. J., and Snyder, S. H. Unique high affinity uptake systems for glycine, glutamic and aspartic acids in central nervous tissue of the rat. *Nature* 234:297–299, 1971.

20. Snyder, S. H. The glycine synaptic receptor in the mammalian central nervous system. *Br. J. Pharmacol.* 53:473–484, 1975.

21. Lam, D. M., et al. Retinal organization: Neurotransmitters as physiological probes. *Neurochem. Int.* 1:183–190, 1980.

22. Lund-Karlsen, R. The toxic effect of sodium glutamate and DL-α-aminoadipic acid on rat retina: Changes in high affinity uptake of putative transmitters. *J. Neurochem.* 31:1055–1061, 1978.

23. Wofsey, A. R., Kuhar, M. J., and Snyder, S. H. A unique synaptosomal fraction which accumulates glutamic and aspartic acids in brain tissue. *Proc. Natl. Acad. Sci. U.S.A.* 68:1102–1106, 1971.

24. McGeer, P. L., Eccles, J. C., and McGeer, E. G. (eds.). *Molecular Neurobiology of the Mammalian Brain.* New York: Plenum, 1978.

25. McGeer, E. G., and McGeer, P. L. Localization of glutaminase in the rat neostriatum. *J. Neurochem.* 32:1071–1075, 1979.

26. Johnston, G. A. R. Central nervous system receptors for glutamic acid. In L. J. Filer, Jr., et al. (eds.), *Glutamic Acid: Advances in Biochemistry and Physiology.* New York: Raven Press, 1979. Pp. 177–185.

27. Davies, J., et al. Antagonism of excitatory amino acid-induced synaptic excitation of spinal neurones by *cis*-2,3-piperidinedicarboxylate. *J. Neurochem.* 36:1305–1307, 1981.

28. McGeer, E. G., Olney, J. W., and McGeer, P. L. (eds.). *Kainic Acid as a Tool in Neurobiology.* New York: Raven Press, 1978.

29. Curtis, D. R., and Watkins, J. C. The excitation and depression of spinal neurons by structurally related amino acids. *J. Neurochem.* 6:117–141, 1960.

30. Jasper, H. H., and Koyama, I. Rate of release of amino acids from the cerebral cortex of the cat as affected by brain stem and thalamic stimulation. *Can. J. Physiol. Pharmacol.* 47:889–905, 1969.

31. Huxtable, R., and Barbeau, A. (eds.). *Taurine.* New York: Raven Press, 1976.

32. Guidotti et al. Biochemical evidence for two classes of GABA receptors in rat brain. *Brain Res.* 172:566–571, 1979.

33. Placheta, P., and Karobath, M. Regional distribution of Na$^+$-independent GABA and benzodiazepine binding sites in rat CNS. *Brain Res.* 178:580–583, 1979.

34. Simmonds, M. A. A site for the potentiation of GABA-mediated responses by benzodiazepines. *Nature* 284:558–560, 1980.

35. Sharif, N., and Roberts, P. J. L-Aspartate binding sites in rat cerebellum: A comparison of the binding of L-[^{3}H]aspartate and L-[^{3}H]glutamate to synaptic membranes. *Brain Res.* 211:293–303, 1981.

36. Massotti, M., Guidotti, A., and Costa, E. Characterization of benzodiazepine and γ-aminobutyric recognition sites and their endogenous modulators. *J. Neurosci.* 1:409–418, 1981.

37. Gavish, M., and Snyder, S. H. Benzodiazepine recognition sites on GABA receptors. *Nature* 287:651–652, 1980.

Eric J. Simon
Jacob M. Hiller

Chapter 13. Opioid Peptides and Opiate Receptors

Opium is one of the oldest medications known to man. Its efficacy in relieving pain and diarrhea has been known for thousands of years. Morphine was recognized during the nineteenth century to be the major alkaloid responsible for most of the beneficial effects of opium, as well as for its undesirable side effects, in particular the development of addiction upon chronic use.

This chapter discusses recent exciting developments in the neurochemical and neuropharmacological aspects of opiate research. The field has been moving so rapidly that this summary is, of necessity, incomplete. For a fuller discussion of aspects of this work, the reader is referred to a number of books and reviews [1–5]. There, the reader will also find a much more complete bibliography than it is possible to supply in this chapter. After a brief historical discussion of the discovery of the opiate receptor and the endogenous opioids, we deal in somewhat greater depth with both topics.

Historical Summary

The hypothesis that specific receptors for opiates exist in the central nervous system of animals and man arose from pharmacological studies of narcotic analgesics and from the large-scale efforts mounted in many industrial, governmental, and university laboratories to attempt synthesis of a nonaddictive analgesic. Many very useful compounds were synthesized, some of which are in clinical use, but synthesis of the perfect nonaddictive analgesic has not yet been achieved. However, a large body of information on the structural requirements for pharmacological action came out of this work. It was recognized that analgesic action and addiction liability are highly stereospecific,

that is, these activities are present in only one of the enantiomers of a racemic mixture. It was also shown that relatively small alterations in parts of the morphine molecule result in drastic changes in its pharmacology. Perhaps the most interesting and important such change is the substitution of the methyl on the tertiary amino group by an allyl or cyclopropylmethyl group that endows the resulting molecule with potent and specific antagonistic activity against many of the pharmacological actions of morphine and related opiates. Some of these antagonists (e.g., nalorphine, cyclazocine) retain some of their analgesic or "agonist" potency, whereas others (e.g., naloxone and naltrexone) become "pure" antagonists, devoid of detectable agonist activity.

The remarkable stereospecificity and structural constraints placed upon many of the actions of opiates was most easily explained by the existence of highly specific binding sites in the central nervous system to which narcotic analgesic drugs must attach to exert their effects. Binding to these sites, or "receptors" (in analogy to endocrine receptors), is presumed to trigger a series of chemical or physical reactions, or both, that result in the observed responses. Antagonists are thought to be analogs that can bind to the receptors with high affinity but are unable to trigger one or more of the subsequent events.

Though the receptor postulate has existed for several decades, the biochemical demonstration of its validity did not occur until 1973. Using modifications of a method for measuring stereospecific binding of opiates in brain homogenates developed by Goldstein and coworkers [6], Terenius at Uppsala, Sweden [7], Pert and Snyder at The Johns Hopkins University [8], and Simon and coworkers at New York University [9] simultaneously and independently reported the existence of stereospecific opiate binding that represented the major portion of total binding to animal brain homogenates. *Stereospecific binding* is defined as that portion of the bound, labeled opiate that is replaceable by excess of an unlabeled opiate but not by its inactive enantiomer. Typical stereospecific binding data are presented in Table 13-1. Evidence that these binding sites are likely to be the long-sought opiate receptors is summarized in the next section.

Once the existence of opiate receptors was firmly established, a phylogenetic survey showed that such receptors exist in the brains of all vertebrates from hagfish to man [10]. The question was then raised as to why vertebrates should be endowed with highly specific receptors for alkaloids produced by opium poppies, and why such receptors should have survived the eons of evolution. A physiological function that confers a selective advantage on the organism that possesses them seemed probable. Such a function required the existence of endogenous ligands, the binding of which was the real reason for the existence of the receptors. The possibility of an endogenous analgesic was also supported by the observation, known since 1969 [11, 12], that electrical stimulation of the central gray region of the brain could produce powerful analgesia, suggesting activation of an endogenous pain-modulating system.

Because none of the known neurotransmitters or hormones was active in bioassays specific for opiates or bound to opiate receptors with high affinity, the search for new endogenous substances with opioid activity began. First reports of the existence of such substances came simultaneously from John Hughes [13] in Hans Kosterlitz's laboratory in Aberdeen, Scotland, and Terenius and Wahlström [14] in Uppsala, Sweden. The presence of opioid activity in the pituitary gland was first reported by Goldstein and his group [15].

The identification of the first endogenous opioids was accomplished by Hughes and coworkers [16], who found that the opioid activity present in aqueous extracts of pig brain was due to two pentapeptides, Tyr-Gly-Gly-Phe-*Met* and Tyr-Gly-Gly-Phe-Leu, which the authors named *methionine* (*Met*) enkephalin and *leucine* (*Leu*) enkephalin, respectively (*enkephalin*, Greek, "in the head").

The finding of opioid activity in the pituitary and the observation by Hughes and coworkers that the Met-enkephalin sequence is present in the pituitary hormone, β-lipotropin (β-LPH), as residues 61–65, led to the discovery of three longer peptides with potent opioid activity, all representing sequences present in β-LPH [17–19]. These peptides, LPH_{61-76}, LPH_{61-91}, and LPH_{61-77}, were named α-, β-, and γ-*endorphin*, respectively, in accordance with a suggestion by the senior author of this chapter that the term *endorphin* (a contraction of endogenous and morphine) might be an appropriate and useful term for endogenous substances with opioid activity.

Table 13-1. Typical Results of Stereospecific Binding Assays by Filtration Procedure*

Drug	Concentration (M)	D (cpm)	L (cpm)	D-L (cpm)	pmole bound per mg protein
Etorphine	2.5×10^{-10}	4100	540	3560	0.09
	1.0×10^{-9}	7800	2000	5800	0.15
Naltrexone	1.0×10^{-9}	3013	560	2453	0.08
	2.5×10^{-9}	5360	1340	4020	0.17

*Membranes derived from rat brain P_2 fraction were preincubated with $10^{-6} M$ dextrorphan (D) or $10^{-6} M$ levorphanol (L) for 5 min. Samples were then incubated with [^{3}H]etorphine (20 Ci/mmol) or [^{3}H]naltrexone (15 Ci/mmol) for 15 min at 37°C. Samples were filtered through Whatman GF/B filters. Filters were washed twice with 4 ml cold TRIS buffer, pH 7.4, dried, and counted in a liquid scintillation spectrometer in a toluene-based scintillation cocktail.

Opiate Receptors

PROPERTIES AND DISTRIBUTION

During the years following their discovery, much work was done on the properties and distribution of the stereospecific opiate-binding sites, both to enhance our understanding of their function and to provide evidence as to whether they represent pharmacological opiate receptors.

The binding sites are found in the central nervous system and in the innervation of certain smooth-muscle systems (the isolated ileum of the guinea pig and the vas deferens of the mouse have served as extremely useful bioassays for opiates). They are tightly attached to cell membranes, and cell fractionation studies suggest that they exist predominantly in the synaptic region. Stereospecific binding is saturable and of high affinity (10^{-11} to $10^{-7} M$) for drugs that exhibit moderate to strong opiate activity. The pH optimum for binding occurs in the physiological range (pH 7–8).

Biochemical studies have indicated that opiate binding is highly sensitive to various proteolytic enzymes and to a large number of reagents capable of reacting with amino acids and functional groups present in proteins. Thus, opiate binding is inhibited by various sulfhydryl reagents, such as N-ethylmaleimide and iodoacetate. All these studies suggest that one or more proteins play an essential role in the specific binding of opiates. The evidence for other structural components is less conclusive. Binding is highly sensitive to some preparations of phospholipase A, but not to others, nor to phospholipases C and D. Phospholipids may have a role in holding the receptor in its proper conformation in the membrane lipid bilayer. No evidence for the presence of carbohydrates in the binding sites has yet been obtained.

Detailed studies of the distribution of opiate-binding sites within the CNS have been carried out in human autopsy material [20], monkeys [21], and other animals by dissecting and homogenizing brain and spinal cord regions and measuring binding of labeled opiates to the homogenates, as well as by autoradiography of brain and spinal-cord slices after injecting the animals with labeled opiates (mainly [³H]etorphine and [³H]diprenorphine). These studies can be summarized by saying that large differences in levels of binding sites exist between different regions of the CNS. The regions rich in opiate-binding sites are in the limbic system and in all of the areas that have been implicated in pathways of pain perception and modulation, including the substantia gelatinosa of the dorsal spinal cord, the nucleus raphe magnus, the medial thalamus, and the periaqueductal and periventricular gray regions.

The question of the presynaptic or postsynaptic location of opiate receptors has been attacked in a variety of approaches. In monkeys, after dorsal rhizotomy, a reduction in opiate binding in the dorsal horn of the spinal cord was observed. This indicates a presynaptic location for these receptors but does not exclude transsynaptic effects on opiate receptors localized on postsynaptic cord neurons. Other data supportive of a presynaptic localization of receptors comes from autoradiographic studies that demonstrate labeling of small, unmyelinated, visceral afferent fibers of the vagus and glossopharyngeal nerves. Stereospecific depression by opiates of potassium-evoked release of the peptide, substance P, from slices of rat trigeminal nucleus, adds further support to a presynaptic localization. The most direct evidence for presynaptic localization of opiate receptors comes from the finding of stereospecific opiate-binding sites in explant cultures of fetal mouse spinal cord with attached dorsal root ganglia and in simpler cultures of dorsal root ganglia. A high level of opiate receptors was found in the neuritic outgrowth from dorsal root ganglia, even when cultured in the absence of spinal cord. This demonstrated the presence of opiate receptors on nerve fibers destined to provide presynaptic afferent input into the spinal cord.

However, not all published data point to a presynaptic site for opiate binding. Thus, microiontophoretic studies demonstrating that morphine blocks stereospecifically the excitatory effect of glutamate strongly point to a postsynaptic site of opiate action. It could well be that opiate receptors are located both presynaptically and postsynaptically. Such a conclusion has recently been reached for dopamine receptors.

All of the properties, as well as the distribution of the stereospecific opiate binding sites, are consistent with the notion that they are the pharmacological opiate receptors. The best evidence in support of this hypothesis, and perhaps the only evidence that gives us the right to speak of "opiate receptors," is the excellent correlation observed in several laboratories between the pharmacological potency of a large number of opiates (differing in potency by several orders of magnitude) and their binding affinity to brain homogenates.

EVIDENCE FOR CONFORMATIONAL CHANGES IN OPIATE RECEPTORS

The interesting, and possibly important, observation has been made that opiate receptors can exist in at least two conformational states. An apparent discrepancy between results in Snyder's laboratory [8] and in Simon's laboratory [9] led to the realization that the presence of sodium ions during the binding assay permits distinction between agonists and antagonists. Whereas agonist binding is inhibited by sodium salts, the binding of antagonists is either unaffected or, in many instances, augmented by the presence of sodium. This remarkable discrimination by a small ion between closely related molecules (e.g., morphine and nalorphine, oxymorphone and naloxone) is highly specific. It is exhibited, though less effectively, by lithium, but by none of the other alkali metals. In fact, no other inorganic or organic cations have been found that exhibit this effect. A study of the mechanism of this sodium effect has produced evidence that sodium is an allosteric effector, the binding of which produces a conformational change in the receptor. The sodium conformer has a higher affinity for antagonists and a markedly reduced affinity for agonists than does the sodium-free conformer.

The best evidence for an alteration in receptor conformation by sodium ions came unexpectedly from a study of the kinetics of receptor inactivation by the sulfhydryl alkylating reagent, N-ethylmaleimide (NEM), by Simon and Groth [22]. When a membrane fraction from rat brain was incubated

with NEM for various periods and this was followed by inactivation or removal of unreacted NEM, there was a progressive decrease in the ability of the membranes to bind opiates stereospecifically. The rate of receptor inactivation followed pseudo first order kinetics consistent with the existence of one SH-group per receptor, essential for binding. Protection against inactivation was achieved by the addition of low concentrations of opiate agonists or antagonists during the preincubation with NEM; this suggests that the SH-group is located near the opiate-binding site of the receptor.

Considerable protection was observed (half-time of inactivation was increased to 30 min from 8 min) when inactivation by NEM was carried out in the presence of 100 mM NaCl. Since sodium salts were without effect on the alkylation of model SH-compounds, such as cysteine or glutathione, this suggested that the SH-groups were made less accessible to NEM by a conformational change in the receptor protein. The fact that this protection exhibited the same ion specificity (Na^+ protects; Li^+ protects partially; K^+, Rb^+, and Cs^+, not at all) and the same concentration-response to Na^+ as the differential changes in receptor-ligand affinities, indicates that the same conformational change is involved in the two events.

These studies illustrate that the opiate receptor can alter its shape. The physiological function of this plasticity is not yet clear. A role in the coupling of opiate binding to subsequent physical or chemical events has been suggested, as has a role for sodium ions and sodium channels in the action of opiates.

The simple model for the allosteric effect of sodium ions on opiate receptors shown in Fig. 13-1 encompasses the various changes in receptor properties discussed above. One additional property, the evidence for which is not discussed here, is positive cooperativity of opiate binding, which is the reason for representing the receptor as an oligomer.

Heterogeneity of Opiate Receptors

Receptors for various neurotransmitters usually exist in multiple forms. Thus, there are muscarinic

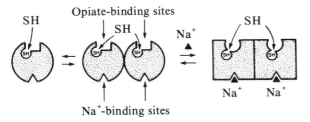

Fig. 13-1. Model for the allosteric effect of sodium ions on the conformation of the opiate receptor.

and nicotinic receptors for acetylcholine, at least two receptors for norepinephrine (α and β), and multiple receptors for dopamine and serotonin. It was therefore of interest to determine whether a similar heterogeneity exists for opiate receptors.

The earliest evidence came from experiments of Martin and coworkers [23] in chronic spinal dogs. Striking differences in pharmacological responses to different types of narcotic analgesics and their inability to substitute for each other in the suppression of withdrawal symptoms in addicted animals led to the postulate that at least three receptor types exist in the CNS of the dog. These were named for the prototype drugs that gave rise to the distinction: μ for morphine, κ for ketocyclazocine and σ for SKF 10047. The data are very convincing but suffer from the obvious drawback that the interpretations could be incorrect: in experiments involving the whole animal, differences ascribed to multiple receptors could occur elsewhere in the complicated sequence between drug binding and pharmacological response.

Kosterlitz's group has published results suggesting that the receptors present in the mouse vas deferens are different from those present in the guinea pig ileum. Evidence for heterogeneity of opiate receptors in guinea pig brain, based on binding studies, has been reported by this group [24]. These experiments show that opiate alkaloids, such as naloxone and morphine, are considerably more effective in displacing labeled alkaloids than are labeled enkephalins, whereas the enkephalins are more effective in displacing labeled enkephalins. These results could be explained either by differences in the way peptides and alkaloids bind to the same receptors or by the existence of different

receptor types. If there are indeed "enkephalin receptors" and "opiate receptors," one may well ask what the endogenous ligand is for the latter. It should be noted that binding is not exclusive: "opiate" receptors will bind enkephalins, albeit with tenfold lower affinity. The possibility is being explored that the opiate receptors may be preferential binding sites for β-endorphin because β-endorphin competes equally well for binding with enkephalins and opiates.

PROGRESS IN RECEPTOR SOLUBILIZATION AND PURIFICATION

We cannot conclude a discussion of opiate receptors in a book on neurochemistry without a brief discussion of attempts to isolate the receptor molecule.

Progress in solubilization and purification has been even slower for the opiate receptor than for some of the other neurotransmitter and hormone receptors. One of the major reasons for this is the extreme sensitivity of the receptor to detergents, including the nonionic variety. Binding of opiates is inhibited by very low concentrations of Triton X-100 and other, usually relatively harmless, detergents.

The most promising advance is the solubilization of an etorphine macromolecular complex that has properties suggesting that it may be an etorphine-receptor complex [25]. To date, the conditions have not been found under which binding of opiates can occur in solution. Moreover, the morphine-receptor complex is sufficiently unstable for its purification to be virtually impossible. A recent extension of this solubilization procedure by Zukin and Kream [26] may prove very useful. They showed that the identical procedure can be used for solubilization of an enkephalin-receptor complex. The solubilized complex was then covalently cross-linked by the use of dimethylsuberimidate. This covalent enkephalin-receptor complex may lend itself to purification and further study.

Endogenous Opioid Peptides

As we noted in the first section, the discovery of the opiate receptors was followed within about two years by the discovery of at least five endogenous peptides that possess opiatelike characteristics, including high affinity for the receptor. This lent a new dimension to research in the field by raising the possibility that this new receptor-ligand system, perhaps analogous to the known receptor-neurotransmitter systems, may provide information on hitherto obscure aspects of brain function and behavior. The most important task facing investigators is the demonstration of the physiological role of these opioid peptides and their receptors. Proof of such a role is always difficult; it has not yet been achieved.

Current evidence suggests that, of the five well-characterized opioid peptides, three are likely to have physiological functions, namely Met- and Leu-enkephalin and β-endorphin. α- and γ-endorphin may be breakdown products of β-endorphin or artifacts of its isolation [27]. The following discussion will therefore be restricted to the enkephalins and β-endorphin. For brevity, when speaking collectively of the endogenous opioid peptides, we shall frequently refer to them as the *endorphins*.

A number of approaches have been used to try to delineate the physiological role of the endorphins. These include (1) mapping of the distribution of the peptides in the CNS and determination of tissue levels and how these are affected by physiological and environmental changes; (2) administration of endorphins to animals and human subjects to study their pharmacological effects; and (3) study of the biosynthesis and metabolism of the endorphins. The results of these approaches will be summarized, and this will be followed by a statement of the current hypotheses regarding the action of endorphins and their possible implication in various physiological and pathological states.

DISTRIBUTION AND TISSUE LEVELS OF ENDORPHINS

This approach requires highly specific and sensitive methods for the identification and quantitation of endorphins. The earliest methods used were the radioreceptor assay and bioassays involving the use of the isolated guinea pig ileum and mouse vas deferens. The radioreceptor assay measures the amount of opioid activity in a tissue extract by the extent to which it can compete for receptor binding with radioactive opiates. This assay is quite sensitive but has the disadvantage of not distinguishing between the different opioid peptides. In fact, great caution must be exercised in the interpretation of data, because an observed decrease in labeled opiate binding could also be due to the presence of nonendorphin inhibitors or even to heat-resistant degradative enzymes.

The bioassays are very useful for demonstrating the presence of functional opioids. Both the ileum and the vas deferens can be made to contract by electrical stimulation, and these contractions are inhibited by low concentrations of opiates or opioid peptides; inhibitory efficacy is well correlated with analgesic potency. Specificity is confirmed by determination of the reversibility of the inhibition by opiate antagonists such as naloxone or naltrexone. The method has the disadvantage of having relatively low sensitivity, and like the binding assay, it cannot distinguish between different endorphins.

The most sensitive and specific assays are those that make use of highly specific antibodies generated against endorphin-protein conjugates in rabbits or other suitable animals. Radioimmunoassays (RIAs) have been developed for both enkephalins and for β-endorphin. They measure the amount of peptide present in a tissue or plasma extract by competition with radiolabeled peptide for binding to the antibody. RIAs that can detect femtomoles of a given peptide have been developed. Like all assays, this one too has its drawbacks. They involve mainly the problem of immunological cross-reaction. Thus, most antisera to Met-enkephalin cross-react with Leu-enkephalin but not with the longer-chain endorphins. The antisera to β-endorphin cross-react with β-lipotropin and the 31K precursor (see Biosynthesis and Metabolism). These peptides differ in size, so they can be separated by high-pressure liquid chromatography before the assay is carried out.

Finally, for mapping the distribution of the opioid peptides, the immunohistochemical techniques have proved extremely useful. These methods consist of treating freeze-dried slices of

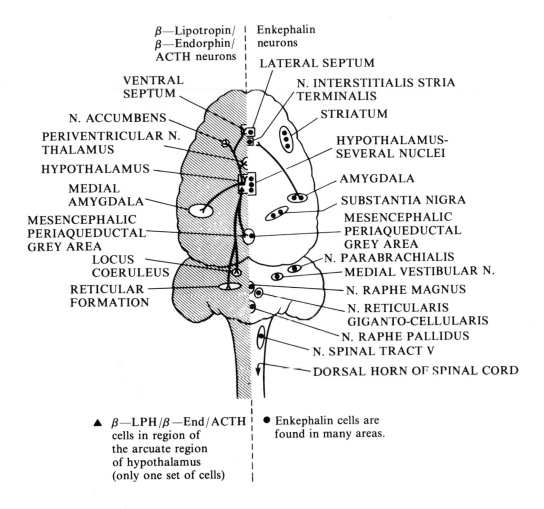

Fig. 13-2. Localization of the enkephalins and of β-endorphin in rat brain. (From Barchas et al., Science 200:964–973, 1978. Reprinted by permission, courtesy of A.A.A.S.)

tissue with antiserum to the peptide that is to be measured. The antigen-antibody complex is then visualized by the use of a second antibody (against the first) conjugated with a fluorescent marker or by the peroxidase-antiperoxidase (PAP) method of Sternberger.

Using both immunohistochemical techniques and RIAs, detailed mapping of opioid peptides in the CNS has been carried out in several laboratories [28–31]. The results are summarized schematically in Fig. 13-2.

The enkephalins are widely distributed throughout the brain and spinal cord. Their distribution closely mirrors that of the opiate receptors, with some exceptions, notably in the globus pallidus, which has the highest levels of enkephalin immunoreactivity but is relatively low in opiate receptors. Areas of high enkephalin concentration include the limbic system and the regions involved in the transmission and modulation of pain impulses, such as the central gray region, nucleus raphe magnus, nucleus reticularis gigantocellularis, nucleus caudalis of the spinal tract of the trigeminal nerve, and the substantia gelatinosa of the spinal cord. Neither rhizotomy nor spinal transsection causes depletion of the enkephalin content of the substania gelatinosa. This suggests that enkephalinergic terminals may be located primarily on interneurons rather than on long, ascending or descending pathways. No difference has yet been found between the distribution of the two enkephalins, but in all areas, the level of Leu-enkephalin is lower than that of Met-enkephalin. There is even some suspicion that the two pentapeptides may be located in the same cells. In addition to finding enkephalins in nerve terminal areas, special techniques (inhibition of axonal transport with colchicine) have permitted visualization of enkephalin-containing cell bodies. It is estimated that there may be twenty or more separate groups of enkephalin-containing cells.

The distribution of β-endorphin is quite different from that of the enkephalins, as depicted in Fig. 13-2. β-Endorphin is restricted to a single group of cell bodies in the arcuate nucleus of the basal hypothalamus and carried by processes emanating from this region to the midline areas near the ventricular surfaces. Thus, β-endorphin-containing nerve tracts are seen projecting from the basal hypothalamus forward through the preoptic area, around the anterior commisure and into the periaqueductal region of the diencephalon and pons. Midline structures containing β-endorphin include the anterior paraventricular nucleus, the dorsal raphe, and the locus coeruleus. The distinctive distribution patterns of enkephalins and β-endorphin in the CNS implies separate physiological roles for these peptides.

High concentrations of β-endorphin are found in the pituitary gland. In the rat pituitary, the highest concentrations of β-endorphin are found in the pars intermedia and pars distalis, with much lower levels in the pars nervosa.

In the gastrointestinal tract, one of the target areas of opiate action, the presence of enkephalins has been demonstrated. Immunoreactive fibers are found throughout the tract, with highest concentration in the stomach, duodenum, and rectum [32].

PHARMACOLOGY

Upon intracerebral or intraventricular injection, the opioid peptides exhibit the various activities characteristic of the opiate alkaloids. These include analgesia, hypothermia, respiratory depression, antidiuretic effects, changes in electroencephalogram patterns, and a variety of behavioral changes, including the induction of catatonia. The endorphins can substitute for morphine in the suppression of withdrawal symptoms in morphine-dependent animals. Chronic infusion of enkephalin or β-endorphin was found to produce tolerance and physical dependence. Cross-tolerance with morphine was demonstrated.

Analgesia produced by the enkephalins is very short-lived, whereas analgesia elicited by β-endorphin lasts for several hours. The short action of the enkephalins appears to be the result of their high sensitivity to degradation by peptidases. β-Endorphin is much more resistant, presumably due to its conformation, which appears to make its terminals less accessible to exopeptidases.

The well-known effects of narcotic analgesics on pituitary hormone release are also observed with the endorphins. For these responses, the peptides can be injected either intraventricularly or parenterally. Like morphine, they stimulate the release of growth hormone, prolactin, ACTH, and antidiuretic hormone and inhibit the release of luteinizing hormone, follicle-stimulating hormone, and thyrotropin. All these effects are reversible by naloxone. In fact, this is one of the few instances in which the administration of the antagonist to a naive animal produces effects. These are opposite to those seen when opiates or endorphins are administered. The mechanism of opioid effects on pituitary hormone secretion is not understood. However, the evidence points to an action at the level of the hypothalamus, rather than effects directly on the pituitary gland.

In organotypic cultures of fetal mouse spinal cord with attached dorsal root ganglia, it has been demonstrated that the sensory evoked electrical response of the synaptic network in the dorsal horn region of the cultures can be selectively depressed by exposure to low concentrations of enkephalins ($10^{-6}M$) and β-endorphin ($10^{-7}M$) in a naloxone-reversible manner [33].

When endorphins are applied iontophoretically and single-cell electrical activity is recorded in various regions of the CNS, inhibition is observed in most brain regions. The exceptions are the hippocampus and the Renshaw cells of the spinal cord, where endorphins and opiates produce excitation. However, at least in the case of the hippocampus, there is good evidence that the excitation results from disinhibition, that is, inhibitory effect of opioids on inhibitory nerve terminals. All these effects are reversible by naloxone, indicating that they are mediated through opiate receptors.

Observation of the short-lived effects of the enkephalins gave impetus to the search for analogs with greater stability and perhaps concomitantly increased potency. Numerous analogs of the enkephalins have been synthesized. The most significant finding was that substitution of D-alanine for the glycine in the 2-position resulted in both increased stability as well as increased potency and duration of action [34]. The increased stability is consistent with degradation of the natural enkephalins by an aminopeptidase, which possibility is further supported by the release of free tyrosine when enkephalins are incubated with tissue homogenates. Substitutions at position 5 further increase stability; this suggests that carboxypeptidases are also involved in enkephalin breakdown. A number of enkephalin analogs stable enough to exhibit potency after parenteral administration have been synthesized. Of particular interest is FK 33-824, synthesized at Sandoz, Ltd. (Tyr-D-Ala-Gly-MePhe-Met(O)-ol); this is a potent, long-acting analgesic that has been found to be effective even upon subcutaneous and oral administration. This compound is currently undergoing clinical trials.

BIOSYNTHESIS AND METABOLISM

Beta Endorphin
Knowledge of how the endorphins are synthesized, where they are stored, and when and how they are released and broken down is of considerable interest and should also help in elucidating the mode of action and function of these peptides.

The finding that β-LPH contains the sequences of β-endorphin and Met-enkephalin suggested that β-LPH may represent a prohormone precursor of these peptides, as well as of β-melanocyte-stimulating hormone (β-MSH), which sequence is also present in β-LPH as residues 37–58. The hydrolysis of β-LPH to β-endorphin and γ-endorphin by a trypsinlike enzyme has been observed.

The observation was made in Guillemin's laboratory that various types of stress led to the simultaneous and proportional secretion of ACTH and β-endorphin into the blood of rats [35]. Hypophysectomy abolished this response, indicating that both peptides are of pituitary origin. Cultured cells or fragments of neoplastic or hyperplastic (Nelson's disease) pituitary glands were also found to secrete ACTH and β-endorphin.

These observations, together with the knowledge that many polypeptide hormones are made through large precursor molecules, led Mains and Eipper [36] to search for a common precursor to ACTH and β-LPH. In a mouse pituitary cell line, AtT20, they found strong evidence that a glycoprotein of M_r 31,000 is such a precursor. They named this simply the *31K protein,* but the term *pro-opiocortin,* suggested by S. Udenfriend, is also used.

Recently, Nakanishi and coworkers [37] purified the messenger RNA that codes for the 31K polypeptide. In collaboration with S. N. Cohen's laboratory [38], they prepared the cDNA, cloned it in *E. coli,* and established the nucleotide sequence of the entire 1091-base cDNA molecule. The biosynthesis of pituitary β-endorphin, which already has been worked out in considerable detail, is discussed further in Chap. 14. Recently, evidence has been found [39] that a similar biosynthetic pathway exists in the hypothalamus. This is consonant with the previous observations by several laboratories that hypophysectomy has no effect on levels of brain enkephalins or β-endorphin.

The metabolism of β-endorphin is also under study. γ-Endorphin appears to be a breakdown product, and little Met-enkephalin seems to be formed. *N*-acetylated β-endorphin has been found, and this suggests that acetylation may be a way by which this peptide is inactivated.

Enkephalins
Our knowledge of enkephalin biosynthesis is in an embryonic state. However, some interesting

observations are being made. As mentioned earlier, the level of enkephalins in the CNS is unchanged even several months after hypophysectomy; this indicates that enkephalins are made somewhere in the brain and spinal cord, rather than imported from the pituitary.

Hughes and coworkers [40] have obtained evidence that enkephalins are synthesized through a large precursor. In studies of tyrosine-^3H incorporation into enkephalins in isolated preparations of guinea pig myenteric plexus and slices of guinea pig striatum, linear incorporation was observed after a lag period of 1 to 2 hours. Incorporation was blocked when such inhibitors of protein synthesis as cycloheximide or puromycin were added during the labeling period, but these agents had no effect when added after the lag period. This suggests the ribosomal synthesis of a polypeptide precursor during the lag period and subsequent proteolytic processing to form enkephalins. Several laboratories have isolated large molecules that give rise to tryptic peptides with opioid activity. These putative precursors appear to be different from any of the molecules involved in the biosynthesis of β-endorphin. This finding has led to the suggestion that enkephalins may be synthesized by a pathway quite different from the ACTH−β-LPH pathway that produces β-endorphin in the pituitary and in the hypothalamus. Evidence supporting this suggestion is now available (see below).

The origin of Leu-enkephalin has long puzzled investigators. Kangawa and coworkers in a very interesting paper that bears on the question [41] report the isolation of a 15-amino-acid peptide with potent opioid activity from the extracts of 30,000 pig hypothalami. Partial amino acid sequencing indicates that Leu-enkephalin represents the N-terminal portion, followed by three basic amino acids; this makes it a good candidate for a precursor of Leu-enkephalin. The peptide has been named *α-neoendorphin*. A peptide of 50,000 M_r, found in bovine adrenal medulla, contains sequences of both Met-enkephalin and Leu-enkephalin in a ratio of 7 copies to 1. This is similar to ratios of enkephalins found in tissues. This peptide may be a common precursor of both enkephalins in the same cells [42].

Two recent developments in enkephalin metabolism should be mentioned briefly. One is the important finding in several laboratories that high potassium evokes a calcium-dependent release of enkephalins from synaptosomal preparations of rabbit striatum and from slices of rat striatum and globus pallidus.

A second report of considerable interest came from Malfroy and coworkers [43] and has been confirmed by others; it suggests that there exists a membrane-bound carboxypeptidase, which appears to be a specific enkephalinase. This enzyme also appears to increase during development of morphine tolerance.

MODE OF ACTION OF ENDORPHINS

The enkephalins fulfill many of the criteria for a neurotransmitter function. They are located at nerve terminals, are readily degraded, and have been shown to be released by high K^+ concentration from brain slices and by electrical stimulation from the myenteric plexus of the guinea pig ileum [44]. The finding that both opiates and endorphins inhibit the release of various neurotransmitters, along with the demonstration that opiate receptors can have a presynaptic location, has given rise to the concept that the enkephalins and, perhaps, brain β-endorphin are neuromodulators, that is, the degree to which they are released modulates the release of classical neurotransmitters. A model that illustrates this idea is presented in Fig. 13-3. There is some evidence that, in the neurons which conduct nociceptive impulses in the spinal cord, the neurotransmitter involved may be the peptide substance P. Thus, the enkephalins may exert analgesic effects in the spinal cord by inhibiting the release of substance P.

The role of pituitary β-endorphin is even more obscure. Its release during stress argues for a function in stressful situations, but the real mode of action and the target on which it acts are unknown. The amount of β-endorphin released even under severe stress is well below the concentration that can produce analgesia. Moreover, retrograde transport of pituitary β-endorphin into the brain, though not ruled out, is held to be unlikely. The finding that β-endorphin secretion is increased by

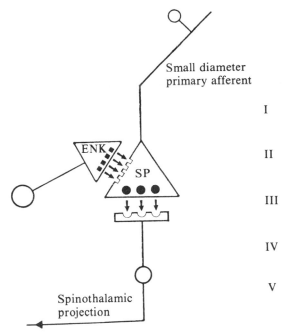

Fig. 13-3. Schematic representation of a possible mechanism for opiate-induced suppression of SP release. SP is shown localized within the terminal of a small-diameter afferent fiber, which forms an excitatory axodendritic synapse with the process of a spinal cord neuron originating in lamina IV or V and projecting rostrally. A local enkephalin-containing inhibitory interneuron (ENK), confined to laminae II and III, forms a presynaptic contact on the terminal of the primary afferent. Opiate receptor sites are depicted presynaptically. Roman numerals on the right refer to the laminae of Rexed. (From Jessel and Iversen, Nature 268:549–551, 1977. Reprinted by permission, courtesy of Macmillan Journals, Ltd.)

adrenalectomy and decreased by corticosteroids suggests that it may in some manner interact with ACTH in its effect on the adrenal cortex.

POSSIBLE ROLES OF CNS ENDORPHINS
The wide distribution of the enkephalins has convinced most investigators that their role may go well beyond that suggested by their opiatelike activities, that is, in pain modulation and the development of tolerance to and dependence on narcotics. Such a general role in brain functions involving mood, emotion, and behavior is further supported by the numerous side effects of the opiate alkaloids.

Many reports have already appeared, and similar ones continue to be published, concerning the involvement of the endorphin-opiate receptor system in a variety of physiological, behavioral, and pathological states. These studies have frequently been done by showing that a given phenomenon is affected by specific opiate antagonists, such as naloxone or naltrexone, or by the administration of endorphins or their analogs. In this manner, the endorphin system has been implicated in memory, overeating, sexual activity, and several mental diseases, including schizophrenia and manic-depressive psychosis. The direct demonstration of changes in endorphin levels or turnover is frequently still lacking.

Probably the best evidence for involvement of the endorphin-opiate receptor system exists for pain modulation. The opioid properties of the peptides and their presence in high concentrations in all brain regions known to be concerned with the conduction and modulation of pain impulses led very early to research activity in this area. Moreover, as mentioned earlier, the intracerebral injection of each known opioid peptide produces analgesia.

Attempts to show that the administration of naloxone lowers pain thresholds or exacerbates the intensity of pain have been surprisingly devoid of success in human volunteers, but a lowering of pain threshold has been found in rats [45].

Several types of analgesia that do not involve the use of drugs have been found to be reversible by naloxone. These include analgesia produced by electrical stimulation of the periaqueductal gray area and acupuncture, in animals as well as in humans. There is an intriguing report [46] that administration of naloxone to patients in pain reverses analgesia produced by placebo. In individuals not susceptible to the placebo effect, the antagonist had no effect.

Reports on the direct demonstration of changes in endorphin levels during pain or relief from pain are also beginning to appear. Terenius's group [2] reported a decrease in opioid activity in the spinal fluid of patients suffering chronic pain due to trigeminal neuralgia. They also reported an increase in level of opioid activity after analgesia by electroacupuncture in patients with intractable pain. These reports have the drawback that the altered opioid activity has not yet been characterized and seems to differ from the known endorphins.

Richardson [47] has reported good success in relieving intractable pain in patients by electrical stimulation with electrodes implanted in the periventricular gray region. The method has been found useful for pain relief through periodic self-stimulation by the patient over a period of months or even years. Akil and coworkers [48] have observed a modest but significant release of Met-enkephalin into the ventricular CSF of these patients 15 to 20 minutes after stimulation. They also found a large release of β-endorphin. Thus, an impressive array at least of circumstantial evidence points to involvement of enkephalins and probably also of brain β-endorphin in pain modulation.

Attempts to implicate the endorphin system in the development of tolerance and dependence have met with much less success. Studies of changes in either the opiate receptors or endorphin levels in chronically morphinized rats have proved largely negative. There is, of course, a strong conviction that the chronic effects of opiates must involve changes in the endorphin-opiate receptor system, but presently there is relatively little evidence to support this attractive notion. One report [49] indicates that the intravenous administration of 4 mg of β-endorphin to human addicts led to dramatic improvement in their severe abstinence syndrome. This relief lasted for several days. Suppression of abstinence symptoms by opiates lasts for only a period of hours; this result suggested to the authors that the endorphins may indeed have an important role in the development of tolerance to and dependence on opiate drugs.

The speculations concerning a possible role of endorphins in mental disease derive largely from the finding that the intracerebral injection of small amounts of β-endorphin causes catatonia in rats. Catatonia is an important component of certain types of schizophrenia. Virtually all of the research to date involves the treatment of schizophrenic patients with naloxone. The results from different laboratories have been contradictory. It certainly has no effect on the catatonic component, but some investigators have reported a decrease in auditory hallucination. The situation is both intriguing and controversial. The most optimistic statement that can be made at this time is that relatively large doses of naloxone may diminish auditory hallucinations in a subclass of schizophrenic patients. It is hoped that in a future edition of this book it will be possible to report significant progress in this important area.

Concluding Remarks

This hitherto unsuspected receptor-peptide system may rival or even surpass in importance such now-classical receptor-neurotransmitter systems as the cholinergic, catecholaminergic, and serotoninergic. However, it cannot be emphasized strongly enough that to date no physiological role has been clearly established for any of the endorphins. There is sufficient circumstantial evidence to permit the hypothesis that the CNS endorphins are neurotransmitters or modulators that may play important roles in pain modulation, opiate addiction, and various aspects of emotion and behavior. Claims that endorphins play a role in sexual activity, appetite, pleasure, and a variety of mental disorders are very exciting, but require substantiation. The role of pituitary β-endorphin and of opioid peptides found in other tissues, such as the intestinal tract and adrenal gland, is even more mysterious at the present time.

A great deal has been learned about the binding site of the opiate receptor by using crude membrane preparations. Much of what remains unknown about its structure and function awaits the isolation of a purified receptor molecule.

One of the many challenges facing scientists in this area is the elucidation of the transducing portion of the receptor and the post-binding events triggered by it that lead to the physiological and pharmacological effects. Reports have appeared suggesting the involvement of adenylate cyclase, and there is some evidence for a role of conformational changes in the receptor or the surrounding membrane. However, the sequellae of the binding of opiates and endorphins to their receptors remain "a black box," into which, we hope, some light will soon be shed.

Recently there has been progress in the solubilization of active opiate receptors. Success has been reported for receptors from toad brain [50], rat brain [51, 52] and neuroblastoma glioma cultures [51]. The properties of the solubilized receptors are similar to those bound to membranes.

New endogenous opioid peptides have also been isolated. One of these, dynorphin [53], has very potent opioid activity in a number of assays. It contains 15 to 17 amino acids, the sequence of which is not found in βLPH.

Acknowledgments

The research carried out in the authors' laboratory was supported by grant DA-00017 from the National Institute on Drug Abuse. We thank Dr. James King for critical reading and Irene Simon for proofreading of the manuscript.

References

*1. Simon, E. J., and Hiller, J. M.   The opiate receptors. *Annu. Rev. Pharmacol. Toxicol.* 18:371–394, 1978.

*2. Terenius, L.   Endogenous peptides and analgesia. *Annu. Rev. Pharmacol. Toxicol.* 18:189–204, 1978.

*3. Beaumont, A., and Hughes, J.   Biology of opioid peptides. *Annu. Rev. Pharmacol. Toxicol.* 19:245–267, 1979.

4. Miller, R. J., and Cuatrecasas, P.   Enkephalins and endorphins. *Vitamin. Horm.* 36:297–382, 1978.

*5. Herz, A. (ed.).   *Developments in Opiate Research. Modern Pharmacology-Toxicology,* vol. 14. New York and Basel: Dekker, 1978.

6. Goldstein, A., Lowney, L. I., and Pal, B. K.   Stereospecific and nonspecific interactions of the morphine congener levorphanol in subcellular fractions of mouse brain. *Proc. Natl. Acad. Sci. U.S.A.* 68:1742–1747, 1971.

7. Terenius, L.   Stereospecific interaction between narcotic analgesics and a synaptic plasma membrane fraction of rat cerebral cortex. *Acta Pharmacol. Toxicol.* (Copenhagen) 32:317–320, 1973.

*8. Pert, C. B., and Snyder, S. H.   Opiate receptor: Demonstration in nervous tissue. *Science* 179:1011–1014, 1973.

*9. Simon, E. J., Hiller, J. M., and Edelman, I.   Stereospecific binding of the potent narcotic analgesic [^{3}H]etorphine to rat brain homogenate. *Proc. Natl. Acad. Sci. U.S.A.* 70:1947–1949, 1973.

10. Pert, C. B., Aposhian, D., and Snyder, S. H.   Phylogenetic distribution of opiate receptor binding. *Brain Res.* 75:356–361, 1974.

11. Reynolds, D. V.   Surgery in the rat during electrical analgesia induced by focal brain stimulation. *Science* 164:444–445, 1969.

*12. Liebeskind, J. C., Mayer, D. J., and Akil, H.   Central Mechanisms of Pain Inhibition: Studies of Analgesia from Focal Brain Stimulation. In J. J. Bonica (ed.), *Advances in Neurology.* International Symposium on Pain. New York: Raven Press, 1974. Vol. 4, pp. 261–268.

13. Hughes, J.   Isolation of an endogenous compound from the brain with pharmacological properties similar to morphine. *Brain Res.* 88:295–308, 1975.

14. Terenius, L., and Wahlström, A.   Search for an endogenous ligand for the opiate receptor. *Acta Physiol. Scand.* 94:74–81, 1975.

15. Teschemacher, H., et al.   A peptidelike substance from pituitary that acts like morphine. I. Isolation. *Life Sci.* 16:1771–1776, 1975.

*16. Hughes, J., et al.   Identification of two related pentapeptides from the brain with potent opiate agonist activity. *Nature* 258:577–579, 1975.

17. Li, C. H., and Chung, D.   Isolation and structure of an untriakontapeptide with opiate activity from camel pituitary glands. *Proc. Natl. Acad. Sci. U.S.A.* 73:1145–1148, 1976.

18. Guillemin, R., Ling, N., and Burgus, R.   Endorphines, peptides, d'origine hypothalamique et neurohypophysaire à activité morphinomimetique. Isolement et structure moléculaire de l'endorphine. *C. R. Acad. Sci. [D]* (Paris) 282:783–785, 1976.

19. Bradbury, A. F., et al.   C fragment of lipoprotein has a high affinity for brain opiate receptors. *Nature* 260:793–795, 1976.

20. Hiller, J. M., Pearson, J., and Simon, E. J.   Distribution of stereospecific binding of the potent narcotic analgesic etorphine in the human brain: Predominance in the limbic system. *Res. Commun. Chem. Pathol. Pharmacol.* 6:1052–1062, 1973.

*21. Kuhar, M. J., Pert, C. B., and Snyder, S. H.   Regional distribution of opiate receptor binding in monkey and human brain. *Nature* 245:447–450, 1973.

22. Simon, E. J., and Groth, J.   Kinetics of opiate receptor inactivation by sulfhydryl reagents: Evidence for conformational change in presence of sodium ions. *Proc. Natl. Acad. Sci. U.S.A.* 72:2404–2407, 1975.

*Key reference.

23. Martin, W. R., et al.   The effects of morphine- and nalorphine-like drugs in the nondependent and morphine-dependent chronic spinal dog. *J. Pharmacol. Exp. Ther.* 197:517–532, 1976.

*24. Lord, J. A. H., et al.   Endogenous opioid peptides: Multiple agonists and receptors. *Nature* 267:495–499, 1977.

*25. Simon, E. J., Hiller, J. M., and Edelman, I.   Solubilization of a stereospecific opiate-macromolecular complex from rat brain. *Science* 190:389–390, 1975.

26. Zukin, R. S., and Kream, R. M.   Chemical cross-linking of a solubilized enkephalin macromolecular complex. *Proc. Natl. Acad. Sci. U.S.A.* 76:1593–1597, 1979.

27. Rossier, J., et al.   Radioimmunoassay of brain peptides. Evaluation of a methodology for the assay of β-endorphin and enkephalin. *Life Sci.* 21:847–852, 1977.

*28. Hokfelt, T., et al.   The distribution of enkephalin immunoreactive cell bodies in the rat central nervous system. *Neurosci. Lett.* 5:25–31, 1977.

29. Yang, H.-Y., Hong, H. S., and Costa, E.   Regional distribution of Leu and Met enkephalin in rat brain. *Neuropharmacology* 16:303–307, 1977.

*30. Watson, S. J., et al.   Immunocytochemical localization of methionine enkephalin: Preliminary observations. *Life Sci.* 21:733–738, 1977.

*31. Bloom, F., et al.   Neurons containing β-endorphin in rat brain exist separately from those containing enkephalin: Immunocytochemical studies. *Proc. Natl. Acad. Sci. U.S.A.* 75:1591–1595, 1978.

32. Polak, J. M., et al.   Enkephalin-like immunoreactivity in the human gastrointestinal tract. *Lancet* 1:972–974, 1977.

33. Crain, S. M., et al.   Selective depression by opioid peptides of sensory-evoked dorsal-horn network responses in organized spinal cord cultures. *Brain Res.* 157:196–201, 1978.

34. Pert, C. B., et al.   [D-Ala^2]-Met-enkephalinamide: A potent, long lasting synthetic pentapeptide analgesic. *Science* 194:330–332, 1976.

35. Guillemin, R., et al. β-Endorphin and adenocorticotropin are secreted concomitantly by the pituitary. *Science* 197:1367–1369, 1977.

36. Mains, R. E., Eipper, B. A., and Ling, N.   Common precursor to corticotropins and endorphins. *Proc. Natl. Acad. Sci. U.S.A.* 74:3014–3018, 1977.

37. Nakanishi, S., et al.   Construction of bacterial plasmids that contain the nucleotide sequence for bovine corticotropin–β-lipotropin precursor. *Proc. Natl. Acad. Sci. U.S.A.* 75:6021–6025, 1978.

38. Nakanishi, S., et al.   Nucleotide sequence of cloned cDNA for bovine corticotropin–β-lipoprotein precursor. *Nature* 278:423–427, 1979.

39. Liotta, A. S., et al.   Biosynthesis in vitro of immunoreactive 31,000 dalton corticotropin–β-endorphinlike material by bovine hypothalamus. *Proc. Natl. Acad. Sci. U.S.A.* 76:1448–1452, 1979.

40. Hughes, J., Kosterlitz, H. W., and McKnight, A. T.   The incorporation of [^{3}H]tyrosine into the enkephalins of striatal slices of guinea-pig brain. *Br. J. Pharmacol.* 63:396P, 1978.

41. Kangawa, K., Matsuo, H., and Igarashi, M. α-Neoendorphin: A "big" Leu-enkephalin with potent opiate activity from porcine hypothalami. *Biochem. Biophys. Res. Commun.* 86:153–160, 1978.

42. Lewis, R. V., et al.   An about 50,000-dalton protein in adrenal medulla: A common precursor of [Met]- and [Leu]enkephalin. *Science* 208:1459–1461.

43. Malfroy, B., et al.   High-affinity enkephalin-degrading peptidase in brain is increased after morphine. *Nature* 276:523–526, 1978.

44. Puig, M. M., et al.   Endogenous opiate ligand: Electrically induced release in the guinea pig ileum. *Eur. J. Pharmacol.* 45:205–206, 1977.

45. Jacob, J. J., Tremblay, E. C., and Colombel, M. C.   Facilitation de réactions nociceptives pour la naloxone chez la souris et chez le rat. *Psychopharmacologia* 37:217–223, 1974.

46. Levine, J. D., Gordon, N. C., and Fields, H. L.   The mechanism of placebo analgesia. *Lancet* 2:654–657, 1978.

47. Richardson, D. E.   Brain stimulation for pain control. *IEEE Trans. Biomed. Eng.* BME-23:304–306, 1976.

48. Akil, H., et al.   Elevation of enkephalin levels in the ventricular CSF of pain patients upon analgetic focal stimulation. *Science* 201:463–465, 1978.

49. Su, C.-Y., et al.   Effects of β-endorphin on narcotic abstinence syndrome in man. *J. Formosan Med. Assoc.* 77:133–141, 1978.

50. Ruegg, U. T., Hiller, J. M., and Simon, E. J.   Solubilization of an active opiate receptor from *Bufo marinus*. *Eur. J. Pharmacol.* 64:367–368, 1980.

51. Simonds, W. F., Koski, G., Streaty, R. A., Hjelmeland, L. M., and Klee, W. A.   Solubilization of active opiate receptors. *Proc. Natl. Acad. Sci. U.S.A.* 77:4623–4627, 1980.

52. Bidlack, J. M., and Abood, L. G.   Solubilization of the opiate receptor. *Life Sci.* 27:331–340, 1980.

53. Goldstein, A., Tachibana, S., Lowney, L. I., Hunkapiller, M., and Hood, L.   Dynorphin (1-13), an extraordinarily potent opioid peptide. *Proc. Natl. Acad. Sci. U.S.A.* 76:6666–6670, 1979.

Harold Gainer
Michael J. Brownstein

Chapter 14. Neuropeptides

Several independent avenues of work have led to the recognition that peptides are involved in nervous system function. The discovery of the peptidergic neurosecretory cell in vertebrates by Ernst Scharrer [1] led to the proposal of the "peptidergic neuron" concept [2] and its subsequent amplification [3, 4]. Initially, the term *peptidergic neuron* referred to those neurosecretory cells in the hypothalamus that released oxytocin and vasopressin directly into the circulation from their nerve terminals in the posterior pituitary. However, two major lines of investigation have been largely responsible for the subsequent broadening of this concept. The first relates to the development of the "releasing-factor" concept by G. W. Harris and coworkers [for historical development, see 5], and the culmination of this conceptual revolution in the isolation and characterization of a tripeptide-releasing factor, that is, thyrotropin-releasing factor [6, 7]. The latter effort represented a landmark event in the field of neuroendocrinology and provided the impetus for the discovery of other peptide-releasing factors [6–8]. The second major development was the detection of substance P by von Euler and Gaddum in 1931 [9] and its isolation and characterization by Leeman and coworkers [10]. The significance of the finding was that this peptide was clearly concentrated in specific extrahypothalamic areas (e.g., sensory ganglia); hence, physiologists were alerted to the possibility that peptides might act as neurotransmitters [10].

Peptidergic neurons commonly occur throughout the animal kingdom [11]. In fact, in lower invertebrates, such as annelids, at least one-half of the cerebral ganglion consists of such neurons [4]. Amino acid sequences are known for several of the invertebrate neuropeptides, for example, the red chromatotropin of crustaceans [12], the locust adipokinetic hormone [13], and a putative neurotransmitter peptide called *proctolin* [11, 14] in insects. Many peptide structures appear to be phylogenetically conserved, since vertebrate peptides have been detected in invertebrates, and vice versa. In addition, there appear to be significant redundancies of peptide structures in different tissues of a single species. For example, there are many analogies and homologies between neuropeptides and peptides isolated from the endocrine system, gastrointestinal tract, and frog skin [6, 15]. To explain this redundancy, Pearse has proposed the APUD concept [15, 16]. The acronym APUD means "amine content and/or amine precursor uptake decarboxylation." Pearse postulates that all peptide hormone–producing cells have a common ontogenetic origin, that is, they derive from the same neuroectodermal precursor cells. If this hypothesis is correct, then the common biochemical [15, 16] and electrophysiological [17] properties of peptidergic neurons and endocrine cells could be related to their developmental history.

Ever since the discovery of the endogenous opioid peptides (see Chap. 13), neuropeptide research has become one of the most rapidly expanding areas in neurobiology. Several books providing both background and current information on the subject have been published [18–21]. We shall attempt to give an overview of the field, which should provide the reader with a basis for further study. Much of our understanding of the functional organization of peptidergic neuronal systems comes from studies of the hypothalamus and pituitary, and therefore, we shall begin with an exposition of this area.

Peptides Involved in Hypothalamic and Pituitary Function

The pituitary is comprised of anterior or distal, intermediate, and posterior or neural lobes. The posterior lobe is of neural origin and comes from the floor of the hypothalamus. It is connected to the median eminence of the hypothalamus by a stalk (Fig. 14-1). The anterior and intermediate parts of the pituitary arise from epithelial cells that migrate up from the roof of the embryonal mouth cavity (Rathke's pouch). The three parts of the pituitary eventually join one another and take up residence beneath the diencephalon, those derived from Rathke's pouch becoming most rostral.

THE POSTERIOR PITUITARY

Axons of large neurons in the supraoptic and paraventricular hypothalamic nuclei travel through the median eminence and stalk to the posterior pituitary, where they terminate near blood vessels. They discharge the peptide hormones vasopressin and oxytocin into these vessels (Fig. 14-1). Separate populations of neurons manufacture the two peptide hormones along with their so-called carrier proteins, the neurophysins [22].

Vasopressin, or antidiuretic hormone, inhibits water diuresis. Without this hormone animals have to consume large amounts of water each day in order to replace their fluid losses. If water is not freely available, depletion of body fluids and cardiovascular collapse rapidly ensue. Vasopressin also increases arterial blood pressure, but this pressor effect is of uncertain physiological importance because much more vasopressin is needed to increase blood pressure than to inhibit diuresis.

Moderate to severe dehydration is associated with an outpouring of vasopressin. Theoretically, this outpouring could be triggered either by the decrease in plasma volume that is associated with dehydration or the increase in osmolarity; the latter seems to be the more important factor. *Osmoreceptor* cells in the central nervous system are concerned with regulating vasopressin release. Cells elsewhere in the body that are sensitive to changes in osmolarity or blood pressure also influence vasopressin secretion.

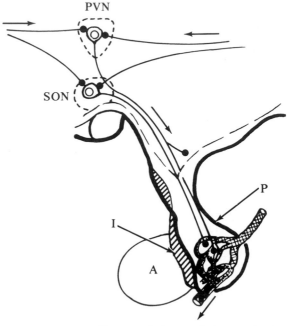

Vasopressin/oxytocin/neurophysins

Fig. 14-1. The hypothalamoneurohypophysial system. Magnocellular neurons in the supraoptic nucleus (SON) and paraventricular nucleus (PVN) of the hypothalamus project via the median eminence to the posterior pituitary (P). There they release their hormones into capillaries. The magnocellular neurons are influenced both by ascending and descending afferents. Note that the axons of some neurons in the paraventricular nucleus terminate in the zona externa of the median eminence and release their contents into the portal capillary plexus. A, anterior lobe; I, intermediate lobe.

A number of pharmacological agents alter the firing patterns of vasopressin-producing neurons and affect the release rate of the hormone. Acetylcholine and histamine are especially potent in releasing vasopressin; norepinephrine has the opposite action. Many other neurotransmitters present in a variety of ascending and descending central pathways probably participate in controlling vasopressin secretion, mediating changes in its release in response to pain, stress, hemorrhage, transfusion, orthostasis, and anoxia.

Oxytocin, the second neurohypophysial hormone to be characterized, plays important roles in reproduction and lactation. The word *oxytocin* ("quick birth") was coined because the hormone stimulates uterine contractions. There is no doubt that oxytocin is secreted during parturition, but its precise role in promoting the ordered evacuation of the fetus from the uterus is still debated.

The part played by oxytocin in milk ejection is clearer. When suckling commences, afferent stimuli from the teats cause reflex release of oxytocin from the posterior pituitary. The oxytocin activates a contractile mechanism, and alveolar milk is expressed through the lactiferous ducts into the sinuses or cisterns connecting to the teat ducts. In the absence of oxytocin, only the milk stored in the cisterns is available to the infant.

It has been suggested that oxytocin influences sperm transport in the female genital tract, milk secretion, male reproductive function, and the estrous cycle of certain animals, but these suggestions are not yet universally accepted.

THE ANTERIOR AND INTERMEDIATE LOBES OF THE PITUITARY

The anterior pituitary contains several types of cells that secrete hormones (see Table 14-1). The intermediate lobe is made of melanotropes and small, nonsecretory satellite cells.

Growth hormone and prolactin have similar primary structures and, to an important degree, similar functions. Growth hormone probably affects metabolic processes in all tissues of the body. Its most obvious action is to cause growth of the immature animal by stimulating elongation of long bones and by stimulating protein biosynthesis at the expense of sugar and fat stores. Some of the actions of growth hormone are mediated by another group of peptides, the somatomedins, which are 6,000 M_r molecules made in the liver. The effects of prolactin, on the other hand, seem to result from the direct influence of this hormone on target cells. Although prolactin can stimulate protein biosynthesis just as growth hormone does, its only certain physiological function is to stimulate lactation in the breast that has been primed with estrogen, progesterone, glucocorticoids, insulin, and thyroxine.

Thyroid-stimulating hormone (TSH), luteinizing hormone (LH), and follicle-stimulating hormone (FSH), as well as human chorionic gonadotropin (CG) are glycoproteins formed from two peptide subunits called α and β *chains*. Fifteen to 30 percent of the total weight of the molecules is contributed by their sugar moieties (polymers of fucose, mannose, galactose, *N*-acetylglucosamine, *N*-acetylgalactosamine, and sialic acid), the rest by the peptide chains. The amino acid sequence of the α chain, which is not biologically active, seems to be the same in the four hormones. The biologically active β chains differ in primary structure.

TSH increases the volume and vascularization

Table 14-1. Cells of the Anterior Pituitary

Cell Type	Percentage of Cells in the Anterior Pituitary	Hormone Produced
Somatotrope	50–60	Growth hormone
Mammotrope	5	Prolactin
Corticotrope	5	Adrenocorticotropic hormone β-Lipotropin β-Endorphin
Thyrotrope	10	Thyrotropin
Gonadotrope	10–15	Luteinizing hormone, follicle-stimulating hormone
Nonsecretory cells (folliculostellate cells)	5	—

of the thyroid gland and stimulates the synthesis and release of thyroid hormones. It also promotes lypolysis in adipose tissue, but the physiological importance of this extrathyroid effect is not understood.

In women, FSH causes growth and development of the ovarian follicle. Subsequently, LH acts upon the follicle, causing it to mature and secrete estrogens. LH then induces ovulation and participates in transforming the follicle into the progesterone-secreting corpus luteum. In men, FSH promotes spermatogenesis, and LH stimulates androgen production by the testis (Leydig cells).

Adrenocorticotropic hormone (corticotropin or ACTH), α-melanocyte-stimulating hormone (α-MSH), β-MSH, β-lipotropic hormone (β-LPH) and β-endorphin comprise a family of peptides that are synthesized as parts of a common precursor molecule, pro-opiocortin, [23] which has a molecular weight of about 31,000. This glycoprotein has β-LPH (β-endorphin and β-MSH) on its carboxyterminal end, ACTH (α-MSH) in the middle, and "γ-MSH" on the N-terminal end.

In all species studied, ACTH has 39 amino-acid-residues. Its first 24 amino acids are constant from species to species. The first 13 amino acids of ACTH are required for the only significant physiological action of the hormone, adrenocorticotropic activity. Adding the next 7 amino acids one at a time progressively enhances the molecule's potency. The remaining 19 amino acids are not required for optimum biological activity.

α-MSH is the first 13 amino acids of ACTH. It is N-acetylated and carboxy-amidated, and, consequently, quite resistant to most peptidases.

β-MSH, β-LPH, α-MSH, and ACTH have 7 amino acids in common (ACTH residues 4 to 10). These residues are the minimum required for melanotropic activity in amphibians and reptiles. The role of melanocyte-stimulating hormones in mammals is still unknown. In fact, the human has a vestigial intermediate pituitary and has little or no circulating α-MSH.

REGULATION OF ANTERIOR PITUITARY FUNCTION

The posterior pituitary is best thought of as a part

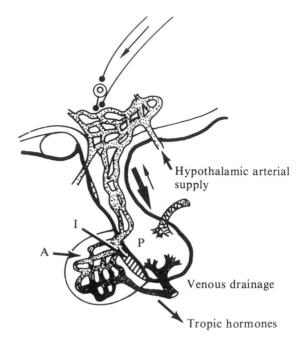

Fig. 14-2. Control of anterior pituitary function. Releasing hormones and release-inhibiting hormones are secreted into portal capillaries in the zona externa of the median eminence. The hormones travel to the anterior pituitary; there they act on tropic hormone-producing cells. These cells secrete into the general circulation; tropic hormones may also travel back to the brain through the portal vessels. Cells that make releasing or release-inhibiting hormones are excited or inhibited by other neurons. Furthermore, release of hypothalamic hormones may be modulated at the median eminence level by a presynaptic mechanism.

of the brain that secretes into the peripheral circulation. The anterior pituitary is an organ that is separate from, but controlled by, the brain. It is connected to the hypothalamus by a special portal vascular system [24] (Fig. 14-2). This system consists of two connected capillary beds, one in the external zone of the median eminence, the other in the pituitary. Axons of a variety of neurons terminate adjacent to portal capillaries in the median eminence. Some of the nerve endings in the median eminence release *hypothalamic hormones* that enter the portal vessels and travel to the anterior pituitary (undiluted by blood from the general circulation). Others release neurotransmitters that probably influence by presynaptic mechanisms the secretion of the hypothalamic hormones.

Upon reaching the anterior pituitary, the hypothalamic hormones stimulate (release hormones or factors) or inhibit (release-inhibiting hormones or factors) the synthesis and secretion of tropic hormones made in the pituitary. A number of releasing hormones and release-inhibiting hormones are likely to be present in the hypothalamus, for example, growth hormone–releasing factor, corticotropin-releasing factor(s), and prolactin-releasing factor.

Two releasing hormones—thyrotropin-releasing hormone (TRH) [25, 26] and luteinizing hormone–releasing hormone (LHRH) [27, 28]—and one release-inhibiting hormone (growth hormone release-inhibiting hormone, or somatostatin) [29] have been isolated and characterized. (See Table 14-2 for the amino acid sequences of these and other peptides.)

The general properties of the hypothalamic hormones were defined by Harris [30]. It is noteworthy that the properties of a releasing factor (or release-inhibiting factor) are quite similar to those of a neurotransmitter (Table 11-3). Indeed, the releasing factors are best thought of as a special class of neurotransmitters that act on a variety of cells, among which are cells in the anterior pituitary.

TRH stimulates the secretion of thyrotropin and prolactin; LHRH stimulates the secretion of LH and FSH. Somatostatin inhibits the secretion of growth hormone, thyrotropin, and prolactin in vitro, but it seems unlikely that somatostatin participates in regulating prolactin in vivo. Dopamine, on the other hand, is a potent inhibitor of prolactin secretion and is found in high concentrations in the median eminence. Hence, it has been suggested that dopamine is a prolactin release-inhibiting hormone.

There is evidence that, in addition to controlling anterior pituitary function, the hypothalamic hormones may act at various loci in the central nervous system distant from the median eminence. Furthermore, somatostatin has been shown to play important roles outside the brain in the pancreas and gastrointestinal tract. It inhibits the secretion of insulin, glucagon, and gastrin and decreases gastric acidity.

FEEDBACK CONTROL OF NEUROENDOCRINE FUNCTION

Figure 14-3 summarizes the information in the preceding sections of this chapter. It should be evident that the neuroendocrine system is a hierarchy with higher centers regulating lower ones. This hierarchical control of secretory activity involves *feedback loops.* That is, some change related to secretory activity is detected by a control center, and the information is used to adjust the output of the control mechanism in an appropriate way. Consequently, Fig. 14-3 could be redrawn with many extra arrows pointing upward to indicate feedback.

Negative, or inhibitory, feedback is the usual means of maintaining a particular level of output in the face of uncontrolled or unpredictable disturbances. For example, an increase in the blood level of adrenocorticosteroids causes a decrease in the release of adrenocorticotropic hormone (ACTH) from the anterior pituitary. This, in turn, results in a decrease in the secretion rate of corticosteroids, and they return toward their original level. Gonadal steroids and thyroxine also exert negative feedback control over their respective tropic hormones.

There is evidence for *positive,* or stimulatory, feedback as well as negative feedback. Implantation of estrogen in the rat pituitary during a critical period of the estrous cycle causes advancement of ovulation, which is probably due to an increase in the plasma level of LH. By acting on the developing ovarian follicle, the LH causes a further increase in estrogen level. Unlike negative feedback systems, positive feedback controls are inherently unstable. Once set in motion, they rapidly produce a high level of activity. For example, estrogen stimulation of LH secretion seems responsible for the peak of LH output that triggers ovulation when the follicle is mature. Inhibitory mechanisms are required for turning off positive feedback control loops. Inhibition by LH of its own secretion may provide such a mechanism in the example cited above.

In general, the higher a regulatory center is in the

Table 14-2. Amino Acid Sequences of Biologically Active Peptides

β-Endorphin
H-Tyr-Gly-Gly-Phe-Met-Thr-Ser-Glu-Lys-Ser-Gln-Thr-Pro-Leu-Val-Thr-Leu-Phe-Lys-Asn-Ala-Ile-Ile-Lys-Asn-Ala-Tyr-Lys-Lys-Gly-Glu-OH

Met-enkephalin
H-Tyr-Gly-Gly-Phe-Met-OH

Leu-enkephalin
H-Tyr-Gly-Gly-Phe-Leu-OH

Somatostatin
H-Ala-Gly-Cys-Lys-Asn-Phe-Phe-Trp-Lys-Thr-Phe-Thr-Ser-Cys-OH

Luteinizing hormone-releasing hormone
pGlu-His-Trp-Ser-Tyr-Gly-Leu-Arg-Pro-Gly-NH$_2$

Thyrotropin-releasing hormone
pGlu-His-Pro-NH$_2$

Substance P
H-Arg-Pro-Lys-Pro-Glu-Glu-Phe-Phe-Gly-Leu-Met-NH$_2$

Neurotensin
pGlu-Leu-Tyr-Glu-Asu-Lys-Pro-Arg-Arg-Pro-Tyr-Ile-Leu-OH

Angiotensin I
H-Asp-Arg-Val-Tyr-Ile-His-Pro-Phe-His-Leu-OH

Angiotensin II
H-Asp-Arg-Val-Tyr-Ile-His-Pro-Phe-OH

Angiotensin III
H-Arg-Val-Tyr-Ile-His-Pro-Phe-OH

α-Melanocyte–stimulating hormone
Acetyl Ser-Tyr-Ser-Met-Glu-His-Phe-Arg-Trp-Gly-Lys-Pro-Val-NH$_2$

Adrenocorticotropic hormone
H-Ser-Tyr-Ser-Met-Glu-His-Phe-Arg-Trp-Gly-Lys-Pro-Val-Gly-Lys-Lys-Arg-Arg-Pro-Val-Lys-Val-Tyr-Pro-Asn-Gly-Ala-Glu-Asp-Glu-Leu-Ala-Glu-Ala-Phe-Pro-Leu-Glu-Phe-OH

L-Carnosine
N-β-alanyl-L-histidine

Bombesin
pGlu-Glu-Arg-Leu-Gly-Asn-Glu-Trp-Ala-Val-Gly-His-Leu-Met-NH$_2$

Oxytocin
H-Cys-Tyr-Ile-Glu-Asn-Cys-Pro-Leu-Gly-NH$_2$

Lysine vasopressin
H-Cys-Tyr-Phe-Glu-Asn-Cys-Pro-Lys-Gly-NH$_2$

Arginine vasopressin
H-Cys-Tyr-Phe-Glu-Asn-Cys-Pro-Arg-Gly-NH$_2$

Arginine vasotrocin
H-Cys-Tyr-Ile-Glu-Asn-Cys-Pro-Arg-Gly-NH$_2$

Vasoactive intestinal peptide
H-His-Ser-Asp-Ala-Val-Phe-Thr-Asp-Asn-Tyr-Thr-Arg-Leu-Arg-Lys-Glu-Met-Ala-Val-Lys-Lys-Tyr-Leu-Asn-Ser-Ile-Leu-Asn-NH$_2$

Bradykinin
H-Arg-Pro-Pro-Gly-Phe-Ser-Pro-Phe-Arg-OH

Cholecystokinin octapeptide
Glu-Ala-Tyr-Gly-Trp-Leu-Asp-Phe-NH$_2$

Table 14-3. Criteria for Assessing the Physiological Role of Any Proposed Substance as a Releasing Factor

1. The putative releasing factor must be extractable from hypothalamic or stalk–median eminence tissue
2. It must be present in hypophysial portal blood in greater amounts than in systemic blood (i.e., it is released into the portal capillaries)
3. Varying concentrations of the substance in portal vessel blood should be related to varying secretion rates of one of the anterior pituitary hormones under a number of different experimental and environmental conditions

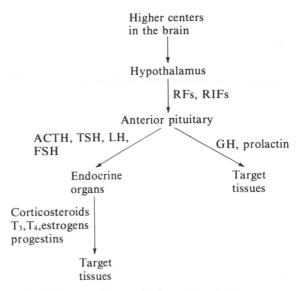

Fig. 14-3. *Neural control of anterior pituitary function. RF, releasing factor; RIF, release-inhibiting factor.*

neuroendocrine hierarchy, the more opportunities it has to be fed back upon, positively or negatively. Theoretically, the feedback control of a center can be mediated by the secretory product of the center itself (this sort of feedback by releasing hormones onto the very cells that make them is termed *ultrashort feedback*), by the secretory products of lower centers, or by reflexes triggered by these secretory products. Cells in the anterior pituitary and in the hypothalamus are sensitive to peripheral hormone levels. These hormone-brain and hormone-pituitary interactions are responsible for so-called long feedback effects. For example, repeated injection of exogenous thyroxine into an animal with an isolated pituitary will cause atrophy of its thyroid gland, just as in the intact animal. This is taken to indicate that the isolated pituitary gland, in addition to maintaining a low rate of TSH secretion, is sensitive to the level of thyroxine in the general circulation. Increasing the thyroxine level inhibits the TSH release and produces atrophy of the target organ. After stalk section, however, the system is unresponsive to many of the stimuli that would have increased thyroid activity in the intact animal, such as environmental stress. The input to the pituitary-thyroid axis from these stimuli is neural and is mediated by the hypophysial portal system. Similar observations have been made for ACTH and the gonadotropic hormones.

Feedback control of brain centers by adenohypophysial tropic hormones is referred to as *internal* or *short feedback*. There is evidence that each of the tropic hormones except prolactin may

act on the hypothalamus in such an inhibitory short loop. Since the pressure in pituitary portal vessels is low, blood flow in this vascular system is probably bidirectional, although predominantly towards the pituitary (Fig. 14-2). Therefore, pituitary secretions can return to the median eminence, to the cerebrospinal fluid, and, finally, to the rest of the brain either directly by this route or indirectly (and much diluted) through systemic circulation. Peripheral hormones must be carried to the brain through the general circulation. Once there, these peripheral hormones act, along with pituitary tropic hormones, on a variety of neurons that are involved in neuroendocrine regulation.

Experimental Approaches to the Study of Neuropeptides
There is no single best approach to the detection and isolation of biologically active neuropeptides. However, one general paradigm that has been used with success [31] is presented in Table 14-4. In this approach, the biochemist is directed by the biological phenomenon of interest, that is, the bioactivity of the peptide. The biological assay may be either a physiologically relevant one (e.g., as was

the case for the hypothalamic releasing factors, see above) or a reproducible response to the peptide in a neural or nonneural tissue that may have no apparent relationship to its actual physiological role in the nervous system (as was the case for substance P and the sialogogic bioassay, see [1]). In some cases, if it is feasible, even a complex behavioral response can be used as the basis for a bioassay.

The development of a quantitative bioassay is not a trivial endeavor. To some extent it depends upon an effective procedure for extraction of the peptide from the tissue. The extraction should be done under conditions that protect the peptide from degradative processes (e.g., proteolytic enzymes), and a solvent should be used in which the peptide is highly soluble. Methods for preventing degradation of the peptide during extraction include microwave treatment or freezing of the tissue with liquid nitrogen, adding protease inhibitors (e.g., Trasylol [aprotinin]) to the extraction solvent, and boiling the tissue in dilute acid. In addition to the problems of degradation, one must also attend to the problem of recovery. Peptides tend to bind to glass surfaces, may be associated with binding proteins, and may be destroyed by such processes as oxidation and esterification of sensitive amino acid residues during extraction. Obviously, the initial extraction step is critical and often must be tailored to the specific peptide being extracted and to the specific tissue from which it is to be extracted [31].

Even with a good extraction procedure, one may find that the biological activity in the extract was altered or masked by other substances that were co-extracted. Only by sequential separation steps and bioassay at each step can one determine if this is indeed the case. Herein lies the major value of the quantitative bioassay. The bioassay provides a major criterion for purity of the peptide as it is being fractionated. The aim is to subject the extract to a variety of sequential separation procedures until the isolated peptide is at maximum and constant specific activity (i.e., where the units of biological activity per amount of peptide is maximal and constant). In addition, the bioassay can be

Table 14-4. Steps in the Analysis of a Neuropeptide*

1. Development of a quantitative bioassay
2. Evidence that the biologically active material is peptidic in nature
3. Development of extraction and separation procedures for maximum yields of the purified peptide
4. Chemical and physical characterization of the pure peptide (e.g., molecular weight determination and amino acid composition)
5. Obtain amino acid sequence of the peptide
6. Chemical synthesis of the peptide (which is then tested for bioactivity using quantative bioassay)
7. Produce antibodies to peptide
8. Characterization of antibodies using synthetic analogs of the peptide (purification of antibodies)
9. Development of immunological assays and procedures for use on neural tissues (e.g., radioimmunoassay and immunocytochemistry)

*Although it is highly desirable to have, at the outset, a biological activity of the peptide that can be monitored by a quantitative bioassay, not all studies on peptides begin with this step. However, the value of a bioassay is emphasized by its role in the establishment of purity criteria for the isolated and the synthetic peptides.

used early to determine whether the bioactive substance is a peptide. Preliminary evidence of its peptidic nature can be obtained by evaluating its size by molecular filtration chromatography and by determining whether it maintains activity after boiling at neutral pH (most, but not all, peptides do) and whether the bioactivity is destroyed by incubation of the material with proteolytic enzymes (e.g., pronase, trypsin, etc.) or by acid hydrolysis.

A variety of separation procedures can be used to isolate the purified peptide. These include molecular filtration chromatography (which also provides information about the size of the peptide), selective extractions in diverse solvents, ion exchange chromatography, thin layer chromatography, high-voltage electrophoresis, and, where possible, specific affinity chromatography. The last procedure is particularly efficacious, as it provides a large purification in a single step because of a specific property of the peptide (i.e., it may bind specifically to a protein and will be eluted from a column on which this protein is attached only in the presence of an excess of a competing ligand). A recently developed separation technique having very high resolution and speed and known as *high-performance liquid chromatography* (HPLC) has been applied successfully to peptide separation. The point of using these separation procedures is to generate a pure peptide. One criterion of purity has already been discussed, that is, the peptide is at maximum and constant specific biological activity. Several other criteria should also be fulfilled: N-terminal and C-terminal analysis of the peptide shows that there is only one N-terminal and one C-terminal amino acid, and analysis of the amino acid composition of the peptide demonstrates that the molar ratios of its constituent amino acids remain constant integrals throughout sequential fractionation procedures.

Given an isolated pure peptide in sufficient quantity, analysis of its amino acid sequence can then be performed, and ultimately, chemical synthesis of the peptide can be done in large quantities. The purity and fidelity of the chemically synthesized neuropeptides must be tested by the above chemical and bioassay procedures.

IMMUNOLOGICAL PROCEDURES

Immunological techniques have become the methods of choice for the study of neuropeptide distributions and cellular compartmentation. This is because the radioimmunoassay (RIA) technique can detect extremely low levels of peptides (femtomoles). Immunological reactions are quite specific, and RIAs require relatively little technical investment [32]. Similarly, the techniques of immunocytochemistry provide a unique morphological approach to the cellular and subcellular localization of peptides even in a tissue as heterogeneous as the brain.

The production of antibodies to the peptide involves the immunization of rabbits, goats, or guinea pigs with a peptide that has been emulsified in Freund's adjuvant. Relatively impure peptides can be used for immunization, and slight denaturation of the antigens may actually improve their immunogenicity. Small peptides that may not be antigenic can be made so by coupling them to larger proteins, such as bovine serum albumin or thyroglobulin. Usually, several animals are immunized simultaneously with the antigen, since it is not possible to predict which animal will produce the best antiserum with regard to concentration, specificity, and sensitivity of their antibodies. Antibody concentration tends to increase with repeated immunizations, reaching a maximum after about 3 to 5 immunizations. The presence and characteristics of the antibody are usually tested, using RIA methods, after each reimmunization.

Approaches to the development and validation of an RIA procedure have been discussed extensively [32]. In addition, kits for RIA of certain peptides are now available commercially, although they are generally quite expensive per assay. Despite the obvious power of RIA for the analysis of peptides, there are many potential pitfalls and sources of artifacts that may confront the naive user. It must be remembered that, even in the best of cases, the unique value of RIA is in its extraordinary sensitivity and simplicity. Its specificity, however, is based on immunological reactions with antigenic determinants that may be shared by diverse molecules (e.g., prohormones versus peptide hormones). Hence, in a strict sense, peptides cannot be shown to exist in a tissue by means of immunological procedures. What is measured is specific peptidelike immunoreactivity, and definitive proof of a specific peptide's presence in the tissue still remains a biochemical one.

The principle of immunocytochemistry is to detect the antigen in tissue by light and electron microscopy by using a labeled antibody. The various markers for antibodies include covalently bound fluorescent molecules, ferritin, enzymes (peroxidase), and radioactive substances [33]. The recent uses of enzymatic [10] and radioactive [34] markers in antigen-antibody complexes have greatly enhanced the sensitivity of this method and have reduced some of the problems inherent in covalent labeling of the antibodies [33, 34]. Although immunocytochemical techniques are extremely useful and provide a unique approach to the cellular localization of peptides, proof of specificity of the immunoreaction is very difficult to obtain. It is generally agreed that the specificity manifested by antiserum in a RIA does not guarantee specificity in an immunocytochemical procedure that uses the same antiserum, partly because of the much higher antisera dilutions used in RIA [34]. One approach used to deal with this problem is to purify the antibodies by means of affinity chromatography, that is, to produce so-called monospecific antibodies. In this approach, purified antigen is covalently coupled to Sepharose beads. Specific antibody will attach to the beads in a column and, after washing the nonspecific antibodies out of the column, the specific antibody can be selectively eluted and used. Another approach is to absorb out the specific antibody in the immunocytochemical procedure by the addition of excess antigen as a control for nonspecific labeling. Although both of these approaches are employed by various investigators, their limitations have been discussed by others [35]. In any case, evidence for the detection of a "specific" peptide by immunocytochemistry is usually regarded as less compelling than evidence obtained by the RIA methods. As with RIA, the peptide visualized immunocytochemically is referred to as "specific-peptidelike immunoreactivity."

Peptide Distribution in the Nervous System

One reason for studying the distribution of peptides in the central nervous system is to determine whether they are present in neurons. This is the first thing that must be shown if a peptide is to be considered a neurotransmitter candidate. By examining the neuroanatomy of peptidergic systems, one does much more than satisfy this criterion, however. If one function of a peptide is known, its distribution can hint at the role of brain areas where it is found. For example, the presence of LHRH in the septum and preoptic areas suggested (but certainly did not guarantee) that these regions might be involved somehow in reproduction. Indeed, these regions may provide the anatomical substrate for LHRH-induced lordotic behavior [36].

If the central role of a peptide is a mystery, as with substance P, looking at its distribution may provide clues about its actions. The presence of large amounts of substance P in the dorsal part of the spinal cord hinted that it might mediate pain sensation [37]. In addition to providing a starting point for physiological and behavioral studies, neuroanatomical studies are necessary as first steps for biochemical and cell biological investigations. Conversely, the demonstration that specific cells in which a peptide has been visualized are capable of manufacturing the peptide provides a final vindication of the anatomical data (see Table 14-5).

Each peptide studied to date has its own unique distribution reflecting the location of the neuronal perikarya that produce it and the processes that store and release it. Axons and nerve endings are especially rich in peptides. The cell bodies seem to manufacture peptide precursors and send them down the axons rather rapidly, so that peptide levels in perikarya are normally not very high. For this reason, peptidergic cell bodies have proven difficult to visualize immunocytochemically. Agents such as colchicine that block axonal transport have been used by immunohistochemists to promote the build-up of peptides in cell bodies. After colchicine treatment, peptide-containing perikarya that are impossible to see otherwise can sometimes be visualized.

There is nothing about the anatomy of central peptidergic neurons that distinguishes them from other classes of neurons. Some are large, and some are small; some are local-circuit neurons and others project to distant regions. Consequently, in the absence of immunological staining techniques, peptide-producing neurons cannot be separated from their nonpeptide-producing neighbors. In fact, it has been suggested recently that such peptides as substance P and somatostatin can coexist with monoamines in certain neurons [38–41]. Moreover, diverse peptides can be made by neurons as parts of single precursors. In theory, ACTH, α-MSH, β-MSH, and the endorphins could all be made by and released from the same cell. What determines how a precursor will be processed re-

Table 14-5. Immunocytochemical Localization of Peptides in the CNS*

Peptide	Localization
LHRH	*Perikarya* (higher mammals and humans): scattered cells in the arcuate (2–5% of the neurons); ventral premammillary, ventromedial, and dorsomedial nuclei *Processes:* median eminence *Perikarya* (rodents): scattered neurons in the periventricular, suprachiasmatic, medial preoptic, lateral septal, and diagonal band nuclei plus the interstitial nucleus of the stria terminalis. *Processes:* axons can be traced to the median eminence, supraoptic crest. Other processes visualized in the posterior pituitary, telencephalon, septum, thalamus, mammillary body, ventral tegmental area, habenula, and amygdala
TRH	*Perikarya:* dorsomedial and periventricular nuclei, possibly *Processes:* median eminence; paraventricular, anterior hypothalamic, and medial preoptic nuclei; medial forebrain bundle; lateral septal nucleus; nucleus accumbens; zona incerta; nucleus intercalatus; cranial motor nuclei (III, V, VII, XII); ventral horn of the spinal cord
Somatostatin	*Perikarya:* near the third ventricle in the preoptic and paraventricular nuclei and scattered in the ventromedial and paraventricular nuclei, thalamus, and spinal ganglia *Processes:* throughout the central nervous system. Especially rich in fibers are the hypothalamus (median eminence; ventromedial, arcuate dorsomedial, and ventral premammillary nuclei); amygdala; lateral septum; brain stem; and substantia gelatinosa of the spinal cord
Vasopressin Oxytocin Neurophysins	*Perikarya:* large cells in the supraoptic and paraventricular nuclei, small cells in the dorsal pole of the suprachiasmatic nuclei (vasopressin) *Processes:* posterior pituitary; median eminence (axons and terminals); choroid plexus; supraoptic crest; diagonal band; medial amygdaloid nucleus; lateral septum; medial dorsal thalamus; epithalamus; periventricular area; mesencephalic central gray; ventral tegmental area; locus coeruleus; parabrachial and vagal nuclei; area postrema; dorsal spinal cord
Substance P	*Perikarya:* spinal and cranial sensory ganglia (20% of the cells); periaqueductal gray; nucleus raphe magnus; medial habenular nucleus; basal ganglia; and nucleus of the spinal trigeminal tract *Processes:* spinal cord; reticular part of the substantia nigra; central gray; and ventral tegmental area
Neurotensin	*Perikarya:* hypothalamus; interstitial nucleus of the stria terminalis; amygdala; and midbrain tegmentum *Processes:* Substantia gelatinosa of the spinal cord; nucleus of the spinal trigeminal tract; central amygdaloid area; anterior pituitary; median eminence; and preoptic and basal hypothalamic areas
α-MSH	*Perikarya:* Arcuate nucleus *Processes:* septum; interstitial nucleus of the stria terminalis; medial preoptic, anterior hypothalamic, dorsomedial, and periventricular nuclei. Moderate numbers of fibers are in the paraventricular and arcuate nuclei; amygdala; tractus diagonalis; mammillary body; central gray; cuneiform nucleus; and nucleus of the solitary tract
β-Lipotropin	*Perikarya:* scattered cells in the arcuate nucleus and along the ventral surface of the hypothalamus *Processes:* hypothalamic periventricular nucleus; zona incerta; ansa leuticularis; stria terminalis; nucleus accumbens; medial amygdaloid nucleus; nucleus periventricularis thalami; mesencephalic central gray; and locus coeruleus

Table 14-5 (Continued)

Peptide	Localization
ACTH	*Perikarya:* arcuate region *Processes:* hypothalamus; thalamus; amygdala; periaqueductal gray; and reticular formation (the distribution parallels that of β-lipotropin)
Enkephalins	*Perikarya:* hypothalamus; central gray; nucleus raphe magnus; nucleus of the spinal trigeminal tract; and dorsal horn of the spinal cord *Processes:* spinal cord (laminae I, II, V, VII; the area around the central canal; the substantia gelatinosa of the spinal cord and medulla); medulla (nucleus of the olitary tract, cranial motor nuclei, dorsal vagal nucleus, lateral reticular nucleus); pontine tegmentum; mesencephalon (central gray, compact part of the substantia nigra, raphe nuclei); thalamus (rostral, dorsal and medial nuclei); hypothalamus (periventricular area; ventromedial, dorsomedial, arcuate, supraoptic, suprachiasmatic nuclei; median eminence; mammillary body); medial preoptic nucleus; bed nucleus of the stria terminalis; globus pallidus; nucleus accumbens; and central amygdala
Angiotensin	*Perikarya:* unknown *Processes:* fibers containing an angiotensin II-like material are scattered throughout the brain and spinal cord
Bradykinin	*Perikarya:* overlying the periventricular and dorsomedial nuclei of the hypothalamus *Processes:* periaqueductal gray; hypothalamus; perirhinal and cingulate cortices; the ventral portion of the striatum; and lateral septal area
Prolactin	*Perikarya:* unknown *Processes:* hypothalamus (periventricular, arcuate, dorsomedial, ventral pre-mammillary, dorsal premammillary nuclei; medial forebrain bundle); preoptic area (periventricular, suprachiasmatic nuclei); periventricular nucleus of the thalamus; Forel's H_2 field; mammillothalamic tract; and supramammillary decussation
Cholecystokinin	*Perikarya:* periaqueductal gray; dorsal raphe; dorsomedial hypothalamus; cerebral cortex; hippocampus *Processes:* mensencephalon; diencephalic periventricular area; lateral thalamus; pyriform cortex; hippocampus; central amygdala; lateral septal area (no cells or fibers detected in the cerebellum, spinal cord, medulla, or pons)
Vasoactive intestinal polypeptide	*Perikarya:* limbic cortex; neocortex (1–5%) *Processes:* limbic cortex; neocortex; central amygdaloid nucleus; suprachiasmatic nucleus; medial preoptic nucleus; and anterior hypothalamic nucleus

Other peptides have been detected in the brain but mapping studies are too preliminary to describe: insulin, bombesin-like peptide, growth hormone, carnosine, and glucagon.

*See special reference list related to distribution of peptides in the CNS, page 294.

mains to be seen. Whether neurons can release different biologically active peptides at different times, under different circumstances, is also unknown.

Many peptides have been found in unexpected places. Pituitary tropic hormones such as prolactin and growth hormone have been shown to be present in the brain and seem to be there in specific populations of neurons. Insulin has also been detected in brain extracts. Hormones present in the blood or in structures that are in close proximity to the brain, such as the pituitary or pineal, may not be made by central neurons; they may be taken up and stored by them. Alternatively, part of the hormone in the brain may be made endogenously, and part may be provided by an outside source. Until more is known about the biosynthesis of peptides by central neurons, it will not be possible to prove that the "peripheral" hormones in the brain are indeed made there.

In addition to demonstrating that numerous gut and pituitary hormones are widely distributed in the central nervous system, workers in this field have shown that hypothalamic hormones are not as narrowly distributed as they were once thought to be. Somatostatin, for example, is found both inside the hypothalamus and outside it. In fact, only about one-quarter of the somatostatin in the brain is in the hypothalamus. Therefore, it has been suggested that somatostatin may act as a neurotransmitter at sites other than the median eminence. Similarly, based on its widespread distribution, it has been said that TRH may be a central neurotransmitter. This suggestion has been called into question recently, however [41]. Much of the radioimmuno-assayable TRH outside the hypothalamus, septum, and preoptic area does not cochromatograph with pyroglutamylhistidylprolinamide (TRH), and may be a closely related substance, which may or may not be biologically active. Clearly, much more work needs to be done to develop simple methods for the extraction, separation, detection, and characterization of the peptides.

Biosynthesis of Neuropeptides

Much of our understanding of peptide biosynthesis in general comes from studies on tissues other than brain. To date, the mechanisms for the biosynthesis of neuronal peptides appear to be similar to those mechanisms found in other eukaryotic tissues. Two major alternatives exist: (1) the synthesis of oligopeptides by enzymatic mechanisms, that is, synthetases; and (2) synthesis by conventional ribosomal protein synthesis mechanisms, usually as a *prohormone*, which is degraded by limited proteolysis to specific peptide products in the cell before release. The mechanism (1) is used for small peptides, such as carnosine (β-alanyl-L-histidine) and glutathione (γ-L-glutamyl-L-cysteinylglycine), which are found in various eukaryotic tissues (including brain) and are synthetized by such enzymes as carnosine synthetase and γ-glutamyl-L-cysteine (plus tripeptide) synthetase, respectively. Larger peptides, such as insulin, nerve growth factor, ACTH, endorphin, vasopressin, and oxytocin, appear to be synthesized as prohormones.

A number of approaches to the study of peptide biosynthesis have evolved in recent years. The first issue to be considered is which of the above biosynthetic mechanisms is relevant. If various eukaryotic protein synthesis inhibitors (e.g., cycloheximide, puromycin) inhibit the synthesis of the peptide, there is presumptive evidence for the prohormone mode of synthesis. If this is not the case, a search for a specific enzymatic mechanism is in order. Another approach is to employ radioimmunoassays for the peptide to see whether upon biochemical separation (e.g., gel filtration), higher molecular weight, heterogeneous immunoreactive forms of the peptide can be detected. This also represents presumptive evidence, but not proof, of a prohormone ("big" forms of insulin, ACTH, growth hormone, calcitonin, and other peptides have been detected by this method). The key experiment is to demonstrate biosynthesis of the peptide (and prohormone) from isotopically labeled amino acids in a pulse-chase labeling paradigm. In such a paradigm, a tissue known to contain substantial quantities of the peptide of interest is exposed to radioactive amino acids for a short time (*pulse*). During this pulse, a larger form of the peptide should be detected. The tissue, having been pulsed in this manner, is then exposed to a large excess of nonradioactive amino acids to dilute out the radioactive ones (*chase*) or, alternatively, to protein synthesis inhibitors to block further de novo protein synthesis, and is incubated for various periods. The minimum requirement in these experiments is to show that the higher molecular weight precursor (or prohormone) decreases in radioactivity with time after the chase or addition of inhibitor. Concurrently, there is an increase in the radioactivity of the peptide product. To demonstrate this, it is necessary in many cases (particularly with heterogeneous tissue such as brain) to use an antibody to the peptide that also reacts with the precursor in a quantitative immunoprecipitation procedure to resolve the relevant labeled molecules. Labeled presumptive precursors can be purified from the immunoprecipitates and evaluated for the presence of the peptide sequence by limited proteolysis mapping in vitro and by analysis of amino acid sequences. Finally, the use of cell-free protein-synthesizing systems (e.g., wheat germ and reticulocyte in vitro systems) and polyribosomes from the tissue of interest can lead to the synthesis of the prohormone in vitro. This approach has the advantage of also identifying the preprohormone, that is, the prohormone with a characteristic peptide still attached to its N-terminus that is used as a signal to direct the prohormone into the cisternae of the endoplasmic reticulum, as well as representing the first step in the isolation of the mRNA and, ultimately, the gene for the prohormone.

DEVELOPMENT OF THE PROHORMONE CONCEPT

The discovery in 1967 by Steiner and coworkers that insulin is synthesized in a larger precursor form as proinsulin [42] provided the impetus for further studies, which have shown that this is a common mode of biosynthesis of eukaryotic peptides destined for secretion. The continuing studies on proinsulin offer a useful intellectual and experimental paradigm [43]. Proinsulin is a single polypeptide chain ordered as follows: NH₂-B chain-Arg-Arg-C peptide-Lys-Arg-A chain-COOH. The presumed function of the C peptide is to ensure the correct folding and sulfhydryl oxidation between the A and B chains in proinsulin. The higher rate (15 times) of mutation in the C peptide as compared to the insulin moiety, suggests that the C peptide may not have a physiological function. However, studies indicate that immunoassay of C peptide may be a useful differential diagnostic procedure for hypoglycemia [44]. The transformation of pro-

insulin to insulin in the β cells begins in the Golgi apparatus, where new secretory granules are formed, and continues in the granules thereafter. The half-time of conversion is about 1 hr. Two major processing enzymes have been identified in the granules, a trypsinlike endopeptidase and a carboxypeptidase B-like exopeptidase. The insulin is maintained in the granule in a crystalline form (in combination with zinc). These studies provided several important generalizations: (1) peptide hormones can be synthesized in larger precursor forms (i.e., as prohormones); (2) posttranslational processing of the prohormone occurs in the secretory granule; and (3) peptides other than the known biologically active one(s) will emerge from this biosynthetic mechanism, and, if processing occurs intragranularly, all will be released simultaneously by the cell.

The intracellular organization involved in the biosynthesis of proteins destined for secretion has been known for some time [45]. More recently, it has been discovered that the intracellular compartmentation following synthesis of the protein on the rough endoplasmic reticulum (RER) is determined, in part, by the translational process itself. The initial N-terminal amino acid sequence of the protein serves as a signal for the protein to transverse the RER membrane and enter the cisternae, where the signal sequence is immediately cleaved off. Similar signal sequences exist for secreted proteins and intrinsic membrane protein (Chap. 3). The prohormone, plus its transient N-terminal sequence, which usually contains 20 to 30 amino acids, is referred to as a *preprohormone* [for examples, see 46].

The enzymatic mechanisms involved in the conversions of protein precursors (prohormones) to peptides (hormones) are poorly understood. In virtually all cases where it has been studied [46], the enzyme activity appears to be similar to the insulin model described above. The conversions appear to be due to combined actions of trypsinlike endo-peptidases and carboxypeptidase B-like exopeptidases. Analysis of the primary structures of various prohormones [46] indicate that they contain sequences of 2 to 3 basic amino acids (lysine or arginine) at the cleavage sites and, therefore, would be susceptible to appropriate cleavage by the above enzymes. In all cases, pancreatic trypsin appears to mimic the endogenous protease activity. However, in no case has the enzyme activity been inhibited by specific inhibitors of pancreatic trypsin (e.g., soybean trypsin inhibitor or TLCK). It is not known whether the trypsinlike enzyme is a specific enzyme in each system.

Recently, a precursor form of β-nerve growth factor (β-NGF) has been detected in pulse-chase biosynthesis experiments [47]. The precursor has an apparent molecular weight of 22,000, and is subsequently converted to the biologically active form of β-NGF (M_r 13,260) by a trypsinlike enzyme. Especially interesting is that the biologically active β-NGF is extracted from mouse salivary gland, where it is found in high concentration, in a stable 7S complex [48]. The 7S NGF complex has a molecular weight of 130,000, and is composed of dimers of each of three subunits: β-NGF (M_r 13,260), an α subunit (M_r 26,500), and a γ subunit (M_r 26,000). The γ subunit is believed to be the arginine-specific esteropeptidase that converts the precursor to β-NGF [47, 48]. The significance of the continued binding of the enzyme, or γ subunit, to the product in the 7S complex after cleavage of the precursor has been suggested as a mechanism to prevent further degradation by other intracellular proteases. That this 7S complex enzyme is not specific for the cleavage of β-NGF precursor has been shown by its ability to promote fibrinolysis by converting plasminogen to plasmin [49].

THE CORTICOTROPIN-ENDORPHIN PRECURSOR

The existence of large immunoreactive forms of corticotropin (ACTH) has been known for many years [50]. In addition, it has been known that the sequences of β-MSH and β-LPH are contained in β-LPH, and that α-MSH is a tridecapeptide identical to the N-terminal sequence of ACTH [51]. Because of these and similar observations, it was suspected that precursor, β-MSH, and endorphin were all derived from β-LPH.

A major advance in this field was recently made by studies on an ACTH-secreting pituitary tumor cell line of mice, which demonstrated that there was a 31,000 M_r common precursor for both ACTH and β-LPH [23, 52]. These elegant studies involved the use of quantitative pulse-chase experiments, immunoprecipitation by specific ACTH and endorphin antisera, and peptide-mapping procedures after limited proteolysis. In addition, the common precursor has been shown to be a glycoprotein, with one of the two carbohydrate chains potentially attached to the carboxyl-terminal half of the ACTH$_{1-39}$ peptide. The tentative structure of this precursor and the potential peptide products generated from it are illustrated in Fig. 14-4. Note that there are at least six known biologically active peptides—ACTH, α-MSH, β-LPH, β-MSH, β-endorphin, and Met-enkephalin—contained within the precursor's sequence. Evidence exists for the biological relevance of this biosynthetic pathway for all but β-MSH and Met-enkephalin [53, 54]. Note also that, in addition to yielding ACTH-like and endorphinlike peptides, the processing of the 31,000 M_r precursor produces a large N-terminal glycopeptide fragment (M_r 11,200) of unknown function, quite reminiscent of the C peptide and proinsulin.

When mRNA that encodes for the common precursor is translated in a cell-free protein-synthesizing system, an unglycosylated form (M_r 28,500) of the precursor is synthesized [52, 55, 56]. The carbohydrate attached to the precursor posttranslationally in the RER and Golgi appears to be important in regulating its subsequent intracellular processing [57]. Recently, cDNA synthesized from the mRNA that encodes the common precursor in the bovine neurointermediate lobe was inserted into bacterial plasmids and cloned. Sequence analysis of the cDNA has demonstrated that it contains the entire coding sequence for both ACTH and β-LPH and that these two sequences are separated by a 6-base pair sequence encoding lysine and arginine [58]. Because the carboxyl terminus of the ACTH in the precursor is linked to the amino terminus through two basic amino acids, it is likely that the converting enzymes will be similar to the trypsinlike and carboxypeptidase B-like activities described above for other prohormones.

Nakanishi and coworkers [58] have obtained the complete nucleotide sequence of cloned cDNA encoding bovine corticotropin–β-lipotropin precursor mRNA. The N-terminal segment shown in Fig. 14-4 also contains a melanotropin sequence (γ-MSH), and all the component peptides of the precursor are separated by pairs of lysine and arginine residues.

PEPTIDE BIOSYNTHESIS IN NEURONS

It is not commonly recognized that the first hypothesis for the existence of a prohormone derived from studies on the nervous system. In 1964, Sachs and Takabatake [59] hypothesized that vasopressin, a nonapeptide, and neurophysin, a protein of about 10,000 M_r [see review of neurophysins in 60], were formed by posttranslational processing of a common precursor protein. Two precursors of neurophysin (about 20,000 M_r each), one associated with vasopressin synthesis and the other with oxytocin synthesis, have been identified in pulse-chase and immunoprecipitation experiments on the rat hypothalamoneurohypophysial system [61–63]. Direct evidence that these neurophysin precursors exhibit close homology and contain the nonapeptides oxytocin and vasopressin has been obtained in peptide-mapping (limited proteolysis) studies. Because the precursor is 20,000 M_r and the known peptide products sum to only about 11,000 M_r, it is expected that, as with proinsulin and the corticotropin-endorphin precursor, physiologically "extraneous" peptides may be generated during posttranslational processing of the precursor. The nature of these peptides is unknown at present.

Conversion of these precursors appears to occur in the secretory granules during axonal transport [61, 62]. Given this site of conversion, one would expect that the unknown peptides would also be released during the stimulus-induced exocytosis of the neurophysins and their respective nonapeptides. A hypothetical model of a peptidergic neuron is illustrated in Fig. 14-5.

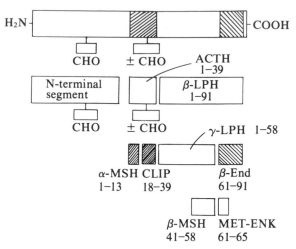

Fig. 14-4. *Structure of the corticotropin-lipotropin (endorphin) precursor, showing the biologically active peptide products that are theoretically possible.*

Secretion of Neuropeptides

The neuropeptide secretion mechanism appears to be similar to that of conventional neurotransmitter secretion [64]. Most studies on the mechanism of neuropeptide secretion have focused on the neural lobe of the posterior pituitary [64]. The principle events in the release of neuropeptides occur as follows: The propagated action potential depolarizes the nerve terminal and induces an influx of Ca^{2+}, which produces exocytosis and extrusion of secretory granule (or vesicle) contents into the extracellular space. The dependence of the stimulus-secretion coupling on extracellular calcium is well established [65, 66], and various morphological features of the exocytotic process have been visualized in freeze-fracture studies [67]. Retrieval of the granule membranes after exocytosis is in large vacuoles [68, 69], but, in contrast to cholinergic terminals, where recycling of vesicle membrane occurs (Chap. 8), little is known at present about the fates of the retrieved peptidergic granule membranes.

In view of the above information about the calcium dependency of peptide secretion from nerve terminals, this feature of the basic mechanism has been used as a criterion for the physiological

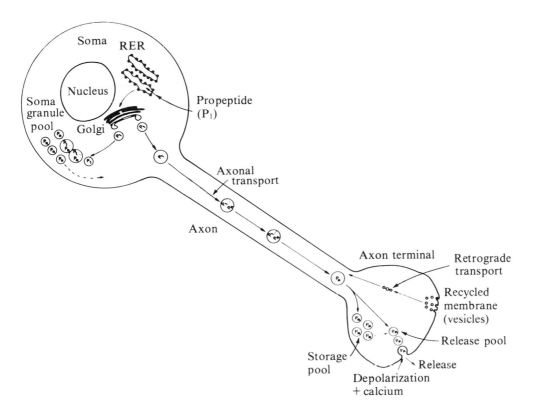

Fig. 14-5. Hypothetical model of biosynthesis, translocation, processing, and release of peptides in a peptidergic neuron. RER, rough endoplasmic reticulum; P_1, propeptide or precursor molecule; $P_1 \ldots P_n$, intermediates between P_1 and P_n; (P_n), final peptide products of processing. (From Mains et al., Proc. Natl. Acad. Sci. U.S.A. *74:3014–3018, 1977.)*

relevance of stimulation-induced release of peptides from a variety of experimental preparations. The release experiments are usually performed on either thin tissue slices, or blocks, or on synaptosomes, isolated nerve endings, prepared from a specific brain area and incubated in a well-oxygenated physiological medium. After an initial washing of the tissue by repeated changes of medium, the stimulus is given. The stimulus may be field electrical stimulation, depolarization by an excess of K^+ or by the addition of veratridine (Na^+ channel activation) to the medium. In all cases, removal of Ca^{2+} from the medium should prevent secretion of the peptides. In some cases, the membrane depolarization step is bypassed by direct application of a Ca^{2+} ionophore (e.g., A23187), which causes an increase in intracellular Ca^{2+}, and thus induces exocytosis. In some cases, release experiments can be done in the intact animal by using either push-pull cannulae in specific brain regions [70], or by monitoring the CSF for peptide release after specific brain areas have been stimulated. Examples of such paradigms are given in Table 14-6.

The temporal pattern of release in vivo, although poorly understood, is significant. There is a tendency for peptidergic neurosecretory cells to fire in bursts, each burst followed by inactivity. This suggests that the periodicity is particularly efficacious for secretory activity in these cells [71]. The periodicity may also be important to the target organ; this has been elegantly demonstrated in a recent study [72] in which monkeys with hypothalamic lesions that abolish LH and FSH release

Table 14-6. Neuropeptide Secretion

Peptide	Experimental Preparation	Stimulus	Footnote Reference
Substance P	Hemisected rat spinal cord	Electrical (lumbar roots) K^+ depolarization	A
Substance P	Rat hypothalamic slices	K^+ depolarization	B
Somatostatin	Rat hypothalamic slices	K^+ depolarization, Ca^{2+} ionophore	C
CRF	Rat hypothalamic synaptosomes	Electrical field stimulation	D
Enkephalin	Rat globus pallidus slices	K^+ depolarization	E, F
Enkephalin	Human CSF, in vivo	Periventricular brain site electrical stimulation	G
β-Endorphin	Human CSF, in vivo	Periaqueductal gray electrical stimulation	H

A. Otsuka, M., and Konishi, S. *Nature* 264:83–84, 1976.
B. Jessell, T., Iversen, L. L., and Kanazawa, I. *Nature* 264:81–83, 1976.
C. Berelowitz, M., et al. *J. Neurochem.* 31:1537–1539, 1978.
D. Edwardson, J. A., and Bennett, G. W. *Nature* 251:425–427, 1974.
E. Iversen, L. L., et al. *Nature* 271:679–681, 1978.
F. Bayon, A., et al. *Proc. Natl. Acad. Sci. U.S.A.* 75:3503–3506, 1978.
G. Akil, H., et al. *Science* 201:463–465, 1978.
H. Hosobuchi, Y., et al. *Science* 203:279–281, 1979.

by the pituitary were infused with LHRH. Constant infusion of LHRH failed to restore LH and FSH secretion, whereas once-hourly infusion of LHRH reestablished normal hormone release. Thus, the cyclic pattern of LHRH delivery to the target organ was more important than the amount delivered. We suggest that the intermittent delivery may avoid "down-regulation" or "desensitization" of the LHRH receptors in the target tissue.

Inactivation Mechanisms

The time course and extent of neurotransmitter action is determined, in part, by the mechanisms involved in the reduction of the neurotransmitter concentration around the receptor. This can occur either by diffusion of the substance away from the receptor; reuptake by the presynaptic terminals or surrounding glia, or both (as for the catecholamines and GABA); or by enzymatic degradation of the substance (analogous to acetylcholine-

esterase action on acetylcholine). Thus far, there have been no convincing data to indicate that reuptake of neuropeptides takes place, and enzymatic degradation appears to be the principle mechanism for inactivation of neuropeptides.

The classification of tissue proteinases (and peptidases) is in flux, and several alternative schemes have been proposed. In general, proteolytic enzymes are described as either exopeptidases or endopeptidases (proteinases). Exopeptidases hydrolyze peptides from either their C- or N-terminal regions by removal of single amino acids (or dipeptides). Endopeptidases cleave internal bonds of proteins and peptides. They often show specificity with regard to the nature of the peptide bond—for example, trypsin hydrolyzes exclusively at basic amino acid, lysine, and arginine residues—but rarely are specific to only one substrate. The reason probably is that the specificity of limited proteolysis is determined by the three-dimensional structure (conformation) of the peptide substrate *and* of the protease [73]. The substrate region containing the susceptible peptide bond must match the active site of the enzyme for hydrolysis to occur. Thus, proteases may degrade diverse substrates with conformational homologies, much as receptors will bind diverse substances with common conformations (e.g., morphine and enkephalin).

Keeping the above caveats about protease specificity in mind, we note with interest that enzymes that show selective degradation of various biologically active peptides have been found in various tissues, including brain (see Table 14-7). Many of the neuropeptides in Table 14-7 have groups blocked by N-terminal acetylation, C-terminal amidation, or by addition of N-terminal pyroglutamate. These prevent the action of exopeptidases. Therefore, relatively specific endopeptidases are involved in their degradation.

Peptide Receptors

A great deal can be learned about the affinity and specificity of a biological receptor for its natural ligand by means of dose-response measurements either in the whole animal or in isolated organs in vitro. Alternatively, binding of radiolabeled agonists or antagonists to whole cells, suspension of plasma membranes, or solubilized membrane components can be studied. The last-named are fast and relatively simple to perform and, additionally, serve as a first step in receptor purification. They must be undertaken cautiously, however, because not all binding is to biologically relevant sites (i.e., receptors). Several criteria must be satisfied to establish that the interaction of a ligand with any given preparation represents binding to a receptor (Table 14-8).

Ideally, the binding studies should be conducted first in a homogeneous population of viable cells. In this way, quantitative comparisons between binding and biological effects can be made. The activation of a ligand-dependent, membrane-localized enzyme, such as adenylate cyclase or phosphatidylethanolamine *N*-methyltransferase, might be measured at the same time that binding is determined. Similar sets of parallel measurements

can sometimes be made on isolated membrane preparations, but there is no guarantee that ligand-induced modulation of enzyme activity is the same in the intact cell as it is in an isolated membrane.

It should be obvious that intact, homogeneous cells cannot easily be obtained from the brain for direct comparisons of binding and biological activity. Nevertheless, it is possible to compare binding of a variety of agonists and antagonists and, in this way, to determine the structural specificity of central binding sites. Thus, most of the criteria listed in Table 14-8 can be met. To the extent that cells or membranes harvested from the central nervous system are heterogeneous, though, little can be learned by comparing receptor contents of different brain regions. Meaningful comparisons of this sort can be made only by isolating purified populations of plasma membranes from cells and measuring the number of receptors per milligram of membrane.

Only a few of the biologically active peptides characterized to date have been successfully labeled and used in binding studies. This is due to several common problems encountered in studies of peptide receptors: (1) difficulties in labeling the peptide may occur; iodinated peptide may be inactive (e.g., TRH, LHRH, substance P); tritiation may prove difficult or may yield a product with too low a specific activity; (2) enzymatic degradation of the labeled peptide may take place; and (3) the half-life of the peptide-receptor complex may be so short that the bound ligand cannot be separated from the unbound.

Solutions to these problems have been found for a few peptides. Insulin [74], for example, can be iodinated without losing its biological activity, and its degradation by peptidases in membrane preparations can be inhibited by bacitracin. Although the density of insulin receptors on cells is low, specific binding of insulin to cells and membranes can be detected by using radioiodinated insulin (1,000 Ci/mmole). It would be difficult, if not impossible, to study insulin binding by using a tritiated ligand, but tritiated ligands have been used successfully to study other classes of receptors, among them the receptors for the opioid peptides (Chap. 13). These

Table 14-7. Peptidases in Brain and Other Tissues

Peptide Substrate	Tissue Source of Peptidase	Footnote Reference
Insulin	Liver	C, D
Glucagon	Liver	C, E
Bradykinin	Brain, liver, kidney, lung, etc.	F, G
Angiotensin	Liver, brain	A, B, H
TRH	Blood plasma	I
	Brain, pituitary	A, J, K
LHRH	Hypothalamus	L, M
	Whole brain	N
Somatostatin	Brain	O, P
Substance P	Brain, hypothalamus	P, Q
Neurotensin	Brain homogenate	A
MIF	Blood, brain, kidney	R
	Hypothalamus, pituitary	S
Vasopressin	Kidney	A, T
Oxytocin	Brain	U
	Uterus, brain, kidney, blood	V, W
MSH	Brain	A
ACTH		
Opiate peptides		

A. Marks, N. In H. Gainer (ed.), *Peptides and Neurobiology.* New York: Plenum, 1977. Pp. 221–258.
B. Marks, N. In A. Lajtha (ed.), *Handbook of Neurochemistry.* Vol. 3. New York: Plenum, 1970. Pp. 133–171.
C. Ansorge, S., et al. *Eur. J. Biochem.* 19:283–288, 1971.
D. Burghen, G. A., Kitabchi, A. E., and Brush, J. S. *Endocrinology* 91:633–642, 1972.
E. McDonald, J. K., et al. *J. Biol. Chem.* 244:6199–6208, 1969.
F. Camargo, A. C. M., Ramalho-Pinto, F. J., and Green, L. J. *J. Neurochem.* 19:37–49, 1972.
G. Cicilini, M. A., et al. *Biochem. J.* 163:433–439, 1977.
H. McDonald, J. K., et al. *J. Biol. Chem.* 249:234–240, 1974.
I. Neary, J. T., et al. *Science* 193:403–405, 1976.
J. Mudge, A. W., and Fellows, R. E. Bovine pituitary pyrrolidone carboxylpeptidase. *Endocrinology* 93:1428–1434, 1973.
K. Prasad, C., and Peterkofsky, A. *J. Biol. Chem.* 251:3229–3234, 1976.
L. Griffiths, E. C., et al. *Brain Res.* 85:161–164, 1975.
M. Koch, Y., et al. *Biochem. Biophys. Res. Commun.* 61:95–103, 1974.
N. Marks, N., and Stern, F. *Biochem. Biophys. Res. Commun.* 61:1458–1463, 1974.
O. Marks, N., and Stern, F. *FEBS Lett.* 55:220–224, 1975.
P. Akopyan, T. N., et al. *J. Neurochem.* 32:629–631, 1979.
Q. Benuck, M., and Marks, N. *Biochem. Biophys. Res. Commun.* 65:153–160, 1975.
R. Walter, R., Nerdle, A., and Marks, N. *Soc. Exp. Biol. Med.* 148:98–103, 1975.
S. Marks, N., et al. *J. Neurochem.* 22:735–739, 1974.
T. Levi, J., Rosenfeld, S., and Kleeman, C. R. *J. Endocrinol.* 62:1–10, 1974.
U. Hooper, K. C., and Hopkinson, C. R. N. *Acta Endocrinol.* 75:636–646, 1974.
V. Walter, R., et al. *Science* 173:827–829, 1971.
W. Walter, R., and Simmons, W. H. In A. M. Moses and L. Share (eds.), *Neurohypophysis.* Basel: Karger, 1976. Pp. 167–188.

Table 14-8. Characteristics of
Ligand-Receptor Interactions

Biological activity
  The labeled ligand should have the same biological
  potency as its unlabeled parent compound
High affinity
  Concentrations of ligand as low as those that are bio-
  logically effective should specifically bind to receptors
Reversibility
  Agonists with rapidly reversible biological actions
  should dissociate rapidly from their binding sites
Structural or steric specificity
  Binding of a labeled ligand and displacement of this
  ligand by other agonists or antagonists should quan-
  titatively reflect the biological potencies of the agonists
  and antagonists treated
Saturability
  A biologically relevant concentration of ligand should
  saturate specific binding sites

are unique, in that they can be occupied by members
of a large group of well-characterized, nonpeptide agonists and antagonists. Labeled antagonists
with high affinities for the opiate receptor and with
conveniently long receptor-antagonist half-lives
have been used in lieu of the peptides to study
binding sites in the brain and elsewhere.

More and more superpotent, nondegraded peptide agonists and antagonists are being synthesized.
Some of these should prove useful ligands for
binding studies.

Peptides and Neuronal Function
Although it is apparent that hypothalamic peptides
are physiologically important messengers in the
regulation of the anterior pituitary (see Regulation
of Anterior Pituitary Function), the situation for
the rest of the brain is less clear. Extensive pharmacological evidence suggests that there are a variety
of peptide receptors in extrahypothalamic areas.
In addition, exposure of the nervous system to
specific peptides often produces profound changes
in the biochemistry and physiology of the nervous
system as well as specific modifications of behavior
(see Table 14-9). Immunocytochemical procedures

can demonstrate that neurons containing biologically active peptides are distributed throughout the brain. Nevertheless, it is still not possible
to state whether peptides play a unique role in
neural function.

Can neuropeptides act as neurotransmitters? The
work on proctolin, an insect neuropeptide [14],
suggests that they can. Although the criteria for
the identification of a neurotransmitter are well
established (Chap. 8), it is often difficult to satisfy
them in any specific case. The case of substance P is
instructive. Although substance P fulfilled many of
the desiderata of a candidate for primary afferent
transmitter [10], its time course of action was too
slow in comparison to natural afferent activity, and
hence, its candidacy as the primary afferent transmitter was not credible. However, recent evidence
suggests substance P might be associated specifically with slower-conducting fibers in pain pathways [75]. The point is that unless the neural
circuit, in which the peptide may be involved, is
understood and amenable to experimental analysis,
it is extremely difficult to evaluate the status of any
putative transmitter. Because of this difficulty, and
because the morphology of peptidergic synapse is
poorly understood, the term *neuromodulatory* is
often ascribed to a peptide's action. It should be
apparent that the criteria for identification of
"neuromodulators" are identical to those of neurotransmitters and that the use of this term does not
obviate the necessity for rigorous analysis of the
action mechanisms of the substance in question.
Whether neuromodulators and neurotransmitters
are distinct entities is still a matter of debate.

To evaluate the physiological role of a peptide or
any other chemical substance, it is necessary first
to identify the neural circuit and critical synapse(s)
where the peptide is acting. Given this information,
a physiological analysis of its mechanisms of action
(see Table 14-10) is then possible.

Ten years after von Euler showed (1946) that
norepinephrine is the transmitter released by
sympathetic neurons, interest in that monoamine
began to grow rapidly. Several things contributed
to this growth: the introduction of the fluorescence

Table 14-9. Peptide Actions in the Nervous System

Peptide	Action	Footnote References
Substance P	Depolarizes motor neurons	A(1–3)
	Excites cuneate neurons	A4
	Excites Betz cells	A5
	Depolarizes mesenteric neurons	A6
	Excitatory in A10 dopaminergic area	A7
	Modulates somatostatin release	A8
	Involved in Huntington's disease	A9
Neurotensin	Modulates release of growth hormone, prolactin, TRH	B1
	Hypothermia, neurotransmitter modulation	B2, 3
TRH	Influences psychomotor action of L-dopa (Parkinson's disease)	A9; I1
	Depresses CNS neuron firing	A9; C1, 2
	Influences turnover of catecholamines, serotonin and acetylcholine	A9; B3
LHRH	Initiates mating behavior, lordosis	A9; D1, 2
	Depresses CNS neuron firing	A9; C2
Angiotensin	Intraventricular injection: pressor response	E1, 2
	Dipsogenic action	E3, 4
	Releases ADH	E5
	Increases firing rates of subfornical and SON neurons	E6, 7
	Increases turnover of acetylcholine	B3
	Presynaptic facilitation	E8
	Involved in Huntington's disease	A9
Bradykinin	CNS injection: motor excitation, sedation	F1, 2
	Excites peripheral nerve terminals	F3
Bombesin	Hypothermia, hyperglycemia	A9; G1, 2
	Inhibits TRH secretion	
Oxytocin	Modifies hypothalamic neuron firing	H1, 2
Vasopressin	Induces pacemaker activity	H3, 4
	Attenuation of amnesia	H5
	Influences learning, memory	H6–8
MIF	Potentiates L-dopa antagonism of oxotremorine-induced tremors	I1–3
	Influences memory	A9; H5
ACTH	Effects on conditioned avoidance	H8
MSH	Involved in Parkinson's disease	A9
	Tropic hormone in fetus (MSH)	J1
	ACTH intracerebral produces hyperactivity	J2
	Modulates behavior	H8; J3, 4
	Influences dopamine turnover	J5
Endogenous opiates (enkephalin, endorphin)	Analgesia influences behavior	A9; J2
	Antidiuretic effects	K1
	Heat adaptation	K2
	Inhibits somatostatin release	A8
	Depresses dorsal horn potentials	K3

A 1. Konishi, S., and Otsuka, M. *Brain Res.* 65:397–410, 1974.
  2. Konishi, S., and Otsuka, M. *Nature* 252:734–735, 1974.

histochemical technique for monoamines; the development of sensitive and specific assays for catecholamines and the enzymes involved in their synthesis and metabolism; the availability of radiolabeled norepinephrine and of radiolabeled sympathetic agonists and antagonists; and the synthesis of a variety of drugs that could be used as probes of sympathetic function. A wealth of new data about catecholamines in central and peripheral nerves was generated in the 1960s and 1970s and contributed to a flourishing of ideas.

Today, neurochemists are as excited about neuropeptides as they were about monoamines in the early 1960s. This is in part because the peptides are so potent biologically, and in part because they are present in discrete systems of neurons. Undoubtedly many peptides remain to be discovered and characterized. In fact, the number of peptides

Table 14-9 (Continued)

    3. Otsuka, M., Konishi, S., and Takahashi, T. *Proc. Jpn. Acad.* 48:342–346, 1972.
    4. Krjnevic, K., and Morris, M. *Can. J. Physiol. Pharmacol.* 52:736–744, 1974.
    5. Phillis, J. W., and Limacher, J. J. *Brain Res.* 69:158–163, 1974.
    6. Katayama, Y., and North, R. A. *Nature* 274:387–388, 1978.
    7. Stinus, L., Kelley, A. E., and Iversen, S. D. *Nature* 276:616–618, 1978.
    8. Sheppard, M. C., Kronheim, S., and Pimstone, B. L. *J. Neurochem.* 32:647–649, 1979.
    9. See ref. 75.
B 1. Maeda, K., and Frohman, L. A. *Endocrinology* 103:1903–1909, 1978.
    2. Bissette, G., et al. *Life Sci.* 23:2173–2182, 1978.
    3. Malthe-Sorenssen, D., et al. *J. Neurochem.* 31:685–691, 1978.
C 1. Reneaud, L. P., and Martin, J. B. *Brain Res.* 86:150–154, 1975.
    2. Reneaud, L. P., Martin, J. B., and Brazeau, P. *Nature* 255:233–235.
D 1. Moss, R. L., and McCann, S. M. *Science* 181:177–179.
    2. Pfaff, D. W. *Science* 182:1148–1149, 1973.
E 1. Bickerton, R. K., and Buckley, J. P. *Proc. Soc. Exp. Biol. Med.* 106:834–836, 1961.
    2. Smookler, H. H., et al. *J. Pharmacol. Exp. Ther.* 153:485–494, 1966.
    3. Epstein, A. N., Fitzsimons, J. T., and Rolls, B. J. *J. Physiol.* (London) 210:457–474, 1970.
    4. Simpson, J. B., and Routtenberg, A. *Science* 181:1172–1175, 1973.
    5. Peck, J. W., and Epstein, A. N. *Fed. Proc.* 30:113, 1971.
    6. Felix, D., and Akert, K. *Brain Res.* 76:350–353, 1974.
    7. Nicoll, R. A., and Barker, J. L. *Nat. New Biol.* 233:172–174, 1971.
    8. Lokhandwala, M. F., Amelang, E., and Buckley, J. P. *Eur. J. Pharmacol.* 52:405–409, 1978.
F 1. DaSilva, G. R., and Rocha e Silva, M. *Eur. J. Pharmacol.* 15:180–186, 1971.
    2. Krauthamer, G. M., and Whitaker, A. H. *Brain Res.* 80:141–145, 1974.
    3. Franz, M., and Mense, S. *Brain Res.* 92:369–383, 1975.
G 1. Brown, M., Rivier, J., and Vale, W. *Science* 196:998–1000, 1977.
    2. Moody, T. W., et al. *Proc. Natl. Acad. Sci. U.S.A.* 75:5372–5376, 1978.
H 1. Moss, R. L., Dyball, R. E. J., and Cross, B. A. *Exp. Neurol.* 34:95–102, 1972.
    2. Nicoll, R. A., and Barker, J. L. *Brain Res.* 35:501–511, 1971.
    3. Barker, J. L., and Gainer, H. *Science* 184:1371–1373, 1974.
    4. Barker, J. L., Ifshin, M. S., and Gainer, H. *Brain Res.* 84:501–513, 1975.
    5. Flexner, J. B., et al. *Brain Res.* 134:139–144, 1977.
    6. Greidamus, T. B. W., and DeWied, D. *Behav. Biol.* 18:325–333, 1976.
    7. Greidamus, T. B. W., Bohus, B., DeWied, D. *Prog. Brain Res.* 42:135–141, 1975.
    8. DeWied, D., and Gispen, W. H. In H. Gainer (ed.), *Peptides in Neurobiology.* New York: Plenum, 1977. Pp. 397–448.
I 1. Castensson, S., et al. *FEBS Lett.* 44:101–105, 1974.
    2. Plotnikoff, N. P., et al. *Life Sci.* 10:1279–1283, 1971.
    3. Plotnikoff, N. P., et al. *Proc. Soc. Exp. Biol. Med.* 140:811, 1972.
J 1. Challis, J. R. G., and Torosis, J. D. *Nature* 269:818–819, 1977.
    2. Jacquet, Y. F. *Science* 201:1032–1034, 1978.
    3. Martin, J. T. *Science* 200:565–567, 1978.
    4. Gispen, W. H., et al. *Life Sci.* 17:645–652, 1976.
    5. Lichtensteyer, W., Lienhart, R., and Kopp, H. G. *Psychoneuroendocrinology* 2:237–248, 1977.
K 1. Tseng, L. F., Loh, H. H., Li, C. H. *Int. J. Pept. Protein Res.* 12:173–176, 1978.
    2. Holaday, J. W., et al. *Proc. Natl. Acad. Sci. U.S.A.* 75:2923–2927, 1978.
    3. Crain, S. M., et al. *Brain Res.* 157:196–201, 1978.

Table 14-10. Potential Sites and Mechanisms
of Neuropeptide Action

I. Acts as a conventional neurotransmitter in a synaptic pathway
II. Influences a synaptic pathway by its:
  A. Presynaptic action:
    1. Effects amount and time course of transmitter release
    2. Effects transmitter reuptake at synapse
    3. Alters "releasable" and "nonreleasable" transmitter pools
    4. Effects transmitter biosynthesis
  B. Postsynaptic action on receptor:
    1. Alters receptor sensitivity
    2. Effects receptor-ionophore coupling
      a. Kinetics
      b. Specific ionic conductances
  C. Effects on electrogenesis:
    1. Change in electrically excitable membrane properties
      a. Resting conductance
      b. Spike threshold
      c. Intracellular electrical resistance (length constant)
      d. Current-voltage relations of membrane
      e. Coupling resistance at electrotonic junctions
      f. Alters electrogenic pump activity
    2. Excitation-coupled phenomena
      a. Muscle contraction
      b. Metabolic processes

---

2 to 10 amino acids long that might theoretically exist is astronomical ($>10^{13}$). There are 10^{10} neurons in the human brain, so it is easy to imagine—although this is unlikely—that each neuron makes its own unique peptide.

References

1. Scharrer, E. Die Lichtempfindlichkeit blinder Erlitzen (Untersuchungen über das Zwischenhirn der Fische. I.). *Z. Vergleich. Physiol.* 7:1–38, 1928.
2. Bargmann, W., Lindner, E., and Andres, K. H. Über Synapsen an endokrinen Epithelzellen und die Definition sekretorischer Neurone. Untersuchungen am Zwischenlappen der Katzenhypophyse. *Z. Zellforsch.* 77:282–298, 1967.
3. Zetler, G. The peptidergic neuron: A working hypothesis. *Biochem. Pharmacol.* 25:1817–1818, 1976.

*Key reference.

4. Scharrer, B. Peptidergic neurons: facts and trends. *Gen. Comp. Endocrinol.* 34:50–62, 1978.
*5. Fink, G. The development of the releasing factor concept. *Clin. Endocrinol.* 5 (Suppl.):245s–260s, 1976.
*6. Guillemin, R. Peptides in the brain: The new endocrinology of the neuron. *Science* 202:390–402, 1978.
*7. Schally, A. V. Aspects of hypothalamic regulation of the pituitary gland. *Science* 202:18–28, 1978.
*8. Guillemin, R. The expanding significance of hypothalamic peptides, or, is endocrinology a branch of neuroendocrinology? *Prog. Horm. Res.* 33:1–28, 1977.
9. Von Euler, U. S., and Gaddum, J. H. An unidentified depressor substance in certain tissue extracts. *J. Physiol.* (London) 72:74–87, 1931.
10. Leeman, S., and Mroz, E. A. Substance P. *Life Sci.* 15:2033–2044, 1974.
11. Frontali, N., and Gainer, H. Peptides in Invertebrate Nervous Systems. In H. Gainer (ed.), *Peptides in Neurobiology.* New York: Plenum, 1977. Pp. 259–294.
12. Fernlund, P., and Josefsson, L. H. Crustacean color-change hormone: Amino acid sequence and chemical synthesis. *Science* 177:173–175, 1972.
13. Stone, J. V., et al. Structure of locust adipokinetic hormone, a neurohormone that regulates lipid utilization during flight. *Nature* 263:207–211, 1976.
14. Starratt, A. N. Proctolin, an insect neuropeptide. *Trends Neurosci.* 2:15–17, 1979.
15. Pearse, A. G. E. Peptides in brain and intestine. *Nature* 262:92–93, 1976.
*16. Pearse, A. G. E., and Takor, T. T. Neuroendocrine embryology and the APUD concept. *Clin. Endocrinol.* (Oxf.) 5 (Suppl.): 229s–244s, 1976.
17. Tischler, A. S., et al. Neural properties of cultured human endocrine tumor cells of proposed neural crest origin. *Science* 192:902–904, 1976.
18. Gainer, H. (ed.). *Peptides in Neurobiology.* New York: Plenum, 1977.
19. Porter, J. C. (ed.). Hypothalamic peptide hormones and pituitary regulation. *Adv. Exp. Med. Biol.* Vol. 87. New York: Plenum, 1977.
20. Costa, E., and Trabucchi, M. (eds.). *The Endorphins. Adv. Biochem. Psychopharmacol.* Vol. 18. New York: Raven Press, 1978.
21. Gotto, A. M. (ed.). *Brain Peptides.* New York: Elsevier North-Holland, 1979.
22. Acher, R., and Fromageot, P. The Relationship of Oxytocin and Vasopressin to Active Proteins. In H. Heller (ed.), *The Neurohypophysis.* London: Butterworth, 1957. Pp. 39–50.
23. Mains, R. E., Eipper, B. A., and Ling, N. Com-

mon precursor to corticotropins and endorphins. *Proc. Natl. Acad. Sci. U.S.A.* 74:3014–3018, 1977.

24. Green, J. D., and Harris, G. W. The neurovascular link between the neurohypophysis and adenohypophysis. *J. Endocrinol.* 5:136–146, 1947.

25. Bøler, J., et al. The identity of chemical and hormonal properties of the thyrotropin-releasing hormone and pyroglutamylhistidylprolineamide. *Biochem. Biophys. Res. Commun.* 37:705–710, 1969.

26. Burgus, R., et al. Structure moleculaire du facteur hypothalamique TRH d'origine ovine: Mise en evidence par spectrometrie de masse de la sequence pGlu-His-Pro-NH$_2$. *C. R. Acad. Sci. [D]* (Paris) 269:1870–1873, 1969.

27. Matsuo, H., et al. Structure of the porcine LH- and FSH-releasing hormone. I. The proposed amino acid sequence. *Biochem. Biophys. Res. Commun.* 43:1334–1339, 1971.

28. Burgus, R., et al. Structure moleculaire du facteur hypothalamique (LRF) d'origine ovine controlant la secretion de l'hormone de goandotrope hypophysaire de luteinisation. *C. R. Acad. Sci. [D]* (Paris) 273:1611–1613, 1971.

29. Brazeau, P., et al. Hypothalamic peptide that inhibits the secretion of immunoreactive pituitary growth hormone. *Science* 179:77–79, 1973.

30. Harris, G. W. Humours and hormones. *J. Endocrinol.* 53:ii–xiii, 1972.

31. Leeman, S. E., Mroz, E. A., and Carraway, R. Substance P and Neurotensin. In H. Gainer (ed.), *Peptides in Neurobiology*. New York: Plenum, 1977. Pp. 99–144.

*32. Yalow, R. S. Radioimmunoassay: A probe for the fine structure of biological systems. *Science* 200: 1236–1242, 1978.

33. Sternberger, L. A. Immunocytochemistry of neuropeptides and their receptors. In H. Gainer (ed.), *Peptides in Neurobiology*. New York: Plenum, 1977. Pp. 61–97.

34. Petrusz, P., et al. Specificity in immunocytochemical staining. *J. Histochem. Cytochem.* 24: 1110–1115, 1976.

35. Swaab, D. F., Pool, C. W., and Van Leeuwen, F. W. Can specificity ever be proved in immunocytochemical staining? *J. Histochem. Cytochem.* 25: 388–389, 1977.

36. Moss, R. L. Role of hypophysiotropic neurohormones in mediating neural and behavioral events. *Fed. Proc.* 36:1978–1983, 1977.

37. Lembeck, F. Zur Frage der zentralen Übertragung afferenter Impulse. III. Mitteilung. Das Vorkommen und die Bedeutung der Substanz P in den dorsalen Wurzeln des Ruckenmarks. *Naunyn-Schmiedebergs Arch. Exp. Path. Pharmak.* 219: 197–213, 1953.

38. Hokfelt, T., et al. Occurrence of somatostatin-like immunoreactivity in some peripheral sympathetic noradrenergic neurons. *Proc. Natl. Acad. Sci. U.S.A.* 74:3587–3591, 1977.

39. Chan-Palay, V., Jonsson, G., and Palay, S. L. On the coexistence of serotonin and substance P in neurons of the rat's central nervous system. *Proc. Natl. Acad. Sci. U.S.A.* 75:1582–1586, 1978.

40. Hokfelt, T., et al. Immunohistochemical evidence of substance P-like immunoreactivity in some 5-hydroxytryptamine–containing neurons in the rat central nervous system. *Neuroscience* 3: 517–538, 1978.

41. Youngblood, W. W., Lipton, M. A., and Kizer, J. S. TRH-like immunoreactivity in urine, serum, and extrahypothalamic brain: Non-identity with synthetic Pyroglu-Hist-Pro-(NH$_2$) (TRH). *Brain Res.* 151:99–116, 1978.

42. Steiner, D. F., and Oyer, P. E. The biosynthesis of insulin and a probable precursor of insulin by a human islet cell adenoma. *Proc. Natl. Acad. Sci. U.S.A.* 57:473–480, 1967.

43. Steiner, D. F. Insulin today. *Diabetes* 26:322–340, 1976.

44. Rubinstein, A. H., et al. Clinical significance of circulating proinsulin and C-peptide. *Recent Prog. Horm. Res.* 33:435–475, 1977.

45. Palade, G. Intracellular aspects of the process of protein synthesis. *Science* 189:347–358, 1975.

46. Habener, J. F., and Kronenberg, H. M. Parathyroid hormone biosynthesis: Structure and function of biosynthetic precursors. *Fed. Proc.* 37:2561–2566, 1978.

47. Berger, E. A., and Shooter, E. M. Evidence for pro-B-nerve growth factor, a biosynthetic precursor to B-nerve growth factor. *Proc. Natl. Acad. Sci. U.S.A.* 74:3647–3651, 1977.

48. Mobley, W. C., et al. Nerve growth factor. *N. Engl. J. Med.* 297:1096–1104, 1977.

49. Orenstein, N. S., et al. Nerve growth factor: A protease that can activate plasminogen. *Proc. Natl. Acad. Sci. U.S.A.* 75:5497–5500, 1978.

50. Yalow, R. S., and Berson, S. A. Characteristics of "big ACTH" in human plasma and pituitary extracts. *J. Clin. Endocrinol. Metab.* 36:415–423, 1973.

51. Scott, A. P., et al. Pituitary peptide. *Nat. New Biol.* 244:65–67, 1973.

52. Roberts, J. L., and Herbert, E. Characterization of a common precursor to corticotropin and β-lipotropin: Identification of β-lipotropin peptides and their arrangement relative to corticotropin in

the precursor synthesized in a cell free system. *Proc. Natl. Acad. Sci. U.S.A.* 74:5300–5304, 1977.

53. Eipper, B. A., and Mains, R. E. Existence of a common precursor to ACTH and endorphin in the anterior and intermediate lobes of the rat pituitary. *J. Supramol. Struct.* 8:247–262, 1978.

54. Loh, Y. P. Immunological evidence for two common precursors to corticotropins, endorphins, and melanotropin in the neurointermediate lobe of the toad pituitary. *Proc. Natl. Acad. Sci. U.S.A.* 76:796–800, 1979.

55. Roberts, J. L., and Herbert, E. Characterization of a common precursor to corticotropin and β-lipotropin: Cell-free synthesis of the precursor and identification of corticotropin peptides in the molecule. *Proc. Natl. Acad. Sci. U.S.A.* 74:4826–4830, 1977.

56. Nakanishi, S., et al. A large product of cell-free translation of messenger-RNA coding for corticotropin. *Proc. Natl. Acad. Sci. U.S.A.* 73:4319–4323, 1976.

57. Loh, Y. P., and Gainer, H. The role of glycosylation in the biosynthesis, degradation, and secretion of the ACTH-lipotropin common precursor and its peptide products. *FEBS Lett.* 96:269–272, 1978.

58. Nakanishi, S., et al. Nucleotide sequence of cloned cDNA for bovine corticotropin-β-lipotropin precursor. *Nature* 278:423–427, 1979.

59. Sachs, H., and Takabatake, Y. Evidence for a precursor in vasopressin biosynthesis. *Endocrinology* 75:943–948, 1964.

60. Pickering, B. T., and Jones, C. W. The Neurophysins. In C. H. Li (ed.), *Hormonal Proteins and Peptides*. New York: Academic, 1978. Pp. 103–158.

61. Gainer, H., Sarne, Y., and Brownstein, M. J. Neurophysin biosynthesis: Conversion of a putative precursor during axonal transport. *Science* 195:1354–1356, 1977.

62. Gainer, H., Sarne, Y., and Brownstein, M. J. Biosynthesis and axonal transport of rat neurohypophysial proteins and peptides. *J. Cell Biol.* 73:366–381, 1977.

63. Brownstein, M. J., Robinson, A. G., and Gainer, H. Immunological identification of rat neurophysin precursors. *Nature* 269:259–261, 1977.

64. Douglas, W. W. How do neurones secrete peptides? Exocytosis and its consequences, including "synaptic" vesicle formation, in the hypothalamoneurohypophysial system. *Prog. Brain Res.* 39:21–39, 1973.

65. Dreifuss, J. J. A review of neurosecretory granules: Their contents and mechanisms of release. *Ann. N.Y. Acad. Sci.* 248:181–201, 1975.

66. Thorn, N., et al. Calcium and neurosecretion. *Ann. N.Y. Acad. Sci.* 307:618–639, 1978.

67. Theodosis, D. T., Dreifuss, J. J., and Orci, L. A freeze-fracture study of membrane events during neurohypophysial secretion. *J. Cell Biol.* 78:542–553, 1978.

68. Nordman, J. J., and Morris, J. F. Membrane retrieval at neurosecretory axon endings. *Nature* 261:723–725, 1976.

69. Theodosis, D. T., et al. Secretion-related uptake of horseradish peroxidase in neurohypophysial axons. *J. Cell Biol.* 70:294–303, 1976.

70. Gaddum, J. H. Push-pull cannulae. *J. Physiol.* (London) 155:1–2, 1961.

71. Gainer, H. Input-Output Relations of Neurosecretory Cells. In P. J. Gaillard and H. H. Boer (eds.), *Comparative Endocrinology*. New York: Elsevier North-Holland, 1978. Pp. 293–304.

72. Belchetz, P. E., et al. Hypophysial responses to continuous and intermittent delivery of hypothalamic gonadotropin-releasing hormone. *Science* 202:631–633, 1978.

73. Neurath, H., and Walsh, K. A. Role of proteolytic enzymes in biological regulation (a review). *Proc. Natl. Acad. Sci. U.S.A.* 73:3825–3832, 1976.

74. Cuatrecasas, P. Insulin receptor of liver and fat cell membranes. *Fed. Proc.* 32:1838–1846, 1973.

75. Collu, R., et al. (eds.). *Central Nervous System Effects of Hypothalamic Hormones and Other Peptides*. New York: Raven Press, 1979.

References Related to CNS Peptide

LHRH

Immunocytochemical Evidence

Barry, J., and Carette, B. *Cell Tissue Res.* 164:163–178, 1975; Barry, J., Dubois, M. P., and Carette, B. *Endocrinology* 95:1416–1423, 1974; Barry, J., Dubois, M. P., and Poulain, P. Z. *Zellforsch. Microskop. Anat.* 146:351–366, 1973; Barry, J., et al., *C. R. Acad. Sci. [D]*(Paris) 276:3191–3193, 1973; Hoffman, G. E. *Anat. Rec.* 184:429–430, 1976.

Bioassay Evidence

McCann, S. M. *Am. J. Physiol.* 202:395–400, 1962; Schneider, H. P. B., Crighton, D. B., and McCann, S. M. *Neuroendocrinology* 5:271–280, 1969.

RIA Evidence

Palkovitz, M., et al. *Endocrinology* 96:554–558, 1974; Wheaton, J. E., Krulich, L., and McCann, S. M. *Endocrinology* 97:30–38, 1975; Kizer, J. S., Palkovits, M., and Brownstein, M. *Endocrinology* 98:309–315, 1976; Brownstein, M., et al. *Endocrinology* 98:662–665, 1976a.

TRH

Immunocytochemical Evidence

Hökfelt, T., et al. *Eur. J. Pharmacol.* 34:389–394, 1975; Hökfelt, T., et al. *Neurosci. Lett.* 1:133–139, 1975; Elde, R. P., and Parsons, J. A. *Am. J. Anat.* 144:541–548, 1975; Alpert, L. C., et al. *Endocrinology* 98:255–258, 1976; Hökfelt, T., et al. *Acta Endocrinol.* 80(Suppl.):5–41, 1975; Hökfelt, T., et al. *Neuroscience* 1:131–136, 1976.

RIA Evidence

Brownstein, M. J., et al. *Science* 185:267–269, 1974; Brownstein, M., et al. *Proc. Natl. Acad. Sci. U.S.A.* 72:4177–4179, 1975; Jackson, I. M. D., and Reichlin, S. *Endocrinology* 95:854–862, 1974; Oliver, C., et al. *Endocrinology* 95:540–553, 1974; Winokur, A., and Utiger, R. D. *Science* 185:265–267, 1975; Youngblood, W. W., Lipton, M. A., and Kizer, J. S. *Brain Res.* 151:99–116, 1978.

SOMATOSTATIN

RIA Evidence

Brownstein, M. J., et al. *Endocrinology* 96:1456–1461, 1975; Brownstein, M. J., et al. *Endocrinology* 100:246–249, 1977; Epelbaum, J., et al. *Endocrinology* 101:1495–1502, 1977; Kobayashi, R., Brown, M., and Vale, W. *Brain Res.* 126:584–588, 1977.

Bioassay Evidence

Vale, W., et al. *Endocrinology* 94:Λ128, 1974.

VASOPRESSIN, OXYTOCIN, NEUROPHYSIN

Immunocytochemical Evidence

Swanson, L. W. *Brain Res.* 128:346–353, 1977; Zimmerman, E. A. In L. Martini and W. F. Ganong (eds.), *Frontiers in Neuroendocrinology.* New York: Raven Press, 1976. Vol. 4, pp. 25–62.

RIA Evidence

George J. M., and Jacobowitz, D. *Brain Res.* 93:363–366, 1975; George, J. M., Staples, S., and Marks, B. *Endocrinology* 98:1430–1433, 1976.

SUBSTANCE P

Immunocytochemical Evidence

Hökfelt, T., et al. In U. S. van Euler and B. Pernow (eds.), *Substance P.* New York: Raven Press, 1977. Pp. 117–145; Hökfelt, T., et al. *Science* 190:889–890, 1975; Ljungdahl, A., Hökfelt, T., and Nilsson, B. *Neuroscience* 3:861–944, 1978; Nilsson, G., Hökfelt, T., and Pernow, B. *Med. Biol.* 52:424–427, 1974.

RIA Evidence

Cuello, A. C., et al. In J. Hughes (ed.), *Centrally Acting Peptides.* New York: Macmillan, 1978. Pp. 135–156; Brownstein, M. J., et al. *Brain Res.* 116:299–305, 1976; Brownstein, M. J., et al. *Brain Res.* 135:315–323, 1977; Mroz, E. A., Brownstein, M. J., and Leeman, S. E. *Brain Res.* 113:597–599, 1976; Mroz, E. A., Brownstein, M. J., and Leeman, S. E. *Brain Res.* 125:305–311, 1977.

NEUROTENSIN

Immunocytochemical Evidence

Uhl, G. R., Kuhan, M. S., and Snyder, S. H. *Proc. Natl. Acad. Sci. U.S.A.* 74:4059–4063, 1977.

RIA Evidence

Kobayashi, R., Brown, M., and Vale, W. *Brain Res.* 126:584–588, 1977; Uhl, G. R., and Snyder, S. H. *Life Sci.* 19:1827–1832, 1976; Carraway, R., and Leeman, S. E. *J. Biol. Chem.* 251:1045–1052, 1976.

α-MSH

Immunocytochemical Evidence

Dube, D., et al. *Endocrinology* 102:1283–1291, 1978; Jacobowitz, D. M., and O'Donohue, T. L. *Proc. Natl. Acad. Sci. U.S.A.* 75:6300–6304, 1978.

RIA Evidence

Eskay, R. L., et al. *Brain Res.* 178:55–67, 1979; Oliver, C., and Porter, J. C. *Endocrinology* 102:697–705, 1978.

β-LIPOTROPIN

Immunocytochemical Evidence

Watson, S. J., Barchas, J. D., and Li, C. H. *Proc. Natl. Acad. Sci. U.S.A.* 74:5155–5158, 1977; Zimmerman, E. A., Liotta, A., and Krieger, D. T. *Cell Tissue Res.* 186:393–398, 1978; Pelletier, G., et al. *Life Sci.* 22:1799–1804, 1978.

RIA Evidence

Krieger, D. T., et al. *Biochem. Biophys. Res. Commun.* 76:930–936, 1977.

ACTH

Immunocytochemical Evidence

Watson, S. J., Richard, III, C. W., and Barchas, J. D. *Science* 200:1180–1182, 1978; Larsson, L.-I., *Lancet* II:1321–1323, 1977.

RIA Evidence

Krieger, D. T., Liotta, A., and Brownstein, M. J. *Brain Res.* 128:575–579, 1977; Krieger, D. T., Liotta, A., and Brownstein, M. J. *Proc. Natl. Acad. Sci. U.S.A.* 74:648–652, 1977.

ENDOGENOUS OPIATES

Immunocytochemical Evidence

Hökfelt, T., et al. *Neurosci. Lett.* 5:25–32, 1977; Simantov, R., et al. *Proc. Natl. Acad. Sci. U.S.A.* 74:2167, 1977.

RIA Evidence

Matsukuma, S., et al. *Brain Res.* 159:228–233, 1978; Rossier, J., et al. *Proc. Natl. Acad. Sci. U.S.A.* 74:5162–5165, 1977; Hong, J. S., et al. *Brain Res.* 134:383–386, 1977; Yang, H.-Y., Hang, J. S., and Costa, E. *Neuropharmacology* 16:303–307, 1977; Hughes, J. *Brain Res.* 106:189–197, 1976; Simantov, R., et al. *Brain Res.* 106:189–197, 1976.

ANGIOTENSIN

Immunocytochemical Evidence

Fuxe, K., et al. *Neurosci. Lett.* 2:229–234, 1976.

VASOACTIVE INTESTINAL POLYPEPTIDE (VIP)

Immunocytochemical Evidence

Fuxe, K., et al. *Neurosci. Lett.* 5:241–246, 1977; Larsson, L.-I., et al. *Proc. Natl. Acad. Sci. U.S.A.* 73:3197–3200, 1976.

RIA Evidence

Samson, W. K., Said, S. I., and McCann, S. M. *Neurosci. Lett.* 12:265–269.

CHOLECYSTOKININ

Immunocytochemical Evidence

Innis, R. B., et al. *Proc. Natl. Acad. Sci. U.S.A.* 76:521–525, 1979; Straus, E., et al. *Proc. Natl. Acad. Sci. U.S.A.* 74:3033–3034, 1977.

RIA Evidence

Van der Hagghen, J. J., Signeau, J. C., and Gepts, W. *Nature* 257:604–605, 1975; Straus, E., and Yalow, R. S. *Proc. Natl. Acad. Sci. U.S.A.* 75:486, 1978.

OTHER PEPTIDES

Immunocytochemical Evidence

Correa, F. M. A., et al. [bradykininlike peptides] *Proc. Natl. Acad. Sci. U.S.A.* 76:1489–1493, 1979; Fuxe, K., et al. [prolactinlike peptides] *Science* 196:889–900, 1977.

RIA Evidence

Havrankova, J., et al. [insulin] *Proc. Natl. Acad. Sci. U.S.A.* 75:5737–5741, 1978; Margolis, F. L. [carnosine] *Science* 184:909–911, 1974; Facold, S. T., et al. [pituitary hormones] *Science* 199:804–806, 1978; Brown, M., et al. [neurotensinlike and bombesinlike peptides]. In S. R. Bloom (ed.), *Gut Hormones.* London: Churchill Livingston, 1978. Pp. 515–558.

James A. Nathanson
Paul Greengard

Chapter 15. Cyclic Nucleotides and Synaptic Transmission

Many of the biochemical and physiological responses of target cells to circulating hormones depend on adenosine 3',5'-monophosphate (cyclic AMP). Cyclic AMP is viewed as a "second messenger" that translates extracellular messages into an intracellular response. Because the receptors for neurotransmitters show many similarities to those for systemic hormones, one important role of cyclic AMP in the nervous system is analogous to its role in nonneuronal tissues—the translation of certain synaptic chemical messages into responses of receptor cells. Recent evidence suggests that cyclic AMP may also regulate certain other neuronal functions, such as neurotransmitter synthesis and release, intracellular movements, carbohydrate metabolism, and trophic and developmental processes.

The cyclic AMP molecule is part of a complex system of cellular regulation and represents one link in a chain of biochemical reactions, each chain having its own substrates, enzymes, and control mechanisms. The variation in one or more of the components of this system allows cyclic AMP to exert diverse effects on the cellular functions of different tissues. A less extensive body of evidence suggests that another cyclic nucleotide, guanosine 3',5'-monophosphate (cyclic GMP) may also be involved in translating certain hormonal and neurotransmitter signals into appropriate cellular responses. In this chapter we try to explain the action mechanism of these cyclic nucleotide systems and their relationship to neuronal function.

Role of Cyclic AMP in Hormone Action

RELATIONSHIP BETWEEN HORMONE RECEPTORS AND ADENYLATE CYCLASE

The actions of many hormones on their target cells are mediated through an increase in the intracellular concentration of cyclic AMP [1, 2]. It is thought that the membrane receptors for this class of hormones may be intimately associated with the regulatory subunit of adenylate cyclase, the membrane-bound enzyme that catalyzes the formation of cyclic AMP from adenosine triphosphate (ATP) [3]. Thus, when the proper hormone binds with the regulatory subunit of the enzyme, the catalytic subunit, thought to be located on the inner surface of the cell membrane, is stimulated to form cyclic AMP at an increased rate. It is the resulting increase in cyclic AMP that mediates the intracellular effects of the hormone. Cyclic AMP is broken down in the cell by another enzyme, cyclic nucleotide phosphodiesterase, which hydrolyzes cyclic AMP to 5'-AMP [4, 5].

Although many hormones stimulate adenylate cyclase, others have no effect on the enzyme, while a few may mediate their effects by inhibiting adenylate cyclase, thereby decreasing the intracellular concentration of cyclic AMP.

ACTION MECHANISM OF CYCLIC AMP

Once formed inside a cell, cyclic AMP exerts its effects on intracellular processes through activation of cyclic AMP–dependent protein kinases [6–8]. These enzymes catalyze the phosphorylation, by ATP, of protein substrates, according to the reaction:

$$ATP + protein \longrightarrow ADP + phosphoprotein$$

Cyclic AMP stimulates this enzymatic reaction. Protein kinases that are cyclic AMP–dependent are composed of a regulatory (inhibitory) subunit and a catalytic subunit. By binding to the regulatory subunit, cyclic AMP leads to dissociation of the enzyme, resulting in activation of the catalytic subunit and an increase in the rate of phosphorylation of the appropriate substrate. Phosphorylation usually occurs on serine residues, but occasionally on threonine residues, of the substrate protein. This phosphorylation of the substrate protein leads to an alteration of intracellular physiology. Phosphate is removed from the substrate protein by another enzyme, phosphoprotein phosphatase, which cleaves phosphate from the serine or threonine residues. The intracellular action mechanism of cyclic AMP appears, in almost all instances studied so far, to be through a change in the level of phosphorylation of substrate proteins.

The nature of the proteins phosphorylated in cyclic AMP–dependent reactions varies considerably. The protein may be a known enzyme, such as phosphorylase b kinase (Chap. 17); a nuclear protein, such as histone; or a membrane-bound protein, such as those found in synaptic-membrane fractions. This last type of substrate may be important in relation to the possible role of cyclic AMP in synaptic transmission, for it provides a means through which cyclic AMP could regulate the ion permeability of membranes (see Action Mechanism of Cyclic AMP in Synaptic Transmission).

DETERMINANTS OF SPECIFICITY
OF HORMONE ACTION
Viewed overall, specificity of hormone action resides at several levels. First, the nature of the membrane receptor (regulatory subunit of adenylate cyclase) will determine if the hormone will increase (or decrease) cyclic AMP levels. Even though a cell has an adenylate cyclase, the enzyme will not respond to a particular hormone unless it has a receptor site that can bind and be activated by that hormone. Second, the nature of the cyclic AMP–dependent protein kinases (or phosphoprotein phosphatases) present in the cell will determine the pattern of protein substrates phosphorylated. Third, the nature of the substrate(s) present will determine the ultimate physiological response. For instance, a liver cell does not have the synaptic membrane proteins that are present in a nerve cell, so it cannot be subject to the same phosphorylation

reaction that might affect membrane permeability in the neuron.

Cyclic AMP and Neuronal Function
Figure 15-1 illustrates a possible role of cyclic AMP in mediating synaptic transmission in neurons. A variety of experimental criteria useful in evaluating whether cyclic AMP (or cyclic GMP) mediates a postsynaptic permeability change are presented in Table 15-1.

ENZYMATIC MACHINERY
IN NERVOUS TISSUE
Part of the evidence that cyclic AMP may mediate the actions of certain neurotransmitters is the presence in excitable tissue of the enzymes and substrates necessary for cyclic AMP–mediated reactions [9–13].

Adenylate Cyclase
The adenylate cyclase activity of neural tissue is almost entirely particulate. The enzyme utilizes ATP as the preferred substrate (K_m 0.3–1.5 mM) and needs a divalent cation, such as magnesium, manganese, or cobalt. Certain additional cofactors, such as guanosine triphosphate (GTP) and calcium, exert important regulatory effects on adenylate cyclase activity.

GTP exerts its effects on adenylate cyclase through interaction with a guanine nucleotide regulatory protein that is essential for the coupling of the hormone receptor to the catalytic subunit of adenylate cyclase. The action of calcium appears to occur through its binding to a protein called *calmodulin,* which has important regulatory actions, not only on adenylate cyclase but also on phosphodiesterase and protein kinase.

Relevant to its possible role in neuronal function is the fact that adenylate cyclase activity is higher in brain than in most other tissues. The exact distribution of activity among the various regions of the brain varies in different species, although in all species the activity is greater in gray than in white matter. Subcellular distribution studies have shown that the highest levels of adenylate cyclase are found in those fractions rich in synaptic mem-

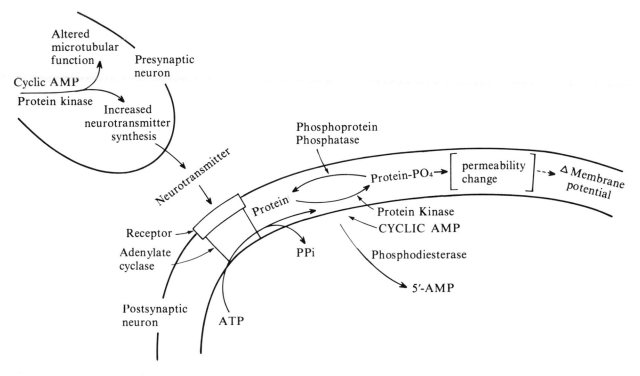

Fig. 15-1. Model of a proposed mechanism by which cyclic AMP may mediate synaptic transmission at certain types of synapses. Also shown are possible presynaptic effects of cyclic AMP. (From Greengard, Cyclic Nucleotides, Phosphorylated Proteins, and Neuronal Function, New York: Raven Press, 1978.)

branes, strengthening the belief that cyclic AMP found in the brain may have relevance to neurons and to synaptic function.

The adenylate cyclase activity of neural tissue is regulated by a number of neurotransmitters, including norepinephrine, dopamine, serotonin, histamine, octopamine, prostaglandins, opiates, and certain other peptides. Close similarities have been found between the physiological receptor for a particular neurotransmitter and the regulatory subunit of the adenylate cyclase with which it interacts. Such similarities constitute important evidence that a particular neurotransmitter-sensitive adenylate cyclase may mediate the physiological action of that neurotransmitter. This is discussed in detail later in this chapter.

Recent studies indicate that frequently there may exist more than one type of physiological receptor for each neurotransmitter. Each of these so-called receptor subtypes (which can be distinguished by their somewhat different pharmacological properties) may mediate a different action in the presence of the same neurotransmitter. Thus, for example, norepinephrine can affect both α-adrenergic and β-adrenergic receptors, which are found in different proportions in different tissues. (In blood vessels, for example, α-adrenergic receptors cause vasoconstriction and β-receptors cause vasodilitation.) Some receptors and receptor subtypes regulate adenylate cyclase activity while others do not. The action of dopamine at dopamine-1 (D1) receptors is associated with a stimulation of adenylate cyclase while dopamine's action at D2 receptors is not.

Many of the neurotransmitter receptors or receptor subtypes (e.g., D1, β-adrenergic, H$_2$-histaminergic) that regulate adenylate cyclase do so through stimulation of the enzyme. Other neurotransmitter receptors or receptor subtypes (e.g.,

Table 15-1. Some Criteria for Mediation by a Cyclic Nucleotide of a Postsynaptic Permeability Change

A. Synaptic activation and cyclic nucleotide levels
   1. Electrical stimulation of the presynaptic input should increase tissue levels of the cyclic nucleotide
   2. This increase in cyclic nucleotide level should be antagonized by pharmacological agents that block the post-synaptic permeability change
   3. The increase should not occur when transmitter release is prevented with low Ca^{2+} and high Mg^{2+}
   4. The increase should not occur when the postsynaptic cells are antidromically activated
B. Neurotransmitters and cyclic nucleotide levels
   1. Levels of the cyclic nucleotide should increase when the intact tissue (or blocks or slices of the tissue) is exposed to the neurotransmitter thought to be responsible for the postsynaptic permeability change
   2. This increase should be antagonized by agents that block the neurotransmitter-induced postsynaptic permeability change
C. Neurotransmitters and adenylate (or guanylate) cyclase
   1. A neurotransmitter-sensitive adenylate cyclase (or guanylate cyclase; however, see text) should be demonstrated in cell-free preparations of the tissue
   2. Activation by the neurotransmitter of this neurotransmitter-sensitive adenylate (or guanylate) cyclase should be blocked by the same antagonists referred to in sections A2 and B2 of this table
D. Cytochemistry
   1. Cytochemical techniques should demonstrate that cyclic nucleotide levels increase specifically in the postsynaptic cells in response to synaptic activation
   2. Similarly, cytochemical techniques should demonstrate that cyclic nucleotide levels increase specifically in the postsynaptic cells in response to the appropriate neurotransmitter
E. Phosphodiesterase inhibitors
   1. Phosphodiesterase inhibitors should potentiate the effects of activating the synaptic pathway and of applying the putative neurotransmitter on the increase in cyclic nucleotide levels
   2. Phosphodiesterase inhibitors should potentiate the effects of activating the synaptic pathway and of applying the putative neurotransmitter on the postsynaptic permeability change
F. Application of cyclic nucleotides
   1. The cyclic nucleotide injected intracellularly should mimic the physiological effects of activating the synaptic pathway and of applying the putative neurotransmitter

Source: Beam, K. G., and Greengard, P. *Cold Spring Harbor Symp. Quant. Biol., The Synapse* 40:157–168, 1976.

opiates, α-adrenergic, muscarinic cholinergic) lead to an inhibition of adenylate cyclase activity. Both neurotransmitter-induced activation and neuro-transmitter-induced inhibition of adenylate cyclase require the presence of GTP.

Brain adenylate cyclase activity is also affected by calcium and fluoride ions. Although the effect of fluoride, which acts directly on the catalytic sub-unit of the enzyme, is primarily of theoretical interest, the action of calcium has important physiological implications. Thus, if calcium can regulate adenylate cyclase activity, it is possible that normal (or drug-induced) depolarization of nerve cells, resulting in transmembrane movements of calcium, could affect cyclic AMP–mediated pro-

cesses (such as protein phosphorylation) inde-pendently of direct neurotransmitter actions. Recent evidence indicates that, in some cases, cal-cium is able to regulate protein phosphorylation through a calcium-dependent protein kinase [6].

Phosphodiesterase
Cyclic-nucleotide phosphodiesterase converts cyc-lic AMP to 5′-AMP and thus serves to terminate reactions initiated by the cyclic nucleotide [4, 5]. Like adenylate cyclase, magnesium or manganese ion is required for activity. Phosphodiesterase is stimulated by imidazole and is inhibited by the methyl xanthines, including caffeine, theophyl-line, and theobromine. Inhibition of phosphodies-

terase has the effect of augmenting and prolonging certain cyclic AMP-mediated reactions. There appear to be multiple forms of phosphodiesterase, each with different properties, including substrate specificities. In rat cerebrum and cerebellum, for example, there are at least four separable forms, some of which can be stimulated and inhibited differentially. Certain of the phosphodiesterases from brain can be activated by an endogenous, heat-stable, calcium-binding protein known as *calmodulin.*

Phosphodiesterase activity is greater in brain than in most other tissues. Subcellular distribution studies show a high concentration of the enzyme in synaptic membrane fractions. Histochemical studies have revealed intense phosphodiesterase activity at the postjunctional thickening of synapses in the cerebral cortex of the rat. This localization tends to support a role for cyclic AMP in neurotransmission: a phosphodiesterase at the postjunctional site would have access to, and would thus be able to degrade, cyclic AMP that had been synthesized as a result of stimulation of adenylate cyclase by a neurotransmitter.

Protein Kinase and Phosphoprotein Phosphatase
Protein kinase activity dependent on cyclic AMP has been found in all excitable and nonexcitable tissues so far examined. Under appropriate conditions, the activity of this enzyme is stimulated as much as twentyfold in the presence of cyclic AMP [6–8]. The level of cyclic AMP normally found in brain is about 0.3 μM—the same concentration that is needed for half maximal stimulation of protein kinase of brain. This means that small changes in the usual brain concentrations of cyclic AMP may regulate the activity of the enzyme. In subcellular distribution studies, the highest specific activity of the enzyme is found in synaptic membrane fractions, as is that of adenylate cyclase and phosphodiesterase.

A phosphoprotein phosphatase also has been demonstrated in brain tissue. This enzyme is able to hydrolyze the phosphate from phosphoserine residues of proteins that have previously been phosphorylated in cyclic AMP–dependent reactions. In this way, the enzyme may serve to terminate the action of cyclic AMP. Under certain conditions, the rate at which endogenous protein phosphatase can remove phosphate from substrate proteins in the synaptic membrane fraction can be stimulated by cyclic AMP, thereby hastening the return of the protein to its dephosphorylated form. Like protein kinase, the highest concentration of phosphoprotein phosphatase is found in synaptic membrane fractions.

Substrates for Cyclic AMP–Dependent Phosphorylation Reactions
Ultimately, the identity of the phosphorylated substrates determines the outcome of cyclic AMP–dependent reactions. A number of studies have shown that synaptic membrane fractions from brain are excellent substrates for endogenous cyclic AMP–dependent protein kinases and phosphoprotein phosphatases. In fact, the subcellular distribution of substrates for the protein kinases and phosphatases parallels that of the protein kinases and phosphatases themselves. The phosphorylation of synaptic membrane proteins by endogenous protein kinase(s) exhibits considerable specificity with respect to the individual substrate proteins that are phosphorylated. In rat cerebral cortex, for example, separation of phosphorylated synaptic membrane proteins by sodium dodecyl sulfate–polyacrylamide gel electrophoresis reveals that, out of several dozen protein bands, the phosphorylation of only a few is markedly affected by cyclic AMP. These experiments also suggest that the phosphorylated proteins may be situated in the immediate vicinity of a cyclic nucleotide—dependent protein kinase in the synaptic membrane (see Action Mechanism of Cyclic AMP in Synaptic Transmission).

Certain protein components in brain other than those in synaptic membranes also can be phosphorylated in cyclic AMP–dependent reactions. For example, synaptic vesicles, neurotubules, myelin membranes, and ribosomes all contain proteins that serve as effective substrates for intrinsic cyclic AMP–dependent protein kinases (see Other Actions of Cyclic AMP in Neural Tissues).

CYCLIC AMP LEVELS IN WHOLE BRAIN, BRAIN SLICES, AND CULTURED CELLS

Whole Brain

The levels of cyclic AMP in intact vertebrate brain are higher than those in almost any other tissue. In most unstimulated nonneural tissues, the cyclic AMP concentration is on the order of 0.5 to 2.5 picomoles per milligram of protein. In mammalian brain, the range is from 10 to 20 picomoles per milligram of protein. The hypothalamus and striatum have the highest levels; those in the cerebellum and hippocampus are somewhat lower, although the range is not great. Immunohistochemical techniques for localizing cyclic AMP have shown that in the cerebellum the nucleotide is present mostly in the granule and Purkinje cells.

Endogenous cyclic AMP levels are markedly affected by the method of tissue fixation used. After decapitation of the rabbit, for example, cyclic AMP levels in rabbit brain rise as much as eightfold within 90 seconds. The mechanism of this post-decapitation rise is not understood, although it may be related to nerve terminal depolarization induced by anoxia, with a resultant release of some endogenous activator of cyclic AMP synthesis.

Brain Slices

EFFECTS OF PUTATIVE NEUROTRANSMITTERS. Many laboratories have studied the effects of putative neurotransmitters on cyclic AMP levels in respiring slices of brain tissue [13–15].

Norepinephrine, epinephrine, dopamine, serotonin, histamine, adenosine, glutamate, aspartate, and a variety of analogs of these suspected neurotransmitters have been shown to increase the cyclic AMP content of cortical brain slices from 2- to 10-fold or more. In some cases, there is substantial variation among different species. Histamine, for example, causes large increases of cyclic AMP in slices from rabbit cerebral cortex, cerebellum, or striatum, but has little effect in the rat. Regional differences also exist, and the reader is referred to several recent reviews for further details [11–16].

The use of brain slices has the advantage over broken-cell preparations of more nearly approximating the condition of the intact brain but also has some disadvantages for the study of adenylate cyclase receptors. First, levels of cyclic AMP in brain slices represent the net difference between synthesis by adenylate cyclase and degradation by phosphodiesterase. If there is an increase in cyclic AMP level in response to a hormone, it is not always clear whether the increase is a result of activation of adenylate cyclase, inhibition of phosphodiesterase, or some indirect effect such as a change in the ATP content of cells. Second, it is difficult to ascertain if the putative neurotransmitter being tested is the immediate cause of the increase in cyclic AMP content observed. For example, it may be that the putative neurotransmitter that is applied depolarizes certain neurons, which then release a second, endogenous (and unidentified) neurotransmitter, and it is this one that actually interacts with the adenylate cyclase receptor responsible for the observed change in cyclic AMP. These studies with brain slices have produced important, but indirect, evidence for the presence of hormone-sensitive adenylate cyclase in neuronal tissue.

EFFECT OF ELECTRICAL PULSES AND DEPOLARIZING AGENTS. The cyclic AMP content of brain slices can be elevated severalfold either by stimulating the slices electrically or by applying depolarizing agents, such as high extracellular potassium, ouabain, batrachotoxin, or veratridine. The increase in cyclic AMP brought about by these procedures is blocked by low-calcium and high-magnesium media, by membrane-stabilizing agents such as tetrodotoxin or local anesthetics, and (paradoxically) by theophylline. It is thought that electrical stimulation and depolarizing agents may cause release of endogenous substances, which then stimulate adenylate cyclase receptors. Specifically, it has been proposed that adenosine may be the mediator of some depolarization-induced increases in cyclic AMP. It has been shown that endogenous adenosine is released during depolarization and that exogenous adenosine is potent in increasing cyclic AMP levels in brain slices. In addition, the effect of adenosine in elevating cyclic AMP levels is blocked by theophylline. It is uncertain whether adenosine can be considered a neurotransmitter, but current evidence certainly does suggest that it may have a role in cyclic AMP metabolism.

Cultured Cells

Several putative neurotransmitters, including norepinephrine, histamine, adenosine, and prostaglandins, stimulate very large accumulations of cyclic AMP in intact- and broken-cell preparations of cells grown in culture. It has been found that the cyclic AMP content of glial tumor lines is elevated by catecholamines, histamine, and adenosine, whereas neuroblastoma cells respond primarily to certain prostaglandins and only weakly to other agents.

NEUROTRANSMITTER-SENSITIVE ADENYLATE CYCLASES AND THEIR POSSIBLE ROLE IN NEURONAL FUNCTION

If cyclic AMP does mediate the postsynaptic action of a particular neurotransmitter, the adenylate cyclase and the physiological receptor should share properties in common that are specific for that neurotransmitter. That is, agents that activate the adenylate cyclase should also activate the physiological receptor, and conversely, agents that antagonize the activation of the receptor. (There should be a corresponding correlation for receptors whose activation is associated with a decrease in adenylate cyclase activity.) It appears that several neurotransmitters—dopamine, norepinephrine, serotonin, histamine, and octopamine—fulfill these criteria, suggesting that some of their actions may be mediated through cyclic AMP [6, 13, 17, 18]. There is similar, but less complete, evidence that the actions of certain prostaglandins and peptide neurohormones, including the endogenous opiates, may, at least in part, be mediated through cyclic AMP (see Chaps. 13, 14, and 16).

Dopamine

A dopamine-sensitive adenylate cyclase has been identified in several mammalian tissues, including the sympathetic ganglion, retina (see Chap. 10), caudate nucleus, limbic and certain cortical areas of the brain, as well as in invertebrate ganglia. This enzyme has its highest specific activity in synaptic membrane fractions of the mammalian brain, is activated by dopamine at concentrations of $1 \mu M$ or less, and is inhibited by many agents known to block certain dopamine receptors. Those dopamine receptors which regulate the activity of adenylate cyclase have been termed *type 1*, or *D1, receptors*. Other dopamine receptors (termed *D2*) do not appear to be associated with adenylate cyclase.

A variety of evidence suggests that dopamine may also function as a neurotransmitter in the caudate nucleus and limbic areas of the mammalian brain. Hypoactivity of the dopaminergic pathway to the caudate nucleus is thought to be involved in the etiology of Parkinson's disease, and hyperactivity of the dopaminergic pathway to the limbic forebrain has been implicated as a possible cause of schizophrenia. In the treatment of Parkinson's disease (see Chap. 36), L-dopa, which is converted to dopamine in the brain, is used. Conversely, antipsychotic agents such as the phenothiazines, which are known to block dopamine receptors, are used to treat schizophrenia.

The dopamine-sensitive adenylate cyclase which is present in the caudate and limbic areas of the brain has properties very similar to those of some of the dopamine receptors in brain. The enzyme is stimulated by low concentrations of dopamine and apomorphine, and the activation by dopamine is blocked by a variety of antipsychotic drugs in a fashion correlated with the known clinical potency of these agents. Such antipsychotic agents as fluphenazine competitively inhibit activation of the enzyme by dopamine at extremely low concentrations ($K_i = 5$–$8 nM$), similar to those present in brain after therapeutic doses. Compounds structurally related to fluphenazine, but lacking antipsychotic effectiveness, show only a slight ability to block enzyme activation. Results such as these suggest that both the therapeutic effects and the extrapyramidal side effects of certain antipsychotic agents may be caused, at least in part, by their ability to block the activation by dopamine of certain dopamine-sensitive adenylate cyclases in the brain. This same concept of interference with adenylate cyclase-associated receptors may also apply to the mechanism of action of other psychoactive drugs, such as LSD (see under Serotonin) and certain antidepressant agents (see under Histamine).

Norepinephrine

In the cerebellum, a norepinephrine-sensitive adenylate cyclase has been identified that may mediate the inhibitory effect of norepinephrine on Purkinje cells [12]. This enzyme is stimulated by low concentrations of norepinephrine, and such stimulation is antagonized by β-adrenergic blocking agents. Electrophysiological studies have demonstrated that norepinephrine applied iontophoretically results in a hyperpolarization and slowing in the firing rate of Purkinje cells. This effect is potentiated by phosphodiesterase inhibitors, and is blocked by prostaglandin E_1 (see Chap. 16). The same effect can be produced by iontophoretically applied cyclic AMP. Furthermore, the ability of various cyclic AMP analogs to mimic the effect of norepinephrine correlates with the ability of these analogs to activate cyclic AMP–dependent protein kinase from brain: those analogs which are the most effective activators of the kinase likewise cause the greatest slowing of firing rate.

Electrical stimulation of the locus coeruleus also causes slowing in the firing rate of Purkinje cells through norepinephrine-containing projections, which terminate on Purkinje cell dendrites. The effect of such locus coeruleus stimulation is potentiated by phosphodiesterase inhibitors and blocked by prostaglandin E_1. Furthermore, histochemical localization studies have shown that locus coeruleus stimulation results in a dramatic increase in the number of Purkinje cells that show cyclic AMP staining. Evidence similar to that just described supports a role for cyclic AMP in mediating the effects of norepinephrine on the firing rate of hippocampal and cerebral cortical pyramidal cells.

Serotonin

There is much evidence that serotonin may function as a neurotransmitter in various invertebrate ganglia, as well as in the central and peripheral nervous systems of mammals (see Chap. 11). The actions of serotonin are blocked by various antiserotonergic agents, including such hallucinogens as LSD. In insect thoracic ganglia, an adenylate cyclase sensitive to low (<1 μM) concentrations of serotonin has been identified. This enzyme has characteristics similar to those of certain known invertebrate serotonin receptors. Activation of the enzyme by serotonin is blocked in a competitive manner by extremely low concentrations of LSD ($K_i = 5$ nM), 2-bromo-LSD ($K_i = 5$ nM), and the structurally unrelated serotonin blocker, cyproheptadine ($K_i = 0.25$ μM). The effect of these blockers on the serotonin-sensitive adenylate cyclase is specific, as evidenced by the fact that a dopamine-sensitive adenylate cyclase and an octopamine-sensitive adenylate cyclase present in the same ganglion are blocked only poorly by the same antiserotonergic agents. Serotonin is known to increase cyclic AMP levels in other invertebrate ganglia as well. In molluscs, serotonin-stimulated cyclic AMP accumulation appears to trigger a sequence of events leading to an increase in neurotransmitter release that, in turn, alters a simple behavior in the animal.

A serotonin-sensitive adenylate cyclase has been identified in several areas of immature rat brain, as well as in neuroblastoma cells in tissue culture. In the rat, the response of adenylate cyclase to serotonin is greatest in the colliculi and hypothalamus and declines substantially during early development.

Histamine

Electrophysiological evidence supports the existence of histamine receptors that, when activated by this amine, result in a change in the neuronal firing rate (see Chap. 11). There are two types of histamine receptors in both brain and peripheral tissues; those that are blocked by classical antihistaminics (H_1) and those that are not (H_2). A specific H_2-sensitive adenylate cyclase has been identified in rat and guinea pig brain. This enzyme is activated by histamine and H_2-receptor agonists, and the stimulation by histamine is blocked by H_2-antagonists such as metiamide, but not by H_1-receptor antagonists such as mepyramine. Recent studies have shown a correlation between the therapeutic effects of various drugs as antidepressants and the ability of these drugs to inhibit H_2-stimulated adenylate cyclase; this raises the possibility that antidepressants may exert some of their clinical effects through interaction with histaminergic neurotransmission.

Octopamine

Octopamine, found in both vertebrates and invertebrates, is a phenethylamine that lacks the catechol structure of norepinephrine and dopamine. Recent studies have shown the existence in arthropod and molluscan ganglia of neuronal receptors for octopamine that are distinct from those for dopamine and norepinephrine. An octopamine-sensitive adenylate cyclase, distinct from adenylate cyclases activated by dopamine or serotonin, has been identified in insect thoracic ganglia, supporting the possibility that octopamine may be a neurotransmitter. This enzyme is activated by low concentrations ($<0.1 \ \mu M$) of octopamine. The activation is blocked by α- but not by β-adrenergic antagonists. As yet, an octopamine-sensitive adenylate cyclase has not been identified in mammalian nervous tissue.

Peptides and Prostaglandins

Recent findings indicate that certain peptides that have been proposed as putative neurotransmitters in the nervous system may exert some of their effects through regulation of cyclic AMP metabolism. For example, substance P, an undecapeptide that may function as a neurotransmitter for primary sensory afferents, has been reported to activate adenylate cyclase in both human and rat brain homogenates.

The endogenous opiates, which have been proposed as natural pain-suppressing neurotransmitters, appear also to have important interactions with cyclic AMP (see Chap. 13). In cultured neuroblastoma glioma cell hybrids, morphine and other narcotic analgesics inhibit both basal and prostaglandin E_1–stimulated adenylate cyclase activity. (By itself, prostaglandin E_1 also stimulates adenylate cyclase activity in rat brain homogenates.) The narcotic antagonist, naloxone, blocks the effect of morphine. After chronic administration of morphine, there is a compensatory increase in the amount of adenylate cyclase in these cells.

This latter finding has led to the suggestion that certain of the symptoms of opiate dependence may be due to the increase in the amount of adenylate cyclase secondary to chronic inhibition of the enzyme by morphine.

ACTION MECHANISM OF CYCLIC AMP IN SYNAPTIC TRANSMISSION

Cyclic AMP–Regulated Phosphorylation of Specific Membrane Proteins

Phosphorylation of membrane proteins that is cyclic AMP–dependent represents a possible mechanism for producing the ion permeability changes associated with activation of certain neurotransmitter-sensitive adenylate cyclases. In the mammalian brain, the endogenous phosphorylation of three synaptic membrane proteins has been found to be markedly affected by cyclic AMP. Phosphorylation of these proteins is rapid, reaching maximal levels in less than 5 seconds. Two of these proteins (designated *proteins Ia and Ib*), have been observed to be present only in neural tissues that contain synapses, such as cerebral cortex, cerebellum, and caudate nucleus. Peripheral tissues such as lingual nerve, liver, lung, kidney, and spleen contain very little of this protein, and that which is present appears localized to areas where efferent nerves make synaptic contact. In the brain, during development, proteins Ia and Ib increase markedly during synaptogenesis. Recent biochemical and histochemical studies suggest that these same proteins are localized in synaptic vesicles.

In addition to occurring in broken-cell preparations, phosphorylation of specific proteins has been demonstrated in intact neural tissue. In slices of brain, for example, the phosphorylation of proteins Ia and Ib is stimulated by depolarizing agents such as potassium and veratridine, by phosphodiesterase inhibitors, and by 8-bromo cyclic AMP, a potent cyclic AMP analog. Furthermore, in intact brain, pharmacological agents that elevate the rate of neuronal firing increase the phosphorylation of these proteins, and agents that suppress neuronal firing decrease their phosphorylation. In intact *Aplysia* ganglia, both serotonin and octopamine cause a delayed (22 hr) phosphorylation of a specific membrane protein. In addition, intracellular injection of the active catalytic subunit of protein kinase mimics certain of the effects of serotonin in *Aplysia* ganglia. In slices of guinea pig cerebral cortex, norepinephrine has been reported to stimulate the phosphorylation of total protein of neuronal, but not of glial, fractions.

Correlation Between Membrane Permeability and the State of Phosphorylation of Membrane Proteins

Cyclic AMP is known to cause a slow hyperpolarization of neurons in several regions of the nervous system. These areas include the cerebellum, caudate nucleus, hippocampus, cerebral cortex, and sympathetic ganglion [12]. In the cerebellum, where the hyperpolarization of Purkinje cells has been studied by intracellular electrode techniques, it appears that cyclic AMP–induced hyperpolarization is consistently associated with an increase in transmembrane resistance (decrease in conductance). This is different from the classical mechanism of inhibitory postsynaptic potentials, in which the hyperpolarization is associated with an increased conductance to potassium or chloride ions. The increased membrane resistance observed with cyclic AMP may possibly be the result of a decrease in the resting conductance to sodium or calcium ions.

If protein phosphorylation is responsible for changes in ionic permeability, a correlation should exist between the state of phosphorylation of (a) particular membrane protein(s) and the state of ion permeability of the membrane. In the nervous system, the short duration of permeability changes in membrane has made it difficult to establish such a correlation. However, in at least three vertebrate tissues (avian erythrocytes, amphibian bladder epithelium, and mammalian heart muscle), where the duration of hormone-induced permeability changes is much longer, it appears that a correlation does exist. In the avian erythrocyte, for example, catecholamines have been shown to increase passive sodium and potassium transport, apparently through a mechanism involving cyclic AMP. Activation of β-adrenergic receptors is known to cause an increase in the cyclic AMP

content of the erythrocytes, and exogenous cyclic AMP mimics the effect of the catecholamines in increasing cation transport. Both β-adrenergic agonists and cyclic AMP have been shown to stimulate the rapid phosphorylation of a single, high molecular weight protein located in the erythrocyte plasma membrane. The time course and the dose-response relationship of the catecholamine-stimulated phosphorylation of this protein agree well with the time course and dose-response relationship for the catecholamine-induced increase in cation transport. In addition, certain agents that block the catecholamine-induced increase in phosphorylation also block the catecholamine-induced increase in sodium transport. These findings suggest that the phosphorylation of this membrane protein may be causally linked with the increased permeability of the erythrocyte membrane to cations.

Other Actions of Cyclic AMP and Protein Phosphorylation in Neural Tissue

The above sections describe the possible involvement of cyclic AMP in certain types of synaptic transmission. Recent evidence indicates that this nucleotide may also have other important functions in the nervous system.

NEUROTRANSMITTER SYNTHESIS. Cyclic AMP–dependent protein phosphorylation can affect the state of activation of certain neurotransmitter synthetic enzymes. For example, both cyclic AMP and protein kinase increase the activity of tyrosine hydroxylase (TH) in supernatant fractions from areas of brain rich in catecholamine nerve terminals. This activation occurs without the synthesis of new enzyme.

Cyclic AMP can also alter enzyme activity through the de novo synthesis of protein. In the adrenal gland, transsynaptic stimulation of medullary cells results in a delayed increase in TH activity. Following nerve stimulation, there is first an increase in cyclic AMP in the cytosol, followed by activation of protein kinase. It is thought that this protein kinase is translocated to the cell nucleus, where it causes gene derepression and the synthesis of new TH. In the pineal gland, cyclic AMP is involved in the regulation of melatonin synthesis (see Chap. 10).

OTHER PRESYNAPTIC FUNCTIONS. In intact synaptosomes, agents that depolarize and increase calcium transport across the membrane of nerve terminals also stimulate the phosphorylation of an endogenous membrane-bound protein. This calcium-dependent (but cyclic AMP–independent) phosphorylation appears to require the presence of a calcium-dependent protein regulator (calmodulin). Though it has not been proven, this phosphorylation might be linked to neurotransmitter release.

CELL GROWTH AND DIFFERENTIATION. Cyclic AMP and its synthetic derivatives slow the division of nerve and glial cell lines in culture and cause them to express differentiated morphology (see Chap. 23).

MICROTUBULE FUNCTION. Cyclic AMP stimulates neurite outgrowth and elongation in cultured sensory ganglia through a mechanism apparently unrelated to that used by nerve growth factor. Moreover, when highly purified preparations of neurotubules are used, a protein component of high molecular weight is capable of undergoing phosphorylation catalyzed by an endogenous cyclic AMP–dependent protein kinase.

CEREBRAL VASCULATURE. Both the larger superficial vessels as well as the deep intraparenchymal microvessels of the brain contain adenylate cyclase activated by norepinephrine and histamine. It has been postulated that cyclic AMP in these vessels could be related to changes in vascular resistance, permeability, or both.

GLIAL CELL FUNCTION. Catecholamines, histamine, and adenosine cause large increases in cyclic AMP levels in various glial tumor cell lines. The function of these increases is not yet known.

CARBOHYDRATE METABOLISM. Cyclic AMP may be involved in the activation of brain phosphorylase (see Chap. 17).

VISION. A light-dependent activation of cyclic nucleotide phosphodiesterase has been observed that may regulate the sensitivity of photoreceptors to incident illumination (see Chap. 7).

LONG-TERM CHANGES IN NEURONAL FUNCTION. Electrophysiological studies in invertebrate and sympathetic ganglia have implicated cyclic AMP in long-term alterations of synaptic function. From a biochemical point of view, such alterations are consistent with the long-term changes in membrane ion permeability that can accompany cyclic AMP–dependent phosphorylation.

Cyclic GMP and Neuronal Function

Evidence gathered in recent years has suggested that a second cyclic nucleotide, cyclic GMP, may be important in regulating cellular metabolism and function [19]. Although, in general, much less is known about the physiological role of cyclic GMP than of cyclic AMP, it appears that cyclic GMP may be involved in nervous system function. Specifically, a number of reports suggest that cyclic GMP may mediate certain of the effects of acetylcholine acting at muscarinic receptors and of histamine acting at H_1 receptors.

CYCLIC GMP AND ASSOCIATED ENZYMES IN NERVOUS TISSUE

In general, in both the brain and the peripheral tissues, levels of cyclic GMP are only 2 to 10 percent of those of cyclic AMP. The cyclic GMP levels in brain are similar to those in several nonneural tissues. In the cerebellum, however, concentrations of cyclic GMP are 10 times higher and nearly equal to those of cyclic AMP.

Guanylate cyclase, which catalyzes the formation of cyclic GMP from GTP, is found to a substantial degree in the soluble cellular fraction (in contrast to adenylate cyclase, which is almost entirely particulate). Brain guanylate cyclase isolated from the soluble fraction of osmotically shocked synaptosomes has been reported to have an especially high specific activity. Particulate fractions do have significant enzyme activity, nevertheless, and it has been shown that this activity can be increased substantially by nonionic detergents. In the nervous system, as in nonneuronal tissues, it has not yet been possible to demonstrate stimulation by hormones or neurotransmitters of guanylate cyclase activity in broken-cell preparations.

Cyclic GMP is hydrolyzed to 5'-GMP by cyclic nucleotide phosphodiesterase. Although the several identified molecular species of phosphodiesterase will hydrolyze both cyclic AMP and cyclic GMP to a significant degree, some forms of the enzyme are more active against one nucleotide, and some against the other.

Specific cyclic GMP–dependent protein kinases have also been identified. These enzymes, which have been found in both vertebrate and invertebrate neural and nonneural tissue, are selectively stimulated by low concentrations of cyclic GMP but not of cyclic AMP. Endogenous substrates for cyclic GMP–dependent protein kinase have been found in the cerebellum as well as in membrane fractions from each of several types of mammalian smooth muscle.

Taken together, the above evidence suggests that cellular regulation by cyclic GMP may involve a set of enzyme reactions generally similar to those of the cyclic AMP system. Thus, the presence of guanylate cyclase, cyclic GMP phosphodiesterase, cyclic GMP–dependent protein kinase, and specific substrates for cyclic GMP–dependent phosphorylation provides the necessary elements for a chain of intracellular reactions that may mediate the physiological effects of cyclic GMP.

CYCLIC GMP STUDIES IN INTACT PREPARATIONS

Central Nervous System

In contrast to the difficulty of demonstrating a hormonal stimulation of cyclic GMP formation in broken-cell systems, investigators have reported neurotransmitter-induced increases in cyclic GMP in intact nerve tissue [11–13]. Several reports have suggested that cyclic GMP may be, either directly or indirectly, involved in the action of acetylcholine in the central nervous system. In mice, systemic administration of oxytremorine, a cholinergic agent, increases the cyclic GMP content of both cerebral cortex and cerebellum, an effect that is blocked by pretreatment with atropine. In slices of rabbit cerebral cortex or cerebellum, low concentrations of acetylcholine and such other muscarinic agonists as bethanechol increase cyclic GMP content; this effect is prevented by the muscarinic antagonist atropine but not by the nicotinic antagonist hexamethonium. The acetylcholine-induced increase in cyclic GMP requires the presence of calcium ions in the extracellular medium. It has been sug-

gested that an increase in intracellular calcium, which occurs in response to the applied acetylcholine, stimulates guanylate cyclase activity, and that this causes the observed increase in cyclic GMP level.

Depolarizing agents, such as veratridine, ouabain, and potassium, also increase cyclic GMP levels in slices. This rise in cyclic GMP also requires the presence of calcium. The effect is not blocked by atropine, indicating that acetylcholine is probably not involved in this phenomenon. The amino acids glutamate and glycine increase cerebellar cyclic GMP when applied to slices or when given by intraventricular injection. Gamma-aminobutyric acid (GABA), on the other hand, causes a decrease in cerebellar cyclic GMP when given intraventricularly.

Electrophysiological studies of neurons in the rat cerebral cortex have shown that iontophoretically applied cyclic GMP, like acetylcholine, increases the firing rate of certain pyramidal cells. Cortical pyramidal cells which are unaffected by acetylcholine show no response to cyclic GMP. These latter cells often display a decrease in firing rate in response to norepinephrine, an effect mimicked by cyclic AMP.

Peripheral Nervous System

In both frog and rabbit sympathetic ganglia, stimulation of the preganglionic fibers causes a slow excitatory (depolarizing) postsynaptic potential, which is blocked by atropine. The same effect can be produced by applying acetylcholine or bethanechol. Substantial evidence suggests that cyclic GMP metabolism may be linked to the muscarinic effects of acetylcholine in these peripheral sympathetic ganglia. In the frog ganglion, brief presynaptic stimulation at physiological rates causes a twofold increase in cyclic GMP content. This increase in cyclic GMP is blocked by the muscarinic antagonist atropine. When the release of neurotransmitter is prevented by a high-magnesium, low-calcium Ringer's solution, the same preganglionic stimulation no longer raises cyclic GMP levels.

In slices of bovine superior cervical ganglion, both acetylcholine and bethanechol increase cyclic

GMP content. This effect is blocked by atropine, but not by the nicotinic blocking agent hexamethonium. Histochemical evidence also shows that the increase in cyclic GMP caused by acetylcholine takes place in the postganglionic neurons.

Electrophysiological studies in the rabbit have shown that the dibutyryl derivative of cyclic GMP mimics electrical stimulation and acetylcholine in causing a slow depolarization of the sympathetic ganglion.

Muscarinic cholinergic end organs, such as intestine, heart, and ductus deferens, all display increases in cyclic GMP when exposed to acetylcholine, as does the sympathetic ganglion. Furthermore, these increases are blocked specifically by muscarinic antagonists. Electrical stimulation of the vagus nerve has been shown to increase cyclic GMP in stomach mucosa, and this effect, too, is abolished by atropine. A cyclic GMP–dependent protein kinase found in intestine, ductus deferens, and uterus causes the phosphorylation of specific membrane proteins. It is not as yet known whether the membrane-permeability changes that occur in response to activation of muscarinic receptors in cholinergically innervated tissues are mediated through an acetylcholine-induced increase in cyclic GMP and the stimulation of cyclic GMP–dependent phosphorylation of specific membrane proteins.

Recent studies in vertebrate skeletal muscle have shown that nicotinic cholinergic stimulation can also increase cyclic GMP. Such increases may result indirectly from membrane depolarization, rather than through activation of a neurotransmitter-sensitive guanylate cyclase.

Conclusion

The available evidence supports a role for cyclic AMP in several aspects of neuronal function. One of the most important of these is as a mediator of the postsynaptic effects of a number of neurotransmitters. Through this mechanism, neurotransmitter diffusing across the synaptic cleft and contacting the postsynaptic membrane is thought to activate a specific adenylate cyclase located in that membrane. The resulting increase in cyclic AMP in the receptor cell activates a cyclic AMP–dependent

protein kinase (or phosphoprotein phosphatase) that changes the level of phosphorylation of a particular membrane-bound protein (or proteins). It is postulated that the phosphorylated protein then causes a change in ion permeability of the nerve membrane. In some cases, this change in ion permeability may be relatively long lasting, and it is possible that, under certain circumstances, such a mechanism could form the basis for plastic changes in the nervous system. Less extensive data suggest a role for cyclic GMP as mediator of certain of the postsynaptic effects of some other neurotransmitters. In addition, recent evidence suggests that cyclic nucleotides may play a role in presynaptic events.

The full extent of the involvement of cyclic AMP and cyclic GMP in neuronal function is not yet known. It seems likely that these nucleotides are involved in several aspects of the functioning of the nervous system. The nature and extent of this involvement represent important areas for future study.

Acknowledgment

Preparation for this chapter was supported in part by H.E.W. grants DA-01627, MH-17387, NS-16356, and NS-08440, and grants from the McKnight Foundation. J.A.N. is the recipient of a PMAF Faculty Development Award in Clinical Pharmacology.

References

*1. Robison, G. A., Butcher, R. W., and Sutherland, E. W. *Cyclic AMP.* New York: Academic, 1971.
*2. Greengard, P. Phosphorylated proteins as physiological effectors. *Science* 199:146–152, 1978.
3. Birnbaumer, L., and Iyengar, R. Coupling of receptors to adenylate cyclase. In J. A. Nathanson and J. W. Kebabian (eds.), *Biochemistry of Cyclic Nucleotides.* New York: Springer-Verlag, 1981.
4. Appleman, M. M., Ariano, M. A., Takemoto, D. J., and Whitson, R. H. Cyclic nucleotide phosphodiesterases. In J. A. Nathanson and J. W. Kebabian (eds.), *Biochemistry of Cyclic Nucleotides.* New York: Springer-Verlag, 1981.
5. Amer, M. S., and Kreighbaum, W. E. Cyclic nucleotide phosphodiesterases: Properties, acti-

*Key reference.

vators, inhibitors, structure-activity relationships, and possible role in drug development. *J. Pharm. Sci.* 64:1–37, 1975.

*6. Greengard, P. *Cyclic Nucleotides, Phosphorylated Proteins, and Neuronal Function.* New York: Raven Press, 1978.

*7. Beavo, J. A., and Mumby, M. C. Cyclic AMP-dependent phosphorylation. In J. A. Nathanson and J. W. Kebabian (eds.), *Biochemistry of Cyclic Nucleotides.* New York: Springer-Verlag, 1981.

8. Langan, T. A. Protein kinases and protein kinase substrates. *Adv. Cyclic Nucleotide Res.* 3:99–153, 1973.

9. Beam, K. G., and Greengard, P. Cyclic nucleotides, protein phosphorylation and synaptic function. *Cold Spring Harbor Symp. Quant. Biol., The Synapse* 40:157–168, 1976.

10. Drummond, G. I., Greengard, P., and Robison, G. A. (eds.), Second International Conference on Cyclic AMP. *Adv. Cyclic Nucleotide Res.* 5, 1975 (several articles).

*11. Dunwiddie, T. V., and Hoffer, B. J. Physiological role of cyclic nucleotides in the nervous system. In J. W. Kebabian and J. A. Nathanson (eds.), *Pharmacology and Physiology of Cyclic Nucleotides.* New York: Springer-Verlag, 1981.

*12. Bloom, F. E. The Role of Cyclic Nucleotides in Central Synaptic Function. In *Reviews of Physiology, Biochemistry, and Experimental Pharmacology.* New York: Springer-Verlag, 1975.

*13. Nathanson, J. A. Cyclic nucleotides and nervous system function. *Physiol. Rev.* 57:158–256, 1977.

*14. Daly, J. W. Role of Cyclic Nucleotides in the Nervous System. In L. L. Iversen, S. D. Iversen, and S. H. Snyder (eds.), *Handbook of Psychopharmacology.* New York: Plenum, 1975. Pp. 47–130.

15. George, W. J., and Ignaro, L. J. (eds.). Third International Conference on Cyclic Nucleotides. *Adv. Cyclic Nucleotide Res. 9,* 1977 (several articles).

16. McIlwain, H. Cyclic AMP and Tissues of the Brain. In B. R. Rabin and R. B. Freedman (eds.), *Effects of Drugs on Cellular Control Mechanisms.* New York: Macmillan, 1972. P. 281.

*17. Greengard, P. Possible role for cyclic nucleotides and phosphorylated membrane proteins in postsynaptic actions of neurotransmitters. *Nature* 260: 101–108, 1976.

*18. Kebabian, J. W. Biochemical regulation and physiological significance of cyclic nucleotides in the nervous system. *Adv. Cyclic Nucleotide Res.* 8: 421–508, 1977.

*19. Goldberg, N. D., and Haddox, M. K. Cyclic GMP metabolism and involvement in biological regulation. *Annu. Rev. Biochem.* 46:823–896, 1977.

Chapter 16. Prostaglandins and Thromboxanes in the Nervous System

The discovery of the prostaglandins dates back to 1933, when von Euler and Goldblatt described active principles in human seminal fluid and extracts of sheep seminal vesicular glands that stimulated isolated intestinal and uterine muscle and lowered the blood pressure in intact animals. It was shown that these activities were due to highly potent acidic lipids, and von Euler proposed the name "prostaglandin" because, initially, they were thought to derive from the prostate gland.

Intensive work on the purification and elucidation of the structure of these active principles was carried out by Bergström and his team in Sweden during the years 1956 to 1963 [1]. Two classes of prostaglandins were separated by solvent partition between ether and phosphate buffer. The compounds more soluble in ether were called *prostaglandin E* and those more soluble in the phosphate buffer were called *prostaglandin F* (after *Fosfat*). Elegant chemical degradation studies and the powerful techniques of gas-liquid chromatography combined with mass spectrometry, which also were being developed in Sweden at that time, resulted in the elucidation of the structures of this new group of compounds, even though only a few milligrams of the purified compounds were then available. The prostaglandins were found to be a family of oxygenated, unsaturated, 20-carbon cyclopentane carboxylic acids, in which individual members differ in the positions and types of oxygenation and unsaturation.

Immediately after the structures were established, the origins of the prostaglandins from certain essential fatty acids was demonstrated by two groups of scientists—those of Bergström in Sweden and van Dorp in Holland—who showed that microsomal fractions from sheep vesicular glands bioconverted arachidonic acid ($\triangle^{5,8,11,14}$ all *cis*-eicosatetraenoic acid) into PGE_2. Subsequently, it was shown that $PGF_{2\alpha}$ also was formed from arachidonic acid; that $\triangle^{8,11,14}$ eicosatrienoic acid (homo-γ-linolenic acid) was the precursor of PGE_1 and $PGF_{1\alpha}$; and that $\triangle^{5,8,11,14,17}$ eicosapentaenoic acid was the precursor of PGE_3 and $PGF_{3\alpha}$ [1]. These transformations are illustrated in Fig. 16-1.

The capacity for biosynthesis of prostaglandins is widely distributed in the animal kingdom. In most mammalian tissues (including nervous tissue, particularly in the human), arachidonic acid is quantitatively the most important precursor for local endogenous biosynthesis of prostaglandins.

In the older literature, one finds that different names have been given to the biological activity of lipid extracts of tissues, including *slow-reacting substance C, Darmstoff, intestinal stimulant acid lipids, irin, menstrual stimulant, vasodepressor lipid, medullin, and unsaturated hydroxy fatty acid fractions from brain*. It is now known that the lipid extracts owe many of their biological activities to the presence of one or more of the prostaglandins, prostaglandin endoperoxides, and lipoperoxides [1, 2].

Dramatic changes have taken place in research on the prostaglandin system as the result of the isolation and determination of the structure of two prostaglandin endoperoxides, PGG_2 and PGH_2, in 1973 [3]. In addition to their conversion into the primary, stable prostaglandins, PGE_2, PGD_2, and $PGF_{2\alpha}$, these endoperoxides also are converted enzymatically in certain tissues into thromboxane A_2 (identical to rabbit aorta-contracting substance) and prostacyclin, or PGI_2 [4–9], both highly biologically active, unstable derivatives. These path-

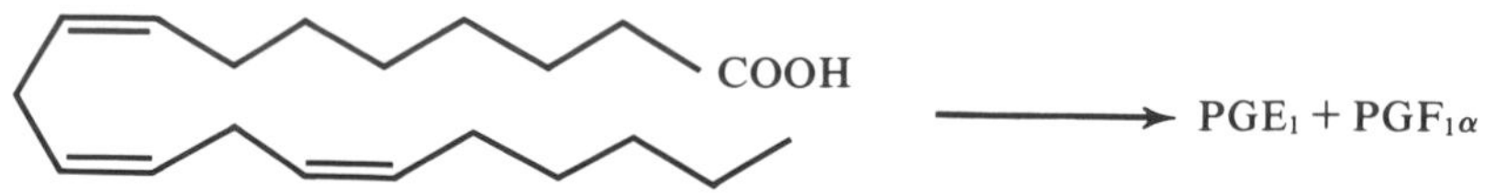

8,11,14-Eicosatrienoic acid → $PGE_1 + PGF_{1\alpha}$

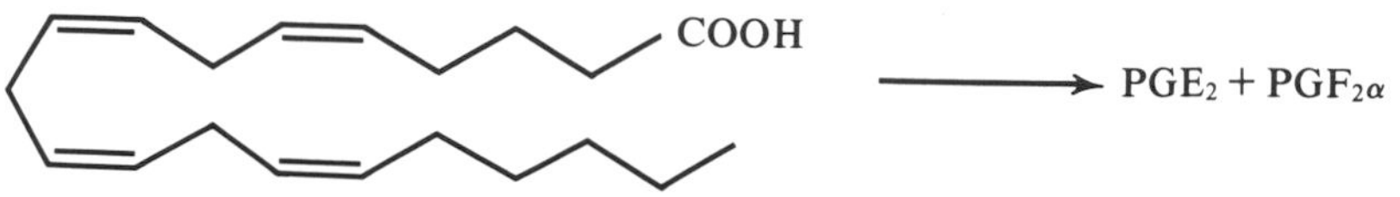

Δ 5,8,11,14-Eicosatetraenoic acid
(arachidonic acid) → $PGE_2 + PGF_{2\alpha}$

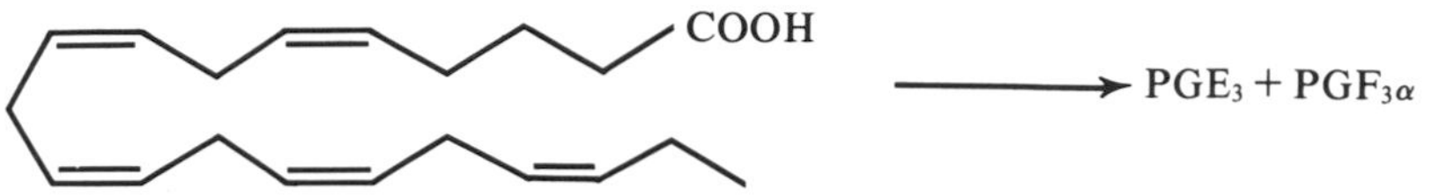

5,8,11,14,17-Eicosapentaenoic acid → $PGE_3 + PGF_{3\alpha}$

Fig. 16-1. Formation of prostaglandins from poly-unsaturated fatty acids. Note that unsaturated bonds are all cis *and are located from the carboxyl end. Thus, arachidonic acid (Δ 5, 8, 11, 14) is also ω 6, 9, 12, 15.*

ways are discussed below in greater detail. It now seems that in a number of tissues the formation of thromboxane A_2 and prostacyclin from arachidonic acid is quantitatively more important than formation of the primary prostaglandins.

A wide range of physiological and pathophysiological stimuli (hormones, neurotransmitters, enzymes, peptides, trauma, inflammation, pyrogens, immune and allergic reactions, neoplasia) activate the plasma-membrane enzymes in mammalian cells and so lead to the formation of the prostaglandin endoperoxides, prostaglandins, and thromboxanes. The biologically active compounds do not accumulate intracellularly and, therefore, occur only in trace amounts in tissues and body fluids. After formation, action, and release, they are converted rapidly into inactive metabolites, which appear in the blood and urine. The pharmacological actions of the prostaglandins and thromboxanes are exeedingly diverse and may differ according to tissue, species, and depending upon whether their action is studied in vivo or in vitro. The physiological importance of these compounds, although still far from clear, is growing rapidly at the present time, particularly in the areas of vascular homeostasis, platelet function,

and hormone secretion. They can be regarded as mediators or bioregulators of many processes that couple stimulus and secretion. The primary prostaglandins and thromboxane A_2 are regarded as local hormones, although evidence is growing that prostacyclin is truly a circulating hormone released from the vascular endothelium into the circulation and controls the ability of platelets to aggregate. The decreased or excessive formation of prostaglandins and thromboxanes may modify cellular homeostasis profoundly and may be an important factor in many human diseases [9–16].

Mechanism of Biosynthesis

The multienzyme system required for the biosynthesis of the prostaglandin endoperoxides from arachidonic acid is outlined in Fig. 16-2. The prostaglandin endoperoxides and their metabolites cannot be formed from precursor fatty acids that are esterified to complex lipids. Unesterified fatty

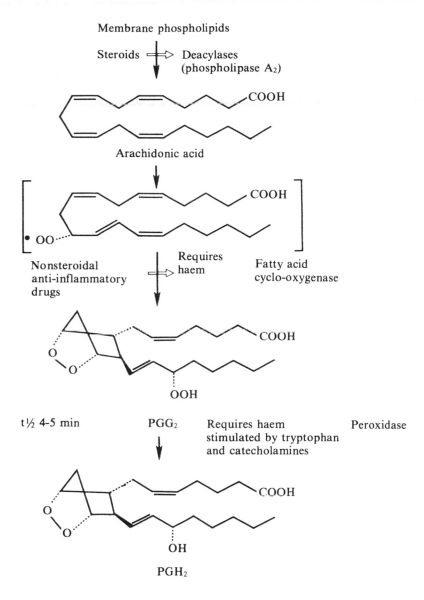

Membrane phospholipids

Steroids ⟹ Deacylases
(phospholipase A₂)

Arachidonic acid

Nonsteroidal
anti-inflammatory
drugs

Requires ⟹ haem   Fatty acid
cyclo-oxygenase

t½ 4-5 min   PGG₂   Requires haem   Peroxidase
                              stimulated by tryptophan
                              and catecholamines

PGH₂

Fig. 16-2. Pathway for the biosynthesis of the prosta-glandin endoperoxides, PGG₂ and PGH₂. The rate of endogenous biosynthesis is controlled by the activity of acyl hydrolases that release free arachidonic acid from complex lipids.

acids, such as arachidonic acid, are virtually un-detectable in most tissues in vivo, so a controlled release from complex membrane lipids by acyl hydrolases or deacylases is required to provide sub-strate for the first step in the formation of the pros-taglandin endoperoxides. There is evidence that the most likely deacylase is a membrane phospho-lipase A₂ activity, although other enzymes, such as cholesterol esterase and diglyceride lipase, may be involved in certain tissues. Knowledge of the overall mechanism for prostaglandin endoperoxide syn-thesis is largely the result of investigations of

Samuelsson and coworkers in Sweden [6, 17]. The initial step is the removal by a lipoxygenaselike reaction of a prochiral hydrogen in the S configuration at C13 of the polyunsaturated fatty acid (e.g., arachidonic acid) substrate. The Δ^{11} double bond isomerizes into the Δ^{12} position, and molecular oxygen is inserted at C11 to form the 11-peroxy-5,8,12,14-eicosatetraenoic acid. This intermediate is converted by cyclization to form the cyclopentane ring and by the further addition of molecular oxygen at C15 into the 15-S-hydroperoxy prostaglandin endoperoxide, PGG$_2$. The enzyme(s) that carry out these transformations is (are) now termed *fatty acid cyclo-oxygenase(s)* and require(s) heme as a cofactor. The reduction of the 15-hydroperoxy group of PGG$_2$ by a peroxidase produces PGH$_2$, the 15-hydroxy prostaglandin endoperoxide. The peroxidase activity is intimately coupled with the cyclo-oxygenase, also requires heme, and is stimulated by tryptophan and such catecholamines as norepinephrine and dopamine. Solubilization, purification, and characterization of these two enzymes from membranes has been achieved only recently [6, 18, 19].

It had been known for some time that the biosynthesis of prostaglandins can be inhibited by several fatty acids that are not substrates for the cyclo-oxygenase (e.g., γ-linolenic acid or eicosatetraynoic acid). In 1971, Vane and coworkers made the important discovery that nonsteroidal anti-inflammatory drugs, such as acetylsalicylic acid (aspirin), indomethacin, and the fenamates were potent, irreversible inhibitors of the fatty acid cyclo-oxygenase [20–22]. This discovery has been of great importance in determining physiological and pathophysiological processes that involve mediation of the prostaglandin system. The inhibitory action of aspirin appears to be due to the irreversible acetylation of the cyclo-oxygenase [23, 24]. There is evidence that the anti-inflammatory action of certain steroids resides in their ability to generate an inhibitor of the release of the precursor fatty acids from membrane phospholipids [25].

When isolated from several tissues (seminal vesicles, platelets, and lung), PGG$_2$ and PGH$_2$ have a half-life in aqueous solutions of about 5 minutes, but can be stored for several weeks in dry, nonpolar solvents at low temperatures. When formed in tissues, the endoperoxides are metabolized further by three principal routes: (1) the primary prostaglandin pathways, (2) the thromboxane pathway, and (3) the prostacyclin pathway. These transformations are illustrated in Fig. 16-3. In the primary prostaglandin pathway, specific isomerases form PGE$_2$ and PGD$_2$. Reduced glutathione added to reaction mixtures favors PGE$_2$ formation. The enzymic nature of PGF$_{2\alpha}$ formation from PGH$_2$ by reduction is unresolved at the present time. It is of interest and of potential physiological importance that PGE$_2$ and PGF$_{2\alpha}$ are interconvertible by dehydrogenase and reductase activities in some tissues.

The thromboxane pathway was first discovered by Hamberg and Samuelsson in platelets stimulated to aggregate by arachidonic acid, collagen, or thrombin. Thromboxane A$_2$ has a unique, bicyclic, oxane-oxetane ring structure and is very unstable in aqueous solutions, where it has a half-life of 30 seconds and is hydrolyzed nonenzymatically into the stable compound thromboxane B$_2$ [4, 6]. The formation of thromboxane A$_2$ greatly stimulates platelet aggregation and is a powerful arterial vasoconstrictor, as well. The thromboxane pathway is also present in several other tissues (i.e., leukocytes, lung, spleen, umbilical artery, and brain). Imidazole and its methyl and butyl derivatives, as well as certain chemically synthesized endoperoxide analogs, are selective inhibitors of the thromboxane synthetase [14, 22]. A further reaction that is of some importance is the generation of the chemically reactive compound malondialdehyde, and 12-L-hydroxy-5,8,10-heptadecatrienoic acid (HHT) by either the decomposition of thromboxane A$_2$ or directly from the endoperoxides.

The prostacyclin pathway was discovered in 1976, when Vane and coworkers found that incubated rings of aortic tissue released a labile substance, at that time called *PGX*, which strongly inhibited platelet aggregation. Collaboration with chemists of the Upjohn Company soon led to the complete characterization of prostacyclin (PGI$_2$), the cyclic enol-ether prostaglandin [8, 15, 16]. This prostaglandin is the most potent inhibitor of platelet aggregation known, and it stimulates platelet cyclic AMP formation dramatically. It is also a potent vasodilator of all vascular beds, including cerebral arterioles. Many tissues have now been shown to synthesize PGI_2, often in much greater amounts than they synthesize the primary prostaglandins [see 16].

In 1971, Pace-Asciak and Wolfe postulated the origin of this compound from the endoperoxides in studies on prostaglandin synthesis in the rat stomach [26]. The PGI_2 synthetase is inhibited by 15-hydroperoxyarachidonic acid, and it has been reported that tranylcypromine, the monoamine oxidase inhibitor, can also inhibit PGI_2 synthesis or action in some circumstances [22]. PGI_2 is unstable in neutral and acidic conditions but is much more stable above pH 8.0. PGI_2 is hydrolyzed non-enzymatically into the stable, biologically inactive compound 6-keto-$PGF_{1\alpha}$. Much research is now concentrating on the chemical synthesis of selective inhibitors of both the PGI_2 and thromboxane pathways.

Catabolism

Studies with tritium-labeled prostaglandins have shown that both the E and F types are converted extremely rapidly into inactive metabolites when injected into the systemic circulation; these metabolites are excreted principally in the urine [27–29]. Four main types of transformation take place:

1. Oxidation of the allylic alcohol group at carbon 15 to the 15-keto-prostaglandins by a specific, NADH-dependent, 15-hydroxyprostaglandin dehydrogenase. The highest activities of this enzyme are found in the lung, spleen, and kidney cortex and the lowest are in brain.
2. Reduction of the Δ^{13} double bond to form dihydro compounds. There is much variability in the activity of the reductase in different tissues, in different animal species, and in different stages of development.

3. β Oxidation, principally in the liver, occurs to form dinor or tetranor prostaglandins.
4. ω Oxidation by microsomal enzymes transforms the metabolites further into ω-1, ω-2 hydroxylated compounds, and then to dicarboxylic acids.

The major urinary metabolites in man from $PGF_{1\alpha}$ and $PGF_{2\alpha}$ are 5α,7α-dihydroxy-11-keto-tetranor-prostane-1,16-dioic acid. The analogous metabolite from PGE_1 and PGE_2 is 7α-hydroxy-5, 11-diketo-tetranor-prostane-1,16-dioic acid. Figure 16-4 illustrates these interconversions. Many other urinary metabolites exist that vary with the animal species. A 9-keto reductase activity and a 9-hydroxy dehydrogenase activity that would lead to the interconversions of E and F type prostaglandins (see Fig. 16-3) have been reported in a number of tissues and species. Details of these activities can be obtained from the literature [15, 29]. An interesting finding is that, each day, males excrete considerably more prostaglandin metabolites in the urine than do females; this indicates a greater total body synthesis [9].

The catabolic pathway of thromboxane B_2, PGI_2, and 6-keto-$PGF_{1\alpha}$ is essentially similar to that of the E and F prostaglandins. All the metabolites of these compounds have not as yet been determined. Precise measurements of the major metabolites in blood or urine by either radioimmunoassay or gas chromatography–mass spectrometry methods is of key importance in determining altered synthesis of prostaglandins or thromboxanes in physiological cycles or in disease [6]. Because little catabolism takes place in brain, the biologically active compounds can be measured as such in the cerebrospinal fluid [30].

Formation and Release of Prostaglandins from the Central Nervous System

Release of prostaglandins into superfusates of cerebral cortex, cerebellum, spinal cord, and the cerebral ventricles in vivo and increased synthesis and release after stimulation of neural pathways has been clearly demonstrated [9, 30, 31]. It has been reported that PGE_1 and $PGF_{1\alpha}$ occur in the

A. The primary prostaglandin pathways

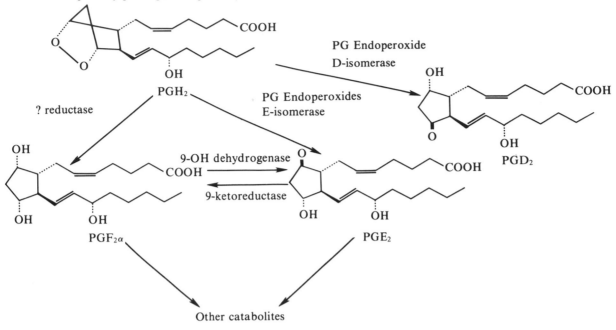

PG Endoperoxide
D-isomerase

PG Endoperoxides
E-isomerase

? reductase

PGH₂

9-OH dehydrogenase

9-ketoreductase

PGD₂

PGF₂α

PGE₂

Other catabolites

B. The thromboxane pathway

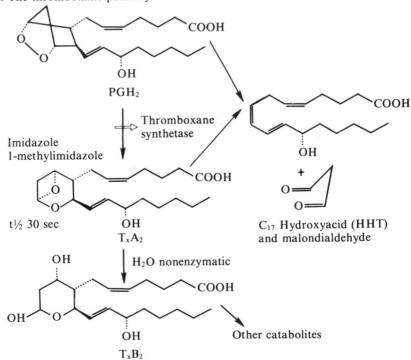

PGH₂

Thromboxane
synthetase

Imidazole
1-methylimidazole

t½ 30 sec

TxA₂

H₂O nonenzymatic

C₁₇ Hydroxyacid (HHT)
and malondialdehyde

OH

+

TxB₂

Other catabolites

C. The prostacyclin pathway

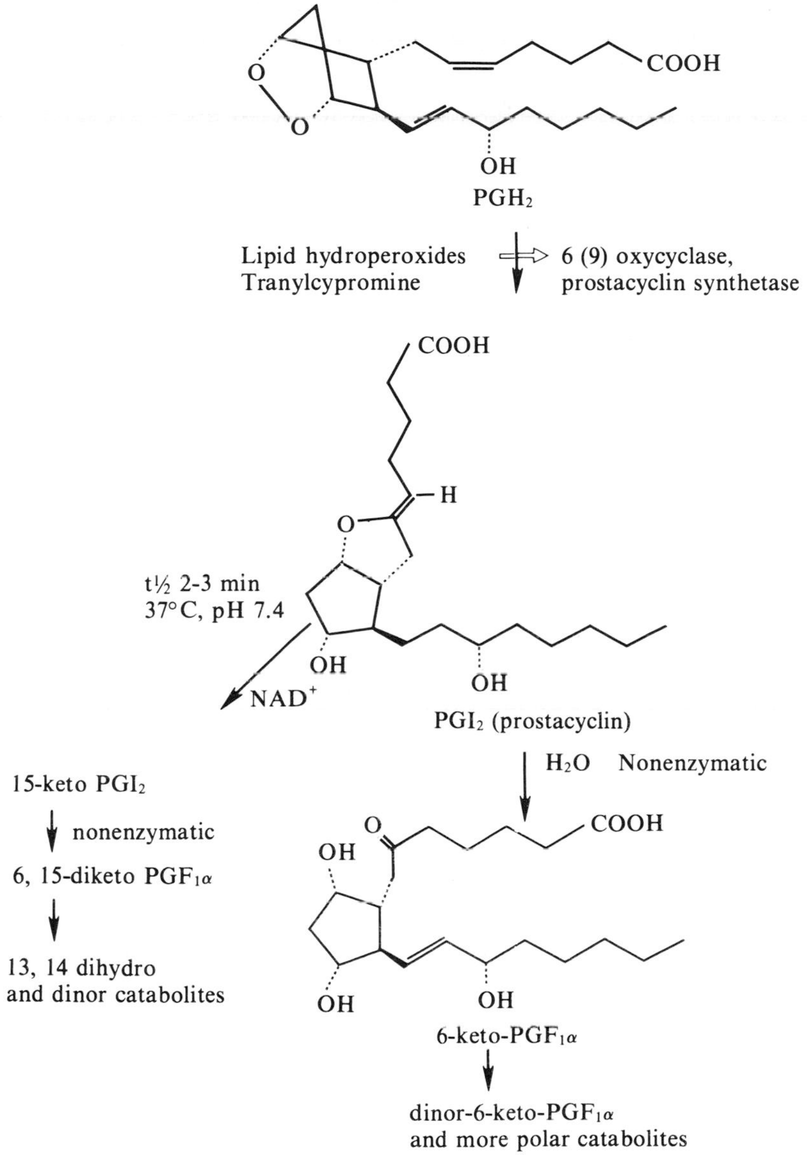

PGH$_2$

Lipid hydroperoxides   ⇒   6 (9) oxycyclase,
Tranylcypromine   prostacyclin synthetase

COOH

t½ 2-3 min
37°C, pH 7.4

NAD$^+$

PGI$_2$ (prostacyclin)

H$_2$O   Nonenzymatic

15-keto PGI$_2$

↓ nonenzymatic

6, 15-diketo PGF$_{1\alpha}$

↓

13, 14 dihydro
and dinor catabolites

COOH

6-keto-PGF$_{1\alpha}$

↓

dinor-6-keto-PGF$_{1\alpha}$
and more polar catabolites

*Fig. 16-3. The three major pathways for the bio-
synthesis of the primary prostaglandins, thromboxanes
(Tx), and prostacyclin (PGI$_2$) from the prostaglandin
endoperoxides.*

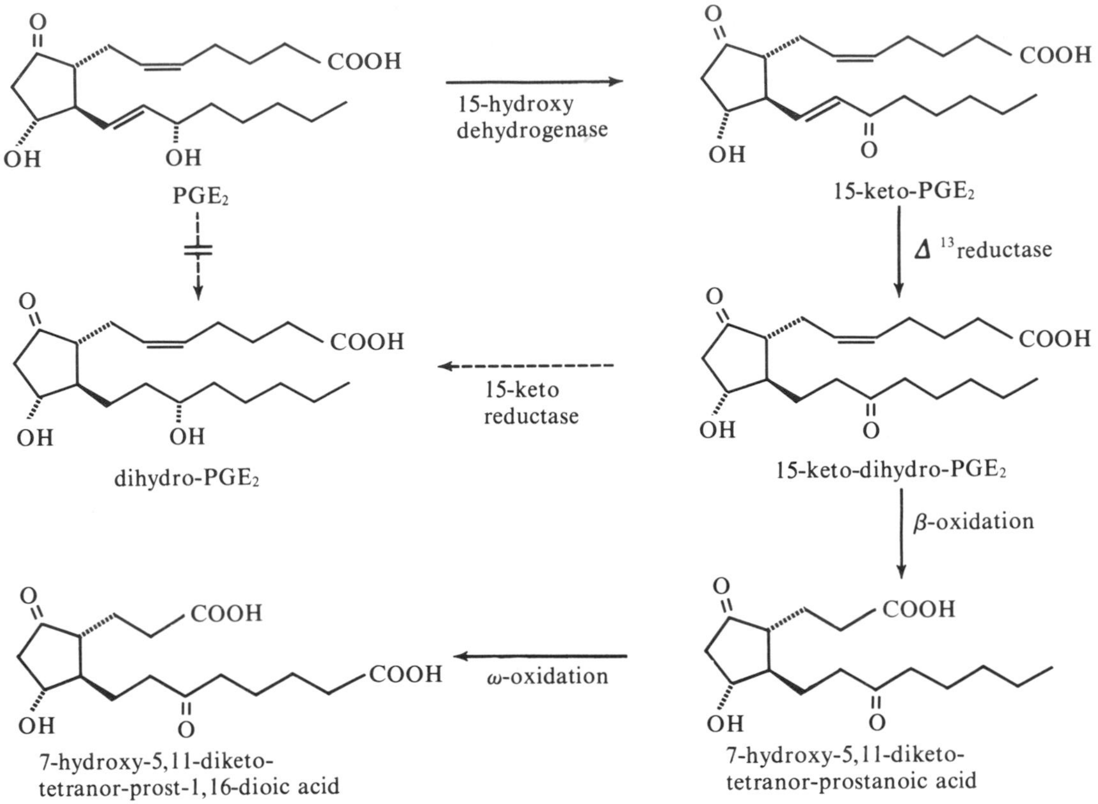

Fig. 16-4. *Major pathways in the catabolism of PGE₂ in man. The tetranor dicarboxylic acids are found in the urine. Essentially similar reactions occur in the catabolism of thromboxane B₂ and PGI₂ and 6-keto-PGF₁ₐ.*

mammalian central nervous tissue; however the $\triangle^{8,11,14}$ eicosatrienoic acid precursor is not found in either brain-complex lipids or in the unesterified fatty acid fraction [28, 30]. When chemically specific methodology is used and precautions are taken against post mortem changes in prostaglandin synthesis, the endogenous levels of PGE₂ and PGF₂ₐ are about 10 nanograms per gram of fresh tissue weight. Incubation of brain homogenates or tissue slices reveals considerable biosynthetic capacity to form PGF₂ₐ, PGE₂, PGD₂, and thromboxanes from an endogenous pool of free arachidonic acid [32–34]. Table 16-1 illustrates this point for several species. It is important to appreciate that the prostaglandin endoperoxide product that predominates varies with both the mammalian species and the brain region studied. Most studies show a predominance of PGF₂ₐ synthesis in cerebral cortex, but the reason is unclear,

since most studies also indicate few biological effects of this prostaglandin on brain function, as compared with PGE₂. It is of considerable interest that the median eminence has been shown to synthesize predominantly PGE₂. It has been demonstrated that PGE₂ stimulates the release of pituitary hormones, probably through stimulating the release of the hypothalamic releasing factors [35].

Recent work has shown the synthesis of thromboxane B₂ (and hence thromboxane A₂) in brain, although there are species differences; for example, the guinea pig shows a higher synthetic

Table 16-1. Endogenous Biosynthesis of Prostaglandins and Thromboxanes by Brain Tissue in Vitro (μg/g tissue*)

Species and Region	$PGF_{2\alpha}$	PGE_2	PGD_2	TxB_2
Rat				
Cerebral cortex slices	0.6	0.2	0.5	—
Cerebral cortex homogenate	0.8	0.3	1.2	0.2
Cerebral cortex homogenate + norepinephrine 1 mM	2.5	0.4	—	0.4
Cerebellum homogenate	0.2	0.2	0.3	—
Hippocampus homogenate	0.9	0.8	1.6	—
Guinea pig				
Cerebral cortex homogenate	0.6	0.1	1.4	1.7
Cerebellum homogenate	0.4	0.1	0.5	—
Hippocampus homogenate	1.2	0.2	1.1	—
Cat				
Cerebral cortex homogenate	2.0	0.8	0.2	—
Cerebellum homogenate	0.7	0.8	0.1	—
Hippocampus homogenate	0.9	1.6	0.2	—

*The prostaglandins and thromboxanes (Tx) were measured by gas chromatography–mass spectrometry, using deuterated compounds as carriers and internal standards. Values are means of 4–6 determinations for 45–60 minute incubations in Ringer's-bicarbonate-glucose (RBG) or phosphate buffer at pH 7.4.
Sources: Wolfe, Rostoworowski, and Pappius, *Can. J. Biochem.* 54:629–640, 1976; Wolfe, Rostoworowski, and Marion, *Biochem. Biophys. Res. Commun.* 70:907–913, 1976; Abdel-Halim et al., *Prostaglandins* 14:633–643, 1977 and 17:411–418, 1979.

capacity than does the rat [36]. There are some indications that thromboxanes may be synthesized by the glial cells. Prostaglandin D_2 is also formed in brain, and this may have functional implications, because it is a more potent stimulator of adenylate cyclase than is PGE_2 [33]. Prostacyclin is formed in small amounts in brain, but it probably originates from vascular elements, because isolated cerebral microvessels synthesize this prostaglandin.

The rate-controlling step in prostaglandin endoperoxide synthesis is thought to be the release of arachidonic acid from a plasma-membrane lipid pool. Evidence exists that a nonlysosomal-membrane phospholipase A_2 is the lipolytic enzyme which, after activation, provides substrate to the fatty acid cyclo-oxygenase. Extrinsic stimuli to cells and the associated deacylation reaction are thought to be related to the release of free calcium and a change in the structural arrangement of phospholipids in the plasma membrane [37]. Brain tissue in vivo contains very small amounts of unesterified fatty acids. Hypoxia, ischemia, trauma,

electroconvulsive shock, and convulsive drugs cause a rapid increase in the free fatty acid level, and arachidonic acid is released initially at a faster rate than are other fatty acids. These conditions also are associated with an increase in $PGF_{2\alpha}$ and PGE_2 synthesis. However, caution is needed in accepting the view that the synthetic enzymes of the prostaglandin system in brain are closely coupled to a phospholipase A_2–mediated release of arachidonic acid. The amount of this fatty acid released is about 100 times greater than the amount converted to prostaglandins and thromboxanes. If there is close coupling of prostaglandin synthesis to substrate release, a highly specific compartment must be involved.

The prostaglandins and thromboxanes formed during normal neuronal activity or in response to other stimuli diffuse into the cerebrospinal fluid. They then are transported out to the circulation by the choroid plexus and are inactivated in extraneural tissues. Thus, measurement of prostaglandin levels in cerebrospinal fluid can give a good indication of conditions that cause increased prostaglandin formation in vivo. Normally, human cerebrospinal fluid contains less than 100 picograms per milliliter $PGF_{2\alpha}$ and PGE_2 (range 30–140 pg/ml). Greatly increased levels are found in patients with epileptic seizures and after cerebral infarction, meningoencephalitis, or surgical brain trauma [38]. Recently, 6-keto-$PGF_{1\alpha}$ has been found in CSF, and the measurement of this prostaglandin could be a good indicator of damage to cerebral blood vessels. Prostaglandin levels are also significantly elevated in ventricular CSF of cats made febrile by administration of bacterial pyrogens [38].

Release from Autonomic Nerve Synapses and Regulation of Neurotransmission

Stimulation of sympathetic or parasympathetic nerves is associated with release of prostaglandins, principally PGE_2 and $PGF_{2\alpha}$. The release rate is, in general, related to the stimulus frequency and decreases to spontaneous levels on cessation of stimulation. The postsynaptic effector-cell membrane is most likely the site of synthesis, because receptor blockade by drugs (hyoscine, atropine, phenoxybenzamine, dibenzyline) inhibits prostaglandin release. Addition of the neurotransmitter also stimulates prostaglandin release. The many investigations of Hedqvist and coworkers on sympathetic nerve stimulation to various organs (heart, oviduct, spleen, vas deferens) have shown that the effector responses are inhibited by PGE_1 and PGE_2 but not by the PGF series of prostaglandins [39–41]. The inhibition can be produced by picogram and nanogram amounts well within the range of physiological concentrations.

Hedqvist put forward a working hypothesis that endogenous PGE_2 formed in and released from the postsynaptic effector membrane during stimulation inhibits the release of norepinephrine from presynaptic terminals. Evidence for this negative feedback-control hypothesis was obtained by using specific inhibitors of endogenous prostaglandin synthesis, namely, 5,8,11,14-eicosatetraynoic acid and indomethacin [21, 39]. In the presence of these compounds, the overflow of norepinephrine from

sympathetic nerve terminals is increased with a corresponding increase in the effector responses. The influx of calcium into nerve terminals is an essential part of stimulus-coupled exocytosis of norepinephrine, together with the adenine nucleotides and dopamine β-hydroxylase from sympathetic nerve terminals, and it is thought that this process is inhibited by the E-type prostaglandins. The Hedqvist hypothesis is diagrammatically represented in Fig. 16-5.

Release of PGE_2 from adrenergic pathways in the central nervous system may also be involved in the regulation of neurotransmitter release. The stimulated release of norepinephrine and dopamine from rat cerebral cortex and neostriatum in vitro is reduced by PGE_2. The disappearance time of dopamine histofluorescence in the neostriatum of rats pretreated with a tyrosine hydroxylase inhibitor is decreased when PGE_2 is infused into the carotid artery.

Although much evidence favors a role for E-type prostaglandins in the control of autonomic neurotransmission, there is some evidence that the F-type prostaglandins also are involved but appear to have a facilitatory action [30, 42]. Prostaglandin $F_{2\alpha}$ is known to potentiate the action of norepinephrine on vascular systems. Thus, two primary prostaglandins, PGE_2 and $PGF_{2\alpha}$, may have competitive interactions at monoaminergic synapses, analogous to the opposite effects of thromboxane A_2 and prostacyclin on platelet aggregation and vascular smooth muscle. There is no evidence that prostaglandins have any action on the release of acetylcholine or on the effector responses at nicotinic cholinoreceptors in sympathetic ganglia or at the neuromuscular junction.

Effects of Prostaglandins on Cyclic Nucleotides

Cyclic nucleotides play an important role in the mediation of postsynaptic effects of several neurotransmitters in both central and peripheral synapses (see Chap. 15). Prostaglandins of the E and D types stimulate cyclic adenosine monophosphate (cyclic AMP) formation in many tissues, including cerebral cortex slices in vitro and in cultured neural

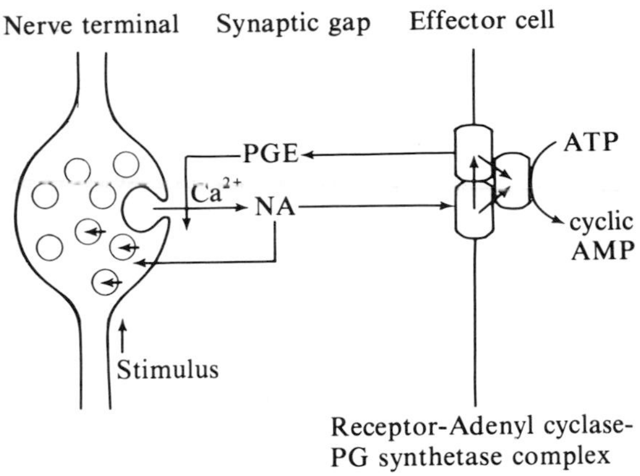

Nerve terminal   Synaptic gap   Effector cell

Receptor-Adenyl cyclase-
PG synthetase complex

Fig. 16-5. Feedback control of the release of norepinephrine by E-type prostaglandins (Hedqvist hypothesis).

cells [6, 43–45]. Which brain cell types—neuronal or glial—are specifically affected is not certain. Synergism of action on adenylate cyclase occurs with combinations of hormones and prostaglandins, but the meaning of these complex interactions is far from clear. Some evidence suggests that PGE_2 modifies the postsynaptic action of norepinephrine and dopamine, but there are many points of contention, particularly regarding this role in central synapses [38]. Future work must take into consideration effects of the prostaglandin endoperoxides, thromboxanes, and prostaglandins D_2 and PGI_2 (prostacyclin). PGI_2 is the most potent stimulator of platelet adenylate cyclase known, but a similar action on neurons has not been shown so far. Prostacyclin synthesis in brain appears to take place predominantly in vascular elements. Prostaglandin D_2 may be far more important in brain parenchyma as a stimulator of adenylate cyclase.

It is known that increases in intracellular cyclic AMP are associated with inhibited cell growth of various cell lines in culture. Mouse neuroblastoma cells in culture, for example, respond to dibutyryl cyclic AMP and prostaglandins E_1 and E_2 with a striking morphological differentiation and the development of axonlike processes. Is this solely a pharmacological response, or does it truly reflect action of brain PGE_2 on the cellular differentiation

process? It has also been reported that morphine and related drugs inhibit the stimulation of cyclic AMP formation by E-type prostaglandins. Opiates—as well as the endogenous peptides, endorphins—are known to decrease intracellular cyclic AMP levels, and the inhibition of the action on cyclic AMP levels produced by prostaglandins in the brain may be physiologically important [44].

High activities of guanylate cyclase take place in brain. It is interesting that the cholinergic agonists serotonin and $PGF_{2\alpha}$ elevate tissue levels of cyclic guanosine 5′-phosphate (cyclic GMP). It has been suggested that $PGF_{2\alpha}$ formation in brain facilitates excitation of cholinergic and serotoninergic pathways by activating guanylate cyclase, but as yet no solid evidence exists. It has been hypothesized that cyclic AMP and cyclic GMP have opposing actions in intracellular events and constitute an important control system (the Yin-Yang hypothesis, see [6] and [46]).

Effects on CNS Function

Direct intraventricular injections of E-type prostaglandins in experimental animals have a marked sedative effect, which may progress to a stuporous and catatonialike state. The effect of barbiturates is potentiated and animals are protected to some degree against the convulsions produced by pentylenetetrazol or electroshock. The effects of injected prostaglandins are prolonged and are present long after the injected prostaglandins have been removed through the choroid plexus. The mechanism of the sedative effects is unclear, but it is likely a slowly reversible depression of neurotransmission in certain central pathways through the reduction of neurotransmitter release, as has been demonstrated in peripheral adrenergic pathways.

Prostaglandins of both E and F types have complex actions on spinal cord reflexes and brain stem cardioregulatory and respiratory centers. Inhibitory and excitatory effects have been found, the results varying with the animal species and type of prostaglandin studied. The interested reader should consult the literature for details of these pharmacological actions and their relationships to neurophysiological mechanisms [30, 31, 40, 47]. Clearly, both excitatory and inhibitory actions are produced, and the effects are prolonged. Such prolonged changes are inconsistent with a transmitter-like role of prostaglandins and favor a modulatory action on synaptic transmission.

Fever and Temperature Regulation

Three neurotransmitters, 5-hydroxytryptamine (5HT), norepinephrine (NE), and acetylcholine, are involved in temperature regulation in the hypothalamus. Body temperature is controlled through antagonistic relationships (thermogenic or thermolytic) of 5HT and NE on neurons in the anterior hypothalamic-preoptic area. Acetylcholine is considered the transmitter in the temperature-raising pathway.

In recent years, convincing evidence has implicated stimulated endogenous biosynthesis of prostaglandins by the anterior hypothalamus in the genesis of fever caused by bacterial pyrogens and endotoxins [10, 21, 30, 31, 38]. This is based on the following results:

1. Prostaglandins of both E and F types are synthesized by hypothalamic tissue in vitro.
2. The E-type prostaglandins, injected intraventricularly, raise the temperature in a dose-dependent fashion in all animal species examined so far. PGE_1 is the most powerful pyretic agent known when injected directly into the anterior hypothalamus.
3. Fever is produced in unanesthetized cats by microinjections directly into the anterior hypothalamus of as little as 2 ng of PGE_1. This fever is unaffected by paracetamol (4-acetamidophenol) or aspirinlike drugs.
4. Pyrexia produced by intracerebral injections of pyrogens is inhibited by potent prostaglandin synthetase inhibitors, for example, indomethacin.
5. The amounts of PGE_2 in cerebrospinal fluid are greatly increased during fever produced by bacterial pyrogens and endotoxins.

Current knowledge indicates that pyrogens of exogenous origin—foremost among them bacterial endotoxins—as well as pathological conditions causing tissue inflammation elicit the formation of an endogenous pyrogen in neutrophils and cells of the reticular endothelium. This pyrogen is carried to the rostral region of the hypothalamus by the circulation. Activation of the prostaglandin-generating system occurs either at the level of the cerebral vessels or within the hypothalamus to form prostaglandin endoperoxides and PGE_2, which act on the thermoregulatory pathways to elevate the "set-point" for temperature regulation, thus causing fever. Although a large body of evidence supports the existence of a prostaglandin link in the central action of endogenous pyrogen, it should be clearly understood that some forms of pyrogenic fever do not seem to involve the prostaglandin system. For further details, the reader should consult recent reviews [38, 48]. Prostaglandins in the role of mediators are involved only in fevers sensitive to antipyretic drugs that inhibit prostaglandin endoperoxide biosynthesis, and prostaglandins probably do not contribute to normal body temperature regulation.

Release of Anterior Pituitary Hormone

Another area of much current interest, in which a sizable amount of evidence indicates that prostaglandins are involved, is the regulation of the synthesis and secretion of hormones by the anterior pituitary, mediated through peptide neurohormones (releasing factors) that are synthesized and released by hypothalamic neurons into the hypophyseal portal blood vessels (Chap. 14 and refs. 38, 49, 50). Inhibitors of prostaglandin synthesis are known to interfere with anterior pituitary hormone secretion. Microinjections or implantation of prostaglandin E_2 into the hypothalamus or injections into the ventricular system effectively stimulate the release of luteinizing hormone, follicle-stimulating hormone, prolactin, gonadotropin, and adrenocorticotropic hormone, most probably through their respective releasing hormones [50]. Prostaglandin E_2 elevates luteinizing hormone–releasing hormone (LHRH) in blood, and this PGE_2-evoked release is suppressed by antibodies to the releasing hormone. The medial basal hypothalamus and, in particular, the median eminence form and release PGE_2 in response to catecholaminergic stimulation, whereas blockade of PGE_2 synthesis by indomethacin suppresses the release of LHRH by catecholamines. Indomethacin also lowers the elevated levels of luteinizing hormone of castrated rats and prevents steroid-induced gonadotropin release in both rats and sheep. The action of PGE_2 appears to be directly on the neurons that release the hypophysiotropic hormones, because neurotransmitter receptor blockers do not prevent the increase in anterior pituitary hormone release. As mentioned previously, PGE_2 can stimulate cyclic AMP formation, and the effects on releasing-hormone release could be exerted through changes in the production of this cyclic nucleotide.

All the results mentioned here, plus many others, strongly suggest an important regulatory role of prostaglandins on hypothalamic neurons. Thus, we come back to a recurring theme in the physiological role of prostaglandins in nervous tissue: that the local formation of prostaglandins in the nervous system, when triggered by specific stimuli, can interact with specific neurons and change the release of monoamines, hypothalamic peptides, and pituitary hormones.

Cerebral Circulation

Much recent interest centers on the contributions that prostaglandins and thromboxanes might make to both normal and pathophysiological responses of cerebral blood vessels. Agents that constrict cerebral blood vessels are present in platelet-rich plasma. Serotonin is one of these, but its vasoconstrictive action is short lived. Of much greater importance is the release of thromboxane A_2, which is the most potent vasoconstrictor of cerebral vessels known at the present time. There is mounting evidence that thromboxane A_2 formation is important in the generation of vasospasm after subarachnoid hemorrhage. Both PGE_2 and $PGF_{2\alpha}$ have vasoconstrictive effects on cerebral arterioles and reduce cerebral blood flow, and their effects are prolonged [38]. In cerebral ischemia and cerebral thromboembolism (stroke), the release of these prostaglandins and thromboxane A_2 could contribute significantly to the expansion of the ischemic damage to the brain and further compromise the already tenuous local blood flow in these clinical situations. It is of considerable interest that experiments with dogs pretreated with indomethacin before they are subjected to a period of global ischemia indicate a facilitation of postischemic perfusion of the brain [51]. Prophylaxis with drugs that inhibit the fatty acid cyclooxygenase may have beneficial effects in patients predisposed to cerebral ischemia. Indeed, clinical trials with aspirin in patients with transient ischemic attacks indicate a significant protection against subsequent stroke in male subjects but, curiously, not in female [52]. The vascular endothelium of cerebral blood vessels synthesizes principally prostacyclin, known to be a potent vasodilator of cerebral blood vessels, as well as an inhibitor of platelet aggregation [16]. The formation of this prostaglandin within small vessels and capillaries of the brain may be important in the maintenance of vascular homeostasis and efficient cerebral perfusion. Damage to the cerebral endothelium, such as occurs in the formation of cerebral aneurisms, could locally disrupt prostacyclin formation and thus predispose to local thrombogenesis. It seems clear that, in the future, the prostaglandin system will have important clinical implications, particularly in neurological diseases associated with vascular insults.

Acknowledgment
Supported by the Medical Research Council of Canada.

References
*1. Bergström, S., Carlson, L. A., and Weeks, J. R. The prostaglandins: A family of biologically active lipids. *Pharmacol. Rev.* 20:1–48, 1968.
2. Vargaftig, B. B. Search for Common Mechanisms Underlying the Various Effects of Putative Inflammatory Mediators. In P. W. Ramwell (ed.), *The Prostaglandins*. New York: Plenum, 1974. Vol. 2, pp. 205–276.

*Key reference.

3. Hamberg, M., and Samuelsson, B. Detection and isolation of an endoperoxide intermediate in prostaglandin biosynthesis. *Proc. Natl. Acad. Sci. U.S.A.* 70:899–903, 1973.

*4. Hamberg, M., Svensson, J., and Samuelsson, B. Thromboxanes: A new group of biologically active compounds derived from prostaglandin endoperoxides. *Proc. Natl. Acad. Sci. U.S.A.* 72:2994–2998, 1975.

5. Samuelsson, B., et al. Prostaglandins and Thromboxanes: Biochemical and Physiological Considerations. In F. Coceani and P. M. Olley (eds.), *Prostaglandins and Perinatal Medicine. Advances in Prostaglandin and Thromboxane Research.* New York: Raven Press, 1978. Vol. 4, pp. 1–25.

*6. Samuelsson, B., et al. Prostaglandins and thromboxanes. *Annu. Rev. Biochem.* 47:997–1029, 1978.

7. Moncada, S., et al. An enzyme isolated from arteries transforms prostaglandin endoperoxides to an unstable substance that inhibits platelet aggregation. *Nature* 263:663–665, 1976.

*8. Moncada, S., and Vane, J. R. The Discovery of Prostacyclin (PGX). A Fresh Insight into Arachidonic Acid Metabolism. In N. Karash and J. Fried (eds.), *Biochemical Aspects of Prostaglandins and Thromboxanes.* New York: Academic, 1977. Pp. 155–177.

*9. Samuelsson, B., and Paoletti, R. (eds.). *Advances in Prostaglandin and Thromboxane Research.* Vols. 1 to 8. New York: Raven, 1976–1980.

10. Bergström, S. (ed.). International Conference on Prostaglandins. *Advances in Biosciences 9.* Oxford: Pergamon-Vieweg, 1973.

11. Karim, S. M. M. (ed.). *Prostaglandins: Physiological, Pharmacological and Pathological Aspects.* Baltimore: University Park Press, 1976.

12. Silver, M. J., Smith, J. B., and Kocsis, J. J. (eds.). *Prostaglandins in Hematology.* New York: Spectrum Publications, 1976.

*13. Ramwell, P. W. (ed.). *The Prostaglandins.* Vols. 1, 2, 3. 1973, 1974, 1977.

*14. Kharash, N., and Fried, J. (eds.) *Biochemical Aspects of Prostaglandins and Thromboxanes.* New York: Academic, 1977.

*15. Ramwell, P. W. (ed.). *Prostaglandins* (Los Altos, Ca.) Geron-X. [Numerous papers in this journal, particularly from Vol. 12, 1976 on.]

*16. Vane, J. R., and Bergström, S. (eds.). *Prostacyclins.* New York: Raven Press, 1979.

*17. Samuelsson, B. Structure, Biosynthesis and Metabolism of Prostaglandins. In S. J. Wakil (ed.), *Lipid Metabolism.* New York: Academic, 1970. Pp. 107–153.

18. Miyamoto, T., et al. Purification of prostaglandin endoperoxide synthetase from bovine vesicular gland microsomes. *J. Biol. Chem.* 251:2629–2636, 1976.

19. Ogino, N., et al. Purification of prostaglandin endoperoxide E isomerase from bovine vesicular microsomes, a glutathione requiring enzyme. *J. Biol. Chem.* 252:890–895, 1977.

20. Vane, J. R. Inhibition of prostaglandin synthesis as a mechanism of action of aspirinlike drugs. *Nat. New Biol.* 231:232–235, 1971.

*21. Robinson, H. J., and Vane, J. R. (eds.). *Prostaglandin Synthetase Inhibitors.* New York: Raven Press, 1974.

*22. Vane, J. R. Inhibitors of Prostaglandin, Prostacyclin and Thromboxane Synthesis. In F. Coceani and P. M. Olley (eds.), *Prostaglandins and Perinatal Medicine. Advances in Prostaglandin and Thromboxane Research.* New York: Raven Press, 1978. Vol. 4, pp. 25–44.

23. Roth, G. J., Stanford, N., and Majerus, P. W. Acetylation of prostaglandin synthetase by aspirin. *Proc. Natl. Acad. Sci. U.S.A.* 72:3073–3076, 1975.

24. Burch, J. W., et al. Sensitivity of fatty acid cyclooxygenase from human aorta to acetylation by aspirin. *Proc. Natl. Acad. Sci. U.S.A.* 75:5181–5184, 1978.

25. Flower, R. J., and Blackwell, G. J. Anti-inflammatory steroids induce biosynthesis of a phospholipase A_2 inhibitor which prevents prostaglandin generation. *Nature* 278:456–458, 1979.

26. Pace-Asciak, C., and Wolfe, L. S. A novel prostaglandin derivative formed from arachidonic acid by rat stomach homogenates. *Biochemistry* 10:3657–3669, 1971.

*27. Samuelsson, B., et al. Prostaglandins. *Annu. Rev. Biochem.* 44:669–695, 1975.

*28. Berti, F., Samuelsson, B., and Velo, G. P. (eds.) *Prostaglandins and Thromboxanes.* New York: Plenum, 1976.

*29. Lands, W. E. M. The biosynthesis and metabolism of prostaglandins. *Annu. Rev. Physiol.* 41:633–652, 1979.

30. Wolfe, L. S. Possible Roles of Prostaglandins in the Nervous System. In B. W. Agranoff and M. H. Aprison (eds.), *Advances in Neurochemistry.* New York: Plenum, 1975. Vol. 1, pp. 1–49.

*31. Coceani, F. Prostaglandins and the central nervous system. *Arch. Intern. Med.* 133:119–129, 1974.

32. Wolfe, Leonhard S., Rostworowski, K., and Pappius, H. M. The endogenous biosynthesis of prostaglandins by brain tissue in vitro. *Can. J. Biochem.* 54:629–640, 1976.

33. Abdel-Halim, S., et al. Identification of prostaglandin D_2 as a major prostaglandin in homogenates of rat brain. *Prostaglandins* 14:633–643, 1977.

34. Abdel-Halim, S. Regional and species differences

in endogenous prostaglandin biosynthesis by brain homogenates. *Prostaglandins* 17:411–418, 1979.

35. Ojeda, S. R., Naor, Z., and McCann, S. M. Prostaglandin E levels in hypothalamus, median eminence, and anterior pituitary of rats of both sexes. *Brain Res.* 149:274–277, 1978.

36. Wolfe, L. S., Rostworowski, K., and Marion, J. Endogenous formation of the prostaglandin endoperoxide metabolite, thromboxane B_2, by brain tissue. *Biochem. Biophys. Res. Comm.* 70:907–913, 1976.

*37. Galli, C., Galli, G., and Porcellati, G. (eds.). Phospholipases and prostaglandins. *Adv. Prostaglandin Thromboxane Res.,* vol. 3, 1978.

*38. Wolfe, L. S., and Coceani, F. The role of prostaglandins in the central nervous system. *Annu. Rev. Physiol.* 41:669–684, 1979.

39. Hedqvist, P. Autonomic Neurotransmission. In P. W. Ramwell (ed.), *The Prostaglandins.* New York: Plenum, 1973. Vol. 1, pp. 101–132.

*40. Horton, E. W. The Prostaglandins. In T. W. Goodwin (ed.), *Biochemistry of Lipids,* MTP International Review of Science. Baltimore: University Park Press, 1974. Pp. 237–270.

41. Hedqvist, P. Action of prostacyclin on adrenergic neuroeffector transmission in the rabbit kidney. *Prostaglandins* 17:249–258, 1979.

*42. Brody, J. J., and Kadowitz, P. J. Prostaglandins as modulators of the autonomic nervous system. *Fed. Proc.* 33:48–60, 1974.

43. Bergström, S. Prostaglandins: Members of a new hormonal system. *Science* 157:1–10, 1967.

*44. Kebabian, J. W. Biochemical Regulation and Physiological Significance of Cyclic Nucleotides in the Nervous System. In P. Greengard and G. A. Robison (eds.), *Advances in Cyclic Nucleotide Research.* New York: Raven Press, 1977. Vol. 8, pp. 421–508.

*45. Harris, R. H., Ramwell, P. W., and Gilmer, P. J. Cellular mechanisms of prostaglandin action. *Physiol. Rev.* 41:653–668, 1979.

46. Goldberg, N. D., O'Dea, R. F., and Haddox, M. K. Cyclic GMP. In P. Greengard and G. A. Robison (eds.), *Advances in Cyclic Nucleotide Research.* New York: Raven Press, 1973. Vol. 3, pp. 155–223.

47. Potts, W. J., East, P. F., and Mueller, R. A. Behavioural effects. *Prostaglandins* 2:157–173, 1974.

*48. Veale, W. L., Cooper, K. E., and Pittman, Q. J. Role of prostaglandins in fever and temperature regulation. *Prostaglandins* 3:145–167, 1977.

*49. Behrman, H. R. Prostaglandins in hypothalamo-pituitary and ovarian function. *Annu. Rev. Physiol.* 41:685–700, 1979.

50. Ojeda, S. R., Negro-Vilar, A., and McCann, S. M. Release of prostaglandin Es by hypothalamic tissue. *Endocrinology* 104:617–658, 1979.

51. Furlow, T. W., and Hallenbeck, J. M. Indomethacin prevents impaired perfusion of the dog's brain after global ischemia. *Stroke* 9:591–594, 1978.

52. Barnett, H. J. M., McDonald, J. W. D., and Sackett, D. L. Aspirin—effective in males threatened with stroke (editorial). *Stroke* 9:295–298, 1978.

Addendum

Since this chapter was prepared, new knowledge on the mechanisms of arachidonic acid release from membrane phospholipids and new pathways of arachidonic acid metabolism have been discovered. Activation of membrane receptors by a variety of stimuli is associated with the transmethylation of a specific pool of phosphatidyl ethanolamine to phosphatidylcholine followed by the release of arachidonic acid by phospholipase A_2 [53]. In some cells, activation of a phosphatidylinositol-specific phospholipase C occurs, followed by arachidonic acid release by diglyceride lipase or by conversion of the 1,2-diacylglycerides to phosphatidic acid and then transesterification to other phospholipids and deacylation [54, 55]. Metabolic studies in leukocytes led to the discovery of a new class of oxygenated metabolites of arachidonic acid named *leukotrienes* [56, 57]. The formation of these compounds is initiated by a specific lipoxygenase reacting at the 5-carbon of arachidonic acid to form a 5-hydroperoxy acid which loses water to become an unstable 5,6-oxido-7,9,11,14-eicosatetraenoic acid. This latter intermediate is converted either to 5,12-dihydroxy acids with potent chemotactic activity or through the action of glutathione S-transferase to 5(S)-hydroxy-6(R)-S-glutathionyl-7,9-*trans*,11,14-*cis*-eicosatetraenoic acid identified as one of the components of slow-reacting substance of anaphylaxis (SRS-A). This leukotriene elicits a prolonged excitatory action on cerebellar Purkinje neurons [58]. Two articles update the synthesis and roles of prostaglandins in cerebral blood vessels and the microcirculation [59, 60].

*53. Hirata, F., and Axelrod, J.   Phospholipid methylation and biological signal transmission. *Science* 209:1082–1090, 1980.

54. Lapetina, E. G., Billah, M. M., and Cuatrecasas, P. Rapid acylation and deacylation of arachidonic acid into phosphatidic acid of horse neutrophils. *J. Biol. Chem.* 255:10966–10970, 1980.

55. Marshall, P. J., Boatman, D. E., and Hokin, L. E. *J. Biol. Chem.* 256:844–847, 1981.

*56. Samuelsson, B.   The leukotrienes: A new group of biologically active compounds including SRS-A. *Trends Pharmacol. Sci.* 1:227–230, 1980.

*57. Borgeat, P., and Sirois, P.   Leukotrienes: A major step in the understanding of immediate hypersensitivity reactions. *J. Medicinal Chem.* 24:121–126, 1981.

58. Palmer, M. R., Mathews, R., Murphy, R. C., and Hoffer, B. J.   Leukotriene C elicits a prolonged excitation of cerebellar Purkinje neurons. *Neurosci. Lett.* 18:173–180, 1980.

59. Goehlert, U. G., Ny Ying Kin, N. M. K., and Wolfe, L. S.   Biosynthesis of prostacyclin in rat cerebral microvessels and the choroid plexus. *J. Neurochem.* 36:1192–1201, 1981.

*60. Kontos, H. A.   Regulation of the cerebral circulation. *Annu. Rev. Physiol.* 43:397–407, 1981.

Section IV. Metabolism

Abel L. Lajtha
Howard S. Maker
Donald D. Clarke

Chapter 17. Metabolism and Transport of Carbohydrates and Amino Acids

This chapter outlines aspects of carbohydrate and amino acid metabolism that are important for brain. Alterations in energy and carbohydrate metabolism, which are produced by varying functional demands of the nervous system and by pathological conditions, are discussed in Chaps. 24, 29, 30, and 36.

Although it is sometimes stated that brain is unique among tissues in its high rate of oxidative metabolism, overall brain metabolic rate (CMRO₂) is of the same order as unstressed heart and renal cortex [1]. However, regional metabolic fluxes in brain may greatly exceed the overall metabolic rate, and they are closely coupled to fluctuations in metabolic demand (Chap. 24).

Energy Metabolism

Oxidative steps of carbohydrate metabolism normally contribute 36 of the 38 high-energy phosphate bonds (~P) generated during the aerobic metabolism of a single glucose molecule. Approximately 15 percent of brain glucose is converted to lactate and does not enter the citric acid cycle. There are indications, however, that this might be matched by a corresponding uptake of ketone bodies. The total net gain of ~P is 33 equivalents per mole of glucose utilized. The steady state level of adenosine triphosphate (ATP) is high and represents the sum of a very rapid synthesis and utilization. Half of the terminal phosphate groups of ATP turn over in about 3 seconds, on the average, and probably in considerably shorter periods in certain regions [2]. The level of ~P is kept constant by regulation of adenosine diphosphate (ADP) phosphorylation in relation to ATP hydrolysis. The active adenylate kinase reaction, which forms equal amounts of ATP and adenosine monophosphate (AMP) from ADP, prevents any great accumulation of ADP.

Only a small amount of AMP is present under steady state conditions; consequently, a relatively small percentage decrease in ATP may lead to a relatively large percentage increase in AMP. AMP is a positive modulator of several reactions that lead to increased ATP synthesis, so such an amplification factor provides a sensitive control for maintenance of ATP levels [3]. Between 37 and 42°C brain metabolic rate increases at a rate of about 5 percent per degree.

The level of creatine phosphate in brain is even higher than that of ATP, and creatine phosphokinase is extremely active. The creatine phosphate level is exquisitely sensitive to changes in oxygenation, providing ~P for ADP phosphorylation and thus maintaining ATP levels. The creatine phosphokinase system may also function in regulating mitochondrial activity. The BB isoenzyme of creatine kinase is characteristic of, but not confined to, brain. Thus, finding this isoenzyme in body fluids does not necessarily indicate disruption of neural tissue.

Currently, it is common to relate metabolism to the *energy charge* of a tissue, which is equal to one-half the average number of anhydride-bound phosphate groups per adenosine moiety [4]: (ATP + ½(ADP)/(ATP) + (ADP) + (AMP). Calculated in this way, the steady state energy charge of most tissues is approximately the same and declines rapidly when energy demand exceeds supply (see Chaps. 24 and 35). It is a convenient shorthand for expressing relative energy states. It ignores nonadenylate energy stores, however, and its application to brain, which possesses finely tuned mechanisms for regulation and coupling of energy supply to utilization, can be misleading. Because brain metabolism actually responds in various ways to changes in the levels of individual nucleotide cofactors, metabolites, and ion fluxes, the calculated energy charge is an oversimplification that may cause overconfidence in one's knowledge of the true energy state and metabolic activity level of the tissue [5–9].

GLUCOSE TRANSPORT

Under ordinary conditions, the basic substrate for brain metabolism is glucose. The brain depends on glucose for energy and as the major carbon source for a wide variety of simple and complex molecules. Although other tissues can utilize glucose, it is not the primary metabolite of most. Heart, renal cortex, and even liver (the carbohydrate storehouse) derive most of their energy from fatty acids. During hypoglycemia these other tissues stop metabolizing glucose, making more available to the brain. Liver glycogen metabolism is under neural as well as hormonal control, allowing a sensitive provision for the needs of the brain. Stimulation of a cholinergic pathway in the lateral hypothalamus causes increased glycogen synthesis and decreased liver gluconeogenesis (through the vagus nerve), and stimulation of the ventromedial hypothalamus causes increased glucogenolysis and gluconeogenesis by a process not mediated by cyclic AMP [10].

A transient decline in the oxidative metabolism of glucose may lead to an abrupt disruption of brain function. Despite this dependence on glucose, the brain at rest extracts only about 10 percent of the glucose from the blood flowing through it—about 5 mg (28 μmol) glucose/100 g/min. If the flow of blood is slowed, a relatively greater fraction of both the oxygen and the glucose of the blood is taken up by the brain (see Chap. 24). The entry of most water-soluble substances into brain from blood is restricted. Even small molecules the size of glucose or fructose do not simply diffuse across this anatomicophysiological barrier. For selected metabolites important to brain metabolism, however, specific mechanisms exist to carry these molecules across the barrier (see Chap. 25). Although many glycolytic metabolites and substances that can be transformed into these metabolites can sustain brain metabolism in vitro, they fail to do so in the intact animal simply because they cannot penetrate into brain at sufficient rates. Although mannose may sustain brain metabolism in vivo, most other sugars, such as fructose, cannot be taken up rapidly enough, and brain metabolism cannot continue at normal rates when dependent on fructose alone. The capacity of fructose to sustain metabolism in the immature brain may be related to an incomplete barrier or to a lower metabolic demand before the brain matures [11].

Glucose crosses the barrier by a carrier mechanism specific to D-glucose. Certain analogs, such as 2-deoxyglucose, can be used to study this transport process, because they are not metabolized beyond the hexokinase step [12]. The use of radiolabeled deoxyglucose to delineate regional glucose metabolism is discussed below (Regional Differences) and in Chap. 24. When used to indicate rates of metabolism, it is probable that the rate-limiting step actually determined is that of hexose phosphorylation. Despite active transport, the concentration of glucose in brain is lower than it is in structures lacking a barrier, for example, sympathetic ganglia or peripheral nerve [13].

The affinity of the transport system for glucose may be expressed as a K_m analogous to enzyme activity. The K_m of glucose uptake into mammalian brain is 7 to 8 mM, approximately the level of plasma glucose. Although isolated brain capillary endothelial cells possess a glucose transport system with an affinity many times greater than that of in vivo transport [14], transport into endothelial cells evidently does not regulate transport into brain.

With a concentration at or below the K_m of the system, small changes in plasma glucose cause significant changes in the amount transported. Thus, within limits, glucose and glycogen levels in brain vary directly with blood glucose concentrations. The rate of influx of glucose increases linearly up to about 7 mM plasma glucose and at a lesser rate to about 20 mM. Brain glucose is always lower than blood glucose. There is, then, no safety device to supplement such a small carbohydrate reserve during hypoglycemia. Beyond the blood-brain barrier, brain tissue itself takes up glucose much more avidly. Glucose can be taken up into nerve terminals by carrier processes that possess an affinity for glucose 30 times higher than that of the blood-brain barrier transport system [12]. These terminals may be able to function despite low overall brain glucose levels. Brain tissue beyond the barrier is apparently sensitive to insulin, and an increase in glucose uptake and glycogen storage can be demonstrated in vitro. Although at present there is no report of a definite effect of circulating insulin on the intact brain, insulin has been detected in CSF [7, 15].

GLYCOGEN

Although present in relatively low concentration in brain (3.3 mmol per kilogram brain in rat), glycogen is a unique energy reserve that requires no energy (ATP) for initiation of its metabolism. As with brain glucose, glycogen levels in brain appear to vary with plasma glucose concentrations. Brain biopsies have shown that human brains contain much higher glycogen levels than do rodent brains, but the effects of anesthesia and pathological change in the tissue may have contributed to the high levels in biopsies. Glycogen granules have been seen in electron micrographs of glia and neurons of immature animals, but only in astrocytes of adults [16]. This may have been because neurons and oligodendroglia lack glycogen or because the methods used failed to preserve the granules. Barbiturates decrease brain metabolism and increase the number of granules that can be found, particularly in astrocytes of synaptic regions. Astrocyte glycogen may form a store of carbohydrate, made available to neurons by as yet undefined mechanisms. Associated with the granules are enzymes concerned with glycogen synthesis and, perhaps, degradation. The increased glycogen found in areas of brain injury may be due to glial changes or to decreased utilization during tissue preparation. The accepted role of glycogen is that of a carbohydrate reserve utilized when glucose falls below need. However, there is a rapid, continual breakdown and synthesis of glycogen (17 μmol/kg/min) [17]. This is approximately

2 percent of the normal glycolytic flux in brain and is subject to elaborate control mechanisms. This suggests that, even under steady state conditions, local carbohydrate reserves are important for brain function. If glycogen were the sole supply, however, the normal glycolytic flux in brain would be maintained for less than 5 minutes.

The enzyme systems that synthesize and catabolize glycogen in other tissues also are found in brain, but their kinetic properties and modes of regulation appear to differ [18]. Glycogen levels in liver are regulated to reduce blood glucose (through insulin) below the renal threshold after a carbohydrate meal and to maintain blood glucose levels (through decreased insulin, glucagon, and epinephrine) at other times. Resting aerobic muscles utilize glucose and fatty acids for energy, but a large store of glycogen is utilized under the relatively hypoxic conditions present during strong rapid contractions. Glycogenolysis in muscle is linked to contraction by sensitivity to the same changes in ionized calcium that couple muscle-membrane excitation to contraction. Circulating epinephrine also will increase muscle glycogenolysis controlled by the cyclic AMP system. Liver glycogen is stored for use by the entire body, and the regulation of muscle glycogen reflects its use during brief periods of intense activity. Glycogen metabolism in brain, however, is controlled locally. This metabolism is isolated from the tumult of systemic activity, evidently because of the blood-brain barrier. Although glucocorticoid hormones that penetrate the brain will increase glycogen turnover, circulating protein hormones and biogenic amines are without effect [17]. Beyond the barrier, cells are sensitive to local amine levels, so drugs that penetrate the barrier and modify amine levels or membrane receptors cause metabolic changes [19].

Separate systems for the synthesis and degradation of glycogen provide a greater degree of control than would be the case if glycogen were degraded simply by reversing the steps in its synthesis (see Fig. 17-1). The level of glucose 6-phosphate, the initial synthetic substrate, usually varies inversely with the rate of brain glycolysis because of a greater

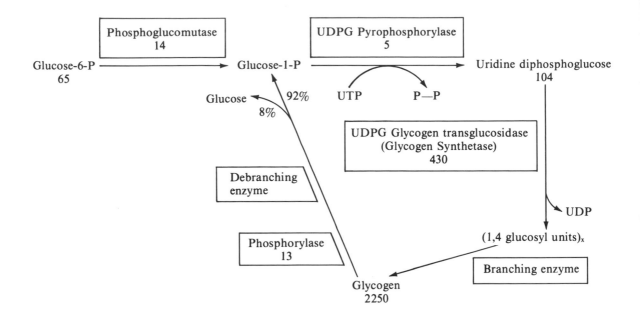

facilitation of the phosphofructokinase step relative to glucose transport and phosphorylation. Thus, the decline in glucose 6-phosphate at times of energy need decreases glycogen formation.

The glucosyl group of uridine diphosphate (UDP) is transferred to the terminal glucose of the nonreducing end of an amylose chain in an α-1,4-glycosidic linkage (Fig. 17-1). This reaction is catalyzed by glycogen synthetase and is the rate-controlling reaction in glycogen synthesis [18]. In brain, as in other tissues, glycogen synthetase occurs in both a phosphorylated (D) form, which is dependent for activity on glucose 6-phosphate as a positive modulator, and as a dephosphorylated, independent (I) form sensitive to, but not dependent on, the modulator. Although in brain the independent form of the glycogen synthetase requires no stimulator, it has a relatively low affinity for UDP-glucose. At times of increased energy demand, there is a change not only from the D to the I form, but an I form with an even lower affinity for the substrate develops. The inhibition of glycogen synthesis is enhanced, and this increases the availability of glucose 6-phosphate for energy needs. Goldberg and O'Toole [18] hypothesize that, in brain, the I form is associated with inhibition

Fig. 17-1. Glycogen metabolism in brain. Enzyme data from mouse brain homogenates. The figures under each enzyme represent V$_{max}$ at 38° C in mmol per kilogram wet weight per minute. Metabolite levels from quick-frozen adult mouse brain are indicated in micromoles per kilogram wet weight. (Metabolite data from Passonneau et al., J. Biol. Chem. 244:902, 1969. Enzyme data from Breckenridge and Gatfield, J. Neurochem. 3:234, 1961.)

of glycogen synthesis under conditions of energy demand, whereas the D form is responsible for a relatively small regulated synthesis under resting conditions. The regulation of the D form may be responsible for reducing the rate of glycogen formation in brain to about 5 percent of its potential rate. In liver, where large amounts of glycogen are synthesized and degraded, the I form of the synthetase is associated with glycogen formation. At the present time, it appears that the two tissues use the same biochemical apparatus in different ways in relation to differences in overall metabolic patterns.

Under steady state conditions, it is probable that less than 10 percent of phosphorylase in brain (Fig. 17-1) is in the unphosphorylated *b* form (requiring AMP), which is inactive at the very low

AMP concentrations present normally. When the steady state is disturbed, there may be an extremely rapid conversion of the enzyme to the *a* form, which is active at low AMP levels. Brain phosphorylase *b* kinase is indirectly activated by cyclic AMP and by the micromolar levels of ionized calcium released during neuronal excitation (see Chap. 15). Brain endoplasmic reticulum, like that in muscle, is capable of taking up this calcium to terminate its stimulatory effect. These reactions provide energy from glycogen during excitation and when cyclic AMP–forming systems are activated. It has not been possible to confirm directly, however, that the conversion from phosphorylase *b* to *a* is a control point of glycogenolysis in vivo. Norepinephrine and (probably) dopamine activate glycogenolysis through cyclic AMP; but epinephrine, vasopressin, and angiotension II do so by another mechanism, possibly involving calcium or a calcium-mediated proteolysis of the phosphorylase kinase [19]. The hydrolysis of the α-1,4-glycoside linkages leaves a limit dextrin that turns over at only half the rate of the outer chains [17]. The debrancher enzyme that hydrolyzes the α-1,6-glycoside linkages may be rate-limiting if the entire glycogen granule is to be utilized. Because one product of this enzyme is free glucose, approximately one glucose molecule for every eleven of glucose 6-phosphate is released if the entire glycogen molecule is degraded (Fig. 17-1). α-Glucosidase (acid maltase) is a lysosomal enzyme whose precise function in glycogen metabolism is not known. In Pompe's disease (the hereditary absence of the enzyme), glycogen accumulates in brain lysosomes as well as in those elsewhere (Chaps. 27 and 29). The steady state level of glycogen is regulated precisely by the coordination of synthetic and degradative processes through enzymatic regulation at several metabolic steps [6, 7].

GLYCOLYSIS

The terms *aerobic* and *anaerobic glycolysis* may be misleading. Since the time when metabolism began to be studied in the Warburg apparatus, workers usually have referred to the production of lactate under conditions of "adequate" oxygen as *aerobic glycolysis,* and that under anoxia as *anaerobic glycolysis.* Aerobic glycolysis, thus defined, measures only a small portion of total glycolysis [20]. Recently it has become common to refer to the Embden-Meyerhoff glycolytic sequence from glucose (or glycogen glucosyl) to pyruvate by the term *glycolysis*. Changes in the activity of the sequence at various oxygen levels have been termed *aerobic* or *anaerobic glycolysis*. Failure to differentiate between these definitions may lead to confusion, particularly if one is examining data pertinent to neurochemistry derived from more recent methods, such as cell and tissue culture. *Glycolytic flux* is defined indirectly: it is the rate at which glucose must be utilized to produce the observed rates of ADP phosphorylation.

Figure 17-2 outlines the flow of glycolytic substrates in brain. Glycolysis first involves phosphorylation by hexokinase. The reaction is essentially irreversible and is a key point in the regulation of carbohydrate metabolism in brain. The electrophoretically slow-moving (type 1) isoenzyme of hexokinase is characteristic of brain. In most tissues hexokinase may exist in the cytosol (soluble), or it may be firmly attached to mitochondria [21]. Under conditions in which no special effort is made to stop metabolism while isolating mitochondria, 80 to 90 percent of brain hexokinase is bound. In the live steady state, however (i.e., when availability of substrates keeps up with metabolic demand and end products are removed), an equilibrium exists between the soluble and the bound enzyme. Binding changes the kinetic properties of hexokinase and its inhibition by glucose 6-phosphate, so that the bound enzyme on mitochondria is more active. The extent of binding is inversely related to the ATP/ADP ratio, so conditions in which energy utilization exceeds supply shift the solubilization equilibrium to the bound form and produce a greater potential capacity for initiating glycolysis to meet the energy demand. This mechanism allows ATP to function both as a substrate of the enzyme and, at another site, as a regulator to decrease ATP production through its influence on enzyme binding. It also confers

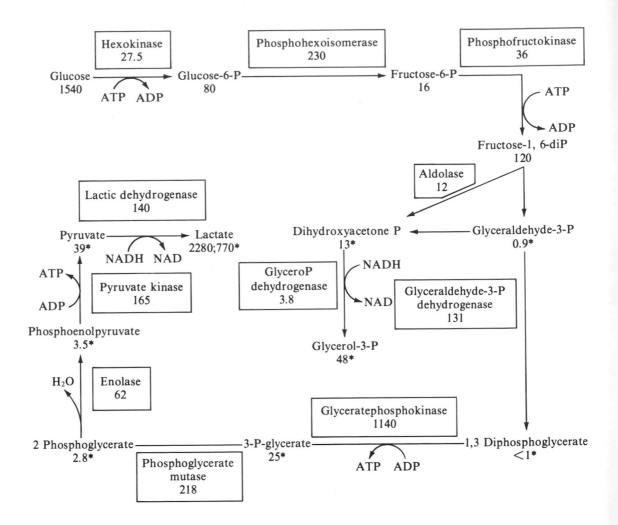

preference on glucose in the competition for the MgATP^{2-} generated by mitochondrial oxidative phosphorylation. Thus a process that will sustain ATP production continues at the expense of other uses of energy. Because energy reserves are rapidly exhausted postmortem, it is not surprising that brain hexokinase is found to be almost entirely bound.

The significance of reversible binding of other enzymes to mitochondria is not clear. The measured glycolytic flux, when compared to the maximal velocity of hexokinase, indicates that, in the steady state, the hexokinase reaction is 97 percent inhibited. Brain hexokinase is inhibited by its

Fig. 17-2. Glycolysis in brain. Enzyme and metabolite data expressed as in Figure 17-1. (Data from McIlwain, Biochemistry and the Central Nervous System. Boston: Little, Brown, 1966, pp. 1–26.) Asterisk indicates 10-day-old mouse brain [40].

product, glucose 6-phosphate, and to a lesser extent by ADP, and allosterically by 3-phosphoglycerate and several nucleoside phosphates, including cyclic AMP and free ATP^{4-}. The ratio of ATP to magnesium may also have a regulatory action. In addition to acting on enzyme kinetics, glucose 6-phosphate solubilizes hexokinase, thus reducing the enzyme's efficiency when the reaction product accumulates. The sum total of these mechanisms is a fine tuning of the activity of the initial enzyme of glycolysis in response to changes in the cellular environment to increase glycolytic flow when needed and suppress it when demands for its eventual products (energy and glycolytic metabolites) are less. Glucokinase (low-affinity hexokinase), a major component of liver hexokinase, has not been found in brain.

Glucose 6-phosphate represents a branch point in metabolism because it is a common substrate for enzymes involved in glycolytic, pentose-phosphate shunt, and glycogen-forming pathways. There is also slight, but detectable, glucose 6-phosphatase activity in brain, the significance of which is not clear. The liver requires this enzyme to convert glycogen to glucose. The differences between the liver and brain hexokinase and the differences between the modes of glycogen metabolism of these two tissues can be related to the function of liver as a carbohydrate storehouse for the body, whereas brain metabolism is adapted for rapid carbohydrate utilization for energy needs.

In glycolysis, glucose 6-phosphate is the substrate of phosphohexose isomerase. This is a reversible reaction (small free-energy change), whose 5:1 equilibrium ratio in brain favors glucose 6-phosphate.

Fructose 6-phosphate is the substrate of phosphofructokinase, a key regulatory enzyme controlling glycolysis [3]. The other substrate is $MgATP^{2-}$. Like other regulatory reactions, it is essentially irreversible. It is modulated by a large number of metabolites and cofactors, whose concentrations under different metabolic conditions have great effects on glycolytic flux. Prominent among these are availability of $\sim P$ and citrate levels. Brain phosphofructokinase is inhibited by ATP, magnesium, and citrate and is stimulated by NH_4^+, K^+, Pi, 5'-AMP, 3',5'-cyclic AMP, ADP, and fructose 1,6-diphosphate. Possibly its inhibition by reduced pyridine nucleotides can be overcome by an increase in pH. The effects of NH_4^+, inorganic phosphate, and AMP are additive, and there is evidence for several different allosteric

sites on this complex enzyme. In general, activity is inhibited by ATP and enhanced by substances that accumulate under conditions in which $\sim P$ reserves are diminished. Activity is also increased by 3',5'-cyclic AMP, the presence of which leads ultimately to increased energy use. Inhibition by citrate would amount to an end-product inhibition if acetate, its precursor, is considered the final product of glycolysis. The concentration of NH_4^+, a product of amino acid and amine metabolism, is controlled by transamination reactions coupled to citric acid cycle intermediates, as well as by glutamic dehydrogenase and glutamine synthetase. Increase of glycolysis, by raising pyruvate and α-ketoglutarate levels, would tend to reduce NH_4^+ levels. The stimulation by NH_4^+ is unaffected by high ATP levels, allowing acceleration of glycolysis to increase the availability of α-ketoglutarate and pyruvate for transamination even when $\sim P$ levels are adequate.

When oxygen is admitted to cells metabolizing anaerobically, utilization of O_2 increases, and utilization of glucose and lactate production drops (Pasteur effect). Modulation of the phosphofructokinase reaction can account directly for the Pasteur effect. In the steady state, ATP and citrate levels in brain apparently are sufficient to keep phosphofructokinase relatively inhibited as long as the level of positive modulators (or disinhibitors) is low. When the steady state is disturbed, activation of this enzyme produces an increase in glycolytic flux that takes place almost as fast as the events changing the internal milieu.

Fructose 1,6-diphosphate is split by brain aldolase to glyceraldehyde 3-phosphate and dihydroxyacetone phosphate. Dihydroxyacetone phosphate is the common substrate for both glycerophosphate dehydrogenase, an enzyme active in NADH oxidation and lipid pathways (see Chap. 18), and triose phosphate isomerase, which maintains an equilibrium between dihydroxyacetone phosphate and glyceraldehyde 3-phosphate; the equilibrium strongly favors accumulation of dihydroxyacetone phosphate.

After the reaction with glyceraldehyde phosphate dehydrogenase, glycolysis in the brain proceeds through the usual steps. Brain enolase (D-2-phosphoglycerate hydrolase), which catalyzes dehydration of 2-phosphoglycerate to phosphoenolpyruvate, is present as two related dimers, one of which (γ) is specifically associated with neurons, and the other (α) with glia. The neuronal γ subunit is identical to the neuron-specific protein 14-3-2 that was isolated from brain several years ago. Differential sensitivities of the enolases to temperature and salts may make them useful in determining neuron/glia ratios in tissue samples. It is of interest that brain phosphoenolpyruvate kinase controls an essentially irreversible reaction, which requires not only Mg^{2+} (as do several other glycolytic enzymes) but also K^+ or Na^+. This step also may be regulatory.

Brain tissue, even when it is at rest and well oxygenated, produces a small amount of lactate, which is removed in the venous blood. This amount is derived from 13 percent of the pyruvate produced by glycolysis. The measured lactate level in brain depends on the success of halting brain metabolism rapidly during tissue processing. Five isoenzymes of lactate dehydrogenase are present in adult brain. The one that moves electrophoretically most rapidly toward the anode (band 1) predominates. This isoenzyme is generally higher in those tissues that are more dependent on aerobic processes for energy; the slower-moving isoenzymes are relatively higher in tissues such as white skeletal muscle, which is better adapted to function at suboptimal oxygen levels (see Chap. 27). The activities of lactate dehydrogenases and their distribution in various brain regions, layers of the retina, brain neoplasms, brain tissue cultures, and during development indicate that the synthesis of these isoenzymes might be controlled by oxygen levels in the tissues. Lactate dehydrogenase functions in the cytoplasm as a means of oxidizing NADH, which accumulates as the result of the activity of glyceraldehyde phosphate dehydrogenase in glycolysis. It thus permits glycolytic ATP production to continue under anaerobic conditions. Lactate dehydrogenase also functions under aerobic conditions because NADH cannot easily penetrate the mitochondrial membrane. The oxidation of NADH in the cytoplasm depends on this reaction and on the activity of *shuttle mechanisms* that transfer reducing equivalents to the mitochondria.

Glycerol phosphate dehydrogenase is another enzyme indirectly associated with glycolysis that participates in the cytoplasmic oxidation of NADH. This enzyme reduces dihydroxyacetone phosphate to glycerol 3-phosphate, oxidizing NADH in the process. Under hypoxic conditions, the levels of α-glycerophosphate and lactate increase initially at comparable rates, although the amount of lactate produced greatly exceeds that of α-glycerophosphate. The relative levels of the oxidized and reduced substrates of these reactions indicate much higher local levels of NADH in brain than are found by gross measurements. In fact, the relative proportions of oxidized and reduced substrates of the reactions that are linked to the pyridine nucleotides may be a better indicator of local oxidation-reduction states ($NAD^+/NADH$) in brain than is provided by the direct measurement of the pyridine nucleotides themselves ([5–8, 15], and Chap. 35).

An aspect of glucose metabolism that has led to much confusion among neurochemists is the observation that labeled glucose appears in carbon dioxide much more slowly than might be suggested from a cursory examination of the glycolytic pathway plus the citric acid cycle [22]. Glucose flux is ~ 0.5 to 1.0 μmol/min/g wet weight of brain in a variety of species. The level of glycolytic plus tricarboxylate cyclic intermediates is ~ 2 μmol/g. Hence these intermediates might be predicted to turn over every 2 to 4 min, and $^{14}CO_2$ production might be predicted to reach a steady state in 5 to 10 min. This is not observed experimentally. In addition, large quantities of radioactivity are trapped in amino acids related to the Krebs (TCA) cycle (70 to 80 percent) from 10 to 30 min after a glucose injection. This is due to the high activity of transaminase in comparison with the flux through the citric acid cycle, and the amino acids developed by transamination behave as if they were a part of the Krebs cycle. When the pools of these amino acids (approx. 20 μmol/g) are added to the levels of TCA cycle components plus glycolytic intermediates, the time for $^{14}CO_2$ evolution is increased by a factor of ten, and this agrees with the values observed experimentally.

In contrast, in tissues such as the liver, the amino acids related to the Krebs cycle are present at much lower steady state values, and 20 percent of the radioactivity from administered glucose is trapped in these amino acids at short times after injection. As a result, ignoring the radioactivity trapped in amino acids has a relatively small effect on estimates of glycolytic fluxes in liver but makes an enormous difference in brain. Immature brains more nearly resemble liver in this respect. The relationship of the Krebs cycle to glycolysis undergoes a sharp change during development, coincident with the development of the metabolic compartmentation of amino acid metabolism that is characteristic of adult brain.

PYRUVATE DEHYDROGENASE COMPLEX
Pyruvate dehydrogenase (14 nmol/min/mg protein in rat brain), which controls the entry of pyruvate into the citrate acid cycle as acetyl coenzyme A (acetyl-CoA), is actually a mitochondrial multienzyme complex that includes the enzymes pyruvate dehydrogenase (decarboxylase), lipoate acetyl transferase, and lipoamide dehydrogenase, and the coenzymes thiamine pyrophosphate, lipoic acid, CoA, and flavine and nicotinamide dinucleotides. It is inactivated by being phosphorylated at the decarboxylase moiety by a tightly bound $MgATP^{2-}$-dependent protein kinase and activated by being dephosphorylated by a loosely bound Mg^{2+}- and Ca^{2+}-dependent phosphatase. About half the brain enzyme is usually active. Pyruvate protects the complex against inactivation by inhibiting the kinase. ADP is a competitive inhibitor of Mg^{2+} for the inactivating kinase. Under conditions of greater metabolic demand, increases in pyruvate and ADP and decreases in acetyl CoA and ATP make the complex more active. Pyruvate dehydrogenase is inhibited by NADH, decreasing formation of acetyl-CoA during hypoxia and allowing more pyruvate to be reduced by lactate dehydrogenase, thus forming the NAD necessary to sustain glycolysis. Several investigators have reported abnormalities of the complex (particularly lipoamide dehydrogenase) in some hereditary ataxias, but not all studies have confirmed these findings and the relationship remains tenuous [23–25].

Although acetylcholine synthesis is normally controlled by the rate of choline uptake and cholineacetyltransferase activity (see Chap. 9), the supply of acetyl-CoA can be limiting under adverse conditions. Choline uptake is, however, independent of acetyl-CoA concentration. A cytoplasmic pyruvate dehydrogenase specifically associated with acetylcholine synthesis has been suggested, but the data used are open to other interpretations and the hypothesis is as yet unverified. The mitochondrial membrane is not permeable to the acetyl-CoA produced within it but there is efflux of its condensation product, citrate. Acetyl-CoA can then be formed from citrate in the cytosol by ATP citrate lyase. The acetyl moiety of acetylcholine is formed in a compartment with rapid glucose turnover, presumably the synaptosome. The cytosol of cholinergic endings is rich in citrate lyase, and it is probable that the citrate shuttles the acetyl-CoA from the mitochondrial compartment. During hypoxia or hypoglycemia, acetylcholine synthesis can be inhibited by failure of the acetyl-CoA supply [26, 27].

CITRIC ACID CYCLE
The energy output and oxygen consumption in adult brain are associated with high levels of enzyme activity in the citric acid cycle [8]. The actual flux through the citric acid cycle (Krebs cycle) depends on glycolysis and active acetate production, which can "push" the cycle, the possible control at several enzymatic steps of the cycle, and the local ADP level, which is known to be a prime activator of the mitochondrial respiration to which the citric acid cycle is linked. The steady state level of citrate in brain is about one-fifth that of glucose. This is relatively high as compared with levels of glycolytic intermediates or with that of isocitrate.

As in other tissues, there are two isocitrate dehydrogenases in brain. One is active primarily in the cytoplasm and requires nicotinamide-adenine dinucleotide phosphate (NADP) as cofactor; the other, bound to mitochondria and requiring NAD, is the enzyme that participates in the citric acid cycle. The NAD-linked enzyme catalyzes an essentially irreversible reaction, has allosteric properties, is inhibited by ATP and reduced NAD (NADH), and may be stimulated by ADP. The function of cytoplasmic NADP isocitrate dehydrogenase is uncertain, but it has been postulated that it supplies the reduced NADP (NADPH) that is necessary for many reductive synthetic reactions. The relatively high activity of this enzyme in immature brain and white matter is consistent with such a role. α-Ketoglutarate dehydrogenase, which oxidatively decarboxylates α-ketoglutarate, requires the same cofactors as does the pyruvate decarboxylation step.

Succinate dehydrogenase, the enzyme that catalyzes the oxidation of succinate to fumarate, is tightly bound to mitochondrial membrane. In brain, succinate dehydrogenase may also have a regulatory role when the steady state is disturbed. Isocitrate and succinate levels in brain are little affected by changes in the flux of the citric acid cycle, as long as an adequate glucose supply is available. The highly unfavorable free-energy change of the malate dehydrogenase reaction is overcome by the rapid removal of oxaloacetate, which is maintained at low concentrations under steady state conditions by the condensation reaction with acetyl-CoA [5–7, 15, 28].

Malic dehydrogenase is one of several enzymes in the citric acid cycle that is present in both the cytoplasm and mitochondria. The function of the cytoplasmic components of these enzyme activities is not known, but they may function in the transfer of hydrogen from the cytoplasm into mitochondria.

Another source of much misunderstanding in the interpretation of the citric acid cycle is the distinction between its function as an oxidative scheme for energy production and its function as a biosynthetic process for the production of amino acids, for example, glutamate, glutamine, γ-aminobutyric acid (GABA), aspartate, and asparagine, as well as other amino acids needed for protein synthesis. To export net amounts of α-ketoglutarate or oxaloacetate from the Krebs cycle, the supply of dicarboxylic acids must be replenished. The major route for this seems to be the fixation of CO_2 to pyruvate or another substrate at this three-carbon level. Thus, the rate of CO_2 fixation sets the upper limit at which biosynthetic reactions can occur. This has been estimated as approximately 0.15 μmole per gram of wet weight of brain per minute in studies of acute ammonia toxicity in cats, or approximately 10 percent of the flux through the citric acid cycle. Liver, on the other hand, appears to have 10 times the capacity of brain for CO_2 fixation, as is appropriate for an organ geared to making large quantities of protein for export.

The activity of pyruvate dehydrogenase seems to be the rate-limiting step for the entry of pyruvate from glycolysis into the Krebs cycle.

INTRACELLULAR MESSENGERS

The action of many hormones and some neural transmitters is indirect. These substances act at membranes of specific receptor cells to cause the intracellular release of an active molecule (*second messenger*), which in turn modifies cellular metabolism and function. Ionic calcium is such a substance; 3′,5′-cyclic AMP is another (see Chap. 15).

In sensitive cells, epinephrine activates the membrane-associated adenylate cyclase system that converts ATP into 3′,5′-cyclic AMP. This substance, unlike 5′-AMP, retains a high-energy phosphate bond and can activate various protein kinases, among which is phosphorylase *b* kinase kinase. This enzyme catalyzes the phosphorylation of phosphorylase *b* kinase, which in turn stimulates the conversion of phosphorylase *b* to the *a* form; this facilitates the breakdown of glycogen. Also 3′,5′-cyclic AMP activates the kinase that converts glycogen synthetase to the regulated D form. Relatively high levels of 3′,5′-cyclic AMP are found in brain and may function postsynaptically in interneural transmission, particularly at adrenergic synapses. Preganglionic sympathetic stimulation increases cyclic AMP in the postsynaptic cell in proportion to the rate of stimulation.

PENTOSE PHOSPHATE SHUNT

Controversy exists concerning the proportion of brain glucose that is metabolized along the pentose phosphate shunt. The most common technique for determining that proportion has been to compare $^{14}CO_2$ release or ^{14}C appearing in triose phosphates, lactate, or glycogen from glucose 6-^{14}C to that from glucose 1-^{14}C. The C-1 carbon of glucose is lost to CO_2 during flow along the shunt, so equal yields of $^{14}CO_2$ from glucose labeled with C-1 and C-6 may indicate that glucose metabolism occurs primarily by the glycolytic route, whereas a high relative yield of $^{14}CO_2$ from glucose labeled with C-1 suggests a greater flow along the shunt. Such procedures are known to be approximations that are subject to a variety of errors that have produced estimates of pentose-phosphate flow ranging from 0 to 21 percent of glycolysis. The shunt pathway is definitely active in brain, and it is probable that, under basal conditions in the adult, at least 5 to 8 percent of brain glucose is metabolized through the shunt [29]. Both shunt enzymes and metabolic flux have been found in isolated nerve endings. The pathway has relatively high activity in developing brain, reaching a peak during myelination. Its main contribution probably produces the NADPH required for the reductive reactions necessary for lipid synthesis (Chap. 18). The shunt pathway also provides pentose for nucleotide synthesis; however, only a small fraction of the activity of this pathway would be required to meet such a need (see in Chap. 19). In other tissues, shunt activity is linked to the reduction of glutathione, and this protective mechanism against toxic products of oxidative metabolism may also function in brain. As with glycogen synthesis, turnover in the pentose-phosphate pathway decreases under conditions of increased energy need, for example, during and after high rates of stimulation [30]. Pentose phosphate flux apparently is regulated by the concentrations of glucose 6-phosphate, NADP, glyceraldehyde 3-phosphate, and fructose 6-phosphate [30]. Transketolase, one of the enzymes in this pathway, requires thiamine pyrophosphate as a cofactor. Poor myelin maintenance in thiamine deficiency may be due to the failure of the pathway to provide sufficient NADPH for lipid synthesis ([5–7] and Chap. 33).

METABOLIC COMPARTMENTATION

Clearly, protein synthesis has a major requirement for amino acids in all tissues, and brain is no exception. However, there is increasing evidence that many of the amino acids derived from the Krebs cycle also function as neurotransmitters (Chap. 12). If one were to assume that the difference in glutamate levels in brain and other tissue (an estimated 8 $\mu mol/g$) is related to the special function of glutamate as a neurotransmitter, it might be expected that glutaminergic nerve endings would predominate in certain brain areas, particularly cortex. (This estimate of the quantity of glutamate that functions as a neurotransmitter is probably an upper limit.) Because GABA and glutamate are intimately related, not only metabolically but also as opposing neurotransmitters (inhibitory versus excitatory), another estimate of the quantity of glutamate that functions as a neurotransmitter is similar to the level of GABA, that is, approximately 2 $\mu mol/g$. Of course, this would vary according to the particular brain area and is probably at lower-limit estimate. The work of Snyder and coworkers does in fact suggest that glutamate and GABA may be among the major neurotransmitters in the CNS [31].

The compartmentalization in brain of glutamate into separate pools that equilibrate only slowly is a vital factor in regulating separately such special functions of glutamate as neurotransmission and such general functions as protein biosynthesis [17]. This does not mean that glutamate metabolism may not be compartmented in other tissues, but that the characteristics of such pools may be quite different.

Not only is glutamate metabolism in brain characterized by the existence of at least two distinct pools; the Krebs cycle intermediates associated with these pools are also distinctly compartmented [32–34]. A mathematical model to fit data from radiotracer experiments that require separate Krebs cycles to satisfy the hypotheses of compartmentation has been developed [32, 35]. A key assumption of the current models is that GABA is metabolized at a site different from that at which it is synthesized. The best fit of the kinetic data is obtained when glutamate, from a small pool that is actively converted to glutamine, flows back to the large pool that is converted to GABA. An enzymatic basis for such predictions is now developing; it has been shown that glutamic acid decarboxylase (GAD) (E.C. 3.1.1.15) is localized at or near nerve terminals, whereas GABA transaminase, the major degradative enzyme, is mitochondrial [36].

Increasing evidence points to the small pool of glutamate as probably glial. Thus it seems that glutamate released from nerve endings is taken up by glia (and by presynaptic and postsynaptic terminals, or both), converted to glutamine, and recycled to glutamate and GABA. Various estimates of the proportion of glucose carbon that flows through the GABA shunt (Chap. 12) have been published, but the most definitive experiments show the value to be approximately 10 percent [15] of the total glycolytic flux. Although this may seem small, it should be understood that the portion of the Krebs cycle flux that is used for energy production (ATP synthesis, maintenance of ionic gradients) does not require CO_2 fixation, but that the portion used for biosynthesis of amino acids does. By recycling the carbon skeleton of glutamate through glutamine and GABA to succinate, the need for dicarboxylic acids to replenish intermediates of the Krebs cycle is diminished when export of α-ketoglutarate takes place.

It is difficult to get good estimates of the extent of CO_2 fixation in brain, but estimates of the maximum capability obtained under conditions of ammonia stress, when glutamine levels increase rapidly, suggest that CO_2 fixation occurs at 0.15 μmol/g/min (in cat) and 0.33 μmol/g/min (in rat), that is, at about the same rate as for the GABA shunt.

For comparison, it should be pointed out that only about 2 percent of the glucose flux in whole

brain goes toward lipid synthesis and approximately 0.3 percent is used for protein synthesis. Thus the turnover of neurotransmitter amino acids is a major biosynthetic effort in brain.

Metabolic compartmentation of glutamate is usually observed when ketogenic substrates are administered to animals. Interestingly enough, acetoacetate and β-hydroxybutyrate do not show this effect. Apparently this is because ketone bodies are a normal substrate for brain and are taken up into all types of cells. Acetate and similar substances, which are not taken up into brain efficiently, appear to be more readily taken up or activated in glia, or both. This may lead to the abnormal glutamate/glutamine ratio that is observed. Similarly, metabolic inhibitors, such as fluoroacetate, appear to act selectively in glia and produce their neurotoxic action without marked inhibition of the overall Krebs cycle flux in brain.

A nonuniform distribution of various compounds in living systems is of wide occurrence. Steady state levels of GABA are well documented as varying over a fivefold range in discrete brain regions (2 to 10 mM), and it has been estimated that GABA may be as high as 50 mM in nerve terminals. Observations in brain indicate the existence of pools with half-lives of many hours for mixing, which is most unusual. The discovery of a subcellular morphological compartmentation, that is, that there are different populations of mitochondria in cerebral cortex that have distinctive enzyme complements, may provide a somewhat better perspective by which to visualize such separation of metabolic function. We still do not know if different mitochondrial populations are present within single cells or are characteristic of different cell populations. The heterogeneity of brain tissue fosters the latter as the simpler explanation, but there is no positive evidence for either assumption.

Tapia [37] has proposed that, in addition to the phasic release of both excitatory and inhibitory transmitter, there is a continuous tonic release of GABA, dependent only on the activity of the enzyme responsible for its synthesis and independent of the depolarization of the presynaptic membrane. Such inhibitory neurons could act tonically by constantly maintaining an elevated threshold in the excitatory neurons so that the latter would start firing when a decrease occurs in the continuous release of GABA acting upon them. This is consistent with a good correlation between the inhibition of GAD and the appearance of convulsions after certain drug treatments. GABA levels have been observed to be depleted by some convulsant drugs and elevated by others. Wood and coworkers [38] introduced the concept of a critical GABA factor that combines the activity of GAD and the level of GABA because the degradation of GABA is not the rate-limiting step in the overall process that determines the availability of GABA at the synapse; rather, it is the activity of GAD. To describe the relative excitability of the CNS, this formula uses the change in GAD activity combined with an empirical factor (0.4) times the square root of the change in the GABA concentration. Such notions fit well with the observation that the so-called GABA shunt involves a significant part (about 10 percent) of the total glycolytic flux in brain. The role of amino acids as neurohumoral agents and transmitters is more fully described in Chap. 12.

MITOCHONDRIA

As in other tissues, brain mitochondria apparently are self-replicating bodies, although most of their active enzymes depend on the cell's chromosomal-ribosomal apparatus for synthesis. As noted above, not all mitochondria are identical in enzyme complement or function. Brain mitochondria have an affinity for oxygen several times that of liver mitochondria and also react differently to osmolar changes both morphologically and biochemically. Because current methods of separating mitochondria from other cell components depend on sedimentation from homogenates (Chap. 3), differences related to function and intracellular provenance are difficult to define. Furthermore, mitochondrial size and function do change during maturation. Therefore, functional heterogeneity among brain mitochondria may be related to their location in perikarya, synaptosomes, or various glial cells.

The mitochondrial membranes and matrix form metabolic compartments separate from the cytosol so that the entry and egress of metabolites and ions are selective. This allows a degree of metabolic control that is not possible otherwise. For example, mitochondrial membranes are not freely permeable to pyridine nucleotides. The brain contains several enzymes that could function in postulated shuttle systems that transfer hydrogen generated in the cytosol (e.g., NADH) to the mitochondria to be oxidized by the electron-transport system. These enzymes include mitochondrial and cytoplasmic malate dehydrogenases (NAD) as well as cytoplasmic (NAD) and mitochondrial (flavoprotein) glycerol phosphate dehydrogenases.

The sine qua non of brain metabolism is its high rate of respiration. In the coupled, controlled state, the level of mitochondrial function depends on local concentrations of ADP. The entry of ADP into mitochondria is restricted insofar as it must exchange with intramitochondrial ATP. The high steady state mitochondrial respiration in brain is related to local availability of substrates and the ratio of ADP to ATP. This may not be reflected in the average ratio of ADP to ATP in whole brain, which is quite low. Brain mitochondria also differ from those in other tissues because they contain higher concentrations of certain "nonmitochondrial" enzymes. Hexokinase, creatine kinase, and perhaps lactic dehydrogenase are partially mitochondrial. Hexokinase and creatine kinase may function to maintain local levels of ADP by transferring ~P from ATP to creatine or glucose [5–7, 28].

RELATION OF CARBOHYDRATES
TO LIPID METABOLISM

The principal source of lipid carbon in brain is blood glucose. Carbohydrate intermediates and related metabolites—such as acetate (fatty acid and cholesterol), dihydroxyacetone phosphate (glycerol phosphate), mannosamine, pyruvate (neuraminic acid), glucose 6-phosphate (inositol), galactose, and glucosamine—supply the building blocks of the complex lipids (Chap. 18). NADPH is also necessary for the reductive synthesis of lipids. When a few polyunsaturated fatty acids and sulfate are supplied, immature brain slices readily form all the lipids of myelin and cell membrane, using glucose as the only substrate. Energy supply through the carbohydrate pathways in the form of ATP is also required to supply nucleoside phosphates for lipid assembly [6, 30].

CARBOHYDRATE IN NEURONAL FUNCTION

The high functional requirement of nervous tissue for ~P is probably related to energy demands for transmitter synthesis, packaging, secretion, uptake, and sequestration; for ion pumping to maintain ionic gradients; for intracellular transport; and for synthesis of complex lipids and macromolecules in both neuronal and glial cells. The manner in which metabolism is coupled to function is conceptualized easily from the discussion of the regulatory mechanisms that control carbohydrate metabolism and can be illustrated by $(Na^+ + K^+)$-ATPase, which functions in the $Na^+ - K^+$ exchange pump so essential for maintaining electrolyte gradients (see also Chap. 6). This enzyme is particularly active in regions with high concentrations of synaptic membranes, for example, gray matter and synaptosomes. This membrane-associated, topographically oriented enzyme is stimulated by extracellular K^+ and intracellular Na^+, so its activity is increased by the ionic changes that accompany depolarization (Chap. 5). The ADP that is released intracellularly is an activating modulator for mitochondria and several rate-limiting reactions: glycolytic (hexokinase, phosphofructokinase), Krebs cycle (NAD-dependent isocitric dehydrogenase), and glycogenolytic (phosphorylase). The changes accompanying the consequently increased metabolic flux lead to inhibition of other pathways, such as that of glycogen synthesis and the pentose phosphate shunt, whereas the lowered ~P levels and NADPH levels inhibit various synthetic reactions. Because the products of reactions that use ~P are accelerators of reactions leading to ~P formation, energy supply as ATP is regulated by utilization. The set-points of this regulation may be altered in certain toxic-metabolic states. Under many adverse conditions, for example hypoxia, energy utilization is decreased in brain, heart, and other tissues. The mechanisms of this apparently protective response are unknown but may be related to changes in hydrogen-ion or calcium fluxes. Although the linkage of neuronal function to energy metabolism has been emphasized, it should be pointed out that physiological failure during hypoxia, ischemia, or hypoglycemia in brain (and other tissues) begins before overall energy levels fall below those expected to be adequate to support function. Among the suggested causes of the dysfunction are defects in acetylcholine (see Pyruvate Dehydrogenase Complex, above) and catecholamine synthesis. The affinity of tyrosine hydroxylase for oxygen is several orders of magnitude less than that of the mitochondrial enzymes; this makes amine synthesis relatively more vulnerable to hypoxia.

REGIONAL DIFFERENCES

There are two major techniques for studying regional metabolism. The first, developed by Lowry and coworkers [3, 8], measures changes in carbohydrate metabolites and energy cofactors during a few seconds of ischemia in microdissected samples and assumes that their rates of change reflect those before ischemia. The second (see Chap. 24) is based on the measurement of grain density by autoradiography of freeze-dried sections after isotopically labeled deoxyglucose has been administered, and assumes instantaneous and sustained isotopic equilibrium throughout brain tissue and plasma. The normal glucose flux estimated by the former method is usually more than twice that of the deoxyglucose method. Estimations based on the Lowry technique are increased by the stimulation resulting from decapitation, but are much closer to the glucose consumption calculated from the oxygen consumption. The deoxyglucose method of Sokoloff [39] underestimates the true flux, because of failure to attain equilibrium conditions, but gives accurate relative values in different regions. Moreover, it is a more practical method for comparing glucose phosphorylation in many different regions simultaneously and under different conditions. The highest glucose phosphorylation rates are found in the inferior colliculi and the auditory cortex. This rate is so closely coupled to neuronal function that it has been possible to map a region of decreased flux in the visual cortex that corresponds to the optic disc interruption of the retinal photoreceptors (*physiological blind spot*). In general, those regions of brain with higher metabolic requirements have both higher enzyme activity in the glycolytic series and the citric acid cycle and higher levels of respiration. Several glycolytic and mitochondrial enzymes are more active in regions with large numbers of synaptic endings (*neuropil*) than in areas rich in neuronal cell bodies. On the other hand, the activity of glucose 6-phosphate dehydrogenase (a rate-limiting enzyme of the pentose phosphate pathway) is high in myelinated fibers and tends to vary with the degree of myelination. Phosphofructokinase and phosphorylase are distributed in a relatively constant ratio in different brain regions; this suggests a relationship between glycolysis and glycogenolysis. Hexokinase distribution is more closely linked to mitochondrial enzymes than to glycolytic enzymes [40]. The oligodendroglial cell that maintains myelin in the CNS probably ranks, along with the neuron and its processes, as one of the cells with the highest known metabolic requirements.

METABOLISM OF THE RETINA

The rabbit retina is avascular and depends almost entirely on diffusion from choroidal capillaries. The primate retina, however, is vascularized from the vitreal surface as far as the bipolar cell layer. The rabbit retina shows high rates of glucose and oxygen consumption and also of lactate formation. The high rate of aerobic lactate formation might be due to segregation of glycolytic and oxidative processes as well as to the adaptation of the poorly vascularized inner layers to a relatively anoxic existence. The rod inner segment contains packed mitochondria and has high levels of all mitochondrial enzymes and hexokinase. This is the region closest to the choroidal nutrient supply.

In the vascularized inner layers of the monkey retina, hexokinase activity is almost twice that in the homologous layers of the rabbit retina. Several

glycolytic enzymes, including phosphofructokinase and glyceraldehyde phosphate dehydrogenase, as well as lactic dehydrogenase and glycogen phosphorylase, tend to be higher toward the vitreous surface in rabbit than in monkey retina. The total energy reserves (especially high glycogen levels) and lactate levels increase as the avascular vitreous surface of the rabbit retina is approached. Malate dehydrogenase and NAD-dependent isocitrate dehydrogenase, the citric acid cycle enzymes, vary with the relative density of mitochondria, which is high in the layer of rod inner segments and in the synaptic layers. Data such as these suggest that adaptive changes occur in carbohydrate enzymes and metabolism and that these changes are dependent on the local availability of substrates and oxygen. As in brain, however, continued electrical responsiveness of the retina depends upon oxidative metabolism. The response to light is dependent on metabolic processes and control mechanisms that are similar to those described for the maintenance of electrical activity in brain ([4] and Chap. 7).

PERIPHERAL NERVE

In mice, the metabolic rate of peripheral nerve is about 7 percent of that in brain. As in brain, carbohydrate reserves are low. In the sympathetic system, as in brain, glucose is the major metabolite of both nerve and ganglion. But the system differs from brain in that there is no apparent barrier to glucose uptake in ganglia, and glucose levels are close to those of blood. Glucose levels in peripheral nerve are intermediate between those of brain and the ganglia. The patterns of substrate distribution and utilization in stimulated nerve differ from those in nerve at rest. Depletion of energy reserves leads to the failure of synaptic transmission before failure of conduction. Transmission in sympathetic ganglia can fail after carbohydrate reserves (glucose and glycogen) are depleted, despite maintenance of high levels of ~P. The situation is similar to that in hypoglycemic brain (see in Chap. 24), and similar mechanisms may be involved [24].

The Composition of the Free Amino Acid Pools

SOURCE OF AMINO ACIDS FOR BRAIN

The Levels of Amino Acids and Related Compounds

It is clear that brain cannot make carbon skeletons of the amino acids that are essential in the diet and must depend on transport of these amino acids from the blood. On the other hand, the amino acids that are made in the animal body also appear to be synthesized in brain. There is no convincing evidence that amino acids made in the liver or other organs are transported by the blood to the brain in significant quantities. Ammonia is taken up actively by brain if circulating ammonia levels are increased, either artificially or when liver function is impaired. The uptake of ammonia from normal circulatory ammonia levels probably is sufficient to maintain the brain in nitrogen balance, although the portion of nitrogen supplied as ammonia versus that available as preformed amino acids is not well established. Glucose metabolism appears to be adequate to replenish the carbon supply for the skeletons of nonessential amino acids.

Most of the amino acid content of brain, like that of other tissues, is present as protein. Essential free amino acids in brain are present at low level; their level as protein components is several hundred times higher. Because of this concentration difference, a net growth of less than 1 percent protein would exhaust the available free amino acid content of the brain if it were not replenished from the circulation.

Neurochemists noted early that the composition of the free amino acid pool in the brain is different from that of other tissues; the biggest difference is the relatively high content of glutamic acid and related amino acids, including aspartate, glutamine, and GABA. These compounds comprise more than half of the total free amino acid content in brain.

The concept of a special position of glutamate was affirmed by the finding that glutamate can support the respiration of incubated slices of brain and that radioactivity rapidly accumulates in brain glutamic acid after the administration of radioactive glucose. Although many studies have measured changes in glutamate under hypoglycemic and ischemic conditions, the role of glutamate in energy production in the brain has not been clearly established. This concept led to unsuccessful trials of glutamate feeding as a treatment for mental illness; it was demonstrated that such feedings are unable to elevate cerebral glutamate levels because of an effective blood-brain barrier to the entry of this amino acid. In acute ammonia toxicity, the conversion of glutamate to glutamine is the main form of removal of cerebral ammonia; under such conditions local glutamate formation has been shown.

The content of free amino acids in the brain is maintained at fairly constant levels under most conditions and is a characteristic of that organ. In general, three groups can be distinguished: (1) the essential amino acids, which are present at fairly low levels—close to those in plasma; (2) the nonessential amino acids, which are present at concentrations several times higher than the essential ones; and (3) compounds that are specifically present in brain, such as GABA and acetylaspartic acid [41].

The composition of the free amino acid pool as shown in Table 17-1 is similar in most species [42]. The amino acid level in the spinal fluid is much lower than in brain. CSF amino acid levels are also lower than those in plasma. The amino acid composition of spinal fluid is not parallel to that of brain; for example, note the high glutamine and low glutamate in the CSF, and the brain/CSF concentration ratio for glutamate of approximately 800. The free pool in brain also does not reflect the amino acid composition of the cerebral proteins. The amino acids are present at much higher levels in the protein-bound than in the free form. The concentration ratio of protein-bound to free amino acids in brain varies from 10 for glutamic acid to 1,800 for isoleucine. The amino acids present at high level (glutamate, taurine, GABA, and glycine) are the most active pharmacologically. The amino acids are not all evenly distributed in the brain. For example, taurine and glutamic acid are

Table 17-1. Levels of Free Amino Acids and Related Substances*

	Brain			Human		
	Cat	Rat	Carp	Brain	CSF	Plasma
Glutamic acid	790	1160	550	600	0.8	2
Taurine	230	660	480	93	0.6	6
N-acetylaspartic acid	600	560	80	490		0
Glutamine	280	450	770	580	50	60
Aspartic acid	170	260	350	96	0.02	0.2
γ-Aminobutyric acid	140	230		42		0
Glycine	78	68	62	40	0.7	22
Alanine	48	65	66	25	2.6	35
Serine	48	98	33	44	2.5	11
Threonine	17	66	36	27	2.5	14
Lysine	8	21	34	12	2.1	19
Arginine		11	14	10	1.8	8
Histidine	2	5	36	9	1.3	9
Valine	6	7	15	13	1.6	23
Leucine	7	5	22	7	1.1	12
Isoleucine	3	2	13	3	0.4	6
Phenylalanine	2	5	13	5	0.8	5
Tyrosine	3	7	9	6	0.8	5
Proline	3	8	12	10		18
Methionine	2	4		3	0.3	2
Ornithine	1	2	7	3	0.6	5
P-ethanolamine	120	200	62	110		0.2
Cystathionine	14	2	32	200		
Homocarnosine	0.4	6		23	0.3	0
Glutathione	49	260		200		

*The values presented, which are averages from many publications, are expressed as μmoles of amino acid per 100 grams of brain or 100 milliliters of CSF or plasma.

much lower and glycine is much higher in the midbrain and pons than in other areas. There are further indications of differences among various cells, but this is not easy to establish: the methods for separation and isolation of cells and of particulate fractions such as synaptosomes include procedures that result in losses or redistribution of the soluble amino acids. The physiological activity of these amino acids is further discussed in Chap. 12.

The composition of the protein-free amino acid pool in peripheral nerve is different from that in the brain; most amino acids in mammalian nerve are lower than in brain. GABA is nearly absent in vertebrate peripheral nerve. In some crustacean species, a few specific compounds are at very high level (e.g., aspartate, glycine, and alanine). In other species, the levels (e.g., taurine) are 10 to 100 times higher in peripheral nerve than in brain.

Much less is known about the distribution of peptides in the organism, principally because methods are not as well developed for separation and detection of these compounds, which usually are present at very low levels. Only a few peptides, such as glutathione, are at high levels in the brain. Interest in this class of compounds is great because of their physiological activity. There are indications that a number of peptides are present exclusively in brain. Many γ-glutamyl peptides are found, including γ-glutamyl derivatives of glutamate, glutamine, glycine, alanine, β-aminoisobutyric acid, serine, and valine. These peptides are present at levels of 10 to 700 micrograms per gram of fresh tissue, and they may be formed by transpeptidation reactions from glutathione. In fairly large amounts, N-acetyl-α-aspartylglutamic acid is present (about 10 to 30 milligrams per 100 grams of fresh brain). No function has been attributed to this peptide, but it is known that it forms the N-terminal sequence of the actin molecule in muscle, and it may play a similar role in some brain protein.

Homocarnosine and homoanserine, two peptides of histidine, are also unique to brain. Homocarnosine is γ-aminobutyrylhistidine, the homolog of the long-known muscle constituent, β-alanyl-L-histidine (carnosine). Homoanserine, the γ-aminobutyryl homolog of anserine (β-alanyl-1-methyl-L-histidine) is also present. These histidine peptides are at much higher levels in this tissue than are their more widely distributed relatives, carnosine and anserine. Carnosine is restricted primarily to the olfactory areas of the brain; in the rest of the brain, mainly homocarnosine is present. Since destruction of nasal epithelium results in a marked decrease of olfactory bulb carnosine, this compound might have a role in olfaction. More recently, the distributions of a number of functionally important peptides have been reported (see Chap. 14).

Developmental Changes

The levels of most components, including the components of the free amino acid pool, undergo complex changes during the naturation of the brain. These changes are not strictly parallel in all brain regions. Some are illustrated in Table 17-2. Quantitatively, the greatest changes are a decrease in taurine and an increase in glutamic acid. These are gradual, compared with the rapid de-

Table 17-2. Changes in Amino Acid Levels During Development*

	Fetal (15 day)	Newborn (1 day)	Adult
Taurine	14	16	8.0
Glutamic acid	7.5	5.0	12
Aspartic acid	2.4	2.3	3.8
Threonine	4.3	0.90	0.56
Proline	0.89	0.57	0.15
Glycine	2.26	2.30	1.27
Alanine	5.08	0.80	0.56
Leucine	0.53	0.18	0.06
Tyrosine	0.24	0.20	0.08
Phenylalanine	0.24	0.13	0.07
γ-Aminobutyric acid	0.50	1.62	2.37
Arginine	0.45	0.14	0.11

*Values are from mouse brain, expressed as μmoles of amino acid per gram of brain tissue.

crease in alanine near the time of birth. Although such changes indicate developmental changes in metabolism (in the relative rates of various metabolic pathways), the connection between substrate levels and metabolism is not clear. It is tempting to theorize that the decrease in essential amino acids parallels the decrease in the rate of protein turnover, for example, but one does not necessarily lead to the other. Changes in amino acid levels, for example after low-protein diets, result in changes in protein metabolism in a number of organs, such as muscle and liver. Brain protein metabolism seems to be resistant to changes in amino acid levels, although specific (myelin) proteins may be affected in phenylketonuria by high phenylalanine levels. In spite of such difficulties, developmental studies are helpful in understanding the function of amino acids in the nervous system [43].

Alterations of Amino Acid Levels

The composition of the free amino acid pool remains constant under most conditions. The amino acids are in a dynamic equilibrium, even though many are undergoing rapid metabolism and rapid exchange with plasma amino acids. Flux of the essential amino acids is especially high, with a *half-life* (time for half of the brain content to be exchanged) of a few minutes. Isotopic equilibrium is reached rapidly; this indicates that these amino acids do not have an inaccessible, nonexchangeable fraction.

The daily rhythm of increase in plasma tryptophan after meals is not reflected in brain, because other related amino acids also increase in plasma, competing for the same transport system and jointly inhibiting each other's uptake. Although such changes in amino acid levels in plasma do not produce comparable changes in brain, nutritional and pathological changes in plasma can affect brain amino acids. A selective increase of tryptophan, especially when accompanied by a decrease in the level of competing amino acids, increases the cerebral levels of tryptophan and of its metabolic products, such as serotonin [45]. Although a general increase (for example, after a meal) of all related amino acids does not increase their brain levels, a selective increase in the blood of an amino acid that is a neurotransmitter precursor can result in increasing the cerebral level of both that amino acid and its product, the neurotransmitter. Although variations in the level of essential amino acids in the brain may occur under special or extreme conditions, the penetration of nonessential amino acids into brain is much slower and no change in brain content occurs, even during extreme blood level alterations of these compounds.

In severe malnutrition, the changes of the brain amino acid pools are rather specific: there is a large increase in histidine and homocarnosine [46], whereas some amino acids decrease (valine, serine, aspartate). Among endocrine influences, the effects of insulin in particular have been studied ever since insulin was first used in the treatment of depressive states. In insulin hypoglycemia, the major changes are a decrease of nonessential amino acids; most likely this reflects the changes in the activity of the citric acid cycle. Hyperthyroidism increases most of the nonessential amino acids. In general, relatively small changes in the

reaction rates involved in carbohydrate or energy metabolism do not affect the levels of cerebral amino acids, but major changes do shift the levels of nonessential amino acids, primarily those that react (through amino transfer) with the intermediates of energy metabolism (glutamate, aspartate, alanine) and GABA. For example, in ischemia, hypoxia, and hypothermia, glutamate and aspartate decrease and GABA increases. Similar changes may be found in hibernating animals; upon arousal, levels return to normal [50].

The changes are somewhat different in convulsions. In human epileptogenic brain tissue, the most consistent changes reported were decreases in glutamic acid and taurine and an increase in glycine; these changes were localized in areas of pathological changes; in surrounding areas, aspartate and GABA also were lowered. Such changes could be reproduced in experimentally induced convulsive states. Upon the administration of taurine, amino acid levels tended to return to normal [51]. In induced convulsions, such changes also depend on the convulsant used: pentamethylenetetrazole causes an increase in alanine (interference with the entry of pyruvate into the citric acid cycle); inhibitors of glutamic acid decarboxylase result in increased levels of glutamate.

Drugs, especially at high dosages, also have been reported to affect the levels of nonessential amino acids; the relation of such changes to any of the pharmacological effects of the drugs has not been established. Chlorpromazine lowers glutamate, aspartate, and GABA; drugs altering catecholamine metabolism (reserpine, 6-hydroxydopamine) have similar effects; ethanol was reported to lower GABA levels [52].

Elevated levels of circulating ammonia are known to cause large increases in the level of glutamine in the brains of animals. Loss of liver function in humans, which prevents the normal detoxification of ammonia, leads to ammoniagenic coma and increased levels of glutamine in the CSF. It has sometimes been suggested that this causes a depletion of Krebs cycle intermediates in brain, and thus leads to decreased oxidation and energy production. However, the demonstration that ammonia stimulates the flux of glucose through the Krebs cycle in brain negates such claims. In ammonia-intoxicated animals there is distinct swelling of the glial cells; this has been taken as additional evidence for associating with glial cells the small pool of glutamate active in glutamine formation [47]. However, estimates of the size of the glutamate pool active in glutamine formation seem to indicate that it is too small to be associated with all the glia [48]. It is well established that drugs that affect this pool of glutamate, for example, ouabain, also inhibit ion pumping. However, the pumping of sodium and potassium ions probably represents too large a proportion of the flux of energy through the Krebs cycle to be directly associated with the glutamate cycle. A somewhat more attractive hypothesis beginning to develop is that the glutamate active in glutamine formation may be associated with the pumping of chloride ions and the hyperpolarization of neurons [49].

Transport of Amino Acids

It was already mentioned that related amino acids interfere with each other's uptake from plasma into brain. This can happen only if uptake occurs by mediated transport rather than by passive diffusion. Active transport processes are also present in brain cells: upon incubation, brain slices accumulate amino acids; at the end of the incubation, tissue levels are several times higher than those in the surrounding medium. This uptake against a concentration gradient is higher in slices from brain than in slices from most other organs. The present concept is that the distribution of most physiological metabolites in the brain is governed by mediated transport, rather than by passive diffusion [53].

MECHANISMS

Mediated transport implies the presence of specific membrane components that have an affinity for the transported substrate and that facilitate movement of the substrate. The specificity of the

transport, described below (Specific Systems), indicates that there is participation of membrane proteins. Such transport can be *specific,* affecting only one or a few compounds, and can be *active,* occurring against a concentration gradient (net transport of a substrate into brain from plasma, for example, even if its level in brain is higher than in the plasma). Specific mediated exit of metabolites from the brain also occurs; that is, exit of a compound from the brain is observed even when the level of this compound is higher in plasma than in brain. Factors that influence transport do not necessarily affect uptake and exit similarly, and the sites at which uptake is most active differ from those of exit.

Although specific amino acid "binding proteins" have been isolated from bacterial membranes, the precise mechanism of transport of metabolites through membranes is not well understood. Important differences exist in transport systems of capillaries, neurons, glia, choroid plexus, nerve endings, peripheral nerve, vesicles, mitochondria, and ganglia.

Recently, an enzymatic mechanism for amino acid transport was proposed, involving γ-glutamyl peptide formation of the transported amino acid from glutathione by γ-glutamyltranspeptidase, with subsequent hydrolysis of the peptide and resynthesis of glutathione [54]. The enzyme γ-glutamyltranspeptidase is low in the brain but high in the brain capillaries and in choroid plexus. However, our understanding of its function in transport remains speculative.

Exchange is a third aspect of transport that differs somewhat from simple mediated transport and may be important. If heteroexchange occurs, the uptake of one compound drives the countertransport of a structurally related compound. Heteroexchange has been observed in isolated systems from brain, and it may be quantitatively significant in some pathological cases, such as the aminoacidurias. The half-life (50 percent exchange) for most amino acids through exchange of brain and plasma free pools is in minutes.

Active protein metabolism of the brain results in a very high rate of exchange between the free and the protein-bound forms. The half-life through exchange of free amino acids to protein-bound forms in brain is usually a few hours.

SPECIFIC SYSTEMS

When uptake of one amino acid is studied in the presence or absence of another, inhibition by related compounds is found. This shows that related compounds are transported by the same system and can compete for carrier sites. In brain cells, ten or more transport classes can be identified, with some overlap; some of these have not yet been observed in other tissues. Some are specific for one type of amino acid—for small neutral, large neutral, acidic, or basic; others are fairly specific for a single amino acid—glycine, proline, GABA, taurine, or lysine [53]. In vivo, the transport by brain capillaries appears to utilize only three classes, large neutral, large basic, and acidic; the others are absent or too weak to be detected in measurements of capillary transport rates. This does not completely exclude the nontransported amino acids, but their diffusion into brain is a much slower process than is transport, and it can occur only in the direction from higher to lower concentration. Transport classes exist for many other metabolites, as well. They have been identified for hexoses; pentoses; carboxylic acids; monoamines, diamines, and polyamines; and nucleotides. The high rate of cellular transport for the nonessential amino acids, combined with low capillary transport of the same compounds, is specific for brain.

There is some overlap among the classes because some amino acids have an affinity for another carrier in addition to their own. In substrate specificity, the transport classes in brain are similar to, but not identical with, those described in other systems. In bacteria, classes with narrower specificity are found; in other organisms, there are multiple classes. For example, there are three systems for the large basic amino acids: one specific for lysine alone; another for lysine, arginine, and ornithine; still another for basics and some neutrals.

In addition to the transport classes discussed above, which have relatively low affinity, amino acid transport classes with high affinity and high substrate specificity have been described in brain. These were found primarily in synaptosomal preparations. It was proposed that the low-affinity (K_m approx. 10^{-3} M), more generally distributed transport systems serve metabolic functions; the high-affinity (K_m approx. 10^{-5} M) systems remove the physiologically active (neurotransmitter) amino acids. This high-affinity transport was suggested as another criterion for assignment of neurotransmitter function. It was found for a number of amino acids in the brain, including glutamate, aspartate, GABA, glycine, proline, tryptophan, and taurine, each of which is also a substrate for low-affinity transport. The participation of exchange in these studies must be determined because exchange can simulate high-affinity transport but cannot remove neurotransmitters [55]. Although the suggestion of high-affinity transport as a special mechanism for the removal of neurotransmitters in instances where metabolic inactivation is not sufficient is very attractive, there are indications of other functions for this process. The distribution of high-affinity systems does not seem to be highly specific; for example, high-affinity tryptophan uptake does not follow the serotonergic system or serotonin receptor binding, and a number of high-affinity systems, such as that for taurine, are present in glial and in neuronal cells. Furthermore, high-affinity uptake was found for such non-neurotransmitter amino acids as leucine and in such other tissues as liver and heart [56].

The requirements of structure are fairly strict; decarboxylated amino acids (*amines*) are not transported by the amino acid transport systems. The stereospecificity is not absolute: D amino acids are transported in most cases, but to considerably lower levels than are the L isomers. Despite this, some D amino acids can penetrate the brain because, although their uptake is slower, so is their exit, and this allows slow accumulation. This, again, illustrates that uptake and exit both influence the level of compounds. Some compounds—related to amino acids, although not normal components of biological fluids (such as synthetic amino acid analogs)—have affinity for the various carriers; nonmetabolized analogs are useful in studying transport independent of metabolism.

REQUIREMENTS

Transport against a concentration gradient requires energy. The primary source of the energy that fuels amino acid transport is not known. Inhibitors of metabolic energy also inhibit amino acid uptake, and in many cases, but not all, the decrease in ATP levels is accompanied by a decrease in uptake. Such inhibition, however, may be indirect.

Amino acid uptake in brain, as in other systems, is dependent on Na^+. Inhibition of the Na^+ pump or the absence of Na^+ abolishes most (but not all) of the amino acid transport. These and other indications strongly support the idea that Na^+ electrochemical gradients may be the driving force for transport. Not all compounds show the same dependence on Na^+: diamine uptake is independent, and basic amino acid uptake is only partially dependent on Na^+ levels. Thus, lowering Na^+ does not affect all amino acids to the same degree. The Na^+ dependence of high-affinity uptake appears to be greater than that of low-affinity uptake. The Na^+ dependence of the low-affinity systems is variable, those participating more in exchange having lower or no Na^+ dependence. Although other ions (probably K^+, possibly Ca^{2+}) also may influence transport, Na^+ seems to be a primary factor [57].

CHANGES IN DEVELOPMENT

The composition of the brain, including the free amino acid pool, undergoes large changes during development (Table 17-2). Permeability for most compounds is greater in young than in adult brain. The developing brain therefore is less protected than the mature brain from fluctuations in plasma metabolite levels and from foreign compounds, such as drugs. Although developmental changes in the free pool and in permeability to amino acids have been studied in detail, changes in amino acid transport are not as well known.

Elevation of most amino acids in plasma causes a greater elevation of levels in brain in young, as compared with adult, animals. Despite this, barriers and transport processes are not absent in the immature brain. For example, amino acid levels in fetal brain differ from those in fetal blood. As in adults, the barrier to nonessential amino acid penetration into the brain is stronger in young animals than is the barrier to essential amino acids. Capillary permeability is greater in the immature brain; this may be caused by less tight junctions of the endothelial cells. Extracellular spaces are also larger, facilitating diffusion. Many transport processes develop rapidly and are present at early developmental stages. The transport systems for neurotransmitters develop somewhat later. Transport properties, such as apparent affinity (K_m), usually show no developmental alterations, with GABA an exception to this rule. Important metabolic changes affect amino acid movements during development: protein turnover—both synthesis and breakdown—is higher in young brain; during growth, the net protein deposition utilizes in a few hours as much amino acid as is equivalent to the contents of the free pool (Chap. 23).

REGIONAL ASPECTS OF TRANSPORT

Distribution, especially of nonessential amino acids, is heterogeneous within the brain. Only gross distribution has been studied, but there are indications that the amino acid pool in neurons is different from that in glia and that additional differences exist between nuclear and mitochondrial compartments. Lysosomes, in which protein degradation takes place, and the nerve ending region, where release and removal of neurotransmitter amino acids take place, also represent special compartments.

The active cellular transport of glycine and proline seems to be absent in capillaries; glutamate uptake from capillaries is also low when compared with that of brain slices. This indicates a difference between the capillaries and the cellular membranes in the quantitative distribution of amino acid transport systems. There seems to be heterogeneity within the capillary wall, as well, in that one system (for small neutral amino acids) is absent from the luminal (blood) side.

The choroid plexus, a structure with still different transport properties, influences the composition of spinal fluid and brain (Chap. 25). In vivo and in vitro amino acid transport have been observed in choroid plexus, which contains additional and specialized transport mechanisms, one for organic acids and one for bases. These are absent in brain, but present in kidney [58, 59]. There are indications of other specific systems in the choroid plexus that are not present in other brain areas, such as those for some peptides.

Perhaps the most heterogeneous distribution of transport systems is represented by the high-affinity transport in synaptosomes. Synaptosomes containing the high-affinity glutamate system were separated from those containing the GABA system; and synaptosomes from spinal cord, but not those from brain, contained the glycine system [31].

INFLUENCES OF TRANSPORT
The best-studied alterations of transport occur when a plasma amino acid is increased. Increase of one member of a transport class inhibits the uptake by the brain of the other members of that class. Under pathological conditions (aminoacidurias), the situation is more complex, since the elevation of a particular amino acid in plasma also causes an increase of that amino acid in the brain (see Chap. 28). The increased tissue level, by inhibiting exit or stimulating heteroexchange, may partially counteract the inhibition of uptake by the same increased amino acid in plasma. It was proposed that the increased plasma phenylalanine in phenylketonuria lowers several amino acids in brain. Among these is tryptophan; this results in a lowered brain serotonin and may play a role in the development of mental retardation. The lowering of an amino acid such as tryptophan may also be the cause of a permanently decreased brain protein level if malnutrition persists throughout brain development. It seems that the most sensitive period is when cell division takes place; this is also the period during which recovery can occur. Protein deficiency throughout the active mitotic period results in permanent decrease in cell number and protein content [60]. Learning deficiency can also

be detected; such a deficiency may carry over to the next generation, even if it is well nourished [61]. In contrast, in adult protein deficiency, brain protein content is maintained despite decreasing proteins of most other organs. This is thought to be the consequence of the more active amino acid transport in the adult brain that maintains the free amino acid pool to a greater degree than in other organs [41]. Pathological changes in protein metabolism could alter the free amino acid pool because the major portion of amino acids is protein bound; for example, a net 1 percent breakdown of proteins would increase most amino acids several-fold. An important, but yet undecided, question is what effect an altered amino acid pool has on brain function. In particular, the effects of an increased phenylalanine concentration have been studied with regard to cerebral protein, lipid, and energy metabolism. At present, there are indications that the changes are specific, rather than general. Not all proteins are affected, and changes in some myelin components have been observed ([62, 63] and Chaps. 28 and 32).

References

*1. Maker, H. S. and Nicklas, W. Biochemical responses of body organs to hypoxia and ischemia. In E. D. Robin (ed.), *Extrapulmonary Manifestations of Respiratory Disease*. New York: Dekker, 1978. Pp. 107–150.

*2. Gatfield, P. D., et al. Regional energy reserves in mouse brain and changes with ischaemia and anaesthesia. *J. Neurochem.* 13:185–195, 1966.

*3. Lowry, O. H., and Passonneau, J. V. The relationships between substrates and enzymes of glycolysis in brain. *J. Biol. Chem.* 239:31 32, 1964.

4. Atkinson, D. E. The energy charge of the adenylate pool as a regulatory parameter. *Biochemistry* 7:4030–4034, 1968.

*5. Bradford, H. F. Carbohydrate and Energy Metabolism. In A. N. Davison and J. Dobbins (eds.), *Applied Neurochemistry*. Philadelphia: Davis, 1968. Pp. 222–250.

*6. Lehninger, A. L. *Biochemistry*. New York: Worth, 1970. Pp. 267–564.

*7. McIlwain, H., and Bachelard, H. S. *Biochemistry and the Central Nervous System*. Baltimore: Williams & Wilkins, 1971. Pp. 1–170.

*Key reference.

*8. Gorell, J. M., et al. Levels of cerebral cortical glycolytic and citric acid metabolites during hypoglycemic stupor and its reversal. *J. Neurochem.* 29:187–192, 1977.

*9. Cremer, J. E., and Heath, D. F. Glucose and ketone-body utilization in young rat brains: A compartmental analysis of isotopic data. In S. Berl, D. D. Clarke, and D. Schneider (eds.), *Metabolic Compartmentation and Neurotransmission. Relation to Brain Structure and Function.* New York: Plenum, 1975. Pp. 545–558.

10. Shimazu, T., Matushita, H., Ishikawa, K. Cholinergic stimulation of the rat hypothalamus: Effects on liver glycogen synthesis. *Science* 194:535–536, 1976.

11. Seta, K., Sershen, H., and Lajtha, A. Cerebral amino acid uptake in vivo in newborn mice. *Brain Res.* 47:415–425, 1972.

12. Diamond, I. A., and Fishman, R. A. High-affinity transport and phosphorylation of 2-deoxyglucose in synaptosomes. *J. Neurochem.* 20:1533–1542, 1973.

13. Stewart, M. A., and Moonsammy, G. I. Substrate changes in peripheral nerve recovering from anoxia. *J. Neurochem.* 13:1433–1439, 1966.

14. Goldstein, G. W., Csejtey, J., and Diamond, I. Carrier mediated glucose transport in capillaries isolated from rat brain. *J. Neurochem.* 28:725–728, 1977.

*15. Balazs, R. Carbohydrate Metabolism. In A. Lajtha (ed.), *Handbook of Neurochemistry.* New York: Plenum, 1970. Vol. 3, pp. 1–36.

16. Phelps, C. H. Barbiturate-induced glycogen accumulation in brain. An electron microscopic study. *Brain Res.* 39:225–234, 1972.

17. Watanabe, H., and Passonneau, J. V. Factors affecting turnover of cerebral glycogen and limit dextrin in vivo. *J. Neurochem.* 20:1543–1554, 1973.

18. Goldberg, N. D., and O'Toole, A. G. The properties of glycogen synthetase and regulation of glycogen biosynthesis in rat brain. *J. Biol. Chem.* 244:3053–3061, 1969.

19. Quach, T. T., Rose, C., and Schwartz, J. C. [^{3}H]-glycogen hydrolysis in brain slices: Responses to neurotransmitters and modulation of noradrenaline receptors. *J. Neurochem.* 30:1335–1341, 1978.

*20. Van Eys, E. Regulatory Mechanisms in Energy Metabolism. In D. M. Bonner (ed.), *Control Mechanisms in Cellular Processes.* New York: Ronald, 1961. Pp. 141–166.

21. Knull, H. R., Taylor, W. F., and Wells, W. W. Effects of energy metabolism on in vivo distribution of hexokinase in brain. *J. Biol. Chem.* 248:5415–5417, 1973.

22. Sacks, W. Phenylalanine metabolism in control subjects, mental patients, and phenylketonurics. *J. Appl. Physiol.* 17(6):985–992, 1962.

23. Booth, R. F. G., and Clark, J. B. The control of pyruvate dehydrogenase in isolated brain mitochondria. *J. Neurochem.* 30:1003–1008, 1978.

24. Jope, R., and Blass, J. P. The regulation of pyruvate dehydrogenase in brain in vivo. *J. Neurochem.* 26:709–714, 1976.

25. Ngo, T. T., and Barbeau, A. Steady state kinetics of rat brain pyruvate dehydrogenase multienzyme complex. *J. Neurochem.* 31:69–75, 1978.

26. Sterling, G. H., and O'Neill, J. J. Citrate as the precursor of the acetyl moiety of acetylcholine. *J. Neurochem.* 31:525–530, 1978.

27. Gibson, G. E., Shimada, M., and Blass, J. P. Alterations in acetylcholine synthesis and cyclic nucleotides in mild cerebral hypoxia. *J. Neurochem.* 31:757–760, 1978.

*28. Abood, L. G. Brain Mitochondria. In A. Lajtha (ed.), *Handbook of Neurochemistry.* New York: Plenum, 1970. Vol. 2, pp. 303–326.

29. Hostetler, K. Y., et al. Contribution of the pentose cycle to the metabolism of glucose in the isolated perfused brain of the monkey. *J. Neurochem.* 17:33–39, 1970.

30. Kauffmann, F. C., et al. Effect of changes in brain metabolism on levels of pentose phosphate pathway intermediates. *J. Biol. Chem.* 244:3647–3653, 1969.

*31. Snyder, S. H., et al. Synaptic biochemistry of amino acids. *Fed. Proc.* 32:2039–2047, 1973.

32. Van den Berg, C. J., and Garfinkel, D. A simulation study of brain compartments. *Biochem. J.* 123:211–218, 1971.

33. Gaitonde, M. J., Dahl, D. R., and Elliott, K. A. C. Entry of glucose carbon into amino acids of rat brain and liver in vivo after injection of uniformly ^{14}C-labeled glucose. *Biochem. J.* 94:345–352, 1965.

34. Waelsch, H., et al. Quantitative aspects of CO_2 fixation in mammalian brain in vivo. *J. Neurochem.* 11:717–728, 1964.

35. Garfinkel, D. A simulation study of the metabolism and compartmentation in brain of glutamate, aspartate, the Krebs cycle, and related metabolites. *J. Biol. Chem.* 241:3918–3929, 1966.

36. Wu., J. Y., and Roberts, E. Properties of brain L-glutamate decarboxylase: Inhibition studies. *J. Neurochem.* 23:759–767, 1974.

*37. Tapia, R. The Role of γ-Aminobutyric Acid Metabolism in the Regulation of Cerebral Excitability. In R. D. Myers and R. R. Drucker-Colin (eds.), *Neurohumoral Coding of Brain Function.* New York: Plenum, 1974. Pp. 3–26.

38. Wood, J. D., and Peesker, S. J. Development of an expression which relates the excitability of the brain to the level of GAD activity and GABA con-

tent, with particular reference to the action of hydrazine and its derivatives. *J. Neurochem.* 23: 703–712, 1974.

39. Sokoloff, L.   Relation between physiological function and energy metabolism in the central nervous system. *J. Neurochem.* 29:13–26, 1977.

40. Matschinski, F. M.   Energy metabolism of the microscopic structures of the cochlea, the retina, and the cerebellum. *Adv. Biochem. Psychopharmacol.* 2:217–243, 1970.

*41. Gaull, G. E., et al.   Pathogenesis of Brain Dysfunction in Inborn Errors of Amino Acid Metabolism. In G. E. Gaull (ed.), *Biology of Brain Dysfunction.* New York: Plenum, 1974. Vol. 3, pp. 47–143.

*42. Himwich, W. A., and Agrawal, H. C.   Amino Acids. In A. Lajtha (ed.), *Handbook of Neurochemistry.* New York: Plenum, 1969. Vol. 1, pp. 33–52.

*43. Himwich, W. A. (ed.).   *Biochemistry of the Developing Brain.* Vol. 1. New York: Dekker, 1973.

*44. Lajtha, A.   Alterations in the Amino Acid Content of the Brain. In D. B. Tower and R. O. Brady (eds.), *The Nervous System.* New York: Raven Press, 1975. Vol. 1, pp. 575–584.

45. Fernstrom, J. D., et al.   Nutritional Control of the Synthesis of 5-Hydroxytryptamine in the Brain. In *Aromatic Amino Acids in the Brain, CIBA Foundation Symposium 22.* New York: American Elsevier, 1974. Pp. 153–173.

46. Enwonwu, C. O., and Worthington, B. S.   Regional distribution of homocarnosine and other ninhydrin-positive substances in brains of malnourished monkeys. *J. Neurochem.* 22:1045–1052, 1974.

47. Cremer, J. E., et al.   An Experimental Model of CNS Changes Associated with Chronic Liver Disease: Portocaval Anastomosis in the Rat. In S. Berl, D. D. Clarke, and D. Schneider (eds.), *Metabolic Compartmentation and Neurotransmission. Relation to Brain Structure and Function.* New York: Plenum, 1975. Pp. 461–478.

48. Berl, S., Nicklas, W. J., and Clarke, D. D.   Glial Cells and Metabolic Compartmentation. In E. Schoffeniels et al. (eds.), *Dynamic Properties of Glia Cells.* New York: Pergamon Press, 1978. Pp. 143–149.

49. Raabe, W., and Gumnit, R. J.   Disinhibition in cat motor cortex by ammonia. *J. Neurophysiol.* 38:347–355, 1975.

50. Palladin, A. V., Belik, Ya. V., and Polyakova, N. M.   *Protein Metabolism of the Brain.* New York: Plenum, 1976.

51. Van Gelder, N. M., Sherwin, A. L., and Rasmussen, T.   Amino acid content of epileptogenic human

brain: Focal versus surrounding regions. *Brain Res.* 40:385–393, 1972.

52. Himwich, W. A., and Davis, J. M.   Free amino acids in the developing brain as affected by drugs. *Adv. Behav. Biol.* 8:231–241, 1974.

*53. Lajtha, A.   Amino Acid Transport in the Brain in Vivo and in Vitro. In *Aromatic Amino Acids in the Brain, CIBA Foundation Symposium 22.* New York: American Elsevier, 1974. Pp. 25–49.

54. Meister, A.   Glutathionine: Metabolism and function via the γ-glutamyl cycle. *Life Sci.* 15:177–190, 1974.

*55. Iversen, L. L.   Neuronal Uptake Processes. In B. A. Callingham (ed.), *Drugs and Transport Processes.* Baltimore: University Park Press, 1974. Pp. 275–286.

56. Bondy, S. C., and Harrington, M. E.   Widespread occurrence of specific, high-affinity binding sites for amino acids. *Biochem. Biophys. Res. Commun.* 80:161–168, 1978.

*57. Banay-Schwartz, M., Teller, D. N., and Lajtha, A.   Energy Supply and Amino Acid Transport in Brain Preparations. In G. Levi, L. Battistin, and A. Lajtha (eds.), *Advances in Experimental Biology and Medicine.* New York: Plenum, 1976. Pp. 275–286.

58. Franklin, G. M., Dudzinski, D. S., and Cutler, R. W. P.   Amino acid transport into the cerebrospinal fluid of the rat. *J. Neurochem.* 24:367–372, 1975.

59. Lorenzo, A. V., Smoly-Caruthers, J., and Greene, E.   Development of amino acid transport mechanisms in the choroid plexus. In H. F. Cserr, J. D. Fenstermacher, and V. Fencl (eds.), *Fluid Environment of the Brain.* New York: Academic, 1975. Pp. 167–180.

60. Winick, M.   Malnutrition and the developing brain. *Res. Publ. Assoc. Res. Nerv. Ment. Dis.* 53: 253–261, 1974.

61. Bresler, D. E., Ellison, G., and Zamenhof, S.   Learning deficits in rats with malnourished grandmothers. *Dev. Psychobiol.* 8:315–323, 1975.

62. Agrawal, H., and Davison, A. N.   Myelination and Amino Acid Imbalance in the Developing Brain. In W. A. Himwich (ed.), *Biochemistry of the Developing Brain.* New York: Dekker, 1973. Vol. 1, pp. 143–186.

63. Roberts, S.   Effects of Amino Acid Imbalance on Amino Acid Utilization, Protein Synthesis, and Polyribosome Function in Cerebral Cortex. In *Aromatic Amino Acids in the Brain, CIBA Foundation Symposium 22.* New York: American Elsevier, 1974. Pp. 299–324.

Kunihiko Suzuki

Chapter 18. Chemistry and Metabolism of Brain Lipids

Studies of lipids in the nervous system form an important part of neurochemical investigations. There are several obvious reasons for the importance of brain lipids, both as structural constituents and as participants in the functional activity of the brain. Among various body organs, the brain is one of the richest in lipids. It contains a unique structure, the myelin sheath, which has the highest lipid concentration of any normal tissue or subcellular components, except for adipose tissue, and which has been the subject of intensive and extensive studies in recent years. Another important reason is the existence of a number of genetically determined metabolic disorders involving brain lipids. Identification of abnormally stored lipids and the search for underlying enzymatic defects have been giving strong impetus not only to the investigations of these pathological conditions but also to the study of the chemistry and metabolism of brain lipids in general. There is increasing evidence, furthermore, that lipid molecules play important functional roles within the membrane. Some of the postulated physiological functions of membrane lipids include the site for the cell-to-cell recognition process, specific cell-surface antigens, and specific receptors for toxins or other physiological compounds.

This chapter is designed to provide basic reference regarding brain lipids. The chapter, therefore, will cover only the most basic and elementary aspects of brain lipid, its chemistry, the lipid composition of normal brain, the peculiarities of brain lipids, and the major metabolic pathways. Many important aspects of the biochemistry of brain lipids are covered elsewhere in this volume, such as the lipid and its metabolism in myelin (Chap. 4), developmental changes (Chap. 23), demyelinating diseases (Chap. 32), or inborn errors of sphingolipid metabolism (Chap. 30). There are also several excellent and reasonably up-to-date review articles on the general subject of brain lipids. They are given at the beginning of the reference list for this chapter and are recommended for more details on brain lipids and as a source of additional references [1–8].

Chemistry of Major Brain Lipids

The lipid composition of the brain is unique in both the high total lipid concentration and in the types of lipids present. Three major categories include almost all of the lipids of normal brain: cholesterol, sphingolipids, and glycerophospholipids.

CHOLESTEROL

Cholesterol (formula 18-1) is the only sterol present in normal adult brain in significant amounts. The alcohol group at position 3 may be esterified with a long-chain fatty acid. Esterified cholesterol is present in normal brain only at very low concentrations. Desmosterol, which is the immediate metabolic precursor of cholesterol and has an additional double bond at C-24 (Fig. 18-5), is present in substantial amounts in normal developing brain. Careful examination with highly sensitive analytical methods indicates the presence in normal brain of other sterols and their precursors, such as squalene. The amounts of these other compounds found in normal brain, however, are minute.

SPHINGOLIPIDS

Sphingosine

The basic building block of all sphingolipids is *sphingosine,* which is a long-chain amino diol with one unaturated bond (formula 18-2). The

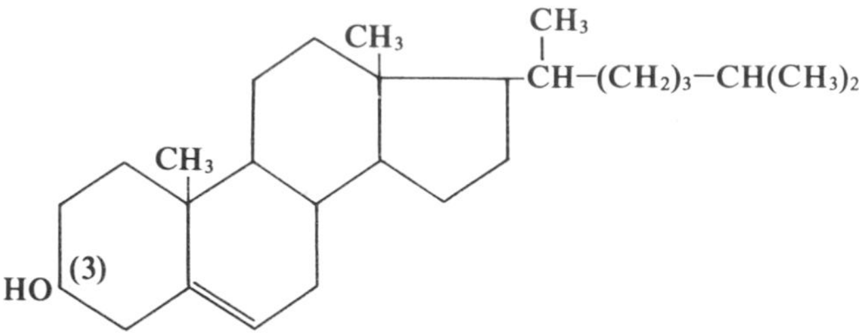

Formula 18-1. Cholesterol

major sphingosine in the brain is C_{18}-sphingosine, but smaller amounts of C_{16}-, C_{20}-, and C_{22}-sphingosines are known to occur. Also, a small portion exists in the saturated form as dihydrosphingosine. Psychosine is sphingosine with additional galactose at the primary alcohol group at C-1 (galactosylsphingosine). Although psychosine is a potentially important metabolic intermediate, it is essentially undetectable in normal brain.

$$CH_3(CH_2)_{12}-CH=CH-CH-CH-CH_2-O-A$$
$$\underset{HO}{|} \quad \underset{NH_2}{|}$$

Formula 18-2. Sphingosine

Ceramide
The amino group of sphingosine is almost always acylated with a long-chain fatty acid, ranging from C_{14} to C_{26}. *N*-Acylsphingosine is generically called *ceramide* (formula 18-3).

$$CH_3(CH_2)_{12}-CH=CH-CH-CH-CH_2-O-A$$
$$\underset{HO}{|} \quad \underset{NH}{|}$$
$$\underset{C=O}{|}$$
$$R = -(CH_2)_n CH_3 \qquad \underset{R}{|}$$

Formula 18-3. Ceramide (*N*-acylsphingosine)
(A = H)

A variety of compounds can be substituted for the C-1 alcohol group of ceramide to form different sphingolipids. "Ceramide A" is any sphingolipid characterized by a substituent, A, at the terminal hydroxyl group of ceramide. We can now define individual sphingolipids in the brain by defining the substituent A.

Sphingomyelin
This is the only phospholipid in the brain that is also a sphingolipid; in this case, A is phosphorylcholine, so sphingomyelin may be defined as ceramide-phosphorylcholine.

Cerebroside and Sulfatide
Cerebroside is a generic term for monohexosylceramide, that is, the substituent A is a hexose. Galactosylceramide is also known as *galactocerebroside,* and glucosylceramide as *glucocerebroside.*

All the cerebroside in normal adult brain is galactocerebroside. Glucocerebroside occurs in the brain in small amounts in certain pathological conditions, as well as in the immature brain. Sulfatide is galactocerebroside with an additional sulfate group at C-3 of the galactose moiety, that is, sulfatide is ceramide-galactose-SO_4^-.

A few glycosphingolipids structurally related to cerebroside are known to occur in small amounts in the brain. One is cerebroside plasmalogen in which the normally unsubstituted hydroxy group at C-3 of sphingosine is substituted with a fatty aldehyde with the α,β-unsaturated ether linkage. The other two are acylated galactocerebrosides, one at C-3, and the other at C-6 of galactose.

Ceramide Oligohexosides (2–4 Sugars)
A series of sugar-containing sphingolipids is known. Unlike cerebroside, all ceramide oligohexosides in the brain have a glucose moiety linked to ceramide. Although these compounds are virtually absent in normal adult brains, they are present in measurable amounts in immature brains

and in some pathological conditions. They are important in relation to the metabolism of brain ganglioside. Some of these substances are ceramide-Glc-Gal, or ceramide dihexoside, also called ceramide lactoside; ceramide-Glc-Gal-GalNAc, or ceramide trihexoside; and ceramide-Glc-Gal-GalNAc-Gal, or ceramide tetrahexoside (Glc = glucose; Gal = galactose; GalNAc = N-acetylgalactosamine). Several other oligohexosylceramides have been reported in the brain in certain pathological conditions.

Gangliosides
Gangliosides are defined as sphingoglycolipids that contain sialic acid. *Sialic acid* is a generic name for N-acylneuraminic acid, and the acyl group of sialic acid in gangliosides of human brain is always the acetyl form. N-Acetylneuraminic acid is commonly abbreviated as NeuNAc (formula 18-4).

Formula 18-4. *N*-Acetylneuraminic acid (Neu*N*Ac)

The series of gangliosides in the brain has the above ceramide oligohexosides as the backbone, with one or more NeuNAc moieties attached. Major gangliosides of the brain are depicted in Fig. 18-1. Several other minor gangliosides have been identified in the nervous system. They include G_{D3}, which is the disialo form of G_{M3}, G_{D2} which is the disialo form of G_{M2}, and sialylgalactosylceramide. The last is unusual in that the hexose residue on ceramide is galactose rather than glucose. It is therefore *sialylated galactocerebroside*.

This compound is attracting attention as a specific component of myelin, particularly in human brain. In the peripheral nerve, a substantial portion of G_{M1} ganglioside contains N-acetylglucosamine in place of N-acetylgalactosamine.

The monosaccharide units of the series of glycosphingolipids described above are linked together with the glycosidic linkage, which is defined as a covalent linkage of the reducing aldehyde group of a sugar to a hydroxy group. Because the configuration around C-1 of hexose defines the anomeric forms, these monosaccharide units are linked together with fixed anomeric configurations. Essentially all glycosidic linkages known to occur in the major brain glycolipids have β configuration. This consideration becomes important in relation to genetic disorders of sphingolipid metabolism (Chap. 30), because hydrolytic enzymes are specific with respect to the anomeric configuration.

GLYCEROPHOSPHOLIPIDS
Glycerophospholipids with two acyl ester linkages are termed phosphatidyl lipids (formula 18-5). In formula 18-5, R_1 and R_2 represent long-chain fatty acids that form ester linkages to two alcohol groups of the parent glycerol molecule. The third alcohol group of the glycerol molecule is linked to a phosphate group. As in sphingolipids, one of the hydroxyl groups of phosphate is substituted with a substituent, A, to form various phosphatidyl substances. When substituent A is hydrogen, the formula is that of phosphatidic acid. Other groups that may be substituted for A are listed in formula 18-5(a).

Formula 18-5. The phosphatidyl moiety (Phosphatidic acid when A = H)

Phosphatidylethanolamine:
$A = -CH_2-CH_2-\overset{+}{N}H_3$

Phosphatidylcholine (lecithin):
$A = -CH_2-CH_2-\overset{+}{N}(CH_3)_3$

Phosphatidylserine:
$A = -CH_2-CH-(\overset{+}{N}H_3)-COOH$

Phosphatidylinositol (monophosphoinositide):
$A =$

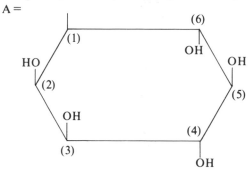

Formula 18-5(a). Additional phosphate groups may be present at position 4, or at positions 4 and 5. The lipids are called *phosphatidylinositol 4-phosphate* (diphospho-inositide) and *phosphatidylinositol 4,5-diphosphate* (triphosphoinositide), respectively.

Another group of glycerophosphatides of potential importance is characterized by the presence of an α,β-unsaturated ether linkage, which replaces the acyl ester at C-1 of phosphatidyl compounds. These are termed *phosphatidal compounds* or *plasmalogens* (formula 18-6).

Although substituent A may be any one of those described for phosphatidyl compounds, almost all of the phosphatidal lipid in the brain is phosphatidalethanolamine, with much smaller amounts of phosphatidalcholine and phosphatidalserine.

$$H_2-C-O-\overset{\overset{\textstyle H}{|}}{C}=\overset{\overset{\textstyle H}{|}}{C}-R_1$$

$$\overset{\overset{\textstyle O}{\|}}{R_2-C}-O-CH$$

$$H_2-C-O-\overset{\overset{\textstyle O}{\|}}{P}-O---A$$
$$|$$
$$OH$$

Formula 18-6. A plasmalogen, possessing the 1-alkenyl-2-acylglycerophosphate structure.

Ceramide——Glc——Gal G_{M3}, hematoside
                |
               NeuNAc

Ceramide——Glc——Gal——GalNAc —— G_{M2}, Tay-Sachs ganglioside
                |
               NeuNAc

Ceramide——Glc——Gal——GalNAc——Gal G_{M1}
                |
               NeuNAc

Ceramide——Glc——Gal——GalNAc——Gal G_{D1a}
                | |
               NeuNAc   NeuNAc

Ceramide——Glc——Gal——GalNAc——Gal G_{D1b}
                |
               NeuNAc
                |
               NeuNAc

Ceramide——Glc——Gal——GalNAc——Gal G_{T1}
                | |
               NeuNAc   NeuNAc
                |
               NeuNAc

Fig. 18-1. Major gangliosides of the brain. The nomenclature of gangliosides is that of Svennerholm (J. Neurochem. 10:613–623, 1963), probably most widely used. For other nomenclatures, refer to Ledeen, J. Am. Oil Chem. Soc. 45:57–66, 1966.

In addition to the major glycerophospholipids above, many glycerolipids are known to be present in small amounts in the brain. Mono-, di-, and triglycerides, which are major lipids in many systemic organs, are present in the brain only in small amounts. Monogalactosyldiglyceride, although present as a minor constituent, appears to be highly localized in the myelin sheath. Other glycerolipids known to occur in the brain include cardiolipin (diphosphatidylglycerol), phosphatidic acid, phosphatidylglycerol, and phosphatidylglycerophosphate. Very small amounts of lyso-

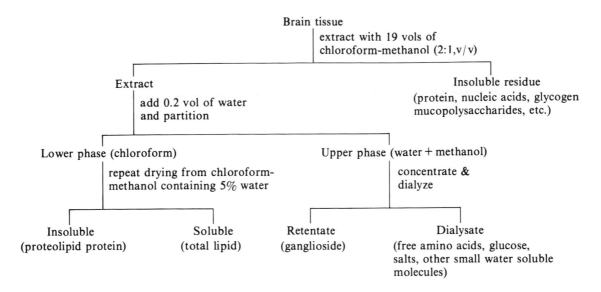

Fig. 18-2. A typical scheme of brain lipid analysis.

phosphatidyl compounds, which result from removal of one of the two acyl groups from glycerophosphatides, also appear to occur as normal constituents of the brain.

Lipid Composition of Normal Adult Human Brain

GENERAL ANALYTICAL SCHEME

Although there are numerous minor modifications, the method of Folch, Lees, and Sloane-Stanley [9] is the conventional starting point for any investigation of lipids in the nervous system. The basic analytical scheme now being used in our laboratory for general analysis of brain lipid is depicted in Fig. 18-2.

Polyphosphoinositides are not extracted by this procedure unless the insoluble residue is reextracted with an acidic mixture of chloroform and methanol. In order to extract ganglioside completely, it is necessary to reextract the chloroform-methanol–insoluble residue with a mixture of chloroform-methanol of a reversed ratio (1:2, v/v) containing 5% water [10]. Otherwise, the procedure is sufficiently quantitative for most pur-

poses, so the final chloroform-methanol–soluble fraction can be used for detailed lipid analysis, and the retentate of the upper phase can be used for ganglioside analysis. When analysis of specific lipid types is intended, the methodology for general survey analysis may be inadequate. For example, quantitative determination of nonpolar gangliosides requires column chromatographic separation of the total lipid extract because the solvent partition procedure does not recover nonpolar gangliosides quantitatively [11].

The proteolipid protein-free lipid fraction and the ganglioside fraction are then ready for detailed analysis of individual lipids. It is not the purpose of this chapter to describe the analytical methods for individual lipids in any detail. Colorimetry and column and thin-layer chromatography are used extensively. Thin-layer chromatography has become established in the analytical investigations of lipids as one of the most convenient and rapid procedures. Figures 18-3 and 18-4 show separations of total lipid and gangliosides in gray and white matter. The compounds have been separated by thin-layer chromatography in some of the routine solvent systems.

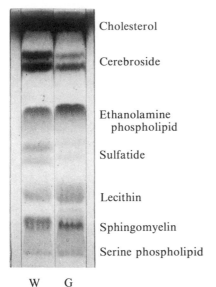

Fig. 18-3. *Thin-layer chromatogram of the total lipid fractions of normal gray (G) and white (W) matter. Approximately 250 µg of total lipid was spotted on a silica gel G plate 250 µ in thickness. Solvent system: chloroform-methanol-water (70:30:4, by volume). Spots were visualized by spraying with 50% sulfuric acid and heating. Note the greater amounts of cerebroside and sulfatide and lesser amounts of phospholipids in white matter. Serine phospholipid streaks from the origin to the area of sphingomyelin in this solvent.*

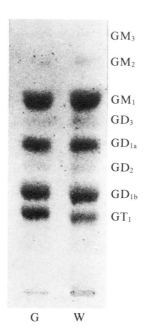

Fig. 18-4. *Thin-layer chromatogram of the ganglioside fraction of normal gray (G) and white (W) matter. The dialyzed upper phase containing approximately 30 µg of NeuNAc was spotted on a silica gel G plate 250 µ in thickness. Chromatography was run in two solvent systems successively: the first solvent was chloroform-methanol-2.5 N ammonia (60:40:9, by volume), and the second solvent, n-propanol and water (7:3 by volume). Spots were visualized by 50% sulfuric acid spray and heating. The four major gangliosides are clearly visible, but other minor gangliosides also are present in very small amounts in normal brain.*

Gas-liquid chromatography is now used extensively for the analysis of almost every constituent moiety of brain lipids. The combination of gas-liquid chromatography with mass spectrometry promises to be a useful tool for simultaneous definitive identification and quantitative determination of such compounds. In recent years, high-performance liquid chromatography has been used increasingly for analysis of lipids because of its speed and high sensitivity.

LIPID COMPOSITION
Typical analytical results for normal adult human brain are given in Tables 18-1 and 18-2. Because the lipid compositions of gray and white matter differ both in total concentration and in the distribution of individual lipids, it is usually important to treat them separately. Depending on the purpose of investigation, selection of specific regions of the nervous system could become of fundamental importance. Equally important is the selection of the basis of reference, such as whole brain, wet weight, dry weight, protein, DNA, or, in cases of lipid studies, total lipid. No single basis of reference is satisfactory or proper in all situations. In Table 18-1 values are given according to three bases of reference commonly used in analytical studies of brain lipids: fresh weight, dry weight, and lipid weight. Fresh weight is often the most appropriate reference standard in pathological conditions involving lipids because lipids are major consti-

Table 18-1. Typical Lipid Composition of Normal Adult Human Brain

Constituents	Gray Matter			White Matter		
	% fresh wt.	% dry wt.	% lipid	% fresh wt.	% dry wt.	% lipid
Water	81.9	—	—	71.6	—	—
Chloroform-methanol– insoluble residue	9.5	52.6	—	8.7	30.6	—
Proteolipid protein	0.5	2.7	—	2.4	8.4	—
Total lipid	5.9	32.7	100	15.6	54.9	100
Upper phase solids	2.2	12.1	—	1.7	6.0	—
Cholesterol	1.3	7.2	22.0	4.3	15.1	27.5
Phospholipid, total	4.1	22.7	69.5	7.2	25.2	45.9
Ethanolamine phospholipid	1.3	7.2	22.7	2.3	8.2	14.9
Lecithin	1.6	8.7	26.7	2.0	7.0	12.8
Sphingomyelin	0.4	2.3	6.9	1.2	4.2	7.7
Monophosphoinositide	0.16	0.9	2.7	0.14	0.5	0.9
Serine phospholipid	0.5	2.8	8.7	1.2	4.3	7.9
Plasmalogen	0.7	4.1	8.8	1.8	6.4	11.2
Galactolipid, total	0.4	2.4	7.3	4.1	14.5	26.4
Cerebroside	0.3	1.8	5.4	3.1	10.9	19.8
Sulfatide	0.1	0.6	1.7	0.9	3.0	5.4
Ganglioside, total*	0.3	1.7	—	0.05	0.18	—

*The amounts of ganglioside were calculated from the total sialic acid, on the assumption that sialic acid constitutes 30 percent of ganglioside weight in a typical ganglioside mixture of normal brain.
Note: Polyphosphoinositides are not included in this table.

Table 18-2. Composition of Major Gangliosides in Juvenile Human Brain*

Constituents	Gray Matter		White Matter	
	Average	Range	Average	Range
Total Neu$N$Ac (μg/g wet wt.)	812	744–918	110	80–180
G_0	3.9	3.2–4.8	4.8	2.8–6.1
GT_1	19.7	15.8–25.7	19.1	14.1–21.2
GD_{1b}	16.7	14.3–19.9	14.8	12.2–18.1
GD_2	3.0	1.2–4.2	1.6	1.2–3.1
GD_{1a}	38.0	29.1–43.7	36.2	30.0–38.2
GD_3	2.0	1.0–2.8	3.2	1.2–5.0
GM_1	14.2	13.0–15.6	18.8	14.6–21.2
GM_2	1.7	1.5–2.0	1.0	0.6–2.0
GM_3	<1	–	<1	–

*Values are expressed as percent of total Neu$N$Ac in each ganglioside, except for total Neu$N$Ac. G_0 represents all sialic acid which has mobility slower than G_{T1}. G_{D2} is Tay-Sachs ganglioside (G_{M2}) with an additional Neu$N$Ac. G_{D3} is hematoside (G_{M3}) with an additional Neu$N$Ac.

tuents of the brain and often decrease drastically, thus substantially altering dry weight. When the water content of the tissue is in question, as is often the case in casually stored, frozen specimens, dry weight may be the reference of choice. To compare relationships among various lipids, total lipid weight often provides the clearest picture.

White matter contains less water and much more lipid and proteolipid than does gray matter. On the basis of wet weight, there is almost three times as much lipid in white matter as in gray matter. There is almost twice as much on a dry-weight basis. As a consequence, there is more of each of the individual lower-phase lipids in white than in gray matter on the basis of wet weight, with the possible exception of monophosphoinositide. In contrast, gangliosides are characteristically gray-matter lipids. Gray matter is ten times richer in gangliosides than is white matter, on dry-weight basis.

When the lipid compositions of gray and white matter are compared, the most conspicuous difference is that white matter is relatively much richer in galactolipids and relatively poor in phospholipids. Galactolipids constitute 25 to 30 percent of the lipids in white matter, whereas they are only 5 to 10 percent of those in gray matter. Phospholipids account for two-thirds of the total lipids in gray matter, but less than half of those in white matter. Plasmalogen constitutes 75 to 80 percent of ethanolamine phospholipid in white matter, but less than half of this phospholipid in gray matter. Sphingoglycolipids, other than galactosylceramide and sulfatide, are present at much lower concentrations in normal adult human brain. These glycolipids are primarily localized in white matter. In contrast, gangliosides are highly localized in neuronal membranes and consequently in gray matter, although the molecular distribution pattern is similar in gray and white matter (see Table 18-2).

Except for the enrichment of ganglioside in gray matter, all other differences in the lipid composition between gray and white matter appear to be due mostly to the presence of myelin in the latter. Myelin constitutes half or more of the total dry weight of white matter, and it is poor in water content and rich in proteolipid protein and galacto-

lipids. Readers are referred to Chap. 4 for details of composition and metabolism of myelin lipids.

The lipid composition of the brain is relatively stable throughout adult life, and the above data may serve as a basis for judging conditions that are altered pathologically. It is essential to keep in mind, however, that substantial changes in lipid composition take place during early development, particularly during the period of active myelination. Before myelination, both gray and white matter have a similar lipid composition, which resembles adult gray matter composition. During active myelination, the brain loses water, predominantly in white matter, the lipid content increases rapidly, and the differences between gray and white matter become more apparent. Characteristically, galactocerebroside is virtually nonexistent before myelination begins and increases concomitantly with the amount of myelin formed [12–15]. Ganglioside is also known to undergo substantial developmental changes [16]. For more details of developmental changes, the reader should refer to Chaps. 4 and 23.

In addition to myelin, the lipid composition of specific subcellular fractions, such as nuclei, mitochondria, synaptic elements, or microsomes, have been investigated [17–20]. With the recent development of procedures to isolate relatively intact neurons and glial cells the lipid compositions of different cell types are also being investigated actively [21].

Although the three major classes of lipids described above constitute most of the lipids found in normal brain, varieties of other lipids are present in small quantities. It should be kept in mind that the small amounts of such lipids do not necessarily mean functional insignificance. Some lipids present in minute amounts could be very important in normal brain function. Recently, *alkanes,* a series of long-chain hydrocarbons, have been reported in the brain [22]. While their physiological significance is still uncertain, they are present at a relatively high concentration in myelin, at nearly 1% of the total lipid fraction. The whole brain or other brain subcellular fractions examined contain less than one-tenth the amount found in myelin. Present also in very minute amounts, but possibly of great functional significance, are dolichols, very long-chain isoprenol polymers, and their derivatives [23]. Sugar-linked dolichols play an important role in biosynthesis of the carbohydrate chains of some glycoproteins [24]. The retina is dependent on retinol not only for its normal function but, quite possibly, for its normal development. Retinol receptors also have been reported in other parts of the brain; this suggests that they may have wider functional significance. Abnormal metabolism of retinol and retinoic acid may well be the underlying cause for the genetic disorder Spielmeyer-Vogt-Batten disease (ceroid lipofuscinosis) [25].

CHARACTERISTICS OF BRAIN LIPIDS

The lipid of the brain possesses several unique characteristics. As mentioned earlier, the brain is one of the richest portions of the body in total lipid content; approximately half the dry weight of the entire brain is lipid. Although by no means constant, the lipid composition of the brain tends to remain relatively unaffected by various external factors, such as the nature of dietary intake, malnutrition, and other conditions that would alter drastically the lipid composition of systemic organs or plasma.

The brain is unique in its lack of certain lipids that are abundantly present elsewhere in the body. Triglycerides and free fatty acids constitute, at the most, only a few percent of the total lipid of the brain. Some of these are probably contributed by blood and blood vessels, rather than by neural tissues. Esterified cholesterol is always much less than 1 percent of the total cholesterol in normal brain, although it is present in slightly higher amounts just prior to active myelination. In pathological conditions in which massive myelin breakdown occurs, esterified cholesterol is often present in high concentrations. Because of this characteristic, the sum of cholesterol, phospholipid, and glycolipid comprises nearly the total lipid, an often useful criterion for judging analyses of brain lipid. If the sum of the three major classes of lipids is substantially less than total lipid weight (e.g., less than

85 percent), the analysis is technically faulty, unless it can be explained otherwise.

Glycolipids of the brain are unique in many ways. Normal adult brain contains only galactocerebroside, whereas almost all systemic organs contain glucocerebroside primarily and very little galactocerebroside. The kidney is the only systemic organ known to contain approximately equal amounts of galactocerebroside and glucocerebroside, but even in this organ the actual amount is almost negligible compared to that in the brain. Brain galactolipids contain high proportions of long-chain fatty acids, including odd carbon members, predominantly C_{24} to C_{26}, which are rarely found in systemic organs. Also, there are high proportions of α-hydroxy fatty acids in brain galactolipids: approximately two-thirds of cerebroside and one-third of sulfatide. α-Hydroxy fatty acids are very unusual in systemic organs.

Brain gangliosides are also unique in their high concentration and molecular distribution. The level of total ganglioside in the brain is rarely approached by any systemic organs; hematoside (G_{M3}) is usually the only ganglioside-related lipid present in significant amounts in most systemic organs.

Biosynthesis and Catabolism of Major Lipids

The biosynthetic and catabolic pathways of brain lipids are generally similar to those in systemic organs. The general references at the beginning of the reference list contain excellent chapters on details of the metabolic pathways of individual lipids. Only the basic outline will be reviewed here.

FATTY ACIDS

Although free fatty acids are very minor constituents of brain, they are important components of all complex brain lipids. The mechanism of fatty acid biosynthesis in the brain appears to be essentially identical with that in other organs, such as liver [26]. De novo synthesis of palmitic acid ($C_{16:0}$) involves acetyl-CoA and malonyl-CoA, and further elongation takes place in mitochondria. Although the brain is capable of synthesizing most fatty acids, it cannot synthesize certain of them, which therefore must be provided from dietary sources and be transported into the brain [27]. These are known as *essential fatty acids* and include linoleic acid (ω-6C$_{18:2}$) and linolenic acid (ω-3C$_{18:3}$). In the nomenclature of fatty acids, the number following ω indicates the position of the first double bond, counting the carbon atoms from the methyl end; the number before the colon is the number of carbon atoms; and the number after the colon, the number of double bonds. Since the brain contains relatively large amounts of polyunsaturated fatty acids, the essential fatty acids are metabolically significant. Desaturation of fatty acids appears to occur at the stage of acyl-CoA. In systemic organs, α-hydroxylation of fatty acids is an intermediate step in C-1 degradation of fatty acids through dehydrogenation and decarboxylation. In the brain, α-hydroxy fatty acids are found as such in galactocerebroside and sulfatide. Prostaglandins are C-20 hydroxylated cyclic fatty acids and derive metabolically from arachidonic acid (ω-6C$_{20:4}$) (Chap. 16). Phytanic acid is a C-20 branched fatty acid (3,7,11,15-tetramethylhexadecanoic acid) which derives only from chlorophyll in dietary sources. Genetic inability to degrade this fatty acid results in Refsum's disease (Chap. 30).

CHOLESTEROL METABOLISM

Although not every step of the biosynthetic pathway of cholesterol known to occur in other tissues has been demonstrated in brain, it is safe to assume that cholesterol synthesis takes place in brain through the same pathway as in systemic organs. Acetate and its precursors are transformed through mevalonic acid to cholesterol (Fig. 18-5).

Desmosterol, the immediate precursor of cholesterol, is known to be present in brain in measurable amounts just prior to myelination [28, 29] and also in the myelin sheath itself in the early stage of myelination [30]. Biosynthesis of cholesterol in brain is most rapid during the period of active myelination, but adult brain retains the capacity to synthesize cholesterol when precursors such as acetate or mevalonate are available. Although most of the cholesterol in brain appears to be synthesized from endogenous precursors, experimental evidence indicates that a small amount of systemically injected cholesterol can be taken up intact and that the rate of uptake is greatest when the rate of cholesterol deposition in brain is most rapid, i.e., during active myelination [31]. Once deposited in brain, cholesterol, particularly that incorporated into myelin, is relatively inert metabolically [32, 33]. When radioactive cholesterol is injected into newly hatched chicks, considerable radioactivity remains in cholesterol of brain, whereas that of liver and plasma virtually disappears within 3 to 8 weeks. This finding is consistent with the apparent lack in brain of an enzyme system for cholesterol degradation.

PHOSPHOLIPID METABOLISM

Metabolic pathways of phospholipid in brain are similar to those in systemic organs [34]. Figure 18-6 depicts the main pathways involving major brain diacylglycerophospholipids (phosphatidylphospholipid) and sphingomyelin.

There are two major synthetic pathways: one involves diglyceride and cytidine 5'-diphosphate choline (CDP-choline) or CDP-ethanolamine for the formation of phosphatidylethanolamine, lecithin, and sphingomyelin; the other passes through CDP-diglyceride to form phosphoinositide and possibly phosphatidylserine (I and II in Fig. 18-6). The formation of phosphatidic acid is an important preliminary pathway common to both the major pathways (III in Fig. 18-6). Choline or ethanolamine is first phosphorylated and is then converted to an active form, CDP-choline or CDP-ethanolamine, by a reaction with cytidine triphosphate. This activated form of choline or ethanolamine then forms phosphatidylcholine (lecithin) or phosphatidylethanolamine by a reaction with diglyceride derived from phosphatidic acid. The direct conversion of phosphatidylethanolamine to lecithin by methylation apparently does not occur in the brain, although it has been demonstrated in some systemic organs. CDP-choline also reacts with ceramide to form sphingomyelin (ceramide-phosphorylcholine) [35]. At least in the brain, an alternate pathway appears to exist in which the first reaction is the formation

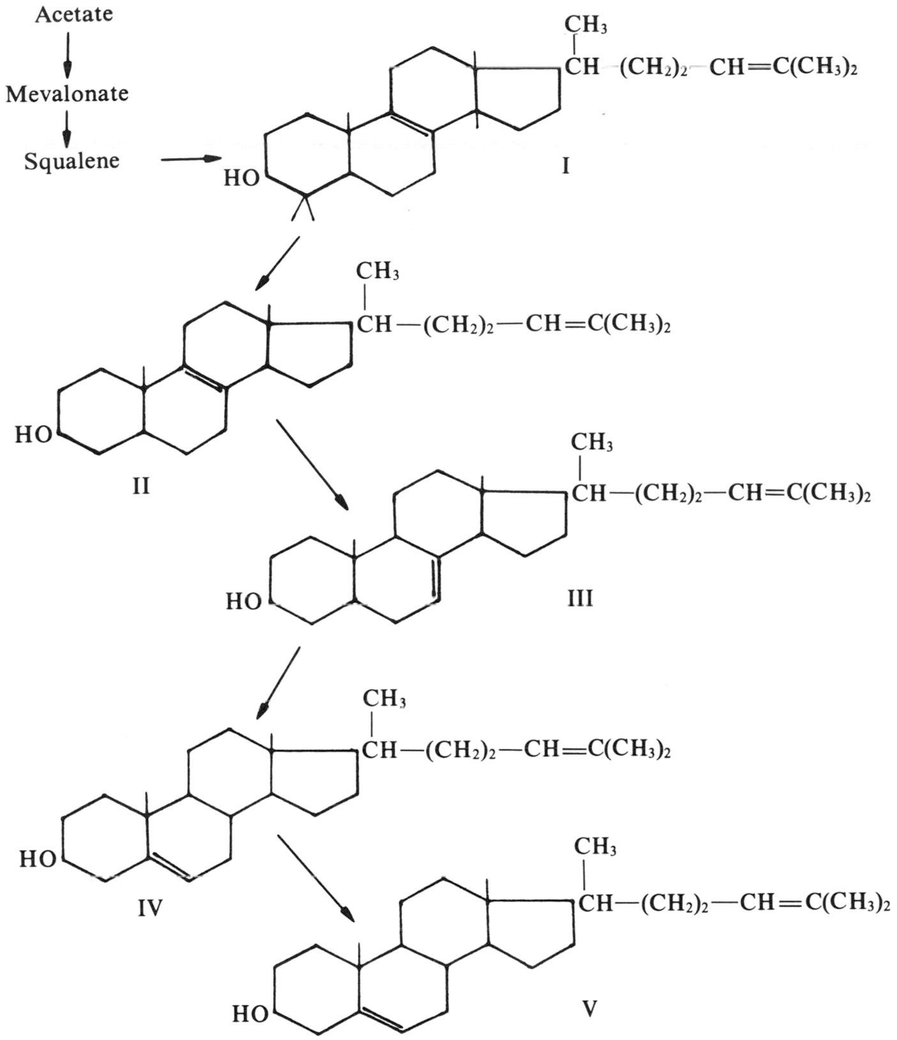

Fig. 18-5. Outline of cholesterol biosynthesis. I, lanosterol; II, zymosterol; III, cholesta-7,24-dienol; IV, desmosterol (24-dehydrocholesterol); V, cholesterol.

of sphingosine phosphorylcholine, followed by its acylation [36]. Direct transfer of phosphoryl-choline from lecithin to ceramide has been demonstrated, and this pathway may well be the most important for synthesis of brain sphingo-myelin [37].

Phosphoinositides are synthesized through a dif-ferent mechanism (II in Fig. 18-6). Instead of form-ing CDP compounds of inositol, CTP reacts with phosphatidic acid to form CDP-diglyceride, which, in turn, reacts with free inositol to form phospha-tidylinositol. Polyphosphoinositides are synthe-sized by stepwise phosphorylation of mono-phosphoinositide. Interconversion of phospha-tidylethanolamine is known to take place in brain [38–40].

There are probably several hydrolytic enzymes in the brain that deacylate phosphatidyl com-

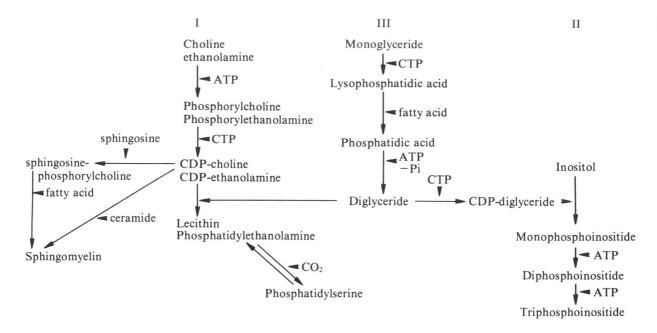

Fig. 18-6. Major pathways of phospholipid biosynthesis.

pounds to lysophosphatidyl compounds. Phospholipase A deacylates the β position of phosphatidylethanolamine, phosphatidylserine, or lecithin. A specific enzyme to deacylate the α' position of these compounds has also been reported [41]. On the other hand, the lyso compounds can be reacylated by acyl-CoA to the original phosphatidyl compounds. This mechanism makes it possible for fatty acids of these phospholipids to turn over independently of the whole phospholipid molecule.

The first step of sphingomyelin degradation is catalyzed by sphingomyelinase, which cleaves sphingomyelin into ceramide and phosphorylcholine. The lack of this enzyme is the cause of at least some forms of Niemann-Pick disease (see Chap. 30).

The high metabolic activity of phosphoinositides is well documented and at present is the focus of intensive investigations regarding their physiological role in brain function.

Biosynthesis of plasmalogen in the brain has not been completely elucidated, but it appears that the pathway is similar to that for the diacyl form of glycerophospholipids [42]. However, plasmalogens might also be formed by reduction of phosphatidyl compounds [43].

CEREBROSIDE AND SULFATIDE

As stated earlier, the normal adult brain contains only galactocerebroside, and alternative pathways have been proposed for its biosynthesis. One is through psychosine, which is formed from sphingosine and uridine 5'-phosphate galactose (UDP-galactose) (I of Fig. 18-7). Psychosine, in turn, may be acylated by acyl-CoA to form galactocerebroside [44]. More recent experimental data indicate, however, that galactocerebroside can be formed through ceramide and UDP-galactose, and the investigators were unable to confirm the acylation of psychosine [45, 46]. At present it appears more likely that the main biosynthetic pathway of brain galactocerebroside is pathway II of Fig. 18-7. Biosynthesis of sulfatide occurs through cerebroside with the "active sulfate," 3'-phosphoadenosine 5'-phosphosulfate (PAPS), as the sulfate donor.

The initial step of sulfatide degradation is removal of the sulfate group and its conversion back to galactocerebroside. The reaction is catalyzed by cerebroside sulfate sulfatase. The lack of this

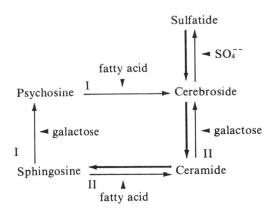

Fig. 18-7. Outline of galactocerebroside biosynthesis.

enzyme characterizes metachromatic leukodystrophy, in which excess sulfatide accumulation occurs (Chap. 30). Then galactocerebroside is degraded to ceramide and galactose by galactocerebroside β-galactosidase, the genetic lack of which causes Krabbe's globoid cell leukodystrophy (Chap. 30). Ceramide is further degraded to sphingosine and fatty acid by ceramidase. Metabolic pathways of neutral glycosphingolipids have been reviewed in some detail [7].

As mentioned earlier, galactocerebroside is almost nonexistent in the brain before myelination. The rate of biosynthesis parallels that of myelin deposition and declines in adult brains. Once deposited, most of the brain cerebroside undergoes only slow turnover, as compared to that of many other phospholipids.

GANGLIOSIDE METABOLISM

Biosynthesis of brain gangliosides occurs by sequential additions of monosaccharides or NeuNAc to the carbohydrate chain, starting from ceramide (Fig. 18-8) [47, 48]. There is no experimental evidence that chains of disaccharides or longer carbohydrates are first synthesized and then transferred in toto to ceramide. The major biosynthetic pathway from lactosylceramide appears to go to G_{M3} ganglioside (ceramide-Glc-Gal-NeuNAc; bold arrow in Fig. 18-8). G_{M2} and G_{M1} gangliosides are then synthesized by sequential addition of N-acetylgalactosamine and galactose. Those polysialo-

gangliosides with only one NeuNAc on the internal galactose are synthesized from G_{M1} by sequential addition of NeuNAc. However, the in vivo pathway for synthesis of the polysialogangliosides with more than one NeuNAc on the internal galactose remains uncertain. In vitro, two pathways seem to exist, one in which the second NeuNAc to the internal galactose is introduced to G_{M3} ganglioside before the additions of N-acetylgalactosamine and galactose, and the other which proceeds through G_{M1} ganglioside. Which pathway is preferred in vivo has not been clarified. The unusual ganglioside, sialylgalactosylglucosylceramide, is synthesized from galactocerebroside and CMP-NeuNAc by a sialyl transferase [49].

These biosynthetic steps are catalyzed by either sialyl or glycosyl transferases that are generally specific for the respective reactions. The active forms of the monosaccharides are UDP derivatives, whereas sialyl transfer occurs through CMP-NeuNAc. Although the bulk of the synthetic activities is localized in the microsomal fraction, there is evidence to suggest that some ganglioside sialyltransferase may also be present in nerve endings.

Degradation of brain gangliosides also proceeds by sequential removal of monosaccharide and NeuNAc by glycosidases and neuraminidases [8, 48]. Most of these hydrolytic enzymes are localized in lysosomes, where the catabolic processes of cellular constituents are believed to take place. Again, some neuraminidase activities are also found in the nerve endings. Although there are still some minor points of uncertainty, the pathway indicated in Fig. 18-8 by bold arrows appears to be the main degradative pathway. Catabolism of brain gangliosides is of fundamental importance to the understanding of some of the most important genetic sphingolipidoses, including G_{M2}- and G_{M1}-gangliosidosis. The topic of genetic sphingolipidoses is covered in Chap. 30.

Some gangliosides appear to act as specific receptors for certain bacterial toxins [48]. The most firmly established is the highly specific binding of G_{M1} ganglioside with cholera toxin, an essential initial event in the sequence of processes through

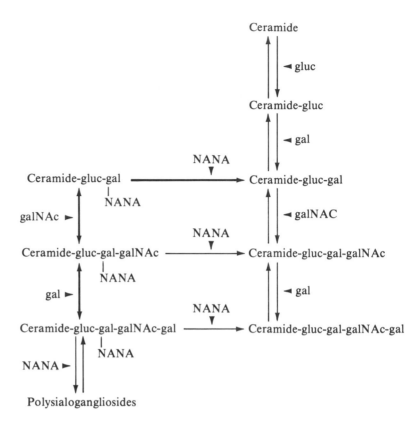

Fig. 18-8. Simplified outline of ganglioside metabolism. In the direction of synthesis, hexose intermediates occur in the form of UDP esters. NeuNAc is incorporated through CMP-NeuNAc. Free sugars are released in the degradative pathways.

which the toxin exerts its effect. Binding of certain polysialogangliosides with tetanus toxin has been often reported. The specificity of the binding has not yet been as firmly established as has the G_{M1} ganglioside–cholera toxin binding. *Botulinum* toxin also binds gangliosides, but the nature of the gangliosides involved and the specificity of the reaction are not well established.

Because of the high concentration in the neuronal membrane [50] and the unusual chemical structure of both hydrophilic and hydrophobic chains, the physiological functions of brain gangliosides— such as their static role as membrane constituents, and their possible involvement in ion transport or in nerve transmission—have been the subject of speculation, but for the most part, they have not been substantiated experimentally. Some experimental information is now beginning to appear concerning the possible role of gangliosides as receptors for such natural cellular constituents as hormones [51].

References

*1. Davison, A. N.   Lipid Metabolism of Nervous Tissue. In A. N. Davison and J. Dobbing (eds.), *Applied Neurochemistry*. Philadelphia: Davis, 1968. Pp. 178–221.

*2. Brady, R. O.   Sphingolipid Metabolism in Neural Tissues. In S. Ehrenpreis and O. C. Solnitzky (eds.), *Neurosciences Research*. New York: Academic, 1969. Vol. 2, pp. 301–315.

*3. Eichberg, J., Hauser, G., and Karnovsky, M. L. Lipids of Nervous Tissue. In G. H. Bourne (ed.), *The Structure and Function of Nervous Tissue*. New York: Academic, 1979. Vol. 3, pp. 185–287.

*4. Lajtha, A. (ed.).   *Handbook of Neurochemistry*. New York: Plenum. See in particular:

*Key reference.

D'Adamo, A. F., Jr. Fatty acids. Vol. 3, 1970, pp. 525–546.

Davison, A. N. Cholesterol Metabolism. Vol. 3, 1970, pp. 547–560.

Hawthorne, J. N., and Kai, M. Metabolism of Phosphoinositides. Vol. 3, 1970, pp. 491–508.

Paoletti, R., Grossi-Paoletti, E., and Fumagalli, R. Sterols. Vol. 1, 1969, pp. 195–222.

Radin, N. S. Cerebrosides and Sulfatides. Vol. 3, 1970, pp. 415–424.

Rapport, M. M. Lipid Haptens. Vol. 3, 1970, pp. 509–524.

Rosenberg, A. Sphingomyelin: Enzymatic Reactions. Vol. 3, 1970, pp. 453–466.

Rossiter, R. J., and Strickland, K. P. Metabolism of Phosphoglycerides. Vol. 3, 1970, pp. 467–489.

Rouser, G., and Yamamoto, A. Lipids. Vol. 1, 1969, pp. 121–169.

Svennerholm, L. Gangliosides. Vol. 3, 1970, pp. 425–452.

*5. Ansell, G. B., Hawthorne, J. N., and Dawson, R. M. C. *Form and Function of Phospholipids.* Amsterdam: Elsevier, 1972.

*6. Stanbury, J. B., Wyngaarden, J. B., and Frederickson, D. C. (eds.). *The Metabolic Basis of Inherited Disease* (4th ed.). New York: McGraw-Hill, 1978. [A standard reference book for biochemistry of inherited metabolic diseases, including those involving brain lipids.]

*7. Morell, P., and Braun, P. Sphingolipid metabolism: Biosynthesis and metabolic degradation of sphingolipids not containing sialic acid. *J. Lipid Res.* 13:293–310, 1972.

*8. Ledeen, R., and Yu, R. Structure and Enzymatic Degradation of Sphingolipids. In H. G. Hers and F. van Hoof (eds.), *Lysosomes and Storage Diseases.* New York: Academic, 1973. Pp. 105–145.

9. Folch-Pi, J., Lees, M., and Sloane-Stanley, G. H. A simple method for the isolation and purification of total lipids from animal tissues. *J. Biol. Chem.* 226:497–509, 1957.

10. Suzuki, K. The pattern of mammalian brain gangliosides. II. Evaluation of the extraction procedures, postmortem changes and the effect of formalin preservation. *J. Neurochem.* 12:629–638.

11. Ledeen, R. W., Yu, R. K., and Eng, L. F. Gangliosides of human myelin: Sialosylgalactosylceramide (G₇) as a major component. *J. Neurochem.* 21:829–839, 1973.

12. Wells, M. A., and Dittmer, J. C. A comprehensive study of the postnatal changes in the concentration of the lipids of developing rat brain. *Biochemistry* 6:3169–3175, 1967.

13. Cuzner, M. L., and Davison, A. N. The lipid composition of rat brain myelin and subcellular fractions during development. *Biochem. J.* 106:29–34, 1968.

14. Norton, W. T., and Poduslo, S. E. Myelination in rat brain: Changes in myelin composition during brain maturation. *J. Neurochem.* 21:759–773, 1973.

*15. Morell, P. (ed.). *Myelin.* New York: Plenum, 1977.

16. Suzuki, K. The pattern of mammalian brain gangliosides. III. Regional and developmental differences. *J. Neurochem.* 12:969–979, 1965.

17. Eichberg, J., Whittaker, V. P., and Dawson, R. M. C. Distribution of lipids in subcellular particles of guinea pig brain. *Biochem. J.* 92:91–100, 1964.

18. Seminario, L. M., Hren, H., and Gomez, C. J. Lipid distribution in subcellular fractions of the rat brain. *J. Neurochem.* 11:197–207, 1964.

19. Lapetina, E. G., Soto, E. F., and DeRobertis, E. Lipids and proteolipids in isolated subcellular membranes of rat brain cortex. *J. Neurochem.* 15:437–445, 1968.

20. Breckenridge, W. C., Gombos, G., and Morgan, I. G. The lipid composition of adult rat brain synaptosomal plasma membranes. *Biochim. Biophys. Acta* 266:695–707, 1972.

*21. Norton, W. T., et al. The lipid composition of isolated brain cells and axons. *J. Neurosci. Res.* 1:57–75, 1975.

22. Darriet, D., Cassagne, C., and Bourre, J. M. Distribution patterns of alkanes in whole brain mitochondria, microsomes, synaptosomes, and myelin isolated from normal mouse. *Neurosci. Lett.* 8:77–81, 1978.

23. Waechter, C. J., Kennedy, J. L., and Harford, J. B. Lipid intermediates involved in the assembly of membrane-associated glycoproteins in calf brain white matter. *Arch. Biochem. Biophys.* 174:726–737, 1976.

24. Waechter, C. J., and Lennarz, W. J. The role of polyprenol-linked sugars in glycoprotein synthesis. *Annu. Rev. Biochem.* 45:95–112, 1976.

25. Wolfe, L. S., et al. Identification of retinoyl complexes as the autofluorescent component of the neuronal storage material in Batten's disease. *Science* 195:1360–1362, 1977.

*26. Olson, J. A. Lipid metabolism. *Annu. Rev. Biochem.* 35:559–598, 1966.

*27. Guarnier, M., and Johnson, R. M. The essential fatty acids. *Adv. Lipid Res.* 8:115–174, 1970.

28. Kritchevsky, D., et al. Desmosterol in developing rat brain. *J. Am. Oil Chem. Soc.* 42:1024–1028, 1965.

29. Paoletti, R., Fumagalli, R., and Grossi, E. Studies in brain sterols in normal and pathological conditions. *J. Am. Oil Chem. Soc.* 42:400–404, 1965.

30. Smith, M. E., Fumagalli, R., and Paoletti, R.   The occurrence of desmosterol in myelin of developing rats. *Life Sci.* 6:1085–1091, 1967.

31. Dobbing, J.   The entry of cholesterol into rat brain during development. *J. Neurochem.* 10:739–742, 1963.

32. Davison, A. N., et al.   The deposition of [4-^{14}C] cholesterol in the brain of growing chickens. *J. Neurochem.* 3:89–94, 1958.

33. Khan, A. A., and Folch-Pi, J.   Cholesterol turnover in brain subcellular particles. *J. Neurochem.* 14:1099–1105, 1967.

*34. Rossiter, R. J.   Biosynthesis of Phospholipids and Sphingolipids in the Nervous System. In K. Rodahl and B. Issekutz (eds.), *Nerve as a Tissue.* New York: Harper & Row, 1966. Pp. 175–194.

35. Sribney, M., and Kennedy, E. P.   The enzymatic synthesis of sphingomyelin. *J. Biol. Chem.* 233:1315–1322, 1958.

36. Brady, R. O., et al.   An alternative pathway for the enzymatic synthesis of sphingomyelin. *J. Biol. Chem.* 240:PC 3693–3694, 1965.

37. Ullman, M. D., and Radin, N. S.   The enzymatic formation of sphingomyelin from ceramide and lecithin in mouse liver. *J. Biol. Chem.* 249:1506–1512, 1974.

38. Borkenhagen, L. F., Kennedy, E. P., and Fielding, L.   Enzymatic formation and decarboxylation of phosphatidylserine. *J. Biol. Chem.* 236:PC 28–30, 1961.

39. Ansell, G. B., and Spanner, S.   The incorporation of the radioactivity of [3-^{14}C] serine into brain glycerophospholipids. *Biochem. J.* 84:12P–13P, 1962.

40. McMurray, W. C.   Metabolism of phosphatides in developing rat brain. I. Incorporation of radioactive precursors. *J. Neurochem.* 11:287–299, 1964.

41. Gatt, S.   Purification and properties of phospholipase A$_1$ from rat and calf brain. *Biochim. Biophys. Acta* 159:304–316, 1968.

42. McMurray, W. C.   Metabolism of phosphatides in developing rat brain. II. Labeling of plasmalogens and other alkali-stable lipids from radioactive cytosine nucleotides. *J. Neurochem.* 11:315–326, 1964.

43. Ansell, G. B., and Spanner, S.   The metabolism of labeled ethanolamine in the brain of the rat in vivo. *J. Neurochem.* 14:873–886, 1966.

44. Brady, R. O.   Studies on the total enzymatic synthesis of cerebrosides. *J. Biol. Chem.* 237:PC 2416–PC 2417, 1962.

45. Morell, P., and Radin, N. S.   Synthesis of cerebroside by brain from uridine diphosphate galactose and ceramide containing hydroxy fatty acid. *Biochemistry* 8:506–512, 1969.

46. Morell, P., Costantino-Ceccarini, E., and Radin, N. S.   The biosynthesis by brain microsomes of cerebrosides containing nonhydroxy fatty acids. *Arch. Biochem. Biophys.* 141:738–748, 1970.

47. Kaufman, B., Basu, S., and Roseman, S.   Studies on the Biosynthesis of Gangliosides. In B. W. Volk and S. M. Aronson (eds.), *Inborn Disorders of Sphingolipid Metabolism.* Oxford: Pergamon, 1967. Pp. 193–213.

48. Ledeen, R. W., and Mellanby, J.   Gangliosides as Receptors for Bacterial Toxins. In A. W. Bernheimer (ed.), *Perspectives in Toxicology.* New York: Wiley, 1977. Pp. 15–42.

49. Yu, R. K., and Lee, S. H.   In vitro biosynthesis of sialosylgalactosylceramide (G$_7$) by mouse brain microsomes. *J. Biol. Chem.* 251:198–203, 1976.

50. Ledeen, R. W.   Ganglioside structure and distribution: Are they localized at the nerve ending? *J. Supramol. Struct.* 8:1–17, 1978.

51. Dreyfus, H., et al.   *Structure and Function of Gangliosides.* New York: Plenum, 1979.

52. Svennerholm, L.   Chromatographic separation of human brain gangliosides. *J. Neurochem.* 10:613–623, 1963.

53. Ledeen, R.   The chemistry of gangliosides: A review. *J. Am. Oil Chem. Soc.* 43:57–66, 1966.

Henry R. Mahler

Chapter 19. Nucleic Acid and Protein Metabolism

Nucleic Acids and Brain Function

Any attempt to formulate neurobiological phenomena in molecular terms must take cognizance of the nature, organization, expression, and regulation of the genetic capabilities of the nervous system and its component parts. At one level, this entails systematic studies of neurological and behavioral mutants and of how alterations in the genome affect defined functions of the nervous system. Such studies can provide very important clues concerning the contributions of single, defined gene products to complex and integrated brain function and behavior. At one level, one deals with emergent properties as a function of time as the independent variable. These include qualitative or quantitative changes in the pattern of the proteins present within a given cell, in a population of cells linked to one another structurally and functionally, or in even more complex systems. By their intervention as enzymes and as essential structural and functional constituents of their membranes, these proteins, in turn, influence all other components of the affected cells.

But such changes in protein patterns are themselves the consequence of shifts in gene expression and its regulation. This is the problem we need to solve. Our concern is not just with those hypothetical or actual changes in response to electrical activity, sensory inputs, and behavioral challenges that produce or reflect specific products in, and alter the properties of, certain families of neurons and the synapses between them [1–4], itself a formidable task. We must also be concerned with the events responsible for the ontology of neuronal formation, localization, and connectivity in the course of development. In biochemical terms, the questions posed constitute an inquiry into the parameters that govern the biosynthesis and degradation of DNA and RNA in brain and nerve, and that is the topic of the first half of this chapter; protein metabolism proper is discussed in the second half.

DNA Versus RNA Metabolism

DNA synthesis and turnover in all somatic cells usually reflect the cell's ability to undergo division and to effect the excision and repair of structural damage. At first glance, these capabilities appear to be directly correlated with the mitotic index of the cells, that is, their rate of division. Although there is now good evidence that certain brain cells (interneurons, astrocytes, glia) continue to divide beyond the fetal stage into infancy or even adulthood, the ordinary long-axoned neurons (*macroneurons*) of mammals cease dividing and proliferating shortly after birth or in early infancy (see [5] and Chap. 23). For instance, in rat cerebral cortex there is no net increase in DNA beyond day 20 after birth, and in humans there is an analogous cut-off around day 50. Furthermore, the amount and kind of DNA have been thought to be constant in all cells of any individual. Only recently has it become apparent that they may be different in germ line and some somatic cells [6]. Most of the literature until now has dealt almost exclusively with the metabolism and functional involvement of various species of RNA formed in the nervous system [7].

This chapter reflects this state of the art and finds its justification in the compelling evidence in favor of the continuity, stability, and identity of the gene complement in all cells of a metazoan organism in contrast to their structural and functional diversity, which, in turn, is subject to further modification with time. All these effects must reflect qualitative or quantitative changes in the expression of the genetic information. In biochemical terms, we are dealing with the transcription of DNA base sequences into RNA and the translation of some of the RNA into the amino acid sequences of polypeptides. Although we might expect patterns of RNA synthesis and nucleic acid metabolism in brain to be generally similar to those of other tissues, quantitative differences should exist. In particular, we might anticipate that the presence of the blood-brain barrier would place serious preferential constraints on the entry of certain precursors for macromolecular biosynthesis. Additional features are due to the inordinate cellular and regional complexity of brain tissue.

Metabolism of Nucleic Acid Precursors
SYNTHESIS OF PURINE AND PYRIMIDINE NUCLEOTIDES

De Novo Synthesis
Qualitatively, the pathways established for the de novo biosynthesis of the purine and pyrimidine nucleotides in other tissues also appear to be operative in nerve and brain. The pathways are shown in Chap. 11. This assertion rests on the demonstration of (1) the conversion of labeled precursors to the expected intermediates in the correct time course, (2) the presence of certain critical enzymes characteristic of and exclusive to the two pathways, and (3) the proper blocks by specific and characteristic inhibitors of key steps, such as the glutamine antagonists azaserine (*O*-diazoacetyl-L-serine) and DON (6-diazo-5-oxo-L-norleucine) for purine, and azauridine for pyrimidine biosynthesis.

Quantitatively, most of the nucleic acid purines probably arise de novo [8], although the operation of other routes (see Salvage Pathways) appears to be of great regulatory significance. For pyrimidines, the situation may be different: the rate of flux through the small pool of orotate actually present is probably insufficient to satisfy the demand for pyrimidines for nucleic acid and coenzyme synthesis, and the block by azauridine can be effectively circumvented by raising the level of available uridine. Furthermore, uridine, but not

orotate, can serve as an adequate precursor of nucleic acid pyrimidines with brain preparations in vitro [9].

Salvage (Reutilization) Pathways and Orotic Acidurias
These observations direct attention to the possibility that a substantial portion of the bases do not arise de novo in the brain but, instead, originate in the liver and are then transported by the circulation in the form of nucleosides—mainly uridine, in the case of pyrimidines. This, the so-called salvage pathway, appears to be of importance in both normal function and certain pathological states of the brain [10].

Administration of uridine and cytidine protect the perfused cat brain from degradation and allow it to exhibit normal carbohydrate metabolism and electrical activity for periods of up to 4 hours. Repeated injections of azauridine block the de novo formation of pyrimidine nucleotides [11]; a similar, but permanent, defect is characteristic of the autosomally inherited, recessive genetic lesion in humans called *orotic aciduria* [8]. Azauridine, after conversion to the nucleotide, specifically inhibits orotidylate decarboxylase; in type I orotic aciduria, both this enzyme and orotidylate pyrophosphorylase—the enzyme that catalyzes the preceding step in the de novo pathway—drop to undetectable levels. (In type II, only the decarboxylase is missing). Severe neurological and electrophysiological disturbances are observed in both instances. These effects can be circumvented or reversed by the administration not only of uridine monophosphate (UMP), the absent direct product, but also of uridine, and this observation permits the inference that the salvage pathway is indeed operative.

These hereditary orotic acidurias, although quite rare, are exceedingly interesting genetic diseases for the following reasons:

1. They constitute the only described instances of blocks in pyrimidine biosynthesis, not just in man, but in higher organisms in general.

2. Because their effects can be overcome by administration of pyrimidines, they also constitute the clearest evidence of auxotrophism in such organisms.

3. Type II may be the result of a lesion in a structural gene; type I, the result of a lesion in a regulatory gene.

4. These defects result in a breakdown of the regulatory machinery of the cells affected, which leads both to overproduction of orotic acid and to the pattern of "pyrimidine starvation" previously observed in pyrimidine auxotrophs in microorganisms.

5. Their consequence—and alleviation—can be mimicked by a synthetic pharmacological agent.

Lesch-Nyhan Syndrome

Even more striking are the manifestations in male children of another genetic lesion that leads to a loss or diminution in hypoxanthine-guanine phosphoribosyltransferase, one of the enzymes of the salvage pathway for purines, responsible for the conversion of hypoxanthine and guanine into their respective nucleotides. Individuals who carry this defect on their X chromosomes exhibit the *Lesch-Nyhan syndrome* [12], which is characterized by an elevated uric acid level in blood and urine (*hyperuricemia*), spastic cerebral palsy (*choreoathetosis*), aggressive and destructive behavior leading to self-mutilation, and mental retardation. Details can be found in Chap. 11.

Nucleotides and Behavior

Finally, it has been claimed that distinct behavioral effects can be elicited in animals and humans by feeding heterologous RNA, an entity that is almost certainly degraded to nucleotides and nucleosides either prior to or in the course of administration. Because the most striking results were the correction of a memory defect in aged subjects, it is not impossible that upon stress or aging the demand on the salvage pathway becomes so great that it can no longer be satisfied wholly by endogenous sources, and dietary supplementation might indeed prove beneficial.

NATURE OF PRECURSOR POOLS

For practical purposes, the only nucleic acid synthesis with which we need to concern ourselves takes place in the nucleus. Thus, the immediate precursor pools involved are constituted by the various nuclear (not the total cellular) nucleoside triphosphates, and the information we require is their concentration both in the steady state and in its more-or-less transient response to a particular stimulus. Unfortunately, this information is not yet available. There are indications that the nuclear pools can be refilled from cytoplasmic nucleoside 5'-phosphates, but whether the diphosphates and triphosphates can also be transported across the nuclear membrane and whether intranuclear phosphotransferases have to intervene are unknown factors, as are the levels and rates of the various enzymatic reactions involved. The relative total concentrations in whole rat brain for the four triphosphates are $ATP \gg GTP \approx UTP \gg CTP$ at all ages, but whereas the concentrations of the first three remain relatively invariant during maturation (at about 200, 30, and 30 μmoles per 100 grams of wet weight, respectively), the last drops to very low levels (less than 1 μmole per 100 grams) in the adult.

FUNCTIONAL CHANGES

General Considerations in Tracer Experiments

The usual, and frequently the only practical, method for investigating the effect of perturbations on the rate and extent of synthesis of cellular, cytoplasmic, or nuclear RNA—either in its totality or in any of its subpopulations—consists in measuring the difference in uptake of some radioactive precursors, for example, uridine. The scheme shown in Fig. 19-1, though simplified, depicts the flow of this precursor into various species of RNA.

Clearly, what needs to be done [13] is (1) to establish the complete kinetics of the flux of label in the unperturbed state and its relevance to RNA synthesis, assuring that what is measured is indeed synthesis, rather than transfer or the filling of one or more of the precursor pools, and (2) to extend this study to the much more difficult problem posed by the introduction of the perturbation. Very few

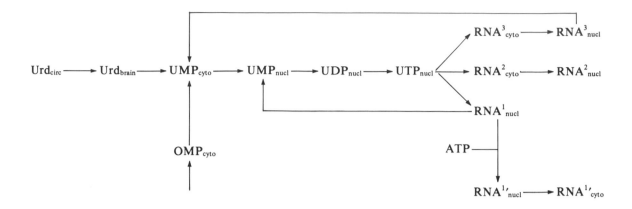

Fig. 19-1. *Flow of uridine into various species of RNA. Urd, uridine; UMP, uridine monophosphate; UDP, uridine diphosphate; UTP, uridine triphosphate; OMP, orotidine 5'-phosphate.*

of the studies that will be discussed meet these stringent criteria. What is commonly done is to take one or, at the most, a selected few time points subsequent to the administration of label and to compare the appearance of the label in some RNA (and, in the better investigations, in one or more of the intermediates) in appropriately selected experimental and control groups. The only permissible inference to be drawn from studies of this type is the rather trivial one that any differences observed indicate differences in the net rate of appearance of label in the RNA, but they cannot be interpreted in terms of differences in the rate of synthesis of this species. In fact, more often than not, the differences may be due to differences in the interconversion of precursors, in transport phenomena, or in rates of degradation of short-lived intermediates or products.

Electrical Stimulation

Electrical stimulation—either briefly at high intensity during electroshock in vivo, or at low intensity, but for a sustained period, of slices in vitro—elicits profound effects on the metabolism of the total nucleotide pools in these systems. The most striking results of electric shock in vivo are relatively persistent alterations in the concentrations of uridine triphosphate (UTP) and guanosine triphosphate (GTP), as well as in their rates of turnover. Investigations with slices have been restricted so far to measurements of the conversion of uridine to its phosphorylated derivatives. A diminution of some 40 percent coincident with

maintenance of the total uridine-containing pool was found, and this was ascribed to effects on the cation pump that resulted in disturbances in the rate of influx of Na^+ into, and efflux of K^+ from, the cells.

To what extent such phenomena are relevant to control of nuclear RNA synthesis in vivo is uncertain. In general, one might expect that the RNA polymerases would respond only if some ribonucleoside triphosphates either dropped to or rose from (1) extremely low levels (less than 10 percent of the K_m), in which case the regulation would be of the "on-off" variety, or (2) the region around its K_m, in which case the rate would be directly proportional to concentration. In view of the results already cited, it might prove fruitful to explore the response of nuclear GTP levels to stimulation in some well-defined system. At all events, any such regulation by availability of a critical substrate may be expected to be nonselective and to effect the transcription of all active genes by any one polymerase to the same extent.

Synthesis and Turnover of DNA

LOCALIZATION AND SPECIES

The only well-authenticated sites at which DNA is found in all animal cells, including brain and nerve, are the nucleus (this includes the nucleolus) and the mitochondria. It has been assumed that various types of DNA sequences, while species specific, are conserved and identical in all somatic cells of the same organism. This may in fact not be so, since certain sequences may be subject to developmentally regulated events such as rearrangements—as in genes for immunoglobulins [14]—or selective methylation of some of their bases [14a]. The latter modification may be of significance in regulating the expression of certain genes in developmental or other schedules for neurogenesis, synaptogenesis, or synaptic modification.

The DNA content of diploid mammalian cells, including neurons and other brain cells, is of the order of 6.5 picograms per cell (or about 1 microgram per milligram of wet brain weight). Virtually all of it is nuclear. This corresponds to a mass of 3.8×10^{12} daltons for the total chromosomal complement of such cells. Thus the maximal (haploid) content of genetic information available to these cells is about 800 times that of *E. coli,* or 100 times that of yeast, encoded in 1.5×10^9 base pairs. The numbers for other animals are lower and subject to much greater variation. The base composition of all animal DNA is close to 60% guanine plus cytosine (G + C). This DNA in nondividing (interphase) nuclei is present as a complex or aggregate called chromatin, which consists of approximately 30% DNA, 10% RNA, and 60% protein by weight. The proteins are composed of both basic species (the five histone species, H1, H2a, H2b, H3, and H4, account for about 80 percent of the total) and acidic species. The DNA of different chromosomes differs with respect to size, base composition, and redundancy of its constituent or subunit segments.

Nucleolar DNA is much more homogeneous with respect to all these criteria: its base composition is also different (about 70% G + C). These properties reflect its principal function of serving as the depository for the information that encodes several hundred copies of the 45S (4×10^6 daltons) precursor of ribosomal RNA.

Mitochondrial DNA accounts for less than 0.1 percent of total cellular DNA. Its base composition is close to that of nuclear DNA, but it is much smaller, more uniform in size (5 μ in length or a particle weight of 10×10^6 daltons), and highly homogeneous with regard to base composition and lack of redundancy. Mitochondrial DNA is present in many ($> 10^3$) copies per cell, an amount corresponding, on the average, to several molecules per mitochondrion; it is not tightly complexed with proteins. It can be isolated as a covalently closed, twisted circle (superhelix), and this configuration probably corresponds to that actually existing inside the cell.

ORGANIZATION

Recent studies have revealed details of the molecular organization of chromosomal DNA and its associated histones: this consists of a tandemly repeated array of particles (nucleosomes) that contain 140 base pairs of DNA wrapped around a tightly associated core of histones, separated by regions of less highly structured—and hence more nuclease-sensitive—DNA, referred to as *linkers* or *spacers*. This organization is characteristic of all chromatin, whether in transcriptionally competent or active (*euchromatic*) or inactive (*heterochromatic*) regions of the chromosome. This also is the organization established for the chromatin of cells from nerve and brain [15, 16]. Rather surprisingly, the repeat length of the linker DNA segments in neurons from the cerebral cortex of adult rodents appears to be significantly shorter (160 base pairs) than that characteristic of cortical glial or kidney cells from the same animals (200 base pairs). This shortened repeat is absent from fetal or newborn neurons and makes its appearance at days 3 and 5 after birth in rabbit and mouse brain, respectively.

TURNOVER

As already mentioned, the rate of turnover of nuclear DNA of mature macroneurons is low, and was, until recently, controversial. It now appears that, although replicative, semiconservative synthesis is certainly absent from the nuclei of such cells, in contrast to a high level of replicative activity in perinatal neurons [17], mature neurons are indeed capable of a significant level of repair synthesis [18, 19]. In fact, its absence in individuals suffering from the hereditary lesions in scleroderma pigmentosum may be the cause of a characteristic neurological abnormality (de Sanctis-Cacchione syndrome). However, at least some of the components of the repair system do appear to be present at significantly lower levels in neurons than elsewhere [19], as shown by the persistence of the modified base O^6-methylguanine (introduced by the neuro-oncogenic agents N-ethyl-N-nitrosourea and N-methyl-N-nitrosourea [20]. Little is known concerning the nature of the responsible enzymes, but the nuclear polymerases in immature neurons appear similar to those studied in and isolated from other eukaryotic cells [17]. Three such enzymes, called α, β, and γ, have been characterized, of which the γ also appears responsible for DNA synthesis in mitochondria [21]. Mitochondrial DNA is known to be susceptible to relatively rapid turnover with a half-life of 31 days in brain and 7.5 days in liver [22]. Nuclear DNA turnover in mouse brain has been reported to be stimulated upon infection by scrapie [20] and inhibited by electroshock [23].

DNA AND NEUROGENESIS

Autoradiographic Studies

Altman and his collaborators [24] have used autoradiography of cell nuclei labeled with ^{3}H-thymidine to determine the nature and extent of postnatal neurogenesis in rodents. By this technique, they were able to demonstrate that considerable DNA synthesis (or at least turnover) and cell proliferation, migration, and differentiation take place in the brain of infant rats (see Chap. 23), and that these events appear to be initiated by the cells of the outer granular layers of the cerebellum, hippocampus, olfactory bulb, and ventral cochlear nucleus. The formation and differentiation of cells classified as microneurons continues during infancy, although at declining rates in most structures. Thus, in the cerebellum, almost all the cells of the granular and molecular layers that form the precursors of granule, stellate, and basket cells are formed and completed during infancy; the basket are earlier than the granule and stellate types, but most of them complete their differentiation and migration by 21 days after birth. In contrast, almost all Golgi cells have already been formed at birth. In the wall of the olfactory ventricle, cell multiplication continues at very high rates for 6 days and declines dramatically by 13 days, but it is still detectable even in the young adult. In the hippocampus, the bulk of the cell population is formed postnatally, and the neurogenesis of granule and stellate cells in the dentate gyrus may continue over a prolonged span of time.

From these observations, Altman [24] has concluded that the long-axoned neurons, or macroneurons, of the brain are formed prenatally but that many of the short-axoned or axonless neurons (microneurons) are formed postnatally. He further proposes that this continued genesis of microneurons may be required for the modulation and feedback regulation of (1) the transmission of sensory information in primary afferent relay areas, (2) the execution of motor action in the cerebellar cortex, and (3) the motivational efficacy of need-catering (appetitive and consumatory activities) in the hippocampus and limbic system in general.

Enzyme Activities

In rat cerebellum, the level of maximum activity of a number of enzymes required for DNA synthesis is not reached until 6 days after birth, whereas the corresponding peaks of activity in cortex, its neurons, and whole brain are observed around 15 to 16 days of gestation [5, 17]. Among the activities tested were DNA polymerase, particularly enzyme α, ribonucleotide reductase, thymidine kinase, carbamylphosphate synthetase, and aspartate transcarbamylase. Similarly, in our laboratory (unpublished results), S. Norton and G. Crawford observed that DNA methylating enzymes and microtubule protein accumulation in cortex (presumably for function of the mitotic apparatus) also reached their peaks around day 15 of gestation.

DNA Content and Ploidy

Perhaps related to some of these considerations is the fact that the chromosome number (*ploidy*), and hence the DNA content, of certain neuronal types in the higher integrative centers is about twice that of the ordinary diploid brain cells (i.e., 13 pg DNA per cell). The nuclei of these unusual cells also are larger than their standard counterparts: among them are the Purkinje cells of the cerebellum and the pyramidal cells of the hippocampus, but not their granule, interneurons, and glial cells [5].

Effects of Growth Hormone

The weight of the brain, its total DNA content (i.e., its *cell number*), as well as the relative proportions of its neurons and glia in newborn or infant rats can be significantly increased if the mother is injected subcutaneously or intravenously with purified growth hormone (from bovine pituitary glands) during the period between days 7 and 20 of pregnancy. The significance of these findings and their generality as to strain and species remain to be explored.

Oligoamines

The oligoamines spermine and spermidine, as well as their precursor, putrescine, are ubiquitous constituents of living cells, where they usually occur in close association with DNA. As organic cations they can and do serve to neutralize some of the charges and stabilize the polyanion. Whether their actual or potential role (as in the regulation of transcription) transcends these features, which are analogous to those exerted by Mg^{2+}, the other principal counterion associated with nucleic acids, is under active investigation in many systems [26]. The occurrence and concentrations of these compounds have been studied in animal and human brain as a function of both isolated brain regions and ontogeny. In one comprehensive study of the rat nervous system, Seiler and Schmidt-Glenewinkel [27] found spermidine/DNA ratios to be nearly constant and equal to 0.11 ± 0.02 $\mu mol/\mu mol$ DNA-P) in the diencephalic and telencephalic regions investigated, whereas they were significantly lower (0.05 ± 0.02 μmol DNA-P) in brain stem, cerebellum, and spinal cord. The spermidine/spermine ratio increased as follows: olfactory bulb 0.6; cerebral cortex 1.3; cerebellum 1.7; hippocampus 2.2; hypothalamus 2.3; caudate nucleus and pons 2.5; thalamus and septum pellucidum 2.7; midbrain 4.7; medulla 16, spinal cord 21; that is, this parameter is directly correlated with content of white matter. The dis-

tribution pattern of putrescine (which, however, is present at a concentration some 100 times lower than spermidine) is similar to that just described for spermidine, except in hypothalamus, which contains an unusually high putrescine concentration. Finally, the distribution of spermidine correlates well with that of RNA (at a ratio of approx. 1:10); however, it is significantly higher in medulla, spinal cord, and peripheral nerve. In the ontogenetic studies on human brain [28], the changes in oligoamine concentration paralleled those of nucleic acid accumulation. The concentration of putrescine in human brain—unlike that of rat brain—was much higher than oligoamine concentrations in all sets of measurements, and there was a marked increase in this component in the brain stem at the time of most rapid myelination. Putrescine also increased markedly in the fetal forebrain at the time of neuroblast multiplication. In aging rats, spermine levels again exhibit a remarkable constancy with age and brain region; spermidine levels increase with age in cerebral cortex, midbrain, and hippocampus [29].

Inhibitors

Arabinosylcytosine (cytosine arabinoside), an analog in which arabinose takes the place of deoxyribose, is an effective and selective inhibitor of DNA synthesis in animals in vivo and in their cells in culture. This inhibition is probably elicited after the nucleoside has been converted to the triphosphate. Since it blocks the uptake of radioactive thymidine into various areas of goldfish brain, it probably functions in the expected manner in this system also. The block is, however, without any effect on certain behavioral parameters that are affected by blocks of protein synthesis (Chap. 40). Thus, neurogenesis or other concomitants of DNA synthesis do not appear involved in these particular behavioral tasks.

The alkylating agents cyclophosphamide and methylazoxymethanol act as inhibitors of mitosis of stem cells in the fetal or newborn animal and block subsequent neurogenesis and development of specific brain areas, depending on the time of their administration (i.e., at 14 to 16 days of development for cerebellum) [11].

Biosynthesis of RNA

LOCALIZATION

In every cell not infected by an RNA virus, all RNA synthesis is absolutely dependent on the presence of a DNA template and is catalyzed by a family of enzymes called *DNA-dependent RNA polymerases* [30]. Therefore, we would expect RNA synthesis to be localized at only two intracellular sites in all cells of the nervous system: in the nucleus, including the nucleolus, and in the mitochondria [31], with the nucleus providing the bulk of this material in both variety and amounts. All the evidence so far available bears out these expectations.

PROPERTIES

Isolated nuclei of brain cells, particularly those of neurons, are capable of effective incorporation of radioactive precursors into RNA at rates at least equal to those observed in the nuclei of cells with a much higher mitotic index [32]. These and other properties of the incorporation reaction, as observed with intact and disrupted nuclei, as well as with different enzyme preparations at various stages of solubilization and purification, suggest a strong analogy (if not an identity) between the responsible enzymes in neuronal tissue [17] and those in such other tissues as liver. The enzymes responsible are now known to consist of at least three species that differ in localization, requirements, inhibition pattern, type of product synthesized, and, presumably, function. Type I (or A) polymerases are localized in the nucleolus, type II (or B) and type III (or C) polymerases in the nucleoplasm. The former are active at low ionic strength and can utilize either Mg^{2+} or Mn^{2+} as a divalent cation cofactor; the second exhibit optimal activity only at higher salt concentrations, 0.1 to 0.2 M $(NH_4)_2SO_4$ being usually employed, and Mn^{2+} is the preferred cofactor. The reactions of all three enzymes are inhibited by actinomycin D, with enzymes of type I the most sensitive (<1 μg per milliliter), and they are resistant to the action of antibiotics of the rifamycin, streptovaricin, and streptolydigin groups, as well as to intercalating dyes (ethidium bromide, acridines) at low concentrations. Only polymerase II is inhibited (with a

$K_i \approx 10^{-8}$ M) by α-amanitin, a bicyclic octapeptide isolated from the poisonous mushroom *Amanita phalloides*. The product of polymerase I appears to be the large, guanine-rich, unmethylated precursor of ribosomal RNA (rRNA), its sedimentation coefficient equal to or less than 45S in most animals. The product of polymerase II is much more heterogeneous, in agreement with its probable function as the principal enzyme responsible for the transcription of active genes in chromatin. The function of polymerase III is probably the synthesis of tRNA and 5S RNA.

At present, there is little information concerning the details of mitochondrial RNA synthesis in brain. By analogy with other cells, one might expect it to be highly susceptible to inhibition by ethidium bromide and resistant to α-amantin [32] and, in intact particles, to actinomycin D; its stable products would then be the mitochondrial tRNAs (≥ 20), the ribosomal RNAs, with sedimentation coefficients of about 12S and 18S, and the ten or so messenger RNAs (mRNAs) for the small number of polypeptides specified by this DNA [31, 33].

TRANSPORT OF RNA

Nucleus to Cytoplasm

Most of the RNA of neurons is localized in the perikaryon and there, as is true in all cells, the majority forms an integral constituent of ribonucleoprotein particles that are themselves aggregated into polymeric structures (polyribosomes, polysomes). These structures exist either free in the cytosol or attached to membranes of the endoplasmic reticulum. They are held together by mRNA and, in conjunction with the soluble transfer RNA (tRNA) of the cytosol, constitute the protein-synthesizing machinery of the cell. After administration of a radioactive precursor, nuclear and nucleolar RNA are the first to become labeled, as might be expected. The latter provides the precursor of ribosomal RNA, the former of mRNA, in the form of an exceedingly polydisperse group of molecules known as *heterogeneous nuclear RNA* (hnRNA). Most of the polynucleotide sequences in these molecules never leave the nucleus and are degraded there, but a minority are excised from their intervening sequences, spliced together, and subjected to further modification at both their 5' and 3' ends; the 5' end is modified by the addition of a characteristic "cap" structure and the 3', by polyadenylation. After these processing events [3, 34], they enter the cytoplasm within a few minutes, probably in association with some proteins (informosomes). This flux of mRNA species is followed within 30 minutes to 1 hour by the stable ribosomal RNAs already integrated into ribonucleoprotein particles.

Nucleus to Axons

In addition to their perikarya, certain neurons also may contain some RNA in their axons, including the *presynaptic thickening* (nerve ending, bouton). In peripheral nerve, particularly in the giant Mauthner neurons of fish or the stretch receptor of the lobster, this axonal RNA may contribute some 0.5 mg per gram of wet weight, although in most other instances the values are considerably lower [35]. The origin and significance of this axonal RNA are open to question. Because in addition to 4S RNA it consists of the usual ribosomal 18S and 28S species and because its synthesis is blocked by actinomycin D, a mitochondrial origin of these stable species is unlikely.

Similar considerations apply to the labeled RNA that makes its appearance in and down the axon shortly after a labeled precursor has been administered to the cell bodies of neurons that have been the object of investigation of axoplasmic flow, such as the sciatic and other peripheral nerves of mammals or the optic nerves of fish, birds, and amphibians (see also Chap. 22). It remains uncertain to what extent this labeled RNA represents macromolecules synthesized in the cell body and then transported down the axon, as contrasted to RNA synthesized in the immediate vicinity by supporting cells (glia) from low molecular weight precursors that have been so transported [35–39]. Even more controversial is whether RNA in or on axons and nerve endings participates in protein synthesis [11]. Although it is generally accepted that these structures do not contain any free ribosomes and polysomes, such ribonucleoprotein particles

present in low concentration and tightly integrated into the axonal or presynaptic membrane might have escaped detection (see Chap. 21).

CHANGES IN RNA SYNTHESIS RELATED TO FUNCTION

Electrical Stimulation in Vivo

The sea hare, *Aplysia*, provides a particularly useful system for correlating electrophysiological and biochemical findings. Certain giant neurons are readily identifiable in its abdominal ganglia; these structures or individual neurons can be removed, stimulated, and monitored electrophysiologically and, at the same time, be exposed to radioactive precursors of RNA. The products formed from them can be isolated subsequently, and the extent and the nature of the incorporation can be explored. Prolonged (about 90 min) stimulation of the ganglion, sufficient to elicit postsynaptic spikes in cell R2, results in a significant increase in the incorporation of labeled nucleosides into RNA as compared with that of unstimulated controls. The newly formed material is found in both the nucleus and the cytoplasm; both ribosomal and hnRNA (presumably mRNA precursors) appear to be affected [40, 41, 41a].

Changes in the specific activity of the precursor pool or in the rate of degradation might serve as alternate explanations for the results obtained. Their interpretation in terms of an increase in the rate of synthesis, however, is consistent with many reports on net increases of stable RNA as a result of stimulation in many species, including earthworm neurons, rat Purkinje cells, frog retinal ganglion, and cat sympathetic ganglion cells.

Electrical Stimulation in Vitro

Contrary to the results obtained in vivo, electrical stimulation of slices of rat or cat cerebral cortex in vitro [41] decreases the rate of incorporation of labeled uridine into RNA by about 50 percent. This effect is blocked by 5 μM tetrodotoxin, a neurotoxin known to inhibit Na^+ influx. An inhibition of the conversion of labeled UMP into UDP + UTP can be demonstrated to accompany the inhibition of RNA labeling, so the most likely explanation, consistent with a number of additional experiments, is that electrical activity affects the Na^+ pump, and a disturbance in the balance between Na^+ and K^+ is responsible for affecting the rate of phosphorylation and, thereby, the availability of labeled nucleoside triphosphates for RNA synthesis. Similar effects may also account for some of the reported decreases in RNA and its synthesis that result from gross stimulation of the cortex in vivo, particularly during electroshock.

Visual Stimulation

When the incorporation of orotate into the RNA in the visual cortex of a totally blind strain of rats is compared with that of normally sighted rats [44], the blind strain exhibits both a delay and a decrease in the rate of labeling of ribosomal RNA and a heterogeneous 5S to 8S RNA. There are no differences in the labeling of these RNAs in the motor cortex; and the difference in the visual cortex is enhanced if a flashing light stimulus is used. Thus, in this instance, there appears to be a positive correlation between neuronal activity and the kinetics of RNA labeling. Since the visual system of the blind animals might be expected to have suffered atrophy long before the start of the experiment, the ability of the system to synthesize certain enzymes required for the incorporation reaction also may have been impaired. In fact, it is known that blinded animals or those kept in the dark from birth show RNA deficits in various cells of the visual system. The dynamics of RNA and protein synthesis have also been reported for the visual cortex of young rats upon first exposure to light after having been reared for 7 weeks in the dark from birth [45].

Visual imprinting of day-old chicks by flashing light is also reported to coincide with a relatively profound and rapid stimulation of RNA (as well as protein) synthesis, particularly in the forebrain roof, as compared with slower increases elicited by continuous illumination, which does not result in imprinting [46].

Olfaction

Catfish brains in vivo, or the experimental half of split-brain preparations in vitro, have been shown to respond in a specific manner to odorants such as morpholine by affecting the amount, as well as the base ratios, of nuclear RNA, but not of cytoplasmic RNA.

Drugs

Earlier reports concerning possible specific effects of 1,3-dicyanoaminopropene and magnesium pemoline (magnesium hydroxide plus 2-amino-5-phenyl-4-oxazolidionone) on RNA synthesis have not been substantiated and should be discounted. On the other hand, administration of LSD (D-lysergic acid diethylamide) to young rabbits appears to elicit enhanced RNA synthesis in nuclei isolated from the cerebral cortex and brain stem 2.5 hours later [46a]. This enhanced activity appears to involve transcription of both ribosomal and messenger RNA. It is not yet certain whether this stimulation bears any causal relation to the stimulation of nuclear histone acetylation, shown by the same investigators to occur within 30 minutes of drug administration.

Development

During the early stages of postnatal development, rapid cellular proliferation is dependent on high levels of the nucleolar polymerase I and extensive synthesis of rRNA. As maturation, accompanied by myelination, progresses, this pattern is replaced by one geared to the production of hnRNA and mRNA that requires high levels of polymerase II [17, 47]. Complementary patterns are also observed for tRNA methyltransferases(s) [48]. Possible alterations in the levels of the polyamines, which can act as specific activators for the polymerases [26], must also be considered, as must the synthesis of chromatin proteins [48a].

Nerve Growth Factor

When nerve growth factor (NGF) is added to embryonic sensory or sympathetic nerve fibers in vivo or in vitro, their growth and proliferation are enhanced but remain largely restricted to axonal processes that are free of myelin sheaths (see Chap. 23). Under these conditions, autoradiography shows rapid incorporation of labeled uridine into the RNA of both the perikaryon and the axon, with a time course consistent with uridine being one of the precursors of the RNA.

Training

Carefully controlled experiments [49] seem to indicate that in mice the acquisition of a new behavioral pattern, at least in response to certain tasks, or of a specific emotional response elicited by or associated with this performance, results in an increased flux of labeled pyrimidines into nucleotide pools and thence into RNA [49]. These increases are restricted to the nuclei of the neurons of the limbic system, whereas decreases are observed in those of the outer layer of the neocortex. The increases in radioactivity do not appear to be restricted to any one type of RNA and do not involve any changes in base ratio. Similar results have also been reported for rats, including actual increases in the amount (not just the rate of labeling) in the RNA of hippocampal nuclei [50]. In contrast, acquisition of a new swimming skill by goldfish is not accompanied by any change in tRNA amino acid acceptor activity or methylation. (Additional discussion can be found in Chap. 40.)

Molecular Species of RNA and their Turnover

If the internal or external milieu can bring about more-or-less selective effects on RNA synthesis, this will generate a qualitative or quantitative alteration of the profile of the various RNA species in the population. Some of the effects observed have already been mentioned in earlier sections: here we address ourselves to this problem in a more explicit fashion.

HYBRIDIZATION

With prokaryotic organisms (bacteria and viruses), it is possible, at least in principle, to determine by appropriate DNA-RNA hybridization techniques the nature and the length of a specific section of the total genome represented by any given RNA transcribed either in vivo or in vitro. The much greater sequence complexity and the large number of partially overlapping, moderately and highly reiterated sequences in the nuclear DNA of metazoan animals impose severe constraints on similar quantitative hybridization experiments, as well as formidable hazards in their interpretation.

As ordinarily performed (i.e., at high RNA/DNA ratios on membrane filters), the restrictions mentioned virtually assure that what are measured are not the locus-specific, unique sequences expected for mRNAs of structural genes. Instead, they assess either or both (1) the sequences present in multiple copies and (2) the extent of overlap between sequences that are partially homologous structurally, but are unrelated functionally. These reservations do not hold for properly performed determinations on such entities as sequences coding for histone mRNAs, 5S RNAs, or ribosomal RNAs, or their precursors, precisely because they are specified by clusters containing more than 100 tandemly reiterated genes for the various species. The values of these particular parameters obtained for brain agree reasonably well with those for other tissues.

In addition, controlled experiments to assess the extent of transcription of unique sequences have been reported for mouse, rat, and human brain [46a, 49–51] with the following results.

1. The number of unique sequences transcribed from adult brain DNA appears significantly higher (2–4-fold) than that from other tissues in all species, reaching levels up to 40 percent of the total, approximately 7×10^8 bases, specifying 2 to 4×10^5 different polypeptides ($M_r = 50,000$).
2. The heterogeneous nuclear, polyadenylate (poly A)-containing RNA and the cytoplasmic, poly A–containing mRNA account for 25 and 8 percent, respectively, of the total available sequences; their average size corresponds to 4,500 and 1,250 base pairs respectively.
3. In addition, adult brain contains a population of non-poly-A–containing RNA of about 7×10^4 different base sequences (1,500 bases).
4. The total number of both types of mRNA sequences, not yet characterized, appears to be a function of ontogeny, varying by a factor of ≥ 2 between fetal and adult tissue in both mice and men.

5. It also appears to vary as a function of brain region in the following order: left frontal cortex $>$ right frontal cortex; right or left temporal and parietal cortex $>$ brain stem.

6. For at least one class of nuclear transcripts there appears to be a statistically significant difference between brain (but not liver) RNAs isolated from rats reared in an experimentally enriched, compared to an impoverished, environment.

The important inferences drawn from the studies outlined under 4 to 6 above now need to be extended and bolstered by assigning the changes to discrete cell types and to unique and defined species of mRNAs and the polypeptides encoded in them.

RAPIDLY LABELED RNA

As discussed earlier, at short times after administration of label to the brain of an animal or even to an isolated neuron, labeled (i.e., newly synthesized) RNA is restricted to the nucleus and nucleolus. As in other tissues, the RNA appears to be mainly of two kinds: ribosomal precursors that first appear in the nucleolus, with sedimentation coefficients of 45S, 35S, and 32S; and a polydisperse (hnRNA) species, with sedimentation coefficients varying from about 50S to about 5S and a base composition close to that of DNA. This is also the species capable of effective hybridization with DNA. Before being able to function as mRNA, the hnRNA has to be processed—segmented and respliced to molecules on the average one-third to one-fourth their original size—"capped" at its 5' terminus and polyadenylated at its 3' end; these events probably take place while the RNA is already complexed to proteins in the form of informofer particles. (*Informofer particles* are mRNA · protein complexes in transit.)

After processing, the population of mRNA molecules is exported into the cytoplasm, where it becomes detectable within a few minutes after the completion of transcription. While traversing the cytoplasm, the RNA molecules remain attached to protein as informosome particles and eventually interact with 80S ribosomes to form polysomes to discharge their function in translation. The labeling rate of the ribosomal RNA proper exhibits a lag and, although slower, proceeds for a longer time relative to mRNA before reaching an isotopic steady state.

POLYSOME TURNOVER AND STATE OF AGGREGATION

In both structure and function, brain and neuronal polysomes exhibit properties similar to those of other tissues and cells. Maintenance of their proper state of aggregation and configuration, and hence their activity, appears to be particularly finely poised and responsive to changes in environment. These parameters appear to be modulated in vitro by the level of Mg^{2+}, the presence and proper balance of K^+ and Na^+, and the concentrations of various amino acids (e.g., phenylalanine) and such transmitters as γ-aminobutyrate.

Such effects may also be operative in vivo, where they may find their explanation in terms of decreased polysomal stability owing either to a reduction in the rate of polypeptide chain initiation or an increase of mRNA degradation by activation of lysosomal nuclease(s), or both of these mechanisms [52]. So far, studies have been restricted to whole brain, cerebral cortex, or derived neuronal and glial populations. Extensions of these studies to more localized areas and small families of homogeneous neurons are sorely needed.

In cortex, polysomes are present in both glial and neuronal perikarya. In the latter, they appear both free and attached to endoplasmic reticulum; both types are capable of and responsible for effective protein synthesis. In adult rats, the turnover rate of both the RNA and the proteins of the various constituent ribosomes is 12 days. Thus, the particles are subject to turnover as a unit. Protein synthesis is very active in brain preparations of young rats and mice shortly after birth (it reaches a maximum at about 10 weeks for rats) and declines as the animals mature. This decline in activity is correlated with adenosine triphosphate (ATP) levels in cortex slices; it is also correlated, at least in part, with a decrease in polysomal RNA, a change in the size distribution in favor of smaller aggregates, and decreased stability of isolated polysomes. Much of this synthetic capacity is devoted to the formation of tubulin subunits and actin. The mRNAs for these species have been isolated from chick embryo brain and shown to consist of molecules about 2,000 nucleotides long [53]. In contrast, mRNAs from polysomes dedicated to the synthesis of the brain-specific proteins S100 and 14-3-2 appear to increase with brain maturation [54].

Coincident with the changes in synthetic rates there is a change in the base composition [3] as reflected in the ratio of guanine + cytosine (G + C) to adenine + uracil (A + U): this ratio has been reported to rise during maturation from 1.30 to 1.50 in whole rat brain, and from 1.41 to 1.66 in single pyramidal cells of the hippocampus. In the latter, the amount of RNA per cell is reported to increase from 24 pg to 110 pg for mature rats and to drop to 53 pg per cell in very old rats, coincident with a rise in the (G + C)/(A + U) ratio to 1.95.

The proportion of total ribosomal RNA found in polysomes has been reported to increase as a function of environmental or behavioral stimulation. For instance, when adult rats were first kept in the dark for 3 days and then exposed to the lights and sounds of the laboratory for 15 min, the polysome-to-monomer ratio increased by 83 percent in cerebral cortex but was unaffected in the liver. On the other hand, electroshock or hyperthermia had the opposite effect: polysomes were dissociated as a result.

Disaggregation of whole-brain polysomes has also been observed in response to the administration to rats of LSD or of the "unnatural" amino acids L-dopa and L-5-hydroxytryptophan, mediated by their conversion to the catecholamine transmitters dopamine and serotonin, respectively, as well as a consequence of hyperphenylalaninemia.

BEHAVIOR AND CHANGES IN BASE RATIOS
The literature contains several reports concerning changes in base ratios resulting from or coincident with the acquisition of new behavioral patterns (see Chap. 40). In general, the experiments have been of two types, and both types are subject to

serious reservations. In the first, total RNA of small cell populations is analyzed by microtechniques; and profound changes are observed, such as formation of RNA with (G + C)/(A + U) ratios in the range of 0.70 to 0.90. These, then, must have been the result of alterations in ribosomal RNA, since it is the only species present in amounts large enough for its base composition to affect cellular base composition. (Messenger RNA accounts for about 5 percent of the total cellular RNA, and in its base composition, it must reflect the average of a large multiplicity of different base sequences. Even under hyperinduction in prokaryotes, a single species never accounts for more than 20 percent of the total population. Thus, total base composition could be altered by 1 percent in the most extreme case.) No such fluctuations in ribosomal RNA have ever been observed in any other system, and they are highly unlikely, in view of the fact that these RNAs are, as we have mentioned, specified by a cluster of highly homogeneous genes.

In the second type of experiment, newly synthesized, rapidly labeled RNA is analyzed by determining the ratio of radioactivity in the uridylate and cytidylate fractions of RNA hydrolysates formed from labeled orotate. However, in the absence of data for nuclear UTP and CTP, the direct precursors, the results are not amenable to any ready interpretations. It is of interest to note in this context that the increased synthesis of RNA, which was discussed in regard to the effects of behavioral training on RNA synthesis (see p. 181), is not accompanied by any changes in base ratio.

Protein Metabolism and Brain Function
Nucleic acids are charged with the hereditary transmission of genetic information and its differential expression, depending on the ontogenetic and functional state of a cell, but the end products of this expression are constituted by that cell's proteins. Their functional versatility is truly protean. They serve the multiple needs of the cell and express its individuality; as structural elements in its membranes and organelles (nuclei, plasmalemma, axonal membranes, synaptic junctions, mitochondria, endoplasmic reticulum, Golgi apparatus,

microtubules, microfilaments, intermediate filaments, etc.); as enzymes; as receptors and transducers for neurotransmitters, hormones, or other regulatory effectors. But proteins are both implements and modulators of the autocatalytic and heterocatalytic system charged with genetic continuity and its expression, that is, as components of the replicative, transcriptional, and translational apparatus.

In this section, we shall discuss how the level of proteins in the nervous system is maintained and controlled. As with nucleic acids, the general features of metabolism of macromolecules in the cells of this highly specialized tissue can be understood in terms developed for other eukaryotic cells, such as the rabbit reticulocyte. However, more interesting and significant are the regulation of synthesis and degradation of specific proteins. This is just beginning to be explored in extraneural systems, and very little hard information is now available with respect to nerve tissue, but our discussion will at least help in pointing out how this might be accomplished in the future.

Steps in Protein Synthesis

GENERAL SCHEME

Protein synthesis on both free and membrane-bound ribosomes in brain perikarya appears similar in all essential features to that established for eukaryotic cells in general. Proteins destined for intracellular use, including peripheral membrane proteins and proteins residing on the cytoplasmic aspect of plasma membranes, are synthesized by polysomal arrays in the cytosol, that is, unattached to membranes. In contrast, proteins destined for export from the cell of origin as well as those plasma membrane proteins that will become part of its external aspect are synthesized by polysomes attached to the membranes of the endoplasmic reticulum (ER). This attachment is twofold: through one of the ribosomal subunits and through the N-terminal segment of the nascent polypeptide chain. Upon chain termination (see under Termination, below), the newly synthesized protein is then discharged into the internal space (*lumen*)

of the ER cisternae in a sequence of reactions usually dependent on the removal of the N-terminal segment (see Processing). It is not yet known to what extent this picture also applies to proteins synthesized in the perikaryon and exported toward the synapse by axoplasmic transport (Chap. 22).

For purposes of subsequent discussion, it is useful to divide the steps in the sequence of reactions into five categories: initiation; elongation; termination; processing; and folding and formation of secondary and higher-order structures.

INITIATION, ELONGATION, AND TERMINATION
Initiation (reactions 1 and 2) and the initial phases of elongation (reactions 3 through 5) are shown in Fig. 19-2. Reaction 3 is the binding of the next (*i* plus 1) aminoacyl-tRNA to the open A site by interaction between its anticodon and the cognate codon on the mRNA. Reaction 4 is the transpeptidation, in which a peptide bond is formed between the amino group of the incoming amino acid and the carboxyl residue of the last (*i*) amino acid on the chain; the last amino acid is still attached to its tRNA. Reaction 5 is the translocation of the growing chain, with the newly added (*i* plus 1) residue from the A to the P site; the (*i* plus 1) residue now constitutes the new C terminus and is still linked to its tRNA; the tRNA of the preceding (*i*) amino acid is released, the A site is vacated, and a new (*i* plus 2) cognate codon is exposed on the mRNA. The process is then repeated until the last (C terminal) amino acid has been added to the growing chain.

Polypeptide synthesis is terminated when the progression of the growing chain along the mRNA exposes a termination codon (UAA, UAG, UGA) to the ribosomal A site. In a reaction requiring GTP and the presence of a specific release factor, the completed chain is detached from the ribosome. The ribosome simultaneously dissociates, ready to initiate another cycle beginning with the attachment of the small ribosomal subunit to the mRNA; this primes it for reaction 1. Between termination and reinitiation, the mRNA is particularly sensitive to hydrolysis catalyzed by nucleases, or to other modifications.

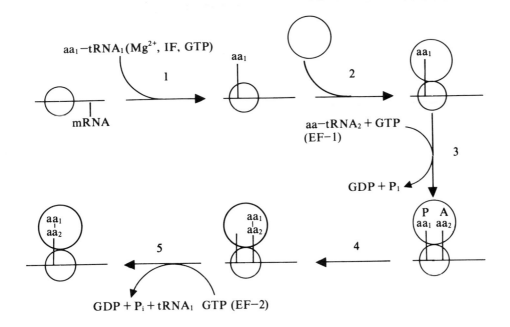

Fig. 19-2. Reactions involved in initiation and elongation. IF, initiation factors; EF, elongation factors. (From H. Weissbach and S. Ochoa, Annu. Rev. Biochem. *45:191–216, 1976. By permission.)*

It can readily be demonstrated that the rate of protein synthesis is susceptible to regulation through the rate of chain initiation. We assume the following simplified model

$$m + R^* \xrightarrow{k_i} P_1 \xrightarrow{k_e} P_2 \xrightarrow{k_e} \xrightarrow{k_e} P_n \xrightarrow{k_r} P_r$$

Here m is mRNA; R^* is the rate-limiting component in the chain initiation, usually the [Met-$tRNA_f$-40S ribosome] complex formed by reaction 1 in Fig. 19-1; k_i is the rate constant for chain initiation; k_e is the rate constant for chain elongation as each amino acid from 2 to n is added; and k_r is the rate constant for release of the chain. If we assume $k_r = k_e$, then the overall rate of synthesis, q, for any given protein equals

$$mR^*k_i[1-L/(k_e/k_iR^*) + (L-1)]$$

where L is the number of codons covered by any ribosome. Computed solutions given by Lodish to this equation are shown in Fig. 19-3.

PROCESSING

Recent studies have disclosed that many proteins are subject to the posttranslational modification by controlled proteolysis of defined segments of the newly synthesized polypeptide chain [55]. These processing reactions are of two types: (1) the well-established conversion of inactive *pro*enzymes (e.g., proinsulin, chymotrypsinogen) or *pro*proteins to their biologically active forms; and (2) the removal of a specific N-terminal "signal" fragment of a *pre*protein (or even of a *prepro*protein) required for the interaction with and penetration of a membrane [25]. This principle applies to many proteins synthesized on membrane-bound polysomes and/or destined for intimate association with exterior or interior cellular membranes, such as the plasmalemma or the inner mitochondrial membrane. So far, there has been no actual demonstration of such processing events in vertebrate brain, but there is no reason to question the relevance of the model to this tissue. It has been verified for protein synthesis in *Aplysia*, in discrete neurons and neuronal clusters with defined function [56, 57].

FOLDING AND FORMATION OF HIGHER-ORDER STRUCTURES

In certain cases (e.g., proinsulin → insulin) secon-

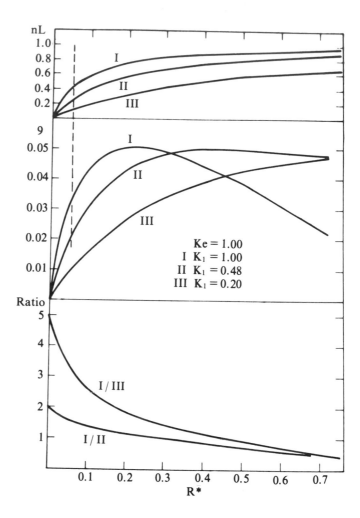

Fig. 19-3. Theoretical calculation of parameters of protein synthesis as a function of R*. A value of 1 is assumed for k_e (rate constant for elongation) and 12 is taken for L, the number of codons covered by one ribosome. Rate constants for chain initiation, k_i, are taken as 1.0 (curve I), 0.48 (curve II), and 0.20 (curve III). The top panel shows the fraction of codons occupied by a ribosome, plotted as a function of R*; the middle panel shows the amount of protein synthesized per mRNA, $q = Qm^{-1}$ plotted as a function of R*; and the bottom panel shows the ratio of amount of protein synthesized by the different mRNAs, plotted as a function of R*. Translation of β- and α-globin mRNAs can be approximated by curves I and II, respectively. The dashed line represents the conditions obtaining in the normal reticulocyte for β-globin mRNA (curve I) and α-globin mRNA (curve II). (From H. E. Lodish, Annu. Rev. Biochem. 45:39–72, 1976. By permission.)

dary structure is assumed and cross-linking occurs after the completion of the primary sequence. In other instances (e.g., pancreatic ribonucleases), the correct secondary structure can be imposed in vitro on the completely unfolded molecules. However, evidence is beginning to accumulate that folding (i.e., formation of secondary and tertiary structures) may be kinetically controlled. In this model, polypeptide chain elongation and folding, at least in their grossest aspects, are coordinate events, and a polypeptide chain assumes some characteristic features by the time its primary structure has been completed [58]. In terms of Fig. 19-4, at least part of the first three steps are pictured with the nascent chain still attached to the ribosome.

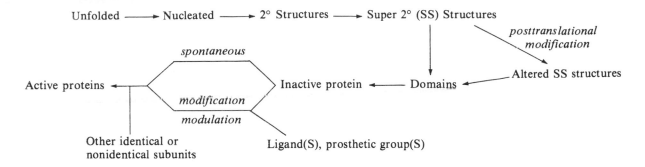

Fig. 19-4. A generalized pathway to active proteins.

ATTACHMENT OF CARBOHYDRATE SIDE CHAINS

Many of the important proteins of nerve tissues, including entities at the synapse, are *glycoproteins,* that is, they contain oligosaccharide side chains attached to selected aspartate, and perhaps serine and threonine, residues of their polypeptide chains [59]. What is the sequence and the location of the enzymatic reactions responsible for this attachment of prosthetic groups? In general, it is believed [60] that the polypeptide is assembled on ribosomes attached to the endoplasmic reticulum. Coincident with its release into the interior lumen of these membrane channels, or soon thereafter, a reaction that may require the participation and subsequent hydrolysis of an N-terminal signal sequence, the incorporation of the first carbohydrate residue at these attachment points may take place. The proteins then traverse the intramembrane channels and cisternae of the endoplasmic reticulum on their way to the Golgi apparatus, and are further modified in the course of this transport by a firmly membrane-bound multi-glycosyl transferase system, which sequentially attaches additional glycosyl residues at appropriate sites. (The molecules UDP-glucose, UDP-glucosamine, GDP-mannose, and CMP-sialic acid, etc., act as glycosyl donors in these reactions.) The terminal residues (fucose, galactose, and sialic acid) of the side chain are added to the glycoprotein at or near the Golgi apparatus, which then modifies [61a] and packages the completed glycoprotein into granules. Some of them may be transported down the axon by axonal flow (Chap. 22). Others are moved to the plasma membrane and fuse with it by a process of exocytosis. This event has two, sometimes linked, consequences. It results in the secretion of some of the newly synthesized glycoproteins and in the incorporation of others into the plasma membrane proper. This group of newly formed membrane proteins can be modified further by the attachment of oligosaccharide chains transferred from the membrane-associated lipid-carrier molecule dolichol phosphate (with dolichol-P-P[Glc]$_n$[Glc′]$_m$ as the actual donor; here Glc and Glc′ are two different monosaccharide units) [61].

INHIBITORS

Protein synthesis by the two systems active in brain—cytoplasmic and mitochondrial ribosomes—appears to be susceptible to inhibition by the same classes of inhibitors previously documented in other animal tissues [62–64]. These are summarized in Table 19-1.

Measurements of Protein Turnover

GENERAL CONSIDERATIONS

Consider a particular protein that is formed from its precursors in a process that does not depend on its concentration in a given cell or tissue but the degradation of which is directly proportional to this concentration. The synthesis then follows zero-order kinetics, while the degradation follows first-order kinetics. Net change in a protein subject to synthesis and degradation can be expressed by equation 19-1.

Table 19-1. Inhibitors of Protein Synthesis

Acting on Cytoribosomal Systems (80S Type)	Acting on Ribosomal Systems of the 70S and 80S Types	Acting on Ribosomal Systems of 70S (Prokaryotic) Type	Acting on Mitochondrial Ribosomes
Anisomycin[a]	Actinobolin	Aminoglycosides	Aminoglycosides[b]
Diphtheria toxin	Aurintricarboxylic acid	Chloramphenicol	*Chloramphenicol*
Emetine	Blasticidin S	Lincomycin	Lincomycin
Glutarimide group	Bottromycin A$_2$	Macrolides	Macrolides
Actiphenol	Edeine	Carbomycin	Carbomycin[c]
Cycloheximide	Fusidic acid	Erythromycin	Erythromycin[c]
Streptimidone	Gougerotin	Spiramycin	Spiramycin[c]
Streptovitacin A	Nucleocidin	Tylosin[d]	
Pederin	Polydextransulphate	Siomycin	Siomycin
Phenomycin	Puromycin	Thiostrepton	*Thiostrepton*
Tenuazonic acid	Sparsomycin	(Bryamycin)	(Bryamycin)
Tylophora alkaloids[e]	Tetracycline group	Kirromycin	
Cryptopleurine	Chlortetracycline		
Tylocrebine	Deoxycycline		
Tylophorine	Oxytetracycline		
	Tetracycline		

[a]The most generally useful inhibitors are in italics.

[b]Incompletely studied; in yeast, neomycin and paromomycin appear to be relatively effective and discriminating mitochondrial inhibitors in vitro—they are ineffective with animal mitochondria; other common members of this group (e.g., streptomycin, kanamycin) are generally ineffective.

[c] Much less effective (requires 100 times higher concentration) with animal mitochondria.

[d] Virtually ineffective with animal mitochondria.

[e] May inhibit some mitochondrial system.

Source: Dunslow and O'Brien, *Eur. J. Biochem.* 91:441–448, 1978; Mahler, *CRC Crit. Rev. Biochem.* 1:381–460, 1973; O'Brien, in E. McConkey (ed.), *Protein Synthesis,* New York: Marcel Dekker, 1976. Pp. 249–307; Bueton and Wood (Ref. 64).

$$dp/dt = k_s - k_d P_t \qquad (19\text{-}1)$$

where P_t is the amount of protein at time t, k_s is its amount (or mass) synthesized per unit time, and k_d is the fraction of protein molecules degraded per unit time.

In the steady state,

$$dp/dt = 0$$

and

$$k_s = k_d P_t \qquad (19\text{-}2)$$

and

$$P_t = k_s/k_d \qquad (19\text{-}3)$$

Now, what will be the effect on the concentration of the protein P as a result of hormonal, nutritional, sensory, or other physiological stimulation of the system? There will be an approach to a new steady state defined by new rates of synthesis and degradation, k_s' and k_d'. The amount of protein P_t is then given by

$$P_t = k_s'/k_d' [1-(1-P_o) k_d'/k_s'] \exp(-k_d't) \qquad (19\text{-}4)$$

where P_o is the amount of protein at the start of the experiment; that is, as defined by equations 19-1 through 19-3. If we take $P_o = 1$ to determine the extent of change ("fold" increase or decrease) then equation 19-4 reduces to

$P_t = C[1 - \exp(-k_d'T)]$

where $C = k_s'/k_d'$ (19-5)

These equations provide not only the background for the actual measurement of the parameters governing the synthesis, degradation, and turnover of various proteins, but, as pointed out by Schimke and Doyle [65], they permit certain important inferences in their own right:

1. In prokaryotes, changes in the amount of any given protein are usually due to the induction of its synthesis. In eukaryotic cells and tissues, they may result not only from increased rates of synthesis, but also by effects on k_d, that is, stabilization or labilization of preexisting protein molecules in the presence of a constant rate of synthesis.
2. The fact that an agent or treatment causes an increase in the amount of one specific protein among a population of different protein molecules does not constitute proof of an effect specific to that particular protein. Since, as shown by equation 19-4, the rate of approach to a new steady state is controlled by k_d', and k_d' varies greatly for different proteins, the time course of increase in amount of each protein will be different, even if their rates of synthesis are all increased by the same factor. Thus, an adequate formulation of the kinetics for changes in protein levels would require all the relevant k_i, k_d, k_s', and k_d' terms. If the k_d for any protein is large (or its half-life short), this species is a good candidate for relatively rapid changes in its amount. This is the rationale for searching for proteins with short half-lives. These may be candidates for regulatory processes, such as synaptic modification through use.

MEASUREMENTS OF RATES OF DEGRADATION AND SYNTHESIS

If we inhibit protein synthesis to a substantial extent, as by restricting the supply of precursors, by interfering with any of the component steps of polypeptide synthesis, or by the addition of an appropriate inhibitor, this will permit measurement of the rate of degradation and evaluation of k_d according to equation 19-6, the well-known exponential decay law. Under this condition, k_s is almost zero, or very much smaller than k_d.

$P = P_o' \exp(-k_d t)$, (19-6)

where P_o' is the amount of protein at the moment synthesis is blocked. Equation 19-6 can be recast in the familiar forms

$k_d = (-1/t) \ln P/P_o'$ or $(-2.3/t) \log P/P_o'$ (19-6a)

$k_d = 0.693/\tau_{1/2}$

where $\tau_{1/2}$ is the time at which $P = 0.5\ P_o'$. (19-6b)

The rate constant of degradation or the half-life of the protein can then be determined, provided its decay follows a simple exponential. In this case, these values are independent of the initial concentration, P_o'. The only measurement required is the rate of change of any quantity proportional to P_o', such as enzymatic activity, ligand binding, antibody titer of the total fraction, or radioactivity (of the pure protein). These are all expressed as specific activity (per unit mass of starting material).

Unlike other modes of assay, experiments with radioactive tracers can be designed to furnish a measurement of k_d, even under steady state conditions, without inhibiting synthesis. This is accomplished by performing a so-called pulse-labeling, or pulse-chase, experiment. In pulse-labeling, the tracer dose is ultimately rendered unavailable by its metabolism, while the injection of a "chase," or nonradioactive, precursor shortly after the tracer can abruptly terminate the pulse even sooner. After an initial transient, the decrement of radioactivity in the pure protein fraction now obeys equation 19-6.

There are three principal ways of determining the rate of synthesis, k_s. In the first method, one measures the initial rate of accumulation of a labeled precursor into the protein. One must know both the specific radioactivity of the immediate precursor at the precise site of synthesis (ideally, the particular aminoacyl tRNA) and the mass fraction of the same precursor in the protein. In the second method, one measures the rate of appearance of a labeled precursor into the protein during a continued supply of precursor with constant specific radioactivity. This is accomplished by a single massive dose, continued infusion, or by multiple injections. These first two techniques give synthesis rates in terms of mass fraction incorporated per unit time. For such purposes, it is convenient to define a constant, k_1, as the fraction of protein molecules synthesized per unit time. Then $k_s = k_1 P_t$ and equation 19-1 becomes

$$dP/dt = k_1 P_t - k_d P_t. \qquad (19\text{-}7)$$

Owing to the particular properties of the steady (stationary) state, measurements of the *rate of incorporation* of precursors into *adult* tissues (e.g., of brain or nerve) and their proteins also provide a measure of their *turnover* or *rate of decay* (see equation 19-2) with P ≃ constant): The time required for the protein to reach 50 percent of the isotopic steady state (i.e., for it to attain 50 percent of its maximum specific activity, ideally equal to 50 percent of the specific activity of the actual precursor) means not only that half of the originally unlabeled molecules have now been replaced by their labeled equivalents, but also that half of them have decayed, that is, this time $t = \tau_{1/2}$ (equation 19-6). Even if steady state conditions do not prevail, an average value of k_d, that is, a k_d valid for a particular range of measurement of k_1, can frequently be obtained; what is required for this approach to be valid is that $\triangle P$ be small—this will usually be the case, even during relatively rapid changes in P_o', that is, during development, provided accurate measurements of $\triangle P/\triangle t$ are available for a short interval of $\triangle t$.

The third method requires a knowledge of the steady state values for P and k_d; k_s can then be calculated directly from equation 19-2.

COMPLICATIONS IN THE MEASUREMENT OF DEGRADATION

Accurate measurement of k_d by the decay of a pulse-labeled protein depends on the replacement of the isotopically labeled species P^* by its unlabeled equivalent, P. Two problems are severe obstacles to obtaining true pulse-labeling. The first problem, especially for proteins with short half-lives, is due to a continued supply of labeled precursor from its original source. The second takes place when the labeled protein is degraded, and the

labeled residue is reutilized in repeated cycles. The problem leads to greater inaccuracy for proteins with longer half-lives. In principle, both these processes can be detected and eliminated, or corrected for, by continuous monitoring of the precursor pool. In most reliable studies, care is taken not to begin decay measurements until the radioactivity in the precursor pool has dropped to the desired low level. The problem of reutilization is reduced or eliminated in one of two ways: (1) by measuring not k_d, but k_s (see above), which is not subject to this particular uncertainty, or (2) use of an amino acid as a precursor that is subject to rapid loss of label or equilibration with large pools of metabolites, to insure virtual absence of label, even in the presence of reutilization [66, 67]. Among the labeled amino acid species that have been suggested for this purpose at one time or other are [1-^{14}C]leucine, [1-^{14}C]tyrosine, [guanido-^{14}]arginine; and arginine, lysine, glutamate, or aspartate labeled in various other positions with either ^{14}C or ^{3}H.

THE DOUBLE-ISOTOPE METHOD FOR MEASURING DEGRADATION

Arias, Doyle, and Schimke [67a; see also 68 and 69] have introduced a double-isotope technique for measuring k_d. In this technique, one isotopic form [^{14}C] of an amino acid (usually, uniformly labeled L-leucine) is administered initially and allowed to decay for a defined length of time, usually 3 to 10 days. Then a second form [^{3}H] of the same amino acid, [4,5-^{3}H]L-leucine, is administered and the animal is killed about 30 minutes later. The loss of radioactivity of any one protein labeled with any one isotope will be governed by equation 19-6, with P and P_o' now proportional to their specific radioactivity. However, it also follows that the ratio of specific or total activities with the two isotopes (eq. 19-8) be

$$^3\text{H}/^{14}\text{C} = P_o'/P_t = \exp(-k_d t) \qquad (19\text{-}8)$$

and

$$\ln(^3\text{H}/^{14}\text{C})_i = -k_d^i \triangle t, \qquad (19\text{-}8\text{a})$$

where i refers to the i*th* species and $\triangle t$ to the interval between the administration of the two isotopes.

Thus a plot of the natural logarithm of the isotope ratios against k_d (determined by some independent means) should give a straight line with a slope equal to Δt. This relationship has been verified experimentally [56]. It also follows that knowledge of k_d for one particular reference protein is both necessary and sufficient for the determination of k_d or $\tau_{1/2}$ for a series of proteins (including the reference) by means of the double-isotope technique [70]. The assumptions on which the methodology is based are (1) the isotope is not metabolized into other products that can be incorporated or otherwise contaminate the proteins being counted; (2) the kinetics of degradation for all protein species is described by equation 19-6; (3) all proteins are in a steady state and their decay characteristics remain the same throughout the experiment; and (4) all protein species are undergoing isotopic decay at the time the animal is killed. The first three assumptions have been validated in many instances for liver and brain. However, it is wise to do so anew in any investigation using the method. For instance, Zak and co-workers [69] have shown that the second assumption becomes valid for proteins with long half-lives (>6 days) only after a period of >6 days, and thus requires relatively long intervals between injections. The third assumption is usually verified by showing invariance of incorporation of the tritiated precursor regardless of the time of its administration—prior to, simultaneous with, or subsequent to the [^{14}C]label. Additional parameters that need critical examination are Δt, the time interval between the two injections, and $\Delta t'$, the interval between the second injection and killing the animal. Again, an analysis by Zak and co-workers [70a] has shown that the method provides maximum sensitivity for proteins with $\tau_{1/2}$ between 1.5 and 3 days, but can be used for proteins with longer $\tau_{1/2}$, provided that Δt is long (20 days) and $\Delta t'$ short (30 minutes).

DETERMINATION OF SYNTHESIS RATES
The most direct determination probably depends on the actual measurement of the specific activity of the immediate aminoacyl-tRNA precursor, such as L-[4,5-^{3}H]leucyl tRNA [71]. A frequently employed alternative is to administer a massive amount of a labeled precursor: implanting pellets of L-tyrosine; massive intraperitoneal injection of L-valine [72–74], L-lysine or L-histidine; continued infusion of L-proline [75]; or feeding L-tyrosine [76]. The difficulty with this approach is that it may be stressful, and the solutions used for injection may be hypertonic.

Many investigators still prefer to administer an amino acid precursor in tracer amounts and to determine the nature of the true specific activity in the relevant precursor pool, either experimentally or by solving a set of differential equations defined by a particular model. (For explicit solutions of the pool problem see references 72 and 77 through 79). Reference 72 demonstrates the particular utility of labeled lysine and tyrosine for such studies in nervous tissue. It shows that a fraction of 0.24 of either amino acid injected into the lateral ventricle of young rats is actually available for incorporation into protein, with rates of 2.2 and 0.9 nmol/min^{-1}/g^{-1} of protein for lysine and tyrosine, respectively.

Specific Features of Protein Metabolism in Nerve Tissues
PROTEINS SPECIFIC TO THE NERVOUS SYSTEM
Proteins specific to the nervous system are of interest because they underlie the developmental specialization and differentiation of the system's cells. These proteins are usually assayed in terms of their biological activity, for example, as enzymes or receptors for specific ligands or, more generally, as antigens. These properties are also frequently employed as aids in the isolation and purification of the proteins. Antigens also can be visualized in cells and tissues and in subcellular fractions derived from them by means of immunoglobulins covalently linked to fluorescent probes, such as fluorescein or rhodamine G for light microscopy, or electron-dense probes such as ferritin or horseradish peroxidase (which generates the electron-opaque entity in situ), for electron microscopy [80].

Table 19-2 contains a partial list of proteins that

Table 19-2. Useful Proteins Specific to the Nervous System

Soluble	Membrane-Bound
Somatic cytoplasm, axoplasm, synaptoplasm	Myelin, axonal, pre- and postjunctional
Glutamate decarboxylase (Chap. 12)	Myelin proteins (Chap. 4), including large
Enzymes involved in catecholamine synthesis	(50,000 M_r) and small (18,400 M_r) basic proteins;
(Chap. 10): tyrosine hydroxylase, DOPA-	proteolipid protein (26,000 M_r)
decarboxylase, dopamine-β-hydroxylase,	Postsynaptic density protein [86] (50,000 M_r)
phenylethanolamine-N-methyltransferase	Receptors for neurotransmitters (Chap. 3), and
Catecholamine-O-methyltransferase	other functional ligands (Chaps. 9–14)
Tryptophan hydroxylase (Chap. 11)	Nicotinic acetylcholine (350,000 M_r)
Choline-O-methyltransferase (Chap. 9)	Muscarinic acetylcholine
Protein 14-3-2 (brain-specific enolase, also	Catecholamines
called *NSP-R* and *antigen α*; 42,000 M_r [81])	Serotonin, histamine
Neurofilament (intermediate filament) protein	Purines
(Chap. 20), 200,000, 145,000, and 68,000 M_r	Opiates, enkephalins, and endorphins
[82])	Other neuroactive peptides
Glial proteins	Proteins I_a and I_b (Chap. 15); 85,000 and 80,000 M_r
S-100 (10,500 M_r [83] or 7,000 M_r [84])	
Glial fibrillar acid protein (glial filament protein,	
GFP; 51,000–54,000 M_r [82, 85])	

appear to be specific for, or at least more prevalent in, cells of the nervous system, arranged according to their localization or presumed function. The list specifically excludes neuroactive small (poly) peptides, which are discussed extensively in Chap. 14.

The possible relationships between the glial and neuronal intermediate filament proteins cited in the Table 19-2 and proteins of similar size and amino acid composition found in other cell types (such as desmin in muscle cells) are still under active investigation (see also Chap. 20). In addition to the proteins tabulated, a number of additional species of great potential interest, but less certain molecular provenance, have been described. Among them are synaptin, found in synaptic vesicles [87] with a molecular weight similar to that of actin (45,000), and histocompatibility antigen Thy 1, which has been reported to be concentrated in synaptic membranes [88].

COVALENT MODIFICATION OF PROTEINS RELATED TO NERVOUS SYSTEM FUNCTION

The susceptibility of brain proteins—especially those localized in the synaptic region and its membranes—to covalent modification may provide a means for altering the efficacy of synaptic transmission as a function of neuronal activity. The molecular events that form the basis for a model involving cyclic nucleotides and resulting in the phosphorylation or dephosphorylation of subsets of synaptic proteins have been proposed in Chap. 15. Of particular interest is the demonstration of a cyclic AMP–dependent phosphorylation of some protein(s) of the small ribosomal subunits, which may then fulfill a relatively long-lasting autocatalytic function in stimulating (or inhibiting) the synthesis of a number of proteins subsequent to the initial increase in concentration of the nucleotide [89]. A second, probably nonoverlapping, subset of such proteins is phosphorylated in response to an elevation in the local concentration of Ca^{2+}. The reaction requires the participation of both a specific protein kinase and the Ca^{2+}-dependent regulator protein (calmodulin, or CDR).

Other covalent modification reactions must be considered. The potential involvement of protein methylation in such modification events is suggested by the occurrence of this reaction and the presence of the enzyme responsible (the S-adenosyl-L-methionine:protein carboxyl-O-methyltransferase) in brain and adrenal chromaffin granules [90]. The addition of tyrosine to the α-carboxyl of the C-terminal glutamate residue of α-tubulin in the presence of the responsible ligase is reported to be specific for this acceptor; α-tubulin extracted from synaptic membranes appears to be virtually exclusively in this tyrosylated form [91].

Among the various possible modification reactions of the carbohydrate side chains of synaptic glycoproteins, the one resting on the soundest experimental foundation is the removal of terminal sialic acid residues by a membrane-associated sialidase [92, 93].

Finally, the possibility must be considered that coincident with, or as a result of, synaptic function some of the presynaptic membrane proteins become selectively internalized and degraded proteolytically [94]. Such events may be of particular relevance to the formation of stable synaptic contacts during the ontogeny of the nervous system [95, 96] (see also Chaps. 21 and 40). Prior modification by one of the posttranslational reactions just described, or others yet unknown, may provide proteolytic enzymes with the signal required for recognition of entities to be removed. The occurrence of such reactions is a special case of protein degradation, to which we now address ourselves.

PROTEIN DEGRADATION

Several recent reviews address the subject of protein degradation [97–99]. Some of the features that emerge from these studies are the following:

1. Susceptibility to degradation by intracellular proteases is maximized by an extended conformation (loss of secondary structure) [100].
2. As corollaries, then, proteins in active association with their substrates and cofactors or other stabilizing ligands and integral proteins in their membrane environment are relatively resistant to proteolysis.
3. Only those segments of the polypeptide chain of membrane proteins that protrude into the intracellular (cytoplasmic) space are vulnerable; transmembrane proteins, or those located on the exterior surface, are rendered susceptible by a process of internalization (*endocytosis*).
4. The degradation rates for soluble proteins vary widely, with half-lives in rat liver between 0.2 hr and 100 hr, whereas muscle proteins show half-lives of the order of 48 hr.
5. Rates frequently are found to correlate with size and charge. Larger molecules are hydrolyzed most rapidly, since they present a large target containing a great number of susceptible bonds; molecules with low (acidic) isoelectric points are affected more readily than are those with neutral or basic isoelectric points. Perhaps this is because of the charges or other related properties carried by the enzyme(s) responsible for the rate-limiting step in the degradation.
6. Glycoproteins appear to be degraded especially rapidly.
7. There are reports of uniform degradation rates for the polypeptide subunits of various membranes, but these—if substantiated—may reflect a difference in rate-determining steps, that is, engulfment of the whole membrane by an autophagic vacuole (*phagolysosome*), followed by degradation within that organelle.
8. Introduction of unnatural amino acids or amino acid analogs or of damage (e.g., by irradiation) into proteins increases their rate of degradation.
9. Although many initial degradative events are brought about by lysosomal proteases ("acid" cathepsins), neutral proteases also have a role. The lysosomal reaction, particularly when it involves endocytosis (point 3, above), may require the participation of such mechanoactive cytoskeletal elements as microtubules or microfilaments, or both.
10. Alterations in protein metabolism by changes of nutritional or hormonal states (associated with changes in insulin or glucocorticoid secretion) appear to be controlled principally by regulation of protein breakdown.

Many brain proteases with an apparently restricted or altered specificity have been studied, principally by N. Marks and his collaborators [101]. Among the endopeptidases are a neutral proteinase (cathepsin M), a cathepsin D, and a trypsinlike entity; among the exopeptidases are an arylamidase that attacks the N terminals, a lysosomal carboxypeptidase A, and a carboxamide peptidase that hydrolyzes preferentially the subterminal Pro-Arg-GlyNH$_2$ and Pro-Leu-GlyNH$_2$ bonds of Arg-vasopressin and oxytocin.

Turnover Rates of Brain Proteins and Their Control

BULK PROTEINS

Effects of Development

During development, there is an increase in both content and complexity of the nervous system that requires net accumulation of proteins. Different brain regions and cell types vary in their time course of maximal proliferative activity and maturation. Superimposed on selective maturation events on the tissue level, there are probably analogous changes even on the level of a group of inhomogeneous cells within a larger population of such cells. This results in the selective elaboration (and subsequent shutdown) of characteristic proteins at one or more critical times (e.g., tubulin at day 15 after gestation in the rat, and myelin basic proteins at day 18 after birth in the mouse). We are concerned with three questions: (1) What regulates the accumulation of proteins in these nonsteady state systems: is the principal effect an enhanced rate of synthesis or an absence (or an abnormally low rate) of degradation, or both? (2) Which of these rates is principally affected in the transition to the steady state? (3) If control of protein metabolism during development can be explained in terms of specific quantitative change in one or more of its component steps, how are these general effects modulated or overridden to account for turning on and off of the preferential synthesis of selected proteins? As concerns (1) and (2), it is now generally agreed that both the net rate of accumulation $\Delta P / \Delta t$ and the actual rate of protein synthesis, k_s, is greater in nervous tissue from immature than from mature animals. This is so both in brain as a whole and in individual brain regions; and this difference, which

in rat preparations amounts to factors of two- to threefold, is exhibited in vivo and in vitro in slices, homogenates, and appropriately supplemented preprogrammed polysomal preparations. The precise cause is not known but may well involve more than one factor. For example, there is an increased tendency of polysomes to become disaggregated with age. This may be due either to a decrease in rate of initiation or increase in mRNA degradation (see Fig. 19-2). This, in turn, has been attributed to an imbalance of required tRNAs, or of their state of methylation. More recently, Lajtha and his collaborators have explicitly addressed the question of possible alterations in both k_s (or k_1) and k_d in the course of maturation. They determined k_d, k_1, and k_a in equation 19-7a at 2, 8, 18, and 37 days after birth in midbrain, cerebellum, pons medulla, and spinal cord of rats (Table 19-3).

$$k_d = k_1 - k_a \simeq k_1 - \Delta P / \Delta t, \qquad (19\text{-}7a)$$

where $k_1 - k_d$ is virtually constant and equal to k_a, the fractional rate of deposition (or accretion) over an interval of a few (~ 2) days; k_a was determined by measuring the increase in protein content, and k_1 by injection of a massive dose of $[1\text{-}^{14}C]$L-valine-$1\text{-}^{14}C$. The valine content of brain protein is 437 nmol/mg^{-1} protein. We see that not only k_1, the rate of synthesis, but also k_d, is increased in immature, as compared to mature, nerve tissue.

Of course, the data shown in Table 19-3 represent values only for the average rates of all the proteins present in the various regions; they therefore are not necessarily representative of, or applicable to, any particular protein. It is known that in adult rodent brain proteins (mainly in the soluble fraction) belong to at least three families, with half-lives of about 15 hours, 3 days, and 10 days [66, 102]. Mitochondrial proteins in the same tissue have been reported to exhibit half-lives of 5.6 days for particles in the cell body and 8.4 days in synaptosomes.

Reported half-lives for individual, well-characterized proteins (still heterogeneous as to origin) vary from 2.8 days for acetylcholinesterase, 3.8 days to 5 days for tubulin, and 5.2 days for choline-*O*-acetyltransferase.

Table 19-3. Kinetic Constants for Protein Metabolism in Rat Brain (%/hr)

| Age (days) | 2 | | 8 | | 18 | | 37 | |
Region	k_1	k_d	k_1	k_d	k_1	k_d	k_1	k_d
Midbrain	1.86	0.9	1.43	0.9	1.13	0.9	0.69	0.7
Cerebellum	2.8	1.8	2.5	1.6	1.5	1.2	0.9*	0.9*
Pons medulla	1.83	1.2	1.52	1.1	1.24	1.0	0.70	0.7
Cord	1.90	1.5	1.64	1.1	1.21	0.9	0.71	0.6

*30 days

SPECIALIZED PROTEINS

Receptors

An interesting example of proteins that are specific in function and localization is the nicotinic acetylcholine receptor localized postsynaptically in the neuromuscular junction. In the course of development of chick embryo, this protein and choline-O-acetyltransferase reach their highest specific activity around the day 12 after fertilization. In culture, developing chick or rat myotubes synthesize the protein with a half-life of 16 to 24 hr. (In such preparations, about 50 percent of all the receptor molecules have been newly synthesized and are in transit to incorporation into the plasma membrane, where they will make their appearance some 3 to 4 hr later. More than 60 percent of these molecules are in the Golgi apparatus [103].) Similar kinetic constants also describe the synthesis of the molecule in diaphragm of adult rat; once it is fixed in the subsynaptic region of that tissue, its stability increases dramatically and its half-life rises to 7.5 days [95].

Enzymes

A number of enzyme activities engaged in the biosynthesis of neurotransmitters are increased when the demand for the neurotransmitter is high, and in some instances this induction has been demonstrated to be due to actual increase in their rate of synthesis.

For instance, the activity of glutamine synthetase in the retina of embryonic chicks follows a characteristic developmental pattern typical for this tissue and is temporally and spatially correlated with other aspects of embryonic development. A characteristic rise in enzyme activity that can be induced precociously with 11-β-hydroxycorticosteroids in either the intact animal or isolated retina in culture takes place without any generalized cell proliferation but within the context of other well-defined changes. The effects observed are, therefore, specific and characteristic [104] and involve accumulation of the enzyme. Whether the accumulation is due to an increase in the rate of synthesis, rather than to a decrease in the rate of degradation, remains to be established; use of actinomycin D has established that the process also requires de novo synthesis of some species of RNA (but not protein) during the initial phases. However, later the process becomes resistant to either high or low concentrations of actinomycin D. These observations are consistent with analogous patterns obtained in the induction of a wide variety of enzymes by glucocorticoids and other hormones in many other systems.

Nadler and coworkers [105] removed one side of the entorhinal cortex of 11-day-old rats and studied the resulting formation of new cholinergic septohippocampal synapses in the ipsilateral dentate gyrus. They used the contralateral side as control and examined the structural, cytochemical, and biochemical levels. They found that, within 5 days, the absolute and specific activities of cholineacetyltransferase and acetylcholinesterase became significantly elevated in the outer part of the molecular layer of the operated, relative to the unoperated, side of the brain. These differences disappeared before the animals reached maturity.

Exposure of explanted rat sympathetic ganglia to 3 μg/ml of NGF resulted in a twofold increase in tyrosine hydroxylase activity within 48 hours [106]. This increase could be shown to be the result of a specific increase in the amount of enzyme present and was accompanied by a 2.5-fold increase in the rate of leucine incorporation into the enzyme that then was purified by immunoprecipitation and gel electrophoresis. The presence or absence of NGF had no effect on the k_d of the enzyme.

In contrast, the spectacular induction (50- to 70-fold increase) of serotonin-N-acetyltransferase activity in the explanted rat pineal gland brought about by norepinephrine (or l-isoproterenol) or dibutyryl cyclic AMP resulted in only a modest (<40 percent) increase in incorporation of amino acids into proteins and could not be explained by quantitative increases in enzyme protein [107]. Induction had, however, previously been shown to be absolutely dependent on the occurrence of some form of protein synthesis.

Acknowledgments

I would like to acknowledge receipt of Research Career Award No. GM 05060 from the National Institutes of Health. Research in my laboratory on some of these questions is supported by Research Grant No. NS 08309 from the same source.

References

*1. Ansell, G. B., and Bradley, P. B. (ed.). *Macromolecules and Behavior.* London: Macmillan, 1973.

2. Bourne, B. H. (ed.). *Structure and Function of Nervous Tissue.* New York: Academic, 1971.

*3. Davison, A. N. (ed.). *Biochemical Correlates of Brain Structure and Function.* New York: Academic, 1977.

4. Roberts, S., Lajtha, A., and Gispen, W. H. (eds.). *Mechanisms, Regulation, and Special Functions of Protein Synthesis in the Brain.* New York: Elsevier North-Holland, 1977.

5. Millard, S. A. Deoxyribonucleotide Synthesis and DNA in Brain. *Rev. Neurosci.* 1:115–136, 1974.

6. Brown, D. D. Gene expression in eukaryotes. *Science* 211:667–674, 1981.

7. IBRO/IPCS Symposium on Brain Mechanisms and Learning. New York: Raven Press, 1978.

8. Held, I., and Wells, W. Observations on purine metabolism in rat brain. *J. Neurochem.* 16:529–536, 1969.

9. Appel, S. H., and Silberberg, P. H. Pyrimidine synthesis in tissue culture. *J. Neurochem.* 15:1437–1443, 1968.

*10. Kelley, W. N., and Smith, L. H., Jr. Hereditary Orotic Aciduria. In J. B. Stanbury, J. B. Wyngaarden, and D. S. Fredrickson (eds.), *The Metabolic Basis of Inherited Disease* (4th ed.). New York: McGraw-Hill, 1978. Pp. 1043–1071.

*11. Koenig, H. Neurobiological action of some pyrimidine analogs. *Int. Rev. Neurobiol.* 10:199–230, 1967.

12. Kelley, W. N., and Wyngaarden, J. R. The Lesch-Nyhan Syndrome. In J. B. Stanbury, J. B. Wyngaarden, and D. S. Fredrickson (eds.), *The Metabolic Basis of Inherited Disease* (4th ed.). New York: McGraw-Hill, 1978. Pp. 1011–1036.

*13. Bray, H. G., and White, K. (eds.). *Kinetics and Thermodynamics in Biochemistry* (2nd ed.). New York: Academic, 1966. Chaps. 7 and 8.

14. Davis, M. M., et al. Immunoglobulin class switching: Developmentally regulated DNA rearrangement during differentiation. *Cell* 22:1–2, 1980.

14a. Razin, A., and Riggs, A. D. DNA methylation and gene function. *Science* 210:604–610, 1980.

15. Brown, I. R. Postnatal appearance of a short DNA repeat length in neurons of the cerebral cortex. *Biochem. Biophys. Res. Comm.* 84:285–292, 1978.

16. Thomas, J. O., and Thompson, R. J. Variation in chromatin structure in two cell types from the same tissue: A short DNA repeat length in cerebral cortex neurons. *Cell* 10:633–640, 1977.

17. Hübscher, U., Kuenzle, C. C., and Spadari, S. Identity of DNA polymerase γ from synaptosomal mitochondria and rat-brain nuclei. *Eur. J. Biochem.* 81:249–258, 1977.

18. Vilenchik, M. M., and Tretjak, T. M. Evidence for unscheduled DNA synthesis in rat brain. *J. Neurochem.* 29:1159–1161, 1977.

19. Yoshizawa, K., et al. Induction and repair of stand breaks and 3'-hydroxy terminals in the DNA of mouse brain following gamma irradiation. *Biochim. Biophys. Acta* 521:144–154, 1978.

20. Kimberlin, R. H., Shirt, D. B., and Collis, S. C. The turnover of isotopically labelled DNA in vivo in developing, adult, and scrapie-affected mouse brain. *J. Neurochem.* 23:241–248, 1974.

21. Hübscher, U., Kuenzle, C. C., and Spadari, S. Variation of DNA polymerases α, β, and γ during

*Key reference.

perinatal tissue growth and differentiation. *Nucl. Acid Res.* 4:2917–2929, 1979.

22. Gross, N. J., Getz, G. S., and Rabinowitz, M. Apparent turnover of mitochondrial deoxyribonucleic acid and mitochondrial phospholipids in the tissues of rat. *J. Biol. Chem.* 244:1552–1562, 1969.

23. Giuditta, A., Abrescia, P., and Rutigliano, B. Effect of electroshock on thymidine incorporation into rat brain DNA. *J. Neurochem.* 31:983–987, 1978.

*24. Altman, J. DNA Metabolism and Cell Proliferation. In A. Lajtha (ed.), *Handbook of Neurochemistry,* vol. 2. New York: Plenum, 1969.

25. Blobel, G. Synthesis and Segregation of Secretory Proteins: The Signal Hypothesis. In B. R. Brinkley and K. R. Porter (eds.), *Cell Biology 1966–1967.* New York: Rockefeller University Press, 1977. Pp. 318–325.

*25a. Wickner, W. The assembly of proteins into biological membranes: The membrane trigger hypothesis. *Annu. Rev. Biochem.* 48:23–45, 1979.

*26. Tabor, C. W., and Tabor, H. 1,4-Diaminobutane (putrescine, spermidine, and spermine). *Annu. Rev. Biochem.* 45:285–306, 1976.

27. Seiler, N., and Schmidt-Glenewinkel, T. Regional distribution of putrescine, spermidine and spermine in relation to the distribution of RNA and DNA in the rat nervous system. *J. Neurochem.* 24:791–795, 1975.

28. McAnulty, P. A., et al. Polyamines of the human brain during normal fetal and postnatal growth and during postnatal malnutrition. *J. Neurochem.* 28:1305–1310, 1977.

29. Shaskan, E. G. Brain regional spermidine and spermine levels in relation to RNA and DNA in ageing rat brain. *J. Neurochem.* 28:509–516, 1977.

*30. Chambon, P. Eucaryotic RNA Polymerases. In P. D. Boyer (ed.), *The Enzymes.* (3rd ed.), vol. 10. New York: Academic, 1974. Pp. 261–331.

*31. Chambon, P. Eukaryotic nuclear RNA polymerases. *Annu. Rev. Biochem.* 44:613–638, 1978.

32. Montanaro, N., Novello, F., and Stirpe, F. Effect of α-amanitin on ribonucleic acid polymerase II of rat brain nuclei and on retention of avoidance conditioning. *Biochem. J.* 125:1087–1090, 1971.

33. Anderson, S., et al. Sequence organization of the human mitochondrial genome. *Nature* 290:457–465, 1981.

34. Abelson, J. RNA processing and the intervening sequence problem. *Annu. Rev. Biochem.* 48:1035–1070, 1979.

*35. Koenig, E. Nucleic Acid and Protein Metabolism of the Axon. In A. Lajtha (ed.), *Handbook of Neurochemistry,* vol. 2. New York: Plenum, 1969.

35a. Gunning, P. W., et al. The direct measurement of the axoplasmic transport of individual RNA species: Transfer but not ribosomal RNA is transported. *J. Neurochem.* 32:1737–1745, 1979.

*36. Austin, L., et al. tRNA, its Axonal Transport and Fate. In S. Roberts, A. Lajtha, and W. H. Gispen (eds.), *Mechanisms, Regulation, and Special Functions of Protein Synthesis in the Brain.* New York: Elsevier North-Holland, 1977. Pp. 71–78.

37. Gainer, H. Intercellular transfer of proteins from glial cells to axons. *Trends Natur. Sci.* 1:93–96, 1978.

37a. Lasek, R. J., Gainer, H., and Barker, J. L. Cell-to-cell transfer of glial proteins to the squid giant axon. *J. Cell Biol.* 74:501–523, 1977.

38. Gambetti, P., et al. Quantitative autoradiographic study of labeled RNA in rabbit optic nerve after intraocular injection of [³H]uridine. *J. Cell Biol.* 59:677–684, 1973.

39. Ingoglia, N. A., Grafstein, B., and McEwen, B. S. Effect of actinomycin D on labelled material in the retina and optic tectum of goldfish after intraocular injection of tritiated RNA precursors. *J. Neurochem.* 23:681–687, 1974.

40. Berry, R. W. Ribonucleic acid metabolism of a single neuron: Correlation with electrical activity. *Science* 166:1021–1023, 1970.

41. Peterson, R. P. RNA in single identified neurons of *Aplysia. J. Neurochem.* 17:325–338, 1970.

41a. Peterson, R. P., and Kernell, D. Effects of nerve stimulation on the metabolism of ribonucleic acid in a molluscan giant neuron. *J. Neurochem.* 17:1075–1085, 1970.

42. DeLarco, J., et al. Polyadenylic acid–containing RNA from rat brain. *J. Neurochem.* 24:215–222, 1975.

43. DeLarco, J., et al. Polyadenylic acid–containing RNA from rat brain synaptosomes. *J. Neurochem.* 25:131–317, 1975.

44. Dewar, A. J., and Reading, H. W. Nervous activity and RNA metabolism in the visual cortex of rat brain. *Nature* 225:869–870, 1970.

45. Rose, S. P. R. Early visual experience, learning, and neurochemical plasticity in the rat and the chick. *Philos. Trans. R. Soc. Lond. B. Biol. Sci.* 278:307–318, 1977.

46. Rose, S. P. R. Macromolecular mechanisms and long-term changes in behaviour. *Biochem. Soc. Trans.* 6:844–848, 1978.

46a. Brown, I. R. Analysis of Gene Activity in the Mammalian Brain. In S. Roberts, A. Lajtha, and W. H. Gispen (eds.), *Mechanisms, Regulation, and Special Functions in the Brain.* New York: Elsevier North-Holland, 1977. Pp. 29–46.

47. Banks, S. P., and Johnson, T. C. Maturation-dependent events related to DNA dependent RNA synthesis in intact mouse brain nuclei. *Brain Res.* 41:155–169, 1972; Developmental alterations in RNA synthesis in isolated mouse brain nucleoli. *Biochim. Biophys. Acta* 294:450–460, 1973.

48. Elahi, E., and Sellinger, O. Z. The postnatal methylation of transfer ribonucleic acid in brain. Evidence for the methylation of precursor transfer ribonucleic acid. *Biochem. J.* 177:381–384, 1979.

48a. Heizmann, C. W., et al. Fluctuations of non-histone chromosomal proteins in differentiating brain cortex and cerebellar neurons. *Biol. Chem.* 255:11504–11511, 1980.

49. Grouse, L., Omenn, G. A., and McCarthy, B. J. Studies by DNA-RNA hybridization of transcriptional diversity in human brain. *J. Neurochem.* 20:1063–1073, 1973.

50. Van Ness, J., et al. Complex population of non-polyadenylated messenger RNA in mouse brain. *Cell* 18:1341–1349, 1979.

51. Kaplan, B. B., et al. The sequence complexity of brain ribonucleic acids. *Trans. Am. Soc. Neurochem.* 12:71, 1981.

*52. Roberts, S. Translational control of brain protein synthesis. In S. Roberts, A. Lajtha, and W. H. Gispen (eds.), *Mechanisms, Regulation, and Special Functions of Protein Synthesis in the Brain.* New York: Elsevier North-Holland, 1977. Pp. 3–20.

53. Cleveland, D. W., Kirschner, M. W., and Cowan, N. J. Isolation of separate mRNAs for α- and β-tubulin and characterization of the corresponding in vitro translation products. *Cell* 15:1021–1031, 1978.

54. Murthy, M. R. V., et al. Synthesis of Brain Specific Proteins in Vitro Using Cerebral Cortex Polysomal Components from Young and Old Rats. In S. Roberts, A. Lajtha, and W. H. Gispen (eds.), *Mechanisms, Regulation, and Special Functions of Protein Synthesis in the Brain.* New York: Elsevier North-Holland, 1977. Pp. 21–28.

*55. Lodish, H. E. Translation control of protein synthesis. *Annu. Rev. Biochem.* 45:39–72, 1976.

56. Berry, R. W. Processing of low molecular weight proteins by identified neurons of *Aplysia*. *J. Neurochem.* 26:229–231, 1976.

57. Loh, Y. P., et al. Subcellular fractionation studies related to the processing of neurosecretory proteins in *Aplysia* neurons. *J. Neurochem.* 29:135–139, 1977.

58. Yon, J. M. Some aspects of protein folding. *Biochimie* 60:581–591, 1978.

*59. Mahler, H. R. Glycoproteins of the Synapse. In R. U. Margolis and R. K. Margolis (eds.), *Complex Carbohydrates of Nervous Tissue.* New York: Plenum, 1978.

*60. Sharon, N. (ed.). *Complex Carbohydrates. Their Chemistry, Biosynthesis and Function.* Reading, Mass.: Addison-Wesley, 1975. Pp. 26–29 and 177–190.

61. Lennarz, W. J. Lipid linked sugars in glycoprotein synthesis. *Science* 188:986–991, 1975.

61a. Staneloni, R. J., and Leloir, L. F. The biosynthetic pathway of the asparagine-linked oligosaccharides of glycoproteins. *Trends Biochem. Sci.* 4:65–67, 1979.

62. Denslow, N. D., and O'Brien, T. W. Antibiotic susceptibility of the peptidyltransferase locus of bovine mitochondrial ribosomes. *Eur. J. Biochem.* 91:441–448, 1978.

*63. Mahler, H. R. Biogenetic autonomy in mitochondria. *CRC Crit. Rev. Biochem.* 1:381–460, 1973.

64. Bueton, D. E., and Wood, W. M. The mitochondrial translation system. *Subcell. Biochem.* 5:1–86, 1978.

65. Schimke, R. T., and Doyle, D. Control of enzyme levels in animal tissues. *Annu. Rev. Biochem.* 39:929–976, 1970.

66. Chee, P. Y., and Dahl, J. L. Measurement of protein turnover in rat brain. *J. Neurochem.* 30:1485–1493, 1978.

67. Forgue, S. T., and Dahl, J. L. The turnover rate of tubulin in rat brain. *J. Neurochem.* 31:1289–1297, 1978.

67a. Arias, I. M., Doyle, D., and Schimke, R. T. Studies on the synthesis and degradation of proteins of the endoplasmic reticulum of rat liver. *J. Biol. Chem.* 244:3303–3315, 1969.

68. Glass, R. D., and Doyle, D. On the measurement of protein turnover in animal cells. *J. Biol. Chem.* 247:5234–5242, 1972.

69. Zak, R., Martin, A., and Blough, R. Assessment of protein turnover by use of radioisotopic tracers. *Physiol. Rev.* 59:407–447, 1900.

*70. Weissbach, H., and Ochoa, S. Soluble factors required for eukaryotic protein synthesis. *Annu. Rev. Biochem.* 45:191–216, 1976.

70a. Zak, R., et al. Comparison of turnover of several myofibrillar proteins and critical evaluation of double-isotope method. *J. Biol. Chem.* 252:3430–3435, 1977.

71. Martin, A. F., et al. Measurements of half-life of rat cardiac myosin heavy chain with leucyl-tRNA used as precursor pool. *J. Biol. Chem.* 252:3422–3429, 1977.

*72. Dunlop, D., Lajtha, A., and Toth, J. Measuring Brain Protein Metabolism in Young and Adult Rats. In S. Roberts, A. Lajtha, and W. H. Gispen (eds.), *Mechanisms, Regulation, and Special Functions of Protein Synthesis in the Brain*. New York: Elsevier North-Holland, 1977. Pp. 79–96.

73. Dunlop, D. S., Van Elden, W., and Lajtha, A. Protein degradation rates in regions of the central nervous system in vivo during development. *Biochem. J.* 170:637–642, 1978.

74. Reith, M. E. A., Schotman, P., and Gispen, W. H. Measurements of in vivo rates of protein synthesis in brain, spinal cord, heart, and liver of young versus adult rats. Intact versus hypophysectomized rats. *J. Neurochem.* 30:587–594, 1978.

75. Laurent, G. J., et al. Turnover of muscle protein in the fowl (*Gallus domesticus*): Rates of protein synthesis in fast and slow skeletal, cardiac, and smooth muscle of the adult fowl. *Biochem. J.* 176:393–405, 1978.

76. Maruyama, K., Sunde, M. L., and Swick, R. W. Growth and muscle protein turnover in the chick. *Biochem. J.* 176:573–582, 1978.

77. Coulson, W. F., and Hart, B. Measurement of the rate of incorporation in vivo of amino acid into brain protein. *Biochem. Soc. Trans.* 5:1425–1428, 1977.

78. Lajtha, A., et al. Compartments of protein metabolism in the developing brain. *Biochim. Biophys. Acta* 561:491–501, 1979.

78a. Dunlop, D. S., et al. Brain slice protein degradation and development. *J. Neurochem.* 36:258–265, 1981.

*79. Garlick, P. J., and Swick, R. W. Determination of the Average Degradation Rate of Mixtures of Protein. In V. Turk and N. Marks (eds.), *Intracellular Protein Catabolism, II*. New York: Plenum, 1977. Pp. 103–107.

80. Eng, L. F., and Bigbee, J. W. Immunohistochemistry of nervous system–specific antigens. *Adv. Neurochem.* 3:43–98, 1978.

*81. Zomzely-Neurath, C., and Keller, A. The Different Forms of Brain Enolase: Isolation, Characterization, Cell Specificity and Physiological Significance. In S. Roberts, A. Lajtha, and W. H. Gispen (eds.). *Mechanisms, Regulation, and Special Functions of Protein Synthesis in the Brain*. New York: Elsevier North-Holland, 1977. Pp. 279–298.

82. Liem, R. K. H., et al. Intermediate filaments in nervous tissues. *J. Cell Biol.* 79:637–645, 1978.

83. Isobi, T., and Okuyama, T. The amino acid sequence of S-100 protein (PAP I-b protein) and its relation to the calcium-binding proteins. *Eur. J. Biochem.* 89:379–388, 1978.

84. Dannies, P. S., and Levine, L. Structural properties of bovine brain S-100 protein. *J. Biol. Chem.* 246:6276–6283, 1971.

85. Dahl, D. Glial fibrillary acidic protein from bovine and rat brain degradation in tissues and homogenates. *Biochim. Biophys. Acta* 420:142–154, 1976.

86. Kelly, P. T., and Cotman, C. W. Synaptic proteins. Characterization of tubulin and actin and identification of a distinct postsynaptic density polypeptide. *J. Cell Biol.* 79:173–183, 1978.

87. Bock, E. Nervous system specific proteins. *J. Neurochem.* 30:7–14, 1978.

88. Acton, R. T., et al. Association of Thy-1 differentiation alloantigen with synaptic complexes isolated from mouse brain. *Proc. Natl. Acad. Sci. U.S.A.* 75:3283–3287, 1978.

89. Roberts, S., and Ashby, C. D. Ribosomal protein phosphorylation in rat cerebral cortex in vitro. Influence of cyclic adenosine 3′, 5′-monophosphate. *J. Biol. Chem.* 253:288–296, 1978.

90. Gagnon, C., et al. Enzymatic methylation of carboxyl groups of chromaffin granule membrane proteins. *J. Biol. Chem.* 253:3778–3781, 1978.

91. Nath, J., and Flavin, M. An apparent paradox in the occurrence, and the *in vivo* turnover, of C-terminal tyrosine in membrane-bound tubulin of brain. *J. Neurochem.* 35:693–706, 1980.

92. Cruz, T. F., and Gurd, J. W. Reaction of synaptic plasma membrane sialoglycoproteins with intrinsic sialidase and wheat germ agglutinin. *J. Biol. Chem.* 253:7314–7318, 1978.

93. Yohe, H. C., and Rosenberg, A. Action of intrinsic sialidase of rat brain synaptic membranes on membrane sialolipid and sialoprotein components in situ. *J. Biol. Chem.* 252:2412–2418, 1977.

*94. Silverstein, S. C., Steinman, R. M., and Cohn, Z. A. Endocytosis. *Annu. Rev. Biochem.* 46:669–722, 1977.

95. Changeux, J-P., and Danchin, A. Selective stabilization of developing synapses as a mechanism for the specification of neuronal networks. *Nature* 264:705–712, 1976.

96. Ruffolo, R. R., Jr., et al. Synapse turnover: A mechanism for acquiring synaptic specificity. *Proc. Natl. Acad. Sci. U.S.A.* 75:2281–2285, 1978.

97. Goldberg, A. L., and Dice, J. F. Intracellular protein degradation in mammalian and bacterial cells. *Annu. Rev. Biochem.* 43:835–869, 1974.

98. Goldberg, A. L., and St. John, A. C. Intracellular protein degradation in mammalian and bacterial cell, II. *Annu. Rev. Biochem.* 45:747–803, 1976.

*99. Scanlin, T. F., and Glick, M. C. Turnover of Mammalian Surface Membranes. In G. A. Jamieson and D. M. Robinson (eds.), *Mammalian Cell Membranes: Responses of Plasma Mem-*

branes. Boston: Butterworths, 1976–77. Vol. 5, pp. 1–28.

100. McLendon, G., and Radany, E.   Is protein turnover thermodynamically controlled? *J. Biol. Chem.* 253:6335–6337, 1978.

*101. Marks, N.   Specificity of Breakdown Based on the Inactivation of Active Proteins and Peptides by Brain Proteolytic Enzymes. In V. Turk and N. Marks (eds.), *Intracellular Protein Catabolism, II.* New York: Plenum, 1977. Pp. 85–102.

102. Lajtha, A., Latzkovits, L., and Toth, J.   Comparison of turnover rates of proteins of the brain, liver, and kidney in mouse in vivo following long-term labeling. *Biochim. Biophys. Acta* 425:511–520, 1976.

103. Fambrough, D. M., and Devreotes, P. N.   Newly synthesized acetylcholine receptors are located in the Golgi apparatus. *J. Cell Biol.* 76:237–244, 1978.

104. Sarkar, P. K., and Moscona, A. A.   Glutamine synthetase induction in embryonic neural retina: Immunochemical identification of polysomes involved in enzyme synthesis. *Proc. Natl. Acad. Sci. U.S.A.* 70:1667–1671, 1973.

105. Nadler, J. V., Cotman, C. W., and Lynch, G. S.   Altered distribution of choline acetyltransferase and acetylcholinesterase activities in the developing rat dentate gyrus following entorhinal lesion. *Brain Res.* 63:215–230, 1973.

106. Max, S. R., et al.   Nerve growth factor–mediated induction of tyrosine hydroxylase in rat superior cervical ganglia in vitro. *J. Biol. Chem.* 253:8013–8015, 1978.

107. Morrissey, J. J., and Lovenberg, W.   Protein synthesis in pineal gland during serotonin-*N*-acetyltransferase induction. *Arch. Biochem. Biophys.* 191:1–7, 1978.

Section V. Cell Motility

Raymond J. Lasek

Chapter 20. Cytoskeletons and Cell Motility in the Nervous System

The complex and varied capabilities of the nervous system can be traced to its remarkable cyto-architecture. Nerve cells and glial cells extend processes over long distances to make specific contacts with hundreds or thousands upon thousands of other cells. When looking at the complex forms that neurons and glial cells take, the neuro-chemist may ask, What is the substance of this order? He or she will quickly realize that the extra-cellular connective tissue that gives structure to other tissues is missing from the nervous system. Although encased in layers of connective tissue, the central nervous system lacks the intracellular connective-tissue matrix, which is composed of collagen or elastin in other tissues. Instead, the architecture of nervous systems is based on intra-cellular fibrous skeletons. These *cytoskeletons,* as they are now called, are involved in many of the most fundamental nervous system processes. They are directly involved in the many motile behaviors that cells of the nervous system display; these include such morphogenetic events as the early rolling up of the vertebrate neural tube, em-bryonic cell migration, axonal growth, and myelin wrapping. Cytoskeletal elements are also impor-tant in intracellular motility; examples are axonal transport and secretion, including secretion of neurotransmitters.

Much of our knowledge of cytoskeletons comes from microscope studies. It is interesting from a historical viewpoint that our basic conception of nervous system circuitry arose from the use of selective metallic stains that reveal the intra-cellular fibrillar structures of neurons and glia. It has been more than 100 years since these stains were discovered, and we still do not understand why one metallic stain will reveal one class of neurons and

not another, or stain glial cells, but not neurons selectively. However, with the advent of the elec-tron microscope, we now know much about the detailed structure of the elements that constitute the cytoskeleton. Substantial progress has been made in the chemistry of these structures, so that the subunit proteins of all the major cytoskeletal elements have been identified.

Many excellent reviews exist on the subject of the cytoskeletal elements, including a compre-hensive collection of work on cell motility and cytoskeletons with an excellent bibliography and index [1].

Types of Cytoskeletal Elements

Three major fibrillar elements have been identified in metazoan cells. These are microtubules, inter-mediate filaments, and microfilaments. Each of these fibrous polymers has unique subunits and a characteristic structure. In the following section, some of the salient structural and chemical features will be reviewed. The reader should also refer to Chap. 2 and a text of neurocytology, such as that by Peters, Palay, and Webster [2].

MICROTUBULES

The microtubule, as its name implies, is a tubular structure 25 nm in diameter. The wall of the micro-tubule consists in most cases of 13 protofilaments composed of a globular protein, tubulin. *Tubulin* is a 110,000 dalton dimer made up of two different subunits, α- and β-tubulin (see Chap. 22). Micro-tubules are located in the mitotic spindle, cilia, and nearly all types of cellular extensions in the ner-vous system. These relatively rigid structures are arranged along the long axis of axons and den-drites. They appear to be polarized, and morphological differences have been noted between the distal end of the microtubule and the end nearest the cell body [3]. Although microtubules appear to be greater than 20 or 30 μm in length, they do not extend the length of the axon. Microtubules are often found in parallel arrays and are connected by sidearms or bridges. Some of the accessory proteins that decorate the microtubule and comprise the sidearms have been identified and are called *microtubule-associated proteins* (MAPs) [4, 5].

Cytoplasmic microtubules, such as those in axons and dendrites, are thought to be dynamic structures; in many cases they can be depolymerized by reducing the temperature to 4°C or by treatment with antimitotic drugs such as colchicine [6]. The microtubules repolymerize when the temperature is raised or the drug is removed. In vitro studies with purified microtubule proteins indicate that microtubules are in a dynamic equilibrium between monomeric and polymeric states. This is probably also the case for many of the microtubules in vivo. A great deal of effort has been made to understand the assembly-disassembly reaction [4, 7]. Nearly all of this work has been carried out on tubulin and MAPs obtained from the brains of vertebrates. Brain is an excellent source of tubulin, because tubulin comprises 10 percent or more of the protein that can easily be solubilized with physiological, nondenaturing buffers. The first important breakthrough in the study of microtubule assembly in vitro came from the work of Weisenberg, who discovered that the assembly reaction is severely inhibited by micromolar concentrations of Ca^{2+} [7]. Subsequently, it was found that relatively high concentrations of the buffers PIPES and MES enhance the polymerization reaction. Glycerol is often used to promote polymerization [7]. The capacity of tubulin to polymerize is relatively labile; it is easily lost within hours but can be preserved by storage at −70°C.

The cyclic assembly-disassembly reaction is an important method for purifying tubulin and MAPs [4, 7]. Tubulin is cycled by disassembling microtubules at 0 to 4°C and reassembling into microtubules at 37°C. At each step, the soluble tubulin or microtubules are separated from other

materials by centrifugation. Ca^{2+} is a particularly important factor in the reaction, and its concentration must be controlled by a chelator such as EGTA. Guanosine 5′-triphosphate (GTP) is necessary for the assembly reaction; it apparently interacts directly with a binding site on tubulin. The addition or removal of tubulin subunits takes place at the ends of the microtubules.

Although purified tubulin can be polymerized in vitro, it is thought that polymerization in the cell requires accessory proteins, the MAPs [4, 5]. In the nervous system, two classes of MAPs have been identified and shown to promote microtubule assembly in vitro. These include two high molecular weight proteins, *HMW* (sometimes referred to as *MAP 1* and *MAP 2*), and a fraction of lower molecular weight proteins with molecular weight around 68,000, referred to collectively as the *tau factor*. Antibodies to all of these proteins have been used to demonstrate that the MAPs are incorporated into the microtubule structure during in vitro assembly in their presence. Microtubules polymerized from tubulin in the presence of MAP 2 in vitro are decorated with projections that resemble those found in vivo [8]. Much of the continuing interest in these factors is based on the assumption that the MAPs and other factors are important in controlling assembly of microtubules in specific regions of the cell.

The organization of microtubules in the cell during both cell division and differentiation has been associated with the centrioles [9]. The centriole and pericentriolar material represent a microtubule-organizing center (MTOC). Neurons and glia, like other animal cells, contain two centrioles, which make up the centrosome. This structure is usually located near the nucleus and associated with the Golgi apparatus. The centrioles are replicated during the process of cell division. The mitotic spindle, which is composed of microtubules, is organized by the centrioles during cell division, and microtubules project from the centriolar region in the developing neuron. In vitro studies with detergent-extracted cell ghosts demonstrate that the centriolar region can determine both the length and number of microtubules assembled at these sites [9]. The number of microtubules that form around the centrioles in vitro is related to the number that normally radiate from the centrioles in the living cells. Microtubules extend outward from the centrioles, and it appears that tubulin assembly is associated with the pericentriolar material. Although assembly is initiated at the centriole and the microtubules may extend out into the axon or dendrite during the initial formation of these processes, the centrioles do not appear to determine the polarity of the cell during initial neurite development. Instead, the polarity of the cell is determined by unidentified factors in the periphery of the cell, which are possibly associated with the microfilament network [10]. Thus, the centrioles represent a microtubule assembly site and can be considered one of the centers for organization of the cytoskeleton in the cell. However, other factors must act in concert with microtubules to produce the complex cell shapes.

A number of enzymatic modifications of tubulin and its associated proteins have been noted. One unusual modification, the addition of tyrosine to the carboxy terminal of α-tubulin [4], may be associated with membranes. The phosphorylation of MAP 2 has been studied in some detail [5].

Microtubules generally are found in association with intermediate filaments in cells. There are, of course, many exceptions, including organisms such as crustacea, which do not appear to have intermediate filaments; and certain neuronal processes, such as parallel fibers of cerebellar granule cells, which contain only microtubules. However, the frequent association of microtubules and intermediate filaments suggest that these two cytoskeletal elements have a preferential interaction with each other through their accessory proteins [7, 11].

INTERMEDIATE FILAMENTS
Intermediate filaments (IF) gained their name because their diameter (7–11 nm) is intermediate between microtubules (25 nm) and microfilaments (4 to 6 nm) [7]. IF are found in neurons (*neurofilaments*) and glia (glial *filaments*) and are placed in one category, based primarily on their same size.

Neurofilaments and glial filaments seem related to the general class of IF, which includes tonofilaments of keratinocytes, and IF in fibroblasts and smooth muscle cells [12]. All these filaments are similar, but they are not identical. They differ in some of the details of their morphology and differ substantially in the molecular weight of their protein subunits. Despite these differences, there is reason to suspect that the structures represent a related group of polymers composed of primary subunits that have evolved from a common precursor protein [12].

Neurofilaments
Neurofilaments are particularly abundant in axons and generally increase in proportion to microtubules as axons increase in diameter [13]. They occur in bundles associated by wispy cross-arms, by which they appear to interact with each other and with microtubules [14]. They tend to be situated near the center of the axon. In some unusual cases, such as the giant axon of the marine annelid *Myxicola infundibulum,* the axoplasm consists primarily of neurofilaments and contains very few microtubules [15]. This giant axon has been an extremely useful model for understanding the properties of neurofilaments [15–17].

Neurofilaments have been isolated from the axoplasm of giant axons of *Myxicola* and squid and from mammalian CNS and PNS [20, 22]. Isolated filaments are extremely long, measuring tens of microns in length. They have a ropelike substructure consisting of four protofilaments, which are twisted tightly around each other in a helix. When neurofilaments are dissociated in urea, they unravel into two strands, which then break up into subunits [17]. The subunits are rod shaped, and therefore differ from microtubules and microfilaments, which consist of globular subunits [15]. The subunit structures have not been determined, but they appear to be between 10 and 50 nm in length [17]. The elongated form of the subunit results from the presence of coiled-coil α helix. This feature appears to be a universal property of the IF proteins [12]. The coiled-coil helix of intermediate filament apparently differs from that of many other proteins in that it may be a triple helix consisting of three peptide chains. Other proteins, such as tropomyosin and myosin, have helical regions consisting of two peptide chains.

Although the neurofilament was one of the first intracellular structures to be identified by use of the electron microscope, the study of its chemistry lags behind that of microtubules. The subunits of mammalian neurofilaments were discovered only recently. Progress was hampered initially because the glial filament subunit was confused with that of the neurofilaments [13, 20]. Neurofilament protein (NFP) in mammals consists of three subunit proteins, first recognized by Hoffman and Lasek [21] in studies of the slow component of axonal transport. These three proteins were called the *neurofilament triplet* because they were transported together in the axon at the same rate—about 1 mm/day. The triplet proteins have molecular weights of approximately 70,000, 150,000, and 200,000. However, the exact molecular weights vary from these figures by 10,000 to 15,000 in different mammalian species.

Two basic methods have been developed for purifying NFP. One by Schlaepfer and coworkers [22, 23] involves extracting minced peripheral nerve or spinal cord in a hypotonic solution at room temperature, sedimenting the extracted tissue at low speed, adding salt to isotonic concentration, and sedimenting neurofilaments at high speed. This preparation is enriched in the triplet. Antisera against these proteins stain neurons specifically [23]. The other method evolved from a technique for the preparation of axons from brain, developed by Norton and Shelanski. This "axon-flotation" method, as it was originally employed, produced preparations that were enriched in a 51,000 to 55,000 M_r polypeptide that originally was proposed to be the neurofilament subunit but is now known to be the subunit of glial filaments [20, 24]. Liem and coworkers [20] discovered that salt concentration was extremely important in determining the proportion of glial filaments versus neurofilaments that was obtained by this method. They have adopted the following method for purifying neurofilaments from mammalian brain. The homogenate is centrifuged at high speed in a dense sucrose solution, in which myelinated axons float to the surface. This pellicle of axons is lysed and the filaments are collected by sedimentation. If the axons are lysed in hypotonic solution, glial filaments composed of 51,000 M_r protein sediment. However, if

the axons are lysed with an isotonic solution containing Triton X100, the sedimented filament preparation contains substantial amounts of the neurofilament triplet in addition to the glial filament protein (GFP). Both of these methods are new, and it seems likely that they will be improved.

The identification and purification of invertebrate neurofilaments from annelids and mollusks was simplified by the availability of pure axoplasm, obtained by dissection from the giant axons of the squid and *Myxicola*. Squid neurofilaments contain major proteins with molecular weights of 200,000 and 60,000 [18]. *Myxicola* NFP consists of two polypeptides with molecular weights of 150,000 and 160,000 [18]. Recently, neurofilaments have been purified from squid brain by cyclic assembly-disassembly [25]. By using the strategy originally employed in the purification of fibroblast intermediate filaments, Zakoff and Goldman purified squid brain neurofilaments by disassembling them in 1.0 M KCl, sedimenting the residual material, and reassembling the neurofilaments by dialyzing the supernatant against dilute buffer [25]. The neurofilaments are sedimented and subjected to another cycle of disassembly and assembly. This method has not yet been applied to mammalian neurofilaments. It has been reported that the NFP triplet associates with microtubules during cyclic assembly-disassembly. This is apparently due to the association of NFP with the microtubules through the MAPs [11].

NFP is actively phosphorylated by an endogenous neuronal kinase that was first identified in the squid axon [31]. Polypeptides with molecular weights of 200,000 and 600,000 are phosphorylated in the squid, but the 60,000 M_r protein, which is also a major component of squid neurofilaments, is not. The phosphorus is attached to serine by an ester bond. Phosphorylation is apparently a general property of neurofilaments and has been found in *Myxicola* as well as in mammalian neurofilaments [26]. In *Myxicola,* the 150,000 and 160,000 M_r subunits are phosphorylated, and in mammals all three triplet polypeptides are phosphorylated. The physiological role of neurofilament phosphorylation has not been ascertained.

One interesting property of NFP is its degradation by an endogenous Ca^{2+}-activated protease which is specific for NFP. The proteolytic activity was first discovered in axoplasm from the giant axon of *Myxicola* and also has been identified in squid axoplasm and mammalian nervous tissue [16,

28, 29]. Precautions must be taken against this protease during the purification of NFP; however, the protease requires Ca^{2+} in the millimolar range and is fairly effectively controlled by chelators as well as by a number of protease inhibitors. The neurofilament is otherwise very stable; this stability is apparently the result of a propensity of the protein subunits to associate with each other laterally. The Ca^{2+}-activated protease may reduce the capacity of the subunit to polymerize. This type of proteolytic control mechanism has been proposed for neurofilament disassembly in the presynaptic terminal [21] and also for degradation of the neurofilaments during Wallerian degeneration [29].

Aging human neurons display an abnormal accumulation of silver-stained neurofibrillary tangles in the nerve cell body. These tangles resemble abnormal neurofilaments that are twisted tightly about each other [37]. These structures are also found in neurons of individuals with Alzheimer's disease [37]. Essentially, nothing is known concerning the chemistry of these structures. Antibodies to highly purified NFP or GFP do not stain them.

Glial Filaments
Glial filaments are the intermediate filaments found in large numbers in mammalian astrocytes [14]. Glial filaments can be differentiated from neurofilaments by their morphology, chemistry, and solubility properties [13]. Glial filaments are somewhat smaller in diameter than neurofilaments, are found in tightly packed bundles, and do not have cross-bridges [14]. This morphological distinction between glial filaments also applies to the nervous systems of annelids and mollusks [17]. GFP has been identified in mammals and has a molecular weight from 51,000 to 55,000 M_r [13].

Whereas all NFP have one or more major high molecular weight subunits of 150,000 M_r or greater, proteins from glial filaments and all other nonneuronal IF do not have a major subunit greater than 60,000 M_r [12]. These differences in molecular weight are likely to be related to structural differences in the intermediate filaments. Antibodies to GFP stain astrocytes and not neurons

[13]. Furthermore, antibodies to GFP from brain do not stain Schwann cells, which also contain intermediate filaments [31]. Therefore, both GFP and NFP appear to be cell type specific.

The discovery of GFP can be traced back to the study of glial fibrillary acidic protein by Eng and coworkers [32, 33]. These investigators isolated a highly acidic, water-soluble protein from multiple sclerosis plaques, which consist principally of reactive astrocytes. Electron microscope immunocytochemistry demonstrated that the antibody specifically stained bundles of glial filaments. This glial fibrillary acidic protein increases in regions of the brain undergoing reactive gliosis [33] (see also Chaps. 19, 23, 32).

MICROFILAMENTS
The word *microfilaments* (MFs) refers to the actin-containing 4 to 6 nm filaments that are seen in cells generally [12]. MFs are similar in structure to the actin filaments that interact with myosin thick filaments in skeletal muscle to produce muscle contraction [34] (see Chap. 27). Actin microfilaments have been identified in many cell types, including neurons, by means of decorating them with the heavy meromyosin that forms "arrowheads" with the filaments [12]. In some nonmuscle cells, such as fibroblasts, the microfilaments are arranged in long bundles (*stress fibers*) that are recognizable under the light microscope. However, in the nervous system the microfilaments are generally short and make up a meshwork. This actin-containing meshwork is apparently associated with the plasma membrane of the nerve cell. Studies on the squid giant axon demonstrate that the cytoskeleton is attached to the plasma membrane, possibly by the microfilaments [35]. Microfilaments are likely to be involved in cell locomotion; they are particularly abundant and well developed in the growth cone of elongating axons [36]. The filopodia that extend from the growth cone often contain bundles of microfilaments.

Actin is a globular protein, 3.5 nm in diameter, with a molecular weight of 42,000. (The review by Pollard and Weighing [34] is a useful source of information on the chemistry of actin and myosin.)

Cyclic assembly and disassembly of MF has been used as a final purification step for actin. At least three forms of actin have been identified by two-dimensional polyacrylamide gel electrophoresis [37]. α-, β-, and γ-Actin differ in their isoelectric points. α-Actin is the predominant form in skeletal muscle; the β and γ forms are found in the nervous system. There are separate genes for each of these isomers, and they are expressed differentially during cellular development. The amino acid sequences of brain and muscle actin differ in only a few residues. Actin comprises 6 percent of the protein of adult chicken brain and 8 to 10 percent of that of embryonic chick brain [36].

Evidence is growing that MFs interact with myosin in such cells as fibroblasts. Immuno-cytological studies with antibodies to smooth muscle myosin suggest that myosin is associated with the MF bundles [38]. Neurons also can be stained with antimyosin antibody [39]. In fact, actin was first identified in brain as *actomyosin* by Puszhkin, Berl, and their coworkers [40]. They also first demonstrated actomyosin in nervous tissue, indicating the existence of contractile proteins in nonmuscle cells [see 36 for review].

The mechanisms by which actin-myosin inter-actions are regulated in nonmuscle cells differ from those in skeletal muscle [12], although the protein tropomyosin, which regulates actin-myosin interactions in muscle, has been found in brain. The brain form differs from that of muscle and consists of two 30,000 M_r polypeptide chains [12, 36]. Recently, a mechanism involving the Ca^{2+}-regulated phosphorylation of one myosin light chain has been discovered in smooth muscle. Calmodulin mediates the effect of Ca^{2+} on a specific kinase which regulates the actin-myosin inter-action [41]. This mechanism may also operate in nonmuscle cells. A troponin complex may also exist in brain; however, it remains to be demon-strated that the calcium-regulatory protein in this complex is troponin C and not calmodulin [42].

The evidence supporting the association of myosin with microfilaments adds significantly to the possibility that these structures are involved in contractile events that produce motility in the nervous system. However, until the structural organization of the microfilament-myosin complex and its relationship to the elements that are moved is elucidated, the relevance of the neuronal con-tractile system to that of muscle will remain un-certain.

The drugs cytochalasin and phalloidin have been found to interfere with MF function [37]. Cyto-chalasin prevents polymerization and results in the disassembly of MF. Phalloidin apparently acts by irreversibly stabilizing MF and preventing dynamic changes in the MF network. Although cytochalasin affects other aspects of cell metabolism, it is a useful means of implicating MF in cell motility when it is used at appropriate concentrations. For example, cytochalasin inhibits the elongation of the axon.

The protein α-actinin, found in the Z band of muscle (see Chap. 27), is also present in nonmuscle cells; and antibodies to α-actinin stain the adhesion sites at which cells in tissue culture attach to the substrate [38]. MFs are closely associated with these adhesion sites, and it has been suggested that these sites and the associated MF are involved in cell locomotion.

In neurons, the synapse represents a region of great intercellular adhesivity (Chap. 19). Many synapses have a density associated with the inner surface of the postsynaptic membrane. These post-synaptic densities (PSDs) are composed of fila-mentous and granular material [43]. The major protein of the PSD has a molecular weight of 51,000. The PSDs also contain actin and calmodulin [41]. These observations suggest that the cytoskeleton contains differentiated regions that are associated with specializations in the plasma membrane. Such specializations may be involved in intercellular adhesivity, as well as in organizing proteins, such as receptors, within the membrane.

Cytoskeletons and Cell Motility

Two mechanisms of cell motility have been well described. One, found in skeletal muscle, is based on the actomyosin system; the second, found in cilia, involves the dynein microtubule system [1]. Whereas actomyosin has been demonstrated clearly

Table 20-1. The Components of Axonal Transport and Their Relationship to Cytological Structures

Anterograde Rate Components			Rate (mm/day) in Mammals	Types of Materials	Hypothesized Structures
Fast		I*	200–400	Glycoproteins, glyco-lipids, acetylcholines-terase, serotonin, peptides	Vesicles, agranular reticulum, granules
Intermediate		II	50	Mitochondrial proteins	Mitochondria
		III	15	Myosin-like protein	?
Slow	SCb	IV	2–4	Actin, clathrin, enolase, CPK, calmodulin	Microfilaments, axoplasmic matrix
	SCa	V	0.2–1	Neurofilament triplet proteins, tubulin	Microtubule-neuro-filament network

*Roman numerals refer to the nomenclature developed by Willard, Cowan, and Vagelos (*Proc. Natl. Acad. Sci. U.S.A.* 71:2183–2187, 1974) for the components of transport. In addition, see references 50, 52, 54.

in the cells of the nervous system [36, 39], the evidence for the presence of the contractile protein dynein is incomplete and only suggestive [4]. However, the possibility remains that both these mechanisms may operate within neurons.

Two examples of cell motility in the nervous system are likely to involve an actomyosin system. These are the rolling-up of the neural plate into the neural tube and the active extension of the filopodia from the growth cone during axon elongation [12, 36]. The evidence consists principally of the observation of MF in the contractile regions of these structures and the presence of myosin in the growth cone [36, 43]. However, actomyosin contraction has not been directly demonstrated in these motile regions.

Two aspects of intracellular motility in neurons have been the subject of active research, axonal transport (see Chap. 22) and the associated process of membrane recycling in the presynaptic terminal [39]. Much evidence for the identity and interrelationships of cytoskeletal elements is derived from their rates of axonal transport. Five components of anterograde axonal transport have been recognized in mammalian nerve cells and are summarized in Table 20-1 [44–46]. The cytoskeleton proteins are conveyed in the two subcomponents of slow transport: slow component a (SCa) and slow component b (SCb) [21, 47].

Studies on the transport of proteins in the mammalian visual system indicate that SCa and SCb represent two distinct cytoskeletal networks, the microtubule-neurofilament network and the microfilament network, respectively [47]. SCa has a very simple protein composition and is composed principally of tubulin and the neurofilament triplet. In labeling experiments, the proteins of SCa move coherently within the axon as a bell-shaped wave. The coherent transport of tubulin and NFP suggests that these proteins move as microtubules and neurofilaments, which interact to form the *MT-NF network* [24, 47]. That network is continuously moving within the axon at 0.2 to 1 mm per day from the cell body, where it is assembled, to the axon terminals. In the growing axon, this continued movement is involved in axonal elongation. In the nongrowing axon, the continuous advance is apparently halted at the presynaptic terminal [21]. That is, in nongrowing axons, the proteins of the MT-NF network are not degraded as they move along the axon, but only after they enter the presynaptic terminal. Thus, the life span of tubulin and NFP is determined by the length of the axon. Since SCa moves at 1 mm per day, tubulin and NFP have a life span of a few days in axons that are a few millimeters long, but in axons that are 10 cm long, these proteins have a life span of 100 days. Consequently, average life spans for tubulin or NFP obtained for the whole brain are of questionable significance.

The second subcomponent of slow transport, SCb, moves 4 to 5 times faster than does the MT-NF network in SCa, and contains a more complex constellation of proteins [47]. SCb is the only component of transport that contains actin and clathrin, another cytoskeletal protein [47]. Clathrin is the subunit protein of the basketlike structure that surrounds coated vesicles. These vesicles are involved in the movement of membranes in cells and have been implicated in membrane recycling in the presynaptic terminal. Clathrin binds to filamentous actin and α-actinin; this suggests that it may be complexed with the microfilaments during transport. The presence of actin and clathrin in SCb has led to the suggestion that SCb represents the microfilament network [50, 54, 55].

One puzzling aspect of SCb is that this transport component includes dozens of "soluble" proteins. Yet, the transport characteristics of the SCb proteins indicate that they move together in the axon [45, 52, 53]. These proteins apparently comprise a macromolecular complex that includes the actin microfilaments. It is interesting that many of the SCb proteins appear to be enzymes of intermediary metabolism, such as the nerve-specific enolase and creatine phosphokinase [45, 52]. These enzymes usually are thought to diffuse freely in the cell. However, the axonal transport data raise serious questions about the conventional view. Furthermore, the possibility arises that glycolytic enzymes contribute structural characteristics to the cytoskeleton and that changes in metabolism may lead directly to changes in structure [51].

In summary, studies of axonal transport have distinguished two cytoskeletal networks. SCa consists of the long and linear microtubules and neurofilaments that interact to form the MT-NF network, which moves at 1 mm per day. SCb consists of actin and clathrin in association with a large number of other proteins, including enzymes of intermediary metabolism. These proteins comprise the microfilament network, which moves 4 to 5 times faster in the axon than does the MT-NF network. The presence of actin and clathrin in the presynaptic terminal, and the relative paucity of microtubules and neurofilaments in this region of the neuron, indicate that the microfilament network and its associated proteins may represent the primary cytoskeletal component of the presynaptic terminal. Similarly, other regions of the nerve cell, such as dendritic spines that contain fine filamentous elements, may also have cytoskeletons based on the microfilament network [56].

The characteristics of these networks in the axons and dendrites are determined to some degree in the cell body, where the cytoskeletal proteins are synthesized and assembled. The networks may differ substantially in different processes of the same nerve cell. For example, whereas dendrites generally contain many microtubules and few neurofilaments, axons are often characterized by a large number of neurofilaments. A dramatic example of the differences between two branches of the same axon can be seen in the dorsal root ganglion cell [48]. The central and peripheral branches of this ganglion cell differ in their microtubule-neurofilament content, and this correlates with the axonal transport of the cytoskeleton in the two processes. The differential character of the networks in separate processes apparently arises in the cell body, possibly owing to the presence of separate organizing regions for each primary extension of the nerve cell. This issue is related to the general question of specific routing of materials in the nerve cell [46] (see also Chap. 22).

References

1. Goldman, R. D., Pollard, T., and Rosenbaum, J. *Cell Motility.* Cold Spring Harbor, N.Y.: Cold Spring Harbor Laboratory, 1976.
2. Peters, A., Palay, S. L., and Webster, H. *The Fine Structure of the Nervous System: The Neurons and Supporting Cells.* Philadelphia: Saunders, 1976.

3. Chalfie, M., and Thomson, J. N. Organization of neuronal microtubules in the nematode *Caenorhabditis elegans*. *J. Cell Biol.* 82:278–279, 1979.

4. Kirschner, M. W. Microtubule assembly and nucleation. *Int. Rev. Cytol.* 54:1–71, 1978.

5. Sloboda, R. D., et al. Microtubule-Associated Proteins (MAPs) and Assembly of Microtubules in vitro. In R. Goldman, T. Pollard, and J. Rosenbaum (eds.), *Cell Motility.* Cold Spring Harbor, N.Y.: Cold Spring Harbor Laboratory, 1976.

6. Wilson, L., and Bryan, J. Biochemical and pharmacological properties of microtubules. *Adv. Cell Mol. Biol.* 3:21–72, 1974.

7. Gaskin, F., and Shelanski, M. L. Microtubules and intermediate filaments. *Essays Biochem.* 12:115–146, 1976.

8. Kim, H., Binder, L. I., and Rosenbaum, J. L. The periodic association of MAP 2 with brain microtubules in vitro. *J. Cell Biol.* 80:266–276, 1979.

9. Brinkley, B. R., Cox, S. M., and Fistel, S. H. Organizing centers for cell processes. *Neurosci. Res. Program Bull.* Vol. 19, 1981. In press.

10. Lasek, R. J., Brinkley, B. R., and Solomon, F. Organizing centers: The form and transport of cytoskeletons. *Neurosci. Res. Program Bull.* Vol. 19, 1981. In press.

11. Shelanski, M. Neurofilaments and microtubules. *Neurosci. Res. Program Bull.* Vol. 19, 1981. In press.

12. Goldman, R. D., et al. Cytoplasmic fibers in mammalian cells: Cytoskeletal and contractile elements. *Annu. Rev. Physiol.* 41:703–722, 1979.

13. Shelanski, M. L., and Liem, R. K. Neurofilaments. *J. Neurochem.* 33:5–13, 1979.

14. Wuerker, R. Neurofilaments and glial filaments. *Tissue Cell* 2:1–9, 1970.

15. Gilbert, D. S. Axoplasm architecture and physical properties as seen in the *Myxicola* giant axon. *J. Physiol.* (London) 253:257–301, 1975.

16. Gilbert, D., Newby, B., and Anderton, B. Neurofilament disguise, destruction, and discipline. *Nature* 256:586–589, 1975.

17. Krishnan, N., Kaiserman-Abramof, I. R., and Lasek, R. J. Helical substructure of neurofilaments isolated from *Myxicola* and squid giant axons. *J. Cell Biol.* 82:323–335, 1979.

18. Lasek, R. J., Krishnan, N., and Kaiserman-Abramof, I. R. Identification of the subunit proteins of 10 nm neurofilaments isolated from axoplasm of squid and *Myxicola* giant axons. *J. Cell Biol.* 82:336–346, 1979.

19. Steinert, P. Structure of the three-chain unit of the bovine epidermal keratin filament. *J. Mol. Biol.* 123:49–70, 1978.

20. Liem, R. K. H., et al. Intermediate filaments in nervous tissues. *J. Cell Biol.* 78:637–645, 1978.

21. Hoffman, P. N., and Lasek, R. J. The slow component of axonal transport: Identification of structural polypeptides of the axon and their generality among mammalian neurons. *J. Cell Biol.* 66:351–366, 1975.

22. Schlaepfer, W. W., and Freeman, L. Neurofilament proteins of rat and human peripheral nerve and spinal cord. *J. Cell Biol.* 78:653–662, 1978.

23. Schlaepfer, W. W., and Lynch, R. G. Immunofluorescent studies of neurofilaments in the rat and human peripheral and central nervous system. *J. Cell Biol.* 74:241–250, 1977.

24. Goldman, J. E., Schaumberg, H. H., and Norton, W. T. Isolation and characterization of glial filaments from human brain. *J. Cell Biol.* 78:426–440, 1978.

25. Zackroff, R. A., Goldman, A., and Goldman, R. In vitro reassembly of squid brain intermediate filaments (neurofilaments) and their purification by assembly-disassembly. *Biol. Bull.* 157:403, 1979.

26. Pant, H. C., et al. Neurofilament protein is phosphorylated in squid giant axon. *J. Cell Biol.* 78: R23–R27.

27. Shecket, G., and Lasek, R. J. Phosphorylation of neurofilament protein. *J. Cell Biol.* 83:143a, 1979.

28. Pant, H., and Gainer, H. Properties of a calcium-activated protease in squid axoplasm which selectively degrades neurofilament proteins. *J. Neurobiol.* 11:1–12, 1980.

29. Schlaepfer, W. W., and Micko, S. Calcium-dependent alterations of neurofilaments in transected rat sciatic nerve. *J. Cell Biol.* 78:369–378, 1978.

30. Wisniewski, H., and Terry, R. D. Neuropathology of the Aging Brain. In R. D. Terry and S. Gershon (eds.), *Neurobiology of Aging.* New York: Raven Press, 1976. Vol. 3, pp. 265–280.

31. Schlaepfer, W. W., Freeman, L. A., and Eng, L. F. Studies of human and bovine spinal nerve roots and the outgrowth of CNS tissues into the nerve root entry zone. *Brain Res.* 177:219–229, 1979.

32. Eng, L. F. The Glial Fibrillary Acid (GFA) Protein. In R. Bradshaw and D. Schneider (eds.), *Proteins of the Nervous System.* New York: Raven Press, 1980.

33. Eng, L. F., and Bigbee, J. W. Immunohistochemistry of Nervous System-Specific Antigens. In B. W. Agranoff and M. H. Aprison (eds.), *Advances in Neurochemistry.* New York: Plenum, 1978. Vol. 3, pp. 43–98.

34. Pollard, T. D., and Weighing, R. R. Actin and myosin in cell movement. *Crit. Rev. Biochem.* 2:1–65, 1974.

35. Metuzals, J., and Tasaki, I. Subaxolemmal filamentous network in the giant nerve fiber of the squid (*Loligo pealei L.*) and its possible role in excitability. *J. Cell Biol.* 78:597–621, 1978.

36. Bray, D. Actin and myosin in neurons: a first review. *Biochimie,* 59:1–6, 1977.

37. Korn, E. D. Biochemistry of actomyosin-dependent cell motility (a review). *Proc. Natl. Acad. Sci. U.S.A.* 75:588–599, 1978.

38. Goldman, R. D., et al. The dynamics and interactions of the cytoskeleton and cytomusculature of nonmuscle cells. *Neurosci. Res. Program Bull.* Vol. 19, 1981. In press.

39. Kuczmarski, E. R., and Rosenbaum, J. L. Studies on the organization and localization of actin and myosin in neurons. *J. Cell Biol.* 80:356–372, 1979.

40. Berl, S., Puszhkin, S., and Niklas, W. Actomyosinlike protein may function in the release of transmitter material at synaptic endings. *Science* 179:441–446, 1973.

41. Cheung, W. Y. Calmodulin plays a pivotol role in cellular regulation. *Science* 207:19–27, 1980.

42. Mahendran, C., and Berl, S. Resolution of brain troponin complex. *J. Neurochem.* 33:149–158, 1979.

43. Cohen, R. S., et al. The structure of postsynaptic densities isolated from dog cerebral cortex: Overall morphology and protein composition. *J. Cell Biol.* 74:181–203, 1977.

44. Lasek, R. J., Gainer, H., and Barker, J. L. Cell-to-cell transfer of glial proteins to the squid giant axon. The glial-neuron protein transfer hypothesis. *J. Cell Biol.* 74:501–523, 1977.

45. Lasek, R. J. Axonal transport: A dynamic view of neuronal structure. *Trends Neurosci.* 3:87–91, 1980.

46. Grafstein, B., and Forman, D. S. Intracellular transport in neurons. *Physiol. Rev.* 60:1167–1283, 1980.

47. Black, M. M., and Lasek, R. J. Slow components of axonal transport: Two cytoskeletal networks. *J. Cell Biol.* In press.

48. Lasek, R. J. The dynamic ordering of neuronal cytoskeletons. *Neurosci. Res. Program Bull.* Vol. 19, 1981. In press.

49. Willard, M., Cowan, W. M., and Vagelos, P. R. The polypeptide composition of intra-axonally transported proteins. Evidence for four transport velocities. *Proc. Natl. Acad. Sci. U.S.A.* 71:2183–2187, 1974.

50. Black, M. M., and Lasek, R. J. Axonal transport of actin: Slow component b is the principal source of actin for the axon. *Brain Res.* 171:401–413, 1979.

51. Brady, S. T., and Lasek, R. J. Axonal transport: A cell biological method for studying proteins which associate with the cytoskeleton. *Methods Cell Biol.* In press, 1981.

52. Brady, S. T., and Lasek, R. J. Nerve specific enolase and creatine phosphokinase in axonal transport: Soluble proteins and the axoplasmic matrix. *Cell* 23:523–531, 1981.

53. Brady, S. T., Tytell, J., Heriot, K., and Lasek, R. J. Axonal transport of calmodulin: A physiologic approach to identification of long-term associations between proteins. *J. Cell Biol.* In press, 1981.

54. Ellisman, M., and Porter, K. R. Microtrabecular structure of the axoplasmic matrix: Visualization of the cross-linking structures and their distribution. *J. Cell Biol.* 87:464–479, 1980.

55. Garner, J., and Lasek, R. J. Clathrin is axonally transported as part of slow component b: The axoplasmic matrix. *J. Cell Biol.* 88:172–178, 1981.

56. LeBeux, Y. J., and Willemot, J. An ultrastructural study of microfilaments in rat brain by means of heavy meromyosin labelling. *Cell Tissue Res.* 160:1–36, 1975.

Samuel H. Barondes

Chapter 21. Biochemical Approaches to Cell Adhesion and Recognition

One of the outstanding characteristics of the nervous system is the complexity of interneuronal connections. Although little is presently known about the substances that establish and maintain these specific cellular associations, chemicals are believed to be important in two ways—as chemotactic agents, which guide cell migration, and as cell adhesion molecules, which bind cells together. The purpose of this chapter is to consider what is known about the biochemical basis of specific cell adhesion in the nervous system. First, I will try to formulate the nature of the problem in some detail by considering a popular example—development of connections between the retina and the optic tectum. Next, I will consider strategies for identifying cell adhesion molecules and summarize attempts to identify such molecules in both simpler biological systems and the nervous system. The interested student will find many books to augment this survey. He or she may start with two that cover this field from divergent points of view [1, 2].

Retinotectal Connections—A Model of Specific Neuronal Connections

The formation of specific neuronal connections is frequently studied by examining synapse formation between the processes of retinal ganglion cells and those of optic tectal cells. This system has been favored for a number of reasons. First, the structure of the retina, a two-dimensional sheet of cells with precise projections to the optic tectum, displays specific neuronal connections in a very clear form. Second, individual retinal ganglion cells, or small groups of them, are very accessible to manipulation. These cells can be activated with a highly collimated beam of light, can be injected with radioactive precursors, or can be ablated by microsurgical tech-

niques, allowing for determination of anatomical and functional patterns of connection after experimental treatments. Furthermore, in some vertebrates the retinotectal connections can regenerate after transection of the optic nerve.

Formation of retinotectal connections involves outgrowth of a bundle of retinal axons, migration to the contralateral optic tectum, assumption of correct position on the surface of the optic tectum, and then a further migration perpendicular to the tectal surface into the deeper tectal layers where synapses are formed. In the chick, a common subject for investigation, the axons reach the tectum by about day 9 of embryogenesis, and by about day 12 all of the terminals have assumed their correct position on the tectal surface. At this time, they dive into the deeper tectal layers. When the connections are completed, the dorsal retina innervates the ventral tectum and the ventral retina innervates the dorsal tectum. In the other dimension, the anterior (or nasal) retina innervates the posterior tectum and the posterior (or the temporal) retina innervates the anterior tectum.

How is the specific innervation of retina by tectum brought about? Sperry [3] proposed that this pattern is generated by interaction between substances on the surface of the growth cones of retinal ganglion cells and those on the surface of the tectal neurons. He envisioned a specific chemoaffinity based on the complementarity of the cell-surface molecules. Formation of the pattern of connections could be explained if critical properties of the retina and the tectum were defined by two perpendicular gradients of complementary molecules. The ultimate pattern would be determined by equilibrium positions in which these complementary adhesive reactions were best satisfied.

Because this is one of the most important formulations underlying studies of interneuronal associations, let us consider a version of it in somewhat more detail. One critical idea suggests existence of concentration gradients of regulatory substances that produce critical changes in responsive cells. In specification of retinal cells and tectal cells in the anteroposterior (or nasal-temporal) dimension, a regulatory substance (presumably a small molecule synthesized by a group of cells concentrated in the midline of the embryo) diffuses and influences some critical property of responsive tissues (Fig. 21-1). The anterior (nasal) retinal and tectal cells, which are closer to the midline, would be exposed to a higher concentration of this substance than would be posterior (temporal) cells. A graded change in these cells would be produced, with the biggest effect in the cells closest to the midline, and the smallest on the most remote cells. Another regulatory substance, operating in a dimension perpendicular to the first one, might spread from a dorsal focus, thereby causing changes primarily in the dorsotectal or retinal cells. Retinal cells would then make synapses with tectal cells, which receive inverse relative amounts of regulatory substances. Since the most dorsal and anterior cells of both retina and tectum would have been most strongly influenced by both the midline and the dorsoventral gradients, they would prefer contact with the most posterior and ventral tectal cells that had been least exposed to these influences.

The nature of the cellular changes produced by the putative regulators is not known. Presumably a permanent alteration of gene expression is produced. For the purpose of this discussion, the mechanism by which regulators direct differentiation is not critical; but it is pertinent to consider an example of specific biochemical changes that might be produced by the regulatory gradients. In this hypothetical case, let us assume that oligosaccharides on the surface of retinal and tectal cells represent one of the critical surface properties that determines their association. Let us also assume the following: (1) there are a large number of glycoprotein and glycolipid molecules in the plasma membranes of retinal and tectal cells to which addi-

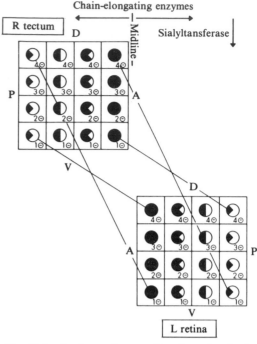

Fig. 21-1. A scheme for specification of retinal ganglion cells and tectal cells by the same gradients of diffusible regulatory substances. One putative regulatory substance spreads from the midline and has a greater influence on cells closer to the midline than those furthest from the midline. Another putative regulatory substance spreads in a dorsoventral direction and has a greater influence on the dorsoretinal and dorsotectal cells, than on the ventral cells. Connections are ultimately made between cells that have complementary surfaces. Symbols: A, anterior (or nasal); D, dorsal; P, posterior (or temporal); V, ventral. (Reprinted from S. H. Barondes [22], with permission from The Rockefeller University Press.)

tional specific saccharides may be added; (2) the probability of addition of the sugars to these cell-surface substances is linearly related to the cellular concentration of one or more glycosyltransferases, referred to here as *chain-elongating enzymes;* (3) the new or elongated polysaccharide chains that are formed by the chain-elongating enzymes bind (with an affinity that is some function of their length or cellular concentration, or both) to the active site of a carbohydrate-binding protein present to a variable extent on the surface of the retinal and tectal cells; and (4) the cellular concentration of this carbohydrate-binding protein varies inversely with the cellular concentration of chain-elongating enzymes.

Given these assumptions, let us now postulate (Fig. 21-1) that the regulatory substance in the anterior-posterior dimension induces the synthesis of chain-elongating enzymes, which direct the incorporation of specific sugars into cell-surface glycoproteins or glycolipids. "Black" cells close to the inducer will have surfaces rich in these specific heterosaccharides. They are shown as completely black in Fig. 21-1. Those most distant from the focus will have fewer sugars and are shown as mostly white. Let us also assume that the same regulatory substance represses synthesis of the cell-surface carbohydrate-binding protein. As a consequence, the concentration of carbohydrate-binding protein is inversely proportional to that of the chain-elongating enzymes. Black cells rich in the specific heterosaccharides would be poor in the carbohydrate-binding proteins, and conversely.

Specification of cells in the dorsoventral dimension could be directed by a regulatory substance that leads to the synthesis of gradient of a sialyltransferase. This enzyme could transfer sialic acid residues to cell-surface glycolipids and glycoproteins. Assuming that the cellular concentration of the sialyltransferase determines the number of negatively charged sialic acid residues on the cell surface and the net cellular surface negativity, this would be distributed as indicated in Fig. 21-1. Cells with many sialic acid residues would be very negative, and are marked as 4 minus, whereas those with few would be less negative, and are marked as 1 minus.

When retinal cell terminals reach the tectum, they would reversibly associate with tectal neuronal processes. The best fit, that is, their equilibrium position, would be determined by relevant molecular interactions. Retinal cells rich in cell-surface oligosaccharides and poor in carbohydrate-binding proteins would tend to make contact with tectal cells, which are poor in cell-surface oligosaccharides and rich in carbohydrate-binding proteins;

and retinal cells with abundant cell surface sialic acids would be repelled by tectal cells with a similar high density of negative residues. The net result would be that black negative cells from retina or tectum would tend to become associated with relatively white positive cells, and so on. Through this comparatively simple scheme, the observed retinotectal relationships could be established.

There is presently little evidence for this working hypothesis. Indeed, even the basic idea that specific retinotectal synapses are due to selective cell-adhesive reactions remains controversial. Selective chemotaxis remains another potential mechanism for guiding retinal axons to their proper tectal destinations. Adhesive interactions mediating the ordering of retinal axons within the optic nerve may also play a role. In addition, trial and error might operate in initial synapse formation, with complex feedback mechanisms based on the consequences of the functioning synapse that could determine whether it will persist. One merit of the scheme proposed is that it is fairly parsimonious, requiring only a few common molecules, rather than a large number of unique molecules to specify the interacting cell surfaces.

Some General Considerations about Cell-Adhesion Molecules

Although there is a lack of agreement even about simple definitions, molecules that bind cells to other cells or to extracellular materials will here be called *cell-adhesion molecules* (CAMs). Such molecules might be "nonspecific," and bind any pair of cells together. Alternatively, they might bind to specific receptors that are expressed only on certain cells. By mediating binding of these specific cells, the CAMs could also be functioning as "cell-recognition molecules," that is, molecules that determine which cells associate. In this regard, it is important to point out that cell-recognition molecules need not be CAMs. Rather, they might be cell-surface molecules confined to certain cells, which, when combined with appropriate complementary molecules, signal that cellular contact should be established by some other molecular interaction. The latter interacting molecules would be CAMs, but need not be cell-recognition molecules.

Because of their versatility, it is generally assumed that many CAMs are proteins. Cell adhesion is thought to result from interactions between a cell-surface protein and some type of complementary cell-surface receptor, which would also be designated as a CAM. The complementary receptor could be either a protein or another type of molecule. As I have indicated above, specific oligosaccharides, which are so abundant on the cell surface as components of glycoproteins and glycolipids, are favorite candidates.

Some common conceptions of the molecular basis of cell-cell adhesion are illustrated in Fig. 21-2. In each case, two cell surfaces are shown bound together by interaction of one or more molecules arising from each cell surface. In A-C, the interacting cell surfaces are indistinguishable, but in D the two cells are different. Note also that the interacting molecules might be identical or different. Both could be integral membrane proteins or glycoproteins that are firmly rooted within the lipid bilayer (Fig. 21-2A, B, D) or peripheral membrane proteins like the complementary bivalent ligand shown in Fig. 21-2C.

The adhesive interactions shown in Fig. 21-2 might bind many different types of cells together, as they might all possess sufficient copies of the interacting molecules to bind to each other. If this were the case, the CAMs might serve no cell-recognition function. However, if there were several complementary pairs of cell-adhesion molecules displayed to greater or lesser extent on different cells, a basis for highly complex specific cellular associations could be established. Even a single complementary pair present on all cells, but present to a variable extent, could provide the basis for complex patterns of selective cellular association. For example, simply varying the number of CAMs on the cell surface or their time of appearance in development could provide some selectivity. Furthermore, the degree to which the specific molecules are ordered or clustered in the membrane could be of importance. Although it is possible that

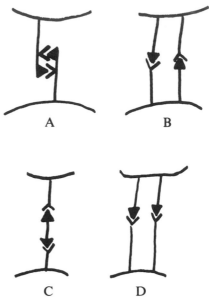

Fig. 21-2. Models of cell-adhesion molecules binding the surfaces of adjacent cells. (A) Single cell-adhesion molecule containing two different and complementary sites. (B) Two distinct complementary cell-adhesion molecules, both bound in the lipid bilayer of the cell surface. (C) Two distinct complementary cell-adhesion molecules, one of which is outside the lipid bilayer. (D) As in B, but each interacting cell contains only one type of cell-adhesion molecule.

CAMs play no role in the specific cellular associations generally referred to as cellular recognition, it is easy to see how they could be employed for this purpose, as already considered in the above discussion of retinotectal connections.

Criteria for Identification of Cell-Adhesion Molecules

The first task in attempting to find CAMs is to establish criteria for their identification. Unfortunately, the phenomenon under consideration— binding of a cell to another cell or to an extracellular material—involves many more variables than the association of two molecules in solution. For molecular analysis, it may be convenient to envision cells as billiard balls coated with various amounts of adhesive material of different degrees of mutual affinity. But cells are obviously more

Table 21-1. Expected Characteristics of (Criteria for) a Cell Adhesion
Molecule (CAM) and False Positives and Negatives

Expected Characteristics of CAM	Reasons for	
	False Positive	False Negative
Located on cell surface	Coincidental	Overlooked; inaccessible
Appearance of CAM correlates with development of adhesiveness	Coincidental	CAM present before adhesiveness, but other factor is limiting
Complementary receptor on cell surface (if CAM is isolated as polyvalent molecule, it will agglutinate test cells)	Binding has other function or is nonspecific	CAM binds poorly when solubilized; receptors saturated
Binding univalent antibodies or haptens to CAM blocks adhesion	Nonspecific effect	Affinity of univalent antibodies or haptens for CAM relatively low
Mutant with impaired cell adhesion has defective CAM	Indirect effect	Defect in CAM not detected by the measurements used

complex than billiard balls. Some characteristics that distinguish cells from such a model include (1) irregular and changing shape; (2) motility, which may be influenced by positive and negative chemotactic systems; (3) continuous reorganization of membrane structure in response to various cues.

Some commonly cited characteristics of (or criteria for) CAMs are listed in Table 21-1. First, a CAM must be shown to be present on the cell surface. Not all copies need be on the cell surface, but some must be. In addition, a CAM must be present on the cell surface when the cell develops adhesiveness. If it appears on the surface after adhesiveness develops, this argues against its role in cell adhesion; if its appearance correlates with the development of adhesiveness, it is taken as supportive evidence. There should also be something on the cell surface to which the CAM binds. We will refer to it as a *complementary receptor*. The receptor would also be a CAM; and, as shown in Fig. 21-2A, it might be identical with the CAM with which it is also complementary. Identification of the receptor might be made by demonstrating that CAM binds in some specific manner to the cell surface. Specificity is generally inferred from high affinity of binding and from saturability of binding, the latter indicating a limited number of specific

binding sites. If the CAM is bivalent, binding might be detected by the agglutination of the cells by CAM, along the lines shown in Fig. 21-2C.

The other two criteria for a CAM are based on measurements of cell adhesion either by in vitro assays or by some more natural method of directly observing cell adhesion. Such adhesion should be blocked by univalent antibodies directed against the CAM, if they are added in sufficient amount and are of sufficient affinity to block the function of the CAM. Addition of haptens that block the active site of CAM (e.g., sugars that bind the site of a CAM which is complementary to a cell-surface heterosaccharide) should also block cell adhesion. Finally, a mutant that shows impaired cell adhesion (for example, in a cultured line of the type of cell under investigation) should have absent or abnormal CAM.

Each of these expected characteristics of a CAM is compatible with the models shown in Fig. 21-2, as well as with more elaborate ones. An additional point, expressed in Table 21-1, is that, in the experimental application of each of these criteria, any result found could be a false positive or a false negative. For example, let us consider the most obvious criterion—that a CAM must be present on the cell surface. This could be shown in many ways.

If an antibody specific for the molecule is available, evidence that the antibody binds to the cell surface establishes the antigen's cell-surface location. Another technique is to incorporate radioactive iodine into cell-surface proteins by a reaction that depends on the enzyme *lactoperoxidase*. The enzyme cannot penetrate the cell membrane, so only cell-surface proteins are accessible to iodination. After the iodination reaction is terminated, the iodinated proteins could be identified by one of a number of techniques, such as polyacrylamide gel electrophoresis (PAGE). If a specific protein is iodinated, this is taken as evidence that it is present on the cell surface.

Establishing by these techniques that a particular molecule is present on the cell surface is not definitive evidence that it plays a role in cell adhesion. In this context, such a result could be called a false positive. On the other hand, the apparent absence of a molecule from the cell surface cannot be taken as incontrovertible evidence that it is not a CAM. There are a number of ways in which this could come about. For example, the molecule might be relatively scarce compared to other cell-surface molecules and could be iodinated so sparsely by the lactoperoxidase technique that it might not be detected on PAGE. The molecule in question also could be hidden from such reagents, or other substances employed as markers, such as antibodies raised against this molecule in a soluble form. It might be capable of interacting as a CAM in this cryptic state, or it might become exposed after a preliminary cellular interaction of another type. The point here is that failure to find a molecule on the cell surface could be a false negative in that it does not preclude its being a CAM.

False-positive and false-negative results are also possible with each of the other criteria listed in Table 21-1. For example, a correlation between the time during differentiation of synthesis of a putative CAM and the time of development of cellular adhesiveness could be coincidental. On the other hand, it is possible that the putative CAM is present long before the cell converts from a nonadhesive to an adhesive form. This could occur if the complementary substance with which it binds is the limiting factor—either in its time of synthesis or of appearance on the cell surface. Another possibility is that some general property of the cell membrane is a limiting factor. Therefore, failure to demonstrate a correlation between the appearance of adhesiveness and the appearance of the putative CAM could be a false negative.

There could also be false positives and false negatives with another relatively straightforward criterion—the presence of complementary cell-surface receptors for the putative CAM. Demonstrating the presence of such receptors could itself be a false positive, in that the molecule-receptor complex might be doing something other than binding cells together. For example, hormones bind to cells, thereby triggering specific reactions—and yet hormones are not CAMs. Even if the putative CAM is polyvalent and binding leads to agglutination of the cells, this could be a false positive. For example, basic proteins normally associated with nucleic acids can agglutinate cells by binding to acidic residues on the cell surface, but it is unlikely that these are CAMs. Failure to demonstrate binding of a putative CAM to a cell, or of agglutination of cells by such molecules, also could be misinterpreted. Once solubilized, the molecule might bind very poorly because it might be in a somewhat denatured form. Another possibility is that receptors present on the surface of the cell are already saturated with CAMs, so adding more does not lead to measurable binding.

The requirement that reagents which bind CAMs should block the adhesion reaction is also subject to misinterpretation. The reagents, whether univalent antibodies or specific ligands, could produce a false positive by nonspecifically affecting cellular interactions. Or there might be a false negative, as the affinity of the antibodies or ligands for a CAM might be so much lower than that of the CAM for its complementary cell-surface receptor that there is little competition and no measurable block in adhesion. Finally, even studies of mutants that show abnormal cell adhesion are subject to misinterpretation. A false positive could be produced if a mutation affected a critical step in differentiation which in turn blocked many subsequent steps in development. These steps could include synthesis of the putative CAM as well as another molecule which is the actual direct mediator of cell adhesion. Even a point mutation in the putative CAM found in cells that showed impaired adhesion could be a false positive, in that the effect could be indirect. By this is meant that the affected molecule might not directly bind cells together but might influence some other process, which itself directly mediates the adhesion. On the other hand, a false negative is possible, in that a mutant cell with impaired cell adhesion could appear to have normal CAMs, because their abnormality might not be detectable by the measurement technique being used. Only determination of the complete structural sequence of the potential CAM might turn up the defect.

How then are we to identify CAMs conclusively? Satisfying any single criterion is not convincing, so multiple experimental approaches are required. Even then, interpretations must be made with caution. They should be heavily dependent on estimates of the validity of the cell-adhesion assays employed for many of these studies.

Criteria for an Assay of Specific Cell Adhesion

An important prerequisite for studying CAMs is to establish some quantitative measurement of cell adhesion that is valid and "meaningful"—that is, measures something identical with, or closely related to, the cell adhesion that occurs in vivo. Establishing valid assays is probably the major stumbling block in this field.

In many cell adhesion assays, a comparison is made of the rate of binding of cells to each other in suspension [for example, see ref. 4]. In some cases, single cells prepared by dissociation of tissues are gyrated together and the rate of formation of clumps of cells is observed. Dissociation itself poses a major problem, in that it might remove or destroy CAMs. Often the cells must be incubated under prescribed conditions to recover from dissociation before the assay is done. Clump formation may then be measured either by microscopic inspection or by the use of an electronic particle counter. The detectors of the counter can be set so

that the disappearance of particles having the dimensions of single cells and the formation of particles of sizes that correspond to clumps of various numbers of cells can all be measured. The rate of clump formation is taken as a measure of the adhesiveness of the cells. The relative adhesiveness of different cell populations can be estimated by using this assay. In addition, the role of potential CAMs can be evaluated. In some cases, the effect of these CAMs on cell adhesion can be studied directly. In others, effects of reagents that react with the CAMS can be evaluated. For example, univalent antibodies raised against purified CAMs would be expected to block cell adhesion. In addition, the assay might be useful in searching for CAMs. For example, if crude antisera raised against whole cells block the measured cell adhesion, the relevant cell-surface antigens, which might be CAMs, could be identified by showing that they adsorbed the blocking activity of the antiserum.

Another commonly used assay measures the binding of a population of single cells to an immobilized layer of cells [5]. The single cells, called *probe cells,* either are labeled with radioactivity or in some other manner, whereas the layer of cells immobilized on a solid support (e.g., a tissue-culture dish) are unlabeled. The rate at which labeled cells bind to the layer is a measure of adhesion of the probe cells to the layered cells. Actual measurement may be made by counting radioactivity or by autoradiography. If the probe cells are labeled with a dye, their binding can be directly observed by microscopy. Relative binding of different types of cells to self or to other cells can be determined by varying the cell type in probe and layer. Applications of this assay are similar to those of the assay measuring clump formation in gyrated suspension.

Such assays have the merit of convenience and reproducibility. However, it is difficult to know the relationship between the characteristics they measure and cell adhesion in vivo. How does binding in a gyrated suspension relate to binding in vivo? How can one decide if the affinity of a cell for a layer of cells bound to a plastic dish is a measure of its adhesiveness in vivo? Adhesion can be measured in these circumstances, but it provides us with little confidence that it is related to the behavior of the cells in the organism.

Some criteria that may be used in attempting to determine whether a cell adhesion assay is valid include tissue-specificity, developmental stage—specificity, and the effects of specific reagents. Each criterion is formulated on the expectation of a correlation between adhesion as measured in the assay and some biological function of the cell. For example, if liver cells stick better to liver cells than to brain cells, and if the latter stick better to brain cells, it indicates cell-type specificity or tissue-specificity, which validates the assay. If selectivity is demonstrated with a wide range of cell types, confidence is increased.

Developmental stage—specificity is another criterion of some value. If cells at a specific embryonic age stick better to like cells than to those of a different age, this is taken as evidence validating the assay. However, it remains possible that the adhesion measured in this assay is due to a property of the cell surface that appears with differentiation, but that normally has nothing to do with cell-cell association; the important cell-adhesion property might not be assayed under the experimental conditions.

The criterion of blockade by specific reagents can also be used to validate a cell-adhesion assay. For example, consider the finding that antibodies (or their univalent derivatives) raised against a tissue-specific, or a developmental stage—specific, cell-surface component blocks the cell-cell adhesion observed in a given assay. This suggests that the specific component is a CAM and that the assay is valid, because it is dependent on the action of this component. However, the finding does not necessarily validate the assay, as binding antibodies to cell-surface molecules not normally involved in cell adhesion might also be inhibitory.

Cellular Slime Molds: A Model System

Given the complexities of the problem of cell adhesion, it is particularly important to choose a favorable system for analysis. Although our ulti-mate concern is cellular association in the nervous system, there may be advantages to a search for generally applicable principles in a system that lends itself more readily to experimentation. One organism used for much pioneering work on cell adhesion is the sponge [reviewed in ref. 2]. Recently, the cellular slime molds have become a popular choice for this work. To understand why, it is first necessary to consider the life cycle of these simple eukaryotic cells.

In the presence of bacteria on which they feed, slime-mold cells exist as unicellular amoebae that divide approximately every 3 to 6 hours. In this condition, the cells are called *vegetative cells;* this part of their life cycle may be called the nonsocial phase, because the cells show no tendency to associate. However, when the food supply is exhausted, the amebas differentiate into an adhesive form over the course of some 9 to 12 hours. The cells then aggregate, in response to pulses of chemotactic agents, generally cyclic AMP, to form a multicellular structure that contains up to 10^5 cells. In the ensuing 12 hours, this aggregate further differentiates into a fruiting body. About 20 percent of the cells in the aggregate become stalk cells and the rest become spore cells. The spore cells are in a dormant state, resistant to unfavorable environments. However, if the spores are exposed to a favorable environment they germinate; the amebas emerge and begin a new life cycle.

The cellular slime molds therefore have a number of advantages for studies of cell adhesion: (1) cells can be isolated in a nonadhesive form and at various stages of cell-cell adhesion; (2) a large number of cells at an identical stage of development can be raised in culture so that considerable material is available for biochemical studies; (3) the culture conditions are simple and resemble the natural environment of these organisms. Therefore, slime-mold cells show normal cell-association properties under defined conditions, where cells from higher organisms might lose them; (4) a number of species of cellular slime molds have been shown to display species-specific cellular association, raising the possibility of studying species-specific cell-cell adhesion.

Given such advantages, some progress has been made in determining the molecular basis of cell-cell adhesion in these organisms. Two potential cell-adhesion molecules have been shown to appear on the surface of slime-mold cells as they differentiate from a vegetative to a cohesive form. One, called *contact site A,* is a cell-surface glycoprotein isolated by Müller and Gerisch [6]. Their experimental strategy was as follows: (1) raise antibodies to cohesive slime mold cells; (2) make univalent antibody fragments (Fab fragments), so that when the antibodies are added to the cells they will not agglutinate them (as would be the case with divalent immunoglobulin), but might inhibit cell adhesion by blocking appropriate cell-surface molecules; (3) identify the cell-surface components to which the Fab binds. Müller and Gerisch indeed found that Fab fragments block cell adhesion and that, when they fractionate the membrane proteins of adhesive slime-mold cells, one glycoprotein adsorbs all this blocking activity. The purified glycoprotein, called *contact site A,* could be a CAM.

As with all such experiments, interpretation must be made with some caution. The finding that Fab binding to contact site A blocks adhesion does not prove that contact site A is a CAM as defined here. It is possible that binding Fab to this antigen (but not other cell-surface antigens) sets in motion a complex cellular response that renders the cell non-adhesive. Were this the case, contact site A, although involved in cell adhesion, might not directly bind cells together and thus, in this sense, would not be a CAM. Another problem with this approach is that contact site A might prove to be a substance that is only immunologically cross-reactive with a critical cell-adhesion molecule, rather than being identical to it. Because contact site A is a glycoprotein, the true CAM may be a rare molecule with an identical oligosaccharide chain on its surface. Binding Fab to the oligosaccharide chain on contact site A might remove this blocking activity, yet contact site A would again not be a CAM.

Another candidate for a CAM in cellular slime molds is a cell-surface lectin [7; reviewed in 1]. This lectin is a polyvalent, carbohydrate-binding protein

absent from vegetative slime-mold cells but synthesized as the cells differentiate to a cohesive form. In cohesive slime-mold cells of some species, it may comprise as much as 2 to 3 percent of the total cellular protein. This potential CAM agglutinates erythrocytes that contain cell-surface oligosaccharides to which the lectin can bind. This provides an easy assay for the presence of the lectin in cell extracts, and suggests that the lectin could be a CAM like that shown in Fig. 21-2C.

Considerable evidence has accumulated in support of this hypothesis [reviewed in 1, 2]. First, the lectin has been demonstrated on the surface of cohesive cells in an active, carbohydrate-binding form. Second, there are complementary receptors on the cell surface to which the purified lectin can bind with high affinity. Third, the purified lectin agglutinates fixed slime-mold cells that have lost their endogenous lectin activity. Fourth, Fab fragments prepared from antibodies raised against the lectin can, under certain experimental conditions, interfere with cell-cell adhesion [8]. Finally, a slime-mold mutant that shows impaired cell adhesion appears to contain an abnormal structural gene for the lectin, so the lectin protein synthesized during development lacks agglutination activity [9].

Some puzzling problems remain. First, Fab fragments directed against the lectin are not very potent blockers of cell-cell adhesion [8]. Although this could occur if Fab binds with a lower affinity to the antigen than the antigen does to its receptor, implication of the lectin as a CAM would be more convincing if the Fab result were stronger. Second, about 98 percent of the lectin is found intracellularly and only 2 percent is on the cell surface. Although it is difficult to understand why a CAM is concentrated intracellularly, the lectin is so abundant that 2 percent represents more than 10^5 molecules per cell surface—a very respectable number. Third, it has recently been shown that there are several genes that direct the synthesis of the major lectin of *D. discoideum,* making interpretation of the mutant studies more difficult. Despite these uncertainties, the bulk of the evidence supports a role for the lectin in cell adhesion and supports the general hypothesis that cell adhesion is mediated by the binding of a cell-surface, carbohydrate-binding protein and its complementary oligosaccharide receptor. Some work in the nervous system is also consistent with this general conclusion.

Studies of Cell Adhesion in the Nervous System

Considerable effort has been devoted to two problems: (1) whether retinotectal associations are indeed due to specific cell adhesion and (2) identification of cell adhesion molecules and determination of their specificity.

SPECIFIC CELL ADHESION IN RETINA AND TECTUM

Marchase and Barbera [10, 11] have sought to determine if there is selective adhesiveness between retinal cells from specific regions and particular parts of tectum. They split tecta of chick embryos into dorsal and ventral halves and fastened a number of each to the bottom of a petri dish. Dissociated, radiolabeled retinal cells from either the dorsal or ventral retina were added, and after reaction for some hours, the relative binding of dorsal or ventral retinal cells to dorsal or ventral tectal halves was determined. Dorsal retinal cells preferentially bound to ventral tecta, whereas ventral retinal cells preferentially bound to dorsal tecta [11]. Effects of a number of glycosidases and simple sugars on these adhesive reactions were studied. Because of specific inhibitory effects either upon addition of N-acetylgalactosamine to the binding assay or pretreatment of retina or tectum with β-N-acetylhexosaminidase, a CAM containing a terminal N-acetylgalactosamine residue was inferred [10]. The data suggested that this molecule, concentrated on dorsal tectal cells and dorsal retinal cells, binds to a specific complementary substance concentrated on ventral retinal and tectal cells. Furthermore, some evidence suggests that the relevant molecule is a glycolipid, G_{M2} ganglioside [10], which has a terminal N-acetylgalactosamine.

Another approach, that taken by Gottlieb, Glaser, and coworkers, supports a difference in cell-surface adhesive properties of dorsal and ventral retinal cells and suggests a gradient of specificity [12]. In these experiments, retinas of chick embryos, either unlabeled or labeled by incorporation of ^{32}P, were separated into 6 equal segments arranged dorsoventrally. The retinal cells were then dissociated, and some were bound to a glass surface and reacted with labeled cells from all the segments. A gradient was demonstrated, in that the most dorsal cells bound best to the most ventral, in a graded fashion. This would be consistent with a model like that already considered in Fig. 21-1. Its molecular basis has not yet been determined.

Taken together, these results support the hypothesis that specific cell-adhesion reactions may play a role in the formation of specific retinotectal synaptic connections. Another important result of the studies is that these selective adhesive reactions may be measurable only at critical stages in embryo development. Cells from very early or very late embryos do not show specific binding, presumably because either they lack the specific CAMs or the action of other CAMs prevails. The adhesive specificity in retina and tectum does not appear to be confined to the retinal ganglion cells and the tectal cell processes with which they associate: retinal ganglion cells comprise only a tiny fraction of the total cellular population of the retina, and yet specific binding apparently is not confined to this small number of cells. Thus, it appears that the retinal cells in the various zones contain the specific properties measured in the binding assay, even though most will never interact with the tectum. Likewise, the part of the optic tectum to which retinal cells are bound in the assay that uses tectal halves is its surface, which is distant from the tectal neurites with which synapses form.

SEARCH FOR CAMS IN THE NERVOUS SYSTEM

Approaches like those employed with cellular slime molds have been used in an attempt to identify CAMs in the nervous system. In one approach, cells of a tissue are dissociated, and the aggregation of those cells, measured in various ways, is determined in the presence and absence of crude materials that are being screened for CAMs. A variety of sources of these materials have been used, including the media of cultured embryo cells, aqueous tissue extracts, or extracts of membrane-associated materials. This approach may be illustrated by work of Hausman and Moscona [13], who isolated a factor from membrane preparations of neural retina cells of 10-day-old chick embryos that markedly increased the size of aggregates formed by gyrating dissociated neural retinal cells from these embryos. It had no effect on aggregate formation with dissociated optic tectal or cerebral cells. The factor, which could not be obtained from neural retina cells of embryos older than 13 days, was shown to be a glycoprotein with molecular weight of approximately 50,000.

Lectins have been identified in embryonic chick brain [14] and muscle [15]. Although there is presently no evidence that these are CAMs, the work with slime molds encourages further exploration of this possibility. In muscle, appearance of a lectin shows a striking degree of developmental regulation [15]. The lectin is low in 8-day-old pectoral muscle, rises to a maximum between 12 and 16 days of embryonic development and declines to very low levels in the adult. In brain, there are also some changes with development, but the maximum level is much lower than in muscle [14]. The lectin interacts with β-galactosides, including lactose, and has been purified by affinity chromatography. It appears to be identical in muscle, brain, and other tissues [16]. It has been localized immunologically to optic tectal neurons during nervous system development, but it is not detected in these cells thereafter [17]. The lectin is predominantly intracellular, but a fraction appears to be detectable on the cell surface, where it might function as a CAM.

Rutishauser, Edelman, and colleagues have raised antibodies to embryonic chick retinal cells and have shown that univalent antibody fragments prepared from such antibodies block aggregation of dissociated retinal cells [18]. By purifying retinal-cell components and searching for the material that adsorbs this blocking activity, they have purified a protein with apparent molecular weight (in sodium dodecylsulfate) of about 140,000 that they believe to be a CAM. Antibody raised against this purified protein also blocks aggregation of dissociated retinal cells. The antibody binds to the surface of retinal neurons but is not completely specific, in that it also binds to cells from brain, spinal cord, sympathetic and dorsal root ganglia. The univalent antibody fragments block the association of axons into bundles when added to spinal ganglion cultures. This novel assay supports a biological function for the antigen, perhaps in axon-axon association [19]. However, as indicated in the discussion of the slime-mold studies, evidence of this type does not conclusively demonstrate that the antigen is a CAM in the sense that the molecule directly binds cells together. Nevertheless, this provocative finding underscores the potentiality of the immunological approach.

The search for other antibodies that influence cell adhesion will be facilitated by further development of valid cell-adhesion assays. It is also encouraged by advances in immunological sophistication, which include the promising monoclonal antibody technique [20]. This procedure allows preparation of large amounts of monospecific antibodies, even when one is starting with a mixture of uncharacterized proteins. In this technique, an animal is immunized with a crude mixture of antigens, such as whole-brain homogenate, and its antibody-forming cells are fused with a cell line that allows propagation of each antibody-forming cell in culture. Clones of individual antibody-forming cells are isolated. Those directed to cell-surface antigens might be identified easily by preliminary screening methods. Then, by testing the effects of each of these antibodies in an appropriate cell-adhesion assay, one might determine the number and nature of CAMs in this system. Recently, the monoclonal antibody technique has been used to demonstrate a very marked topographic gradient of an antigen in the developing chick retina [21]. There were 35 times as much antigen in the dorsoposterior retina as in the ventroanterior retina. However, the possible participation of this antigen in cell adhesion has not yet been examined.

Acknowledgment

Preparation of this chapter was supported in part by grants from the McKnight Foundation and the National Institute of Mental Health.

References

1. Barondes, S. H. (ed.). *Neuronal Recognition.* New York: Plenum, 1976.
2. Garrod, D. R. (ed.). *Specificity of Embryological Interactions* (Receptors and Recognition, Series B., Vol. 4). London: Chapman and Hall, 1978.
3. Sperry, R. W. Chemoaffinity in the orderly growth of nerve fiber patterns and connections. *Proc. Natl. Acad. Sci. U.S.A.* 50:703–710, 1963.
4. Orr, C. W., and Roseman, S. Intercellular adhesion: A quantitative assay for measuring the rate of adhesion. *J. Membr. Biol.* 1:110–116, 1969.
5. Walther, B. T., Ohman, R., and Roseman, S. A quantitative assay for intercellular adhesion. *Proc. Natl. Acad. Sci. U.S.A.* 70:1569–1573, 1973.
6. Müller, K., and Gerisch, G. A specific glycoprotein as the target site of adhesion blocking Fab on aggregating *Dictyostelium* cells. *Nature* 274:445–449, 1978.
7. Rosen, S. D., Kafka, J. A., Simpson, D. L., and Barondes, S. H. Developmentally regulated, carbohydrate binding protein in *Dictyostelium discoideum. Proc. Natl. Acad. Sci. U.S.A.* 70:2554–2557, 1973.
8. Rosen, S. D., Chang, C-M., and Barondes, S. H. Intercellular adhesion in the cellular slime mold *P. Pallidum* inhibited by interactions of asialofetuin or specific univalent antibody with endogenous cell surface lectin. *Dev. Biol.* 61:202–213, 1977.
9. Ray, J., Shinnick, T., and Lerner, R. A mutation altering the function of a carbohydrate binding protein blocks cell-cell cohesion in developing *Dictyostelium discoideum. Nature* 279:215–221, 1979.
10. Marchase, R. B. Biochemical investigations of retinotectal adhesive specificity. *J. Cell Biol.* 75:237–257, 1977.
11. Barbera, A. J., Marchase, R. B., and Roth, S. Adhesive recognition and retinotectal specificity. *Proc. Natl. Acad. Sci. U.S.A.* 70:2482–2486, 1973.
12. Gottlieb, D. I., Rock, K., and Glaser, L. A gradient of adhesive specificity in developing avian retina. *Proc. Natl. Acad. Sci. U.S.A.* 73:410–414, 1976.
13. Hausman, R. F., and Moscona, A. A. Purification and characterization of the retina-specific cell-aggregating factor. *Proc. Natl. Acad. Sci. U.S.A.* 72:916–920, 1975.
14. Kobiler, D., and Barondes, S. H. Lectin activity from embryonic chick brain, heart, and liver: Changes with development. *Dev. Biol.* 60:326–330, 1977.
15. Nowak, T. P., Haywood, P. L., and Barondes, S. H. Developmentally regulated lectin in embryonic chick muscle and a myogenic cell line. *Biochem. Biophys. Res. Comm.* 68:650–657, 1976.
16. Kobiler, D., Beyer, E. C., and Barondes, S. H. Developmentally regulated lectins from chick muscle, brain and liver have similar chemical and immunological properties. *Dev. Biol.* 64:265–272, 1978.
17. Gremo, F., Kobiler, D., and Barondes, S. H. Distribution of an endogenous lectin in the developing chick optic tectum. *J. Cell Biol.* 79:491–499, 1978.
18. Rutishauser, U., Thiery, J.-P., Brackenbury, R., and Edelman, G. M. Adhesion among neural cells of the chick embryo. III. Relationship of the surface molecule CAM to cell adhesion and the development of histotypic patterns. *J. Cell Biol.* 79:371–381, 1978.
19. Rutishauser, U., Gall, W. E., and Edelman, G. M. Adhesion among neural cells of the chick embryo. IV. Role of the cell surface molecule CAM in the formation of neurite bundles in cultures of spinal ganglia. *J. Cell Biol.* 79:382–393, 1978.
20. Kohler, G., and Milstein, C. Continuous cultures of fused cells secreting antibody of predefined specificity. *Nature* 256:495–499, 1975.
21. Trislen, D., Schneider, M., and Nirenberg, M. A topographic gradient of molecules in retina can be used to identify neuron position. *Proc. Natl. Acad. Sci. U.S.A.* 78:2145–2149, 1981.
22. Barondes, S. H. Brain Glycomacromolecules and Interneuronal Recognition. In F. O. Schmitt (ed.), *The Neurosciences: A Second Study Program.* New York: The Rockefeller University Press, 1970. Pp. 747–760.

Chapter 22. Axoplasmic Transport

The long axonal extension of the neuron requires a continual supply of materials synthesized in the cell body—a wide range of soluble proteins, membranous components, and various organelles. Some of the materials transported are needed to replace constituents that turn over in the membrane and organelles of the fiber, others are needed to bring substances participating in energy metabolism. Still other components transported are neurotransmitters or transmitter-related components supplied to the nerve terminals for release and subsequent excitation of postsynaptic cells. Neurotrophic substances and modulators are released as well from the nerve terminals to affect the functional state of juxtaposed cells. The general properties of the transport of material in nerves and its characteristics have been described in recent reviews [1–8].

Methods of Study and Characteristics of Transport

ANTEROGRADE TRANSPORT

If the nerve fibers are interrupted, for example, by cutting or ligating, a bulging of the nerve fibers is seen a few millimeters proximal to the level of interruption. This "damming" was considered by Weiss and Hiscoe [9] to be caused by a continual outward movement of all the axonal contents, that is, their "growth" down within the sheath. EM studies show a growth of fine regenerating fibers forming within a few millimeters of the ends of the interrupted nerve fibers [10], and a differential accumulation of vesicles, mitochondria, soluble proteins, and other components within the fibers [11]. Also accumulated are specific neurotransmitters, such as norepinephrine (NE), that are present in dense-core vesicles (DCVs) and seen as a

fluorescent material in formaldehyde-treated nerve preparations. By this means, Dahlström and her coworkers found that NE accumulates quickly proximal to ligations or crushes, in a manner expected of a fast rate of transport away from the cell body [12]. Brimijoin and Wiermaa used a cold-block technique and found a fast rate of transport of the DCVs as measured by their content of dopamine β-hydroxylase (DBH) and NE, at a rate close to 400 mm/day [13]. This was confirmed by double-ligation studies of nerve, which showed that NE moves at this same fast rate [14]. Those studies also showed that dopamine (DA) moves at a fast rate, as a result of a constant turnover of amines in the DCVs as they are being transported. Acetylcholinesterase (AChE) also moves at a fast rate in mammalian cholinergic fibers [3], at close to 410 mm/day [15]. This same fast rate of AChE transport was also found in frog nerve when the rate was calculated for a temperature of 38°C and the Q_{10} was taken into account [16].

A more direct measure of transport rates and the properties of transport within the fibers is by the use of precursors labeled with radionuclides, such as ^{32}P as orthophosphate, ^{35}S-, ^{3}H-, or ^{14}C-labeled amino acids, [^{3}H]fucose, and various other labeled precursors [1–2, 4–8]. By injecting the precursor directly into the nervous system near the cell bodies, the blood-brain barrier is bypassed, allowing a much higher level of uptake of precursor by the cells with a correspondingly higher level of radioactivity transported into the fibers [2]. This also reduces the adventitious uptake and labeling of Schwann cells and other nonaxonal components of nerve that are seen with systemic injection.

By use of a high concentration of [^{3}H]leucine and the relatively long sciatic nerve available in the cat, a fast outflow of labeled proteins was found when the ventral-horn motoneuron region of the seventh lumbar spinal segment (L7) or the L7 dorsal-root ganglion was injected [2]. The precursor is taken up relatively quickly by the cells and incorporated into labeled proteins and polypeptides. The subsequent movement down the sciatic nerve fibers can be shown by autoradiography. The rate of outflow is determined by removing the nerves at various times after injection and cutting them into small pieces for counting in a scintillation spectrometer. The outflow of radioactivity typically shows a plateau that rises to a characteristic crest distally and then drops steeply to background levels [Fig. 22-1].

The front of radioactivity was found to move outward in cat sciatic nerves linearly with time, at a rate of 410 ± 50 mm/day. This same rate was found in the sciatic nerves of various mammalian species that range in size from the rat to the goat [17]. It does not depend on the function of the nerve, whether sensory or motor, and as shown by autoradiography, the same rate is present in myelinated fibers of 3 to 22 μm diameter, as well as in unmyelinated fibers [5, 17]. The same rate of close to 410 mm/day was computed in the fibers of non-mammalian specimens—the garfish olfactory [18] and frog sciatic nerves [19]—at a temperature of $38°C$, taking into account the Q_{10}. The Q_{10}'s reported vary from 2 to 3.5, with a Q_{10} of 2 found in cat nerve [20].

The cell bodies are not essential for fast transport. Once the labeled proteins gain entry to the fibers, the cell bodies can be destroyed or a proximal ligation can be made without affecting transport in the fibers distal to the ligation [2].

Transport is also widely studied in the visual system by injecting labeled amino acids into the posterior chamber of the eye for uptake by the ganglion cells of the retina [8]. In the fish, bird, and rodent, the optic fibers from each eye cross almost entirely to terminate in the opposite tectum or lateral geniculate. After protein synthesis in the ganglion cells, protein transport in the optic nerve is shown by the pattern of labeled protein in the nerve or by the accumulated radioactivity in the

nerve endings in the tectum (fish and bird) or lateral geniculate (mammal) of the opposite side [8]. However, the precursor also leaks from the eye into the blood circulation to a considerable degree and gains entry directly into optic nerve terminals in the tectum or lateral geniculate, where proteins are also synthesized locally. To control for this uptake and incorporation of precursor locally from the circulation, the radioactivity present in the ipsilateral tectum or lateral geniculate, which do not receive the axonally transported components, is subtracted from that of the side contralateral to the injected eye. [³H]proline is a better precursor to use in the visual system than is [³H]leucine, because proline does not as readily pass the blood-brain barrier to become locally incorporated in the tectum or lateral geniculate [21]. In studies of the visual system, several waves of accumulation of labeled materials have been seen, and this suggests several slow- and fast-transport systems, with the fastest rate close to 200 mm/day [8].

A wide range of labeled proteins and polypeptides are transported. To study this aspect of transport, sciatic nerve, tectum, or lateral geniculate are dissected and homogenized at various times after labeled precursor has been injected. After differential centrifugation of the homogenate, gel-filtration of the high-speed supernatant fractions is used to separate the protein and polypeptide components. Soluble proteins with M_r 10,000 to more than 450,000 and peptides below 10,000 are transported at both fast and slow rates in nerve [22]. Several hours after the injection of the precursor, at a time corresponding to the arrival of substances by fast transport, the particulate fraction of the homogenized tissue is labeled to a greater extent than other components. Later, when nerves or optic tecta are removed one to several days or weeks after injection, a greater proportion of soluble proteins of higher molecular weight are found [8, 22].

Sodium dodecylsulfate–polyacrylamide gel electrophoresis (SDS-PAGE) is a powerful technique used to assess the various monomeric proteins transported [23]. By this method a large number of individual proteins are found to be labeled.

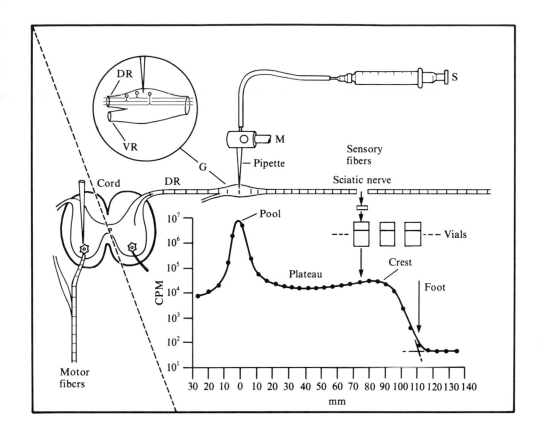

Fig. 22-1. Technique of isotope labeling and outflow pattern of fast transport. The L7 dorsal root (DR) ganglion is shown with a pipette held by a micromanipulator (M) inserted for injection of [³H]leucine, using a polyethylene tube and syringe (S). (Insert shows ganglion with T-shaped nerve cells.) The dorsal root ganglion (G) and sciatic nerve are cut into 5 mm segments. Each segment is placed in a vial and solubilized; scintillation fluid is added and counted. The display of activity in counts per minute (CPM) is shown, using a logarithmic scale on the ordinate and the distance in millimeters on the abscissa, taking zero as the ganglion. A typical pattern for a 6.5 hour downflow is shown. A high level of activity remains in the ganglion and falls distally to a plateau before rising to a crest. A sharp drop is seen at the front of the crest down to the baseline level at its foot. At the left of the slanting dashed line (left), an injection of the L7 ventral horn is shown for uptake of precursor by the motor neurons. The ventral root (VR) and sciatic nerve are cut and measured for outflow, as in the ganglion injection.

Analysis of small segments of nerve taken along its length at different times after injection indicates the apparent rate at which a given polypeptide species is moving. The rates for various peptides so derived in the rabbit visual system are classed as: group I, at least 240 mm/day; group II, 34–68 mm/day; group III, 4–8 mm/day; group IV, 2–4 mm/day; and group V, 0.7–1.1 mm/day [23, 24] (see also Chap. 20, Table 20-1). Much variation in these rates is found, depending on the species and nerve system investigated [8].

This technique has shown that α and β tubulins, the subunits of microtubules, are slowly transported at about 1 mm/day along with a triplet of polypeptides of 200,000, 145,000, and 68,000 M_r, which represent the subunits of the neurofilaments [25, 26]. These polypeptides are discussed in Chap. 20. A calcium-activated protease that degrades the higher molecular-weight components needs to be taken into account when assessing the presence of triplet subunits [27]. Other identified polypeptides transported at a somewhat faster rate of 3 to 4 mm/day include actin [28, 29]. The question of how the various, slowly transported components are carried down the fibers, whether by one or more separate transport mechanisms or by the same mechanism responsible for fast transport (*unitary hypothesis*), is discussed later in this chapter under Unitary Hypothesis.

OTHER CHARACTERISTICS OF ANTEROGRADE TRANSPORT

When [³H]glucosamine or [³H]fucose was used as a precursor, fast downflow of labeled glycoproteins and glycolipids incorporated into membranes was found [30–32]. Rapid transport of sulfated glycoproteins and mucopolysaccharides was found when $^{35}SO_4^{2-}$ was used as the precursor [33]. The fast downflow of phospholipids seen with [³H]choline as a precursor [34], and the transport of [³H]cholesterol following uptake [35], is a further indication of the downflow of membrane or membrane-bound materials. The slower transport of phospholipids [2, 36], shown by using $^{32}P_i$ as a precursor, probably is the result of differences in the time at which lipids are phosphorylated from the phosphate compartment in the cell bodies.

Motion of particles in single fibers is visualized by dark-field or Nomarski optics microscopy [37–39]. These particles include the relatively large mitochondria seen moving both in the anterograde and retrograde directions, with rates at times approaching that of fast transport. On the other hand, biochemical techniques for labeling and measuring the mitochondria have clearly shown that they accumulate at ligations or cut ends of nerve fibers with a slow-transport pattern [1, 2, 40]. The apparent conflict is due to the fact that the mitochondria move only infrequently. This behavior may be expected on the basis of the unitary hypothesis.

Transport of components into the nerve terminals was found by injecting brain with [³H]leucine and isolating the synaptosomes at different times

thereafter by differential centrifugation [41]. Over a period of days, the specific activity of the labeled proteins in the synaptosomal fraction increased, as expected of their slow transport into the terminals. Local synthesis of protein in the terminals is not likely to account for this pattern (see Chap. 19). Studies have shown fast transport of labeled polypeptides into synaptosomes, as well; the major peak has M_r of 60,000 and is precipitable by vinblastine [42]. One identified polypeptide found to be transported at a fast rate into synaptosomes after [³H]leucine has been applied topically to the exposed cortex is a calcium-binding protein (CaBP) [43]. The CaBP (possibly calmodulin) presumably plays an important role in the regulation of Ca^{2+} in the nerve terminals (see Calcium Regulatory Mechanisms, below).

Another interesting technique is the intracellular injection of a labeled amino acid, such as [³H]-glycine, directly into single motoneuron cell bodies. The precursor is rapidly incorporated into labeled proteins which, as shown by autoradiography, are carried down the axon and into the dendrites, as well [44]. Interestingly, after [³H]glycine is injected into single *Aplysia* neurons R3–R14, the amino acid appears to be transported in the nerve as such [45], the glycine acting as a neurotransmitter. Single-cell injections have been used to particular advantage by Schwartz and coworkers [7]. Injection of the *Aplysia* serotonergic R2 cell with [³H]serotonin is followed by an outflow of [³H]serotonin packaged in DCVs into the giant nerve fiber, and the outflow pattern has the same characteristics as those found in mammalian multifiber nerves [46]. The rate of outflow in the *Aplysia* neuron, calculated at 37°C, is close to 410 mm/day.

Many other substances are known to be transported in axons and dendrites [1–8].

RETROGRADE TRANSPORT

Retrograde transport from nerve endings toward the cell body was first seen by Lubinska and coworkers as an accumulation of AChE just distal to nerve ligations [3]. Variations of rates of retrograde transport of AChE have been reported, but when assessed by double ligations in cat sciatic nerve, the rate was found to be close to 220 mm/day [15]. Some substances have even higher rates of retrograde transport [39, 47]. The list of exogenous substances known to be taken up by nerve and transported toward the perikaryon includes tetanus toxin and herpes and polio viruses. The protein horseradish peroxidase (HRP), taken up by nerve terminals and retrogradely transported [40, 48, 49], has been widely employed as a marker to show the paths of fibers in the CNS. The mechanisms by which different substances are taken up by the nerve terminals were studied by using HRP, nerve growth factor (NGF), cholera toxin, wheat germ agglutinin, ricin II, phytohemagglutinin, and concanavalin A [50]. These, when injected into the anterior chamber of the eye, are taken by the terminals of the adrenergic neurons in the iris and carried by retrograde transport to the cell bodies located in the superior cervical ganglion. Nerve growth factor taken up by terminals of sensory and sympathetic nerve fibers in the immature organism and transported to the cell body plays a role in the maturation of the neuron (see Chap. 23).

Dark-field microscopy shows that a larger number of particules move in the retrograde than in the anterograde direction [38, 39]. This is due to limitations of size resolution. Electron microscopy has shown that many of the particles undergoing retrograde transport are relatively large, multilamellated bodies [51, 52]. Most of the smaller vesicular and tubulovesicular bodies carried by anterograde transport and accumulating proximal to nerve interruptions fall below the resolution of light microscopy.

Retrograde transport has a role in the regulation of protein synthesis in the cell bodies. After transection of nerve fibers, chromatolysis of the cells appears in several days, at the time when levels of nucleic acids and proteins increase in the nerve-cell bodies. These changes are related to neuronal regeneration (see Chap. 23). Chromatolysis does not appear to be associated with changes in the rate or the amount of substances carried distally within the nerve fibers by fast transport [53]. The onset of chromatolysis could possibly be caused by the loss of a signal substance which normally is transported proximally in the fibers to act in the perikaryon as a negative-feedback control of synthesis [2]. An alternative possibility, indicated by the work of Bisby [47], is that the earlier return of components to the cell bodies seen after making nerve interruptions [54] may be a positive signal for the initiation of chromatolysis.

Metabolism and Fast Axoplasmic Transport
OXIDATIVE PHOSPHORYLATION
Fast axoplasmic transport is maintained in vitro with the same form and rate as seen in vivo. The precursor [³H]leucine is injected into the L7 dorsal root ganglion and 2 hours of downflow are allowed in vivo before the sciatic nerves are removed and placed into chambers equilibrated with moist 95 percent O_2 + 5 percent CO_2 at a temperature of 38°C or into flasks containing oxygenated Ringer's solution [20]. The similarity of axoplasmic transport in vitro to that in vivo was shown by the same crest advancing at the same rate. Transport in vitro is maintained for 6 hours or more in glucose-free media, indicating that there is an adequate store of endogenous metabolites present in the fibers.

The dependence of transport on oxidative metabolism was shown with in vitro preparations by the replacement of oxygen with nitrogen, which blocks transport within 15 min (Fig. 21-2). Cyanide, azide, or dinitrophenol, inhibitors of mitochondrial oxidative phosphorylation (see Chap. 17), all produce a block in this same period of time [2]. At the time of block, the total ~P (the level of ATP and creatine phosphate) fell from 1.2 μ moles per gram to approximately half that value [55]. The remaining ~P is not available to the fast axoplasmic-transport mechanism and may be sequestered in Schwann cells or in some axonal compartment inaccessible to the transport mechanism. Axoplasmic transport and action potentials fail at approximately the same time after initiating anoxia [56].

GLYCOLYSIS
When sheathed nerves transporting labeled proteins in vitro were exposed to iodoacetic acid (IAA),

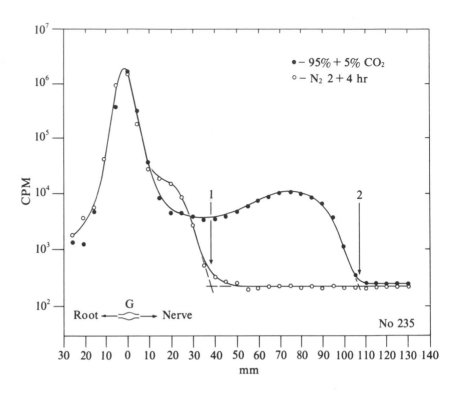

Fig. 22-2. *Block of in vitro downflow by N_2. In vitro transport shown in nerves removed from an animal 2 hours after injecting the L7 dorsal root ganglion with [^3H]leucine. One nerve (o) was placed in a chamber containing moist, 95% O_2 + 5% CO_2 for an additional 4 hours and kept at 38° C. The rate of transport in vitro was that expected of fast transport in the animal (arrow 2). The other nerve (o) was similarly treated, except that it was exposed to N_2 in a chamber for 4 hours. The crest advanced no further than that of the 2 hours of downflow (arrow 1) that had taken place in the animal.*

transport declined slowly; a complete block appeared in 1.5 to 2.0 hours [56]. This delay does not represent slow entry of IAA through the perineural sheaths and the axolemma of the nerve fibers, because a complete inhibition of the key glycolytic enzyme glyceraldehyde-phosphate dehydrogenase (Chap. 17) takes place in the nerve after only 10 minutes of exposure to IAA [55].

The longer time needed to block transport after inhibition of glycolysis than that after interruption of mitochondrial phosphorylation may be explained by the utilization of acetyl-CoA or other metabolites that aid in maintaining that supply of ATP for a time. When those metabolites are exhausted, mitochondrial ATP production fails. Consistent with this interpretation is the finding that the level of $\sim$P in nerve exposed to IAA also fell to about half the control level of 1.5 to 2.0 hours when fast axoplasmic transport was blocked [56]. When pyruvate or lactate was added to the IAA-treated nerves, fast transport was almost normal, and levels of $\sim$P remained close to control values

[57]. Pyruvate was approximately 20 times more effective in maintaining transport with IAA present than was lactate.

Banks and his colleagues found that the interruption of glycolysis with fluoride also blocked fast axoplasmic transport, the addition of pyruvate preventing the block [58].

TRICARBOXYLIC ACID CYCLE
The tricarboxylic acid cycle can be blocked by fluorocitrate derived from added fluoroacetate

(FA). Nerves exposed in vitro to FA in concentrations of 4 to 10 mM, showed a block of fast axoplasmic transport in approximately 1.0 to 1.5 hours [56]. The ~P at the time of block falls to the critical level of 0.5 to 0.6 μmol/g, that is, half the control level. As with the block of glycolysis with IAA, when oxidizable metabolites are exhausted, ATP production fails and fast axoplasmic transport is blocked.

LOCAL ANOXIA AND ENERGY STORES
The supply of ATP is maintained locally all along the nerve fiber. This was indicated by covering a small region of the nerve distal to the advancing crest of labeled protein with a plastic strip spread with petrolatum [59]. The anoxia so produced caused a block of fast axoplasmic transport, as shown by the damming of radioactivity proximal to just the anoxic region and the lack of labeled components distal to it. The front of the dammed radioactivity remained sharp, thus showing no diffusion of labeled materials into the anoxic region of the fibers. Neither oxygen nor ATP appears to diffuse significantly from the oxygenated portion of nerve into the adjacent covered portion. If they did diffuse, the transport mechanism would have been supplied with its needed source of energy and labeled materials would be carried into that region.

When, after a period up to 1.5 hours, the local anoxic block was relieved by removing the petrolatum strips covering the nerves, fast axoplasmic transport resumed without any significant delay. After anoxia lasting 1.75 hours and longer, transport did not recover immediately. Even so, transport can recover if longer recovery times are allowed. By using cuff compression to produce anoxia in vivo, it was found that transport could resume after anoxia lasting up to 7 hours, if some days are allowed for recovery [60]. A long time required for recovery after longer periods of anoxia was also seen in studies where a direct compression of nerves was accomplished [61]. After long periods of anoxia, electrical excitability returns much more quickly than does axoplasmic transport. This phenomenon, termed *dissociation* [60], may possibly be due to an altered Ca^{2+} regulation.

A Model of Axoplasmic Transport and the Role of Calcium

A transport model that accounts for the ATP requirement and the finding that a wide range of materials, including particles such as DCVs and mitochondria, soluble proteins of high molecular weight, polypeptides, and amino acids, all are transported at a fast rate, is the *transport filament hypothesis* [62]. The various materials transported are considered to be bound to hypothetical transport filaments that act as common carriers. It is supposed that the filaments with their bound components move along the microtubules or neurofilaments, or both, by means of side-arms, and that ATP is utilized as the energy source for side-arm movement [63] (Fig. 22-3).

The model is analogous to the sliding-filament model of muscle contraction (see Chap. 27). In axoplasmic transport, the microtubules act as the stationary elements along which the transport filaments are moved. The ATP required for movement of the filaments by the side-arms is considered to be utilized by $(Ca^{2+} + Mg^{2+})$-ATPase, an enzyme found in nerve [64]. Recently, the $Ca^{2+} + Mg^{2+}$-ATPase associated with microtubules has been implicated [65].

We would expect that in accord with this model Ca^{2+} or Mg^{2+} (or both) would be necessary to maintain transport. However, until recently there has been little evidence for dependence of transport on either Ca^{2+} or Mg^{2+}. Transport in vitro was normal even in nerves placed in a Ca^{2+}-free medium. It was demonstrated that this normal transport is due to the low ionic permeability of the perineural sheath. When a desheathed nerve preparation was used, it was found that Ca^{2+} is, in fact, required to maintain transport [66, 67]. For those studies, the L7 dorsal root ganglion was injected with [^{3}H]leucine and, after a period of downflow, the sciatic nerve carrying the labeled proteins was removed. The peroneal branch was desheathed, the tibial branch remained sheathed to serve as a control. This preparation, when placed in a medium containing Ringer's solution, showed axoplasmic transport of the usual pattern in both the desheathed and sheathed branches. However, when nerves so prepared were

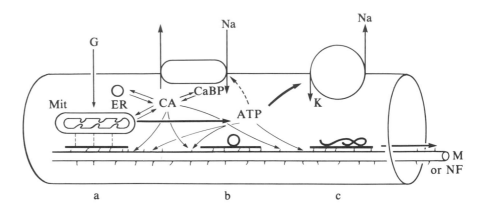

incubated in a Ca^{2+}-free solution (i.e., in an isotonic NaCl or sucrose medium), a block of transport was first seen only in the desheathed peroneal nerve within 30 minutes and was complete within approximately 2.6 hours (Fig. 22-4).

Transport in the sheathed tibial branch remained unaffected because of the low permeability of the perineural sheath and retention of Ca^{2+} within the endoneural space. A similar block of transport was seen in the desheathed branch placed in a Ringer's medium that contained 4 mM EGTA, as would be expected if the lack of Ca^{2+} is critical in causing the block. In support of this interpretation, a normal form and rate of axoplasmic transport was maintained in the desheathed nerve when 5 mM Ca^{2+} was added to either an isotonic saline or sucrose solution as seen in Fig. 22-5.

However, Ca^{2+} is normally present at levels of 1.5 to 2.0 mM in extracellular fluid in the body. With this concentration of Ca^{2+} in the in vitro studies, a partial defect in transport appears in the desheathed nerve. Normal transport can be restored with the addition of 4 mM K^+ to a medium containing 1.5 mM Ca^{2+} [67]. Potassium appears to facilitate Ca^{2+}, but K^+ cannot substitute for Ca^{2+} except at the high levels of 50 to 70 mM [67].

In confirming the requirement of Ca^{2+} for transport in nerve fibers, Hammerschlag and coworkers consider it to have a specific role in the gating of transported components from the cell body to its fiber [68].

Although Mg^{2+} acts somewhat like Ca^{2+} on the transport mechanism, it was not able to replace

Fig. 22-3. Transport filament hypothesis. Glucose (G) enters the fibers, and after oxidative phosphorylation in the mitochondrion (Mit), ATP is produced. A pool of ATP supplies energy to the sodium pump, which controls the level of Na^+ and K^+ in the fiber, and to the microtubule side-arms for the movement of transport filaments (shown as black bars). The various components bound to the filaments and carried down the fiber include (a) the mitochondrion giving rise to a fast, but temporary, movement (with a slow net forward movement); (b) particulates or vesicles; and (c) soluble protein or polypeptides (shown as folded or globular configurations). Thus, a wide range of component types and sizes is carried down the fiber at the same fast rate. Cross-bridges between the transport filament and the microtubules effect the movement when supplied by ATP. In addition, Ca^{2+} is shown participating in transport filament movement. Regulation of Ca^{2+} is shown with sequestration in mitochondria and ER, and binding to CaBP. A Na^+-Ca^{2+} exchange or Ca^{2+} pump (ATP supplied by dashed line) is present in the membrane.

Ca^{2+} in maintaining transport to the same degree in the desheathed cat-nerve preparation [66]. Addition of magnesium ion prolonged transport beyond the time when block was seen in nerves placed in an isotonic saline or sucrose medium (3.5 hours compared to 2.6 hours). Magnesium ion may act to retain Ca^{2+} within the fibers in nerves placed in a low-Ca^{2+} medium.

REGULATION OF CALCIUM AND TRANSPORT
The block of transport seen in a Ca^{2+}-free medium is probably due to its depletion in the nerve fibers. Free Ca^{2+} in a concentration close to 10^{-7} M has

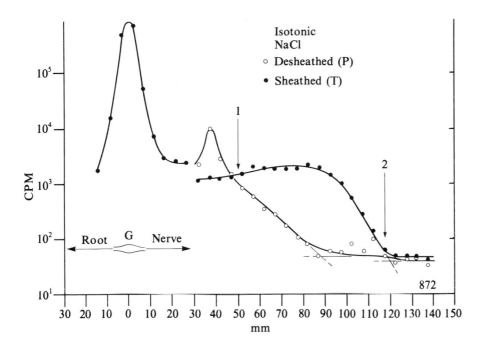

Fig. 22-4. Transport in a Ca^{2+}-free medium. Outflow in a sciatic nerve in vitro and its desheathed peroneal branch (○) and sheathed tibial branch (●) is shown after the L7 ganglion has been injected with [^{3}H]leucine. Downflow was allowed for 2 hours in the animal before the sciatic nerve was removed, the peroneal branch desheathed, and the nerve placed in an in vitro medium containing Ca^{2+}-free isotonic NaCl. Above arrow 1, approximately where the peroneal nerve is desheathed, a peak of dammed activity is seen. This is followed by a steep descent to baseline at about 2.6 hours. The tibial nerve shows typical axoplasmic transport outflow without block to arrow 2, the expected distance.

been measured in the cephalopod giant axon [69], and this level also is believed to be present in the cytoplasm of a wide variety of cells, including the axoplasm of mammalian nerve fibers (see Chap. 6). The total amount of Ca^{2+} is higher; most of it is sequestered in the mitochondria and smooth endoplasmic reticulum (ER). This was shown by means of a histochemical technique that uses pyroantimonate or oxalate to bind to Ca^{2+}; the Ca^{2+} appears as electron-dense granules in these organelles in EM sections of nerves so prepared [70, 71].

The Ca^{2+} that enters nerve fibers, either by diffusion or as a result of electrical activity, eventually is extruded from the fibers by a Na^+-Ca^{2+} exchange mechanism [69, 72] or by an energy-requiring Ca^{2+} pump in the axonal membrane [73]. The desheathed mammalian nerve preparation placed in a medium that contains from 25 to 35 mM Ca^{2+} may still show axoplasmic transport; the regulatory mechanism acts to keep the level of free Ca^{2+} low in the axoplasm. At levels above 50 to 60 mM Ca^{2+}, transport was blocked, but only after a long exposure [67]. A long exposure to high Ca^{2+} activates proteolytic enzymes, with destruction of neuronal structures as shown in small, cut pieces of nerve with their axoplasm exposed to Ca^{2+} in the medium [74].

CALMODULIN AND THE TRANSPORT MECHANISM

The application of $^{45}Ca^{2+}$ to frog dorsal root ganglion neurons is followed by transport of $^{45}Ca^{2+}$ in the fibers of the sciatic nerve [75] at a rate characteristic of fast axoplasmic transport in mammalian nerve. This comparison depends on calculating the transport rate in frog nerve at 37°C. Transport of $^{45}Ca^{2+}$ at the usual rate of 410 mm/day was also observed in the sciatic nerves of cats after injection

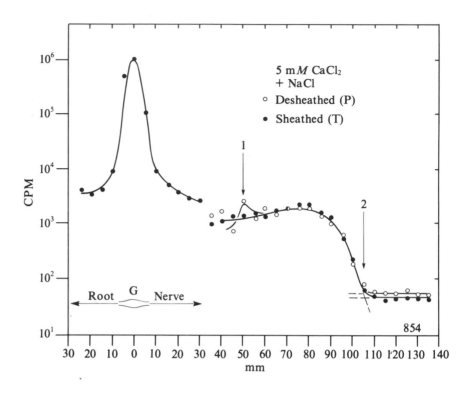

Fig. 22-5. Transport in medium containing 5 mM CaCl₂. Outflow in the desheathed peroneal branch (○) and the sheathed tibial branch (T) is shown. After 2 hours of downflow in vitro, the peroneal nerve was desheathed and the nerve placed in an in vitro medium of 5 mM CaCl₂ and 140 mM NaCl for an additional 4 hours. The points represent labeled materials present in 5 mm segments cut from the dorsal root, L7 ganglion (G), and nerve. Distal to 30 mm from the ganglion, each branch is cut individually, and thus outflow in the tibial (T) and peroneal (P) branches can be shown separately. Arrow 1 indicates the upper end of the desheathed region, and arrow 2 the front of the crests of transported material expected in both nerves. The crests seem to have the same height in this example. It should be noted that the logarithmic scale serves to diminish amplitude differences in the two branches. In general, a greater amount of labeled activity was usually transported in the tibial branch, since it is the larger of the two. A small degree of damming activity is seen above the upper site, where desheathing was initiated (arrow 1).

of the L7 dorsal root ganglia [76]. In those studies, the $^{45}Ca^{2+}$ transported was bound to a calcium-binding protein (CaBP) of approximately 15,000 M_r. Equilibrium dialysis showed that this CaBP has a K_d of 6.66×10^{-5} M for Ca^{2+}, one similar to those of other CaBPs. Calmodulin, a CaBP that activates a wide variety of enzymes, has been recognized as present in many tissues (Chaps. 3, 6, 15). Calmodulin was identified in mammalian nerve [77], and its properties were found to be similar to those of the CaBP previously found in nerve [78]. This is shown by the same molecular weight (15,000 to 17,000), similar Ca^{2+}-binding properties, and similar isoelectric focusing values (pI $\approx$ 4.1).

Fast transport of a small amount of calmodulin raises the possibility that calmodulin is bound to, or part of the transport filament itself. Calmodulin could locally activate the $(Ca^{2+} + Mg^{2+})$-ATPase on the side-arms to utilize the ATP required for movement of the transport filaments. In this regard, it is of interest that a calmodulin-related peptide was reported to be rapidly transported [79].

Alternatively, calmodulin could be closely associated with or be part of the $(Ca^{2+} + Mg^{2+})$-ATPase of the microtubular side-arms. This possibility is based on studies of the $(Ca^{2+} + Mg^{2+})$-ATPase associated with tubulin subunits. These are obtained by purifying tubulin by 2 or 3 cycles of cooling and heating (see also Chap. 20). The tubulin preparations show activation of the enzyme by Ca^{2+} in the range of 10^{-8} to $10^{-6} M$ [65], the concentration of free Ca^{2+} likely to be present in the axoplasm of the nerve. In addition, the $(Ca^{2+} + Mg^{2+})$-ATPase activity was blocked by trifluoperazine, an agent that binds to and interferes with the action of calmodulin.

To substantiate the transport-filament hypothesis, the most pressing need is to identify the transport filament itself. Actin, in its filamentous form (F actin), could possibly play that role. It is of interest that DNase I, which binds to actin and prevents it from acting, blocked axoplasmic transport when injected into the cell body [80]. However, most of the actin is transported at a slow rate [28, 29]. Fast transport of actin or some other polypeptide with an action similar to that of actin has not been identified.

UNITARY HYPOTHESIS
Much of the slow-transported material consists of the tubulins, triplet proteins, and actin (see also Chap. 20). These are viewed as being assembled at the cell body and moved as a coherent structure down the fibers by some mechanism other than that responsible for fast transport [26]. In another view, rather than separate mechanisms, slow transport is presumed to be the result of a drop-off and redistribution of materials from the fast-transport system [81, 82]. According to this extension of the transport filament model, termed the *unitary hypothesis* [81], components are considered to drop off locally in the fibers from the transport filaments. The drop-off of materials from the crest accounts for the decrease in height with distance seen in the garfish olfactory [18] and in the cat sciatic nerves [17, 83]. Those materials and the products of their turnover can return to the transport mechanism for redistribution in both the anterograde and retrograde directions [53], and this accounts for the broadening of the regular slow waves shown by Cancalon in garfish olfactory nerves [84]. Additionally, there is a slower exit of labeled, slow-transported components from the cell bodies that also contributes to the observed pattern of slow downflow. In agreement with the unitary hypothesis, the tubulins, triplet proteins, and other components usually characterized as slow-transported materials are believed to be transported as subunits: these undergo turnover in the neurofilaments, microtubules, and the actin-containing cytoskeleton structures. Some of these subunits appear to be carried in the fibers as fast-transported components [85]. It is necessary, however, to prove that these are not adventitiously bound to other fast-transported components.

MICROTUBULES AND TRANSPORT
In the model presented above, the microtubule side-arms are believed to propel the transport filaments to which the various transported materials are bound, one set of side-arms directed for anterograde transport, another for retrograde transport. The properties of microtubules are described in Chapter 20. Here we note some aspects directly related to their essential role in transport. Since the work of Dahlström and Kreutzberg, colchicine and the vinca alkaloids, vinblastine (VLB) and vincristine (VCR), substances that bind to tubulin and disrupt the microtubules of dividing cells, are known to cause disassembly of microtubules in nerve fibers and also to block axoplasmic transport [86]. A dynamic equilibrium is believed to exist between the tubulin subunits and microtubules. By binding to tubulin, the mitotic-blocking agents cause a shift of tubulin from the microtubules and thus result in their disassembly and an interruption of fast axoplasmic transport.

Disassembly of microtubules into their tubulin subunits, however, may not account for the block of axoplasmic transport in all cases; transport in invertebrate nerve was reported to be blocked without evident disruption of microtubules [87], and similar findings in mammalian nerve were reported after use of halothane [88] and the local anesthetic lidocaine [89]. On the other hand, in a quantitative study in which the mitotic-blocking agent maytansine was used, the block of transport was found to be regularly related to the microtubular disassembly measured [90]. It is possible that some alteration, perhaps random missing segments of microtubule, not readily observed as a decrease in their number in EM cross-sections, can account for the block of transport recorded before obvious evidence of disassembly appears in those preparations.

A factor in determining the effectiveness of these agents is their uptake by the fibers. A comparison of the vinca agents VCR, VLB, and the new derivative vindesine (VDS), has shown that VCR, the most neurotoxic of the three agents [91], is taken up into the fibers most readily [92]. The degree of tubulin-binding and specificity of binding to tubulin must also be considered.

Recently, it has been claimed that transport may continue in sheathed nerves of rat when microtubules are disassembled by high Ca^{2+} [93]. The explanation for this finding is not known. It suggests a permeability to Ca^{2+} that is not evident in the already mentioned studies with sheathed cat nerves [66].

Routing

The dorsal-root ganglion neurons have one fiber branch that enters the spinal cord through the dorsal root and another branch that enters the peripheral nerve. When the L7 dorsal root ganglia of monkeys were injected with [³H]leucine, the same rate of fast axoplasmic transport of labeled activity was found in each of the two branches of its neurons, but 3 to 5 times more labeled material was seen in the crest moving down the peripheral nerve branch as compared to the dorsal root [17]. The difference in the amount of labeled proteins transported could not be accounted for by measured differences in diameters, the density of microtubules, or of neurofilaments in the two branches of these neurons [94]. The asymmetry in outflow could come about by the movement of more transport filaments down the peripheral

nerve branch per unit time as compared to the dorsal root branch.

Such routing of materials in one branch of a neuron as compared to another appears to be of fundamental significance in accounting for neuronal properties. By this process, different kinds of materials can be moved selectively into the branches of the same neuron. This is obviously the case for the dorsal-root ganglion neurons where specific transmitter materials need to be supplied to the presynaptic terminals of the dorsal root branch to effect synaptic transmission in the CNS, while other specific components must supply the sensory receptor terminals for transduction of stimuli. Routing may very well underlie the preferential growth of some nerve fiber branches as compared to others in the course of maturation or regeneration [95].

Axon Membrane in Relation to Transport

Little evidence for dependence of the fast axoplasmic transport mechanism on membrane activity per se has been found. When tetrodotoxin or procaine is used to block the excitability of the membrane, fast axoplasmic transport continues as usual [2, 6]. Depolarizing the membranes of desheathed nerve fibers by replacing Na^+ with K^+ in the medium also had little effect on axoplasmic transport [67]. Local anesthetics, however, can have a more complex action. In low concentrations, lidocaine and halothane can block membrane excitability without affecting transport; at somewhat higher concentrations, they can enter the fibers to block the transport mechanism, and at still higher concentrations, can cause disassembly of microtubules [88, 89].

Repetitive stimulation of nerves in vitro has either no influence on axoplasmic transport or a small (15 percent) decrease after stimulation at rates of 350 pulses per second for 4 hours [96]. Considering that the small decrement in transport could be due to an increase in Na^+, the effect of batrachotoxin (BTX) on transport was studied. This agent, which acts to open Na^+ channels, was found to block fast axoplasmic transport when present in concentrations of less than 0.2 μM [97].

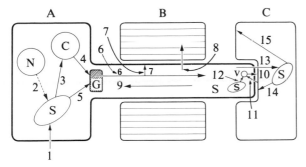

Fig. 22-6. (A) *cell body;* (B) *nerve fiber;* (C) *terminal region with the neuromuscular junction and a muscle fiber shown. In* (A), *upon entry of precursor (1), the nucleus (N) controls (2) synthesis (S); arrow (3) shows a compartmentalization (C) of synthesized material. Materials move from the synthesis site and the compartment into the axon (4, 5). (G) represents a gate, possibly the Golgi apparatus, that controls the egress of materials into the axon. The transport system in the fiber* (B) *moves materials down the nerve fiber (6). Arrows represent some components that supply the membrane (7) and the Schwann cell (8). The myelin sheath is represented by parallel horizontal lines. Retrograde transport is shown by the arrow directed toward the cell body (9). In the terminal region* (C), *vesicles (v) involved in transmission are shown (10) with a reconstitution of their transmitter content (11). Synthesis of components in their terminal is indicated by (S), with some contribution of downflowing control materials (12). An arrow from the nerve terminal that enters the muscle fiber (13) indicates the flow of trophic materials, some of which control synthesis (2) in the muscle fiber. Receptor proteins are shown by arrows (14) and (15) inserted into the membrane at the usual site (14) and, after denervation, at new (15) receptor sites.*

Even lower concentrations were effective on CNS injection [98]. When sheathed nerves were used, decreasing Na^+ in the medium did not appear to affect the BTX block. However, when the de-sheathed nerve preparation was used, most, if not all, of the transport block produced by BTX was eliminated when Na^+ was deleted from the in vitro medium [67]. This effect of BTX has been verified with respect to the saltatory organelle movements seen in neuroblastoma cells [99], movements which are considered to be a model of axoplasmic transport. The block of transport reported earlier for ouabain [62, 100] also could be related to Na^+ entry.

Those experiments, and similar ones made with veratridine, point to an increased entry of Na^+ into the axon as a cause of transport block. Possibly the increase in Na^+ intraaxonally may release Ca^{2+} from the mitochondria [101], and the increased level of free Ca^{2+} in the axoplasm, in turn, blocks transport. Na^+ and Ca^{2+} movements are discussed further in Chap. 6.

NERVE TERMINALS

Vesicles containing neurotransmitters or neurotransmitter-synthesizing enzymes (or both), as well as proteins and other materials, are supplied to the nerve terminals (Fig. 22-6).

In addition to neurotransmitters released from the nerve terminals, trophic materials move out of the nerve terminal to affect the postsynaptic cells [102, 103] (see also Chap. 23). Loss of trophic substances accounts for some of the altered properties of muscle after nerve transection. Evidence for translocation of labeled materials from the nerve to postsynaptic cells has been obtained in autoradiographic studies of muscle [104], and labeled components have been found in the visual cortex of brain after retinal uptake and transport, indicating a transsynaptic passage through the lateral geniculate [105]. The specificity of components transported remains in question.

The demonstration of trophic effects of nerve on muscle must be carefully evaluated because some of the muscle changes seen after nerve transection may be due to decreased activity [106]. Evidence for a neurotrophic factor is the finding that the time of onset of putative trophic changes in muscle depends on whether the nerve was cut close to or far from the muscle [107, 108]. Such changes are the tetrodotoxin-resistant action potentials in the muscle fibers or the early decrease in resting membrane potential. Comparison of the effect of nerve transection with a chronic block of nerve by TTX has indicated that some of the effects on muscle are due to the loss of a neurotrophic substance [109–111].

A neurotrophic factor in nerve appears partly to control the presence of ACh receptors (AChRs) in the muscle membrane. AChRs are usually restricted in the adult muscle fiber to the end-plate region (see Chap. 26). Puromycin, cycloheximide, and actinomycin D prevent the development of new ACh receptors in denervated muscle cultured in vitro [112]. Similar experiments carried out in vivo also indicated that the trophic substance may normally act at the DNA-RNA level, to repress the synthesis of the AChR in the muscle fiber and, in turn, the turnover of the receptors in the membrane [113]. Marked changes in mRNA sequences that appear after denervation have given additional support to this hypothesis [114]. Polypeptides with neurotrophic actions have been isolated from nerve [115]. This is a field of investigation with much promise.

Transport Used as a Tracer for Anatomical Studies

Axoplasmic transport combined with autoradiography is now a valuable technique used to trace fiber pathways within the CNS [116]. After the injection of a labeled amino acid such as [³H]-leucine, its uptake by nerve-cell bodies and incorporation into protein is followed by the transport of the labeled proteins in axons, as has been shown by means of autoradiography. The advantages of the *transport autoradiography* technique over the usual neuroanatomical method, where lesions are made and the degenerated fibers traced by appropriate stains, is that the labeled proteins are not taken up adventitiously by adjacent axons, and the method is more sensitive. Often, for example, fine degenerating fibers cannot be detected by stains. Also, if a relatively brief time is allowed for fast transport to carry labeled materials into the nerve terminals, autoradiographs will show the pattern of presynaptic endings on their cells of termination. And, when more time is allowed for slow transport, labeled activity in the fibers can be used to trace their route from the cell bodies to the synaptic terminations. Both anterograde transport shown by autoradiography and retrograde transport of HRP are often combined in neuroanatomical studies.

Another technique based on axoplasmic transport is used to show the paths of adrenergic,

cholinergic, or serotonergic fibers in the CNS. In this method, one cuts tract fibers and determines the accumulation of neurotransmitter or neurotransmitter-related components in the stumps of fibers connected to the cell bodies and their decrease in the fibers disconnected from their cell bodies (see Chap. 10).

References

*1. Jeffrey, P. L., and Austin, L.   Axoplasmic transport. *Prog. Neurobiol.* 2:205–225, 1973.

*2. Ochs, S.   Systems of material transport in nerve fibers (axoplasmic transport) related to nerve function and trophic control. *Ann. N.Y. Acad. Sci.* 228:202–223, 1974.

*3. Lubinska, L.   On axoplasmic flow. *Int. Rev. Neurobiol.* 17:241–296, 1975.

*4. Helsop, J. P.   Axonal flow and fast transport in nerves. *Adv. Comp. Physiol. Biochem.* 6:75–163, 1975.

*5. Ochs, S., and Worth, R. M.   Axoplasmic Transport in Normal and Pathological Systems. In S. G. Waxman (ed.), *Physiology and Pathobiology of Axons.* New York: Raven, 1978. Pp. 251–264.

*6. Wilson, D. L., and Stone, G. C.   Axoplasmic transport of proteins. *Annu. Rev. Biophys. Bioeng.* 8:27–45, 1979.

*7. Schwartz, J. H.   Axonal transport: Components, mechanisms and specificity. *Annu. Rev. Neurosci.* 2:467–504, 1979.

*8. Grafstein, B., and Forman, D. S.   Intracellular transport in neurons. *Physiol. Rev.* 60:1167–1283, 1980.

*9. Weiss, P., and Hiscoe, H. B.   Experiments in the mechanism of nerve growth. *J. Exp. Zool.* 107:315–395, 1948.

10. Friede, L., and Bischausen, R.   The fine structure of stumps of transected nerve fibers in subserial sections. *J. Neurol. Sci.* 44:181–203, 1980.

11. Martinez, A. J., and Friede, R. L.   Accumulation of axoplasmic organelles in swollen nerve fibers. *Brain Res.* 19:183–198, 1970.

*12. Dahlström, A.   Axoplasmic transport (with particular respect to adrenergic neurons). *Philos. Trans. R. Soc. Lond. B. Biol. Sci.* 261:325–358, 1971.

13. Brimijoin, S., and Wiermaa, M. J.   Direct comparison of the rapid axonal transport of norepinephrine and dopamine-β-hydroxylase activity. *J. Neurobiol.* 8:239–250.

*Key reference.

14. Ben-Jonathan, N., Maxson, R., and Ochs, S. Fast axoplasmic transport of noradrenaline and dopamine in mammalian peripheral nerve. *J. Physiol. (London)* 281:315–324, 1978.

15. Ranish, N., and Ochs, S. Fast axoplasmic transport of acetylcholinesterase in mammalian nerve fibers. *J. Neurochem.* 19:2641–2649, 1972.

16. Partlow, L. M., Ross, C. D., Motwani, R., and McDougal, D. B. Transport of axonal enzymes in surviving segments of frog sciatic nerves. *J. Gen. Physiol.* 60:388–405, 1972.

17. Ochs, S. Rate of fast axoplasmic transport in mammalian nerve fibers. *J. Physiol. (London)* 227:627–645, 1972.

18. Gross, G. W., and Beidler, L. M. Fast axonal transport in the C-fibers of the garfish olfactory nerve. *J. Neurobiol.* 4:413–428, 1973.

19. Edström, A., and Hanson, M. Temperature effects on fast axonal transport of proteins *in vitro* in frog sciatic nerves. *Brain Res.* 58:345–354, 1973.

20. Ochs, S., and Smith, C. J. Low temperature slowing and cold-block of fast axoplasmic transport in mammalian nerves *in vitro*. *J. Neurobiol.* 6:85–102, 1975.

21. Neale, J. H., Neale, E. A., and Agranoff, B. W. Radioautography of the optic tectum of the goldfish after intraocular injection of ^{3}H-proline. *Science* 176:407–410, 1972.

22. Kidwai, A. M., and Ochs, S. Components of fast and slow phases of axoplasmic flow. *J. Neurochem.* 16:1105–1112, 1969.

23. Willard, M., and Cowan, W. M. The polypeptide composition of intra-axonally transported proteins—evidence for four transport velocities. *Proc. Natl. Acad. Sci. U.S.A.* 71:2183–2187, 1974.

24. Willard, M. B., and Hulebak, K. L. The intra-axonal transport of polypeptide H: Evidence for a fifth (very slow) group of transported proteins in the retinal ganglion cells of the rabbit. *Brain Res.* 136:289–306, 1977.

25. Hoffman, P. N., and Lasek, R. J. The slow component of axonal transport identification of major structural polypeptides of the axon and their generality among mammalian neurons. *J. Cell Biol.* 66:351–366, 1975.

*26. Lasek, R. J., and Hoffman, P. N. The Neuronal Cytoskeleton, Axonal Transport and Axonal Growth. In Goldman, R., Pollard, T., and Rosenbaum, J. (eds.), *Cell Motility*. Cold Spring Harbor: Cold Spring Harbor Laboratory, 1976. Pp. 1021–1049.

27. Shelanski, M. L., and Liem, R. K. H. Neurofilaments. *J. Neurochem.* 33:5–13, 1979.

28. Willard, M., Wiseman, M., Levine, J., and Skene, P. Axonal transport of actin in rabbit retinal ganglion cells. *J. Cell Biol.* 81:581–591, 1979.

29. Black, M. M., and Lasek, R. J. Axonal transport of actin: Slow component b is the principal source of actin for the axon. *Brain Res.* 171:401–413, 1979.

30. Karlsson, J. O., and Sjöstrand, J. Rapid intracellular transport of fucose-containing glycoproteins in retinal ganglion cells. *J. Neurochem.* 18:2209–2216, 1971.

31. Forman, D., Grafstein, B., and McEwen, B. S. Rapid axonal transport of (^{3}H) fucosyl glucoproteins in the goldfish optic system. *Brain Res.* 48:327–342, 1972.

32. Elam, J. S., and Agranoff, B. W. Rapid transport of protein in the optic system of the goldfish. *J. Neurochem.* 18:375–387, 1971.

33. Elam, J. W., and Peterson, N. W. Axonal transport of sulfated glycoproteins and mucopolysaccharides in the garfish olfactory nerve. *J. Neurochem.* 26:845–850, 1976.

34. Abe, T., Haga, T., and Kukokawa, M. Rapid transport of phosphatidylcholine occurring simultaneously with protein transport in the frog sciatic nerve. *Biochem. J.* 136:731–740, 1973.

35. Rostas, J. A. P., McGregor, A., Jeffrey, P. L., and Austin, L. Transport of cholesterol in the chick optic system. *J. Neurochem.* 24:295–302, 1975.

36. Miani, N. Analysis of the somato-axonal movement of phospholipids in the vagus and hypoglossal nerves. *J. Neurochem.* 10:859–874, 1963.

37. Kirkpatrick, J. B., Bray, J. J., and Palmer, S. M. Visualization of axoplasmic flow *in vitro* by Nomarski microscopy. Comparison to rapid flow of radioactive proteins. *Brain Res.* 43:1–10, 1972.

38. Cooper, R. D., and Smith, R. S. The movement of optically detectable organelles in myelinated axons of Xenopus laevis. *J. Physiol. (London)* 242:77–97, 1974.

39. Forman, D. S., Padjen, A. L., and Siggins, G. R. Axonal transport of organelles visualized by light microscopy. Cinemicrographic and computer analysis. *Brain Res.* 136:197–213, 1977.

40. Friede, R. L., and Ho, K.-C. The relation of axonal transport of mitochondria with microtubules and other axoplasmic organelles. *J. Physiol. (London)* 265:507–519, 1977.

41. Barondes, S. H. Delayed appearances of labeled protein in isolated nerve endings and axoplasmic flow. *Science* 146:779–781, 1964.

42. Barondes, S. H. Slow and rapid transport of protein to nerve endings in mouse brain. *Acta Neuropath. Berl. Suppl.* V.:97–103, 1971.

43. Iqbal, Z., and Ochs, S.   Calcium binding protein in brain synaptosomes. *Soc. Neurosci. Abstr.* Vol. II, Part 1:47, 1976.

44. Lux, H. D., Schubert, P., Kreutzberg, G. W., and Globus, A.   Excitation and axonal flow: Autoradiographic study on motoneurons intracellulary injected with a ^{3}H-amino acid. *Exp. Brain Res.* 10:197–204, 1970.

45. Price, C. H., McAdoo, D. J., Farr, W., and Okuda, R.   Bidirectional axonal transport of free glycine in identified neurons R3-R14 of Aplysia. *J. Neurobiol.* 10:551–571, 1979.

46. Goldberg, D. J., Schwartz, J. H., and Sherbany, A. A.   Kinetic properties of normal and perturbed axonal transport of serotonin in a single identified axon. *J. Physiol. (London)* 281:559–579, 1978.

*47. Bisby, M. A.   Retrograde axonal transport. *Adv. Cell. Neurobiol.* 1:69–117, 1980.

48. Kristansson, K.   Retrograde axonal transport of horseradish peroxidase. Uptake at mouse neuromuscular junctions following systemic injection. *Acta Neuropathol.* 38:143–147, 1977.

49. LaVail, M. M., and LaVail, J. H.   Retrograde intra-axonal transport of horseradish peroxidase in retinal ganglion cells of the chick. *Brain Res.* 85:273–280, 1975.

50. Dumas, M., Schwab, M. E., and Thoenen, H.   Retrograde axonal transport of specific macromolecules as a tool for characterizing nerve terminal membranes. *J. Neurobiol.* 10:179–197, 1979.

51. Tsukita, S., and Ishikawa, H.   The movement of membranous organelles in axons. Electron microscopic identification of anterogradely and retrogradely transported organelles. *J. Cell Biol.* 84:513–530, 1980.

52. Smith, R. M.   The short term accumulation of axonally transported organelles in the region of localized lesions of single myelinated axons. *J. Neurocytol.* 9:39–65, 1980.

53. Ochs, S.   Retention and redistribution of proteins in mammalian nerve fibers by axoplasmic transport. *J. Physiol.* 253:459–475, 1975.

54. Bisby, M. A., and Bulger, V. T.   Reversal of axonal transport at a nerve crush. *J. Neurochem.* 29:313–320, 1977.

55. Sabri, M. I., and Ochs, S.   Relation of ATP and creatine phosphate to fast axoplasmic transport in mammalian nerve. *J. Neurochem.* 19:2821–2828, 1972.

*56. Ochs, S.   Energy metabolism and supply of $\sim$P to the fast axoplasmic transport mechanism in nerve. *Fed. Proc.* 33:1049–1058, 1974.

57. Ochs, S., and Smith, C. B.   Fast axoplasmic transport in mammalian nerve *in vitro* after block of glycolysis with iodoacetic acid. *J. Neurochem.* 18:833–843, 1971.

58. Banks, P., Mayor, D., and Mraz, P.   Metabolic aspects of the synthesis and intra-axonal transport of noradrenaline storage vesicles. *J. Physiol. (London)* 229:383–394, 1973.

59. Ochs, S.   Local supply of energy to the fast axoplasmic transport mechanism. *Proc. Natl. Acad. Sci. U.S.A.* 68:1279–1282, 1971.

60. Leone, J., and Ochs, S.   Axonic block and recovery of axoplasmic transport and electrical excitability of nerve. *J. Neurobiol.* 9:229–245, 1978.

61. Sjöstrand, J., Rydevik, B., Lundborg, G., and McLean, W. G.   Impairment of Intraneural Microcirculation, Blood-Nerve Barrier and Axonal Transport in Experimental Nerve Ischemia and Compression. In Korr, J. M. (ed.), *The Neurobiologic Mechanisms in Manipulative Therapy.* New York: Plenum, 1978, Pp. 337–355.

62. Ochs, S.   Fast transport of materials in mammalian nerve fibers. *Science* 176:252–260, 1972.

63. Ochs, S.   Calcium Requirement for Axoplasmic Transport and the Role of the Perineural Sheath. In Jewett, D. L., and McCarroll, H. R. (eds.), *Nerve Repair and Regeneration: Its Clinical and Experimental Basis.* St. Louis: Mosby, 1980. Pp. 77–88.

64. Khan, M. A., and Ochs, S.   Magnesium or calcium activated ATPase in mammalian nerve. *Brain Res.* 81:413–426, 1974.

65. Ochs, S., and Iqbal, Z.   Calmodulin and calcium activation of tubulin associated Ca-ATPase. *Soc. Neurosci. Abstr.* 6:501, 1980.

66. Ochs, S., Worth, R. M., and Chan, S. Y.   Calcium requirement for axoplasmic transport in mammalian nerve. *Nature* 27:748–750, 1977.

67. Chan, S. Y., Ochs, S., and Worth, R. M.   The requirement of Ca^{2+} and the effect of other ions on axoplasmic transport in mammalian nerve. *J. Physiol. (London)* 301:477–504, 1980.

68. LaVoie, P. A., Bolen, F., and Hammerschlag, R.   Divalent cation specificity of the calcium requirement of proteins in axons of desheathed nerves. *J. Neurochem.* 32:1745–1751, 1979.

69. Baker, P. F.   Transport and metabolism of calcium ions in nerve. *Prog. Biophys. Mol. Biol.* 24:177–223, 1972.

70. Duce, I. R., and Keen, P.   Can neuronal smooth endoplasmic reticulum function as a calcium reservoir? *Neuroscience* 3:837–848, 1978.

71. Henkart, M. P., Reese, T. S., and Brinley, F. J., Jr.   Endoplasmic reticulum sequesters calcium in the squid giant axon. *Science* 202:1300–1303, 1978.

72. Brinley, F., Spangler, S. G., and Mullins, L. J. Calcium and EDTA fluxes in dialyzed squid axons. *J. Gen. Physiol.* 66:223–250, 1975.

73. DiPolo, R. Ca pump driven by ATP in squid axons. *Nature* 274:390–392, 1978.

74. Schlaepfer, W. W. Experimental alterations of neurofilaments and neurotubules by calcium and other ions. *Exp. Cell Res.* 67:73–80, 1971.

75. Hammerschlag, R., Dravid, A. R., and Chiu, A. Y. Mechanism of axonal transport—a proposed role for calcium ions. *Science* 188:273–275, 1975.

76. Iqbal, Z., and Ochs, S. Fast axoplasmic transport of a calcium-binding protein in mammalian nerve. *J. Neurochem.* 31:409–418, 1978.

77. Iqbal, Z., and Ochs, S. CDR protein in nerve. *Abstr. Fed. Proc.* 38:849, 1979.

78. Iqbal, Z., and Ochs, S. Characterization of a calcium regulator protein in mammalian nerve. Seventh International Society Neurochemistry, 1979. P. 391.

79. Tashiro, T., Kasai, H., and Kurokawa, M. A calmodulin-related polypeptide rapidly migrates within the mammalian nerve. *Biomed. Res.* 1:292–299, 1980.

80. Isenberg, G., Schubert, P., and Kreutzberg, G. W. Experimental approach to test the role of actin in axonal transport. *Brain Res.* 194:588–593, 1980.

81. Ochs, S. A unitary concept of axoplasmic transport based on the transport filament hypothesis. *Excerpta Med. Int. Congr. Ser.* 36:128–133, 1975.

*82. Gross, G. W. The microstream concept of axoplasmic and dendritic transport. *Adv. Neurol.* 12:283–296, 1975.

83. Muñoz-Martinez, E. J., Núñez, R., and Sanderson, A. Axonal transport: A quantitative study of retained and transformed protein fractions in the cat. *J. Neurobiol.* 12:15–26, 1981.

84. Cancalon, P. Influence of temperature on the velocity and on the isotope profile of slowly transported labeled proteins. *J. Neurochem.* 32:997–1007, 1979.

85. Stromska, D. P., Iqbal, Z., and Ochs, S. Fast axoplasmic transport of tubulin and triad proteins. *Soc. Neurosci. Abstr.* 5:63, 1979.

*86. McClure, W. O. Effects of drugs upon axoplasmic transport. *Adv. Pharmacol. Chemother.* 10:185–220, 1972.

87. Fernandez, H. L., Huneeus, J. F. C., and Davidson, P. F. Studies on the mechanism of axoplasmic transport in the crayfish cords. *J. Neurobiol.* 1:395–409, 1970.

88. Kennedy, R. D., Fink, B. R., and Byers, M. R. The effect of halothane on rapid axonal transport in the rabbit vagus. *Anesthesiology* 36:433–443, 1972.

89. Byers, M. R., Hendrickson, A. E., Fink, B. R., Kennedy, R. D., and Middaugh, M. E. Effects of lidocaine on axonal morphology, microtubules and rapid transport in rabbit vagus nerve in vitro. *J. Neurobiol.* 4:124–143, 1973.

90. Ghetti, B., and Ochs, S. Maytansine-induced block of axoplasmic transport and microtubule loss. *Soc. Neurosci. Abstr.* 3:30, 1977.

91. Chan, S. Y., Worth, R. M., and Ochs, S. Block of axoplasmic transport *in vitro* by vinca alkaloids. *J. Neurobiol.* 11:251–264, 1978.

92. Iqbal, Z., and Ochs, S. Uptake of vinca alkaloids into mammalian nerve and its subcellular components. *J. Neurochem.* 34:59–68, 1979.

93. Brady, S. T., Crothers, S. D., Nosal, C., and McClure, W. O. Fast axonal transport in the presence of high Ca^{2+}: Evidence that microtubules are not required. *Proc. Natl. Acad. Sci. U.S.A.* 77:5909–5913, 1980.

94. Ochs, S., Erdman, J., Jersild, R. A., and McAdoo, V. Routing of transported materials in the dorsal root and nerve fiber branches of the dorsal root ganglion. *J. Neurobiol.* 9:465–481, 1978.

95. Ochs, S. Regeneration of Nerve in Relation to Axoplasmic Transport: An Analysis. In Millesi, H., Mingrino, A., and Gorio, A. (eds.), *Posttraumatic Peripheral Neuropathies.* New York: Raven, 1981.

96. Worth, R. M., and Ochs, S. The effect of repetitive electrical stimulation on axoplasmic transport. *Soc. Neurosci. Abstr.* Vol. II, Part *1*:50, 1976.

97. Ochs, S., and Worth, R. Batrachotoxin block of fast axoplasmic transport in mammalian nerve fibers. *Science* 187:1087–1089, 1975.

98. Boegman, R. J., and Albuquerque, E. X. Axonal transport in rats rendered paraplegic following a single subarachnoid injection of either batrachotoxin or 6-aminonicotinamide into the spinal cord. *J. Neurobiol.* 11:282–290, 1980.

99. Forman, D. S., and Shain, W. G., Jr. Batrachotoxin blocks saltatory organelle movement in electrically excitable neuroblastoma cells. *Brain Res.* 212:242–247, 1981.

100. Partlow, L. W., Ross, C. D., Motwani, R., and McDougal, D. B., Jr. Transport of axonal enzymes in surviving segments of frog sciatic nerve. *J. Gen. Physiol.* 60:388–405, 1972.

*101. Carafoli, E., and Crompton, M. The regulation of intracellular calcium. *Curr. Top. Membranes Transp.* 10:151–216, 1978.

*102. Gutmann, E. Neurotrophic relations. *Annu. Rev. Physiol.* 38:177–216, 1976.

103. Guth, L., and Albuquerque, E. X. Neurotrophic regulation of resting membrane potential and extrajunctional acetylcholine sensitivity in mam-

malian skeletal muscle. *Physiol. Bohemoslov.* 27:401–414, 1978.

104. Korr, I. M., Wilkinson, P. N., and Chornock, F. W. Axonal delivery of neuroplasmic components to muscle cells. *Science* 155:343–345, 1967.

105. Specht, S. C., and Grafstein, B. Axonal transport and transneuronal transfer in mouse visual system following injection of (^{3}H)fucose into the eye. *Exp. Neurol.* 54:352–368, 1977.

106. Lømo, T., and Westgaard, R. H. Control of ACh sensitivity in the rat. *Cold Spring Harbor Symp. Quant. Biol.* 40:263–281, 1976.

107. Deshpande, S. S., Albuquerque, E. X., and Guth, L. Neurotrophic regulation of prejunctional and postjunctional membrane at the mammalian motor endplate. *Exp. Neurol.* 53:151–165, 1976.

*108. Thesleff, S. Physiological effects of denervation of muscle. *Ann. N.Y. Acad. Sci.* 228:89–103, 1975.

109. Pestronk, A., Drachman, D. B., and Griffin, J. W. Effects of muscle disease on acetyl choline receptors. *Nature* 260:349, 1976.

110. LaVoie, P. A., Collier, B., and Tenenhouse, A. Comparison of α-bungarotoxin binding to skeletal muscles after inactivity or denervation. *Nature* 260:349–350, 1976.

111. Bray, J. J., Hubbard, J. I., and Mills, R. G. The trophic influence of tetrodotoxin-inactive nerves on normal and reinnervated rat skeletal muscles. *J. Physiol. (London)* 297:479–491, 1979.

*112. Drachman, D. B. Trophic functions of the neuron. *Ann. N.Y. Acad. Sci.* 228:1–406, 1974.

113. Grampp, W., Harris, J. B., and Thesleff, S. Inhibition of denervation changes in skeletal muscle by blockers of protein synthesis. *J. Physiol. (London)* 221:743–754, 1972.

114. Metafora, S., Felsani, A., Cotrufo, R., Tajana, G. F., Del Rio, A., De Prisco, P. P., Rutigliano, B., and Esposito, V. Neural control of gene expression in the skeletal muscle fibre: changes in the muscular mRNA population following denervation. *Proc. R. Soc. Lond. B Biol. Sci.* 209:257–273, 1980.

115. Oh, T. H. Neurotrophic effects of sciatic nerve extracts on muscle development in culture. *Exp. Neurol.* 50:376–386, 1976.

*116. Cowan, W. M., and Cuenod, M. (eds.). *The Use of Axonal Transport for Studies of Neuronal Connectivity.* New York: Elsevier, 1975.

Section VI.
Physiological Integration

Joyce A. Benjamins
Guy M. McKhann

Chapter 23. Development, Regeneration, and Aging of the Brain

The precise cellular and subcellular mechanisms that regulate development have not been clearly defined in any mammalian system, certainly not in one so complex as the nervous system. At present, we know a great deal about biochemical changes that occur in whole brain or nerve during development [1–6; for historical review, see 7]. Some progress has been made in dissecting the origin and development of various cell types in the nervous system and the factors that control their maturation [8, 9].

The first section of this chapter discusses overall changes in composition and metabolism of the developing nervous system and relates them to cellular changes, where possible. In the second section, the maturation of the two major cell populations in the nervous system, neurons and glia, is described, with emphasis on systems in which the biochemical events underlying the morphological and functional changes have been studied.

The events of nervous system development often have been divided into stages for ease of discussion and organization. These stages are artificial, at best, particularly when applied to a dynamic system. In addition, the nervous system is heterogeneous from region to region in the timing of development of cell types and complexity of interaction among those types. The following general scheme [1] serves to indicate major changes applicable to all species:

1. Organogenesis and neuronal multiplication
2. The brain-growth spurt (sometimes called *critical period*)
   a. Axonal and dendritic growth, glial multiplication, and myelination
   b. Growth in size
3. Mature, adult size
4. Aging

Biochemical Changes in Development

The most obvious index of brain growth is weight. The most rapid growth may occur before, after, or at the time of birth, depending on the species (Fig. 23-1). In general, brain weight reaches its maximum before body weight, as illustrated for rat brain in Fig. 23-2. The period of maximal rate of weight increase takes place at various times in different regions of the nervous system, in the following sequence: peripheral nerves, spinal cord, cerebrum, cerebellum. The cerebellum shows the sharpest rate of growth, the spinal cord the most gradual. In general, the increase in weight of a region of the brain corresponds to myelination and the proliferation of neuronal processes. The increase in membranous structures is accompanied by an increase in brain solids and a decrease in brain water. For example, in rat brain, water is 90 percent of the total brain weight at birth and 83 percent at maturity [14].

The developmental changes in four major constituents of brain—DNA, RNA, protein, and lipid—are summarized for the forebrain of rat in Fig. 23-2, with values expressed as percentages of adult levels. In Fig. 23-3, changes in brain weight, DNA, and cholesterol are expressed in terms of rate of change, emphasizing the time of most rapid increase. The sequential changes in these components illustrate the events that take place in the developing nervous system. Early proliferation of cells is indicated by synthesis of DNA. As differentiation occurs, DNA replication is followed by increased transcription of DNA to RNA and then by translation of RNA to protein. With the appearance of cell-specific enzymes and structural proteins, each cell type acquires its unique metabolism and morphology. Maturation of such elements as neuronal processes, synaptic endings, and myelin involves deposition of lipids and proteins into those membranous structures. DNA content of brain is considered a reliable indicator of cell number, and the ratio of protein to DNA indicates cell size. This ratio increases after neuronal division ends, reflecting, in part, the arborization of neuronal processes. Increasing lipid content indicates compartmentation and membrane formation, particularly of axonal, dendritic, and myelin membranes.

These developmental events occur at different ages in various species (Table 23-1). It is impossible to give exact times for the onset or end of these events, but the ages in Table 23-1 are intended to serve as approximate guidelines. Cortex was chosen because more complete data are available for this brain region than for others.

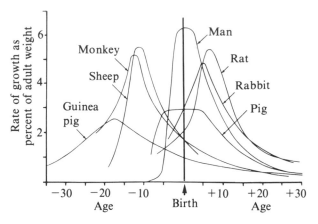

Fig. 23-1. Rate of brain growth (wet weight) in relation to birth in different species. Increments were calculated as percentage of adult weight gained in a given interval. Humans, in months; sheep, monkey, and pig, in weeks; rabbit, guinea pig, and rat, in days. (Reprinted from J. Dobbing and J. Sands [10], with permission.)

NUCLEIC ACIDS

The first increases in brain DNA reflect proliferation of neuronal precursors. Later increases are due primarily to the appearance of glial precursors. In human brain, two major periods of cell proliferation have been detected by measuring DNA levels [10]. The first period begins at 15 to 20 weeks of gestation and corresponds to neuroblast proliferation. The second begins at 25 weeks and continues into the second year of postnatal life. This latter period corresponds to multiplication of glial cells and includes a second wave of neuronogenesis, restricted to microneurons in certain regions of the brain. In the rat, these regions are primarily the granular layer of the cerebellar cortex, the olfactory lobe, and hippocampus [25].

In smaller species, DNA in brain appears to accumulate in a linear manner until the adult level is reached. Perhaps two phases of DNA accumulation have not been detected because of a lack of

Table 23-1. Comparison of Developmental Milestones in Cortex of Several Species*

Species	Rapid Increase in Maturity and Number of Nerve Processes	Histological Appearance of Myelin	DNA at Maximal Level	Protein at Maximal Level
Rat	6–24 days [16, 17]	10–40 days [21]	20 days [12]	99 days [12]
Mouse	2–17 days [18]	9–30 days [22]	16 days [15]	80–90 days [15]
Guinea pig	(41–45 days) [19]	(63 days) to 7 days [19]	7 days [19]	55 days [15]
Man	(6 months) to 3 months [15, 20]	(7 months) to 4 years [23]	6–8 months [24]	2 years [24]

*Values in parentheses represent days or months of gestation, the other values the time after birth. Pertinent references are in brackets.

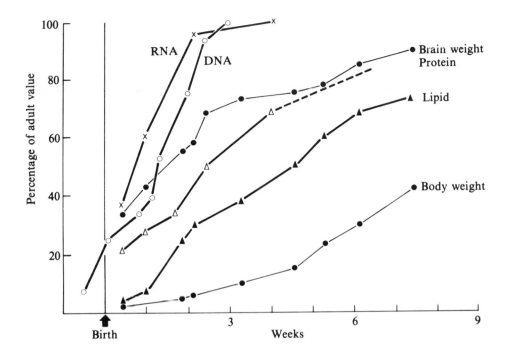

Fig. 23-2. Increases in body weight and in several brain constituents during development in rat. Values are expressed as percentages of maximal (adult) values. Results for body weight, brain weight, and brain lipid have been calculated from the data of Kishimoto, Davies, and Radin [11], DNA values from the data of Fish and Winick [12], RNA values from the data of Mandel [13], and protein values from the data of Himwich [14, 15].

sufficient data during the period of neuronal division. In rat, neuronal division is largely prenatal and glial division is postnatal. The values in Fig. 23-2 suggest two phases of DNA accumulation in rat brain, and one study has demonstrated that the rate of increase in DNA and the activity of DNA polymerase are high at 6 days before birth, lower at birth, then higher again, reaching a peak between 6 and 10 days after birth [26].

As with weight increase, the period of most rapid DNA synthesis and accumulation is earliest in spinal cord, followed by cerebrum, then cerebellum. For example, at birth, rat cerebrum has 50 percent of its adult DNA content, whereas cerebellum has only 3 percent [12]. The rate of increase in cell num-ber is most rapid in cerebellum, slower in cerebrum, and most gradual in cord. Thus, in postnatal rat brain, DNA content increases five times more rapidly in cerebellum than in cerebrum.

The rate of incorporation of radioactive thymidine into DNA [25] and the activity of DNA polymerase [26] increase during periods of cell proliferation in a given region, then decrease as cell division ends; thus, these factors give a reasonable approximation of mitotic activity.

As DNA accumulation ends, the ratio of RNA to DNA increases. On a cellular level [8], most of the newly synthesized RNA remains in the nucleus until cell division has ended. Upon differentiation, the nucleolus matures, with increased RNA synthesis, especially of ribosomal RNA (rRNA) and transfer of RNA into the cytoplasm. In neurons, Nissl substance (rRNA) first becomes prominent at this stage. The rate of RNA synthesis decreases after maturation, together with the activity of RNA polymerase in nuclei of both neurons and glia [27].

Characterization of the RNA in rat brain shows that a larger proportion of RNA synthesis results in messenger RNA (mRNA) synthesis in brain than in liver [28]. In developing brain, RNA characteristics are compatible with the rapid rate of protein synthesis observed. Compared with adult brain: (a) the mRNA turns over more rapidly, (b) more of the ribosomal RNA is polysomal and membrane bound, and (c) these polysomes are more stable [29]. The base ratios of nucleotides in RNA show some changes in development in various regions of brain, but the contributions of individual cell types to these changes are not yet known [30].

The individual ribosomal monomers of rat brain may acquire structural and functional differences by interaction with mRNA and the endoplasmic reticulum. Any factor affecting the proportions of free and membrane-bound ribosomes may change the rate of protein synthesis. There may be qualitative differences as well; ribosomes attached to the membrane may synthesize protein for secretion, membrane expansion, or axoplasmic flow (in the case of neurons), whereas free ribosomes may synthesize proteins for local intracellular use.

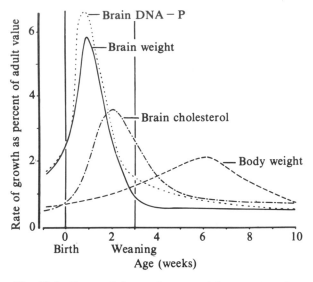

Fig. 23-3. *Rates of change in wet weight, DNA, and cholesterol of developing rat brain, and their relationship to the later bodily growth spurt. Values were calculated as increments (percentage of adult values) at two-day intervals. (Reprinted from J. Dobbing and J. Sands [10], with permission.)*

PROTEINS

In developing rat brain, protein increases more rapidly than does wet weight. As previously mentioned, the ratio of protein to DNA indicates cell size, and this ratio is elevated during development. The time at which the protein content of brain reaches its maximal level in various species is summarized in Table 23-1. As with most other constituents, proteins increase most rapidly in rat cortex during the first 2 to 3 weeks of postnatal life. In this same period, there is a shift from water-soluble to membrane-bound proteins. Compositions of the protein populations also change during development.

A number of brain-specific proteins have been detected by their antigenicity, and their developmental changes have been studied [31, 32]. One example, Thy-1 antigen, is found in both thymus and brain. In mouse brain, the concentration, which is very low until day 7, increases rapidly to the adult level by day 23. The antigen is primarily in gray matter, and its pattern of increase correlates with synaptogenesis [33].

Glial fibrillary acidic protein, localized in astroglial processes [34], shows a peak concentration at 10 to 14 days in mouse brain, reflecting astroglial differentiation at the time of myelination [32]. Three other brain-specific proteins appear about the time myelin formation begins: the acidic S-100 protein, which is primarily glial, and basic protein(s) and proteolipid protein(s) of myelin. The subcellular fraction studied most extensively during development in brain is the myelin membrane (see Chap. 4). Changes in the protein composition of isolated myelin fractions have been demonstrated, with increasing proportions of basic and proteolipid proteins relative to proteins of higher molecular weight.

The amounts of actin and tubulin in rat brain increase after birth but reach a plateau at 10 to 15 days; other proteins continue to increase. By adulthood, the proportions of actin and tubulin relative to other proteins are about half those seen at day 10 [35].

Developmental changes in a number of enzymes have been observed, both histochemically [36] and biochemically [37, 38]. In addition to changes in total enzyme content or in relative amounts of activity, isozyme patterns change for several enzymes, including fructose 1,6-diphosphate aldolase, and lactic dehydrogenase (LDH); the changes in LDH probably are associated with increasing rates of respiration in maturing brain [30].

Incorporation of amino acids into brain proteins is most rapid during fetal and newborn periods, as measured both in vivo and in vitro [39, 40]. Some studies show a continuous decrease from birth to adulthood; others show an intermediate peak of activity during the first or second week after birth. In vivo studies with radioactive precursors are complicated by a number of factors [39–41], including changes in available amino acid pools during development, variability among animals, and sensitivity of protein synthesis in the newborn rat to changes in body temperature. Generally, small amounts of radioactive precursors are used, and values are corrected for the specific activity of the amino acids in brain (which may not reflect the actual pool available for protein synthesis). Investigators have measured brain protein synthesis in vivo by injecting "flooding" amounts of a precursor, which results in a high concentration of that amino acid in brain and a constant specific activity over a 2-hour period [40]. In cerebrum of rat, a rate of 1.9 to 2.1 percent replacement of protein-bound amino acid per hour was found from several days before birth to 4 days after birth. This rate declined gradually to about 0.8 to 0.7 percent per hour by 37 days, then to 0.5 percent per hour by 39 weeks. Rates measured in vitro with brain slices from young animals (3 and 10 days) were comparable to those measured in vivo, but when adult tissue was used, in vitro rates fell to about 10 percent of adult in vivo values.

There is general agreement that rates of ribosomal-directed protein synthesis decrease with maturation of neural tissue, but the factors responsible for the decline in activity have not been defined [41]. Some investigators have found that ribosomal activity measured in vitro decreases with maturation, whereas others have not. Perhaps the discrepancies are caused by variations in methods of ribosome preparation, in the source of mRNA, or in incubation conditions for measurement of protein synthesis. No major structural differences have been detected in brain ribosomes for young as compared to old animals. Possible control mechanisms under investigation include levels of specific mRNAs, which may be the single most important influence for regulation; changes in soluble factors; capacity of ribosomes to bind these factors; and chemical modification of ribosomal proteins (for example, by phosphorylation).

In addition to decreasing rates of protein synthesis with development, the average half-lives of proteins become greater, indicating decreasing rates of breakdown. The activity of brain proteinases, which increases just after birth, decreases with maturation in parallel with the increasing half-life [42]. The average rate of turnover of proteins in 10-day-old rats is estimated to be 1.7 times that in adult rats [43]. This slower turnover with maturation may be due to a change in the turnover of a majority of the proteins or to synthesis of a higher proportion of slowly turning-over proteins in adult brain. In the latter case, the higher ratio of glial cells to neurons and the greater contribution of myelin proteins in mature brains may be factors, because glial fractions are reported to incorporate amino acids at a slower rate than neuronal fractions and the major myelin proteins have relatively long half-lives.

LIPIDS

The most rapid increase in lipid content of brain begins after the periods of greatest increase of DNA and protein. Changes in specific lipids have been well documented [44, 45]. Changes in fatty acid chain length and degree of saturation have been determined for several groups of lipids [44, 46].

The rapid increase in lipid content is closely related to the onset of myelination. About 50 percent of all lipid in white matter, or 30 percent of total brain lipid, has been estimated to belong to myelin sheaths in rat brain (see Chap. 4).

Comprehensive analysis of lipids in developing rat brain [45] indicates that they may be divided into groups on the basis of their period of most rapid change with respect to myelination. Sterol esters and gangliosides undergo marked shifts before myelination begins; other lipids show marked, moderate, or small increases during myelination. In rat brain, total levels of sterol ester increase from birth to 40 days [47]. Unlike other lipids, sterol ester decreases in concentration during this period, except for a transient increase apparently related to onset of myelination [47].

The gangliosides are 27 percent of their adult concentration on day 3, and increase rapidly to 90 percent by day 24. The pattern of gangliosides (see Chap. 18 for nomenclature) in rat brain also changes [48]. G_{M1} and G_{T1} comprise the major proportion at birth and then fall; G_{D1a} increases to become the predominant ganglioside in the adult brain. Similar changes take place in human cortex, although G_{M1} remains a major ganglioside after an initial drop. Increases in gangliosides and in the activity of the enzyme that synthesizes their precursor, glucocerebroside, are related temporally to the outgrowth of axons and dendrites in agreement with the possible localization of much of the ganglioside in nerve processes.

A second category of lipids is characterized by low concentration at 3 days (less than 10 percent of the adult level), followed by dramatic increases between 12 and 18 days. This category includes galactocerebroside, cerebroside sulfate, sphingomyelin, and triphosphoinositide. In keeping with their high degree of localization in the myelin membrane is the low concentration of these lipids at birth and their subsequent increase at the time myelination starts. The activity of the enzymes that synthesize galactocerebroside and cerebroside sulfate also parallels myelination, with low levels at birth and marked peaks of activity at about 17 to 20 days [49, 50].

Lipids in a third category occur at 12 to 34 percent of their adult value at birth and increase during myelination, although the increase is less than in those in the second category. Ethanolamine and choline plasmalogens, cholesterol, and phospha-tidylserine are in this group. These lipids are associated with nonmyelin membranes in the brain of newborn rat, and the increases during the period of myelination are probably due to elaboration of both myelin and nonmyelin membranes.

Three of the major phospholipids—phosphatidylethanolamine, phosphatidylinositol, and phosphatidylcholine—comprise the fourth category. These lipids are 40 to 50 percent of their adult value at 3 days and increase only moderately in concentration during development. They are ubiquitous components of most membrane structures; their temporal pattern of development is not related to any specific morphological change but reflects increasing synthesis of membranes by brain cells.

Maturation is accompanied by an increase in both hydroxy and long-chain saturated fatty acids, due in large part to the abundance of these fatty acids in the lipids of the myelin membrane. Fatty acid aldehydes are found primarily in ethanolamine plasmalogen, which is also enriched in myelin, so fatty acid aldehydes of brain increase with the long-chain saturated fatty acids and the hydroxy fatty acids.

In summary, elevation of the galactolipid and plasmalogen content of brain correlates well with the morphological appearance of myelin, and increases in gangliosides appear to be related to the increasing arborization of neurons. In the rat, the maximal rate of change in ganglioside content takes place at about day 10, and the maximal rate of change in content of galactocerebroside plus sulfatide occurs about day 20 (Fig. 23-4). These times correspond, respectively, to the middle of the periods characterized by the outgrowth of neuronal processes and by the formation of myelin.

OTHER CHANGES IN COMPOSITION
AND METABOLISM
In tissues undergoing rapid growth and differentiation, dramatic increases occur in the levels of polyamines and in the activity of ornithine decarboxylase, the first step in polyamine biosynthesis. Some evidence suggests that the polyamines may influence nucleic acid metabolism. In developing rat brain, changes in levels of the polyamine

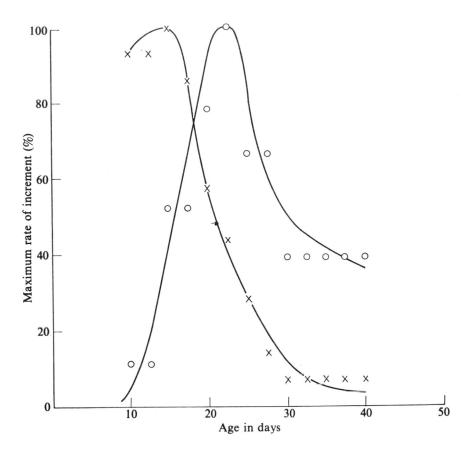

Fig. 23-4. Rates of change in gangliosides and in cerebrosides plus sulfatides in the developing rat brain [1]. Results have been calculated from the data of Kishimoto, Davies, and Radin [11], and are expressed as (o) mg of galactolipid (cerebroside and sulfatide) or as (x) mg of ganglioside stearate per 2.5 days in whole rat brain. Stearate was found to be the major ganglioside fatty acid (83% to 91% of the total fatty acids) [11]. (Reprinted from A. N. Davison and J. Dobbing [1], with permission.)

spermidine and the activity of the enzyme ornithine decarboxylase correlate with the rate of synthesis and accumulation of RNA and DNA [51]. Levels of activity of ornithine decarboxylase in developing rat brain are increased by thyroxine, growth hormone, lactogenic hormone, and insulin, reflecting increased rates of RNA and DNA synthesis. Cortisol decreases both the activity of the enzyme and

nucleic acid synthesis [51]. The activity of the enzyme in brain and heart has been reported to decrease rapidly and reversibly when rat pups are deprived of maternal attention [52].

During maturation of rat brain, levels of the glycosaminoglycans hyaluronic acid, chondroitin sulfate, and heparin sulfate increase after birth, reach a peak at 7 days, then decline to adult levels by 30 days [53]. Hyaluronic acid shows the most dramatic change, decreasing from 3.6 μmol hexosamine per gram of lipid-free dry weight at 8 days to 1.4 μmol at 12 days. Almost 90 percent of the hyaluronic acid is soluble at 7 days, compared to 15 percent in adult brain. This soluble pool appears relatively inactive metabolically. The high levels of soluble hyaluronic acid in the immature brain may function in the extracellular space to retain water and form a penetrable matrix for cell migration [53]. Neuronal cell bodies generally have higher levels of glycosaminoglycans than have glial cells, and the membrane-bound glycosaminoglycans are concentrated in light microsomal fractions, possibly in plasma membranes.

Many of the metabolic changes that take place during development can be placed in one of three categories that emphasize their relation to morphological or functional events: (a) energy availability and substrate utilization; (b) metabolism of compounds related to neural transmission; and (c) myelin formation. These are covered in a number of other chapters in this book.

Regulatory Factors in Development

NERVE GROWTH FACTOR

In concert with the intrinsic genetic program within a given neuronal or glial cell, various extrinsic cellular or humoral factors may act on the cell at different stages of development (see Chap. 21). As discussed by Varon and Bunge [54], we may distinguish between *trophic* (or permissive) influences, defined as extrinsic modulators of the overall metabolic activity of the cell, and *specifying* (or instructive) influences, defined as intrinsic agents that effect selection of distinct programs within the cells.

The best-characterized trophic substance known to have a direct and specific effect on nervous system maturation is nerve growth factor (NGF) [55, 56]. This protein is required at a certain stage of development for the survival and maturation of peripheral sympathetic neurons and for the maturation of some sensory neurons. Thus, antibodies to NGF have a devastating effect on sympathetic neurons in vivo and in culture, whereas administration of excess NGF will cause proliferation and hypertrophy of the neurons. NGF or similar factors may play a role in guiding nerve fibers to a target tissue, in preventing degeneration caused by axotomy, and in stimulating regeneration of damaged axons [55, 57]. Whether the effects of

NGF also extend to the CNS is a subject for investigation. NGF stimulates regeneration of lesioned adrenergic neurons in adult rat brain [58] but apparently does not stimulate these neurons during normal development [59].

The biological activity of NGF has usually been assayed by its ability to induce neurite outgrowth from embryonic ganglia in culture. Several radioimmunoassays to measure NGF have been described. Some of these methods give results in close agreement to those from bioassay; others give higher levels [60].

During development, maturation of adrenergic neurons in sympathetic ganglia, as reflected in increased activities of tyrosine hydroxylase and dopamine β-hydroxylase, is regulated by innervation from the preganglionic cholinergic neurons (see Chap. 10). NGF also can selectively induce these enzymes in the postganglionic neurons in the absence of cholinergic input. This induction is seen whether NGF is applied to the neuronal cell bodies or is taken up by retrograde transport; the effect does not depend on changes in levels of cyclic AMP and cyclic GMP. Glucocorticoids stimulate the induction produced by either the cholinergic neurons or NGF, indicating that a common mechanism may be involved.

In addition to increasing levels of tyrosine hydroxylase and dopamine β-hydroxylase, NGF exerts a number of anabolic effects on receptive neurons. Synthesis of lipids, proteins, and RNA is enhanced, as is the activity of the hexose monophosphate shunt. However, no effects of NGF on levels of cyclic AMP, cyclic GMP, or their respective cyclases have been detected. Neurite outgrowth may progress in culture in the absence of de novo RNA or protein synthesis, but these macromolecular processes are required for NGF-mediated initiation of outgrowth [61].

Nerve growth factor is found in snake venom and in high concentration in the submaxillary gland of male mice. The amino acid sequence of the protein from mouse is now known [56]. Under certain conditions of isolation, the factor consists of three different proteins, designated alpha, beta, and gamma, which interact in specific ways. The beta subunit has the biological activity; the roles of alpha and gamma proteins are not clearly defined. Alpha protein is known to possess endopeptidase activity, which may play a role in processing the beta subunit. Gamma protein protects ganglion cells during dissociation. The active beta protein is similar to insulin in a number of ways: they share many common amino acid sequences; both have a general anabolic effect; and both apparently act by binding to receptors on the cell surface. However, the receptors for NGF are different from those for insulin, and insulin will not substitute for NGF in its biological effects.

The cellular site of action and the mechanism of action of NGF are under intense investigation at present. In culture, the minimum concentration of NGF required for survival of sensory or sympathetic ganglia is about 2×10^{-11} M [62]. At this concentration, it is estimated that 10 to 20 percent of the cell-surface membrane receptors for NGF would be occupied, a value similar to that found for several peptide hormones. NGF also binds to receptors within the neuron. It is taken up at nerve endings and transported to the cell body by retrograde axoplasmic flow (Chap. 22). The relative importance of surface receptors versus retrograde transport of NGF from the periphery may depend on the source of NGF and the stage of development of the cell. The site of action may be intracellular, and the binding sites on the surface may act primarily to internalize the NGF. Alternatively, the site of action may be extracellular, and the surface sites may be coupled to a transducing mechanism. The two mechanisms may coexist. In addition, vesicles containing NGF may fuse with the nuclear envelope; therefore, a nuclear site of action is suggested [63]. Various other factors influencing growth or maturation of neuronal, glial, or neural-tumor cells in culture have been described. Conditioned media from several nonneural tissues contain factors that cause immature sympathetic neurons destined to be adrenergic in vivo to become cholinergic instead [64]. A factor that stimulates glial maturation in culture has been described [65]. Growth of astroglia is stimulated by several substances, including epidermal growth factor,

fibroblast growth factor, osteosarcoma factor, and somatomedin B [66].

HORMONES

During specific critical periods of development, hormones may act directly on the central nervous system to produce permanent changes. The same hormone may have different actions at different times. Most hormones produce changes in the rat brain only when administered in the prenatal or immediate postnatal period [67]. Different regions or cell types may be affected preferentially. For example, testosterone administered to newborn rats apparently acts on the hypothalamus to cause male sexual behavior at maturity; its absence leads to female sexual behavior (see Chap. 39 for additional discussion).

A number of hormones have widespread effects on the developing nervous system; the effects of corticosteroids and thyroid hormone have been the most extensively studied [68, 69]. Administration of either hormone to newborn rats leads to decreased brain weight and cell proliferation (presumably glial cells). Corticosteroids appear to have selective effects on the timing of brain maturation; they reduce dendritic branching transiently and probably decrease myelin formation [70]. The onset of maturation of glucose metabolism and metabolic compartmentation is not affected, but several enzymes can be induced by administration of corticosteroids [67].

The decrease in cell number found after thyroid hormone has been administered may be secondary to an acceleration of maturation which causes cell proliferation to end prematurely. There is an acceleration of dendritic branching, onset of myelination, and biochemical maturation, as indicated by changes in glucose metabolism and metabolic compartmentation. In contrast, hypothyroidism leads to retardation of brain development. There is reduction in brain weight, total cell number, the number and size of neurons, the density of axons and synapses, and the amount of myelin. Further, there is delay in the onset of dendritic branching and myelination. Behavioral changes accompanying these altered hormonal states also have been documented. Receptors for thyroid hormone are found on the inner mitochondrial membrane in brains of rats 12 days old and younger, but not in adult brain [71]; this is in keeping with the lack of response of adult brain to thyroid hormone.

Growth hormone deficiency causes decreased myelination in developing rat brain and its administration can reverse the effects of thyroid deficiency [72]. With the detection of insulin and insulin receptors [73] in the CNS, another hormonal influence on brain development lies ready for investigation.

One caution in interpreting experiments on the effects of hormone deficiency—thyroid, for example—is that any changes observed may be due to nutritional deprivation rather than to a specific effect of the lack of hormone. The effects of undernutrition and other deficiencies on the developing brain are discussed in greater detail in Chap. 33.

Experiments in vivo, in brain slices, and in culture have demonstrated the appearance during development of specific receptors for a number of neurohormones [74]. The action of several of these hormones is apparently mediated through cyclic AMP. Thus, addition of prostaglandins, norepinephrine, isoproterenol, or 5-hydroxytryptamine to brain slices causes rapid accumulation of cyclic AMP. This response appears with development: norepinephrine will not stimulate cyclic AMP accumulation in brain slices from newborn rats, but the response appears at day 4 and is maximal at day 10 [75], apparently due to the appearance of β-adrenergic receptors on the cell surface.

Induction of several enzymes in brain appears to be controlled by specific factors during development. For example, the developmental increase of cytoplasmic glycerol phosphate dehydrogenase depends on the presence of glucocorticoids, both in vivo and in culture, and levels of lactic dehydrogenase can be regulated specifically by catecholamines and cyclic AMP [74]. Indirect evidence and studies in glioblastomas indicate that these responses, and the stimulation of cyclic AMP levels by norepinephrine, reside primarily in glial cells rather than in neurons. Hormonal influences on $(Na^+ + K^+)$-ATPase development are described in Chap. 6.

Changes with Aging

Brain growth in rodents continues slowly, long into adulthood, whereas in primates brain weight and other factors show a plateau. Studies on senescent changes in brain are complicated by these differences in growth patterns, the large individual variation in aging, and the scarcity of samples. Little change in brain weight or water content accompanies aging in rats or mice. In primates, including humans, brain weight decreases and water content increases. Species differences have also been noted in changes of DNA content and neuronal number. Little change in either occurs in aging rodent brain [68]. One study in cerebral cortex of rat showed that neuronal and microglial densities were constant between 100 and 700 days, but that densities of astroglia and oligodendroglia increased [76]. In primate and human brains, levels of DNA and numbers of neurons in cerebral cortex decrease significantly with aging, as much as 50 percent in some regions [8, 77, 78]. Little change is found in other regions, including brainstem [76].

With increasing age, multiple morphological changes take place. Many of these changes have been observed in pathological situations in less mature brains, as well. The most prominent neuronal changes are appearance of senile plaques (areas of degenerating neuronal processes, reactive nonneuronal cells, and amyloid), increasing deposits of lipofuscin, and areas of neurofibrillary tangles (twisted tubules) [79]. The deposition of lipofuscin may be related to increased oxidation of unsaturated fatty acids; whether its accumulation leads to cell death or decreased function is not known. Loss of synapses, dendrites, and dendritic spines also occurs with aging [78].

The effects of aging on neurotransmitter systems in brain have received increasing attention over the past several years. Comprehensive studies on various regions of brain have revealed several changes with aging [80, 81]. Acetylcholinesterase and choline acetyltransferase activities decrease with age, particularly in cerebral cortex, indicating involvement of cholinergic systems. Muscarinic acetylcholine receptors are decreased [82]. Two enzymes involved in metabolism of catecholamines—tyrosine hydroxylase and dopa decarboxylase—show appreciable decreases with age in many of the brain regions studied, as does glutamic acid decarboxylase, a key enzyme in GABA metabolism. However, earlier reports suggested that monoamine oxidase increases with age.

Several investigators report decreased postmortem levels of choline acetyltransferase in human cerebral cortex. In senile dementia, several investigators report decreased postmortem levels of choline acetyltransferase in human cerebral cortex relative to cortex from normal age-matched controls [81, 82]. This observation leads to the hypothesis that cholinergic systems, particularly in hippocampus, may be involved in the functional deficits characteristic of senile dementia. The relative roles of neuronal loss versus synaptic degeneration in aging brain are currently under investigation; several lines of morphological and biochemical evidence suggest that synaptic disability is greater than neuronal loss. Such disability may be related to the formation of senile plaques, which may be primary, rather than secondary, to neuronal death. The possibility exists that enhancing synaptic transmission, particularly in cholinergic systems, may ameliorate some of the mental deficits associated with aging. Some investigators consider that increasing tissue levels of acetylcholine might produce enhancement.

Cellular Development of the Nervous System

The morphogenetic events leading to formation of the mature nervous system are described in detail in a number of books [e.g., 8, 83, 84]. During embryonic development, neural ectoderm is induced at the gastrula stage by interaction of the mesodermal tissue from the dorsal lip of the blastopore with the overlying ectoderm; subsequently, the neural ectoderm cells migrate inward to form the neural plate. This interaction appears to involve a diffusible substance, rather than direct contact [85], and the inductor may act through cyclic AMP [86]. During the gastrula stage, neural induction proceeds caudally and cranially from the blastopore, leading to closure of the neural tube and determination of the major regions of the CNS.

Epithelial cells that line the neural tube give rise to migrating cells, which form the neurons of the CNS. Along the dorsal surface of the neural tube lies the neural crest, a column of cells that also is of ectodermal origin and that gives rise to migrating cells that develop into the neurons of the sensory, sympathetic, and parasympathetic ganglia of the peripheral nervous system (PNS). In the CNS, the astroglia and oligodendroglia originate in the neural tube epithelium; the Schwann cells and satellite cells of the PNS arise from both the neural tube and the neural crest. In most brain regions that have been studied, large neurons arise first, followed by small neurons, then glia. Phylogenetically, older regions of brain develop earlier than do newer regions [8].

NEURONS

Proliferation and Migration

Neurogenesis in the rat cerebrum extends from postconception day 11 or 12 to birth. The cerebral vesicle forms in the rat about day 10 of gestation. Shortly thereafter, the ventricular zone of pseudostratified neuroepithelial cells appears. This zone reaches its maximum thickness at about day 14 of gestation. The sequence of development involves three compartments, or zones, of cells. Two zones, ventricular and subventricular, contain dividing cells, and the third zone contains postmitotic cells in the course of their migration and differentiation [8]. The germinal, or stem, cells in the ventricular zone give rise to the large Golgi type I neurons and to the subventricular cells. The latter cells then proliferate and give rise to the smaller Golgi type II neurons and to glial cells; gliogenesis commences while neurogenesis is still continuing [16]. Once the primitive neuron (neuroblast) leaves the ventricular or subventricular zone, it is no longer capable of further division. This is in contrast to glial cells and to neurons of neural crest origin; both of these types can divide after they have migrated away from their original area of proliferation.

It is not known why neuroblasts lose their ability to divide. The neuroblast may lose some of its DNA irreversibly either by deletion or by permanent repression. However, two lines of study indicate that a cytoplasmic factor may be responsible for DNA stability after neurons have differentiated. Nuclei from cells of adult amphibian brain transplanted to oocytes begin to divide, although at a somewhat slower rate than do nuclei from less mature stages [87]. Fusion of adult neurons with an established fibroblast line results in reactivation of DNA synthesis in the neuronal nuclei [88].

Studies of cells of extraneural origin, such as muscle and cancer cells, indicate that the membrane potential may be involved in control of mitogenesis; cells with low membrane potential are mitogenically active; those with high membrane potential are reversibly inactive. DNA synthesis and mitosis have been induced in cultured, fully differentiated neurons from spinal cords of chick embryos by sustained depolarization caused by various agents, such as ouabain, that produce increased levels of sodium and decreased levels of potassium within the cell [89].

The time of origin and subsequent migration of neurons have been mapped by using tritiated thymidine. After it has been injected into the mother, thymidine is available for DNA synthesis for about 60 minutes [25]. Those cells undergoing DNA replication at the time of injection will incorporate [³H]thymidine. Those cells continuing to divide will dilute the label with each subsequent division. The neurons undergoing their final cell division at the time of injection will remain heavily labeled throughout the life of the animal. These techniques have been used to study both normal neuronal formation and abnormal formation in genetically determined and exogenously induced (x-ray, nutritional deprivation, viral infection) defects of the nervous system [8, 25].

The migration of neurons is a carefully programmed process. The cerebral cortex is formed from the inside out; that is, the early migrating cells form the deeper layers of cortex. The later migrating cells pass through these formed layers to constitute more superficial layers.

In other regions of the nervous system, such as the hypothalamus, this pattern of migration may not take place. Here, first-formed cells migrate distally, and later-forming cells position themselves more centrally. In spinal cord, large neurons arise first. In cortex, the smaller neurons of layers VI and IV clearly arise before the large neurons of layer III.

The events underlying neuronal migration are not clear. Some authors suggest that there is only an intracytoplasmic migration of the nucleus, the cell extending from lumen to pia. This migration might be related to the proliferation of microtubules and microfilaments in migrating neurons. Other theories relate to the role of the axon in directing migration or the guidance of migrating neurons by contact with already formed glial processes or other extracellular factors. These theories are discussed in Chap. 21.

During early embryogenesis, massive cell death occurs as the neural tube is developing. Therefore, the number of neurons formed in many brain regions is greater than the number in the adult structure. Factors that determine which cells will die are not understood, although one may be that survival depends on adequate synapse formation with the appropriate target [8, 9]. Increasing available postsynaptic sites has no effect on neuronal proliferation but does decrease cell death among the maturing neurons.

Maturation

Other than its morphology, the characteristics that distinguish a mature neuron from other cells are its abilities to propagate an action potential and to make specialized contacts, through the synapses, with other neurons.

It is not known precisely when the mature membrane properties of a neuron first appear, but maturation may begin shortly after mitosis or after a long period of growth. Two extreme examples are (1) the motor neurons of chick spinal cord, in which axonal growth begins while the cell is migrating out of the germinal layer, and (2) the retinal ganglion cells, in which axonal outgrowth does not take place until the neuron is in its adult position and has grown in size [8].

On a cellular level, the maturing neuron exhibits (a) decreasing numbers of microtubules and increasing numbers of neurofilaments in the cytoplasm; (b) shifting from multiple nucleoli to one large nucleolus, accompanied by an increase in nucleolar RNA; (c) decreasing amounts of free ribosomes and increasing amounts of rough endoplasmic reticulum and the smooth membrane-bounded cisternae of the Golgi apparatus; and (d) growth in size [8, 90].

Axonal outgrowth accompanies these changes in the neuronal cell body and involves the ameboid movement of the growth cone, with new molecules apparently inserted into the membrane near the growing tip [91].

Synapse Formation

The *growth cone* is the first part of the neuron to contact potential target cells, to recognize an appropriate target, and to interact with the target to form a synaptic complex. However, we know relatively little about the molecular factors that guide axonal growth, sometimes over long distances, or about the factors that direct synapse formation at specific sites on target cells [92]. Both mechanical and chemical signals apparently act to guide the growing axon to its destination. In culture, outgrowth of *neurites* (fine nerve processes) from ganglia is stimulated by the appropriate target tissue by means of unknown substances that act over a distance up to 2 mm [93].

A role for glycoproteins or glycolipids in neuronal recognition has been suggested from observations made of aggregation and adhesion in model systems [94, 95]. These are studies of cell bodies, so the described properties are not necessarily identical to those of axons or growth cones. By mapping the binding of lectins or toxins conjugated to ferritin or horseradish peroxidase, the distribution of glycolipids and glycoproteins on developing neurons has been examined [96]. The lectin-binding studies show that different regions of the same neuron bind the same lectins, whereas neurons from different sources bind different lectins. Lectins, such as concanavalin A, are bound in an even distribution over all regions of the neurons, axon, and growth cone. However, freeze-fracture studies show that the density of intramem-

branous particles (possibly glycoproteins or glycolipids) decreases from the cell body down the axon, with almost no particles near the tip of the growth cone.

Although synaptic vesicles are sparse or absent in the growth cone, neurotransmitters apparently can be released. Like the mature endings, the growth cone has receptors and uptake systems for a number of substances, including NGF and cholera toxin, which are transported to the cell body.

The order of appearance of the various morphological features of the synapse as it matures is not entirely clear. Variations among descriptions may arise because there are differences in sampling a dynamic process, in fixing the tissue, or indeed, because the sequence of events may vary for different synapses. In studies monitoring the initial contact between spinal-cord axons and dissociated sympathetic neurons in culture [97], punctate regions of contact between growth cone and target neuron were seen first. Afterward, hypertrophy of the Golgi apparatus and increased numbers of coated vesicles were seen in the target cell. The coated vesicles appeared to transport new membrane components to the postsynaptic density. In 24 hours, the filopodia of the presynaptic ending had retracted and presynaptic vesicles could be seen. In 48 hours, the dense projections of the presynaptic membrane appeared, and the synapse assumed a mature appearance. The smooth ER, lysosomes, and microfilaments of the growth cone were largely replaced by numerous synaptic vesicles, some dense-core vesicles, and a few mitochondria.

Factors determining the position and distribution of synapses on a given target are little understood [8, 9]. The growth cone does not seem first to contact an area rich in postsynaptic receptors; conversely, at least in muscle, the receptors are added to the postsynaptic surface after synapse formation has started. Further, synapses form in muscle even in the presence of α-bungarotoxin, which binds to acetylcholine receptors. Synapses also develop normally in the presence of curare, indicating that electrical transmission is not required. In a number of systems examined, "hyperinnervation" occurs and is followed by degeneration of many of the synapses. One theory holds that there is competition among incoming growth cones for a trophic factor released in limited amounts by the target tissue, and that the exact sites of synapse formation on a given target are not rigorously specified. This factor may be required by the neuronal cell body for maintenance of the synapse, and if an adequate amount is not transported from the synapse to the perikaryon, that synapse is not maintained.

The biochemical maturation of synapses can be followed by analysis of the processes that mediate synaptic transmission. Thus, appearance of enzymes that synthesize specific neurotransmitters, increased levels of transmitter stored in the nerve ending, and high-affinity uptake systems are used as "specific biochemical markers for quantifying neuronal differentiation" [98]. For example, neurochemical studies in rat striatum show that postsynaptic receptors for dopamine are present and that they receive innervation by dopaminergic neurons at birth, as indicated by the simultaneous increase in tyrosine hydroxylase, dopamine, and high-affinity uptake of dopamine (Fig. 23-5). In the same region, the presynaptic and postsynaptic markers for the cholinergic endings do not increase until later, beginning 1 to 2 weeks after birth.

However, the various presynaptic parameters for a particular class of neurons do not always develop in a parallel or coordinated fashion. As one example, GABAergic endings in striatum contain high concentrations of GABA at birth, but low levels of glutamic acid decarboxylase (GAD). After birth, GABA drops; then, from the first postnatal week to adulthood, it rises in parallel with GAD levels. The GABA-uptake system shows a different pattern, reaching a peak at 2 weeks, then dropping again.

Studies of Neuronal Characteristics

The diversity of neuronal types in cerebrum has inhibited definitive study of the biochemical events accompanying their maturation and interaction with other cells. Studies in simpler systems have allowed more detailed correlation of morpho-

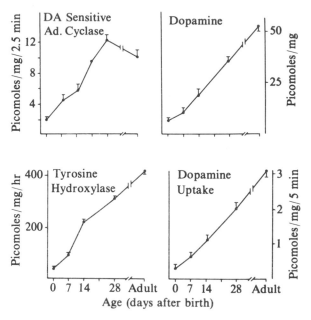

Fig. 23-5. Development of the neurochemical indices of dopaminergic innervation in the striatum of rat. Values are represented in terms of milligrams wet weight of tissue. (Reprinted from J. T. Coyle [98], with permission.)

logical and biochemical changes in developing neurons. Nervous tissue in culture has been used successfully to study neuronal maturation [99].

CELL LINES IN CULTURE. Clonal cell lines derived from the mouse neuroblastoma C 1300 or from chemically induced brain tumors exhibit various combinations of neuronal properties, including electrically excitable membranes, high levels of enzymes involved in transmitter metabolism, receptors for transmitters, and the neuronal specific protein 14-3-2 [100]. These cell lines offer the potential of dissecting the control and interaction of the various genes that give rise to neuron-specific properties.

When cultured neuroblastoma cells attach to a solid substratum, these neuronal characteristics may become more pronounced, and the cells extend neurites, long processes initially containing mitochondria, ribosomes, and dense core vesicles and, later, microtubules and filaments [101]. This differentiation can be stimulated by a variety of conditions, such as decreasing the serum content in the growth medium or exposing cultures to dibutyryl cyclic AMP, acetylcholine, prostaglandins, or bromodeoxyuridine. Multiple changes in protein patterns accompany this differentiation [102].

A number of individual clonal lines, both neuronal and glial in origin, have been derived from rat brain by chemical induction of tumors [103]. In the neuronal lines, low serum content or the presence of dibutyryl cyclic AMP in the culture medium induces process extension, and bromodeoxyuridine causes only cell flattening. Protein synthesis is not required for process extension in either the neuroblastoma C 1300 or induced tumor lines. Colchicine, an alkaloid that dissociates microtubule subunits, causes very rapid retraction of the processes in both systems.

Low serum concentrations and addition of substances of low molecular weight may induce differentiation, in part, by enhancing interaction between the cell surface and the culture dish. Some conditions that induce neurite formation also stop cell division, but several lines of evidence indicate there is no causal relationship between these two events [103].

REAGGREGATING SYSTEMS. Cells dissociated from fetal or developing brain and maintained in rotating flasks aggregate in specific and highly organized patterns [104, 105], and formation of both synapses and myelin has been observed. Abnormal patterns of reaggregation occur with cells dissociated from the brain of the reeler mutant mouse, a mutant characterized by defective orientation and layering of neurons in both cerebral and cerebellar cortex [106].

Under appropriate conditions, some components exhibit biochemical differentiation similar to that in developing brain [105]. For example, three neuronal-enriched enzymes—choline acetyltransferase, acetylcholinesterase, and glutamate decarboxylase—show a pattern of increase similar to that seen in vivo. Receptors for norepinephrine appear in culture, as in vivo, and a shift toward more oxidative metabolism also occurs.

PNS GANGLIA. Superior cervical ganglia (sympathetic) and dorsal root ganglia (sensory) are useful systems for examining neuronal maturation both in vivo and in culture. Morphological and biochemical events during maturation are well documented [54, 57], and the effects of preganglionic and postganglionic manipulation on neuronal maturation and maintenance can be observed readily in a relatively homogeneous system. For example, in superior cervical ganglia of mouse or rat, formation of preganglionic cholinergic synapses correlates well with a 50-fold increase in activity of choline acetyltransferase in the ganglia between birth and 30 days. Maturation of the adrenergic cell body is accompanied by increases in tyrosine hydroxylase and dopamine β-hydroxylase. Preganglionic blockade prevents the increase in tyrosine hydroxylase activity and morphological maturation of the neurons; administration of nerve growth factor at the proper time stimulates maturation. Administration of antiserum to NGF to newborn mice results in destruction of undifferentiated ganglionic neurons, with the earliest lesions occurring in the nucleus. Administration of 6-hydroxydopamine also destroys these young neurons, but apparently by a different mechanism, as the earliest changes are cytoplasmic and NGF cannot reverse the effects. In the adult animal, the differentiated neurons show less severe reversible changes with both insults. In the adults, as well, antiserum to NGF produces nuclear changes and some decrease in cell volume, while 6-hydroxydopamine acts primarily at the adrenergic terminals [55].

RETINAL NEURONS: RECOGNITION AND LOCUS SPECIFICITY. Development of specific synaptic connections has been studied in greatest detail in the visual system of frogs and chicks. Each retinal ganglion cell sends out an axon to a specific location in the optic tectum, so that the spatial pattern of individual retinal axon terminals in the tectum corresponds to the spatial relationship of the corresponding retinal ganglion cells. With electrophysiological techniques, several investigators [8] have mapped the relationship of retinal cells to tectal cells in embryonic frog brain and have found that specification of the gradients that determine the connections takes place after DNA synthesis has ceased and that it precedes fiber outgrowth in retinal neurons. Evidence for recognition and interaction between retinal and tectal cells has come from experiments with dissociated and re-aggregating tissue [107]. Specific changes in glyco-proteins of chick retina have been detected between 7 and 13 days of development. A cell-adhesion molecule, a protein of 140,000 molecular weight, has been purified from neural retina and characterized.

Neuronal Responses in Regeneration

Once differentiated, neurons cannot divide, so their response to injury may be either death, or degeneration of damaged processes followed by regeneration [108, 109]. If a population of neurons dies or is removed, other neurons may be able to reinnervate the same field if the injury occurs early enough in development [8, 9]. Cell death occurs normally during development of the nervous system. Experimentally removing the field into which a group of neurons is sending processes will lead to the death of that group; this suggests a trophic func-tion of the target tissue.

Since the pioneering observations of Ramon y Cajal [108], the central question in regeneration research has been why certain neurons of the mam-malian CNS fail to support sustained axonal growth with normal functional recovery after in-jury [110]. For example, after adult spinal cord or optic nerve in mammals has been severed, limited regeneration of axons may occur, but they rarely cross the site of the lesion and usually degenerate within 2 weeks [111]. Sporadic reports of regeneration and functional recovery have ap-peared but remain to be substantiated.

The nervous systems of most submammalian vertebrate species and selected sites in the mam-malian CNS and PNS exhibit a greater capacity for regeneration. When regeneration does occur after axotomy, lost synapses may be replaced in one of several ways. Germinal epithelium, if still present, can give rise to new dividing neuroblasts, which can send out axons to replace the degenerat-ing ones. Examples of this are found in developing

amphibia [8, 110] and in the olfactory bulb of the mammalian CNS [112]. Axonal regeneration from the injured neuron generally is seen in the nervous systems of amphibians and fish and in the peripheral nervous system of mammals. Within the mammalian CNS, the hypothalamoneuro-hypophyseal system exhibits axonal regeneration after pituitary-stalk section; intrinsic noradrenergic neurons within the locus ceruleus and dopaminer-gic neurons in the mesolimbic and nigrostriatal systems also exhibit regenerative capabilities [113, 114]. A third mechanism, often referred to as col-lateral sprouting, but perhaps more properly termed reactive synaptogenesis [115], involves formation of new synapses by outgrowing branches of appropriate surviving axons that make contacts with the previously denervated sites. This process has been studied extensively at the neuromuscular junction and in the hippocampus.

The problem of why regeneration does not generally occur in mature mammalian CNS has led investigators to examine other systems in which regeneration of neural cells does occur and to de-velop culture systems in which the various factors controlling regeneration may be defined. As in de-velopment, the interplay between the intrinsic determinants in a cell and the extrinsic influences of the cellular environment determine the response of a given cell, that is, full or partial regeneration with normal or abnormal function, dedifferentia-tion and subsequent mitosis, or cell death. Before generalizations can be made, several factors must be considered: the cell type being examined, the kind or extent of injury (for example, transection versus crush), the relative maturity of the cell, and the conditions under which the nerve is regen-erating.

We now realize that the mature CNS has a greater capacity for plasticity and regeneration than was previously recognized. The lack of func-tional recovery in CNS may be because the environ-ment is not conducive, rather than because CNS neurons lack the ability to regenerate. Compared with the PNS, in the CNS (a) there are no neuro-lemmal or endoneurial sheaths to guide regrowth; (b) scarring (growth of astrocytes and connective tissue) is more severe; and (c) an extremely complex level of synaptic connections might have to be reestablished before functional recovery can occur. Possible factors under consideration that might be more specific for a given neuronal type include (a) intrinsic inability of a particular neuron to sustain the metabolism needed for new axonal growth; (b) lack of appropriate trophic factor from target tissue or tissues through which axons are growing; and (c) inhibition of growth by immunological mechanisms elicited by brain autoantigens. Interestingly, supporting cells in fish and amphibia, and in mammalian PNS appear to aid, rather than hinder, regeneration of neurons. One study in mammals suggested that regenerating CNS axons were already retracting before astroglia began proliferating at the lesion site [116]. Recent studies in both lower vertebrates and mammals show that a "conditioning" lesion may increase the capacity of some neurons for axonal regeneration, as outgrowth is more vigorous after the second lesion than after the first [117].

AXONAL REACTION OF REGENERATION. Neurons exhibit a spectrum of morphological and biochemical changes after axotomy [117]. Some neuronal types, such as sympathetic and motor neurons, show classical *chromatolysis* in the cell body (dissolution of Nissl substance or rough endoplasmic reticulum). Other types, such as retinal ganglion cells and noradrenergic interneurons in the CNS, do not show morphological signs of chromatolysis, but undergo the biochemical and structural changes accompanying axonal regeneration. Some signal from the severed axon is presumably transmitted to the perikaryon to trigger these events. Synthesis and turnover of rRNA are increased. Net protein synthesis subsequently may be increased or decreased, but some proteins, such as tubulin, clearly show increased synthesis. Generally, there is a decrease in levels of the enzymes involved in the metabolism of neurotransmitters in the cell. The amount of protein transported by fast axonal transport is increased, with no change in the rate of transport. Changes in slow axoplasmic transport are less well characterized. Synapses on the neuronal cell body itself are removed, and there

is an increase in glia at the old synaptic sites. At about the same time that protein synthesis increases and synaptic boutons disappear from the cell body, axonal outgrowth begins. After the goldfish optic nerve is crushed, outgrowth begins in about 4 days at a rate of 0.34 to 0.42 mm per day. In rat sciatic nerve, the delay after a crush is somewhat shorter (1.3 to 3.2 days) and the rate of outgrowth is about 4 mm per day. The rate of axonal regeneration slows with maturation [118] from 4.7 mm per day in rat pups to 2.4 mm per day in adult rats.

GLIA

Proliferation, Migration, and Turnover

Macroglia, which are composed of oligodendrocytes and astrocytes, have a neuroectodermal origin. Their initial site of proliferation is the ventricular zone; but once active cell division ceases in this zone, the glioblasts migrate into the surrounding nervous tissue and continue to divide in situ [8]. Formation of neurons and glia in a specific region of the CNS may overlap, but this takes place only toward the end of neuronal proliferation. The appearance of astrocytes usually precedes that of oligodendrocytes, but the two cell types continue to form concurrently at later developmental stages [119].

Little is known about the cells responsible for the formation of astrocytes and oligodendrocytes. There are two possibilities. First, there may be a multipotential glial cell [119] that can form both astrocytes and oligodendrocytes. Second, there may be two distinct cell lines, one astrocytic and one oligodendrocytic, that are determined at very early developmental stages. Recent electron-microscope studies support this second possibility, since immature dividing cells with either oligodendroglial or astroglial characteristics can be identified [120]. Astroglia can be traced back to early prenatal stages, when they appear to arise directly from ventricular cells without going through a glioblast stage. The origin of oligodendroglia is less clear; they may arise from undifferentiated glioblasts or poorly differentiated astroblasts. In contrast to neurons, glia arise at scattered sites throughout the tissue and appear to migrate only short distances. One site of glial proliferation throughout the CNS is the subependymal plate, which continues to give rise to glial cells into adult life.

It is uncertain whether there is a turnover of oligodendroglia in mature CNS. Electron-microscope quantitative estimates of neuroglia in cerebral cortex at different ages show no increase in the number of oligodendrocytes in aging rats [121]. It is possible, however, that some oligodendrocytes die and are replaced by new cells.

In developing optic nerve and corpus callosum and in optic nerve undergoing Wallerian degeneration, electron-microscope autoradiographic studies indicate that astrocytes and oligodendrocytes that have differentiated to some degree can still incorporate tritiated thymidine [120]. Immature oligodendroglia that have initiated myelin formation and fibrous astrocytes will still incorporate [³H]thymidine. These data suggest that the long-held tenet that cell division and differentiation are two separate stages of development may not be universally correct.

Throughout the CNS, appearance of oligodendroglia and, subsequently, myelin generally proceeds in a caudocranial direction, with spinal cord first and frontal cortex last. In the corpus callosum and the pyramidal tract of the rat, for example, oligodendroglial proliferation, or "myelination gliosis," begins shortly before birth and reaches a maximum about 4 days after birth [122]. As the rate of cell proliferation decreases, RNA content and protein synthesis increase, and lipid droplets appear in the oligodendroglia. Myelin sheaths first appear in these regions at days 10 to 12. Some cell proliferation continues, though at a lower rate, during the period of myelination.

Interaction between Axons and Myelin-Forming Cells

Oligodendroglial division, migration, and differentiation, as well as the actual attachment of glia to axons and subsequent myelination, are probably all influenced by axons. In the CNS, oligodendroglia migrate toward the unmyelinated axon.

Little is known about the initiation of myelination except that the axon diameter is critical [123]. Speculations about the interrelationship of axons and myelin formation include the suggestion that precursors or formed compounds can be transported from the axon to the forming myelin sheath. Antisera to CNS or galactocerebroside disrupt myelination in CNS organ cultures. When added before myelination, antisera to CNS reversibly prevent differentiation of oligodendroglia [124]. If the serum is heated to remove complement, the oligodendroglia mature and produce membranes, but the membranes accumulate randomly in the culture, rather than in lamellae wrapped around axons. Thus, the interaction between the myelin sheath and axon is disrupted. Cerebroside has been implicated as the molecule involved in both the complement-dependent and complement-independent actions of the antisera, but the mechanisms of these effects are still unknown.

In the peripheral nervous system, Schwann cells myelinate axons. The cell of origin is in the neural crest, and the maturing cell migrates to the axon. Culture systems have been used to analyze the relationship between axons and developing Schwann cells [125]. In cultured explants of dorsal root ganglia, contact of naked neurites with quiescent Schwann cells stimulates the mitogenesis of Schwann cells and subsequent myelination. The presence of collagen is also required for this mitogenic effect [126]. The role of the axon in signaling Schwann cells to myelinate has been demonstrated by transplanting portions of myelinated and unmyelinated nerves [127, 128]. The Schwann cells from myelinated nerve do not myelinate axons growing in from a normally unmyelinated nerve, but the Schwann cells from unmyelinated nerve will myelinate axons from myelinated nerve. These results indicate that the axons contain signals both to stimulate mitogenesis and to induce myelination.

Various agents that raise intracellular levels of cyclic AMP, such as cholera toxin and dibutyryl cyclic AMP, are mitogenic for Schwann cells in culture. Crude extracts of brain and pituitary are also mitogenic for these cells, but apparently stimulate Schwann cell division by a different mechanism, since they do not increase cyclic AMP levels [129].

Myelination

The end point of differentiation of the oligodendrocyte is the formation of myelin. The biochemical events involved in myelin formation are outlined in Chap. 4.

Oligodendroglia may be separated from other cell types in brain, but separation of actively myelinating from myelin-maintaining oligodendroglia is not yet possible. Isolated mature oligodendroglia have a composition different from that of astrocytes or neurons isolated under similar conditions. The oligodendroglial fractions are enriched in myelin components [130]. It is possible to develop the concept that, during myelination, the plasma membrane of the oligodendrocyte changes and new components are added. The composition of isolated oligodendroglial plasma membranes supports this hypothesis [131].

Oligodendroglial Responses in Regeneration

The regenerative response of oligodendroglia is remyelination, with or without preceding proliferation of oligodendroglia. In a number of experimental models, demyelination was followed by remyelination. These models include, in the cat, removal and replacement of cerebrospinal fluid, transient compression of the spinal cord, and cyanide intoxication; in the rat and rabbit, experimental allergic encephalomyelitis; and, in mice, intoxication with cuprizone [132]. In these studies, the criteria of remyelination are morphological, and include altered ratios of myelin-sheath thickness to axon diameter and reduction of internodal length (see Chap. 32).

A viral mode of demyelination and subsequent remyelination in the mouse has been described [133]. Formation of new oligodendroglia occurred, along with remyelination, as judged by incorporation of [^{35}S] sulfate into sulfatide.

It is less certain that remyelination takes place in the human central nervous system. Around the edges of a demyelinative plaque, the so-called shadow plaque in multiple sclerosis, axons with short internodes of myelin are seen. It is not clear if this represents remyelination or partial demyelination (see Chap. 32).

In CNS demyelination induced by disease or by injection with lysolecithin, Schwann cells have been observed to migrate into the CNS and to myelinate axons. Experimentally, Schwann cells can be transplanted into the CNS, where they successfully myelinate CNS axons [134].

Astroglia may play a dual role in remyelination of axons by oligodendroglia [135]. They are active in removal of myelin debris; this removal appears to be necessary for successful remyelination. Subsequently, the presence of astroglia appears necessary for initiation of myelin formation by the oligodendroglia.

Role of Astrocytes in Development

Investigators have suggested a role for "glia" in a number of developmental systems. Often it is not clear what cell types are being described by this term. Presumably the cells are not oligodendroglia, but are mixtures of primitive stem cells and astrocytes.

As previously mentioned, it has been suggested that glial processes form a trellis along which neurons migrate during development. It is not clear what cells would provide this trellis. Rakic and Sidman [136] have suggested that Bergmann astrocytes might play such a role for granular cells migrating from the external granular cell zone to the internal granular cell zone of the cerebellum, and that abnormalities of fiber outgrowth would lead to abnormalities of neuronal migration.

Other possible roles for "glia" that could be important during development are regulation of extracellular concentrations of sodium and potassium (Chap. 6), inactivation of transmitters (Chap. 8), and secretion of substances similar to nerve growth factor. Such hypotheses are difficult to substantiate in the intact nervous system. In tissue-culture systems, however, neuronal-glial interactions can be evaluated. Neuroblasts from chicken cerebrum attach quickly to a monolayer of *astroblasts* (primitive glial cells from a 13-day chick embryo) and differentiate more rapidly than do those cultured on plastic or on layers of fibroblasts or meningeal cells [137]. In the peripheral nervous system, a similar phenomenon has been observed, in that dissociated neurons from dorsal root ganglia of newborn mouse will attach and grow on a layer of nonneuronal cells from the ganglion. Further, neurons that have attached to ganglionic nonneuronal cells have a decreased requirement for nerve growth factor. It has been suggested that, in this system, the growth-promoting effects of nonneuronal ganglionic cells and NGF have a common mechanism [54].

Astrocytes contain a specific protein, glial fibrillary acidic protein (GFAP) [34]. This protein, or a closely related group of proteins, is intracellular and probably is related to glial filaments within fibrous processes. Immunofluorescence, using antisera to GFAP, has been used to detect astrocytic development in cerebellum, cerebral cortex, and spinal cord (see Chap. 20).

Because glial processes are readily detected, antisera to GFAP have been useful in studying the development of Bergmann astrocytes in mouse mutants with cerebellar abnormalities [138]. In all instances, fibers from Bergmann glia appear at the normal time in homozygously affected animals. The subsequent development of fibers, however, is quite different in the particular mutants.

Responses of Astrocytes
It is difficult to comment about age-specific changes in astrocytes because these cells are so sensitive to various stimuli. For example, when one uses the term *gliosis* in a pathological sense, one is referring to the proliferation of astrocytes and microglia. Such responses are seen in a variety of situations, such as trauma, infection, or anoxia. The factors that induce astrocytic proliferation are unknown.

Acknowledgments
This report represents activities supported by funds from the National Institute of Neurological and Communicative Disorders and Stroke.

The authors thank Dr. Robert P. Skoff for his assistance in reviewing comments about morphological aspects of development.

References
*1. Davison, A. N., and Dobbing, J. (eds.). *Applied Neurochemistry.* Philadelphia: Davis, 1968.
*2. Ford, D. H. (ed.). *Neurobiological Aspects of Maturation and Aging.* New York: Elsevier, 1972. Vol. 40.
*3. Himwich, W. A. (ed.). *Developmental Neurobiology.* Springfield, Ill.: Thomas, 1970.
*4. Himwich, W. A. (ed.). *Biochemistry of the Developing Brain.* Vols. 1 and 2. New York: Dekker, 1973, 1974.
*5. McIlwain, H., and Bachelard, S. Chemical and Enzymic Make-up of the Brain During Development. In H. McIlwain, and S. Bachelard (eds.), *Biochemistry and the Central Nervous System.* London: Churchill Livingstone, 1971.
*6. Waelsch, H. (ed.). *Biochemistry of the Developing Nervous System.* New York: Academic, 1955.
*7. Himwich, H. E. Early Studies of the Developing Brain. In W. A. Himwich (ed.), *Biochemistry of the Developing Brain.* New York: Dekker, 1973. Vol. 1, pp. 1–53.
*8. Jacobson, M. *Developmental Neurobiology.* 2nd Edition. New York: Plenum, 1978.
9. Cowan, W. M. Selection and Control in Neurogenesis. In F. O. Schmitt and F. G. Worden, *The Neurosciences: Fourth Study Program.* Cambridge, Mass.: M.I.T. Press, 1979. Pp. 59–79.
10. Dobbing, J., and Sands, J. Comparative aspects of the brain growth spurt. *Early Hum. Dev.* 3: 79–83, 1979.
11. Kishimoto, Y., Davies, W. E., and Radin, N. S. Developing rat brain: Changes in cholesterol, galactolipids, and the individual fatty acids of gangliosides and glycerophosphatides. *J. Lipid Res.* 6:532–536.
12. Fish, I., and Winick, M. Effect of malnutrition on regional growth of the developing rat brain. *Exp. Neurol.* 25:534–540, 1969.
13. Mandel, P., Rein, H., Harth-Edel, S., and Mardell, R. Distribution and Metabolism of Ribonucleic Acid in the Vertebrate Central Nervous System. In D. Richter (ed.), *Comparative Neurochemistry.* New York: Macmillan, 1964. Pp. 149–163.
14. Himwich, W. A. Appendix. In A. Lajtha (ed.), *Handbook of Neurochemistry.* New York: Plenum, 1969. Vol. 1, pp. 469–470.
*15. Himwich, W. A. Biochemistry and neurophysiology of the brain in the neonatal period. *Int. Rev. Neurobiol.* 4:117–158, 1962.
16. Eayrs, J. R., and Goodhead, B. Postnatal development of the cerebral cortex in the rat. *J. Anat.* 93:384–402, 1959.

*Key reference.

17. Aghajanian, G. H., and Bloom, F. E. The formation of synaptic junctions in developing rat brain. A quantitative electron microscopic study. *Brain Res.* 6:716–727, 1967.

18. Kobayashi, T., Inman, O. R., Buno, W., and Himwich, H. E. Neurohistological studies of developing mouse brain. *Prog. Brain Res.* 9:87–88, 1954.

19. Dobbing, J., and Sands, J. Growth and development of the brain and spinal cord of the guinea pig. *Brain Res.* 17:115–123, 1970.

20. Purpura, D. P., Schofer, R. J., Housepian, E. M., and Noback, C. R. Comparative ontogenesis of structure-function relations in cerebral and cerebellar cortex. *Prog. Brain Res.* 4:187–221, 1964.

21. Jacobson, S. Sequence of myelinization in the brain of the albino rat. A. Cerebral cortex, thalamus and related structures. *J. Comp. Neurol.* 121:5–29, 1963.

22. Uzman, L. L., and Rumley, M. K. Changes in the composition of developing mouse brain during early myelination. *J. Neurochem.* 3:171–184, 1958.

23. Yakovlev, P. I., and Lecours, A. R. The Myelogenetic Cycles of Regional Maturation of the Brain. In A. Minkowski (ed.), *Regional Development of the Brain.* Oxford: Blackwell, 1967. Pp. 3–70.

24. Winick, M., Rosso, P., and Waterlow, J. Cellular growth of the cerebrum, cerebellum and brain stem in normal and marasmic children. *Exp. Neurol.* 26:393–400, 1970.

25. Altman, J. DNA Metabolism and Cell Proliferation. In A. Lajtha (ed.), *Handbook of Neurochemistry.* New York: Plenum, 1969. Vol. 2, pp. 137–182.

26. Brasel, J. A., Ehrenkranz, R. A., and Winick, M. DNA polymerase activity in rat brain during ontogeny. *Dev. Biol.* 23:424–432, 1970.

27. Giuffrida, A. M., Cox, D., and Mathias, A. P. RNA polymerase activity in various classes of nuclei from different regions of rat brain during development. *J. Neurochem.* 24:749–755, 1975.

28. Murthy, M. R. V. Membrane-Bound and Free Ribosomes in the Developing Rat Brain. In A. Lajtha (ed.), *Protein Metabolism of the Nervous System.* New York: Plenum, 1970. Pp. 109–127.

29. Rappoport, D. A., Fritz, R. R., and Myers, J. L. Nucleic Acids. In A. Lajtha (ed.), *Handbook of Neurochemistry.* New York: Plenum, 1969. Vol. 1, pp. 101–119.

30. Ford, D. H. Selected maturational changes observed in the postnatal rat brain. *Prog. Brain Res.* 40:1–12, 1973.

31. Bock, E. Immunochemical Markers in Primary Cultures and Cell Lines. In S. Fedoroff and L. Hertz (eds.), *Cell, Tissue and Organ Cultures in Neurobiology.* New York: Academic, 1977. Pp. 407–422.

32. Jaque, C. M., Jorgenson, O. S., Baumann, N. A., and Bock, E. Brain-specific antigens in the quaking mouse during ontogeny. *J. Neurochem.* 27:905–909, 1976.

33. Acton, R. T., and Pfeiffer, S. E. Distribution of Thy-1 differentiation alloantigen in the rat nervous system and in a cell line derived from a rat peripheral neurinoma. *Dev. Neurosci.* 1:110–117, 1978.

34. Bignami, A., and Dahl, D. Astrocyte-specific protein and neuroglial differentiation. An immunofluorescence study with antibodies to the glial fibrillary acidic protein. *J. Comp. Neurol.* 153:27–38, 1974.

35. Schmitt, H., Gozes, I., and Littauer, U. Z. Decrease in levels and rates of synthesis of tubulin and actin in developing rat brain. *Brain Res.* 121:327–342, 1977.

36. Adams, C. W. M. *Neurohistochemistry.* New York: Elsevier, 1965.

37. Van den Berg, D. J. Enzymes in Developing Brain. In W. A. Himwich (ed.), *Biochemistry of the Developing Brain.* New York: Dekker, 1973. Vol. 2, pp. 149–198.

38. Roberts, J., Goldberg, P. B., and Baskin, S. J. Biochemical changes in the central nervous system with age in the rat. *Exp. Aging Res.* 3:61–74, 1977.

39. Johnson, T. C. Regulation of protein synthesis during postnatal maturation of brain. *J. Neurochem.* 27:17–24, 1976.

40. Dunlop, D. S., Van Elden, W., and Lajtha, A. Developmental effects on protein synthesis rates *in vivo* and *in vitro*. *J. Neurochem.* 29:939–945, 1977.

41. Oja, S. S. Comments on the measurement of protein synthesis in the brain. *Int. J. Neurosci.* 5:31–33, 1973.

42. Marks, M., and Lajtha, A. Developmental Changes in Peptide-Bond Hydrolases. In A. Lajtha (ed.), *Protein Metabolism of the Nervous System.* New York: Plenum, 1970. Pp. 39–73.

43. Reith, M. E. A., Schotman, P., and Gispen, W. H. Measurements of in vivo rates of protein synthesis in brain, spinal cord, heart and liver of young versus adult, intact versus hypophysectomized rats. *J. Neurochem.* 24:495–501, 1975.

44. Rouser, G., and Yamamoto, A. Lipids. In A. Lajtha (ed.), *Handbook of Neurochemistry.* New York: Plenum, 1969. Vol. 1, pp. 121–169.

45. Wells, M. A., and Dittmer, J. C. A comprehensive study of the postnatal changes in the concentration of the lipids of developing rat brain. *Biochemistry* 6:3169–3175, 1967.

46. O'Brien, J. S. Lipids and Myelination. In W. A. Himwich (ed.), *Developmental Neurobiology.* Springfield, Ill.: Thomas, 1979. Pp. 262–286.

47. Eto, Y., and Suzuki, K. Cholesterol esters in developing rat brain: Concentration and fatty acid composition. *J. Neurochem.* 19:109–115, 1972.

48. Vanier, M. T., Holm, M., Ohman, R., and Svennerholm, L. Developmental profiles of gangliosides in human and rat brain. *J. Neurochem.* 18:581–592, 1971.

49. Costantino-Ceccarini, E., and Morell, P. Quaking mouse: In vitro studies on brain sphingolipid biosynthesis. *Brain Res.* 29:75–84, 1971.

50. McKhann, G. M., and Ho, W. The in vivo and in vitro synthesis of sulfatides during development. *J. Neurochem.* 14:717–724, 1967.

51. Anderson, T. R., and Schanberg, S. M. Effect of thyroxine and cortisol on brain ornithine decarboxylase activity and swimming behavior in developing rat. *J. Neurochem.* 24:495–501, 1975.

52. Butler, S. R., Suskind, M. R., Schanberg, S. S. Maternal behavior as a regulator of polyamine biosynthesis in brain and heart of the developing rat pup. *Science* 199:445–447, 1978.

53. Margolis, R. V., and Margolis, R. K. Metabolism and function of glycoproteins and glycosaminoglycans in nervous tissue. *Int. J. Biochem.* 8:85–91, 1977.

54. Varon, S. S., and Bunge, R. P. Trophic mechanisms in the peripheral nervous system. *Annu. Rev. Neurosci.* 1:327–362, 1978.

55. Levi-Montalcini, R. The nerve growth factor: Its widening role and place in neurobiology. *Adv. Biochem. Psychopharmacol.* 15:237–250, 1976.

*56. Mobley, W. C., Server, A. C., Ishii, D. N., Riopelle, R. J., and Shooter, E. M. Nerve growth factor. *N. Engl. J. Med.* 297:1086–1104, 1149–1158, 1211–1218, 1977.

57. Black, I. B. Regulation of autonomic development. *Annu. Rev. Neurosci.* 1:183–214, 1978.

58. Bjerre, B., Bjorklund, A., and Stenevi, U. Stimulation of growth of new axonal sprouts of some lesioned neurons in adult rat brain by nerve growth factor. *Brain Res.* 60:161–176, 1973.

59. Konkol, R. J., et al. Evaluation of the effects of nerve growth factor and anti-nerve growth factor on the development of central catecholamine-containing neurons. *Brain Res.* 144:277–285, 1978.

60. Suda, K., Barde, Y. A., and Thoenen, H. Nerve growth factor in mouse and rat serum: Correlation between bioassay and radioimmunoassay determinations. *Proc. Natl. Acad. Sci. U.S.A.* 75: 4042–4046, 1978.

61. Burstein, D. E., and Greene, L. E. Evidence for RNA-synthesis-dependent and independent pathways in stimulation of neurite outgrowth by nerve growth factor. *Proc. Natl. Acad. Sci. U.S.A.* 75: 6059–6063, 1978.

62. Greene, L. A. Quantitative *in vitro* studies on the nerve growth factor (NGF) requirement of neurons. *Dev. Biol.* 58:96–105, 1977.

63. Andres, R. Y., Jeng, I., and Bradshaw, R. A. Nerve growth factor receptors: Identification of distinct classes in plasma membranes and nuclei of embryonic dorsal root neurons. *Proc. Natl. Acad. Sci. U.S.A.* 74:2785–2789, 1977.

64. Patterson, P. H. Environmental determination of autonomic neurotransmitter functions. *Annu. Rev. Neurosci.* 1:1–17, 1978.

65. Lim, R., Turriff, D. E., Troy, S. S., and Kato, T. Differentiation of Glioblasts under the Influence of Glia Maturation Factor. In S. Fedoroff and L. Hertz (eds.), *Cell, Tissue and Organ Cultures in Neurobiology.* New York: Academic, 1977. Pp. 223–235.

66. Pfeiffer, S. E., Betschart, B., Cook, J., Mancini, P., and Morris, R. Glial Cell Lines. In S. Fedoroff and L. Hertz (eds.), *Cell, Tissue and Organ Culture in Neurobiology.* New York: Academic, 1977. Pp. 286–323.

67. Balazs, R., and Richter, D. Effects of Hormones on the Biochemical Maturation of the Brain. In W. A. Himwich (ed.), *Biochemistry of the Developing Brain.* New York: Dekker, 1973. Vol. 1, pp. 253–299.

68. Howard, E. Hormonal Effects on the Growth and DNA Content of the Developing Brain. In W. A. Himwich (ed.), *Biochemistry of the Developing Brain.* New York: Dekker, 1974. Vol. 2, pp. 1–68.

*69. Grave, G. D. (ed.). *Thyroid Hormones and Brain Development.* New York: Raven, 1977.

70. Howard, E., and Benjamins, J. A. DNA ganglioside and sulfatide in brains of rats given corticosterone in infancy, with an estimate of cell loss during development. *Brain Res.* 92:73–87, 1975.

71. Sterling, K. Mitochondrial thyroid hormone receptor: Localization and physiological significance. *Science* 201:1126–1129, 1978.

72. Pelton, E., Grindeland, R., Young, E., and Bass, N. Effects of immunologically induced growth hormone deficiency on myelinogenesis in developing rat cerebrum. *Neurology* 27:282–288, 1977.

73. Havrankova, J., Roth, J., and Brownstein, M. Insulin receptors are widely distributed in the central nervous system of the rat. *Nature* 272:827–829, 1978.

74. DeVellis, J., McGinnis, J. F., Breen, G. A. M., Leveille, P., Bennett, K., and McCarthy, K. Hormonal Effects on Differentiation in Neural Cultures. In S. Fedoroff and L. Hertz (eds.), *Cell,*

Tissue and Organ Cultures in Neurobiology. New York: Academic, 1977. Pp. 485–511.

75. Schmidt, M. H., Palmer, E. C., Dettbarn, W. D., and Robison, G. A. Cyclic AMP and adenyl cyclase in the developing rat brain. *Dev. Psychobiol.* 3:53–67, 1970.

76. Brizzee, K. R. Quantitative histological studies on aging changes in cerebral cortex of rhesus monkeys and albino rats with notes on effects of prolonged low-dose ionizing irradiation in the rat. *Prog. Brain Res.* 40:141–160, 1973.

77. Samorajski, T., and Rolsten, C. Age and regional differences in the chemical composition of brains of mice, monkeys, and humans. *Prog. Brain Res.* 40:253–266, 1973.

78. Terry, R. D. Senile dementia. *Fed. Proc.* 37: 2837–2840, 1978.

79. Wisniewski, H. M., and Terry, R. D. Morphology of the aging brain, human and animal. *Prog. Brain Res.* 40:167–186, 1973.

80. McGeer, E. G., and McGeer, P. L. In R. D. Terry and S. Gershon (eds.), *Neurobiology of Aging.* New York: Raven, 1976. Vol. 3, pp. 386–404.

81. Bowen, D. M., et al. Chemical pathology of the dementias. I and II. *Brain* 100:397–426; 427–453, 1977.

82. Davies, P. Neurotransmitter-related enzymes in senile dementia of the Alzheimer type. *Brain Res.* 171:319–327, 1979.

83. Balinsky, B. I. *An Introduction to Embryology* (4th ed.). Philadelphia: Saunders, 1975.

84. Crelin, E. S. Development of the Nervous System. *Ciba Clin. Symp.* 26(2):1–32, 1974.

85. Toivonen, S., Tarin, D., Saxen, L., Tarin, P. J., and Wartiovaara, J. Transfilter studies on neural induction in the newt. *Differentiation* 4:1–7, 1975.

86. Wahn, H. L., Lightbody, L. E., Tchen, T. T., and Taylor, J. D. Induction of neural differentiation in cultures of amphibian undetermined presumptive epidermis by cyclic AMP derivatives. *Science* 188: 366–369, 1975.

87. Gurdon, J. B. Transplanted nuclei and cell differentiation. *Sci. Am.* 161:24, 1968; Changes in somatic cell nuclei inserted into growing and maturing amphibian oocytes. *J. Embryol. Exp. Morphol.* 20:401–414, 1968.

88. Jacobsen, C.-O. Reactivation of DNA synthesis in mammalian neuron nuclei with cells of an undifferentiated fibroblast line. *Exp. Cell Res.* 53: 316–318, 1968.

89. Cone, C. D., Tongier, M., and Cone, C. M. DNA content of daughter nuclei from ouabain-induced nuclear divisions in central nervous system neurons. *Exp. Neurol.* 57:396–408, 1977.

90. LaVelle, A., and LaVelle, F. W. Cytodifferentiation in the Neuron. In W. A. Himwich (ed.), *Developmental Neurobiology.* Springfield, Ill.: Thomas, 1979. Pp. 117–154.

91. Bray, D. Surface movements during the growth of single explanted neurons. *Proc. Natl. Acad. Sci. U.S.A.* 65:905–910, 1970.

92. Sperry, R. W. Chemoaffinity in the orderly growth of nerve fiber patterns and connections. *Proc. Natl. Acad. Sci. U.S.A.* 50:703–709, 1963.

93. Chamley, J. H., Campbell, G. R., Burnstock, G. An analysis of the interactions between sympathetic nerve fibers and smooth muscle cells in tissue culture. *Dev. Biol.* 33:344–361, 1973.

94. Glaser, L. Cell-cell adhesion studies with embryonal and cultured cells. *Rev. Physiol. Biochem. Exp. Pharmacol.* 83:89–122, 1978.

95. Barondes, S. H., and Rosen, S. D. Cell Surface Carbohydrate-Binding Proteins: Role in Cell Recognition. In S. H. Barondes (ed.), *Neuronal Recognition.* New York: Plenum, 1976. Pp. 331–356.

96. Pfenninger, K. H., and Bunge, R. P. Freeze-fracturing of nerve growth cones and young fibers. A study of developing plasma membrane. *J. Cell Biol.* 63:180–196, 1974.

97. Rees, R. P., Bunge, M. P., and Bunge, R. P. Morphological changes in the neuritic growth cone and target neuron during synaptic junction development in culture. *J. Cell Biol.* 68:240–263, 1976.

98. Coyle, J. T. Biochemical aspects of neurotransmission in the developing brain. *Int. Rev. Neurobiol.* 20:65–103, 1977.

*99. Fedoroff, S., and Hertz, L. (eds.). *Cell, Tissue and Organ Cultures in Neurobiology.* New York: Academic, 1977.

100. Nelson, P. G. Neuronal Cell Lines. In S. Fedoroff and L. Hertz (eds.), *Cell, Tissue and Organ Cultures in Neurobiology.* New York: Academic, 1977. Pp. 347–365.

101. Schubert, D., Harris, A. J., Heinemann, D., Kidkoro, Y., Patrick, J., and Steinbach, J. H. Differentiation and Interaction of Clonal Cell Lines of Nerve and Muscle. In G. Sato (ed.), *Tissue Culture of the Nervous System.* New York: Plenum, 1973. Pp. 55–77.

102. Rosenberg, R. N., Vance, C. K., Prashad, N., and Baskin, F. Specific Protein Species Expressed by Differentiating Neuroblastoma, Glioma and Hybrid Cells in Culture. In S. Fedoroff and L. Hertz (eds.), *Cell, Tissue and Organ Cultures in Neurobiology.* New York: Academic, 1977. Pp. 393–406.

103. Schubert, D. Induced differentiation of clonal rat nerve and glial cells. *Neurobiology* 4:376–387, 1974.

104. Garber, B. Cell Aggregation and Recognition in the Self-Assembly of Brain Tissues. In S. Fedoroff and L. Hertz (eds.), *Cell, Tissues and Organ Culture in Neurobiology.* New York: Academic, 1977. Pp. 515–537.

105. Honegger, P., and Richelson, E. Biochemical differentiation of mechanically dissociated mammalian brain in aggregating cell culture. *Brain Res.* 109:335–354, 1976.

106. DeLong, G. R., and Sidman, R. Alignment defect of reaggregating cells in cultures of developing brains of Reeler mutant mice. *Dev. Biol.* 22:584–600, 1970.

107. Rutishauser, U., Thiery, J.-P., Brackenbury, R., and Edelman, G. Surface Molecules Mediating Interactions among Embryonic Neural Cells. In F. O. Schmitt and F. G. Worden (eds.), *The Neurosciences: Fourth Study Program.* Cambridge, Mass.: M.I.T. Press, 1979. Pp. 735–747.

108. Ramon y Cajal, S. *Degeneration and Regeneration in the Nervous System.* London: Oxford University Press, 1928.

109. Growth and Regeneration in the Nervous System. A Report by the Ad Hoc Subcommittee of the Advisory Council of the NINCDS of the NIH. *Exp. Neurol.* 48(3), part 2, 1975.

110. Guth, L. History of central nervous system regeneration research. *Exp. Neurol.* 48:3–15, 1975.

111. Bernstein, J. J., Wells, M. R., and Bernstein, M. E. Spinal Cord Regeneration: Synaptic Renewal and Neurochemistry. In C. W. Cotman (ed.), *Neuronal Plasticity.* New York: Raven, 1978. Pp. 49–71.

112. Graziadei, P., and Monti Graziadei, G. The Olfactory System: A Model for the Study of Neurogenesis and Axon Regeneration in Mammals. In C. Cotman (ed.), *Neuronal Plasticity.* New York: Raven, 1978. Pp. 131–153.

113. Reis, D. J., Ross, R. A., Gilad, G., and Joh, T. Reaction of Central Catecholaminergic Neurons to Injury: Model Systems for Studying the Neurobiology of Central Regeneration and Sprouting. In C. Cotman (ed.), *Neuronal Plasticity.* New York: Raven, 1978. Pp. 197–226.

114. Raisman, G. Electron microscopic studies of the development of new neurolemmal contacts in the median eminence of the rat after hypophysectomy. *Brain Res.* 55:245–261, 1973.

115. Cotman, B. C., and Nadler, J. V. Reactive Synaptogenesis in the Hippocampus. In C. W. Cotman (ed.), *Neuronal Plasticity.* New York: Raven. Pp. 227–271.

116. Gilson, B. S., and Stensaas, L. J. Early axonal changes following lesions of the dorsal columns in rats. *Cell Tissue Res.* 149:1–20, 1974.

117. Grafstein, B., and McQuarrie, I. G. Role of the Nerve Cell Body in Axonal Regeneration. In C. W. Cotman (ed.), *Neuronal Plasticity.* New York: Raven, 1978. Pp. 155–195.

118. Black, M. M., and Lasek, R. J. Slowing of the rate of axonal regeneration during growth and maturation. *Exp. Neurol.* 63:108–119, 1979.

119. Vaughn, J. E., Hinds, P. L., and Skoff, R. P. Electron microscopic studies of Wallerian degeneration in rat optic nerve. I. The multipotential glia. *J. Comp. Neurol.* 140:175–206, 1970.

120. Skoff, R. P. Neuroglia: A Reevaluation of Their Origin and Development. In S. Fujita (ed.), *Cytogenesis and Cellular Pathology of Neuroglia and Microglia.* Stuttgart: Springer, 1980. Pp. 279–330.

121. Vaughan, D. W., and Peters, A. Neuroglial cells in the cerebral cortex of rats from young adulthood to old age: An electron microscopic study. *J. Neurocytol.* 3:405–429, 1974.

122. Schonbach, J., Hu, K. H., and Friede, R. L. Cellular and chemical changes during myelination: Histologic, autoradiographic, histochemical and biochemical data on myelination in the pyramidal tract and corpus callosum of rat. *J. Comp. Neurol.* 134:21–38, 1968.

123. Friede, R. L. Control of myelin formation by axon caliber (with a model of the control mechanism). *J. Comp. Neurol.* 144:233–252, 1972.

124. Diaz, M., Bornstein, M. B., and Raine, C. S. Disorganization of myelinogenesis in tissue culture by anti-CNS serum. *Brain Res.* 154:231–239, 1978.

125. Wood, P. M., and Bunge, R. P. Evidence that sensory axons are mitogenic for Schwann cells. *Nature* 256:662–664, 1975.

126. Bunge, R. P., and Bunge, M. B. Evidence that contact with connective tissue matrix is required for normal interaction between Schwann cells and nerve fibers. *J. Cell Biol.* 78:943–950, 1978.

127. Aguayo, A., Charron, L., and Bray, G. M. Potential of Schwann cells from unmyelinated nerves to produce myelin: A quantitative ultrastructural and radioautographic study. *J. Neurocytol.* 5:565–573, 1976.

128. Spencer, P. S., and Weinberg, H. J. Axonal Specification of Schwann Cell Expression and Myelination. In S. G. Waxman (ed.), *Physiology and Pathobiology of Axons.* New York: Raven, 1978. Pp. 389–405.

129. Raff, M. C., Abney, E., Brockes, J. P., and Hornby-Smith, A. Schwann cell growth factors. *Cell* 15:813–822, 1978.

130. Poduslo, S. E., and Norton, W. T. Isolation and some chemical properties of oligodendroglia from calf brain. *J. Neurochem.* 19:727–736, 1972.

131. Poduslo, S. E.   The isolation and characterization of a plasma membrane and a myelin fraction derived from oligodendroglia of calf brain. *J. Neurochem.* 24:647–654, 1975.

132. McDonald, W. I.   Remyelination in relation to clinical lesions of the central nervous system. *Br. Med. Bull.* 30:186–189, 1974.

133. Herndon, R. M., Griffin, D. E., McCormick, U., and Weiner, L. P.   Mouse hepatitis virus-induced recurrent demyelination. *Arch. Neurol.* 32:32–35, 1975.

134. Blakemore, W. F.   Remyelination of CNS axons by Schwann cells transplanted from the sciatic nerve. *Nature (London)* 266:68–69, 1977.

135. Blakemore, W. F.   Observations on remyelination in the rabbit spinal cord following demyelination induced by lysolecithin. *Neuropathol. Appl. Neurobiol.* 4:47–59, 1978.

136. Rakic, P., and Sidman, R. L.   Sequence of developmental abnormalities leading to granule cell deficit in cerebellar cortex of Weaver mice. *J. Comp. Neurol.* 152:103–132, 1973.

137. Sensenbrenner, M., and Mandel, P.   Behavior of neuroblasts in the presence of glial cells, fibroblasts, and meningeal cells in culture. *Exp. Cell Res.* 87:159167, 1974.

138. Bignami, A., and Dahl, D.   The development of Bergmann glia in mutant mice with cerebellar malformation: Reeler, Staggerer and Weaver. Immunofluorescence study with antibodies to the glial fibrillary acidic protein. *J. Comp. Neurol.* 155:219–230, 1974.

Louis Sokoloff

Chapter 24. Circulation and Energy Metabolism of the Brain

The biochemical pathways of energy metabolism in the brain are, in most respects, similar to those of other tissues (see Chap. 17). Special conditions that are peculiar to the central nervous system in vivo limit quantitative expression of its biochemical potentialities. In no tissue are the discrepancies between in situ and in vitro results greater, or the extrapolations from in vitro data to conclusions about in vivo metabolic functions more hazardous. Valid identification of the normally used substrates and the products of cerebral energy metabolism, as well as reliable estimation of their rates of utilization and production, can be obtained only in the intact animal; in vitro studies serve to identify pathways of intermediary metabolism, mechanisms, and potential rather than actual performance.

In addition to the usual causes of differences between in vitro and in vivo studies that pertain to all tissues, there are two unique conditions that pertain only to the central nervous system.

First, in contrast to cells of other tissues, nerve cells do not function autonomously. They are generally so incorporated into a complex neural network that their functional activity is integrated with that of various other parts of the central nervous system and, indeed, with most somatic tissues as well. It is obvious, then, that any procedure that interrupts the structural and functional integrity of the network or isolates the tissue from its normal functional interrelationships would inevitably grossly alter at least quantitatively and, perhaps, even qualitatively its normal metabolic behavior.

Second, the phenomenon of the blood-brain barrier (described in Chap. 25) selectively limits the rates of transfer of soluble substances between blood and the brain. This barrier, which probably developed phylogenetically to protect the brain against noxious substances, serves also to discriminate among various potential substrates for cerebral metabolism. The substrate function is confined to those compounds in the blood which not only are suitable substrates for cerebral enzymes but which also can penetrate from blood to the brain at rates adequate to support the brain's considerable energy demands. Substances that can be readily oxidized by brain slices, minces, or homogenates in vitro and that are effectively utilized in vivo when formed endogenously within the brain are often incapable of supporting cerebral energy metabolism and function when present in the blood because of restricted passage through the blood-brain barrier. The in vitro techniques establish only the existence and potential capacity of the enzyme systems required for the utilization of a given substrate; they do not define the extent to which such a pathway is actually utilized in vivo. This can be done only by studies in the intact animal, and it is this aspect of cerebral metabolism with which this chapter is concerned.

Studies of Cerebral Metabolism in Vivo

A variety of suitable methods have been used to study the metabolism of the brain in vivo; these vary in complexity and in the degree to which they yield quantitative results. Some require such minimal operative procedures on the experimental animal that no anesthesia is required, and there is no interference with the tissue except for the effects of the particular experimental condition being studied. Some of these techniques are applicable to normal, conscious human subjects, and consecutive and comparative studies can be made repeatedly in the same subject. Other methods are more traumatic and either require killing the animal or involve such extensive surgical intervention and tissue damage that the experiments approach an in vitro experiment carried out in situ. All, however, are capable of providing specific and relevant information.

BEHAVIORAL PHYSIOLOGICAL AND CHEMICAL CORRELATIONS

The simplest way to study the metabolism of the central nervous system in vivo is to correlate spontaneous or experimentally produced alterations in the chemical composition of the blood, spinal fluid, or both, with changes in cerebral physiological functions or gross CNS-mediated behavior. The level of consciousness, reflex behavior, or the electroencephalogram is generally used to monitor the effects of the chemical changes on the functional and metabolic activities of the brain. For example, such methods first demonstrated the need for glucose as a substrate for cerebral energy metabolism; hypoglycemia produced by insulin or other means altered various parameters of cerebral function that could not be restored to normal by the administration of substances other than glucose.

The chief virtue of these methods is their simplicity, but they are gross and nonspecific and do not distinguish between direct effects of the agent on cerebral metabolism and those secondary to changes produced initially in somatic tissues. Also, negative results are often inconclusive, for there always remain questions of insufficient dosage, inadequate cerebral circulation and delivery to the tissues, or impermeability of the blood-brain barrier.

BIOCHEMICAL ANALYSES OF TISSUES

The availability of analytical chemical techniques makes it possible to measure specific metabolites and enzyme activities in brain tissue at selected times during or after exposure of the animal to an experimental condition. (For details of these extensively used techniques, the reader should consult the first edition of *Basic Neurochemistry,* Boston: Little, Brown, 1972, Chap. 20.) This approach has been very useful in studies of the intermediary

metabolism of the brain. It has permitted the estimation of the rates of flux through the various steps of established metabolic pathways and the identification of control points in the pathways where regulation may be exerted. Such studies have helped to define more precisely the changes in energy metabolism associated with altered cerebral functions produced, for example, by anesthesia, convulsions, or hypoglycemia. Although these methods require killing the animal and analyzing tissue samples, they are in vivo methods in effect since they attempt to describe the state of the tissue while it is still in the animal at the moment of sacrifice. These methods have encountered their most serious problems regarding this point. Postmortem changes in brain are extremely rapid and are not always completely retarded by the most rapid freezing techniques available. These methods have proved to be very valuable, nevertheless, particularly in the area of energy metabolism. (A detailed discussion of results obtained with these methods is presented in Chap. 17.)

RADIOISOTOPE INCORPORATION

The technique of administering radioactive precursors followed by the chemical separation and assay of products in the tissue has added greatly to the armamentarium for studying cerebral metabolism in vivo. Labeled precursors are administered by any one of a variety of routes; at selected later times the brain is removed and the precursor and the various products of interest are isolated. The radioactivity and quantity of the compounds in question are assayed. Such techniques facilitate the identification of metabolic routes and the rates of flux through various steps of the pathway. In some cases, the comparison of the specific activities of the products and precursors has led to the surprising finding of higher specific activities in the products than in the precursors. This is conclusive evidence of the presence of compartmentation [1]. These methods have been used effectively in studies of amine and neurotransmitter synthesis and metabolism, lipid metabolism, protein synthesis, amino acid metabolism, and the distribution of glucose carbon through the various biochemical pathways present in the brain.

The methods are particularly valuable for studies of intermediary metabolism that generally are not feasible by most other in vivo techniques. They are without equal for the qualitative identification of the pathways and routes of metabolism. They suffer, however, from a disadvantage: only one set of measurements per animal is possible because the animal must be killed. Quantitative interpretations are often confounded by the problems of compartmentation. Also, they are all too frequently misused; unfortunately, quantitative conclusions are often drawn on the basis of radioactivity data without appropriate consideration of the specific activities of the precursor pools.

POLAROGRAPHIC TECHNIQUES

The oxygen electrode has been employed for measuring the amount of oxygen consumed locally in the cerebral cortex in vivo [2]. The electrode is applied to the surface of the exposed cortex, and the local PO_2 is measured continuously before and during occlusion of the blood flow to the local area. During occlusion, the PO_2 falls linearly as the oxygen is consumed by the tissue metabolism, and the rate of fall is a measure of the rate of oxygen consumption locally in the cortex. Repeated measurements can be made successively in the animal, and the technique has been used to demonstrate the increased oxygen consumption of the cerebral cortex and the relation between the changes in the EEG and the metabolic rate during convulsions [2]. The technique is limited to the measurements in the cortex and, of course, to oxygen utilization.

ARTERIOVENOUS DIFFERENCES

The primary function of the circulation is to replenish the nutrients consumed by the tissues and to remove the products of their metabolism. This function is reflected in the composition of the blood traversing the tissue. Substances taken up by the tissue from the blood are higher in concentration in the arterial inflow than in the venous outflow, and the converse is true for substances released by the tissue. The convention is to subtract the venous concentration from the arterial concentration so that a positive arteriovenous difference represents net uptake and a negative difference means net release. In nonsteady states there may be transient, but significant, arteriovenous differences that reflect reequilibration of the tissue with the blood. In steady states, in which it is presumed that the tissue concentration remains constant, positive and negative arteriovenous differences mean net consumption or production of the substance by the tissue. Zero arteriovenous differences indicate neither. This method is useful for all substances in blood that can be assayed with enough accuracy, precision, and sensitivity to enable the detection of arteriovenous differences. The method is useful only for the tissues from which mixed representative venous blood can be sampled. Arterial blood has essentially the same composition throughout and can be sampled from any artery. On the other hand, venous blood is specific for each tissue, and to establish valid arteriovenous differences the venous blood must represent the total outflow or the flow-weighted average of all the venous overflows from the tissue under study, uncontaminated by blood from any other tissue. It is not possible to fulfill this condition for many tissues.

The method is fully applicable to the brain, particularly in humans, in whom the anatomy of venous drainage is favorable for such studies. Representative cerebral venous blood, with no more than about 3 percent contamination with extracerebral blood, is readily obtained from the superior bulb of the internal jugular vein. The venipuncture can be made percutaneously under local anesthesia [3, 4] so the measurements can be made during the conscious state, undistorted by the effects of general anesthesia. The monkey is similar, although the vein must be surgically exposed before puncture. Other common laboratory animals are less suitable because extensive communications between cerebral and extracerebral venous beds are present, and uncontaminated representative venous blood is difficult to obtain from the cerebrum without major surgical intervention. In these cases, one can obtain relatively uncontaminated venous blood from the confluence of the sinuses even though it does not contain representative blood from the brain stem and some of the lower portions of the brain.

The chief advantages of these methods are their simplicity and applicability to unanesthetized humans. They permit the qualitative identification of the ultimate substrates and products of cerebral metabolism. They have no applicability, however, to those intermediates that are formed and consumed entirely in the brain without being exchanged with blood, or to those substances that are exchanged between brain and blood with no net flux in either direction. Furthermore, they provide no quantitation of the rates of utilization or production because arteriovenous differences depend not only on the rates of consumption or production by the tissue but also on the blood flow (see below). Blood flow affects all the arteriovenous differences proportionately, however, and comparison of the arteriovenous differences of various substances obtained from the same samples of blood reflects their relative rates of utilization or production.

COMBINATION OF CEREBRAL BLOOD FLOW AND ARTERIOVENOUS DIFFERENCES

In a steady state, the tissue concentration of any substance utilized or produced by the brain is presumed to remain constant. When a substance is exchanged between brain and blood, the difference in its rates of delivery to the brain in the arterial blood and removal in the venous blood must be equal to the net rate of its utilization or production by the brain. This relation can be expressed as follows:

$$CMR = CBF(A - V)$$

where $(A - V)$ is the difference in concentration in arterial and cerebral venous blood, CBF is the rate of cerebral blood flow in volume of blood per unit time, and CMR (cerebral metabolic rate) is the steady-state rate of utilization or production of the substance by the brain.

If both the rate of cerebral blood flow and the arteriovenous difference are known, therefore, the net rate of utilization or production of the sub-

stance by the brain can be calculated. This has been the basis of most quantitative studies of the cerebral metabolism in vivo [5–8].

There are a number of methods for determining the cerebral blood flow, many of them of questionable value or validity. One type of technique involves isolating the cerebral circulation by surgical means; the brain is then perfused at a fixed rate with blood or perfusate, or the rate of flow in the cerebral vascular bed is measured by any one of a variety of flowmeter devices [7, 9]. Such methods are, of course, limited to animals. They can be carried out usually only under general anesthesia and require extensive surgical procedures that make truly normal preparations impossible.

A thorough discussion of the methods for measuring cerebral blood flow is beyond the scope of this chapter, but the subject has been comprehensively reviewed in recent years [6, 7, 10–12].

The most reliable method for determining cerebral blood flow is the inert gas method of Kety and Schmidt [4]. It was originally designed for use in studies of conscious, unanesthetized humans, and it has been most widely employed for this purpose; but it also has been adapted for use in animals [13]. The method is based on the Fick principle, or the law of conservation of matter, and it utilizes low concentrations of a freely diffusible, chemically inert gas as a tracer substance. The original gas was nitrous oxide, but subsequent modifications have substituted other gases, such as ^{85}Kr, ^{79}Kr, or hydrogen [10, 11, 14–16], that can be measured more conveniently in blood. During inhalation of 15% N_2O in air, for example, arterial and cerebral venous blood samples are withdrawn at intervals and analyzed for N_2O content. The cerebral blood flow (in milliliters per 100 g of brain tissue per minute) can be calculated from the equation:

$$CBF = 100\lambda V_{10} / \int_0^{10} (A - V)\, dt$$

where A and V = arterial and cerebral venous blood concentrations of N_2O

V_{10} = concentration of N_2O in venous blood at 10 min

Table 24-1. Cerebral Blood Flow and Metabolic Rate in Normal Young Adult Man

Function	Rate	
	Per 100 g Brain Tissue	Per Whole Brain*
Cerebral blood flow (ml/min)	57	798
Cerebral O₂ consumption (ml/min)	3.5	49
Cerebral glucose utilization (mg/min)	5.5	77

*Brain weight assumed to be 1,400 g.
Source: Based on data derived from literature [8].

$$\lambda = \text{partition coefficient for } N_2O \text{ between brain tissue and blood}$$
$$t = \text{time of inhalation in minutes}$$
$$\int_0^{10}(A - V)\,dt = \text{integrated arteriovenous difference in } N_2O \text{ concentrations over 10 min of inhalation.}$$

The partition coefficient for N_2O is approximately 1 when equilibrium has been achieved between blood and brain tissue. It has been found that at least 10 minutes of inhalation are required to establish equilibrium. At the end of this interval, the N_2O concentration in brain tissue is about equal to the cerebral venous blood concentration.

Because the method requires sampling of both arterial and cerebral venous blood, it lends itself readily to the simultaneous measurement of arteriovenous differences of substances involved in cerebral metabolism. This method and its modifications have provided most of our knowledge of the rates of substrate utilization or product formation by the brain in vivo.

Regulation of Cerebral Metabolic Rate

NORMAL CONSUMPTION OF OXYGEN BY THE BRAIN

The brain is metabolically one of the most active of all the organs of the body. This is reflected in its relatively enormous rate of oxygen consumption, which provides the energy required for its intense physicochemical activity. The most reliable data on cerebral metabolic rate have been obtained in humans although the rates in lower mammals appear to be comparable on a unit-weight basis. Cerebral oxygen consumption in normal, conscious, young men is about 3.5 ml/100 g brain/min (Table 24-1); the rate is similar in young women. The rate of oxygen consumption by an entire brain of average weight (1,400 g) is then about 49 ml O_2 per minute. The magnitude of this rate can be more fully appreciated when it is compared with the metabolic rate of the body as a whole. The average man weighs 70 kg and consumes about 250 ml O_2 per minute in the basal state. Therefore, the brain alone, which represents only about 2 percent of total body weight, accounts for 20 percent of the resting total body oxygen consumption. In children the brain takes an even larger fraction [17].

Oxygen is utilized in the brain almost entirely for the oxidation of carbohydrate [8, 18]. The energy equivalent of the total cerebral metabolic rate is, therefore, approximately 20 watts or 0.25 kcal per minute. If it is assumed that this energy is utilized mainly for the synthesis of high-energy phosphate bonds, that the efficiency of the energy conservation is about 20 percent, and that the free energy of hydrolysis of the terminal phosphate of ATP is about 7 kcal per mole, this energy expenditure then can be estimated to support the steady turnover of close to 7 mmol or about 4×10^{21} molecules of ATP per minute in the entire brain.

The brain normally has no respite from this enormous energy demand. The cerebral oxygen consumption continues unabated day and night. Even during sleep there is no reduction in cerebral metabolic rate; indeed, it may even be markedly increased in rapid eye movement (REM) sleep (see below).

ENERGY-DEMANDING FUNCTIONS

The brain does not do mechanical work, like that of cardiac and skeletal muscle. It does not do osmotic work, as does the kidney in concentrating urine. It does not have the complex energy-consuming metabolic functions of liver, nor, despite the synthesis of some hormones and neurotransmitters, is it noted for its biosynthetic activities. Recently, considerable emphasis has been placed on the extent of macromolecular synthesis in the central nervous system, an interest stimulated by the recognition that there are some proteins with short half-lives in the brain. These represent, however, relatively small numbers of molecules, and, in fact, the average protein turnover and the rate of protein synthesis in the mature brain are slower than in most other tissues except, perhaps, muscle [19]. Clearly, the functions of nervous tissues are mainly excitation and conduction, and these are reflected in the unceasing electrical activity of the brain. The electrical energy is ultimately derived from chemical processes, and it is likely that most of the brain's energy consumption is utilized for active transport of ions to sustain and restore the membrane potentials discharged during the process of excitation and conduction (see Chaps. 5, 6, and 36).

Not all of the oxygen consumption of the brain is used for energy metabolism. The brain contains a variety of oxidases and hydroxylases which function in the synthesis and metabolism of a number of neurotransmitters (see Chap. 10). For example, tyrosine hydroxylase is a mixed-function oxidase which hydroxylates tyrosine to 3,4-dihydroxyphenylalanine (dopa), and dopamine-β-hydroxylase hydroxylates dopamine to form norepinephrine. Similarly, tryptophane hydroxylase hydroxylates tryptophane to form 5-hydroxytryptophane in the pathway of serotonin synthesis. These enzymes are oxygenases, which utilize molecular oxygen and incorporate it into the hydroxyl group of the hydroxylated products. Oxygen also is consumed in the metabolism of these monamine neurotransmitters, which are oxidatively deaminated to their respective aldehydes by monamine oxidase. All of these enzymes are present in brain, and the reactions catalyzed by them utilize oxygen. When, however, the total turnover rates of the neurotrasmitters and the sum total of the maximal velocities of all the oxidases involved in their synthesis and degradation are considered, it is clear that the oxygen consumed in the turnover of the neurotransmitters can account for only a very small, possibly immeasurable, fraction of the total oxygen consumption of the brain.

ROLE OF CEREBRAL CIRCULATION

Not only does the brain utilize oxygen at a very rapid rate, but it is absolutely dependent on continuously uninterrupted oxidative metabolism for maintenance of its functional and structural integrity. There is a large Pasteur effect in brain tissue [20], but even at its maximum rate, anaerobic glycolysis is unable to provide sufficient energy to meet the brain's demands. Since the oxygen stores of the brain are extremely small compared with its rate of utilization, the brain requires the continuous replenishment of its oxygen by the circulation. If the cerebral blood flow is completely interrupted, consciousness is lost within less than 10 seconds, or the amount of time required to consume the oxygen contained within the brain and its blood content [21]. Loss of consciousness as a result of anoxemia, caused by anoxia or asphyxia, takes only a little longer because of the additional oxygen present in the lungs and still-circulating blood. There is evidence that the critical level of oxygen tension in the cerebral tissues, below which consciousness and the normal EEG pattern are invariably lost, lies between 15 and 20 mm Hg [7]. This appears to be so whether the tissue anoxia is achieved by lowering the cerebral blood flow or the arterial oxygen content.

Cessation of cerebral blood flow is followed within a few minutes by irreversible pathological changes within the brain, readily demonstrated by microscopic anatomical techniques. It is well known, of course, that in medical crises, such as cardiac arrest, damage to the brain occurs earliest and is most decisive in determining the degree of recovery.

The cerebral blood flow must be able to maintain the brain's avaricious appetite for oxygen. The average rate of blood flow in the brain as a whole is about 57 ml/100 g tissue/min (see Table 24-1). For the whole brain this amounts to almost 800 ml per minute or approximately 15 percent of the total basal cardiac output. This level must be maintained within relatively narrow limits, for the brain cannot tolerate any major drop in its perfusion. A fall in cerebral blood flow to half of its normal rate is sufficient to cause loss of consciousness in normal, healthy young men [6, 7, 22]. There are, fortunately, numerous reflexes and other physiological mechanisms to sustain adequate levels of arterial blood pressure at the head level and to maintain the cerebral blood flow, even when arterial pressure falls in times of stress [6, 7]. There are also mechanisms to adjust the cerebral blood flow to changes in cerebral metabolic demand.

Regulation of the cerebral blood flow is achieved mainly by control of the tone or the degree of constriction or dilatation of the cerebral vessels. This, in turn, is controlled mainly by local chemical factors, such as PCO_2, PO_2, and pH. High PCO_2, low PO_2, and low pH—products of metabolic activity—tend to dilate the blood vessels and increase cerebral blood flow; changes in the opposite direction constrict the vessels and decrease blood flow [6, 7, 23]. The cerebral blood flow is regulated through such mechanisms to maintain homeostasis of these chemical factors in the local tissue. Their rates of production depend on the rates of metabolism, so cerebral blood flow is, therefore, also adjusted to the cerebral metabolic rate [6, 7, 23].

LOCAL CEREBRAL BLOOD FLOW AND METABOLISM

The rates of blood flow and metabolism presented in Table 24-1 and discussed above represent the average values in the brain as a whole. The brain is not a homogeneous organ, however, but is composed of a variety of tissues and discrete structures that often function independently or even inversely with respect to one another. There is little reason to expect that their perfusion and metabolic rates would be similar. Indeed, experimental evidence clearly indicates that they are not (see Chap. 17). Local cerebral blood flow in laboratory animals has been determined from the local tissue concentrations, measured by a quantitative autoradiographic technique, and from the total history of the arterial concentration of a freely diffusible, chemically inert, radioactive tracer introduced

into the circulation [24, 25]. The results reveal that blood-flow rates vary widely throughout the brain with average values in gray matter approximately 4 to 5 times those of white matter [24–26].

A method has been devised to measure glucose consumption in the discrete functional and structural components of the brain in intact conscious laboratory animals [27]. This method also employs quantitative autoradiography to measure local tissue concentrations but utilizes [14C]deoxyglucose as the tracer. The local tissue accumulation of [14C]deoxyglucose as [14C]deoxyglucose 6-phosphate in a given interval of time is related to the amount of glucose that has been phosphorylated by hexokinase over the same interval, and the rate of glucose consumption can be determined from the [14C]deoxyglucose 6-phosphate concentration by appropriate consideration of (1) the relative concentrations of [14C]deoxyglucose and glucose in the plasma; (2) their rate constants for transport between plasma and brain tissue; and (3) the kinetic constants of hexokinase for deoxyglucose and glucose. The method is based on a kinetic model of the biochemical behavior of 2-deoxyglucose and glucose in brain. The model has been mathematically analyzed to derive an operational equation that presents the variables to be measured and the procedure to be followed to determine local cerebral glucose utilization. The model and the equation are diagrammed in Fig. 24-1. To measure local glucose utilization, a pulse of [14C]deoxyglucose is administered intravenously at zero time, and timed arterial blood samples are then drawn for 30 to 45 minutes for the determination of the plasma [14C]deoxyglucose and glucose concentrations. At the end of the experimental period, the animal is decapitated, the brain is removed and frozen, and brain sections, 20 μm in thickness, are autoradiographed on X-ray film along with calibrated [14C]-methylmethacrylate standards. Local tissue concentrations of 14C are determined by densitometric analysis of the autoradiographs. From the time courses of the arterial plasma [14C]deoxyglucose and glucose concentrations and the final tissue 14C concentration, determined by the quantitative autoradiography, local glucose utilization

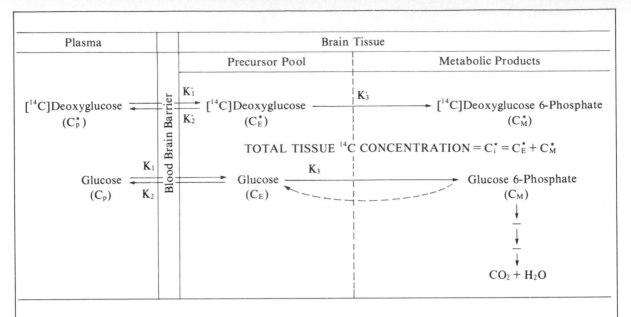

A

General equation for measurement of reaction rates with tracers:

$$\text{Rate of reaction} = \frac{\text{Labeled Product Formed in Interval of Time, 0 to T}}{\begin{bmatrix}\text{Isotope effect}\\\text{correction factor}\end{bmatrix}\begin{bmatrix}\text{Integrated specific activity}\\\text{of precursor}\end{bmatrix}}$$

Operational equation of $[^{14}C]$deoxyglucose method:

Labeled Product Formed in Interval of Time, 0 to T

$$R_i = \frac{\overbrace{C_i^*(T)}^{\substack{\text{Total }^{14}\text{C in tissue}\\\text{at time T}}} - \overbrace{k_i^* e^{-(k_2^* + k_3^*)T}\int_0^T C_p^* e^{(k_2^* + k_3^*)t}\,dt}^{\substack{^{14}\text{C in precursor}\\\text{remaining in tissue at time T}}}}{\underbrace{\left[\dfrac{\lambda \cdot V_m^* \cdot K_m}{\Phi \cdot V_m \cdot K_m^*}\right]}_{\substack{\text{Isotope effect}\\\text{correction}\\\text{factor}}}\underbrace{\left[\underbrace{\int_0^T\left(\dfrac{C_p^*}{C_p}\right)dt}_{\substack{\text{Integrated plasma}\\\text{specific activity}}} - \underbrace{e^{-(k_2^* + k_3^*)T}\int_0^T\left(\dfrac{C_p^*}{C_p}\right)e^{(k_2^* + k_3^*)t}\,dt}_{\substack{\text{Correction for lag in tissue}\\\text{equilibration with plasma}}}\right]}_{\text{Integrated precursor specific activity in tissue}}}$$

B

can be calculated by means of the operational equation for all components of the brain identifiable in the autoradiographs. The procedure is so designed that the autoradiographs reflect mainly the relative local concentrations of [^{14}C]deoxyglucose 6-phosphate. The autoradiographs are, therefore, pictorial representations of the relative rates of glucose utilization in all the structural components of the brain. Autoradiographs of the striate cortex of the monkey in various functional states are illustrated in Fig. 24-2.

This method has demonstrated that local cerebral consumption of glucose varies as widely as blood flow throughout the brain (Table 24-2). In-

Fig. 24-1. Theoretical basis of radioactive deoxyglucose method for measurement of local cerebral glucose utilization.

A. Theoretical model. C_i^* represents the total ^{14}C concentration in a single homogeneous tissue of the brain. C_P^* and C_P represent the concentrations of [^{14}C] deoxyglucose and glucose in the arterial plasma, respectively; C_E^* and C_E represent their respective concentrations in the tissue pools that serve as substrates for hexokinase. C_M^* represents the concentration of [^{14}C]deoxyglucose 6-phosphate in the tissue. The constants k_1^*, k_2^*, and k_3^* represent the rate constants for carrier-mediated transport of [^{14}C] deoxyglucose from plasma to tissue, for carrier-mediated transport back from tissue to plasma, and for phosphorylation by hexokinase, respectively. The constants k_1, k_2, and k_3 are the equivalent rate constants for glucose. [^{14}C]Deoxyglucose and glucose share and compete for the carrier that transports them both between plasma and tissue and for hexokinase which phosphorylates them to their respective hexose 6-phosphates. The dashed arrow represents the possibility of glucose 6-phosphate hydrolysis by glucose 6-phosphatase activity, if any.

B. Functional anatomy of the operational equation of the radioactive deoxyglucose method. T represents the time at the termination of the experimental period; λ equals the ratio of the distribution space of deoxyglucose in the tissue to that of glucose; Φ equals the fraction of glucose which, once phosphorylated, continues down the glycolytic pathway; and K_m^* and V_m^* and K_m and V_m represent the familiar Michaelis-Menten kinetic constants of hexokinase for deoxyglucose and glucose, respectively. The other symbols are the same as those defined in A. (From L. Sokoloff, with permission.)

deed, in the normal animals there is a remarkably close correlation between local cerebral blood flow and glucose consumption [28]. Changes in functional activity produced by physiological stimulation, anesthesia, or deafferentation result in corresponding changes in blood flow [26] and glucose consumption [29] in the structures involved in the functional change. The [^{14}C]deoxyglucose method for the measurement of local glucose utilization has been used recently to map the functional visual pathways and to identify the locus of the visual cortical representation of the retinal "blind spot" in the brain of the rhesus monkey [30] (Fig. 24-2). These results establish that local energy metabolism in brain is coupled to local functional activity and also confirm the long-held belief that local cerebral blood flow is adjusted to metabolic demand in local tissue.

Substrates of Cerebral Metabolism

NORMAL SUBSTRATES AND PRODUCTS

In contrast to most other tissues, which exhibit considerable flexibility in regard to the nature of the foodstuffs absorbed and consumed from the blood, the normal brain is restricted almost exclusively to glucose as the substrate for its energy metabolism. Despite long and intensive efforts, the only incontrovertible and consistently positive arteriovenous differences demonstrated for the human brain under normal conditions have been for glucose and oxygen [8, 18]. One report [31] of glutamate uptake and equivalent release of glutamine has never been substantiated and must at present be considered doubtful. Negative arteriovenous differences, significantly different from zero, have been found consistently only for carbon dioxide, although it is likely that water, which has never been measured, is also produced [8]. Pyruvate and lactate production have been observed occasionally, certainly in aged subjects with cerebral vascular insufficiency [20], but irregularly in subjects with normal oxygenation of the brain [8].

It appears, then, that in the normal in vivo state glucose is the only significant substrate for the brain's energy metabolism. Under normal circumstances no other potential energy-yielding substance has been found to be extracted from the blood in more than trivial amounts. The stoichiometry of glucose utilization and oxygen consumption is summarized in Table 24-3. The normal, conscious human brain consumes oxygen at a rate of 156 μmol/100 g tissue/min. Carbon dioxide production is the same, leading to a respiratory quotient of 1.0, further evidence that carbohydrate is the ultimate substrate for oxidative metabolism. The O_2 consumption and CO_2 production are equivalent to a rate of glucose utilization of 26 μmol glucose/100 g tissue/min, assuming 6 μmol of O_2 consumed and CO_2 produced for each micromole of glucose completely oxidized to CO_2 and H_2O. The glucose utilization actually measured is, however, 31 μmol/100 g/min, which indicates that glucose consumption is not only sufficient to account for the total O_2 consumption but is in excess by 5 μmol/100 g/min. For the complete oxidation of glucose, the theoretical ratio of oxygen-to-glucose utilization is 6.0; the excess glucose utilization is responsible for a measured ratio of only 5.5 μmol of O_2 per micromole of glucose. The fate of the excess glucose is unknown, but it is probably distributed in part in lactate, pyruvate, and other intermediates of carbohydrate metabolism that are released from the brain into the blood, each in insufficient amount to be detectable in significant arteriovenous differences. Probably some of the glucose is also utilized not for the production of energy but for the synthesis of other chemical constituents of the brain.

Some oxygen is known to be utilized for the oxidation of substances not derived from glucose, as, for example, in oxygenase reactions involved in the synthesis of monamine neurotransmitters, as mentioned above. The amount of oxygen utilized for these processes is, however, extremely small and is undetectable in the presence of the enormous oxygen consumption used for carbohydrate oxidation. Also, the amount of amino acids taken up for these purposes is so small as to be undetected in the arteriovenous differences.

The combination of a cerebral respiratory quotient of unity, an almost stoichiometric relationship between oxygen uptake and glucose consumption,

Table 24-2. Representative Values for Local Cerebral Glucose Utilization in the Normal Conscious Albino Rat and Monkey (μmol/100 g/min)

Structure	Albino Rat[a] (10)	Monkey[b] (7)
	Gray Matter	
Visual cortex	107 ± 6	59 ± 2
Auditory cortex	162 ± 5	79 ± 4
Parietal cortex	112 ± 5	47 ± 4
Sensory-motor cortex	120 ± 5	44 ± 3
Thalamus		
lateral nucleus	116 ± 5	54 ± 2
ventral nucleus	109 ± 5	43 ± 2
Medial geniculate body	131 ± 5	65 ± 3
Lateral geniculate body	96 ± 5	39 ± 1
Hypothalamus	54 ± 2	25 ± 1
Mamillary body	121 ± 5	57 ± 3
Hippocampus	79 ± 3	39 ± 2
Amygdala	52 ± 2	25 ± 2
Caudate putamen	110 ± 4	52 ± 3
Nucleus accumbens	82 ± 3	36 ± 2
Globus pallidus	58 ± 2	26 ± 2
Substantia nigra	58 ± 3	29 ± 2
Vestibular nucleus	128 ± 5	66 ± 3
Cochlear nucleus	113 ± 7	51 ± 3
Superior olivary nucleus	133 ± 7	63 ± 4
Inferior colliculus	197 ± 10	103 ± 6
Superior colliculus	95 ± 5	55 ± 4
Pontine gray matter	62 ± 3	28 ± 1
Cerebellar cortex	57 ± 2	31 ± 2
Cerebellar nuclei	100 ± 4	45 ± 2
	White Matter	
Corpus callosum	40 ± 2	11 ± 1
Internal capsule	33 ± 2	13 ± 1
Cerebellar white matter	37 ± 2	12 ± 1

The values are the means plus or minus standard errors from measurements made in the number of animals indicated in parentheses.
[a] From Sokoloff and coworkers [27].
[b] From Kennedy and coworkers [30].

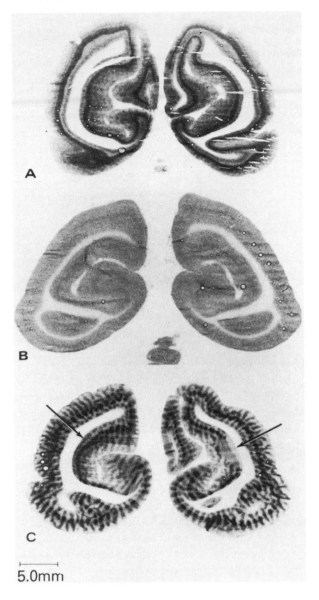

5.0mm

Fig. 24-2. Autoradiographs of coronal brain sections from rhesus monkeys at the level of the striate cortex. A. Animal with normal binocular vision. Note the laminar distribution of the density; the dark band corresponds to layer IV. B. Animal with bilateral visual deprivation. Note the almost uniform and reduced relative density, especially the virtual disappearance of the dark band corresponding to layer IV. C. Animal with right eye occluded. The half-brain on the left side of the photograph represents the left hemisphere contralateral to the occluded eye. Note the alternate dark and light striations, each approximately 0.3 to 0.4 mm in width, representing the ocular dominance columns. These columns are most apparent in the dark lamina corresponding to layer IV but extend through the entire thickness of the cortex. The arrows point to regions of bilateral asymmetry where the ocular dominance columns are absent. These are presumably areas that normally have only monocular input. The one on the left, contralateral to the occluded eye, has a continuous dark lamina corresponding to layer IV that is completely absent on the side ipsilateral to the occluded eye. These regions are believed to be the loci of the cortical representations of the blind spots. (From L. Sokoloff, with permission.)

and the absence of any significant arteriovenous difference for any other energy-rich substrate is strong evidence that the brain normally derives its energy from the oxidation of glucose. In this respect, cerebral metabolism is unique because no other tissue, with the possible exception of the testis [32], has been found to rely only on carbohydrate for energy. This does not imply that the pathways of glucose metabolism in the brain lead, like combustion, directly and exclusively to oxidation. Various chemical and energy transformations occur between the uptake of the primary substrates, glucose and oxygen, and the liberation of the end products, carbon dioxide and water. Various compounds derived from glucose or produced through the energy made available from glucose catabolism are intermediates in the process. Glucose carbon is incorporated, for example, into amino acids, protein, lipids, glycogen, and so on. These are turned over and act as intermediates in the overall pathway from glucose to carbon dioxide and water. There is clear evidence from studies with $[^{14}C]$glucose that the glucose is not entirely oxidized directly, and that at any given moment some of the carbon dioxide being produced is derived from sources other than the glucose that enters the brain at the same moment or just prior to that moment [9, 33]. That oxygen and glucose consumption and carbon dioxide production are essentially in stoichiometric balance and no other energy-laden substrate is taken from the blood means, however, that the net energy made available to the brain must ultimately be derived from the oxidation of glucose. It should be noted that this is the situation in the normal state; as will be discussed later, other substrates may be used in special circumstances or in abnormal states.

OBLIGATORY UTILIZATION OF GLUCOSE

The brain normally derives almost all its energy from the aerobic oxidation of glucose, but this does not distinguish between preferential and obligatory utilization of glucose. Most tissues are largely facultative in their choice of substrates and can use them interchangeably more or less in proportion to their availability. This does not appear to be so

Table 24-3. Relationship between Cerebral Oxygen Consumption and Glucose Utilization in Normal Young Adult Man

Function	Value
O_2 consumption (μmol/100 g brain tissue/min)	156
Glucose utilization (μmol/100 g brain tissue/min)	31
O_2/glucose ratio (mole/mole)	5.5
Glucose equivalent of O_2 consumption (μmol glucose/100 g brain tissue/min)	26*
CO_2 production (μmol/100 g brain tissue/min)	156
Cerebral respiratory quotient	0.97

*Calculated on the basis of 6 moles of O_2 required for complete oxidation of 1 mole of glucose.
Source: Values are the median of the values reported in the literature [8].

in brain. The present evidence indicates that, except in some unusual and very special circumstances, only the aerobic utilization of glucose is capable of providing the brain with enough energy to maintain normal function and structure. The brain appears to have almost no flexibility in its choice of substrates in vivo. This conclusion is derived from the following evidence.

Effects of Glucose Deprivation

It is well known clinically that a drop in blood glucose content, if of sufficient degree, is rapidly followed by aberrations of cerebral function. Hypoglycemia, produced by excessive insulin or occurring spontaneously in hepatic insufficiency, is associated with changes in mental state ranging from mild, subjective sensory disturbances to coma, the severity depending on both the degree and the duration of the hypoglycemia. The behavioral effects are paralleled by abnormalities in EEG patterns and cerebral metabolic rate. The EEG pattern exhibits increased prominence of slow, high-voltage delta rhythms, and the rate of cerebral oxygen consumption falls. In studies of the effects of insulin hypoglycemia in man [34], it was observed that, when the arterial glucose concentration fell from a normal level of 70 to 100 mg per 100 ml to an average level of 19 mg per 100 ml, the subjects became confused and their cerebral oxygen consumption fell to 2.6 ml/100 g/min or 79 percent of the normal level. When the arterial glucose level fell to 8 mg per 100 ml, a deep coma ensued and the cerebral oxygen consumption decreased even further to 1.9 ml/100 g/min.

These changes are not caused by insufficient cerebral blood flow, which actually increases slightly during the coma. In the depths of the coma, when the blood glucose content is very low, there is almost no measurable cerebral uptake of glucose from the blood. Cerebral oxygen consumption, although reduced, is still far from negligible, and there is no longer any stoichiometric relationship between glucose and oxygen uptakes by the brain—evidence that the oxygen is utilized for the oxidation of other substances. The cerebral respiratory quotient remains approximately one, however, indicating that these other substrates are still carbohydrate, presumably derived from the brain's endogenous carbohydrate stores. The effects are clearly the result of hypoglycemia and not some other direct effect of insulin in the brain. In all cases, the behavioral, functional, and cerebral metabolic abnormalities associated with insulin hypoglycemia are rapidly and completely reversed by the administration of glucose. The severity of the effects is correlated with the degree of hypoglycemia and not the insulin dosage, and the effects of the insulin can be completely prevented by the simultaneous administration of glucose with the insulin.

Similar effects are observed in hypoglycemia produced by other means, such as hepatectomy. The inhibition of glucose utilization at the phosphohexoseisomerase step with 2-deoxyglucose also produces all the cerebral effects of hypoglycemia despite an associated elevation in blood glucose content [8]. It appears, then, that when the brain is deprived of its glucose supply in an otherwise normal individual, no other substance present in the blood can satisfactorily substitute for it as the substrate for the brain's energy metabolism.

Other Substrates in Hypoglycemia

The hypoglycemic state provides convenient test conditions to determine whether a substance is capable of substituting for glucose as a substrate of cerebral energy metabolism. If it can, its administration during hypoglycemic shock should restore consciousness and normal cerebral electrical activity without raising the blood glucose level. Numerous potential substrates have been tested in man and animals. Very few can restore normal cerebral functions in hypoglycemia, and of these all but one appear to operate through a variety of mechanisms to raise the blood glucose level rather than by serving as a substrate directly (Table 24-4).

Mannose appears to be the only substance that can be utilized by the brain directly and rapidly enough to restore or maintain normal function in the absence of glucose [35]. It traverses the blood-brain barrier and is converted to mannose 6-phosphate. This reaction is catalyzed by hexokinase as effectively as the phosphorylation of glucose. The mannose 6-phosphate is then converted to fructose 6-phosphate by phosphomannoseisomerase, which is active in brain tissue [35]. Through these reactions mannose can enter directly into the glycolytic pathway and replace glucose.

Maltose also has been found to be effective occasionally in restoring normal behavior and EEG activity in hypoglycemia, but only by raising the blood glucose level through its conversion to glucose by maltase activity in blood and other tissues [8, 35].

Epinephrine is effective in producing arousal from insulin coma, but this is achieved through its well-known stimulation of glycogenolysis and the elevation of blood glucose concentration. Glutamate, arginine, glycine, p-aminobenzoate, and succinate also are effective occasionally, but they probably act through adrenergic effects which raise the epinephrine level and consequently the glucose concentrations of the blood [8].

It is clear, then, that no substance normally present in the blood can replace glucose as the substrate for the brain's energy metabolism. Thus far, the one substance found to do so—mannose—is not normally present in blood in significant

Table 24-4. Effectiveness of Various Substances in Preventing or Reversing the Effects of Hypoglycemia or Glucose Deprivation on Cerebral Function and Metabolism

Effectiveness	Substance	Comments
Effective	Epinephrine	Raises blood glucose concentration
	Maltose	Converted to glucose and raises blood glucose level
	Mannose	Directly metabolized and enters glycolytic pathway
Partially or occasionally effective	Glutamate	Occasionally effective by raising blood glucose level
	Arginine	
	Glycine	
	p-Aminobenzoate	
	Succinate	
Ineffective	Glycerol	Some of these substances can be metabolized to varying extent by brain tissue and could conceivably be effective if it were not for the blood-brain barrier
	Ethanol	
	Lactate	
	Pyruvate	
	Glyceraldehyde	
	Hexosediphosphates	
	Fumarate	
	Acetate	
	β-Hydroxybutyrate	
	Galactose	
	Lactose	
	Inulin	

*Source: Summarized from literature [8].

amounts and is, therefore, of no physiological significance. It should be noted, however, that failure to restore normal cerebral function in hypoglycemia is not synonymous with an inability of the brain to utilize the substance. Many of the substances that have been tested and found ineffective are compounds normally formed and utilized within the brain and are normal intermediates in its intermediary metabolism. Lactate, pyruvate, fructose-1,6-diphosphate, acetate, β-hydroxybutyrate, and acetoacetate are such examples. These can all be utilized by brain slices, homogenates, or cell-free fractions, and the enzymes for their metabolism are present in the brain. Enzymes for the metabolism of glycerol [36] or ethanol [37], for example, may not be present in sufficient amounts. For other substrates, for example, β-hydroxybutyrate and acetoacetate [38–40], the enzymes are adequate, but the substrate is not available to the brain because of inadequate blood level or restricted transport through the blood-brain barrier.

Nevertheless, the functioning of the nervous system in the intact animal depends on substrates supplied by the blood, and no satisfactory, normal, endogenous substitute for glucose has been found. Glucose must, therefore, be considered essential for normal physiological behavior of the central nervous system.

CEREBRAL UTILIZATION OF KETONES IN KETOSIS
Recent developments indicate that the brain may be somewhat more flexible in its choice of nutrients than was once believed and that, in special circumstances, it may fulfill its nutritional needs partly, although not completely, with substrates other than glucose. Normally there are no significant cerebral arteriovenous differences for D-β-hydroxybutyrate and acetoacetate [8, 18], which are "ketone bodies" formed in the course of the catabolism of fat. Owen and coworkers [41] observed, however, that when human patients were treated for severe obesity by complete fasting for several weeks, there was con-

siderable uptake of both substances by the brain. Indeed, if one assumed that the substances were completely oxidized, their rates of utilization would have accounted for more than 50 percent of the total cerebral oxygen consumption—more than that accounted for by the glucose uptake. The uptake of D-β-hydroxybutyrate was several times greater than that of acetoacetate, a reflection of its higher concentration in the blood. The enzymes responsible for their metabolism, D-β-hydroxybutyric dehydrogenase, acetoacetate-succinyl-CoA transferase, and acetoacetylthiolase, have been demonstrated to be present in brain tissue in sufficient amounts to convert them into acetyl-CoA and to feed them into the tricarboxylic cycle at a sufficient rate to satisfy the brain's metabolic demands [38–40].

Under normal circumstances, when there is ample glucose and the levels of ketone bodies in the blood are very low, the brain apparently does not resort to their use in any significant amounts. In prolonged starvation, the carbohydrate stores of the body are exhausted, and the rate of gluconeogenesis is insufficient to provide glucose fast enough to meet the requirements of the brain; blood ketone levels rise as a result of the rapid fat catabolism. The brain then apparently turns to the ketone bodies as the source of its energy supply.

Cerebral utilization of ketone bodies appears to follow passively their levels in arterial blood [42, 43]. In normal adults, ketone levels are very low in blood, and cerebral utilization of ketones is negligible. In ketotic states resulting from starvation, fat-feeding or ketogenic diets, diabetes, or any other condition which accelerates the mobilization and catabolism of fat, cerebral utilization of ketones is increased more or less in direct proportion to the degree of ketosis [42, 43]. Significant utilization of ketone bodies by brain is, however, normal in the neonatal period. The newborn infant tends to be hypoglycemic but becomes ketotic when it begins to nurse because of the high fat content of mother's milk [42, 43]. When weaned onto the normal relatively high carbohydrate diet, the ketosis and cerebral ketone utilization disappear [42, 43]. The studies in infancy have been carried out mainly in the rat, but there is evidence that the situation is similar in the human infant [42]. The first two enzymes in the pathway of ketone utilization are D-β-hydroxybutyrate dehydrogenase and acetoacetyl-succinyl-CoA transferase. These exhibit a postnatal pattern of development in brain that is well adapted to the nutritional demands of the brain. At birth, the activities of these enzymes in brain are low; they rise rapidly with the ketosis that develops with the onset of suckling; reach their peaks just before weaning; and then gradually decline after weaning to normal adult levels of about one-third to one-fourth the maximum levels attained [39, 40, 42–44].

It should be noted that D-β-hydroxybutyrate is incapable of maintaining or restoring normal cerebral function in the absence of glucose in the blood [45]. This suggests that, although it can partially replace glucose, it cannot fully satisfy the cerebral energy needs in the absence of some glucose consumption. One possible explanation may be that the first product of D-β-hydroxybutyrate oxidation, acetoacetate, is further metabolized by its displacement of the succinyl moiety of succinyl-CoA to form acetoacetyl-CoA. A certain level of glucose utilization may be essential to drive the tricarboxylic cycle and provide enough succinyl-CoA to permit the further oxidation of acetoacetate and hence pull along the oxidation of D-β-hydroxybutyrate.

Influence of Age and Development on Cerebral Energy Metabolism

The energy metabolism of the brain and the blood flow that sustains it vary considerably from birth to old age. Data on the cerebral metabolic rate obtained directly in vivo are lacking for the early postnatal period, but the results of in vitro measurements in animal brain preparations [46] and inferences drawn from cerebral blood flow measurements in intact animals [47] suggest that the cerebral oxygen consumption is low at birth, rises rapidly during the period of cerebral growth and development, and reaches a maximal level at about the time maturation is completed (Chap. 23). This rise is consistent with the progressive increase in the

Table 24-5. Cerebral Blood Flow and Oxygen Consumption in Man from Childhood to Old Age and Senility

Life Period and Condition	Age (years)	Cerebral Blood Flow (ml/100 g/min)	Cerebral O_2 Consumption (ml/100 g/min)	Cerebral Venous O_2 Tension (mm Hg)
Childhood	6[a]	106[a]	5.2[a]	—
Normal young adulthood	21	62	3.5	38
Aged				
Normal elderly	71[a]	58	3.3	36
Elderly with minimal arteriosclerosis	73[a]	48[a]	3.2	33[a, b]
Elderly with senile psychosis	72[a]	48[a, b]	2.7[a, b]	33[a, b]

[a]Statistically significant difference from normal young adult ($P < 0.05$).
[b]Statistically significant difference from normal elderly subjects ($P < 0.05$).
Source: From [17] and [49].

levels of a number of enzymes of oxidative metabolism in the brain [44]. The rates of blood flow in different structures of the brain reach peak levels at different times, depending on the maturation rate of the particular structure [47]. In the structures that consist predominantly of white matter, the peaks coincide roughly with the times of maximal rates of myelination [47]. From these peaks, blood flow and, probably, cerebral metabolic rate decline to the levels characteristic of adulthood.

Reliable quantitative data on the changes in cerebral circulation and metabolism in humans from the middle of the first decade of life to old age are summarized in Table 24-5. By 6 years of age, the cerebral blood flow and oxygen consumption have already attained their high levels, and they decline thereafter to the levels of normal young adulthood [17]. A cerebral oxygen consumption of 5.2 ml/100 g brain tissue/min in a 5- to 6-year-old child corresponds to a total oxygen consumption by the brain of approximately 60 ml per minute, or more than 50 percent of the total body basal oxygen consumption, a proportion markedly greater than that occurring in adulthood. The reasons for the extraordinarily high cerebral metabolic rates in children are unknown, but presumably they reflect the extra energy requirements for biosynthetic

processes associated with growth and development.

Despite reports to the contrary [48], cerebral blood flow and oxygen consumption normally remain essentially unchanged between young adulthood and old age. In a population of normal elderly men in their eighth decade of life—who were carefully selected for good health and freedom from all disease, including vascular—both blood flow and oxygen consumption were not significantly different from those of normal young men 50 years younger (see Table 24-5) [49]. In a comparable group of elderly subjects, who differed only by the presence of objective evidence of minimal arteriosclerosis, cerebral blood flow was significantly lower. It had reached a point at which the oxygen tension of the cerebral venous blood declined, which is an indication of cerebral hypoxia. Cerebral oxygen consumption, however, was still maintained at normal levels through removal of larger-than-normal proportions of the arterial blood oxygen. In senile psychotic patients with arteriosclerosis, cerebral blood flow was no lower, but cerebral oxygen consumption had declined. These data suggest that aging of itself need not lower the cerebral oxygen consumption and blood flow, but that when blood flow is reduced, it probably is secondary to arteriosclerosis, which produces cerebral vascular insufficiency and chronic hypoxia in the brain. Because arteriosclerosis is so prevalent in the aged population, most individuals probably follow the latter pattern.

Cerebral Metabolic Rate in Various Physiological States

CEREBRAL METABOLIC RATE AND FUNCTIONAL ACTIVITY

In organs such as the heart or skeletal muscles that perform mechanical work, increased functional activity clearly is associated with increased metabolic rate. In nervous tissues outside the central nervous system, the electrical activity is an almost quantitative indicator of the degree of functional activity, and in structures such as sympathetic ganglia and postganglionic axons [8, 50] increased electrical activity produced by electrical stimulation is definitely associated with increased utilization of oxygen. Within the central nervous system, local energy metabolism is closely correlated with the level of local functional activity. Studies with the [^{14}C]deoxyglucose method [27] have demonstrated pronounced changes in glucose utilization associated with altered functional activity in discrete regions of the CNS specifically related to the function [29]. For example, diminished visual or auditory input depresses glucose utilization in all the components of the central visual or auditory pathways, respectively (Fig. 24-2). Focal seizures increase glucose utilization in components of the motor pathways, such as the motor cortex and the basal ganglia (Fig. 24-3). On the other hand, more complex brain functions involve the electrical activities of heterogeneous units whch are integrated into a composite record; EEG data cannot always be interpreted readily in terms of total functional activity, and the relationship between total brain functional activity and metabolic rate may be obscured.

Convulsive activity, induced or spontaneous, has often been employed as a method of increasing electrical activity of the brain (see Chap. 35). Davies and Remond [2] used the oxygen electrode technique in the cerebral cortex of cat and found increases in oxygen consumption during electrically induced or drug-induced convulsions. Because the increased oxygen consumption either coincided with or followed the onset of convulsions, it was concluded that the elevation in metabolic rate was the consequence of the increased functional activity produced by the convulsive state. Similar results have been obtained in perfused cat brain in which cerebral oxygen consumption was determined from the combined measurements of blood flow and arteriovenous oxygen differences [9].

In the lightly anesthetized monkey, Dumke and Schmidt [51] found an excellent correlation between cerebral oxygen consumption and cerebral functional activity; the latter was judged by muscular movements, ocular reflexes, character of respiration, and level of arterial pressure. Changes in functional activity either occurred spontaneously or were caused (1) by altering cerebral blood flow by means of hemorrhage, transfusions, or epinephrine infusion, or (2) by producing convulsions with analeptic drugs. Cerebral oxygen consumption during the convulsions was double that of the preconvulsive state and fell to half the resting level during the postconvulsive state of depression. Similar increases in cerebral oxygen consumption have been observed in human epileptic patients during seizures [52].

Convincing correlations between cerebral metabolic rate and mental activity have been obtained in humans in a variety of pathological states of altered consciousness [5, 8, 53]. Regardless of the cause of the disorder, graded reductions in cerebral oxygen consumption were accompanied by parallel graded reductions in the degree of mental alertness, all the way to profound coma (Table 24-6). This subject is discussed further in Chap. 35.

Mental Work

It is difficult to define or even to conceive of the physical equivalent of mental work. A common view equates concentrated mental effort with mental work, and it is also fashionable to attribute a high demand for mental effort to the process of problem solving in mathematics. Nevertheless, there appears to be no increased energy utilization by the brain during such processes. From the resting

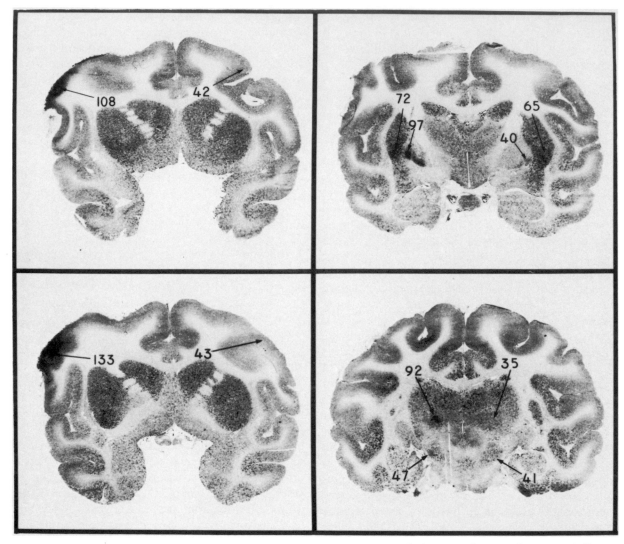

Fig. 24-3. Local glucose utilization during penicillin-induced focal seizures. The penicillin was applied to the hand and face area of the left motor cortex of a rhesus monkey. The left side of the brain is on the left in each of the autoradiographs in the figure. The numbers are the rates of local cerebral glucose utilization in μmol/100 g tissue/min. Note the following: upper left, *motor cortex in region of penicillin application and corresponding region of contralateral motor cortex;* lower left, *ipsilateral and contralateral motor cortical regions remote from area of penicillin applications;* upper right, *ipsilateral and contralateral putamen and globus pallidus;* lower right, *ipsilateral and contralateral thalamic nuclei and substantia nigra. (From L. Sokoloff, with permission.)*

Table 24-6. Relationship between Level of Consciousness and Cerebral Metabolic Rate

Level of Consciousness	Cerebral Blood Flow (ml/100 g/min)	Cerebral O$_2$ Consumption (ml/100 g/min)
Mentally alert Normal young men	54	3.3
Mentally confused Brain tumor Diabetic acidosis Insulin hypoglycemia Cerebral arteriosclerosis	48	2.8
Comatose Brain tumor Diabetic coma Insulin coma Anesthesia	57	2.0

Source: From [5].

Table 24-7. Cerebral Blood Flow and Metabolic Rate in Normal Young Men during Sleep and Mental Work

Condition	Cerebral Blood Flow (ml/100 g/min)		Cerebral O$_2$ Consumption (ml/100 g/min)	
	Control	Exptl.	Control	Exptl.
Deep (slow-wave) sleep	59	65*	3.5	3.4
Mental arithmetic	69	67	3.9	4.0

*Statistically significant difference from control level ($P < 0.05$).
Source: From [54] and [55].

levels, total cerebral blood flow and oxygen consumption remain unchanged during the exertion of the mental effort required to solve complex arithmetical problems (Table 24-7) [54]. It may be that the assumptions that relate mathematical reasoning to mental work are erroneous, but it seems more likely that the areas which participate in the processes of such reasoning represent too small a fraction of the brain for changes in their functional and metabolic activities to be reflected in the energy metabolism of the brain as a whole.

Sleep
Sleep is a naturally occurring, periodic, reversible state of unconsciousness, and the EEG pattern in deep sleep is characterized by high-voltage, slow rhythms very similar to those often seen in pathological comatose states. Nevertheless, in contrast to the depressed cerebral energy metabolism seen in pathological coma, there is surprisingly no change in the oxygen consumption of the brain as a whole in deep, slow-wave sleep (see Table 24-7) [54, 55]. There are no comparable data in man for the state of "paradoxical" sleep (REM sleep), the stage characterized by rapid, low-voltage frequencies in the EEG and believed to be associated with the dream state. However, measurements of local blood flow in most areas of the brain of animals indicate an enormous increase in blood flow throughout the brain in REM sleep [56]. The basis

for this increase is unknown. It cannot be accounted for by any of the known extracerebral factors that could change cerebral blood flow to this degree, and it must be tentatively attributed to a comparable increase in cerebral metabolic rate.

Cerebral Energy Metabolism in Pathological States

The cerebral metabolic rate is normally relatively stable and varies little under physiological conditions. There are, however, a number of pathological states of the nervous system and other organs that affect the functions of the brain either directly or indirectly, and some of these have profound effects on the cerebral metabolism. Some of these disorders are also discussed in Chap. 35.

PSYCHIATRIC DISORDERS

In general, disorders that alter the quality of mentation but not the level of consciousness—for example, the functional neuroses, psychoses, and psychotomimetic states—have no apparent effects on the blood flow and oxygen consumption of the brain. Thus, no changes in either function are observed in schizophrenia [34, 54] or LSD intoxication (Table 24-8) [54]. There is still uncertainty about the effects of anxiety, mainly because of the difficulties in evaluating quantitatively the intensity of anxiety. It is generally believed that ordinary degrees of anxiety or "nervousness" do not affect the cerebral metabolic rate, but severe anxiety or "panic" may increase the cerebral oxygen consumption [5, 54]. This may be related to the level of epinephrine circulating in the blood. Small doses of epinephrine that raise heart rate and cause some anxiety do not alter cerebral blood flow and metabolism, but large doses that are sufficient to raise the arterial blood pressure cause significant increases in the levels of both [54].

Psychosis related to parenchymatous damage in the brain is usually associated with depression of the cerebral metabolic rate. Thus, although normal aging in itself has no effect on cerebral blood flow and oxygen consumption, both are reduced in the psychoses of senility (see Table 24-5) [49, 54, 57]. Senile dementia is always the result of degenerative changes in the brain tissue. In some cases these are secondary to cerebral vascular disease and the ensuing chronic tissue hypoxia. In many cases there is primary parenchymatous degeneration that may even occur prematurely, as in Alzheimer's disease. In either case, cerebral blood flow and metabolic rate are reduced.

CONVULSIVE DISORDERS

Convulsions are discussed above in regard to the relation of cerebral metabolic rate to functional activity. In most types of convulsions studied, the seizures were induced by electroshock or analeptic drugs, or they occurred spontaneously in epileptic disease. In all these, cerebral blood flow and oxygen consumption are significantly increased in the course of the seizure (see Chap. 35 and [52]). Increased energy utilization is not, however, an essential component of the convulsive process. Convulsions may also be induced by impairment of the energy-generating system. Oxygen or glucose deficiency and fluoroacetate poisoning, all associated with a deficient availability or utilization of essential substrates for the brain's metabolism,

Table 24-8. Cerebral Blood Flow and Metabolic Rate in Schizophrenia and in Normal Young Men during LSD-induced Psychotomimetic State

Condition	Cerebral Blood Flow (ml/100 g/min)	Cerebral O_2 Consumption (ml/100 g/min)
Normal	67	3.9
LSD intoxication	68	3.9
Schizophrenia	72	4.0

Source: From [54].

Table 29-9. Cerebral Blood Flow and Metabolic Rate in Humans with Various Disorders Affecting Mental State

Condition	Mental State	Cerebral Blood Flow (ml/100 g/min)	Cerebral O_2 Consumption (ml/100 g/min)
Normal	Alert	54	3.3
Increased intracranial pressure (brain tumor)	Coma	34*	2.5*
Insulin hypoglycemia Arterial glucose level			
74 mg/100 ml	Alert	58	3.4
19 mg/100 ml	Confused	61	2.6*
8 mg/100 ml	Coma	63	1.9*
Thiopental anesthesia	Coma	60*	2.1*
Postconvulsive state			
Before convulsion	Alert	58	3.7
After convulsion	Confused	37*	3.1*
Diabetes			
Acidosis	Confused	45*	2.7*
Coma	Coma	65*	1.7*
Hepatic insufficiency	Coma	33*	1.7*

*Denotes statistical significant difference from normal level ($P < 0.05$).
Source: All studies listed were carried out by Kety and/or his associates, employing the same methods. For references see [8].

cause seizures without increasing cerebral metabolic rate. Hypoglycemic convulsions are, in fact, associated with lowered rates of oxygen and glucose utilization [34], with no apparent depletion of high-energy phosphate stores [52].

Pyridoxine deficiency (see Chap. 33) produces a substrate-deficiency type of convulsion, with reductions in cerebral blood flow and oxygen consumption [52]. The reason is unknown, but since pyridoxine deficiency leads to lowered γ-aminobutyric acid levels in the brain, it has been presumed that the lowered cerebral metabolic rate reflects impairment of the α-ketoglutarate-to-glutamate-to-γ-aminobutyric acid-to-succinic semialdehyde-to-succinate shunt pathway around the α-ketoglutarate-to-succinate step in the tricarboxylic acid cycle in the brain (see Chaps. 12 and 17).

COMA
Coma is correlated with depression of cerebral oxygen consumption; progressive reductions in the level of consciousness are paralleled by corresponding graded decreases in cerebral metabolic rate

(see Table 24-6). There are almost innumerable derangements that can lead to depression of consciousness (Chap. 35). Table 24-9 includes only a few typical examples that have been studied by the same methods and by the same or related groups of investigators.

Inadequate cerebral nutrient supply leads to decreases in the level of consciousness, ranging from confusional states to coma. The nutrition of the brain can be limited by lowering the oxygen or glucose levels of the arterial blood, as in anoxia or hypoglycemia, or by impairment of their distribution to the brain through lowering of the cerebral blood flow, as in brain tumors. Consciousness is then depressed, presumably because of inadequate supplies of substrate to support the energy metabolism necessary to sustain the appropriate functional activities of the brain.

In a number of conditions, the causes of depression of both consciousness and the cerebral metabolic rate are unknown and must, by exclusion, be attributed to intracellular defects in the brain. Anesthesia is one example. Cerebral oxygen consumption is always reduced in the anesthetized state regardless of the anesthetic agent used, whereas blood flow may or may not be decreased and may even be increased [58]. This reduction is the result of decreased energy demand and not an insufficient nutrient supply or a block of intracellular energy metabolism [53]. There is evidence that general anesthetics interfere with synaptic transmission, thus reducing neuronal interaction and functional activity and, consequently, metabolic demands [50, 53].

Several metabolic diseases with broad systemic manifestations are also associated with disturbances of cerebral functions. Diabetes mellitus, when allowed to progress to states of acidosis and ketosis, leads to mental confusion and, ultimately, to deep coma, with parallel proportionate decreases in cerebral oxygen consumption (see Table 24-9) [59]. The abnormalities are usually completely reversed by adequate insulin therapy. The cause of the coma or depressed cerebral metabolic rate is unknown. Deficiency of cerebral nutrition cannot be implicated because the blood glucose level is elevated and cerebral blood flow and oxygen supply are more than adequate. Neither is insulin deficiency, which is presumably the basis of the systemic manifestations of the disease, a likely cause of the cerebral abnormalities since no absolute requirement of insulin for cerebral glucose utilization or metabolism has been demonstrated [8]. Ketosis may be severe in this disease, and there is disputed evidence that a rise in the blood level of at least one of the ketone bodies, acetoacetate, can cause coma in animals [53]. In studies of human diabetic acidosis and coma, a significant correlation between the depression of cerebral metabolic rate and the degree of ketosis has been observed, but there is an equally good correlation with the degree of acidosis [59]. It is possible that ketosis, acidosis, or the combination of both may be responsible for the disturbances in cerebral function and metabolism.

Coma is occasionally associated with severe impairment of liver function, or hepatic insufficiency. In human patients in hepatic coma, cerebral metabolic rate is markedly depressed (see Table 24-9) [53]. Cerebral blood flow is also moderately depressed, but not sufficiently to lead to limiting supplies of glucose and oxygen. The blood ammonia level is usually elevated in hepatic coma, and significant cerebral uptake of ammonia from the blood is observed. Ammonia toxicity has, therefore, been suspected as the basis for cerebral dysfunction in hepatic coma. Because ammonia can, through glutamic dehydrogenase activity, convert α-ketoglutarate to glutamate by reductive amination, it has been suggested that ammonia might thereby deplete α-ketoglutarate and thus slow the Krebs cycle [60]. The correlation between the degree of coma and the blood ammonia level is far from convincing, however, and coma has, in fact, been observed in the absence of an increase in blood ammonia concentration [53]. Although ammonia may be involved in the mechanism of hepatic coma, the mechanism remains unclear, and other causal factors are probably involved [53].

Depression of mental functions and cerebral metabolic rate has been observed in association with kidney failure, i.e., uremic coma [53]. The chemical basis of the functional and metabolic disturbances in the brain in this condition also remains undetermined.

In the comatose states associated with these systemic metabolic diseases, there is depression of both the level of conscious mental activity and cerebral energy metabolism. From the available evidence, it is impossible to distinguish which, if either, is the primary change. It is more likely that the depressions of both functions, although well correlated with each other, are independent reflections of a more general impairment of neuronal processes by some unknown factors incident to the disease.

LOCAL CEREBRAL ENERGY METABOLISM IN HUMANS
The brain is a complex, heterogeneous organ composed of an almost infinite number of structural and functional components. These function more or less independently, subserve widely disparate functions, and exhibit markedly different rates of energy metabolism that are largely independently regulated. Most of the measurements of cerebral energy metabolism in vivo, and all of those in humans,

described above were made in the brain as a whole. The results represented, therefore, the average of the metabolic activities in all its component units. The average, however, often obscures the events in the individual components, and it therefore is not surprising that many of the studies of altered cerebral function, both normal and abnormal, have failed to demonstrate corresponding changes in energy metabolism (see Tables 24-7 and 24-8). The [14C]deoxyglucose method [27] has made it possible to measure glucose utilization simultaneously in all the components of the central nervous system, and it has been used to identify the regions with altered functional or metabolic activities, or both, in a variety of physiological, pharmacological, and pathological states [29]. As originally designed, the method utilized autoradiography of brain sections for localization, which precluded its use in humans. However, recent developments with positron-emission tomography have made it possible to adapt it for human use.

A positron emitted by a positron-emitting isotope is absorbed within a few millimeters of its site of origin, and its mass and that of a neighboring electron are converted into two so-called annihilation gamma rays that exit from the tissue in exactly opposite directions, each with an energy of 0.51 MEV equal to the rest-mass energy of the electron. These γ rays can be measured by externally placed scintillation detectors. With an array of suitably placed detectors and equipment designed to measure only the two γ rays detected in coincidence in detectors aligned at 180°, it is possible to utilize computerized tomography to resolve the concentrations of isotope in specific regions of the brain. In a sense, this technique provides autoradiography in vivo. To adapt the deoxyglucose method for use with this technique, it is necessary, of course, to use a positron-emitting species of radioactive deoxyglucose. [11C]Deoxyglucose would be satisfactory, but the physical half-life of 11C is only 20 minutes, and it is difficult to incorporate 11C into [11C]deoxyglucose sufficiently rapidly to achieve any useful yield. However, 18F is a suitable positron-emitter that can readily be incorporated into 2-[18F]fluoro-2-deoxy-D-glucose, and this analog of deoxyglucose

has been found to retain all the biochemical properties essential for the deoxyglucose method [61]. By the use of this compound, the deoxyglucose method has been adapted for use in humans [61, 62], and it is currently being used in clinical studies. It has already been found useful in localizing epileptogenic foci in patients with seizure states; such foci exhibit low rates of glucose utilization in interictal periods but become metabolically hyperactive during seizures [63]. It is expected that this procedure will make it possible to identify the loci of chemical and functional alterations in both normal and abnormal states of cerebral function in humans.

Acknowledgment
This work was sponsored by the Intramural Research Program of the National Institute of Mental Health and is therefore not subject to copyright.

References

*1. Berl, S., and Clarke, D. D. Compartmentation of Amino Acid Metabolism. In A. Lajtha (ed.), *Handbook of Neurochemistry*. New York: Plenum, 1969. Vol. 2, pp. 447–472.

2. Davies, P. W., and Rémond, A. Oxygen consumption of the cerebral cortex of the cat during metrazole convulsions. *Res. Publ. Assoc. Nerv. Ment. Dis.* 26:205–217, 1946.

3. Myerson, A., Halloran, R. D., and Hirsch, H. L. Technique for obtaining blood from the internal jugular vein and internal carotid artery. *Arch. Neurol. Psychiatry* 17:807–808, 1927.

4. Kety, S. S., and Schmidt, C. F. The nitrous oxide method for the quantitative determination of cerebral blood flow in man: Theory, procedure, and normal values. *J. Clin. Invest.* 27:476–483, 1948.

*5. Kety, S. S. Circulation and metabolism of the human brain in health and disease. *Am. J. Med.* 8:205–217, 1950.

*6. Lassen, N. A. Cerebral blood flow and oxygen consumption in man. *Physiol. Rev.* 39:183–238, 1959.

*7. Sokoloff, L. The action of drugs on the cerebral circulation. *Pharmacol. Rev.* 11:1–85, 1959.

*8. Sokoloff, L. The Metabolism of the Central Nervous System *In Vivo*. In J. Field, H. W. Magoun, and V. E. Hall (eds.), *Handbook of Physiology-Neurophysiology*. Washington, D.C.: American Physiological Society, 1960. Vol. 3, pp. 1843–1864.

*Key reference.

*9. Geiger, A. Correlation of brain metabolism and function by use of a brain perfusion method *in situ*. *Physiol. Rev.* 38:1–20, 1958.

*10. Kety, S. S. The Cerebral Circulation. In J. Field, H. W. Magoun, and V. E. Hall (eds.), *Handbook of Physiology-Neurophysiology*. Washington, D.C.: American Physiological Society, 1960. Vol. 3, pp. 1751–1760.

*11. Sokoloff, L. Quantitative Measurements of Cerebral Blood Flow in Man. In H. D. Bruner (ed.), *Methods in Medical Research*. Chicago: Year Book, 1960. Vol. 8, pp. 253–261.

*12. Betz, E. Cerebral blood flow: Its measurement and regulation. *Physiol. Rev.* 52(3):595–630, 1972.

13. Page, W. F., German, W. J., and Nims, L. F. The nitrous oxide method for measurement of cerebral blood flow and cerebral gaseous metabolism in dogs. *Yale J. Biol. Med.* 23:462–473, 1951.

14. Lassen, N. A., and Munck, O. The cerebral blood flow in man determined by the use of radioactive krypton. *Acta Physiol. (Scand.)* 33:30–49, 1955.

15. Lewis, B. M., Sokoloff, L., Wechsler, R. L., Wentz, W. B., and Kety, S. S. A method for the continuous measurement of cerebral blood flow in man by means of radioactive krypton (^{79}Kr). *J. Clin. Invest.* 39:707–716, 1960.

16. Gotoh, F., Meyer, J. S., and Tomita, M. Hydrogen method for determining cerebral blood flow in man. *Arch. Neurol.* 15:549–559, 1966.

17. Kennedy, C., and Sokoloff, L. An adaptation of the nitrous oxide method to the study of the cerebral circulation in children; normal values for cerebral blood flow and cerebral metabolic rate in childhood. *J. Clin. Invest.* 36:1130–1137, 1957.

*18. Kety, S. S. The General Metabolism of the Brain *in Vivo*. In D. Richter (ed.), *The Metabolism of the Nervous System*. London: Pergamon, 1957. Pp. 221–237.

*19. Waelsch, H., and Lajtha, A. Protein metabolism in the nervous system. *Physiol. Rev.* 41:709–736, 1961.

20. Meyer, J. S., Ryu, T., Toyoda, M., Shinohara, Y., Wiederholt, I., and Guiraud, B. Evidence for a Pasteur effect regulating cerebral oxygen and carbohydrate metabolism in man. *Neurology* 19:954–962, 1969.

21. Rossen, R., Kabat, H., and Anderson, J. P. Acute arrest of cerebral circulation in man. *Arch. Neurol. Psychiatry* 50:510–528, 1943.

22. Finnerty, F. A., Jr., Witkin, L., and Fazekas, J. F. Cerebral hemodynamics during cerebral ischemia induced by acute hypotension. *J. Clin. Invest.* 33:1227–1232, 1954.

*23. Sokoloff, L., and Kety, S. S. Regulation of cerebral circulation. *Physiol. Rev.* 40(Suppl. 4): 38–44, 1960.

24. Landau, W. H., Freygang, W. H., Rowland, L. P., Sokoloff, L., and Kety, S. S. The local circulation of the living brain; values in the unanesthetized and anesthetized cat. *Trans. Am. Neurol. Assoc.* 80: 125–129, 1955.

25. Freygang, W. H., and Sokoloff, L. Quantitative measurements of regional circulation in the central nervous system by the use of radioactive inert gas. *Adv. Biol. Med. Phys.* 6:263–279, 1958.

26. Sokoloff, L. Local Cerebral Circulation at Rest and During Altered Cerebral Activity Induced by Anesthesia or Visual Stimulation. In S. S. Kety and J. Elkes (eds.), *The Regional Chemistry, Physiology and Pharmacology of the Nervous System*. Oxford: Pergamon, 1961. Pp. 107–117.

*27. Sokoloff, L., Reivich, M., Kennedy, C., Des Rosiers, M. H., Patlak, C. S., Pettigrew, K. D., Sakurada, O., and Shinohara, M. The [^{14}C]deoxyglucose method for the measurement of local cerebral glucose utilization: Theory, procedure, and normal values in the conscious and anesthetized albino rat. *J. Neurochem.* 28:897–916, 1977.

28. Sokoloff, L. Local cerebral energy metabolism: Its relationships to local functional activity and blood flow. In M. J. Purves and L. Elliott (eds.), *Cerebral Vascular Smooth Muscle and Its Control*. Ciba Foundation Symposium 56. Amsterdam: Elsevier/Excerpta Medica/North Holland, 1978. Pp. 171–197.

*29. Sokoloff, L. Relation between physiological function and energy metabolism in the central nervous system. *J. Neurochem.* 29(5):13–26, 1977.

30. Kennedy, C., Sakurada, O., Shinohara, M., Jehle, J., and Sokoloff, L. Local cerebral glucose utilization in the normal conscious Macaque monkey. *Ann. Neurol.* 4:293–301, 1978.

31. Adams, J. E., Harper, H. A., Gordon, G. S., Hutchin, M., and Bentinck, R. C. Cerebral metabolism of glutamic acid in multiple sclerosis. *Neurology* 5:100–107, 1955.

32. Himwich, H. E., and Nahum, L. H. The respiratory quotient of testicle. *Am. J. Physiol.* 88:680–685, 1929.

*33. Sacks, W. Cerebral Metabolism *in Vivo*. In A. Lajtha (ed.), *Handbook of Neurochemistry*. New York: Plenum, 1969. Vol. 1, pp. 301–324.

34. Kety, S. S., Woodford, R. B., Harmel, M. H., Freyhan, F. A., Appel, K. E., and Schmidt, C. F. Cerebral blood flow and metabolism in schizophrenia. The effects of barbiturate semi-narcosis, insulin coma, and electroshock. *Am. J. Psychiatry* 104:765–770, 1948.

35. Sloviter, H. A., and Kamimoto, T. The isolated, perfused rat brain preparation metabolizes mannose but not maltose. *J. Neurochem.* 17:1109–1111, 1970.

36. Sloviter, H. A., and Suhara, K. A brain-infusion

method for demonstrating utilization of glycerol by rabbit brain in vivo. *J. Appl. Physiol.* 23:792–797, 1967.

37. Raskin, N. H., and Sokoloff, L. Alcohol dehydrogenase activity in rat brain and liver. *J. Neurochem.* 17:1677–1687, 1970.

38. Itoh, T., and Quastel, J. H. Acetoacetate metabolism in infant and adult rat brain in vitro. *Biochem. J.* 116:641–655, 1970.

39. Pull, I., and McIlwain, H. 3-Hydroxybutyrate dehydrogenase of rat brain on dietary change and during maturation. *J. Neurochem.* 18:1163–1165, 1971.

40. Williamson, D. H., Bates, M. W., Page, M. A., and Krebs, H. A. Activities of enzymes involved in acetoacetate utilization in adult mammalian tissues. *Biochem. J.* 121:41–47, 1971.

41. Owen, O. E., Morgan, A. P., Kemp, H. G., Sullivan, J. M., Herrera, M. G., and Cahill, G. F., Jr. Brain metabolism during fasting. *J. Clin. Invest.* 46:1589–1595, 1967.

*42. Krebs, H. A., Williamson, D. H., Bates, M. W., Page, M. A., and Hawkins, R. A. The role of ketone bodies in caloric homeostasis. *Adv. Enzyme Regul.* 9:387–409, 1971.

*43. Sokoloff, L. Metabolism of ketone bodies by the brain. *Annu. Rev. Med.* 24:271–280, 1973.

44. Klee, C. B., and Sokoloff, L. Changes in D(-)-β-hydroxybutyric dehydrogenase activity during brain maturation in the rat. *J. Biol. Chem.* 242:3880–3883, 1967.

45. Sloviter, H. A. Personal communication, 1971.

46. Himwich, H. E., and Fazekas, J. F. Comparative studies of the metabolism of the brain of infant and adult dogs. *Am. J. Physiol.* 132:454–459, 1941.

47. Kennedy, C., Grave, G. D., Jehle, J. W., and Sokoloff, L. Changes in blood flow in the component structures of the dog brain during postnatal maturation. *J. Neurochem.* 19:2423–2433, 1972.

*48. Kety, S. S. Human cerebral blood flow and oxygen consumption as related to aging. *Res. Publ. Assoc. Nerv. Ment. Dis.* 35:31–45, 1956.

49. Sokoloff, L. Cerebral circulatory and metabolic changes associated with aging. *Res. Publ. Assoc. Nerv. Ment. Dis.* 41:237–254, 1966.

50. Larrabee, M. G., Ramos, J. F., and Bülbring, E. Effects of anesthetics on oxygen consumption and synaptic transmission in sympathetic ganglia. *J. Cell. Comp. Physiol.* 40:461–494, 1952.

51. Dumke, P. R., and Schmidt, C. F. Quantitative measurements of cerebral blood flow in the Macaque monkey. *Am. J. Physiol.* 138:421–431, 1943.

*52. Sokoloff, L. Cerebral Blood Flow and Energy Metabolism in Convulsive Disorders. In H. H. Jasper, A. A. Ward, and A. Pope (eds.), *Basic Mechanisms of the Epilepsies.* Boston: Little, Brown, 1969. Pp. 639–646.

*53. Sokoloff, L. Neurophysiology and Neurochemistry of Coma. In E. Polli (ed.), *Neurochemistry of Hepatic Coma.* New York/Basel: S. Karger, 1971. Pp. 15–33.

*54. Sokoloff, L. Cerebral Circulation and Behavior in Man: Strategy and Findings. In A. J. Mandell and M. P. Mandell (eds.), *Psychochemical Research in Man.* New York: Academic, 1969. Pp. 237–252.

55. Mangold, R., Sokoloff, L., Conner, E., Kleinerman, J., Therman, P. G., and Kety, S. S. The effects of sleep and lack of sleep on the cerebral circulation and metabolism of normal young men. *J. Clin. Invest.* 34:1092–1100, 1955.

56. Reivich, M., Isaacs, G., Evarts, E. V., and Kety, S. S. The effect of slow wave sleep and REM sleep on regional cerebral blood flow in cats. *J. Neurochem.* 15:301–306, 1968.

57. Lassen, N. A., Munck, O., and Tottey, E. R. Mental function and cerebral oxygen consumption in organic dementia. *Arch. Neurol. Psychiatry* 77:126–133, 1957.

*58. Sokoloff, L. Control of Cerebral Blood Flow: The Effects of Anesthetic Agents. In E. M. Papper and R. J. Kitz (eds.), *Uptake and Distribution of Anesthetic Agents.* New York: McGraw-Hill, 1963. Pp. 140–157.

59. Kety, S. S., Polis, B. D., Nadler, C. S., and Schmidt, C. F. Blood flow and oxygen consumption of the human brain in diabetic acidosis and coma. *J. Clin. Invest.* 27:500–510, 1948.

60. Bessman, S. P., and Bessman, A. N. The cerebral and peripheral uptake of ammonia in liver disease with an hypothesis for the mechanism of hepatic coma. *J. Clin. Invest.* 34:622–628, 1955.

*61. Reivich, M., Kuhl, D., Wolf, A., Greenberg, J., Phelps, M., Ido, T., Casella, V., Fowler, J., Hoffman, E., Alavi, A., Som, P., and Sokoloff, L. The [^{18}F]fluoro-deoxyglucose method for the measurement of local cerebral glucose utilization in man. *Circ. Res.* 44:127–137, 1979.

62. Phelps, M. E., Huang, S. C., Hoffman, E. J., Selin, C., Sokoloff, L., and Kuhl, D. E. Tomographic measurement of local cerebral glucose metabolic rate in man with 2-(^{18}F)fluoro-2-deoxy-D-glucose: validation of method. *Ann. Neurol.* 6:371–388, 1979.

63. Kuhl, D., Engel, J., Phelps, M., and Selin, C. Patterns of local cerebral metabolism and perfusion in partial epilepsy by emission computed tomography of ^{18}F-fluorodeoxyglucose and ^{13}N-ammonia. *Acta Neurol. (Scand.)* 60:538–539, 1979.

Transport Mechanisms

Although the brain obtains its required constant supply of oxygen and glucose from the bloodstream, other substances are not readily absorbed from the blood. For example, fructose cannot be substituted for glucose in the treatment of hypoglycemic coma, although brain slices will metabolize it as well as glucose. The central nervous system of mammals appears to require an ultrastable internal environment in order to function effectively, and there are special controls involved in the transport of many materials in the CNS. The sum total of these special transport mechanisms is called the *blood-brain barrier*. Similar special transport mechanisms between blood and cerebrospinal fluid (CSF) constitute the *blood-CSF barrier*. These topics have been reviewed comprehensively [1, 2].

Many substances either do not cross brain capillaries (e.g., acidic dyes) or they cross at a very slow rate (e.g., ions). The classic Experiments of Paul Ehrlich in 1882 are said to be the first to demonstrate that animals given vital dyes become intensely stained by the dye in all parts of the body except the brain. In 1909, Goldman studied the vital staining by trypan blue and noted that, after parenteral administration of a dye, only the brain remains unstained. He found that even after injection of such large amounts of trypan blue, the animal tissues become intensely stained, but the brain remained "snow-white." When he instilled a small amount of trypan blue into the subarachnoid space, however, the brain became intensely stained. The processes that hindered the movement of trypan blue from the bloodstream to the CNS but did not hinder the movement of the dye from the spinal fluid into the brain, became known as the blood-brain barrier. It is now known that trypan blue quickly binds to albumin in the bloodstream. Hence, the impermeant molecule studied by Goldman was the albumin-dye complex. The morphological basis of this blood-brain barrier to proteins will be discussed shortly.

The concentration of many substances in brain and CSF is independent of their concentration in the blood. Homeostatic mechanisms produce an ultrastable internal environment in the brain as other mechanisms maintain the stable internal environment of the body. The stability of the internal environment may be due either to special transport processes (utilizing mediated transport, active clearance, and other mechanisms) or to the dynamic state of cerebral metabolites. It may be worthwhile to review briefly some of the mechanisms involved in transport. (See also [3] and Chap. 6.)

1. *Bulk Flow.* "Bulk flow" means that solutes of various sizes move together with the solvent as a bulk liquid. This concept is important in discussing circulation and absorption in the cerebrospinal fluid. CSF circulates through the ventricular subarachnoid spaces and is absorbed into the bloodstream as a bulk fluid. Because bulk flow implies that solutes of various sizes move collectively with the solvent, all as a single body, it is convenient to measure the bulk absorption of CSF into the bloodstream by measuring the rate of clearance of an inert, large molecular weight tracer, such as blue dextran, radiolabeled serum albumin, or inulin. These tracers do not diffuse into adjacent brain tissue at an appreciable rate. It has been suggested that there may also be bulk flow of brain extracellular fluid through the brain, but this has not yet been demonstrated unequivocally.

2. *Diffusion.* Diffusion consists in the movement

of a solute from a region of higher to one of lower concentration as a result of the random motion of the solute molecule. Diffusion occurs in both the CSF and the extracellular spaces of the brain. In addition, diffusion across plasma membranes is important, especially diffusion across the membranes of the capillary endothelial cells. This is the major route of movement of water, urea, and gases into the brain.

3. *Pinocytosis.* In this process, fluid that includes large molecules and even particles is engulfed by invaginating cell membranes, forming a vesicle which then separates from the membrane. This vesicle can now transport its contents across the cell. Under ordinary conditions, pinocytosis is a slow and uncertain process in brain capillaries and probably moves few molecules.

4. *Mediated Transport.* Mediated transport requires a carrier molecule with specific sites for the substrate involved; this permits the substrate molecule to move readily across either the plasma membrane of a single cell or a cellular membrane composed of a sheet of cells in continuity. When the limited number of sites on the carrier molecule are filled, as for example, when the concentration of substrate molecules on one side of the membrane is sufficient, the number of molecules transported can no longer increase. With further increases of the substrate molecule, the carrier is then saturated and transport is independent of concentration. The kinetics of carrier-substrate transport are identical with those of enzyme-substrate complexing. Moreover, mediated transport implies that another molecule of sufficiently close chemical and steric similarity may occupy the site intended for a given substrate molecule. In the mammalian blood-brain or blood-CSF barrier, such carriers are hypothesized to explain the stereospecificity and concentration independence of transport of hexoses and amino acids, but as yet carrier molecules per se have not been isolated.

5. *Active Transport.* Active transport implies that energy is utilized in the transport of a molecule. To prove the existence of active transport, either the energy-utilizing process must be specifically identified or it must be shown that the molecule is transported against an electrochemical gradient. Although it is possible that the transport of many molecules by carriers does require energy, this must be demonstrated for each molecular species studied. The best examples of active transport are the halides and the small organic molecules, which can be cleared actively from CSF, even though the blood level of such molecules is much higher than that in CSF.

6. *Stability Due to Transport Processes.* The question arises of how the various transport processes can be combined to provide a high degree of stability for the constituents of the CSF and the brain extracellular fluid. Bradbury [4] has defined stability of the blood-CSF systems as follows. If a substance is present in CSF at concentration C_{CSF} and in plasma at concentration C_{pl}, stability occurs when, as a result of a change in plasma concentration, a new steady state is reached so that

$$\Delta C_{CSF} < \Delta C_{pl} \qquad \text{(eq. 25-1)}$$

At steady state, the flux of this substance from plasma to CSF, J_{in}, must equal its flux out, J_{out}, so that for any change in plasma concentration, ΔC_{pl}, stability of CSF will occur when

$$\Delta J_{in} / \Delta C_{pl} < \Delta J_{out} / \Delta C_{CSF} \qquad \text{(eq. 25-2)}$$

J_{in} and J_{out} represent transport processes that need not be identical. For instance, one might be passive and one active. If the carrier involved in J_{in} is saturated at usual plasma concentrations, then the ratio $\Delta J_{in} / \Delta C_{pl}$ will approach zero. Such carrier-mediated transport is probably the most common mechanism controlling the flow of non-lipid soluble substances from the capillary lumen to the brain, but carrier systems have also been found to operate for outward flux. Here, the greatest stability is achieved when the carrier system operates well below saturation, so that the ratio $\Delta J_{out} / \Delta C_{CSF}$ is a positive number. Such asymmetric carrier mechanisms have been implicated in the maintenance of the control of the stability of K^+ in CSF and may also exist for other molecules.

7. *Stability Due to Dynamic State of Cerebral Metabolites.* The processes involved in maintaining constant brain levels of molecules that are metabo-

lized within the brain system are obviously complex and depend on the interplay of dynamic processes. For example, the level of dopamine in brain tissue is relatively constant under normal conditions. This level is the result of an equilibrium between the synthesis of dopamine through tyrosine hydroxylase and DOPA decarboxylase; its degradation by dopamine β-hydroxylase, monoamine oxidase, and catechol-O-methyltransferase; and its storage in granules, which isolates it from these degradative enzymes. Synthesis is usually rate limited by the activity of tyrosine hydroxylase. If this is bypassed by administration of large amounts of the amino acid L-dopa, the brain dopamine will increase. If dopamine in storage granules is released by the administration of reserpine, it will be destroyed quickly by the degradative enzymes, and the total brain level will fall dramatically. Hence, the interplay of factors influencing levels of metabolizable compounds is exceedingly complex and relatively difficult to analyze.

Characteristics of the Blood-Brain Barrier

MORPHOLOGY

For many years there was confusion about the locus of the blood-brain barrier. This is now known to be the capillary endothelium (Fig. 25-1). Ultrastructural studies using markers such as peroxidase, the reaction product of which can be stained in situ with osmium, have shown that the capillary endothelium is a continuous layer, with tight junctions between continuous cells that do not permit the passage of protein markers from the capillary lumen to the basement membrane that surrounds the capillary endothelium [5]. Studies with microperoxidase have shown that molecules with molecular weights as low as 2,000 are excluded by these tight junctions [6]. Although it has not been possible to establish morphologically whether the tight junctions also exclude small hydrophilic molecules of the molecular weight of sugars and amino acids, physiological data suggest that they do and that the primary movement of such substances is by mediated transport. In contrast, if the protein marker enters the extracellular space

of the brain (for example, if it is placed in the subarachnoid or ventricular space), it will diffuse through this extracellular space until it reaches the capillary endothelium. Under these circumstances, the tight junctions will prevent the molecules from diffusing into the capillary lumen. Cerebral capillaries have reduced pinocytosis compared to other blood vessels and lack fenestrations, which serve as the route of the movement of macromolecules in other capillary systems.

As the morphological basis of the blood-brain barrier became evident, physiologists were concerned about the large amount of work that might be required of the capillary endothelium to transport nutrients into the brain. In fact, cerebral capillaries have approximately four times as many mitochondria as do capillary endothelial cells of other tissue [7]. However, as we shall show below, most nutrients are transported by carrier-mediated systems that do not require the expenditure of energy each time a molecule is transported.

DIFFUSION

Water is a most important substance entering the brain by diffusion. When deuterium oxide (D_2O) is administered intravenously as a tracer, the half-time of exchange of brain water varies between 12 and 25 seconds, depending upon the vascularity of the region studied. This rate of exchange is rapid compared with the rate of exchange of most solutes, but it is limited both by the permeability of the capillary epithelium to H_2O and by the rate of cerebral blood flow [8]. In fact, the calculated permeability constant of the cerebral capillary wall to the diffusion of D_2O is about the same as that estimated for the diffusion of water across lipid membranes [9].

Water also moves freely into or out of the brain as the osmolality of the plasma changes. This phenomenon is clinically useful, since intracranial pressure can be reduced by the dehydration of the brain after plasma tonicity has been elevated by such substances as mannitol (Chap. 34). It has been calculated that when plasma osmolality is raised from 310 to 344 mOsm, for example, a 10 percent shrinkage of the brain will result, with half of the

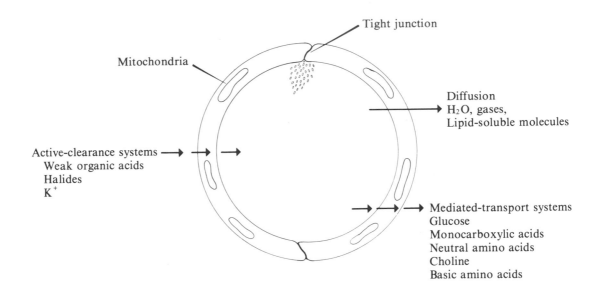

Fig. 25-1. Blood-brain barrier. This diagram depicts the transport processes across capillary endothelial cells in brain parenchyma. The tight junctions between endothelial cells preclude movement of large molecules from the capillary lumen to the extracellular space, and vice versa. Transport from the lumen to the brain extracellular space is primarily by diffusion or by specific carrier-mediated transport systems, which are not energy dependent. Removal of metabolites from brain, however, occurs by active (energy-dependent) transport systems in the endothelial cells. Reflecting their specific transport roles, the brain endothelial cells have an increased number of mitochondria, as compared to those of other capillaries.

shrinkage taking place in 12 minutes. The permeability constant calculated for this osmotic flow of water is slightly larger than that for diffusional flow. However, the movement of water under osmotic load in the example given is slower than diffusional flow because the concentration gradient for the osmotic load is only 34 mOsm, but when D_2O is used to measure diffusion, the gradient is 55 Osm, the same as for H_2O.

Lipid-soluble substances, which include most psychoactive drugs, also move freely, diffusing across the plasma membranes at rates in proportion to their lipid solubility. The permeability of such alcohols as ethanol is especially great. The permeability constants of substances such as thiopental and antipyrine are smaller, barbital is somewhat slower, and urea and salicylic acid are still slower. In a compound such as salicylic acid, only the un-ionized form diffuses across the membranes, and hence the dissociation constant and the pH of the blood are of importance [10]. Whereas many drugs depend on their lipid solubility for entry into the brain, amphetamine is an example of one that may enter the brain by a saturable, but nonstereospecific, mediated-transport system [11].

Because of the failure of proteins to move into the brain, molecules that are bound to protein are,

therefore, impermeant, even if intrinsically lipid-soluble. Examples of these are such dyes as trypan blue and the important molecule bilirubin. If sulfa drugs are administered to an infant or young animal with elevated bilirubin, the bilirubin will be displaced from the albumin by the sulfa drug. This can lead to an increase in kernicterus in jaundiced infants. Some movement of impermeant molecules can occur by pinocytosis, but this is slight in the cerebral capillary endothelium as compared with that in other capillaries.

Gases such as CO_2, O_2, N_2O, Xe, Kr, and volatile anesthetics diffuse rapidly into brain. As a consequence, the rate at which their concentration in brain comes into equilibrium with plasma concentration is limited primarily by the cerebral blood flow. Hence, the inert gases—N_2O, Xe, and Kr— have been widely used to measure cerebral blood flow by both the Kety technique for total blood flow and the Lassen-Ingvar technique for regional blood flow (see Chap. 24).

A good contrast is found between the effects of CO_2, a gas that diffuses freely, and H^+, which moves very slowly into brain. Consequently, the brain pH will reflect blood PCO_2 rather than blood pH. In a patient with a metabolic acidosis and a secondary respiratory alkalosis, the brain will tend to become alkalotic.

MEDIATED TRANSPORT
Glucose is the most rapidly utilized molecule transported across the cerebral capillaries by a specific carrier system. Present evidence is that this is a mediated transport that does not require energy expenditure for each molecule moved.

The steric specificity of the glucose transport system permits D-glucose, but not L-glucose, to enter the brain. Such hexoses as mannose and maltose can also be transported rapidly into the brain; the uptake of galactose is intermediate, whereas fructose is taken up very slowly [12]. 2-Deoxyglucose, on the other hand, is taken up quickly and will competitively inhibit the transport of glucose. The 2-deoxyglucose is then phosphorylated, but not further metabolized. If 2-deoxyglucose is used in tracer quantities, the amount of the phosphorylated tracer in the brain reflects the rate of glucose uptake and metabolism (see Chap. 24).

Monocarboxylic acids, including L-lactate, and such glucose metabolites as acetate and pyruvate are transported by separate stereospecific systems [13]. The rate of entry of these substances is significantly lower than that of glucose [14, 15]. The metabolic significance of these transport systems is not understood.

Neutral amino acids are transported into brain by a well-defined carrier system. The rate of movement of amino acids into brain is variable [12]. Phenylalanine, leucine, tyrosine, isoleucine, tryptophan, methionine, histidine, and dopa may enter as rapidly as glucose, whereas alanine, proline, glutamic acid, aspartic acid, γ-aminobutyric acid, and glycine are virtually excluded. Threonine and serine are intermediate in their rate of uptake. Competitive inhibition is easy to demonstrate. The transport of large neutral amino acids is inhibited by the synthetic amino acid 2-aminonorbornane-2-carboxylic acid (BCH), but not by 2-(methylamino)-isobutyric acid; hence, the transport system is similar to the L (for leucine) transport system defined by Christensen [16] for various mammalian cellular and organic systems [17, 18]. It should be noted that both the essential amino acids and the amino acids serving as precursors for catecholamine and indoleamine synthesis are transported readily, whereas amino acids synthesized readily from glucose metabolites, including those amino acids that act as neurotransmitters, are virtually excluded from the brain.

The L transport system characteristically does not require energy or a Na^+ gradient. A separate transport system is involved in the movement of the basic amino acid arginine into brain [13].

Choline enters the central nervous system through a carrier-mediated transport process that can be inhibited by such molecules as dimethylaminoethanol [19], hemicholinium, and tetraethyl ammonium chloride [20–22].

Simple charged ions will exchange with brain ions, although the exchange is noticeably slower than with other tissues. For example, intravenously administered $^{42}K^+$ exchanges with muscle K^+ in 1 hour, but K^+ exchange in brain is only half completed in 24 to 36 hours. The rate of K^+ flux shows little change as plasma K^+ is varied. Ca^{2+} and Mg^{2+} exchange as slowly as does K^+. Na^+ is somewhat faster, with half-exchange occurring in 3 to 8 hours, but Na^+ exchange is much slower between blood and brain than between blood and the Na^+ of other tissues.

ACTIVE TRANSPORT
There is no evidence that active transport is required for movement of any molecule *into* brain. However, there is indirect evidence that at least three active transport systems operate to remove

molecules from brain. Thus, the active transport of weak organic acids and halides appears to be present in brain tissue as well as CSF [23, 24], since both systems may move molecules out of CSF and brain and into plasma against a concentration gradient presumed to require energy. The removal of excess extracellular K^+ by $(Na^+ + K^+)$-ATPase has been reported [25]; hence, this also represents a form of active transport.

The weak organic acid system that is readily blocked by probenecid is responsible for the transport of such important molecules as prostaglandins, penicillin, and such monoamine metabolites as HVA and 5HIAA [26, 27].

ENZYMATIC BARRIERS IN CAPILLARY ENDOTHELIUM

For at least two molecules, γ-aminobutyrate and L-dopa, transport between blood and brain tissue is retarded by enzymatic degradation of these substances within the capillary endothelium. In both instances, the rate of degradation is such that the administration of very large amounts of γ-aminobutyrate or L-dopa will cause an increase in the amount of these substances that reaches brain tissue [28]. Such enzymatic degradation can be demonstrated histochemically. The enzyme γ-glutamyltranspeptidase, which may function in other tissues in the transfer of amino acids, is present in significant activity in cerebral capillaries. The relationship of this finding to the transport of amino acids across the blood-brain barrier has not yet been established [29].

ISOLATED MICROVESSELS

By using centrifugation techniques, it is possible to isolate cerebral capillaries and other small vessels from brain [30, 31]. These isolated microvessels are active metabolically in vitro and show many of the exchange properties attributed to cerebral capillaries from in vivo preparations. These include carrier-mediated transport of glucose and neutral amino acids and transport of K^+ by $(Na^+ + K^+)$-ATPase [32, 33]. Betz and coworkers have been able to isolate fractions from the microvessel preparations that differ from each other in enzymes present

and represent luminal and antiluminal surfaces [34–36]. According to their data, the neutral amino acid transport system is present in luminal membrane and the $(Na^+ + K^+)$-ATPase in antiluminal.

Influences on Blood-Brain Barrier

DEVELOPMENT

Many of the features of the blood-brain barrier, including the presence of tight junctions in the capillary endothelium and the exclusion of protein molecules, are present in newborn animals. Transport of certain substances—for example, simple ions—is moderately faster in the newborn animal. There is a very great increase in the rate of uptake of certain actively metabolized substances in the rapidly growing brain, which may result either from transport per se or from the high rate of turnover of the metabolites (see Chap. 23).

In fetal and neonatal animals, there is significant movement of transferrin, α-fetoprotein, and albumin into CSF and brain. It is not known to what extent the apparent movement of other molecules in immature animals reflects conjugation of the molecules to the proteins [37].

CHEMICALS AND DRUGS

As already discussed, competitive inhibitors may interfere with carrier-mediated transport of molecules into the brain. Drugs such as dilute mercuric chloride, given intravascularly, may increase the permeability of the blood-brain barrier. There is some possibility that greatly elevated levels of PCO_2 may also increase blood-brain barrier permeability [38].

HYPEROSMOLARITY

Intracarotid injection of extremely hyperosmotic solutions disrupts the blood-brain barrier by osmotic shrinkage of capillary endothelial cells and may produce cerebral edema and focal necrosis. It has been demonstrated, however, that this effect can be controlled and that, by the injection of small amounts of such hyperosmotic solutions as 2 M urea or 5% NaCl, a reversible opening of the blood-brain barrier can be produced [39]. Apparently, there is both opening of tight junctions secondary to the osmotic shrinkage of cell and an increase in pinocytic activity [40, 41]. Such intracarotid injections permit an increased uptake of tracers that ordinarily are excluded (e.g., horseradish peroxidase). Surprisingly, an increase in facilitated transport of glucose has been reported [42]. The uptake of [³H]norepinephrine can be increased three to four times during the osmotic opening of the blood-brain barrier. Similar changes occur with a mechanical disruption produced by rapid injection into the carotid artery [43, 44]. Whether this ability to control the blood-brain barrier reversibly will be important in the use of chemotherapeutic agents normally excluded by the barrier has not yet been determined. Contrast media used routinely for cerebral angiography are perhaps hypertonic enough to produce similar changes during angiography.

PATHOLOGY

A characteristic of almost any focal injury to the brain, whether it is produced by excessive convulsions, knife wounds, freezing, heating, electrical currents, tumors, inflammatory agents, toxins, or other causes, is the breakdown of the blood-brain barrier, with subsequent diffusion of protein molecules into brain tissue. This phenomenon has been used widely to trace such areas of injury, since administration of such dyes as trypan blue bound to protein, or fluorescein bound to protein, enables histological identification of those areas in which the blood-brain barrier has broken down. The mechanism of traumatic injury to the capillary endothelium is still under investigation. Apparently, the tight junctions between cells are sometimes ruptured; in other instances, the capillary endothelial cells are simply torn, so that plasma proteins may pour into the area of injury. But in some instances, at least in certain brain tumors, the capillary endothelium thins out, forming fenestrations across which proteins may move.

Regional Differences in the Blood-Brain Barrier

Movement of substances into given regions depends on such factors as capillary density. More impor-

tant, however, are various regions that are "excluded" from the blood-brain barrier. These are regions in which the capillary endothelium contains fenestrations across which proteins and small organic molecules may move from the blood into the adjacent tissue. Examples of such areas are the area postrema, the median eminence of the hypothalamus, the line of attachment of the choroid plexus, and the pineal gland. These areas may have special functional significance, in that they may be where the brain monitors the contents of the blood. The area postrema is close to what has been called the "vomiting" center of the brain, and the hypothalamus is involved in the regulation of the body's metabolic activity. These areas may be sites at which neuronal receptors may directly sample plasma.

Physiologists have been aware that such substances as radiolabeled serum albumin, which are excluded from entering the brain at the capillary endothelium, nevertheless accumulate throughout the cerebrum in quantities just above those which can be accounted for by the vascular volume of the brain. Recently, it has been demonstrated that some small arterioles (15 to 30 μm in diameter), located primarily near the sulci at the cerebral cortex and scattered through the diencephalon and neighboring regions, will transport such high molecular weight compounds as horseradish peroxidase through their endothelial cells by the process of pinocytosis. These same arterioles possess tight junctions, as does the capillary endothelium [45]. On a quantitative basis, such transport is not sufficient to circumvent the blood-brain barrier, but it may account for the small amounts of serum protein that enter the CSF.

Characteristics of Blood-CSF Barrier

COMPOSITION OF CSF

Cerebrospinal fluid has been characterized as an "ideal" physiological solution. It differs from plasma in that it is almost free of protein, and it differs from an ultrafiltrate of plasma by maintaining the concentrations of various ions at different levels (Table 25-1).

CSF FORMATION

CSF is constantly being formed and removed. The major sites of CSF formation are the choroid plexuses of the ventricles (Fig. 25-2). In addition, a significant extrachoroidal formation of CSF has been demonstrated. In normal subjects, the rate of CSF secretion has been estimated to be 0.3 to 0.4 ml per minute, about one-third the rate at which urine is formed. The fluid elaborated in the ventricles contains only 5 to 10 mg protein per 100 ml.

Histochemical and electron-microscope investigations indicate that the choroid epithelial cells have morphological features similar to those of other secretory cells. Formation of CSF within the ventricles has been deduced from the fact that, if the foramen is obstructed, fluid accumulates rapidly and the ventricle enlarges. From time to time, neurosurgeons have reported seeing drops of fluid form on the surfaces of the choroid plexus.

The formation of CSF by the choroid plexus has been studied more directly. Welch [46] has been able to cannulate the artery and vein of a single choroid plexus in the rabbit. By measuring the average differences of radioisotopes and of the hematocrit, he demonstrated that the formation of CSF and the movement of $^{24}Na^+$ are stopped when a carbonic anhydrase inhibitor is applied to the plexus. Thus, CSF is not simply a serum ultrafiltrate but is controlled by enzymatic processes. Ames and coworkers [47] were able to collect and analyze the fluid formed at the choroid plexus after filling the ventricle with oil. In the cat, they found that the concentration of electrolytes, particularly K^+, Ca^{2+}, and Mg^{2+}, differs from that of a plasma ultrafiltrate. However, the choroid plexus fluid was again found to change very slightly in its electrolytic concentration by the time it reached the cisterna magna.

The rate of formation of CSF has been measured by various means. One simple measurement, carried out more than 30 years ago by Masserman, was to determine the time for CSF replacement after a known amount had been drained. The rate in humans was 0.35 ml per minute. This measurement was criticized on the basis that the drainage altered the intracranial pressure relationships and, there-

Table 25-1. Typical Plasma and CSF Levels of Various Substances*

Substance	Plasma	CSF
Na^+	145.0	150.0
K^+	4.8	2.9
Ca^{2+}	5.2	2.3
Mg^{2+}	1.7	2.3
Cl^-	108.0	130.0
HCO_3^-	27.4	21.0
Lactate	7.9	2.6
PO_4^{3-}	1.8	0.5
Protein	7000.0	20.0
Glucose	95.0	60.0

*Protein and glucose concentrations are in mg/100 ml; all others are in mEq/liter.

fore, probably altered (increased) the rate of CSF formation. Recently, a sophisticated method of measuring CSF formation was introduced by Pappenheimer and coworkers [48, 49]. In this method, simulated spinal fluid is perfused between the ventricle and the cisterna magna, and inulin is added to the perfusion fluid. Because inulin diffuses very slowly into tissue during such a perfusion, the dilution of inulin is taken as a measure of the rate of formation of new spinal fluid. Therefore, if the perfusion at a rate of V_i ml per minute is carried out until a steady state is reached and if the initial concentration of inulin is C_i and the outflow concentration of inulin is C_o, the rate of formation of spinal fluid, V_f, is given by the equation:

$$V_f = V_i(C_i - C_o)/C_o \qquad \text{(eq. 25-3)}$$

Such perfusions have been carried out in a wide variety of species. Typical rates of spinal fluid formation are: rabbit, 0.001 ml per min; cat, 0.02 ml per min; rhesus monkey, 0.08 ml per min; and goat, 0.19 ml per min. Both Cutler and coworkers [50] and Rubin and coworkers [51] carried out measurements in patients undergoing ventriculocisternal perfusion with antitumor drugs and found an average value of 0.37 ml per minute. This corresponds rather closely to the value previously determined from drainage experiments.

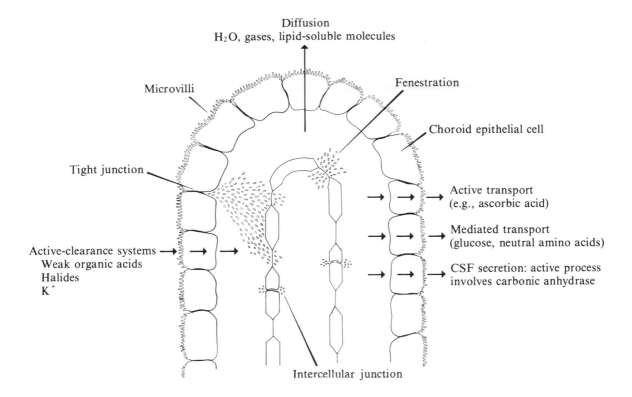

Fig. 25-2. Blood-CSF barrier. The blood-CSF barrier
consists mainly of the choroid plexus. These capillaries differ from those of the brain in that there is free
movement of molecules across the choroid plexus
capillary endothelial cell through fenestrations and
intercellular junctions. The barrier is at the choroid
plexus epithelial cells, which are joined with tight
junctions; there, microvilli may aid in secretion. Active
transport, mediated transport, and diffusion into CSF,
as well as active transport of metabolites from CSF to
blood, have been demonstrated in the choroid plexus.

By use of the ventriculocisternal perfusion
method, it has been found that CSF formation decreases slightly as intracranial pressure increases.
Moreover, CSF is formed at a normal rate and osmolality even when the fluid perfused through the
ventricle is moderately hypertonic or hypotonic.
However, when the perfused fluid is very hypotonic,
CSF formation may cease [52]. CSF formation is
also reduced if serum osmolality is raised.

The total volume of CSF is not precisely measurable. It is estimated to be 100 to 150 ml in normal
adults.

The circulation of CSF begins with the elaboration of fluid in the ventricles. It is aided by arterial
pulsations of the choroid plexuses. These pulsations are transmitted throughout the CSF and can
be seen on the manometer at the time of lumbar
spinal tap. The usual manometer, however, is filled
with spinal fluid, and this displacement of fluid
tends to dampen the pulsations. More prominent
pulsations are recorded if a strain gauge is used.

The fluid circulation is from the lateral ventricles
into the third ventricle and then into the fourth
ventricle. If obstructions are placed at the foramen
between these ventricles, the ventricle upstream
from the obstruction will enlarge significantly, producing obstructive hydrocephalus. Thus, if a
foramen of Monro is obstructed, the lateral ventricle will enlarge. If the aqueduct is obstructed,
both lateral ventricles and the third ventricle will

enlarge. The fluid passes from the fourth ventricle to the cisterna magna and then circulates into the cerebral and spinal subarachnoid spaces.

The CSF is removed at multiple sites. Among the important sites are cranial and spinal nerve root sheaths and the villi and granulations over the large venous sinuses in the skull. There is evidence that the villi act as valves, permitting the one-way flow of CSF from the subarachnoid spaces into sinuses. It has been suggested that some absorption of CSF may occur through pial vessels or by unidirectional pinocytotic activity in capillaries adjacent to the Virchow-Robin spaces at the cortical surface, but this has not been confirmed. Occasionally disease processes will affect these removal sites. For example, obliteration of the subarachnoid space after inflammatory processes or thrombosis of the sinuses will prevent the clearance of fluid. When this occurs, CSF pressure will increase, and hydrocephalus may develop without any obstruction in the ventricular foramina. This is called *communicating hydrocephalus.* Under such circumstances, some CSF absorption may take place across the ventricular ependyma; in addition, some CSF may circulate to the lumbar subarachnoid space through a dilated central canal [53].

Physiologically, absorption appears to be through a valvular mechanism. CSF absorption does not occur until CSF pressure exceeds the pressure within the sinuses. Once this threshold pressure has been reached, the rate of absorption is roughly proportional to the difference between CSF and sinus pressures. A normal human can absorb CSF at a rate up to four to six times the normal rate of CSF formation with only a moderate increase in intracranial pressure. This phenomenon has been used in the development of a constant infusion manometric test for estimation of CSF absorptive capacity [54]. The CSF spaces also show elasticity or distensibility; that is, the volume of the space changes in a nonlinear fashion with changes in CSF pressure.

Some drugs, including anesthetics and CO_2, increase CSF formation. Others, such as carbonic anhydrase inhibitors and norepinephrine, reduce the rate of CSF formation. A well-developed adrenergic and cholinergic nerve supply to the choroid plexus exists. The net effect of sympathetic-fiber stimulation is to reduce the bulk CSF production [44, 55].

Throughout the circulation of CSF, exchange of substances occurs between CSF and blood. This exchange appears to involve metabolic processes that serve to maintain the concentration of substances within the CSF at relatively fixed values.

SIMILARITY TO THE BLOOD-BRAIN BARRIER
The movement of substances from the blood into CSF is, in many ways, analogous to that from blood into brain, even though there are differences in the development of the choroid plexus and of the capillary system in the brain. There is free movement of such molecules as water, gases, and lipid-soluble substances from the blood into the CSF. Substances important for metabolism and maintenance of CSF electrolytes, such as glucose, amino acids, and cations (including K^+, Ca^{2+}, and Mg^{2+}), are transported by saturable carrier-mediated processes. Although it has been supposed that Cl^- content of CSF was determined by passive movement of this anion, it is now evident that a Cl^- pump may exist. The transport of Na^+ from blood into CSF is significantly reduced when carbonic anhydrase is inhibited. With Na^+, however, it has not been possible to demonstrate the phenomenon of saturability, because blood Na^+ cannot be elevated safely much above its usual concentrations. Finally, such macromolecules as proteins, and most hexoses other than glucose, are impermeable and do not enter the CSF.

ACTIVE TRANSPORT FROM CSF AND BRAIN
Active transport from CSF has been especially well studied because it is possible to manipulate the concentration gradient of substances between the CSF and the bloodstream. It has been shown that iodide and thiocyanate, transported from the CSF by saturable carrier mechanisms, can be inhibited competitively (for example, perchlorate inhibits iodide transfer) and must be active because the transport can be carried out against unfavorable electrochemical gradients. A special relationship

for choroid plexus in iodide clearance is proposed, based upon the very active accumulation of anions that occurs in choroid plexus in vitro. The combination of the bulk absorption of CSF and the active transport of molecules from it has been termed the *sink function* of the CSF. This implies that molecules reaching the extracellular fluid of the brain may diffuse into CSF and then be removed either by bulk absorption, by active transport, or by both mechanisms. It has been postulated that this will explain such phenomena as the low concentration of iodide in both brain and CSF, as compared with plasma concentrations. The possibility has now been established for iodide, however, that brain capillaries may transport the same substances out of the brain as the choroid plexus does out of the CSF.

Another important transport system is that involved in clearing weak organic acids out of the CSF. Among the molecules cleared by this mechanism are penicillin, diodrast, and such metabolites as HVA and 5HIAA. This clearance system also shows the phenomenon of saturability and transport against an unfavorable CSF-blood gradient. Probenecid is an effective inhibitor of this system. Again, the choroid plexus can accumulate these molecules in vitro, and there is some suggestive evidence that it plays a role in vivo. In addition, however, rapid clearance of 5HIAA by probenecid-sensitive transport mechanisms is shown in the cerebral subarachnoid space [24]. There is also evidence that amino acids are cleared from CSF to blood by analogous transport processes [56]. Excess K^+ is removed from CSF and brain by an oubain-sensitive system, presumably $(Na^+ + K^+)$-ATPase.

CSF-Brain Interface
The absence of tight junctions between some ependymal and pial cells permits diffusion of proteins and other hydrophilic molecules from the CSF into the brain, and vice versa. Frequently, the diffusional gradients near the interface are very steep, and many substances penetrate only superficially. Some recent evidence shows that the diffusion across the ependyma is slightly faster than that

across the pial-glial surface; however, molecules do move across both surfaces by diffusion.

Quantitative studies of the movement of substances between CSF and brain have led some investigators to postulate that the concentration of ions in extracellular fluid in brain is similar to that in CSF. Because the concentrations of K^+, Ca^{2+}, and Mg^{2+} in CSF are quite different from those in plasma, the verification of this postulate was considered to be of physiological significance. It has now been shown, using specific ion-exchange electrodes that can measure K^+ activity in brain extracellular space, that in fact this postulate was correct, that brain extracellular K is at a concentration of about 3 mM, similar to CSF and different from plasma concentration. Moreover, brain extracellular K is extremely stable, except under such severe experimental conditions as spreading depression or death (when it may rise to values as high as 80 mM) or sustained seizure activity (when it may rise to levels of about 10 to 12 mM). Only small shifts, usually less than 1 mM, are found as a result of local increases in cerebral activity, such as are produced by evoked cortical activity [57]. Thus, one of the functions of CSF, in addition to mechanical protection of the brain and its sink function, may be to provide a reservoir of extracellular fluid.

The CSF-brain interface may play a special role in the regulation of respiration. There is suggestive evidence that some respiratory neurons or their processes are located close enough to the ependymal surface to be responsive both to the HCO_3 level in the CSF and to capillary PCO_2.

Antibiotics
The movement of penicillin, perhaps the most important of the antibiotics, into the brain is controlled largely by the probenecid-sensitive organic-acid transport system in both the choroid plexus and brain capillaries. As a consequence, in the normal state, penicillin concentrations in the CSF are much lower than those in plasma. This is, in fact, of considerable benefit, because penicillin is toxic to cerebral tissue and may produce seizures at relatively low concentrations. During active

bacterial infections of the meninges of the brain, however, there are alterations in the blood-brain barrier, and the penicillin concentrations will increase at the site of inflammation. Similar mechanisms may control such compounds as ampicillin and penicillin G. The low concentration of cephalothin in the CSF might be due to a similar mechanism, but this has not been studied explicitly. However, it is known that the concentration of cephalothin does not increase reliably during infection and, therefore, it is not the optimum drug to use in patients with meningitis. The concentration of gentamicin in CSF is so low that, if this drug is required, it is often given intrathecally. In contrast, certain broad-spectrum antibiotics, such as chloramphenicol and tetracycline, are transported readily into the brain and, in fact, the concentration in brain tissue may be much higher than that in plasma.

References

*1. Katzman, R., and Pappius, H. M. *Brain Electrolytes and Fluid Metabolism*. Baltimore: Williams & Wilkins, 1973.

*2. Lajtha, A., and Ford, D. H. (eds.). *Brain Barrier Systems*. Amsterdam: Elsevier, 1968.

*3. Davson, H. *Physiology of the Cerebrospinal Fluid*. Boston: Little, Brown, 1967.

 4. Bradbury, M. W. B., and Stulcova, B. Efflux mechanism contributing to the stability of the potassium concentration in cerebrospinal fluid. *J. Physiol. (London)* 208:415–430, 1970.

 5. Reese, T. S., and Karnovsky, M. J. Fine structural localization of a blood-brain barrier to exogenous peroxidase. *J. Cell Biol.* 34:207–217, 1967.

 6. Reese, T. S., Feder, N., and Brightman, M. W. Electron microscopic study of the blood-brain and blood-cerebrospinal fluid barriers with microperoxidase. *J. Neuropathol. Exp. Neurol.* 30:137–138, 1971.

 7. Oldendorf, W. H., Cornford, M. E., and Brown, W. J. The large apparent work capability of the blood-brain barrier: A study of the mitochondrial content of capillary endothelial cells in brain and other tissues of the rat. *Ann. Neurol.* 1:409–417, 1977.

 8. Raichle, M. E., Eichling, J. O., and Grubb, R. L. Brain permeability of water. *Arch. Neurol.* 30:319–321, 1974.

*Key reference.

 9. Katzman, R., Schimmel, H., and Wilson, C. E. Diffusion of inulin as a measure of extracellular fluid space in brain. *Proc. Rudolph Virchow Med. Soc. N.Y.* 26:254–280, 1968.

10. Crone, C. The permeability of brain capillaries to non-electrolytes. *Acta Physiol. Scand.* 64:407–417, 1965.

11. Pardridge, W. M., and Connor, J. D. Saturable transport of amphetamine across the blood-brain barrier. *Experientia* 29:302–304, 1972.

12. Oldendorf, W. H. Brain uptake of radiolabeled amino acids, amines, and hexoses after arterial injection. *Am. J. Physiol.* 221:1629–1639, 1971.

13. Pardridge, W. M., and Oldendorf, W. H. Transport of metabolic substrates through the blood-brain barrier. *J. Neurochem.* 28:5–12, 1977.

14. Nemoto, E. M., and Sveringhaus, J. W. Stereospecificity permeability of rat blood-brain barrier to lactic acid. *Stroke* 5:81–84, 1974.

15. Oldendorf, W. H. Carrier mediated blood-brain transport of short-chain monocarboxylic organic acids. *Am. J. Physiol.* 224:1450–1453, 1973.

16. Christensen, H. N. Nature and Roles of Receptor Sites for Amino Acid Transport. In M. S. Ebadi and E. Costa (eds.), *Advances in Biochemical Psychopharmacology*. New York: Raven, 1972. Vol. 4, pp. 39–62.

17. Wade, L. A., and Katzman, R. Rat brain regional uptake and decarboxylation of L-DOPA following carotid injection. *Am. J. Physiol.* 228:352–358, 1975.

18. Yudilevich, D. L., De Rose, N., and Sepulveda, F. V. Facilitated transport of amino acids through the blood-brain barrier of the dog studied in a single capillary circulation. *Brain Res.* 44:569–578, 1972.

19. Millington, W. R., McCall, A. L., and Wurtman, R. J. Deanol acetamidobenzoate inhibits the blood-brain barrier transport of choline. *Ann. Neurol.* 4:302–306, 1978.

20. Cornford, E. M., Braun, L. D., and Oldendorf, W. H. Carrier mediated blood-brain barrier transport of choline and certain choline analogs. *J. Neurochem.* 30:299–308, 1978.

21. Chiueh, C. C., Sun, C. L., Kopin, I. J., Fredericks, W. R., and Rapoport, S. I. Entry of (^{3}H)norepinephrine, (^{125}I)albumin and Evans blue from blood into brain following unilateral osmotic opening of the blood-brain barrier. *Brain Res.* 145:291–301, 1978.

22. Sun, C. L., Chiueh, C. C., Kopin, I. J., Fredericks, W. R., and Rapoport, S. I. Entry of (^{3}H)norepinephrine and (^{125}I)albumin from blood into brain following osmotic opening of blood-brain barrier in the rat. *Abstracts 6th Ann. Meeting Neurosci. Soc.* 2:731, 1976.

23. Davson, H., Domer, F. R., and Hollingsworth, J. R. The mechanism of drainage of the cerebrospinal fluid. *Brain* 96:329–331, 1973.

24. Wolfson, L. I., Katzman, R., and Escriva, A. Clearance of amine metabolites from the cerebrospinal fluid: The brain as a "sink." *Neurology* 24:772–779, 1974.

25. Goldstein, G. W. Relation of potassium transport to oxidative metabolism in isolated brain capillaries. *J. Physiol. (London)* 286:185–195, 1979.

26. Wahlstrom, G. Increased penetration of barbital through the bloodbrain barrier in the rat after pretreatment with probenecid. *Acta Pharmacol. Toxicol. (Copenhagen)* 43:260–265, 1978.

27. Bito, L. Z., and Wallenstein, M. C. Transport of prostaglandins across the blood-brain and blood-aqueous barriers and the physiological significance of these absorptive transport processes. *Exp. Eye Res.* (Suppl.) 25:229–243, 1977.

28. Owman, C., and Rosengren, E. Dopamine formation in brain capillaries—an enzymatic blood-brain barrier mechanism. *J. Neurochem.* 14:547–550, 1967.

29. Orlowski, M., Sessa, G., and Green, J. P. γ-Glutamyl transpeptidase in brain capillaries: Possible site of a blood-brain barrier for amino acids. *Science* 184:66–68, 1974.

30. Mrsulja, B. B., Mrsulja, B. J., Fujimoto, T., Klatzo, I., and Spatz, M. Isolation of brain capillaries: A simplified technique. *Brain Res.* 110:361–365, 1976.

31. Hjelle, J. T., Baird-Lambert, J., Cardinale, G., Spectorm, S. M., and Udenfriend, S. Isolated microvessels: The blood-brain barrier in vitro. *Proc. Natl. Acad. Sci. U.S.A.* 75:4544–4548, 1978.

32. Goldstein, G. W., Wolinsky, J. S., Csejtey, J., and Diamond, I. Isolation of metabolically active capillaries from rat brain. *J. Neurochem.* 25:715–717, 1975.

33. Hansen, A. J., Lund-Andersen, H., and Crone, C. K^+-permeability of the blood-brain barrier, investigated by aid of a K^--sensitive microelectrode. *Acta Physiol. Scand.* 101:438–445, 1977.

34. Betz, A. L., and Goldstein, G. W. Polarity of the blood-brain barrier: Neutral amino acid transport into isolated brain capillaries. *Science* 202:225–227, 1978.

35. Betz, A. L., Firth, J. A., and Goldstein, G. W. Polarity of the blood-brain barrier: Distribution of enzymes between the luminal and antiluminal membranes of brain capillary endothelial cells. *Brain Res.* 192:17–28, 1980.

36. Betz, A. L., Csejtey, J., and Goldstein, G. W. Hexose transport and phosphorylation by capillaries isolated from rat brain. *Am. J. Physiol.* 236:96–102, 1979.

37. Saunders, N. R. Ontogeny of the blood-brain barrier. *Exp. Eye Res.* (Suppl.) 25:523–550, 1977.

38. Mayer, S., Maickel, R. P., and Brodie, B. B. Kinetics of penetration of drugs and other foreign compounds into cerebrospinal fluid and brain. *J. Pharmacol. Exp. Ther.* 127:205–211, 1959.

39. Rapoport, S. I., Hori, M., and Klatzo, I. Testing of a hypothesis for osmotic opening of the blood-brain barrier. *Am. J. Physiol.* 223:323–331, 1972.

40. Brightman, M. W., Hori, M., Rapoport, S. I., Reese, T. S., and Westergaard, E. Osmotic opening of tight junctions in cerebral endothelium. *J. Comp. Neurol.* 152:317–326, 1973.

41. Sterrett, P. R., Thompson, A. M., Chapman, A. L., and Matzke, H. A. The effects of hyperosmolarity on the blood-brain barrier. A morphological and physiological correlation. *Brain Res.* 77:281–295, 1974.

42. Spatz, M., Rap, Z. M., Rapoport, S. I., and Klatzo, I. The Effects of Hypertonic Urea on the Blood-Brain Barrier and on the Glucose Transport in the Brain. In H. J. Reulen and K. Schürmann (eds.), *Steroids and Brain Edema*. Proceedings of an International Workshop. New York: Springer-Verlag, 1972.

43. Hardebo, J. E., Edvinsson, L., Mackenzie, E. T., and Owman, Ch. Regional brain uptake of noradrenaline following mechanical or osmotic opening of the blood-brain barrier. *Acta Physiol. Scand.* 101:342–350, 1977.

44. Hardebo, J. E., Edvinsson, L., and Owman, Ch. Influence of the cerebrovascular sympathetic innervation on blood-brain barrier function. *Acta Physiol. Scand.* 452:65–68, 1977.

45. Westergaard, E., and Brightman, M. W. Transport of proteins across normal cerebral arterioles. *J. Comp. Neurol.* 152:17–44, 1973.

46. Welch, K. Secretion of cerebrospinal fluid by choroid plexus of the rabbit. *Am. J. Physiol.* 205:617–624, 1963.

47. Ames, A., Sakanoue, M., and Endo, S. Na, K, Ca, Mg, and Cl concentrations in choroid plexus of fluid and cisternal fluid compared with plasma ultrafiltrate. *J. Neurophysiol.* 27:672–681, 1964.

48. Pappenheimer, J. R., Heisey, S. R., and Jordan, E. F. Active transport of diodrast and phenolsulfonphthalein from cerebrospinal fluid to blood. *Am. J. Physiol.* 200:1–10, 1961.

49. Heisey, S. R., Held, D., and Pappenheimer, J. R. Bulk flow and diffusion in the cerebrospinal fluid system of the goat. *Am. J. Physiol.* 203:775–781, 1962.

50. Cutler, R. W. P., Page, I., Galicich, J., and Watters, G. V. Formation and absorption of cerebrospinal fluid in man. *Brain* 91:707–720, 1968.

51. Rubin, R. C., Henderson, E. S., Ommaya, A. K., Walker, M. D., and Rall, D. P. The production of cerebrospinal fluid in man and its modification by acetazolamide. *J. Neurosurg.* 25:430–436, 1966.

52. Hochwald, G. M., Wald, A., DiMattio, J., and Malhan, C. The effects of serum osmolarity on cerebrospinal fluid volume flow. *Life Sci.* 15:1309–1319, 1975.

53. Eisenberg, H. M., McLennan, J. E., and Welch, K. Ventricular perfusion in cats with kaolin-induced hydrocephalus. *J. Neurosurg.* 41:20–28, 1974.

54. Katzman, R., and Hussey, F. A simple constant-infusion manometric test for measurement of CSF absorption. 1. Rationale and method. *Neurology* 20:534–544, 1970.

55. Lindvall, M., Edvinsson, L., and Owman, Ch. Histochemical, ultrastructural and functional evidence for a neurogenic control of cerebrospinal fluid production from the choroid plexus. *Acta Physiol. Scand.* (Suppl.) 452:77–86, 1977.

56. Lorenzo, A. V. Amino acid transport mechanisms of the cerebrospinal fluid. *Fed. Proc.* 33:2079, 1974.

57. Katzman, R., and Grossman, R. Neuronal Activity and Potassium Movement. In D. H. Ingvar and N. A. Lassen (eds.), *Brain Work*. Alfred Benzon Symposium VIII. Copenhagen: Munksgaard, 1975. Pp. 149–166.

Part Two. Medical Neurochemistry

Stanton B. Elias
Stanley H. Appel

Chapter 26. Biochemistry of the Myoneural Junction and of Its Disorders

Investigation of neuromuscular transmission has relied heavily on electrophysiological techniques. These have elucidated many properties at the molecular level. The role of calcium in fusion of synaptic vesicles with the nerve terminal plasmalemma; the timing of occupancy of acetylcholine (ACh) receptors; and elementary conductance changes in the postsynaptic membrane have been well described (see Chaps. 5 and 8). The electrophysiological descriptions of the effects of naturally occurring toxins on neuromuscular transmission and the transmission defects in human diseases of neuromuscular transmission have provided a basis for biochemical investigations of normal and pathological functions of the neuromuscular junction. The clearest example has been the use of α-bungarotoxin and α-cobratoxin, which are specific ligands for the nicotinic ACh receptor. These polypeptide toxins have been important tools for the biochemical definition and purification of the ACh receptor. This has had additional importance in the investigation of myasthenia gravis, in which there is a deficiency of ACh receptors at neuromuscular junctions.

This chapter is concerned with the molecular basis of function and dysfunction of neuromuscular junctions and will emphasize toxins that affect certain aspects of neuromuscular transmission (Table 26-1).

Presynaptic Mechanisms

A number of toxins can produce effects on acetylcholine storage and release, and at least one human disorder is manifest by impaired ACh release. Because of their wide range of action, these toxins provide valuable tools for the study of presynaptic mechanisms of ACh storage and release, as well as for the analysis of nerve and muscle trophic interactions.

BOTULINUM TOXIN

Botulinum toxin is a polypeptide neurotoxin with a molecular weight of approximately 150,000. Its subunit structure is not known. The toxin inhibits the release of ACh from cholinergic nerve terminals. This produces marked reductions in frequency and amplitude of miniature end-plate potentials (MEPPs) and end-plate potentials (EPPs), but does not affect postsynaptic ACh sensitivity. In vivo, the actions of botulinum toxin primarily involve neuromuscular junctions and autonomic ganglia, with negligible changes in the central nervous system. The lack of a central effect probably is related to the inability of botulinum toxin to cross the blood-brain barrier.

Botulinum toxin appears to act on the neuromuscular junction in two steps. The first is rapid, temperature-insensitive, and essentially irreversible. Exposure of a neuromuscular junction to botulinum toxin for as little as two minutes, even if followed by extensive washing, will result in paralysis of neuromuscular transmission. This is likely to be a function of the toxin's binding to the presynaptic membrane. The minimum lethal dose of botulinum toxin in the mouse is 1 times 10^{-12} g, or less than 10^8 molecules, so it has been estimated that only 10 molecules of toxin are necessary to block a cholinergic synapse [1]. This necessitates the presence of an extremely specific, high-affinity binding site on the presynaptic membrane. The second step takes place 2 to 3 hours after exposure. Both MEPP frequency and amplitude decline, resulting in a progressive neuromuscular blockade.

Table 26-1. Toxins That Affect Neuromuscular Transmission

	Functional Alteration	Physiological Correlate	Morphological Correlate	Proposed Mechanism
PRESYNAPTIC				
Botulinum toxin	Inhibition of ACh release	Decreased MEPP frequency and amplitude [1]	No alteration in the ultrastructure of the nerve terminal [8]	Binding to a high-affinity presynaptic site Altered sensitivity of ACh release mechanism to calcium ions [5]
β-Bungarotoxin	Initial increase ACh release with subsequent decreased release	Increased MEPP frequency followed by decreased MEPP frequency	May produce destruction of nerve terminal plasma membrane [15]	Binding to a high affinity presynaptic site [13] Phospholipase A activity may produce increased ACh release [25] Inhibition of vesicle fusion with presynaptic membrane and ACh release [8] Activity is calcium sensitive
Black widow spider venom	Massive increase in ACh release followed by cessation of release	Initial increase in MEPP frequency to 300–1,000/sec [18]. Subsequent decline in MEPP frequency to zero	Swollen nerve terminals, devoid of synaptic vesicles [19]. Increase in presumed ACh release sites in freeze-fracture preparations [7]	Binding to high-affinity presynaptic site Formation of cation-selective channels in nerve terminals stimulating transmitter release [20] Inhibition of synaptic vesicle membrane recycling
The myasthenic syndrome (Lambert-Eaton)	Inhibition of ACh release	Decreased quantal contents of EPP, increased by high-frequency stimulation [23]	Presynaptic normal. Increased postsynaptic membrane density (length/area) [22]	Decreased sensitivity of ACh-release mechanism to calcium ion [22] Possible humeral factor from tumors associated with the syndrome [25]
POSTSYNAPTIC				
α-Bungarotoxin	"Irreversible" blockade of ACh receptors	Decreased MEPP and EPP amplitude	No morphological changes	Binding to cholinoceptive site. Irreversibility related to hydrophobic amino acid residues
α-Cobratoxin	"Reversible" blockade of ACh receptors	Decreased MEPP and EPP amplitude	No morphological changes	Binding to cholinoceptive site on ACh receptor

Table 26-1 (Continued)

	Functional Alteration	Physiological Correlate	Morphological Correlate	Proposed Mechanism
Myasthenia gravis	Decreased number of ACh receptors	Decreased MEPP amplitude [32] Decreased sensitivity of motor end-plate to ACh [32]	Decreased post-synaptic membrane density [22] IgG and C_3 bound to motor end-plate and fragments of destroyed junctional folds [42]	Decreased number of ACh receptors in motor end-plate [33] Antibodies against ACh receptor [36] produce this deficiency by (1) membrane lysis [42] and (2) altered ACh-receptor turnover [43-47]
ACETYLCHOLINE DEACTIVATION Acetylcholinesterase deficiency [63]		Decreased MEPP frequency and normal MEPP amplitude. Decreased quantal content of EPP that does not increase with high-frequency stimulation	Decreased size of nerve terminals Postsynaptic-decreased membrane density	Lack of demonstrable 16S ChE at motor end-plate
Acetylcholinesterase inhibition		MEPP frequency and amplitude initially increased but later decreased ACh sensitivity of end-plates decreases with chronic inhibition [60]	Grouped muscle-fiber necrosis [57] Decreased post-synaptic membrane density [58]	Decreased ACh receptors in motor end-plate [60] May reflect down-regulation of receptor synthesis by agonist [62]

Burger and coworkers [2] demonstrated that botulinum toxin prevents release of ACh from nerve terminals of isolated phrenic nerve–diaphragm preparations. When rat phrenic nerve–diaphragm preparations are exposed to botulinum toxin, there is a latent period of 30 to 40 minutes, during which no alterations of neuromuscular transmission are seen. During the next 30 to 40 minutes of exposure, the response to nerve stimulation declines and disappears. If the phrenic nerve is stimulated during toxin exposure, mean paralysis time decreases in proportion to the rate of stimulation. Pharma-cological stimulation of ACh activity also decreases paralysis time. These studies suggest that the rate at which paralysis is produced is a function both of the rate of binding of botulinum toxin and, to some extent, of the rate of ACh turnover in the neuromuscular junction [3].

The first detectable alteration in neuromuscular transmission produced by botulinum toxin is decreased amplitude of MEPPs [1]. However, in nerve terminals incompletely blocked, increasing the calcium ion concentration in the bathing solution reverses some of the effects of the toxin [4].

Neurally evoked EPPs recorded from motor end-plates of poisoned animals are small, consisting of single or few quanta. At a calcium concentration of 2 mM, approximately 95 percent of nerve impulses fail to release transmitter. Reducing calcium concentration below this level results in an increased number of transmission failures. Increasing calcium concentration produces EPPs of greater amplitude and reduces the number of transmission failures. Calcium dependence of botulinum-poisoned synapses, however, differs in two respects from that of normal synapses [5]: (1) the extracellular calcium requirement for maintaining any level of ACh release is much higher in botulinum-poisoned synapses than in normal synapses; (2) the power relationship for calcium dependence of transmitter release in poisoned terminals is much greater in normals (2.8 ± 0.15 versus 1.3 ± 0.18).

Botulinum-treated nerve terminals also are less sensitive to intracellular calcium concentration. Exposure to potassium-free medium, ouabain, or calcium ionophore, A23187, can cause elevations of intracellular calcium concentration. These treatments cause marked elevations of the spontaneous MEPPs recorded in normal neuromuscular junction, but no increase in those treated with botulinum toxin [5]. In calcium-free media, normal nerve terminals respond to ionophore after 15 to 60 minutes to produce MEPP levels greater than 200 per minute. This is presumably due to release of calcium from intracellular storage sites. Toxin-treated junctions do not respond to ionophore in calcium-free medium, but increasing the calcium concentration to 10 mM produces increased MEPP frequency and amplitude. Thus botulinum toxin alters the calcium sensitivity of the transmitter mobilization apparatus, as (a) transmitter release can be induced under extreme conditions, (b) greater than normal concentrations of calcium are required to stimulate transmitter release, and (c) the power relationship between calcium dependency and transmitter release is altered (Fig. 26-1).

The conclusion that botulinum toxin impairs calcium-mediated transmitter release is also supported by studies of the interaction of botulinum toxin with other toxins. Batrachotoxin evokes

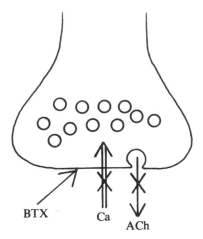

Fig. 26-1. Botulinum toxin (BTX) binds to the nerve-terminal membrane and blocks the calcium-stimulated release of acetylcholine (ACh).

ACh release from motor nerve terminals, and requires calcium ion to be effective. Batrachotoxin produces no effect in botulinum-poisoned terminals [6]. In contrast, the action of the venom of the black widow spider, Latrodectus mactans, is not calcium dependent. Accordingly this venom induces ACh release from nerve terminals pretreated with botulinum toxin, although the release pattern is modified. Freeze-fracture analysis of presynaptic terminal membranes demonstrates spider venom-induced alterations in the sites of transmitter release even when botulinum toxin is present [7]. It appears that botulinum toxin produces neuromuscular blockade through its effects on a calcium-dependent apparatus in the presynaptic membrane that controls fusion and exocytosis of synaptic vesicles. This effect occurs at a time after toxin binds to the nerve terminal and the rate of onset is accelerated by nerve activity. Its major effect appears to be an antagonism of calcium stimulation. Botulinum toxin produces no alterations in the ultrastructure of the presynaptic terminals or in the size and distribution of synaptic vesicles [8].

β-BUNGAROTOXIN

β-Bungarotoxin is a polypeptide with a molecular weight of 21,800. It consists of two subunits;

12,400 M_r and 8,800 M_r. It can be purified from the crude venom of *Bungarus multicinctus* by ion exchange chromatography over CM-Sephadex and CM-cellulose. Although similar neuromuscular blocking activity may be present in a number of peaks from CM-Sephadex chromatography, peak 5 is referred to as β-bungarotoxin [9].

The effect of β-bungarotoxin on neuromuscular transmission is localized to the presynaptic terminal. In rat diaphragm, β-bungarotoxin does not alter the muscle's resting-membrane potential, the contractile response of muscle to direct stimulation or exogenous ACh [10], or the amplitude of nerve action potentials. Total ACh content of hemidiaphragm preparations is also unaltered by β-bungarotoxin.

β-Bungarotoxin activity at nerve terminals occurs in three steps: (1) binding toxin to presynaptic terminal, which occurs within 20 minutes and is not reversible by washing; (2) increased frequency of MEPPs, two to three times normal; and (3) gradual reduction and disappearance of MEPPs. The time required for total paralysis of the nerve-muscle preparation is 4 hours, without nerve stimulation. When the nerve is stimulated, paralysis occurs more rapidly. This pattern of initially increased transmitter release and subsequent blockade of release has been interpreted as an alteration in the parameters that determine the probability of ACh quanta release. The initially increased transmitter release is due to the increased probability of vesicles' fusing with the presynaptic membrane; the

subsequent decreased transmitter release is due to reduced probability of such fusion [8] (Fig. 26-2).

The mechanism through which β-bungarotoxin alters ACh release is unknown. One possibility is the potent phospholipase A_2 activity that this toxin possesses [8]. Highly purified β-bungarotoxin (as monitored by SDS-polyacrylamide electrophoresis, isoelectric focusing, and ion exchange chromatography) catalyzes the hydrolysis of phosphatidylcholine. The phospholipase A_2 activity of β-bungarotoxin raises two questions: (1) Is the phospholipase activity necessary for the neurotoxic effects of the toxin? (2) How does β-bungarotoxin differ from other snake venom phospholipases, such as that of *Vipera russellii*, that do not have neurotoxic activity?

There are two methods by which the phospholipase activity of β-bungarotoxin can be activated. (1) β-Bungarotoxin is calcium-dependent. When strontium is substituted for calcium in bathing solutions, the phospholipase is inactivated [8]. (2) Chemical modification of the toxin can inhibit the phospholipase activity alone, neurotoxic activity alone, or both [11, 12]. This suggests that the phospholipase activity of β-bungarotoxin is neither necessary nor sufficient to produce neurotoxicity. However, the initial increase in transmitter release after exposure to β-bungarotoxin may be a function of the phospholipase activity of the toxin.

The neurotoxic effects of β-bungarotoxin are probably due to the presence of a site on the presynaptic membrane that binds the toxin with a high affinity and high specificity. The affinity of β-bungarotoxin for such a site accounts for its neurotoxic effects and the lack of toxicity of other snake-venom phospholipases. A high-affinity binding site for β-bungarotoxin has been demonstrated in brain tissue [13]. However, presynaptic localization of such binding sites has not been demonstrated in brain or muscle. The ability of β-bungarotoxin to inhibit the action of botulinum toxin in nerve-muscle preparations has been demonstrated [14] and may be due to competition for a particular binding site.

The ultimate mechanism by which β-bungarotoxin produces neuromuscular blockade is unknown. Marked destruction of plasma membranes

Fig. 26-2. β-Bungarotoxin produces alterations in neuromuscular transmission in two steps: (A) binding of β-bungarotoxin (β-BUTX) to the presynaptic nerve terminal is associated with release of ACh. and (B) the calcium-stimulated release mechanism for β-BUTX is blocked.

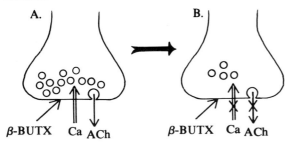

of frog nerve terminals produced by β-bungaro-toxin has been reported [15]. It has been hypothesized that the fatty acids liberated by the phospholipase activity of β-bungarotoxin inhibit oxidative phosphorylation in nerve terminals. Initially, this energy depletion could cause depolarization of the nerve terminal and transmitter release. A late effect of energy depletion would be paralysis of transmitter release [16]. Such a hypothesis has not been confirmed. The inhibitory effects of β-bungarotoxin on the effects of botulinum toxin suggest that these two may have a common site of action that may be important in initiating ACh release.

BLACK WIDOW SPIDER VENOM

Black widow spider venom (BWSV) is another neurotoxin that acts presynaptically. The toxic component of BWSV active at the neuromuscular junction has been characterized as a protein with a molecular weight of approximately 130,000. SDS-PAGE of partially purified BWSV reveals two closely related bands, and isoelectric focusing yields four protein bands. All four are immunologically cross-reactive. Purified venom has no identified enzyme activity and no detectable carbohydrate residues [17].

The effects of BWSV on neuromuscular-junction physiology and morphology are different from those produced by botulinum toxin or β-bungarotoxin. Addition of BWSV to nerve-muscle preparations is followed by a lag period of several minutes during which no alterations of neuromuscular transmission are recorded. The effects of BWSV cannot be reversed by washing. The initial effect is a marked rise in the frequency of spontaneous MEPPs to peak values of 300 to 1,000 per second. MEPP frequency then declines, with an exponential decay to negligible levels in 5 minutes. Evoked EPP amplitude initially is increased during the phase of increased MEPPs, but during the later phase EPPs can no longer be evoked. The effects of BWSV are not sensitive to calcium or magnesium [18].

The physiological effects of BWSV are correlated with marked morphological alterations of the presynaptic nerve terminal. Nerve terminals are

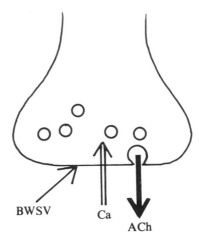

Fig. 26-3. Black widow spider venom (BWSV) binds to nerve-terminal membranes and promotes calcium entry and acetylcholine (ACh) release, thereby depleting the terminal of neurotransmitter and leading to transmission failure.

swollen and contain no synaptic vesicles, although other presynaptic organelles are preserved [18, 19]. Freeze-fracture analysis of presynaptic nerve terminals reveals that BWSV markedly increases the number and concentration of large, intramembraneous particles that are thought to represent sites of vesicle fusion to the presynaptic plasma membrane [17]. In normal nerve terminals, the distribution of such particles is restricted. After treatment with BWSV, these particles are seen over the entire surface of the presynaptic plasma membrane.

The mechanism of action of BWSV has been clarified by a study of its effects on lipid bilayer membranes. BWSV has been demonstrated to interact irreversibly with an artificial membrane to form cation-selective channels [20]. The addition of the venom to the membrane increases conductance in a stepwise fashion over 2 hours. The magnitude of these stepwise increases in conductance (3.6×10^{-10} mho) suggests that BWSV forms discrete channels in the membrane, rather than serving as a cation carrier. Toxin-treated membranes are selective for cations but do not discriminate between sodium and potassium. They are also substantially permeable to calcium (Fig. 26-3).

The biological activity of BWSV can be explained either as the result of formation of cation channels or as a direct consequence of the interaction of the venom with membranes. In the presence of calcium, BWSV could permit entry of extracellular calcium into the nerve terminal, stimulating the release of transmitter. In the absence of calcium, sodium, or potassium, entry could cause the release of calcium from intracellular pools. A second action of toxin may directly alter the distribution of membrane components by affecting the microtubules and microfilaments. This interaction with the membrane cytoskeleton could inhibit recovery of synaptic vesicles from the axolemma. These effects offer the potential for significant clarification of the role of calcium in normal vesicle fusion and membrane recycling.

THE MYASTHENIC SYNDROME (LAMBERT-EATON SYNDROME)

The myasthenic syndrome is a rare disorder of neuromuscular transmission that is sometimes associated with bronchial or oat-cell carcinoma. Approximately 70% of patients with the myasthenic syndrome have carcinoma. The patients experience weakness and fatigability of proximal limb muscles, characterized by a delay in development of maximal strength with voluntary contraction, rather than the loss of strength with exertion that is seen in patients with myasthenia gravis. The diagnostic hallmark of the myasthenic syndrome is a decreased response of muscle to single supramaximal nerve stimulation, but an increased response in muscle to supramaximal nerve stimulation at rates greater than 10 Hz [21].

The site of altered neuromuscular transmission in the myasthenic syndrome is the presynaptic terminal. Postsynaptic structures do not appear to be pathologically altered. Histometric analysis of motor end plates of muscle from patients with the myasthenic syndrome have increased membrane density (length of membrane per area of membrane) with well developed synaptic folds and clefts [22]. The only consistent morphological abnormality seen presynaptically is decreased mean mitochondrial area [22]. Electrophysiological measurements reveal no postsynaptic changes. The major physiological deficit is presynaptic. MEPP frequency is significantly increased (0.28/sec for myasthenic syndrome, versus 0.19/sec in normals). EPP quantum content (1/sec stimulaton) is significantly decreased (9 in myasthenic syndrome; 60 in normals) [23]. Repetitive stimulation at 40 per second produces a significant increase in quantal content of MEPPs. In brief, the defect in the myasthenic syndrome is characterized by decreased release of ACh after a single nerve impulse and may be overcome with repetitive stimulation.

The etiology of the defect in ACh release in the myasthenic syndrome is unknown. Nerve terminals from patients with the myasthenic syndrome do not release ACh in appropriate amounts when depolarized by stimulation or by raising the external potassium concentration to 20 mM. Normal human intercostal muscle shows a 100-fold increase in MEPP frequency when bathed in solutions with 20 mM K$^+$; however, myasthenic syndrome muscle demonstrates only a fourfold increase. Nerve terminals from such patients also demonstrate altered responses to calcium and magnesium. This decreased sensitivity to calcium is reminiscent of the effects of botulinum toxin. Neither respond to elevated external potassium concentrations. However, MEPP amplitudes in botulinum-poisoned junctions are reduced in amplitude, and the distribution of amplitude is skewed toward smaller depolarization potentials. MEPP amplitudes are not reduced in the myasthenic syndrome (Fig. 26-4).

Guanidine hydrochloride has a therapeutic effect in both myasthenic syndrome and botulinum poisoning. Its effect on neuromuscular transmission is to increase the average number of quanta released by presynaptic depolarizations, increasing the quantal content of the EPP measured postsynaptically. It has been hypothesized that guanidine hydrochloride serves as a monovalent cation that is capable of reducing negative charges in membrane. This effect may alter the conductance of calcium channels in the presynaptic membrane in such a way that greater influx of calcium is permitted [24].

The occurrence of the myasthenic syndrome in patients with bronchial carcinoma suggests that such tumors secrete a substance that interferes with neuromuscular transmission.

It has been reported that extracts of tumor tissue from a patient with the myasthenic syndrome are toxic to neuromuscular transmission. Quantal content of EPPs recorded from muscle bathed in tumor extract was 50 percent less than that of control muscles [25]. Clearly, further data are required to confirm these results and to identify this factor.

Postsynaptic Mechanisms

ALPHA-NEUROTOXIN

The discovery that polypeptides from a number of snake venoms possess a specific affinity for nicotinic ACh receptors has revolutionized biochemical approaches to the neuromuscular junction and, more specifically, to postsynaptic receptors. Chang and Lee first reported that α-bungarotoxin binds specifically to the nicotinic ACh receptor. Since that initial report, numerous studies have confirmed the usefulness of α-bungarotoxin and α-cobratoxin as markers for ACh receptors. Lee [26] has recently reviewed the relationship between the structure and function of those polypeptide neurotoxins. Their availability has permitted purification and characterization of mammalian ACh receptors (Table 26-2).

The cobra and sea-snake neurotoxins that bind to ACh receptors consist either of a single polypeptide composed of 61 to 62 amino acid residues cross-linked by four disulfide bridges or of polypeptides with approximately 71 amino acid residues cross-linked by five disulfide bridges. The toxins *Naja naja naja,* and *N. naja simiensis,* commonly used in ACh receptor research, belong to the second category. The primary neurotoxins in the venom of *B. multicinctus,* α-bungarotoxin, are composed of 74 amino acid residues in a single chain, cross-linked by five disulfide bridges. The structures of α-bungarotoxin and type II cobratoxin are markedly similar, with the disulfide bridges occupying the same position in both. Reduction of the disulfide bonds of either results in the loss of toxicity. Certain amino acid residues occupy

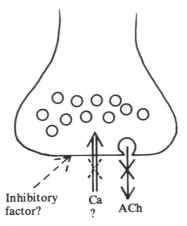

Fig. 26-4. Acetylcholine release is decreased in the myasthenic syndrome, possibly due to the presence of an inhibitory factor which binds to the presynaptic terminal. This effect is reversible by repetitive nerve stimulation or guanidine hydrochloride.

the same position in all the neurotoxins that bind to ACh receptors. These include a tyrosine residue at position 25, lysine at 27, tryptophan at 29, and arginine at 33. It has been suggested that this region is the active site that binds to ACh receptors.

The neuromuscular blockade produced by the α-neurotoxins is a nondepolarizing blockade of postsynaptic ACh sensitivity. Spontaneous MEPPs, evoked EPPs, and sensitivity to exogenous

Table 26-2. Properties of Mammalian ACh Receptor

	Mouse	
Number of receptors per end-plate	87×10^6 [64]	
Receptor density per end-plate	8,500 sites/μm^2 [65]	
Receptor density per crest	20,000 sites/μm^2 [66]	
Receptor density per cultured myotubes	900/μm^2 [67]	
Receptor sedimentation	$9S_{20,\ w}$	
	Rat [68]	*Cat* [69]
Subunit molecular weights	45,000 51,000 (minor 49,000; 56,000; 62,000)	41,000 (minor 58,000; 68,000)

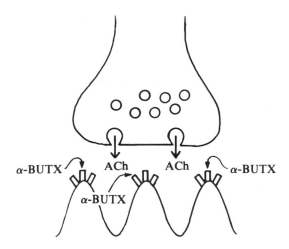

Fig. 26-5. α-Bungarotoxin (α-BUTX) binds to the acetylcholine sites of acetylcholine receptors in the motor end-plates, thereby blocking acetylcholine (ACh) interactions with the receptors.

ACh all are blocked. Presynaptic depolarization and passive membrane properties of muscle are not altered by α-bungarotoxin. α-Bungarotoxin has been reported to enhance transmitter released at the neuromuscular junction after nerve stimulation [27]. The mechanism of this presynaptic effect is unknown.

Binding of α-bungarotoxin to ACh receptors is slowly reversible; binding of cobratoxins is more rapidly reversible because of a more rapid dissociation of toxin-receptor complexes, rather than a more rapid association of toxin with the receptors. These differences are assumed to reflect the differing amino acid compositions of these venoms: α-bungarotoxin has the larger number of hydrophobic amino acids, alanine, and arginine; the reversible type I cobratoxins have fewer hydrophic residues and a greater number of glutamic acid residues; type II cobratoxins have more hydrophobic residues and bind more tightly than do type I venoms (Fig. 26-5).

The relative irreversibility of α-bungarotoxin binding to ACh receptors and the ease of labeling the toxin molecule with radioactive isotopes have made this toxin ideal for the localization of ACh receptors in situ and for the characterization of receptor solubilized from tissue homogenates. The stability of this bond has also enabled researchers to monitor the turnover of ACh receptors in both tissue [28] and organ cultures [29]. The rapid reversibility of cobratoxin binding to ACh receptors has been useful for affinity chromatography purification of the ACh receptor [30].

MYASTHENIA GRAVIS

The α-toxins have been important tools in defining myasthenia gravis as an autoimmune disease in which the number of nicotinic ACh receptors are reduced. Patients with myasthenia gravis (MG) exhibit weakness and fatigability of voluntary skeletal muscles, which result from a defect in neuromuscular transmission. The defect in transmission has been localized to the postsynaptic membrane of the neuromuscular junction. Electron micrographs of muscle biopsies from myasthenia gravis patients reveal marked alterations [22]. Synaptic folds are simplified and membranous debris is present within the synaptic cleft.

Electrophysiological studies have demonstrated that MEPP amplitude is reduced, but MEPP frequency and quantal content are normal [31]. Motor endplates of myasthenic muscle exhibit reduced sensitivity to iontophoretically applied ACh. This observation localizes the site of the neuromuscular conduction defect to the post-synaptic membrane [32].

The results of ^{125}I-α-bungarotoxin autoradiography suggest a deficiency of ACh receptors in MG neuromuscular junctions [33]. This deficiency of ACh receptors has been confirmed by demonstration of a reduced number of ACh receptors in extracts of MG muscle, as determined by ^{125}I-α-bungarotoxin binding [34, 35]. α-Bungarotoxin binding to ACh receptors of normal and MG muscles reveal that the affinity of ACh receptors solubilized from MG muscles is greater than the affinity of normal ACh receptors for α-bungarotoxin [35].

The delineation of MG as an autoimmune disease is based on data from a number of studies. It was initially demonstrated that serum from 5 of 15 patients with MG blocked the binding of ^{125}I-α-bungarotoxin to detergent-solubilized extrajunctional receptors in rat [36]. This blockade was noncompetitive, suggesting that the serum factor, an IgG antibody, was bound to a site on the ACh receptor other than the α-bungarotoxin binding site or the cholinoceptive site.

Maximally serum or IgG produced a 50 percent blockade of bungarotoxin binding. It was subsequently demonstrated that Mg serum blocks binding of α-bungarotoxin to human neuromuscular junctions [37]. A double-antibody radioimmunoassay utilizing ^{125}I-α-bungarotoxin–labeled ACh receptor as antigen has been used increasingly as a diagnostic procedure for MG [38, 39]. When human ACh receptors are used as the antigen source, such an assay can detect ACh receptor antibodies in the serum of up to 88 percent of MG patients, with few, if any, false positive results [39].

The mechanism through which ACh-receptor antibodies produce the ACh-receptor deficiency in MG muscle is still incompletely understood. A number of mechanisms have been proposed:

1. Antibody blocks access of ACh to ACh receptors
2. Antibody induces a complement-dependent membrane lysis
3. Antibody accelerates the degradation of ACh receptors
4. Antibody decreases the synthesis of ACh receptors
5. Antibody alters the ion permeability changes that result from ACh binding to ACh receptors

It is possible that each of these may contribute in greater or lesser degree to the decreased number of functional ACh receptors in MG neuromuscular junctions. Mechanism 1 does not appear to play a significant role in transmission failure. Such antibodies do not alter transmission parameters of nerve-muscle preparations in vitro [40]. Furthermore, noise analysis of MG muscles reveals no difference in single-channel conductance and mean channel lifetime [41].

Mechanisms 2, 3, and 4 appear to play the major roles. The importance of membrane lysis as a significant mechanism for ACh-receptor loss is supported by the presence of IgG and the C_3 component of complement on the postsynaptic membranes of MG muscle. Immune complexes are also present on fragments of membranes apparently extruded into the synaptic cleft [42].

That ACh-receptor antibodies can induce alterations in ACh-receptor turnover has been demonstrated in myotube cultures by utilizing the methods developed by Devreotes and Fambrough [28]. Several laboratories have shown that MG immunoglobulin or serum can significantly increase the degradation rate of ACh receptors [43–45]. In our studies, half-life of ACh receptors in rat myotube cultures was 18.5 hours in the presence of normal serum or globulins, and 6 hours in the presence of MG serum or globulins [43]. The degradation rate of ACh receptors in mature synapses was also accelerated by MG immunoglobulins [46].

Myotube cultures can also be used to estimate the synthesis of ACh receptors. If cultures are incubated with unlabeled α-bungarotoxin at the beginning of the incubation period, subsequent labeling of ACh receptors with ^{125}I-labeled α-bungarotoxin will detect only the receptors that accumulate in the myotube membrane during the incubation period. Because degradation is a first-order reaction, all ACh receptors have equal probability of being degraded at any time. Therefore, the number of receptors that accumulates during the incubation period is a function of both the synthesis rate and the degradation rate. The degradation and accumulation of ACh receptors in myotube cultures has been measured in the continuous presence of normal and MG immunoglobulins and serum. From these values, it is clear that the synthesis rate or the insertion rate (or both) of ACh receptors into the plasma membrane is also decreased [47].

Figure 26-6 summarizes the changes of the neuromuscular junction in MG. Alterations in the rates of synthesis, insertion, and degradation of ACh receptors, as well as alterations in the end-plate membrane, contribute to the pathogenesis of myasthenia gravis and can be explained by the presence of ACh-receptor antibodies. However, the levels of these antibodies do not always correlate with the clinical state of the patient. Other factors that con-

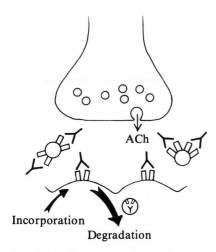

Fig. 26-6. *In myasthenia gravis, antibodies bind to the ACh receptors of skeletal motor end-plates, resulting in a decreased number of receptors through (1) an increased rate of receptor degradation; (2) a decreased rate of receptor incorporation into the end-plate; and (3) membrane lysis, with extrusion of fragments into a widened intersynaptic cleft.*

tribute to ACh-receptor synthesis and turnover must also be making a contribution. These include circulating hormones, the immunological state of the thymus, and the genetic constitution of the patient. More specific mechanisms and additional factors will be defined during the next several years, and these may have far-reaching consequences in effective drug therapy for myasthenia gravis.

ACETYLCHOLINESTERASE

Acetylcholinesterase (AChE) of skeletal muscle is located in the neuromuscular junction, where it hydrolyzes the ACh released from the nerve terminal. Three lines of evidence indicate that AChE is associated with the basal lamina of muscle rather than being an integral part of the postsynaptic plasma membrane. First, mild chemical treatments release AChE from skeletal muscle or the electric organs of *Electrophoris* and *Torpedo*. Tissues treated by mild enzyme hydrolysis [48], or extracted with high ionic strength solutions [49] release AChE. Second, the chemical structure of native AChE suggests that a number of subunits are attached to a filamentous tail that resembles col-

lagen fibrils present in the basal lamina [50]. The tail region contains hydroxyproline, hydroxylysine, and glycine, amino acids found in collagen of the basal lamina. Collagenase treatment of native species of AChE from *Torpedo* (16S, 13.5S or 8S) converts all of the enzyme into a single 11S globular protein that possesses enzyme activity but lacks the fibrous tail portion present in native enzyme. This suggests that the filamentous region of native AChE is not necessary for its enzymatic action and probably serves a structural role in binding the enzyme in situ. Third, AChE activity remains in basal laminar remnants of lysed neuromuscular junction [51].

The levels of AChE present in skeletal muscle have been shown to be dependent on innervation. Muscle AChE, like that of electric organ, exists in three forms: 4S, 10S, and 16S [52]. The 16S form is found exclusively at the neuromuscular junction. Denervation reduces the ChE activity of skeletal muscle with a loss of 16 S AChE [52]. In developmental studies, myotubes cultured from 13- to 14-day-old rat embryo synthesized only 4S and 10S forms of AChE, but myotube cultures from 18-day-old rat embryos contained 16S AChE, in addition to the other forms. Myotube cultures from the younger embryos do, however, develop 16S AChE activity if spinal cord cells are added to the myoblast cultures. Spots of AChE activity can be detected histochemically in nerve-muscle cultures at sites of nerve-muscle contact [53]. Myoblasts from 18-day-old embryos, in which nerve-muscle contacts are made in vivo, maintain the capacity to synthesize 16S AChE in culture without further neuronal influence. These studies could be interpreted as showing that some neural influence alters the capacity of muscle cells to synthesize AChE molecules or to assemble AChE oligomers.

Cholinesterase activity is also present in motor neurons. One report indicated that 10S and 4S AChE are released from nerve terminals into the synaptic cleft [54] at a rate proportional to the frequency of nerve stimulation. This conclusion is based on the assumption that curarized muscle does not release AChE and that the AChE released is of the 4S or 10S form, rather than the 16S that is found in muscle. Although these data support such a conclusion, the possibility that ACh interaction with AChE in the basal lamina results in the release of AChE of the 10S and 4S species cannot be ruled out.

Alterations in AChE activity are relevant to several clinical situations. AChE inhibitors are used as insecticides. Organophosphates are irreversible inhibitors of ChE, and humans exposed to excessive amounts of these substances develop paralysis of all voluntary skeletal muscles, as well as significant autonomic dysfunction. Poisoning with irreversible AChE can be fatal without adequate therapy. In addition, reversible AChE inhibitors—edrophonium, neostigmine, and pyridostigmine—are commonly used in the diagnosis and treatment of myasthenia gravis. Convincing data are now accumulating to suggest that long-term therapy with neostigmne or pyridostigmine can have deleterious, as well as beneficial, effects in this condition. Finally, a metabolic disease has been reported in which the patient had a deficiency of AChE at the neuromuscular junction, resulting in a chronic neuromuscular disease. Each of these circumstances represents a response to deficiency of AChE activity, the first two caused by exogenous inhibitors, the last from an inborn metabolic defect. In all of these situations, it has been possible to demonstrate deleterious effects at the neuromuscular junction when the capacity to deactivate ACh rapidly is lost. Juxtaposing these effects with the loss of AChE activity and other "trophic effects" that occur when muscle is denervated provides a view of nerve-muscle interaction in which regulation of neurotransmitter concentration within a physiological range is necessary for maintenance of neuromuscular junction homeostasis. Too little or too much ACh in the synaptic cleft can markedly alter metabolic events in the postsynaptic muscle membrane, and perhaps in the presynaptic, as well.

It was initially found that single doses of the irreversible inhibitors of AChE could cause marked degeneration of muscle postsynaptic membranes [55]. This finding has been extended by descriptions of morphological, physiological, and biochemical alterations in neuromuscular junctions in animals given single doses of irreversible AChE inhibitors. Similar changes are present in animals chronically treated with reversible AChE inhibitors.

Administration of a single dose of paraoxon (diethyl-p-nitrophenyl phosphate), an organophosphate that is an irreversible AChE inhibitor, produces grouped fiber-muscle necrosis in rat diaphragm [55]. This appears to be due to increased ACh activity. The severity of muscle involvement is decreased by pretreatment of the animal with hemicholinium, a substance that decreases ACh synthesis, or by prior nerve section, which eliminates the source of ACh. When paraoxon-treated rats are also given guanidine, a substance that increases ACh release, the number of affected muscle fibers is increased [56]. The muscle necrosis produced by paraoxon is dose- and time-dependent and is reversible by pyridine-2-aldoxime (2-PAM) [57].

The morphological alterations in paraoxon-induced necrosis are similar to those seen after chronic administration of reversible inhibitors of AChE: postsynaptic motor end-plate alterations are most prominent; there is degeneration of postsynaptic folds, with collapsed residue of preexisting folds present in the synaptic cleft; and the synaptic clefts are widened. In addition, histometric analysis of electron micrographs reveals that the mean postsynaptic membrane profile (membrane length per area) is decreased by as much as 29 percent [58]. Presynaptic alterations indicative of continuous nerve activity also can be seen. Synaptic vesicles are depleted and numerous coated vesicles and membrane cisternae appear [59].

Chronic neostigmine treatment also results in alterations of physiological parameters [60]. Decreased muscle contractility occurs after 3 days of injections; however, this returns to normal in 22 to 25 days. Resting-muscle membrane potential is unaltered for the duration of treatment. Although frequency and amplitude of the miniature end-plate potential are facilitated initially by acute neostigmine injections, chronic injection produces decreased frequency and amplitude. For the most part, the reduced MEPP amplitude is due to postsynaptic alterations. This was demonstrated by measuring ACh sensitivity of affected motor end-plates. The measurements showed that peak ACh sensitivity per end plate in controls was $2,554 \pm 378$ mV per nanocoulomb. Experimental animals treated with neostigmine had peak ACh sensitivity of $1,512 \pm 336$ mV per nanocoulomb after 3 days of treatment and 868 ± 289 mV per nanocoulomb after 20 to 30 days of treatment [60].

It is possible that the reduced MEPP amplitude and ACh sensitivity after inhibition of AChE is the result of reduced concentrations of ACh receptors in the postsynaptic membrane. Chang and co-workers [61] have shown that animals chronically treated with neostigmine had 40 percent fewer ACh receptors (α-bungarotoxin binding sites) than controls. This may be due to increased concentrations of ACh. It has been demonstrated in myotube cultures [62] that high concentrations of cholinergic agonist (carbamyl-choline) produce a down-regulation (reduced synthesis) of ACh receptors. A similar mechanism may be operative in chronic inhibition of AChE, because the resultant increased concentration of ACh and its lengthy exposure could cause a down-regulation ACh-receptor synthesis. This mechanism might be responsible for the postsynaptic alterations after AChE inhibition; however, the membrane lysis produced by acute injections of irreversible inhibitors may be due to some other mechanism.

ACETYLCHOLINESTERASE DEFICIENCY IN MAN

A new syndrome with defective neuromuscular transmission has been described by A. G. Engel and coworkers [63]. The primary abnormality in the patient described by these investigators is a deficiency in the 16S species of AChE at motor end plates. Clinically, this patient had generalized weakness and fatigability reminiscent of myasthenia gravis. However, morphological, electrophysiological, and biochemical studies of the patient's neuromuscular junction have defined the defects as a unique syndrome. In addition to the lack of demonstrable junctional AChE, other differences from myasthenia gravis include the following: (1) ACh receptor concentration was not reduced in the persisting postsynaptic membranes; (2) nerve terminals were markedly reduced, often surrounded by Schwann cells, and the synaptic cleft was widened; (3) MEPP amplitude was normal, but frequency was reduced; (4) although EPP quantum content was markedly reduced at 1 per second, stimulation at 40 per second did not produce an increase such as occurs in the myasthenic syndrome. It is likely that this case is only one of a number of biochemical defects expressed at the neuromuscular junction that may simulate MG clinically.

The AChE abnormality in this patient could be due to lack of neural stimulation of 16S AChE assembly or to some intrinsic abnormality of AChE synthesis or assembly in muscle. In either case, cases such as this suggest that neuromuscular disorders in humans may result from abnormalities of any one of a number of neuromuscular junction constituents.

References

1. Boroff, D. A., del Castillo, J., Evoy, W. H., and Peinhardt, R. A. Observations on the action of Type A botulinum toxin on frog neuromuscular junctions. *J. Physiol.* 240:227–253, 1974.
2. Burgen, A. S. V., Dickens, F., Eatman, L. J. The action of botulinum toxin on the neuromuscular junction. *J. Physiol.* 109:10–24, 1949.
3. Hughes, R., and Whaler, B. C. Influence of nerve ending activity and of drugs on the rate of paralysis of rat diaphragm preparations by Cl. botulinum type A toxin. *J. Physiol.* 160:221–233, 1962.
4. Thesleff, S. Supersensitivity of skeletal muscle produced by botulinum toxin. *J. Physiol.* 151:598–607, 1960.
5. Cull-Candy, S. G., Lundy, H., Thesleff, S. Effects of botulinum toxin on neuromuscular transmission in the rat. *J. Physiol.* 260:177–203, 1976.
6. Simpson, L. L. Pharmacological studies on the subcellular site of action of botulinum toxin type A. *J. Pharmacol. Exp. Ther.* 206:661–669, 1978.
7. Pumplin, D. W., and Reese, T. S. Action of brown widow spider venom and botulinum toxin on the frog neuromuscular junction examined with the free fracture technique. *J. Physiol.* 443–457, 1977.
8. Strong, P. N., Goerke, J., Oberg, S. G., Kelly, R. B. β-bungarotoxin, a presynaptic toxin with enzymatic activity. *Proc. Natl. Acad. Sci. U.S.A.* 73:178–182, 1976.

9. Lee, C. Y., Chang, S. L., Kau, S. T., and Luk, S. H. Chromatographic separation of the venom of *Bungarus multicinctus* and characterization of its components. *J. Chromatogr.* 72:71–82, 1972.

10. Chang, C. C., Chen, T. F., and Lee, C. Y. Studies of the presynaptic effect of β-bungarotoxin on neuromuscular transmission. *J. Pharmacol. Exp. Ther.* 784:339–345.

11. Abe, T., Alema, S., Miledi, R. Phospholipase activity in β-bungarotoxin action. *J. Physiol.* 270: 55P–56P, 1977.

12. Howard, B. D., and Truog, R. Relationship between the neurotoxicity and phospholipase A activity of β-bungarotoxin. *Biochemistry* 16:122–125, 1977.

13. Oberg, S. G., and Kelly, R. B. Saturable binding to cell membranes of the presynaptic neurotoxin, β-bungarotoxin. *Biochim. Biophys. Acta* 433:662–673, 1976.

14. Chang, C. C., Huang, M. C., and Lee, C. Y. Mutual antagonism between botulinum toxin and β-bungarotoxin. *Nature* 243:166–167, 1973.

15. Strong, P. N., Hueser, J. E., and Kelly, R. B. Selective Enzymatic Hydrolysis of Nerve Terminal Phospholipids by β-Bungarotoxin: Biochemical and Morphological Studies. In Z. Hall, R. B. Kelly, and C. F. Fox (eds.), *Cellular Neurobiology*. New York: Alan R. Liss. Pp. 227–249.

16. Wernicke, J. J., Vanker, A. D., and Howard, B. D. The mechanism of action of β-bungarotoxin. *J. Neurochem.* 25:483–496, 1975.

17. Frontali, N., Ceccarelli, B., Gorio, A., Mauri, A., Liekivity, P., Teng, M.-C., and Hurlberg, W. P. Purification from black widow spider venom of a protein factor causing the depletion of synaptic vesicles at neuromuscular junctions. *J. Cell Biol.* 68:462–479, 1976.

18. Longenecker, H. E., Hurlbert, W. P., Mauro, A., and Clark, A. Effects of black widow spider venom on the frog neuromuscular junction. *Nature* 225:701–703, 1970.

19. Clarke, A. N., Mauro, A., Longenecker, H. E., and Hurlbut, W. P. Effects on the fine structure of the frog neuromuscular junction. *Nature* 225:703–705, 1970.

20. Finkelstein, A., Reiken, L. L., and Tzeng, L. L. Black widow spider venom: Effect of purified toxin on lipid bilayer membranes. *Science* 193:1109–1011, 1976.

21. Elmqvist, D., and Lambert, E. H. Detailed analysis of neuromuscular transmission in the myasthenic syndrome. *Mayo Clin. Proc.* 43:689–713, 1968.

22. Engel, A. G., and Santa, T. Histometric analysis of the ultrastructure of the neuromuscular junction in myasthenia gravis and in the myasthenic syndrome. *Ann. N.Y. Acad. Sci.* 183:46–63, 1971.

23. Lambert, E. H., and Elmqvist, D. Quantal components of endplate potentials in the myasthenic syndrome. *Ann. N.Y. Acad. Sci.* 183:183–199, 1971.

24. Matthews, G., and Wickelgren, W. D. Effects of guanidine on transmitter release and neuronal excitability. *J. Physiol.* 266:66–89, 1977.

25. Ishikawa, K., et al. A neuromuscular transmission block produced by a cancer tissue extract derived from a patient with the myasthenic syndrome. *Neurology* 27:140–143, 1977.

26. Lee, C. Y. Chemistry and pharmacology of polypeptide toxins in snake venoms. *Annu. Rev. Pharmacol.* 12:265–286, 1972.

27. Miledi, R. α-Bungarotoxin enhances transmitter "released" at the neuromuscular junction. *Nature* 272:641–643, 1978.

28. Devreotes, P. N., and Fambrough, D. M. Acetylcholine receptor turnover in membranes of developing muscle fibers. *J. Cell Biol.* 65:335–358, 1975.

29. Berg, D. K., and Hall, Z. W. Fate of α-bungarotoxin bound to acetylcholine receptors of normal and denervated muscle. *Science* 184:473–475, 1974.

30. Eldefrawi, M. E., and Eldefrawi, A. T. Purification and molecular characterization of the acetylcholine receptor from *Torpedo* electroplax. *Arch. Biochem. Biophys.* 159:362–373, 1973.

31. Elmqvist, D., et al. An electrophysiological investigation of neuromuscular transmission in myasthenia gravis. *J. Physiol.* 174:417–434, 1964.

32. Albuquerque, E. X., et al. An electrophysiological and morphological study on the neuromuscular junctions in patients with myasthenia gravis. *Exp. Neurol.* 51:536–563, 1976.

33. Fambrough, D. M., Drachman, D. B., Satyamurti, S. Neuromuscular junction in myasthenia gravis: Decreased acetylcholine receptors. *Science* 182:293–295, 1973.

34. Lindstrom, J., and Lambert, E. Content of acetylcholine receptors and antibodies bound to acetylcholine receptor in myasthenia gravis. Experimental autoimmune myasthenia gravis and Eaton-Lambert syndrome. *Neurology* 28:130–138, 1978.

35. Elias, S. B., and Appel, S. H. Acetylcholine receptor in myasthenia gravis: Increased affinity for α-bungarotoxin. *Ann. Neurol.* 4:250–252, 1978.

36. Almon, R. R., Andrew, C. G., and Appel, S. H. Serum globulin in myasthenia gravis: Inhibition of α-bungarotoxin binding to acetylcholine receptors. *Science* 186:55–57, 1974.

37. Bender, A. N., Engel, W. K., Ringel, S. P., Daniels, M. P., and Vogel, Z. Myasthenia gravis: A serum factor blocking acetylcholine receptors of the human neuromuscular junction. *Lancet* 1:607, 1975.

38. Appel, S. H., Almon, R. R., and Levy, N. Acetylcholine receptor antibodies in myasthenia gravis. *N. Engl. J. Med.* 293:760–761, 1975.

39. Lindstrom, J. M., et al. Antibody to acetylcholine receptor in myasthenia gravis: Prevalence, clinical correlates, and diagnostic value. *Neurology* 26:1054–1059, 1976.

40. Albuquerque, E. X., et al. Effects of normal and myasthenic serum on innervated and chronically denervated mammalian muscles. *Ann. N.Y. Acad. Sci.* 274:475–492, 1976.

41. Cull-Candy, S. G., Miledi, R., and Trautmann, A. Acetylcholine-induced channels and transmitter release at human endplates. *Nature* 271:74–75, 1978.

42. Engel, A. G., Lambert, E. A., and Howard, F. M. Immune complexes (IgG and C₃) at the motor endplates in myasthenia gravis. *Mayo Clinic Proc.* 52:267–280, 1977.

43. Appel, S. H., Anwyl, R., McAdams, M. W., and Elias, S. B. Accelerated degradation of cultured rat myotube acetylcholine receptor with myasthenia gravis sera and globulins. *Proc. Natl. Acad. Sci. U.S.A.* 2130–2134, 1977.

44. Kao, I., and Drachman, D. B. Myasthenic immunoglobulin accelerates acetylcholine receptor degradation. *Science* 196:527–529, 1977.

45. Heinemann, S., Merlie, J., and Lindstrom, J. Modulation of acetylcholine receptor in rat diaphragm by anti-receptor sera. *Nature* 274:65–68, 1978.

46. Stanley, E. F., and Drachman, D. B. Effect of myasthenic immunoglobulin on acetylcholine receptors of intact mammalian neuromuscular junctions. *Science* 200:1285–1287, 1978.

47. Appel, S. H., Elias, S. B., and Chauvin, P. The role of acetylcholine receptor antibodies in myasthenia gravis. *Fed. Proc.* 38:2381–2385, 1979.

48. Massoulié, J., Rieger, F., and Tsuji, S. Solubilisation de acétylcholinestérase des organes électriques de gymnote. *Eur. J. Biochem.* 14:430–439, 1970.

49. Hall, Z. Release of neurotransmitters and their interaction with receptors. *Annu. Rev. Biochem.* 41:925–952, 1972.

50. Taylor, P., Lwekuga-Mukasa, J., Lappi, S., and Berman, H. A. Structure of acetylcholinesterase: Its relationship to the post-synaptic membrane. *Adv. Behav. Biol.* 24:239–251, 1977.

51. McMahan, U. J., Sanes, J. R., and Marshall, L. M. Cholinesterase is associated with the basal lamina at the neuromuscular junction. *Nature* 271:172–174, 1978.

52. Hall, Z. W. Multiple forms of acetylcholinesterase and their distribution in endplate and non-endplate regions in rat diaphragm muscle. *J. Neurobiol.* 4:343–361, 1973.

53. Koenig, J., and Vigny, M. Neural induction of the 16S acetylcholinesterase in muscle cell cultures. *Nature* 271:95–77, 1978.

54. Skau, K. A., and Brimijoin, S. Release of acetylcholinesterase from rat hemidiaphragm preparations stimulated through the phrenic nerve. *Nature* 275:224–226, 1978.

55. Arrens, A. T., Metus, E., Wolthius, O. L., and van Bentham, R. M. J. Reversible necrosis at the endplate region in striated muscles of the rat poisoned with cholinesterase inhibitors. *Experientia* 25:57–59, 1969.

56. Fenichel, G. M., Dettbarn, W. D., and Newman, T. M. An experimental myopathy secondary to excessive acetylcholine release. *Neurology* 24:41–45, 1974.

57. Wecker, L., Kiarita, T., and Dettbarn, W. D. Relationship between acetylcholinesterase inhibition and the development of a myopathy. *J. Pharmacol. Exp. Ther.* 206:97–104, 1978.

58. Engel, A. G., Lambert, E. H., and Santa, T. Study of long-term anticholinesterase therapy. Effects on neuromuscular transmission and motor endplate fine structure. *Neurology* 23:1273–1281, 1973.

59. Hudson, C. S., Rush, J. E., Tiedt, T. N., and Albuquerque, E. X. Neostigmine-induced alterations at the mammalian neuromuscular junction. II. Ultrastructure. *J. Pharmacol. Exp. Ther.* 205:340–356, 1978.

60. Tiedt, T. N., Albuquerque, E. X., Hudson, C. S., and Rash, J. E. Neostigmine-induced alterations at the mammalian neuromuscular junction. I. Muscle contraction and electrophysiology. *J. Pharmacol. Exp. Ther.* 205:326–339, 1978.

61. Chang, C. C., Chen, T. F., and Chuang, S.-T. Influence of chronic neostigmine treatment on the number of acetylcholine receptors and the release of acetylcholine from the rat diaphragm. *J. Physiol.* 230:613–618, 1973.

62. Noble, N. D., Brown, T. H., and Peacock, J. H. Regulation of acetylcholine receptor levels by a cholinergic agonist in mouse muscle cell cultures. *Proc. Natl. Acad. Sci. U.S.A.* 75:3488–3492, 1978.

63. Engel, A. G., Lambert, E. H., and Gomez, M. R. A new myasthenic syndrome with endplate cholinesterase deficiency, small nerve terminals, and reduced acetylcholine release. *Ann. Neurol.* 1:315–330, 1977.

64. Hartzell, H. C., and Fambrough, D. M. Acetylcholine receptor production and incorporation into membranes of developing muscle fibers. *Dev. Biol.* 30:153–165, 1973.

65. Porter, C. W., Chiu, T. H., Wieckowski, J., and Barnard, E. A. Types and locations of cholinergic receptor-like molecules in muscle fibers. *Nat. New Biol.* 241:3–7, 1973.

66. Porter, C. W., and Barnard, F. A. Division of cholinergic receptors at the endplate post-synaptic membrane: Ultrastructural studies in two mammalian species. *J. Membr. Biol.* 20:31–49, 1975.

67. Sytkowski, A. J., Vogel, Z., and Nirenberg, M. W. Development of ACh receptor clusters on cultured muscle cells. *Proc. Natl. Acad. Sci. U.S.A.* 70: 270–274, 1973.

68. Froehner, S. C., Reiness, C. G., and Hall, Z. W. Subunit structure of the ACh receptor. *J. Biol. Chem.* 252:8589–8596, 1977.

69. Dolly, J. O. Biochemistry of acetylcholine receptors from skeletal muscle. *Int. Rev. Biochem.* 26:257–309, 1979.

Frederick Samaha
John Gergely

Chapter 27. Biochemistry of Muscle and of Muscle Disorders

The first part of this chapter deals with some key biochemical and ultrastructural aspects of muscle [for recent reviews see 1 through 6]; the second part focuses on selected problems of muscle disorders, based on our current knowledge as portrayed in the first part. The bibliography is by no means complete, and in many instances only recent references have been included. These references, however, can direct the reader to earlier work.

Light microscopists have long known that the physiological unit of muscle, the cell or fiber, contains typical repeating structures along its length. These repeating units are *sarcomeres* and are separated from each other by Z bands. Within each sarcomere can be distinguished the A and I bands; the A band, lying between two I bands, occupies the center of each sarcomere and is highly birefringent. Within the A band, a central lighter zone, the H band, can be seen; and in the center of the H band is the darker M band. The Z discs are at the centers of the I bands. The contractile material is subdivided into smaller units—myofibrils separated by mitochondria and sarcoplasmic reticulum. The muscle cell is surrounded by a plasma membrane, which, together with the various connective tissue elements and collagen filaments, forms the sarcolemma. The interior of the resting cell is maintained by the plasma membrane at an electrical potential about 100 mV more negative than the exterior. When the muscle is stimulated by its nerve, activation of the contractile machinery results in contraction and tension development. One aspect of the coupling of excitation and contraction involves the transverse, or T, tubules, elements of the muscle cell that are continuous with the plasma membrane [2]. These tubules are seen as opening on the surface of the muscle cell, disposed either at the level of the Z

bands or at the junction of the A and I bands, depending on the species; and the depolarization of the membrane spreads activity along the tubules to the interior of the fiber.

At the same time that the ultrastructure of muscle was clarified, a profound change took place in our understanding of the contractile machinery itself [1]. Owing to the work of H. E. Huxley and J. Hanson [7] and A. F. Huxley and R. Niedergerke [8] the typical striation pattern of voluntary muscle can now be attributed to a regular arrangement of two sets of filaments, and contraction can be attributed to the sliding motion of these filaments relative to each other (Fig. 27-1). The thin filaments (diameter about 80 Å) appear to be attached to the Z bands and are found in the I band. The second set of so-called thick filaments (diameter about 150 Å) occupies the A band. The thick filaments seem to be connected crosswise by some material in the M band. In cross section, the thick filaments constitute a hexagonal lattice. In vertebrate muscle, the thin filaments occupy the centers of the triangles formed by the thick filaments. With the acceptance of the existence of two sets of discrete discontinuous filaments came the recognition that (1) the two kinds of filaments become cross-linked only upon excitation, and (2) contraction of muscle does not depend on shortening in the length of the filaments on an ultramicroscopic scale but rather to the relative motion of the two sets of filaments (sliding filament mechanism).

The length of the muscle depends on the length of the sarcomeres, and in turn, the variation in sarcomere length is based upon the variation in overlap between the thin and thick filaments [1]. High-resolution electron micrographs have shown that cross-bridges emanate from the thick filaments, and it is thought that, in active muscle, these structures are responsible for the links with thin filaments.

Table 27-1 shows the protein constituents of the various structures of the contractile apparatus. Myosin is the chief constituent of thick filaments, and actin the chief constituent of thin filaments. A recently discovered component of the thick filaments is the C protein, which, it has been suggested, may play a role in regulating the interaction of myosin cross-bridges with actin [9].

Tropomyosin and a complex of three subunits [16] subsumed under the name *troponin* [17] are present in the thin filaments and play an important role in the regulation of muscle contraction. The proteins constituting the M and the Z bands have not been fully characterized. The presence of creatine kinase in the M line has been demonstrated, but its structural role is not clear, and the role of another component (5S protein) [12] also remains to be elucidated. There is evidence, however, that α-actinin is present in the Z bands and in the rodlike bodies connected to the Z bands that are found in nemaline myopathy [13].

Another constituent of the Z band has been identified as *desmin* (about 50,000 M_r, the subunit of the so-called 10 nm filaments [14]). Filaments in the 10 nm class have been found in a variety of cells and are considered part of the cytoskeleton [15].

The existence of filaments that are continuous throughout the sarcomere has been suggested [16, 17], but in view of the overwhelming evidence

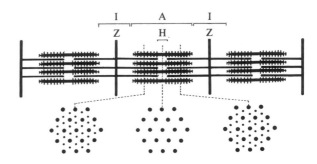

Fig. 27-1. Schematic representation of structure of striated muscle. Actin-containing thin filaments originate at Z lines. Note thick myosin-containing filaments that bear cross-bridges. The M disc lies in the center of the H band. (See text.) (Reproduced with permission from Huxley, H. E., The mechanism of muscle contraction. Science 164:1356, 1969. Copyright 1969. The American Association for the Advancement of Science.)

for the participation of the discontinuous myosin and actin filaments in the contraction process, the former have moved away from the center of attention. Recent reports on an elastic protein filament network in muscle called *connectin* [18], together with the information on 10 nm filaments, will again raise the question of the role of continuous filaments in muscle.

An important development that has taken place over the last few years is the recognition that all cells contain myosin, actin, and other components of the myofilaments, and that a variety of cell func-

Table 27-1. Myofibrillar Proteins

Protein	Localization	Function
Myosin	A band	Contraction; ATPase
C protein	Thick filaments	Structural?
Actin	I band (partial overlap with thick filaments)	Contraction
Tropomyosin	Thin filaments ⎱	⎰ Regulation of actin-myosin interaction; confer Ca^{2+} requirement
Troponin	Thin filaments ⎰	
M protein	Center of thick filaments	Structural?
α-Actinin	Z band	Structural?

tions—including cell motility and probably cell division—depend on these proteins. An important difference between muscle and other tissue is that in nonmuscle the myofibrillar proteins do not form the conspicuous structures found in muscle and that the supramolecular complexes usually have a more fleeting existence [15]. Detailed coverage of nonmuscle cellular "contractile" proteins is outside the scope of this chapter.

Electron micrographs show that thin filaments of muscle contain globular subunits about 55 Å in diameter, arranged in a double-helical structure [19]. These are identified with the protein actin, which can be extracted from muscle that has been treated with acetone. The complete amino acid sequence of actin, which contains 3-methylhistidine, an unusual amino acid, has been determined [20]. The molecular weight of actin is about 42,000. Differences in the amino acid sequence of actins in different cell types—skeletal muscle, cardiac muscle, brain, platelets—have been found in the same organism. However, amino acid replacements in actin are of a very conservative nature in that the character (charge, hydrophobicity) of the residue is preserved, even if species far from each other on the evolutionary scale are compared [21]. Gel electrophoretic differences among actins depend on a few residues at the N terminus; and while these differences correlate with certain broad groupings, the full genetic variety is not revealed by this technique alone [22]. Refinements in recognizing differences among closely related proteins may lead to new insights in the delineation of proteins in diseased muscles.

On addition of salts to a solution of actin, a drastic change in viscosity results, and negatively stained electron micrographs reveal the presence of double-helical filaments that are essentially identical to the thin filaments in appearance. The two physical states of actin characterized by low and high viscosity are called, respectively, *G*- and *F-actin* (G, globular; F, fibrous). The G → F transition is referred to as polymerization. The nucleotide in G-actin is ATP [23]; that in F-actin is ADP. The transformation of ATP to ADP takes place during polymerization, but is not involved in muscle contraction. This reaction presumably takes place

when actin filaments are laid down in the course of development, growth, or regeneration [24].

Myosin

Myosin, the chief constituent of the thick filaments, contrasts with actin in almost every respect. Myosin is a highly asymmetrical molecule with an overall length of about 150 nm and a molecular weight of about 500,000 (Fig. 27-2). Its width varies between about 2 and 10 nm. In contrast to actin, which is made up of a single polypeptide chain, myosin consists of several chains. There are two heavy chains, each with a molecular weight of about 200,000, that run from one end of the molecule to the other. Along most of the length of the molecule, the two chains are intertwined to form a double α helix rod; at one end of the molecule they separate, each forming an essentially globular portion.

By using various proteolytic enzymes, it has been possible to isolate the α-helical portions, including the whole rod and light meromyosin (LMM), which form the core of the thick filaments. One can also isolate segments containing globular portions, heavy meromyosin (HMM), and HMM subfragment 1 (S-1) [25]. The two globular portions contain the sites responsible for the biological activity of myosin; that is, the ability to hydrolyze ATP and to combine with actin. An interesting chemical feature of the heavy chain of myosin is the presence of methylated lysine and histidine. Methylated histidine is present in myosin of adult fast-twitch muscle, but is absent from myosin in embryonic muscle and adult slow-twitch and cardiac muscle [26–28]. It should be noted that the methylated residues present in myosin and actin may open up new possibilities for the study of protein synthesis in normal and abnormal conditions [29], and, in the excreted form, may serve as indicators of muscle breakdown [30].

In addition to the two heavy chains, each myosin molecule contains four light chains with molecular weights of about 20,000. Myosin in fast-twitch muscle contains three types of light chains, designated LC_1, LC_2, and LC_3 in order of increasing speed of migration on sodium dodecylsulfate–polyacrylamide gel electrophoresis (SDS-PAGE). LC_1 and LC_3 are also referred to as A1 and A2, respectively, "A" indicating that they are removable by mild alkali. Myosin in cardiac and slow-twitch muscle contains only two types of light chains, whose mobilities are similar, but distinguishable from, those of LC_1 and LC_2, respectively, of fast-twitch muscle myosin [31, 32].

Each molecule contains two LC_2s. In fast muscle myosin, the sum of $LC_1 + LC_3$ is two per molecule, but they occur in a ratio of about 1.4:0.6, suggesting that some myosin molecules contain pairs of either LC_1 or LC_3 [33]. Recent work [34] utilizing antibodies specific for either LC_1 or LC_3 has succeeded in demonstrating the existence of such homodimers that contain either a pair of LC_1 or a pair of LC_3; more recently, evidence has also been obtained [35] for the existence of molecules containing one LC_1 and one LC_3. In slow-twitch and cardiac muscle myosin, it appears that there are a pair of LC_1s and a pair of LC_2s per molecule.

Light chains in the LC_2 mobility class seem to be related by their ability to undergo phosphorylation by a kinase [36], whose activator is the ubiquitous Ca^{2+}-binding protein calmodulin, formerly known as the calcium-dependent regulatory protein [37]. A light chain that can undergo phosphorylation has been implicated in the regulation of smooth-muscle contraction [38], although this issue has not been finally settled [39]. A regulatory role for LC_2 in cardiac muscle has also been suggested [40]. No direct regulatory function for LC_2 has been found in skeletal muscle, although recently its phosphorylation and dephosphorylation in vivo during contraction and relaxation, respectively, have been reported [41].

It is less clear what possible role the two different nonphosphorylatable light chains—LC_1 and LC_3—may play, although differences in actin-activated ATPase, depending on which of the two chains is present, have been found under some conditions [42].

AGGREGATION OF MYOSIN
Myosin molecules have a tendency to form end-to-end aggregates involving the LMM rods, which then grow into larger structures (the thick filament). The polarity of the myosin molecules is re-

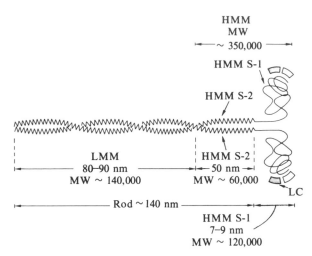

Fig. 27-2. Schematic representation of the structure of the myosin molecule, based chiefly on Lowey, S., Slayter, H. S., Weeds, A. G., and Baker, H. Substructure of the myosin molecule. I. Subfragments of myosin by enzymatic degradation. J. Mol. Biol. 42:1, 1969. The rod portion of the molecule has a coiled α-helical structure. Hinge regions postulated in the mechanism of contraction are at the junction of HMM S-1 and HMM S-2 and of HMM S-2 and LMM. It should be noted that HMM S-1 has one chief polypeptide chain while other fragments have two. Note the light chains (LC) in the head region. The scheme suggests the presence of two different subunits in each HMM S-1. (Reproduced with permission. Walton, J. N. (ed.), Disorders of Voluntary Muscle, 3d ed. Edinburgh: Churchill Livingstone, 1974.)

versed on either side of the central portion of the filament. The globular ends of the molecules form projections on the aggregates similar to those seen on the thick filaments [1]. The central 0.2 μm portion of the thick filament is devoid of cross-bridges (Fig. 27-2). The use of fluorescent antibodies in combination with electron-microscope studies has greatly elucidated the structure of the myosin filaments, and the data suggest that the head pieces are attached to the filaments by means of flexible hinges [43, 44] (Fig. 27-2). Recent physicochemical studies have provided direct evidence for segmental flexibility within the myosin molecule [46–48]. This has important implications for the possible molecular mechanisms of contraction discussed below. According to x-ray data, the cross-bridges on the thick filaments are arranged in a helical fashion [45]. The cross-bridges emerge at levels separated by 143 nm; the number of bridges at each level has not been definitively determined. Estimates range from 2 to 4, the most likely number being 3 [3, 49, 50].

Myosin-Actin Interaction and ATPase Activity

The discovery by Engelhardt and Ljubimova [51] of the adenosine triphosphatase (ATPase) activity of myosin led to the recognition of the important interrelations between the structural and functional aspects of this protein and its role in muscle contraction. The protein originally termed "myosin" was, in the light of our current knowledge, a complex of actin and myosin. The ATPase activity of myosin itself is stimulated by Ca^{2+} and is low in Mg^{2+}-containing media. If purified actin is added to myosin at low ionic strength in the presence of Mg^{2+}, considerable activation of ATPase takes place. This activation is also accompanied by a remarkable change in the physical state of the system. Turbidity increases and, depending on the concentration, superprecipitation results. The latter refers to the appearance of a flocculent precipitate, which often shrinks into a contracted plug. Glycerol-extracted muscle fibers have also been found useful for studying the interaction of myosin and actin without destroying the spatial relation existing in intact muscle. These fibers lack the energy supply system and the excitation-contraction coupling mechanism of intact muscle. Addition of ATP, however, elicits contraction accompanied by the hydrolysis of the ATP.

The combination of actin and myosin can also be observed in solutions of high ionic strength, as indicated by an increase in viscosity. Addition of ATP to this system results in a lowering of viscosity and a decrease of light scattering by the actomyosin solution, both of which are attributable to the dissociation of actomyosin into actin and myosin.

The dissociating effect of ATP, which also can be observed under some conditions at low ionic strength, and the stimulation of the myosin ATPase

activity by actin are important links in our understanding of the mechanism of muscle contraction. Kinetic measurements [6] suggest that, whether actin is present or not, the actual splitting of the phosphate bond in ATP is carried out by myosin without combining with actin. When myosin alone carries out the hydrolysis in the presence of Mg^{2+}, the rate of release of adenosinediphosphate (ADP) and of phosphate, is slow. Combination with actin accelerates the release of ADP. The actomyosin complex is dissociated by ATP and the cycle starts again. It should be noted that, in this view, the direct effect of ATP is always dissociation of actomyosin; the combination of the two proteins results from an inherent affinity between the two. How these processes lead to contraction is discussed later in this chapter (Molecular Events Underlying Muscle Contraction).

Tropomyosin and Troponin

Within recent years it has become apparent that regulatory proteins [52] in the thin filaments exert a great influence on the interaction of actin and myosin. Of these proteins, tropomyosin had been known for a long time, but its role in muscle contraction or its localization had not been elucidated. It is now reasonably clear that *tropomyosin,* an α-helical protein consisting of two polypeptide chains, is associated with the thin filaments.

The other component is *troponin* [52], a complex of three proteins [53] (Fig. 27-3). If the tropomyosin-troponin complex is present, actin cannot stimulate the ATPase activity of myosin unless the concentration of free Ca^{2+} exceeds about 10^{-6} M. The system consisting solely of purified actin and myosin does not show the dependence on Ca^{2+}. Thus the actin-myosin interaction becomes controlled by Ca^{2+} in the presence of the regulatory troponin-tropomyosin complex. This can be demonstrated readily in vitro; the Ca^{2+} concentration can be altered by varying the ratio of total Ca^{2+} added and of chelators such as EGTA. In vivo, the interaction of actin and myosin is regulated by the intracellular concentration of Ca^{2+}. It has been proposed that, of the three proteins in troponin, one, TnT, anchors it to tropomyosin, one,

TnC, is responsible for combination with Ca^{2+}, and the third, TnI, binds to a site made up of actin and tropomyosin when Ca^{2+} is absent [54, 55]. When Ca^{2+} binds to TnC, TnI is released and, as electron microscope and x-ray evidence indicates [56, 57], tropomyosin changes its position within the thin filament to permit the combination of myosin with actin. There are actually two pairs of binding sites for Ca^{2+} on TnC [58]. The pair of sites of higher affinity is specific for Mg^{2+}, and the other pair is specific for Ca^{2+}. It appears that the Ca^{2+}-specific sites play a crucial role in the regulatory process. In recent years, it has been found that the TnI and TnT subunits of troponin [59] can undergo phosphorylation as well as tropomyosin [60]. At present, it is not clear what role these phosphorylation processes play in the regulation of muscle contraction. The structures involved in the regulation of the intracellular Ca^{2+} level are the sarcoplasmic reticulum, a closed compartment within the cell, and the transverse tubules, which play an important role in the mechanism of excitation-contraction coupling.

Excitation-Contraction Coupling

Motor nerve impulses cause the release of acetylcholine at the neuromuscular junction. Acetylcholine initiates depolarization of the muscle cell membrane. Depolarization of the membrane penetrates into the interior of the cell through the transverse tubules that are continuous with the outer membrane (Fig. 27-4). The sarcoplasmic reticulum is in close contact with, but distinct from, the transverse tubules [2, 5]. Together, they are the elements that, in appropriately oriented sections, form the so-called triads noted in electron micrographs. It is currently supposed that the sarcoplasmic reticulum stores Ca^{2+} in relaxed muscle and releases it into the sarcoplasm upon depolarization of the cell membrane and the transverse tubular system. The sarcoplasmic reticulum maintains the low intracellular concentration of resting muscle by means of an ATP-dependent Ca^{2+} pump (Chap. 6). The transport protein of about 100,000 M_r appears to be identical with the ATPase isolated from sarcoplasmic reticulum membrane. Another protein

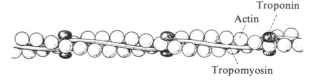

Fig. 27-3. Model of arrangement of actin, tropomyosin, and troponin in the thin filament. Note that troponin itself is a complex of three proteins. Tropomyosin is close to the groove of the actin filaments in relaxed muscle. (Reproduced with permission from Ebashi, S., Endo, M., and Otsuki, I. Control of muscle contraction. Q. Rev. Biophys. 2:351, 1969. Cambridge University Press.)

component of the membrane (the calcium-binding protein calsequestrin) may be important for the Ca^{2+} storage and release process [5, 61]. There has been recent active interest in the biosynthesis and assembly of the sarcoplasmic reticulum in vitro, and in vivo. It appears that, in the course of development, the ATPase enzyme is the last to be inserted into the membrane [62, 63]. A detailed knowledge of these processes is of potential interest for an understanding of various muscle diseases involving membranes.

Muscle Contraction

ENERGETICS

The classic studies on the energetics of muscle contraction have shown that, when muscle shortens under a load, extra energy is liberated in the form of work and that a certain amount of heat is inevitably evolved. This extra energy liberation is known as the Fenn effect. A. V. Hill sought to describe the total energy liberated by a shortening muscle as a sum of three terms: (1) work; (2) activation heat, whose magnitude is independent of both the degree of shortening and the amount of work done; and (3) shortening heat, which is proportional only to the length changes and independent of the load and, hence, of work. Subsequent studies by Hill himself have shown that this analysis of the energy balance may be somewhat oversimplified [64, 65].

There is now general agreement that ATP hydrolysis accompanies muscle contraction and is

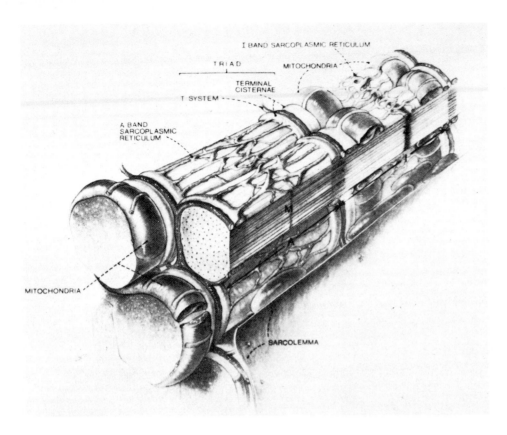

Fig. 27-4. A schematic drawing of part of a mammalian skeletal muscle fiber showing the relationship of the sarcoplasmic reticulum, terminal cisternae, T system, and mitochondria to a few myofibrils. (Reproduced with permission from Eisenberg, B. R., Kuda, A. H., and Peter, J. B. Stereological analysis of mammalian skeletal muscle. I. Soleus muscle of the adult guinea pig. J. Cell Biol. *60:732, 1974.)*

the immediate source of its energy [4, 66]. Although there is good correlation between the amount of ATP plus phosphocreatine broken down and the amount of work performed at various lengths and speeds of contraction, no valid chemical equivalent for the shortening heat in a single twitch has been found. In a series of contractions, the total energy liberated by a muscle, that is, heat and work, agrees well with the calculated energy release (based on in vitro data) from creatine phosphate breakdown. The latter continually rephosphorylates the ADP

resulting from the hydrolysis of ATP. Discrepancies, however, still exist in the early stages of contraction between actual measured chemical energy changes and energy changes calculated from the heat content of compounds known to change during the early phase of contraction [4, 67].

MOLECULAR EVENTS UNDERLYING MUSCLE CONTRACTION

The sliding-filament theory and the role of the cross-bridges in tension production (Fig. 27-5) are supported by the agreement between the experimentally determined tension of single muscle fibers as a function of length and the tension that would follow from the sliding theory on the assumption that tension is proportional to the number of links formed between the thick and thin filaments [68].

X-ray work has shown that the cross-bridges of the thick filaments undergo a transient movement when muscle contracts [45]. Differences in the orientation of the cross-bridges can be seen clearly when electron micrographs of insect relaxed and rigor muscle are compared [69].

That the interaction of the cross-bridges with the actin filaments results in a unidirectional movement, contraction, seems to be based on two things: First, the myosin filaments change their polarity in the middle of the sarcomere owing to the end-to-end aggregation of the constituent molecules; second, there is a built-in polarity in the actin filaments on each side of the Z band, as shown in electron micrographs by the "arrowheads" formed when HMM or subfragment 1 complexes with actin [1].

X-ray diffraction studies indicate that the distances among actin and myosin filaments increase as the sarcomere shortens. The flexible attachments of the myosin heads to the rod portions, discussed earlier, make it possible for the cross-bridges to interact with actin across various distances. The driving force of the contraction is most likely the interaction between actin and the S-1 portion of the myosin molecule [6, 44]. ATP apparently plays a role in the dissociation of the links between actin and myosin. ATP, bound to myosin, is then hydrolyzed, and ADP remains bound. [For a slightly different view, see 70.] A new interaction at a different actin site can then take place, resulting in the displacement of ADP and a small relative movement between the two filaments caused by a changed angle between the attached myosin head and actin. The pitch of the actin helix is slightly different from that of the cross-bridge helix, so a slight movement at an attached bridge would create a favorable situation for attachment of another bridge several actin units away on the same filament (Fig. 27-5). Several theoretical formulations of the cross-bridge model have been given. In earlier models [71], an elastic element has been postulated in the link between the thick filament and the myosin head; in a more recent scheme, the connection is rigid [72].

Muscle Metabolism

Muscle utilizes energy made available in the form of ATP, which is hydrolyzed to ADP and inorganic phosphate. The task of muscle metabolism, apart

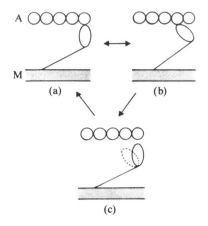

Fig. 27-5. Model of interaction of the myosin head with actin. (a) Attachment of myosin to actin, (b) tilting of myosin head, (c) detachment produced by ATP followed by its hydrolysis. On the basis of in vitro kinetic studies, the myosin species present in (a) + (b) carries the ADP · P product complex. Whether the dissociated myosin head can oscillate between the perpendicular and tilted position or whether it is locked in the perpendicular position is not finally settled. Similarly, the precise point at which the product leaves the actin-myosin complex requires clarification. The attached head may oscillate between positions (a) and (b). Based on Huxley, H. E., The mechanism of muscle contraction. Science 164:1356, 1969, and Huxley, A. F., and Simmons, R. M., Proposed mechanism of force generation in striated muscle. Nature 233:533, 1971. (Reproduced with permission from Watson, J. N. (ed.), Disorders of Voluntary Muscle, 3d ed. Edinburgh: Churchill Livingstone, 1974.)

from the necessity of producing the specific constituents required for the construction of structural components, is to produce ATP. The metabolic pathways involved in the production of ATP in muscle are not essentially different from those present in other tissues, including nerve. There are, however, some features of muscle metabolism that are closely related to the mechanism by which contraction is initiated; others are subject to control by metabolites arising in the course of contraction.

It has long been known that active muscle increases its metabolism by a factor greater than 100. This is particularly true in muscles that contain "fast" fibers, which are involved in rapid bursts of activity. In these muscles, the chief source of energy is the anaerobic breakdown of glycogen, and the enzymatic control of glycogen metabolism furnishes a good illustration of the complex way in which regulation takes place [73]. Apart from specific mechanisms discussed below, the increase in ADP and inorganic phosphate itself serves to increase the rate of ATP synthesis by providing more substrate.

MUSCLE PHOSPHORYLASE
The breakdown of glycogen is catalyzed by the enzyme phosphorylase, the properties and structure of which have been clarified in considerable detail (see Chap. 17). Phosphorylase b, the inactive form, is transformed into phosphorylase a, the active form, by means of phosphorylation. ATP is the phosphate donor, and the reaction is catalyzed by another enzyme, phosphorylase kinase. The latter enzyme exists also in an inactive and an active form, and the activation again is produced by phosphorylation catalyzed by a protein kinase. This enzyme, in turn, is activated by cyclic adenosine monophosphate (cyclic AMP), which is formed from ATP under the influence of adenylate cyclase (Chap. 15). The cyclase responds to hormones and neurohumoral agents such as epinephrine. It has been demonstrated in vivo that stimulation of muscle produces an increase in the active form of phosphorylase a. Although epinephrine stimulates muscles, no actual increase in the phosphorylated form of phosphorylase kinase has been demonstrated.

As we have said, the onset of activity in muscle is mediated by the release of Ca^{2+} from the sarcoplasmic reticulum. It now appears that Ca^{2+}, in roughly the same concentration as that required for the activation of the actomyosin system, also increases the activity of the activated phosphorylase kinase by increasing the affinity to phosphorylase b. Thus, as the actomyosin system becomes active, phosphorylase kinase produces phosphorylase at a higher rate. As muscle activity proceeds, more phosphorylated glucose, which in turn is broken down through the glycolytic pathway, is made available from glycogen. Recent work [74] has shown that calmodulin, the Ca^{2+}-binding protein which, as described above, is involved in the activation of myosin light chain kinase, is also the Ca^{2+}-binding regulatory subunit of phosphorylase kinase. It has also been shown that phosphorylase phosphatase, the enzyme that reverses the activation of phosphorylase, is inactivated by Ca^{2+}. This phosphatase is in turn controlled by an inhibitor, which is itself controlled by cyclic AMP–dependent phosphorylation [73].

GLYCOGEN SYNTHETASE
A different enzyme, glycogen synthetase, catalyzes the biosynthesis of glycogen (see Chap. 17). It exists in two forms, one of which is active under physiological conditions, whereas the other is inactive (see Chap. 17). The same cyclic AMP–dependent protein kinase that activates phosphorylase kinase also phosphorylates glycogen synthetase I. In this case, however, the dephosphorylated form (I) is active and phosporylation by the kinase converts it into an active (D) form. This ensures that, when greater muscle activity requires increased release of phosphorylated glucose units from glycogen, the reverse process catalyzed by the synthetase is shut off [73]. As in the case of phosphorylase, a phosphatase for converting the D to I form is regulated by an inhibitor which, itself, is controlled by cyclic AMP dependent phosphorylation.

PHOSPHOFRUCTOKINASE
Phosphofructokinase is another key enzyme of the glycolytic pathway that introduces a second phosphate into the fructose 6-phosphate molecule prior to its breakdown into trioses. Its activity is under control of the concentration of various metabolites, such as inorganic phosphate, AMP, ATP, and citrate, and even the enzyme's reaction product, fructose 1,6-bisphosphate. This regulation involves an allosteric mechanism, the binding of the so-called effectors taking place at activating and inhibitory sites different from the catalytic site [75, 76]. These regulatory processes are crucial for turning on the metabolism of the active muscle by a

factor of several hundred and again reducing it to the resting level as the demand subsides.

MYOKINASE AND CREATINE KINASE
Myokinase catalyzes the reversible reaction

$$2 \text{ ADP} \rightleftharpoons \text{ATP} + \text{AMP}$$

This reaction assures better utilization of the energy stored in ATP by permitting the hydrolysis of both high-energy phosphate bonds. Creatine kinase catalyzes the reaction

$$\text{creatine phosphate} + \text{ADP} \rightleftharpoons \text{ATP} + \text{creatine}$$

Because creatine phosphate is the chief store of high-energy phosphates in muscle, this reaction permits the rephosphorylation of ADP to ATP, the immediate source of energy in contraction. During rest, the metabolic processes, in turn, replenish the creatine phosphate stores. Interestingly, this reaction created considerable difficulty when attempts were made to demonstrate the breakdown of ATP during single twitch because ATP broken down to ADP was immediately rephosphorylated to ATP, and the small change in creatine phosphate could not be detected. Fortunately, the creatine kinase can be blocked selectively by small amounts of dinitrofluorobenzene, and under that condition a decrease in ATP and formation of ADP could be measured [66].

BIOSYNTHESIS OF SPECIALIZED MUSCLE PROTEINS
The biosynthesis of myofibrillar proteins is a problem of considerable interest for understanding a number of normal and pathological—developmental, adaptive, and regenerative—processes. The basic mechanism of protein synthesis in muscle is the same as in other tissues, including nervous tissue (see Chap. 19). Polysome fractions isolated from embryonic muscle by means of the sucrose gradient technique have been used for in vitro synthesis of myofibrillar proteins. These studies have shown that the heavy and light chains of myosin, actin, and tropomyosin subunits are coded by monocistronic messenger RNAs (mRNAs) [77–79]. Many of the mRNAs coding for myofibrillar pro-

teins have been recently purified [80–82]. It is quite likely that transcriptional control plays a key role [83] in such regulatory events of myofibrillar proteins as muscle differentiation, growth, and transformation. However, it has been suggested that mRNAs are stored as protein-bound complexes in the form of nonpolysomal messenger ribonucleoprotein particles, which are activated for translation of the mRNAs during the terminal differentiation of muscle cells [84]. Clearly, further work is necessary to learn the mechanism of control. A related problem is that of the chemical signal for the increase in protein synthesis in work-induced hypertrophy. Creatine has been suggested as a possible mediator [85]. A recent report indicates the involvement of an RNA-like molecule in the hypertrophy of various organs including those (e.g., heart) that contain muscle tissue [86].

OXIDATIVE METABOLISM
During sustained activity, particularly in those muscles that are rich in mitochondria and in heart muscle, oxidative processes dominate. These involve the oxidation, through the Krebs cycle (see Chap. 17), of pyruvate formed in the anaerobic breakdown of glucose or glycogen and the oxidation of fatty acids, which, as has now been generally recognized, serve as the chief source of energy in oxidative metabolism. Citrate, an intermediate in the Krebs cycle, is an allosteric inhibitor of phosphofructokinase.

Comparison of Muscle Types
It has been known for about a hundred years that striated muscles differ in their velocity of contraction and that correlations exist among the color of the muscle, its velocity of contraction, and the stimulation frequency required to produce a tetanus. In general, red muscles are slower than white and higher frequencies of stimulation are required to produce tetanus in red than in white muscles. However, hardly any muscle as a whole can be considered entirely red or white or slow or fast, and the properties of each individual muscle are determined by the distribution of various fiber types to which the criteria listed in Table 27-2 apply.

Table 27-2. Clinical Description of Familial Periodic Paralyses

Features	Hypokalemic Periodic Paralysis	Hyperkalemic Periodic Paralysis
Onset	Second decade	First decade
Inheritance	Autosomal dominant 10–20% sporadic	Autosomal dominant
Provoking factors	Exercise followed by rest Stress Alcohol Agents lowering serum K^+	Exercise followed by rest Stress Alcohol Agents raising serum K^+
Serum K^+ during attacks	Usually low	Usually rises May be high or low
Myotonia	Rare	Present nearly 100%
High Na^+ intake	Detrimental	Beneficial
Low Na^+ intake	Beneficial	Detrimental
Membrane resting potential	Low	Low
Associated with thyroid disease	Yes	No
Vacuolar myopathy	Yes	Yes
Chronic myopathy	Yes	Yes

There are wide differences when one compares various species. For instance, the soleus muscle in rabbit consists almost entirely of typically slow fibers, whereas in rat and man the soleus contains a mixture of fiber types. Differences in speed of contraction, unless one refers to the intrinsic shortening speed of the sarcomere, are partly due to differences in the contractile apparatus, partly to differences in the speed of Ca^{2+} release and uptake by the sarcoplasmic reticulum [87].

It appears that the differences between types of muscle depend not only on the presence of certain enzymes in large or small amounts: different types of muscle may contain the same enzyme in different forms. The different forms of an enzyme catalyzing the same reaction have been called *isoenzymes,* or *isozymes.* The first molecule thus identified was lactic dehydrogenase [88], which consists of four subunits. Each subunit can be either of the H type, which is predominant in heart muscle, or of the M type, predominant in fast skeletal muscle. A higher content of the H type has been found in embryonic muscle, although differences exist with respect to species and the muscles examined.

Various muscles of the adult contain the two kinds of subunits in various proportions, again with species variations, and the complexes, of which there can be five, differ in their electrophoretic mobility.

Myosin also exists in different forms [89, 90]. The ATPase activity of myosin from a typical slow, or red, muscle is lower than that from fast, or white, muscle, and a striking difference exists with respect to its stability at alkaline pH. Fast muscle myosin can be incubated for 10 min at pH 9 without any loss of activity, whereas myosin from slow muscle loses most of its activity when so treated. More subtle differences exist with respect to stability at low pH. Both kinds of myosin lose activity at acid pH, but the slow muscle type loses less than the fast [89].

In addition to the differences in light chains between slow and fast muscles discussed above, a striking difference between myosin from fast and slow muscles, attributable to a difference in the heavy chain, can be demonstrated also by looking at the electron micrographs of negatively stained aggregates of the rodlike portion of the myosin molecule, LMM [91]. Whereas LMM aggregates from fast muscle myosin show a striated pattern consisting of strongly stained wider segments alternating with lightly stained narrower segments with a main period of 430 A, the situation is reversed in LMM aggregates from slow muscle myosin. The lighter segments are wider than the electron-dense segments, and within the lightly stained zones are four distinct darkly stained lines. More recent work, using electrophoretic separation and peptide maps, provides the most direct evidence for type-specific differences in the heavy chains of myosin [35]. Differences among fiber types have recently been found with respect to other myofibrillar proteins, including tropomyosin and subunits of troponin [92].

Differences in myosin stability at different pHs have become the basis for the histochemical classification of fast and slow fiber types. The degree of correlation between staining for oxidative enzymes and the pH effect on myosin ATPase varies, depending on the species. Slow fibers are rich in mitochondria and, consequently, in mitochondrial enzymes. Most fast fibers are low in mitochondrial and high in glycolytic enzymes; but some fast fibers are rich in mitochondrial oxidative enzymes. Thus, on the basis of four histochemical assays—that is, assays of alkali stable ATPase, acid stable ATPase, succinic dehydrogenase (mitochondrial), phosphorylase (glycolytic)—in principle 16 classes of fibers might exist. Such a survey, recently carried out on cat muscle, actually showed seven distinct types of fiber [93]. These fiber types could be correlated with types described by other authors. Thus, for instance, fibers exhibiting alkali-stable and alkali-labile ATPase and high succinic dehydrogenase activity correspond to the previously described fatigue-resistant fibers. By carrying out acid incubation at slightly different pH, fast fibers can be divided into at least two subgroups [94]. The use of antibodies specific for slow and fast types of myosin and coupled to a fluorescent dye have been found useful in identifying populations of fibers [95, 96]. Further refinements are to be expected from the use of antibodies able to distinguish differences among fibers within the fast group, if such

exist, on the basis of the presence of LC_1 or LC_2 subunits and from gel electrophoretic studies on single fibers [97].

A final word of clarification may be in order. Very often the literature refers to slow muscles as "tonic" and fast muscles as "phasic." This classification is not correct for most vertebrate muscles. Most slow and fast muscles of vertebrates are phasic muscles that exhibit a spread of action potential and exhibit innervation by a single end-plate, the *en plaque* innervation. On the other hand, true tonic muscles, such as the latissimus dorsi anterior of the chicken and some mammalian eye muscles, have multiple innervation, called *en grappe,* and there is no spreading action potential.

Effect of Changes in Activity and Innervation—Trophic Effects

Starting with the work of Eccles and coworkers [98], several authors have reported that, when a fast muscle is cross-reinnervated by a nerve that originally supplied a slow muscle, it acquires properties characteristic of a slow muscle; reciprocal changes take place in a slow muscle that has been cross-reinnervated by a fast muscle nerve. Changes in contractile speed are accompanied by corresponding changes in both the myosin ATPase activity [99, 100] and the protein subunit pattern [101, 102]. Changes have also been observed in the pattern of metabolic enzymes [103–105] and in the activity of the sarcoplasmic reticulum [101, 106]. These changes have been attributed, minimally, to specific influences of fast and slow nerves, maximally, to the elaboration of specific trophic substances (mysterins) by these nerves.

The trophic effects of nerve on muscle [107] have been defined in three ways [108]: (1) the formation of connections—the axon of a motor nerve must grow to and connect with a muscle cell through a neuromuscular junction; (2) the maintenance of integrity—failure of neuronal connection, whether functional or structural, will result in degenerative changes of the muscle; (3) the regulation of metabolic and physiological properties. In a phenomenological sense, such trophic effects cannot be denied. In the sense, however, that the nerve supplies specific trophic substances that not only maintain the integrity of the muscle, but also define its properties, such effects would be questionable, particularly in the light of experiments that show changes in the character of the muscle whose nerve supply has been left intact.

The work of Salmons and Vrbova [109] shows that, even with undisturbed nerve-muscle connections, changes in physiological parameters can be brought about if the pattern of neural activity reaching the muscle is changed. When the motor nerve is stimulated continuously over a period of weeks, imposing on the fast muscle a pattern of activity similar to that normally reaching a slow muscle, a marked slowing of the time course of isometric contraction and relaxation ensues. Such stimulation also produces changes in the subunit pattern of myosin, the ATPase activity of myosin, the staining pattern of LMM paracrystals, and the Ca^{2+} uptake of the sarcoplasmic reticulum. The changes correspond to an essentially constant fast → slow transformation. The biochemical changes in myosin are paralleled by changes in the histochemical ATPase reaction as well as by changes in the glycolytic oxidative enzyme pattern [110–113].

The changeover in the muscle type is attributable to the transformation of the existing fibers by the switching on of normally inactive genes and the switching off of those that had been active, rather than to the destruction of the original fiber population and its replacement by new fibers. This is shown by the fact that [114] early in the course of the transformation of fast muscle, antibodies against both fast and slow myosins react with the same fiber, while in normal fast muscle only the antibody against fast myosin reacts [95, 97]. After complete transformation, again only one type of antibody reacts—that reacting with slow myosin. The same conclusion has been reached from SDS-PAGE studies on single fibers showing the transient presence in the sarcoplasmic reticulum of both fast and slow type of myosin light chains [115]. Other interventions that leave the nerve-muscle connection intact are also able to change the muscle type, as judged by histochemical and biochemical cri-

teria. Thus sectioning of the peroneal nerve caused changes in the ipsilateral soleus from slow to fast type [116]. Removal of the gastrocnemius and soleus muscles in the rat caused the ipsilateral plantaris to change from the relatively fast to the slow type [117].

Clearly, the fact that changes in the activity pattern, with an undisturbed nerve-muscle connection, can alter the physiological and biochemical properties of a muscle raises many interesting questions concerning the trophic effects of the motor nerve. More work will be required to differentiate genuine neural effects related to the type of nerve from those effects originating in the neural activity pattern.

Duchenne Muscular Dystrophy

The muscular dystrophies, which are progressive, genetically determined, primary degenerative myopathies, are at present classified according to clinical, genetic, and histopathological criteria [118]. Readers are referred to Walton's text [118] for a full account of these muscle disorders. Molecular alterations have received intensive study in at least two types of muscular dystrophy—the Duchenne and the myotonic forms, which are discussed in this chapter.

ELEVATIONS OF MUSCLE ENZYMES IN THE SERUM IN DUCHENNE DYSTROPHY

One of the earliest biochemical observations made in patients with Duchenne muscular dystrophy was the discovery that some soluble enzymes are released from the muscle cell into the serum [see in 119]. Soon after Sibley and Lehninger noted the elevation of serum aldolase in patients with muscular dystrophy, other investigators noted serum elevations of other enzymes, including lactate dehydrogenase, glutamic oxaloacetic transaminase, α-glucanphosphorylase, phosphoglucomutase, glycerophosphoisomerase, creatine phosphokinase and pyruvate kinase. Although the serum levels of muscle cell enzymes are elevated in a number of conditions in which muscle fiber degeneration or necrosis occurs, the serum of patients with Duchenne muscular dystrophy, in general, yields the highest levels of enzyme activity. High levels also can be noted in idiopathic rhabdomyolysis, but lower levels are generally observed in cases of myositis, myotonic dystrophy, facioscapulohumeral neuromuscular disease and other conditions.

Creatine phosphokinase (CPK), which is confined mostly to muscle and the central nervous system [119], and the muscle isoenzyme of pyruvate kinase [120] have proven to be the most sensitive enzyme assays in detecting patients with Duchenne muscular dystrophy. With regard to the creatine phosphokinase, the serum enzyme levels are highest early in the disease and decline with its progression. In the advanced stages, the serum creatine phosphokinase may even return to normal levels. Fewer, but similar, observations have been made of pyruvate kinase in Duchenne muscular dystrophy; but there is evidence that the serum pyruvate kinase activity tends to remain elevated in later stages of the disease [120]. The muscle isoenzyme of CPK exists as a dimer (MM) of two identical peptide chains, and the brain CPK isoenzyme consists of a pair of identical peptide chains (BB). A hybrid of these peptides (MB) is the primary isoenzyme found in cardiac muscle. Whereas the MM and MB forms dominate in the serum of patients with muscle disease, the MB isoenzyme is disproportionately elevated in Duchenne dystrophy patients. The MB form may originate from cardiac muscle, even though the evidence for cardiac disease may be minimal in some cases. Another consideration, however, is that the MB isoenzyme is the fetal and early infantile form of muscle CPK. Transition to the MM forms occurs early in life. With a significant incidence of regenerating fibers in Duchenne muscular dystrophy patients, it is not unusual to find the fetal form of a protein such as myoglobin in the muscle cells, and therefore the fetal form of CPK in the serum of patients may also be related to regenerating fibers. The MB form is also elevated in the sera of patients with dermatomyositis, another muscle disease where fiber regeneration is prominent.

Since Duchenne muscular dystrophy is inherited as a sex-linked recessive trait, application of the Lyon principle would indicate that some fraction of carrier female muscle cells are dystrophic, and

hence, carriers of Duchenne muscular dystrophy are expected to have elevated serum enzyme levels. In fact, the serum CPK is elevated in two-thirds of the female carriers; this assay is therefore a useful study in genetic counseling. Since one-third of female carriers of Duchenne dystrophy do not have an elevated CPK, the assay may not be sufficiently sensitive. It is quite likely that the measurement of serum pyruvate kinase in potential carriers will be a more sensitive indicator in detecting the carrier state [120].

Other abnormalities in potential carriers have been found with regard to polyribosomal protein synthesis in muscle [121], erythrocyte membrane protein phosphokinase [122], ultrastructural aspects of muscle and with regard to a number of serum enzyme and electromyographic measurements. In one study [121], Ionasescu assessed the presence of the carrier state with measurements of muscle polyribosomal protein synthesis; and 90 percent of the mothers and 54 percent of the sisters of the patients studied were carriers. It appears that muscle from patients with Duchenne dystrophy or from carriers of this disease exhibits elevated collagen protein synthesis and normal or depressed noncollagen protein synthesis [121]. Ionasescu and coworkers showed a 50 percent decrease in total protein synthesis in muscle cells cultured from patients with Duchenne dystrophy. The addition of calcium chloride or the calcium ionophore A23187 to the muscle cultures completely corrected the decreased protein synthesis [122].

MEMBRANE ABNORMALITIES

A considerable body of data has accumulated indicating the presence of membrane abnormalities in Duchenne dystrophy patients. Because morphological studies of muscle from these patients revealed varying degrees of degenerative changes in most of the muscle fibers, it was reasonable to assume that these changes were responsible for the leakage of muscle enzymes into serum. Some investigators, however, have suggested that, as the serum enzyme levels are at their highest very early in the disease process in Duchenne dystrophy, there may be a primary abnormality in the sarcolemma, with leakage of cellular contents and subsequent degeneration. This idea, though interesting, was without support until Morkri and Engel [123] reported their findings in high-resolution phase-microscope studies of the dystrophic muscle. They demonstrated a population of nonnecrotic fibers with one or more focal lesions. This lesion was wedge-shaped, with the base resting on the fiber's surface. The electron microscope revealed that the plasma membrane overlying the lesion was either absent or disrupted, although the basement membrane was preserved. They suggested that this plasma membrane defect resulted in an ineffective cellular barrier and possibly represented a basic abnormality in the plasma membrane of the muscle fiber in Duchenne dystrophy.

Recently, Schotland and coworkers [124] performed elegant freeze-fracture studies on sarcolemma obtained from patients with Duchenne dystrophy. In both sides of the fractured sarcolemma membrane, the *protoplasmic* and *exoplasmic leaflets,* the dystrophic membrane shows an altered distribution and decreased number of particles that probably represent a variety of proteins.

Another abnormality in the muscle membrane from patients with Duchenne muscular dystrophy was described by Mawatari, Miranda, and Rowland [125]. They studied adenylate cyclase activity in cultured muscle cells from patients with several types of muscle diseases, including Duchenne muscular dystrophy and facioscapulohumeral muscular dystrophy, as well as normal control patients. They found that the basal activity of adenylate cyclase in Duchenne dystrophy myotubes was higher than in all the other studies, and this higher basal activity was not stimulated significantly by epinephrine or isoproterenol. Similar results were noted by Susheela et al. [126].

Abnormalities in red blood cells from patients with Duchenne dystrophy have been described. By using high and low substrate conditions, Mawatari and coworkers [127] found that the basal adenylate cyclase activity in Duchenne dystrophy erythrocyte membranes was about twice that of the controls. Epinephrine stimulated adenylate cyclase activity

of normal membranes two to three times, but did not stimulate the enzyme in Duchenne dystrophy erythrocyte membranes.

In 1975 and 1976, Roses and coworkers [128] described alterations in membrane protein kinase in erythrocytes from patients with Duchenne muscular dystrophy. In studying proteins II and II!, defined as major peaks by electrophoresis on 6% sodium dodecylsulfate–polyacrylamide gels, Roses and his colleagues found an abnormal increase in membrane protein kinase activity compared to that in normal controls. Abnormalities were also described in red blood cell membrane protein kinase from patients with myotonic dystrophy. These alterations, however, were different in that there was a significant decrease in enzyme activity when compared to controls. The importance of this observation in Duchenne dystrophy red blood cells remains to be shown, because in a study carried out by the same laboratory, a group of 21 female potential carriers of Duchenne dystrophy showed abnormalities quantitatively similar to those in male patients, who were clinically affected [129]. Other studies, such as that of Matheson and Howland [130], report specific changes in the shape of the red blood cells; these remain controversial.

Another muscle cell membrane, the sarcoplasmic reticulum, has been studied in Duchenne dystrophy muscle for the last 10 years. Sugita and his collaborators [131] were the first to show that the sarcoplasmic reticulum preparation from Duchenne dystrophy skeletal muscle had a reduced calcium uptake activity. The Mg^{2+}-ATPase activity appeared to be higher than in the controls, but this result must be interpreted with caution, as allowances were not made for effect of changes in Ca^{2+} concentration on ATPase activity. In a study by Samaha and Gergely [132], the calcium uptake process was studied in more detail. The initial rate of uptake over the first 2 minutes was determined in 8 cases of Duchenne dystrophy and in 15 patients without muscle involvement. The initial uptake rate of calcium was exactly one-half that of the normal rate. The total uptake of calcium was approximately one-third of the normal. In the presence of adequate amounts of calcium to allow removal of some calcium by the uptake process, the ATPase activity of the Duchenne dystrophy sarcoplasmic reticulum was half of the normal activity. Unfortunately, the EGTA-sensitive portion of the ATPase activity was not studied in this work. The available data, however, showed that the ratio of calcium taken up to ATP hydrolyzed was actually higher with the dystrophic muscle.

Peter and Worsfold [133] used a different approach to investigate the calcium affinity of sarcoplasmic reticulum. They also observed a reduced rate of uptake and total uptake of calcium by the sarcoplasmic reticulum of Duchenne dystrophy muscle. In their calcium affinity studies, they approached the physiological conditions more closely by studying the sarcoplasmic reticulum's ability to remove calcium as a function of free Ca^{2+} concentration. On incubation with 20 μM calcium, normal sarcoplasmic reticulum vesicles were quickly able to reduce the calcium concentration of the medium to less than 0.3 μM, which is in the range required to induce relaxation of muscle or to inhibit superprecipitation of actomyosin. None of the five cases of Duchenne dystrophy showed normal calcium affinity of the sarcoplasmic reticulum. A similar abnormality was found also in polymyositis and in one patient with the Becker form of the Duchenne dystrophy. Fifteen other cases with various neuromuscular diseases showed no abnormality in calcium affinity.

It is also of interest that in three of the cases where abnormal calcium affinity was observed, the mitochondrial fraction showed normal respiratory rates, acceptor ratios, respiratory control ratios and ADP/oxygen ratios. It is apparent from these studies, therefore, that the sarcoplasmic reticulum is abnormal in Duchenne dystrophy muscle at a time when mitochondrial function appears to be normal. More details on the sarcoplasmic reticulum in Duchenne dystrophy were published by Takagi and coworkers [134] in 1973. This work corroborated the data that both the initial rate of uptake and the total uptake of calcium by the dystrophic sarcoplasmic reticulum were lower than normal. Takagi also found that the Mg^{2+}-ATPase of the sarcoplasmic reticulum was little changed

from the normal and that there were no differences between normal and dystrophic sarcoplasmic reticulum demonstrable by electron microscope study. These investigators also observed that the total lipid, phospholipid, and cholesterol contents of the dystrophic sarcoplasmic reticulum vesicles were within the normal range. There was, however, a significant 40 to 50 percent decrease in phosphatidylcholine. They hypothesized that, since dystrophic muscle is replaced to such an extent by fat and connective tissue, the abnormal composition of the dystrophic sarcoplasmic reticulum membranes could be due to contamination of the fraction by microsomes from adipose and connective tissue. They raised the possibility that the abnormalities in calcium uptake might also be related to the same contamination. The latter point is probably not valid, because Peter and Worsford [133] have shown that, even with the addition of more sarcoplasmic reticulum fraction than used in the normal, the calcium affinity of the dystrophic sarcoplasmic reticulum remains abnormal. It is apparent that even if one takes into account the possibility of contamination of the dystrophic sarcoplasmic reticulum fraction, these membranes are still incapable of lowering free calcium to the same degree as normal sarcoplasmic reticulum membranes.

The reduced calcium uptake by the Duchenne dystrophy sarcoplasmic reticulum is not simply related to the nonspecific degeneration of muscle tissue. The studies by Samaha and Gergely [132] and Peter and Worsford [135] have shown that the calcium uptake and calcium affinity in muscle from patients with myotonic dystrophy are normal, despite the presence of degenerative changes in the muscle.

SARCOPLASMIC RETICULUM MEMBRANE PROTEINS

The studies by Takagi and coworkers [134] on the sarcoplasmic reticulum membrane in Duchenne dystrophy showed no difference from normal tissue in three major proteins. Samaha and Congedo [136] have shown that six proteins in the sarcoplasmic-reticulum fraction of the slow-twitch soleus muscle of rabbit are similar to those in human vastus lateralis muscle. The sarcoplasmic-reticulum membrane proteins from Duchenne dystrophy muscle showed a decrease in the 100,000-dalton ATPase protein and an increase in a 34,000 M_r protein. Because the ATPase protein is involved in calcium transport, a decrease in this protein might be expected if there is, as described, a decrease in calcium transport in Duchenne dystrophy sarcoplasmic reticulum. Further analysis of sarcoplasmic reticulum from ten cases of Duchenne dystrophy suggested two biochemically defined diseases [137]. Six cases had a relatively high and four a relatively low ATPase. No intermediate values were apparent in the ten cases. However, detailed clinical laboratory and myopathological studies did not show any distinguishing features between "high ATPase" and "low ATPase" groups.

CONTRACTILE MECHANISM IN DUCHENNE MUSCULAR DYSTROPHY

The speed of contraction is slow and the contraction time is prolonged in Duchenne dystrophy muscle [138]. In normal muscle there is a correlation between the speed of contraction, actomyosin-ATPase activity, and superprecipitation, so such studies have been performed with isolated actomyosin from patients with Duchenne dystrophy. Studies in two different laboratories [139, 140] have shown that the initial rate of superprecipitation is slow and that the ATPase activity is low. Although the actomyosin-ATPase activity may be the rate-limiting factor in the speed of contraction, there is no evidence that this abnormality of actomyosin is primary. Other properties, such as the pH stability of actomyosin-ATPase and immunological reactions of myosin, have been reported normal [140, 141].

Studies on the regulatory proteins of the myofibril in Duchenne dystrophy muscle showed that the myofibril contained one-third to one-half the normal amount of tropomyosin and troponin. By electrophoresis on sodium dodecylsulfate-containing polyacrylamide gels, there were no abnormalities in migration and no missing or extra proteins [142]. It appears, therefore, that there are no basic abnormalities in the muscle contractile or structural proteins; but there is abundant evidence of membrane abnormalities with the muscle and possibly in other tissues, such as the red blood cell, in patients with Duchenne dystrophy.

The Role of Lysosomal Enzymes

It has long been known that there is a marked elevation of lysosomal enzymes in dystrophic tissue [143]. Whether these enzymes are causative factors in the dystrophic process is unknown. McGowan and coworkers [144] report that low molecular weight protease inhibitors, such as pepstatin, leupeptin, and antipain, delay atrophy and degeneration in normal and dystrophic chicken muscle cultures. Studies by Libby and Goldberg [145] indicated that leupeptin decreased protein degradation in rat skeletal and cardiac muscle inoculated in vitro and lowered protein breakdown in denervated rat skeletal muscles and in muscles from dystrophic mice.

HYPOTHESES

The original classification of the muscular dystrophies was based on the assumption that the abnormality is in the muscle cell. It has been shown, however, that the peripheral nerve exerts profound influence on the properties of the muscle, as alteration in innervation can result in dramatic physiological and structural changes [108]. A new hypothesis suggested that the basic abnormality might lie within the neuron, which may exert an abnormal trophic influence on muscle, causing proteins and organelles to be formed that are not able to function normally and that degenerate earlier than do normal proteins and organelles. It should be pointed out, however, that until recently there has been no evidence of involvement of the peripheral nerve. In addition, no structural abnormalities have been found in motor axon terminals, and a normal number of motor neurons have been found in the spinal cord at autopsy of Duchenne dystrophy patients.

A third hypothesis that has been discussed is that microcirculation of muscle may be the basic cause for Duchenne muscular dystrophy. However, most of the pertinent data come from animal models and there appears to be no substantial evidence of any structural abnormality within the microcirculation of Duchenne dystrophy muscle.

Myotonic Dystrophy

Myotonic dystrophy, first described by Steinert in 1909, is inherited in an autosomal-dominant manner and presents with a unique constellation of abnormalities [118]. Clinically, myotonia appears as a failure of muscles to relax after contraction, or as a delay in the relaxation of a dimple caused by percussion of a muscle (percussion myotonia). Although this phenomenon is described as occurring in the flexors of the fingers, it can take place anywhere, including the tongue, jaw muscles, trunk, and lower extremities. The dystrophic process primarily involves the distal musculature of the upper and lower extremities and the facial and neck muscles. As the process progresses, other muscles become involved.

Myotonic dystrophy is characterized by involvement of organs other than skeletal muscle. For example, cardiac involvement is common and results in 65 percent of the patients showing electrocardiographic abnormalities, usually in the form of conduction defects. Posterior subcapsular cataracts occur in about 90 percent of patients, particularly in the later course of the disease. Impairment of pulmonary vital capacity and maximal breathing capacity results in alveolar hypoventilation. This abnormality is of variable severity: it is of no clinical importance in some cases but appears as apathy, somnolence, and semicomatose states in others. Disturbed esophageal contraction may be shown by contrast radiography. The male testes are often atrophic; the histology resembles that of Klinefelter's syndrome. Females may have abnormalities of menstruation, fertility, and parturition. Additionally present in both men and women may be accelerated breakdown of immunoglobulin G (IgG), an abnormally elevated fasting plasma insulin level, and exaggerated plasma insulin responses to both orally and intravenously administered glucose [146, 147]. A significant incidence of

mental defects occurs in patients with myotonic dystrophy.

Morphometric studies have been carried out on biopsy specimens of muscle and cutaneous branches of the common peroneal nerve in four patients with myotonic dystrophy. The myelinated fiber densities were normal in the superficial and deep peroneal nerves [148]. Internode length and frequency of abnormal axonal fibers were not significantly different from control, nor were the number of myelin lamellae, the number of neural filaments, and number of microtubules per unit area of the axis cylinder abnormal. In another study utilizing ^{125}I-labeled α-bungarotoxin binding to determine the presence of extrajunctional acetylcholine receptor sites, no abnormality was found in nine patients [149]. These data, therefore, do not support the notion of abnormal innervation in myotonic dystrophy.

A GENERALIZED MEMBRANE ABNORMALITY IN MYOTONIC DYSTROPHY

The above discussion indicates that myotonic dystrophy is a pansystemic disease. The current hypothesis suggests that a defect is present in membranes of cells of muscle and other involved tissues. It is apparent that the myotonic phenomenon in muscle tissue is the repetitive firing of the muscle membrane when the patient attempts to relax. It has been shown that if the animal or human muscle is removed from the influence of innervation by excision or by curarization, repetitive firing or myotonia of the plasma membrane persists. It is known that the inhibitor of desmosterol reductase, azacholesterol, can cause myotonia in animals and humans [150, 151]. In one study [151], many of the azacholesterol-treated rats developed severe cataracts, which are reminiscent of those found in myotonic dystrophy. Studies of this chemically induced myotonia showed that the $(Na^+ + K^+)$-ATPase activity was increased in the erythrocyte membrane and the muscle sarcolemma.

In 1973, Roses and Appel demonstrated an abnormality in the membrane-bound protein phosphokinase of erythrocyte ghosts from patients with myotonic dystrophy [152]. The alteration of enzyme activity was reflected primarily in the phosphorylation in one group of proteins identified as band III by SDS-PAGE. It is of interest that these same proteins from erythrocytes of patients with Duchenne dystrophy show an abnormal increase in phosphorylation under the same experimental conditions [153]. However, in the band II protein group of erythrocytes, no abnormality in phosphorylation was noted in the myotonic dystrophy patient, whereas an abnormal increase was seen in the Duchenne dystrophy patient. An abnormal decrease was noted in skeletal muscle membrane phosphorylation in myotonic dystrophy patients. These observations, together with those of the sarcoplasmic reticulum (see earlier, under Duchenne Dystrophy), appear to be the two main biochemical differences between Duchenne and myotonic muscular dystrophy.

Erythrocytes from patients with myotonic dystrophy have shown additional abnormalities. There is a significant decrease in calcium-promoted potassium efflux and in ouabain-sensitive sodium efflux when compared to normal erythrocyte activities [154]. In a study by Butterfield and coworkers [155], electron paramagnetic resonance experiments demonstrated that spin-labeled erythrocyte membranes have spectra recognizably different from those of normal erythrocytes. Further studies by Roses and coworkers [156] have shown that erythrocytes from myotonic dystrophy patients possess increased membrane fluidity; phenytoin "normalizes" the fluidity in these erythrocytes, but has no significant effect on normal erythrocyte spectra.

Mitochondrial Myopathies

A number of reports help to establish the newly emerging group of muscle disorders called *mitochondrial myopathies.*

Luft and coworkers opened up this field when in 1962 they reported the case of a 35-year-old woman with severe hypermetabolism of approximately 28 years' duration [157]. She had profuse perspiration, polydipsia without polyuria, and wasting, despite polyphagia. Creatinuria was present, indicating a decrease in functioning muscle mass. It was

clearly shown that the hypermetabolism was not of thyroid origin. A similar case, reported by Haydar and coworkers [158], was studied in detail by DiMauro and coworkers [158]. This patient was a 20-year-old woman with severe hypermetabolism. Muscle biopsy material revealed an increase in number and total mass of mitochondria; the mitochondria showed abnormally dense crystalline structure. The yield of the mitochondrial fraction in the hypermetabolic patient was approximately twice that of the controls. Although oxidative phosphorylation was normal, the rates of respiration in both cases were maximal, with very little stimulation by ADP. A high rate of basal ATPase activity was observed, with very little activation by dinitrophenol. The respiratory control indexes— activation of respiration by added ADP, with pyruvate and malate as substrates—were close to 1.0 and hence fit the biochemical definition of "loose coupling."

An additional mitochondrial study carried out by DiMauro and coworkers [159] showed that the total calcium taken up was less than normal and that the accumulated calcium could not be retained. The amount of calcium spontaneously released exceeded that taken up, indicating a large amount of endogenous calcium.

In summary, it appeared that the hypermetabolism in these patients was due to loose coupling of mitochondria, a condition in which the control of respiration by phosphate acceptors is lost but the capacity to synthesize ATP is maintained. The basic molecular abnormality in these patients is unknown.

One biochemically defined and lethal mitochondrial myopathy has now been studied in two unrelated male infants. The infants showed failure to thrive from birth, floppy muscles, lactic acidosis, glycosuria, proteinuria, generalized aminoaciduria, and failed to survive four months. Cytochrome c oxidase activity was severely deficient in muscle and kidney tissue [160].

Lipid Myopathy

For years, investigators have paid little attention to the possibility of identifying abnormalities of lipid metabolism in muscle. Recently this uncharted area has been opened by the discovery of two disorders of muscle lipid metabolism. One disorder, which is well characterized, has episodes of myoglobinuria. The second comes under the general heading of *carnitine deficiency* and is not well defined.

LIPID METABOLISM ABNORMALITIES WITH MYOGLOBINURIA

At present, the only completely described cases of lipid metabolism abnormalities with myoglobinuria are those of the brothers studied by DiMauro and coworkers [161]. Their episodes of myoglobinuria began around puberty and usually followed sustained exercise, such as mountain hiking. They had no history of cramps or intolerance of brief exercise, as might occur in the glycogen storage diseases. Fasting, alone or in combination with prolonged exercise, produced myoglobinuria. Clinical laboratory studies carried out during fasting showed that plasma triglycerides rose from their already high levels and serum creatine phosphokinase activity rose tenfold. Myoglobin was detected in the urine. Plasma ketone production was minimal during the fast, but rose promptly after ingestion of medium-chain triglycerides. Muscle morphology was normal, including histochemistry for the presence of fat; and a normal complement of glycogen and phosphorylase and phosphofructokinase enzyme activities were present ruling out glycogen storage disease. The muscle content of carnitine was slightly increased, and the activity of palmitycoenzyme A (CoA) synthetase and acetylcarnitine transferase were normal. Muscle carnitine palmityltransferase activity measured by three different methods in both crude extracts and isolated mitochondria varied from undetectable to 20 percent of normal in both patients. The enzyme defect was also found in leukocytes. Intermediate values were found in white blood cells from their asymptomatic mother. Since both the children were affected and the parents unaffected, an autosomal recessive inheritance is suggested, but an X-linked mode of transmission cannot be ruled out.

The metabolic pathway leading to the conversion of fatty acids into two-carbon fragments used in the citric acid cycle is depicted as follows. Plasma fatty acids enter the cell cytoplasm. Activity of fatty acylthiokinase in the presence of CoA results in the formation of acyl-CoA. The acyl-CoA is converted to acylcarnitine by fatty acylcarnitine transferase I.

$$CH_3—^+N(CH_3)—CH_2—CH(OH)—CH_2—COOH \; +$$

Carnitine

$$R—C(=O)—S—CoA \longrightarrow$$

Acyl-CoA

$$CH_3—^+N(CH_3)—CH_2—CH(O—C(=O)—R)—CH_2—COOH \; + \; HS—CoA$$

Acyl carnitine

The acylcarnitine penetrates the mitochondrial membrane, where it is reconverted to acyl-CoA by fatty acylcarnitine transferase II, and carnitine returns to the extramitochondrial space. The fatty acid chain is broken down to acetyl-CoA by β oxidation, and an activated two-carbon fragment enters the citric acid cycle in which ATP is eventually produced by oxidative phosphorylation.

As mentioned above, fatty acids represent the major source of energy in muscle metabolism. Oleic acid is about 45 percent of free fatty acid in arterial blood, and accounts for more than 45 percent of free fatty acid uptake into muscle. The second most prominent is palmitic acid, which amounts to slightly less than 30 percent of arterial free fatty acid. Complete oxidation of palmitic acid can account for twice as much oxygen utilization as can glucose oxidation.

When muscle carnitine palmityltransferase activity is markedly diminished, the episodes of myoglobinuria may be explained by impairment of long-chain, fatty acid utilization. During normal activity, and on a normal diet, these patients utilize muscle glycogen and blood glucose, and it is apparent that normal activity and moderate or short exercise are well tolerated. After prolonged exercise, and especially with fasting, muscle and liver glycogen supplies probably become depleted and the muscle turns more to the use of fatty acids for energy. The inability to transport palmitic acid into the mitochondria results in severe lack of substrate for the ultimate production of ATP. Although yet to be proved, it appears that ATP depletion results in acute muscle necrosis and myoglobinuria in a fashion similar to that assumed for the glycogen storage diseases.

THE CARNITINE DEFICIENCY SYNDROME

In 1972 Engel and Siekert [162] described a 19-year-old woman with severe generalized weakness; muscle biopsy demonstrated a considerable accumulation of lipid droplets, particularly in type I fibers. This observation alone is sufficient to characterize the disorder as a lipid-storage myopathy. The following year, Engel and Angelini [163, 164] found that in vitro utilization of long-chain fatty acids by a homogenate of the patient's muscle was not effective in the absence of exogenous carnitine but became normal after carnitine was added to the incubation mixture. This led them to measure the concentration of carnitine: values from 8 to 31 percent of normal were found in five different muscle biopsies. Lipid analysis showed a marked increase in triglycerides and diglycerides. Serum triglyceride, cholesterol, and free fatty acid levels were normal. During fasting, ketone bodies were formed normally, and this suggested that liver lipid metabolism was not impaired. In this patient, therapy with corticosteroids was followed by a dramatic improvement. After a year of carnitine administration, together with corticosteroids and low fat diet, the clinical condition of the patient had

not further improved and the concentration of carnitine in skeletal muscle was unchanged.

More than six other cases of carnitine deficiency of muscle have been reported [165–170]. In all these cases, weakness was prominent, serum enzymes were elevated, and muscle pathology was characterized by excess lipid storage, especially in type I fibers. Clinical presentation, age of onset, degree of weakness, involvement of tissue over than muscle, and response to carnitine therapy varied considerably. Therefore, it seems that this syndrome may be due to several different biochemical abnormalities. In a report of Karpati and coworkers [168], the patients had two episodes of acute hepatic encephalopathy at ages 3 and 9, before progressive muscle weakness developed at age 11. Carnitine concentration was much decreased in both liver and plasma, suggesting a defect in carnitine synthesis. A regimen of 2 g per day of DL-carnitine for 5 months resulted in normal plasma carnitine levels and was accompanied by dramatic clinical improvements, although liver carnitine remained low. Angelini and coworkers have reported a 10-year-old girl with insidious muscle weakness, beginning at age 7; histochemical results indicated lipid myopathy. Carnitine deficiency was found in the skeletal muscle, and the patient showed recovery of strength over an 8-month period with 3 g of L-carnitine per day and a medium-chain triglyceride diet. In a case reported by Markesbery and coworkers [165], a 61-year-old woman allegedly had had proximal muscle weakness from age 38. She showed widespread muscle wasting, absent tendon reflexes, and electromyographic findings of a neuropathy. Biopsy revealed a lipid storage myopathy, lipid-containing vacuoles in leukocytes and Schwann cells. The muscle carnitine level was abnormally low, but the serum carnitine level was normal. In a report by Van Dyke [166], an 8-year-old boy with slowly progressive muscle weakness was found to have a lipid myopathy predominantly involving type I muscle fibers. Skeletal muscle carnitine was reduced markedly and serum carnitine was normal. Although the parents were clinically normal, muscle carnitine levels were low in both. There was no clinical evidence of cardiac disease in the patient, but cardiographic studies showed ventricular hypertrophy. Steroid treatment resulted in clinical improvement, but no change in muscle histology. An 11-year-old male patient of Smyth and coworkers [169] had a unique clinical picture characterized by progressive muscle weakness, central nervous system involvement with calcification of basal ganglia, increased cerebrospinal fluid protein concentration, high-tone hearing loss, growth retardation, episodic vomiting, exertional dyspnea, and high levels of serum lactate, pyruvate, and alanine. Liver function was normal and serum carnitine was not measured.

So far, all cases of carnitine deficiency reported show an increased number of lipid droplets in muscle. Not all cases of lipid-storage myopathy, however, are due to carnitine deficiency. Increased numbers of lipid droplets were seen in muscle in a patient with intermittent movement disorder due to pyruvate dehydrogenase deficiency [171]. Twin girls with recurrent myoglobinuria had a lipid myopathy with a postulated carnitine palmityltransferase deficiency [172]. Lipid storage myopathy has been seen in a patient with congenital muscle weakness of unknown etiology, and recently abnormal lipid storage was seen in several tissues including muscle in a patient with congenital ichthiosis as the sole clinical disorder [173]. Accumulations of lipid and abnormal mitochondria in muscle are seen in other syndromes of unknown etiology.

In carnitine deficiency, the biochemical mechanisms are not known. Possibilities for the primary defect include (1) synthesis of carnitine in the liver, (2) the transport of carnitine in the blood, and (3) the uptake of carnitine by muscle tissue.

The Periodic Paralyses
Members of certain families suffer from recurrent attacks of flaccid paralysis known as *familial periodic paralysis.* Within this major syndrome, two clear subcategories have been identified with regard to the alterations in serum potassium levels during the onset of an attack [174]. In one clinical category, attacks are associated with a decrease in serum potassium levels; in the second category,

they are associated with an increase. In view of the many variables that affect the serum potassium level, a single measurement is not always helpful in identifying the hypokalemic and hyperkalemic forms of periodic paralysis. For example, serum potassium may be normal or low during some phase of the weakness in the hyperkalemic forms. A more reliable approach has been to provoke an attack by lowering the serum potassium level with glucose and insulin or by elevating it with the administration of potassium per os. In almost all patients suffering from flaccid paralysis (one exception has been reported), provocative tests permitted categorizaton as hypokalemic or hyperkalemic periodic paralysis.

Whether the alteration in the serum potassium level is the primary event precipitating paralysis in either syndrome is not known. From the clinical point of view, however, the division of the familial periodic paralyses into these two categories allows other distinguishing features to be identified (Table 27-2). The onset of hypokalemic periodic paralysis usually is in the second decade of life. The inheritance is usually autosomal-dominant, but about 10 to 20 percent of cases are sporadic. On rare occasions, myotonia may be identified clinically or by electromyographic studies. In China and Japan, there is a relatively high incidence of sporadic cases of hypokalemic periodic paralysis in association with thyrotoxicosis [175]. Whether the abnormality of thyroid function is the primary factor, or whether the Oriental peoples have a predisposition to developing periodic paralysis that can be triggered by thyrotoxicosis is not known.

The onset of hyperkalemic periodic paralysis is usually in the first ten years of life and almost all case are inherited as an autosomal dominant (Table 27-2). Nearly all patients manifest myotonia on clinical observation or through electromyographic examination. There has been no consistent incidence of cases of hyperkalemic periodic paralysis in association with thyrotoxicosis.

In both syndromes, stress, alcohol, and exercise followed by rest are provoking factors. In addition, a vacuolar myopathy and a chronic progressive myopathy have been described. Several abnormalities associated with and preceding the episodes of flaccid paralysis are known. In both syndromes, the onset of an attack is accompanied by an unresponsiveness of the muscle membrane to nerve stimulation [175]. In patients with hyperkalemic periodic paralysis, at the time of attacks and between attacks, the muscle membrane resting potential is lower than normal [176, 177]. The change of the membrane resting potential from −72 to −45 mV during an attack suggests that the muscle weakness and loss of excitability are a consequence of a depolarizing block of the muscle-fiber membrane. A detailed study of the electrical properties of the muscle membrane in a biopsy sample indicated that in hypokalemic periodic paralysis, the muscle cell was unable to maintain a normal membrane resting potential [178].

These studies suggest a defect in the muscle membrane in both syndromes. In both forms of periodic paralysis, muscle samples obtained between attacks demonstrated normal $(Na^+ + K^+)$-ATPase activity [179]. In addition, in vivo studies on patients with hypokalemic periodic paralysis have shown that between attacks the muscle membrane resting potential may be normal. The work of Engel and Lambert [180] showed that, in hypokalemic periodic paralysis, a paralyzed muscle fiber with the sarcolemma removed can be made to contract by applying calcium directly to the myofibrils. Those studies also indicate that the defect is confined to the muscle membrane and that the molecular mechanism of contraction is intact at the time that paralysis is present. Cardiac arrhythmias have been reported in both syndromes.

Other studies suggest that reversible alterations take place in the sarcoplasmic reticulum membrane during paralysis. Six patients with hypokalemic periodic paralysis were investigated [181–183] and muscle samples obtained during episodes of paralysis. The sarcoplasmic reticulum fraction was isolated from muscle homogenates. The calcium pump ATPase and the calcium-uptake activities were depressed below control values. In one case, it was noted that the amount of sarcoplasmic reticulum was decreased by 50 percent. Studies repeated after patients' recovery from paralysis

showed that the depressed sarcoplasmic reticulum activities had returned toward normal [181].

Although both syndromes seem to involve a pathological change in the muscle membrane, the processes that lead to paralysis in each case appear to be quite different. Potassium ingestion provokes an attack in one patient, and lowering serum potassium provokes an attack in another. Hyperkalemic attacks are less severe and frequent under high-sodium intake and are increased by a low-sodium diet. Hypokalemic attacks are improved by a low-sodium diet and aggravated by high-sodium intake. However, both forms respond with decreased attacks when a diuretic such as acetazolamide is administered.

Glycogen Storage Diseases

In 1952, Cori and Cori [184] demonstrated a specific deficiency of glucose 6-phosphatase in a patient with hepatic form of glycogen storage disease. At present, at least eight groups of inherited glycogen metabolism abnormalities can be defined clinically or biochemically [185]. The inability to metabolize glycogen to lactate can result in a wide variety of clinical problems, depending upon the organ or tissue involved. Muscle is known to be involved in five forms of glycogen storage disease. In types II, V, and VII the muscle symptoms are the sole or predominant manifestation of the disease; in the other two forms, types III and IV, the clinical picture is dominated by liver dysfunction. Additional discussions of glycogen metabolism are found in Chaps. 17 and 29.

TYPE II GLYCOGEN STORAGE DISEASE

Two forms of type II glycogen storage disease have been recognized—the early infantile and the late-onset varieties. In both clinical forms, an acid maltase deficiency has been demonstrated. In the infantile generalized form, the disease is rapidly progressive and death occurs usually before age one. The inheritance pattern appears to be autosomal recessive. Glycogen is increased in muscle, liver, heart, glial cells, the nuclei of brainstem, and anterior horn cells of the spinal cord. With the marked involvement of all these tissues, the clinical disorder presents as a profound weakness attributable to both motor neuron and muscle disease, cardiomegaly with heart failure, and, in some cases, macroglossia. The later-onset forms of the disease could occur in childhood [186–191] or adult life [190–193], and with very few exceptions they are limited to skeletal muscle, simulating muscular dystrophy or polymyositis, with no cardiac or neuronal disorder. Weakness, generally of trunk and proximal limb muscles, is slowly progressive, but involvement of respiratory muscles may cause severe ventilatory insufficiency in about 50 percent of cases [191–193]. These patients show elevated serum creatine phosphokinase, an electromyogram consistent with myotonic discharges in the absence of clinical myotonia, and vacuolar myopathy with an increase in glycogen content.

Urinary excretion of acid maltase is markedly reduced in patients and heterozygotes with late onset acid maltase deficiency [194]. In 1961, Hers [195] demonstrated that tissues from normal persons contain an α-1,4-glucosidase (acid maltase) and that this enzyme is absent in patients with type II glycogen storage disease. Formulating the general concept of inborn lysosomal diseases, Hers stated that the normal mechanism of cellular renewal begins by a process wherein portions of cytoplasm are surrounded by a membrane and physically isolated from the rest of the cell within an autophagic vacuole, or autophagosome. When the autophagic vacuole merges with a primary lysosome containing several acid hydrolases, the autophagic vacuole is transformed into a digestive vacuole. Once all the components of the sequestered cytoplasm have been digested by the appropriate hydrolases, small molecules pass through the lysosomal membrane and are reutilized by the cell; undigested material is retained within residual or dense bodies. In acid maltase deficiency, electron-microscope studies have shown the presence of two fractions of glycogen, one freely dispersed within the cell and the other segregated in vacuoles surrounded by a single membrane.

Detailed morphological examination at autopsy reveals an excessive accumulation of glycogen within a number of organs, including muscle and motor neurons. Glycogen is found free within the cytoplasm, autophagic vacuoles, or lysosomes. The glycogen-loaded cells then die. This explanation, however, is not adequate. Muscle tissue does not normally possess high quantities of lysosomes. The normal degradation of glycogen to glucose 1-phosphate occurs outside of lysosomes and involves enzymes other than acid maltase. The questions that remain unanswered are, Why does the glycogen not surrounded by a membrane accumulate within cells and why is it not degraded through the normal glycogenolytic pathways of the cytoplasm?

Another question concerns the biochemical basis for observed differences between infantile and late-onset acid maltase deficiency cases. In this regard, Angelini and Engel [196, 197] found decreased neutral maltase activity in several tissues from infantile, but not late-onset, acid maltase deficiency. In other studies, Dreyfus and coworkers [198, 199] reported electrophoretic studies suggesting the presence of abnormal isozymes of acid maltase. Mehler and DiMauro [194], using a very sensitive fluorometric assay, found some residual acid maltase activity in muscle from 15 cases with late-onset acid maltase deficiency, but no enzyme activity in 3 infantile cases. The residual activity was 3 to 12 percent of normal and was electrophoretically and kinetically normal. Leukocyte acid maltase is either normal [188, 201] or partially reduced [193, 197, 200] in late-onset acid maltase deficiency cases but is undetectable in the infantile form [201].

Several different therapeutic strategies have been tried, particularly in the infantile form, including labilization of lysosomes, stimulation of glycogenolysis, and enzyme replacement; in no instance was any significant clinical improvement made.

TYPE V GLYCOGEN STORAGE DISEASE (McARDLE'S DISEASE)

The clinical symptoms of patients with McArdle's disease depend on their ages and the severity of the case [185]. From childhood to adolescence, the patients may have few complaints, save increased fatigability. Between 20 and 40 years of age, severe cramps and myoglobinuria develop when patients exercise strenuously. Characteristically, they can carry on moderate exercise over a short period with no problem. If, however, a sudden, vigorous exercise is carried out, they experience muscle stiffness and aching. In association with this cramping and stiffness, the serum levels of such enzymes as creatine phosphokinase, lactate dehydrogenase, and aldolase, as well as myoglobin, rise dramatically, indicating either some membrane incompetence or necrosis of muscle cells. The myoglobinuria may be a severe enough complication to cause renal shutdown. The cramp induced with exercise in McArdle's disease is electrically silent and, therefore, fits the physiological definition of contracture. If patients with McArdle's syndrome continue to exercise after the appearance of fatigue and cramps, the discomfort may disappear as the patient appears to get his "second wind"; increased mobilization of free fatty acids that provide the muscle with alternative fuel and increased blood flow to the exercising muscle may be the basis for this second wind [202, 203]. Patients over age 40 may have progressive wasting and weakness of muscles [204–206].

This disorder was first delineated clinically by McArdle in 1951 when he studied a patient who had no increase in venous blood lactate during ischemic arm exercise [207]. He suggested that a defect was present in the degradation of glycogen to lactate. Subsequently, Mommaerts and coworkers [208] and Schmid and coworkers [205] demonstrated the lack of muscle phosphorylase in this form of glycogen storage disease. Clinical evaluation of these patients with McArdle's disease revealed that ischemic arm exercise does not cause the normal increases in venous blood lactate, that the induced cramp is electrically silent, and that muscle cells accumulate normal glycogen in the sarcoplasm.

Both contracture and myoglobinuria in McArdle's disease are attributed to a critical shortage of ATP during strenuous exercise, as much of the energy for normal muscle contraction derives from glycogen. A deficiency of ATP would impair muscle relaxation by inhibiting the ATP-dependent calcium uptake by the sarcoplasmic reticulum. A more severe depletion of ATP could alter the

integrity of cell membranes with the resultant leakage of myoglobin and enzymes into the serum. The pathogenetic mechanism, however, has not been verified experimentally, and in one study of two patients the concentration of ATP did not change before and during contracture [209]. Alterations were noted, however, in creatine phosphate, creatine, and inorganic phosphate. Permanent damage to the sarcoplasmic reticulum membranes apparently does not accompany a contracture, because calcium uptake or ATPase activities were not found defective in sarcoplasmic reticulum fractions isolated from contractured muscle [210].

McArdle's disease is not a single genetic entity. Although most cases are inherited in an autosomal-recessive manner, one family had this illness transmitted as an autosomal dominant [211], and the genetic basis for the striking prevalence of male patients (4:1) needs to be explained. Further genetic heterogeneity is demonstrated with immunological methods aimed at detecting the phosphorylase protein. In some patients, no enzyme protein was detectable [212–215], whereas in others the enzyme protein was present, although inactive or only partially active [213–215]. Another puzzle is the histochemical demonstration of phosphorylase activity in regenerating cultured muscle fibers from three patients with McArdle's disease [216].

Several therapeutic measures have attempted to bypass the metabolic block and provide muscle with glycolytic fuels. These approaches have not been successful.

TYPE VII GLYCOGEN STORAGE DISEASE

The type VII syndrome is characterized biochemically by a defect in muscle phosphofructokinase (PFK) and is similar to McArdle's syndrome. Since the first case described by Tarui [217], a total of six cases have been reported [217–220]. The clinical picture is one of exercise intolerance, contractures, and myoglobinuria. As is the case in McArdle's disease, a second-wind phenomenon occurs and ischemic exercise results in no increase in venous lactate. Muscle morphology and the degree of glycogen accumulation are also similar in the two diseases. The diagnosis may be suggested by erythrocyte studies, because a partial defect of red blood cell PFK has been found. In normal red blood cells, PFK is composed of both muscle type (M) and red blood cell type (R) subunits. In patients with phosphofructokinase deficiency in muscle, the M subunits are lacking, and because of this partial defect, a mild hemolytic tendency is noted in the red blood cells. Hexosemonophosphate intermediates that precede the metabolic block, including glucose 6-phosphate and fructose 6-phosphate, accumulate; hexosediphosphates, such as fructose 1,6-diphosphate, distal to the block, are diminished [217–220].

A reduction of the muscle form of phosphofructokinase in erythrocytes of parents, the occurrence of the disease in siblings of both sexes, and consanguinity in one set of parents, suggest an autosomal-recessive inheritance.

References

1. Huxley, H. E. Molecular Basis of Contraction in Cross-Striated Muscle. In G. H. Bourne (ed.), *The Structure and Function of Muscle*. New York: Academic, 1972. Vol. 2, pp. 301–387.
2. Franzini-Armstrong, C. Membranous Systems in Muscle Fibers. In G. H. Bourne (ed.), *The Structure and Function of Muscle*. New York: Academic, 1972. Vol. 2, pp. 531–691.
3. Squire, J. M. Muscle filament structure and muscle contraction. *Annu. Rev. Biophys. Bioeng.* 4:137–163, 1975.
4. Homsher, E., and Kean, C. J. Skeletal muscle energetics and muscle metabolism. *Annu. Rev. Physiol.* 40:93–131, 1978.
5. Tada, M., Yamamoto, T., and Tonomura, Y. Molecular mechanism of active calcium transport by sarcoplasmic reticulum. *Physiol. Rev.* 58:1–79, 1978.
6. Taylor, E. W. Mechanism of actomyosin ATPase and the problem of muscle contraction. *Crit. Rev. Biochem.* 6:103–164, 1979.
7. Huxley, H. E., and Hanson, J. Changes in the cross-striations of muscle during contraction and stretch and their structural interpretations. *Nature* 173:973–976, 1954.
8. Huxley, A. F., and Niedergerke, R. Structural changes in muscle during contraction. *Nature* 173:971–973, 1954.
9. Starr, R., and Offer, G. Interaction of C protein with HMM and subfragment 2. *Biochem. J.* 171:813–816, 1978.
10. Ebashi, S., Endo, M., and Ohtsuki, I. Control of muscle contraction. *Q. Rev. Biophys.* 2:351–384, 1969.
11. Greaser, M., and Gergely, J. Reconstitution of troponin activity from three protein components. *J. Biol. Chem.* 246:4226–4233, 1971.
12. Trinick, J., and Lowey, S. M-protein from chicken pectoralis muscle: Isolation and characterization. *J. Mol. Biol.* 113:343–368, 1977.
13. Sugita, H., et al. Staining of the nemaline rod by fluorescent antibody against α-actinin. *Proc. Jpn. Acad.* 50:237–240, 1974.
14. Granger, D. L. and Lazarides, E. The existence of an insoluble Z disc scaffold in chicken skeletal muscle. *Cell* 15:1253–1268, 1978.
15. Goldman, R. D., et al. Cytoplasmic fibers in mammalian cells: Cytoskeletal and contractile elements. *Annu. Rev. Physiol.* 41:703–722, 1979.
16. Guba, F., Harsanyi, V., and Vajda, E. The muscle protein fibrillin. *Acta Biochim. Biophys. Acad. Sci. Hung.* 3:353–365, 1978.
17. McNeal, P., and Hoyle, C. Evidence for superthin filaments. *Am. Zool.* 7:483–498, 1967.
18. Maruyama, K., et al. Connectin. An elastic protein of muscle. Characterization and function. *J. Biochem. Tokyo* 82:317–338, 1977.
19. Hanson, J., and Lowy, J. The structure of F-actin and of actin filaments isolated from muscle. *J. Mol. Biol.* 6:46–60, 1963.
20. Elzinga, M., et al. Complete amino acid sequence of actin of rabbit skeletal muscle. *Proc. Natl. Acad. Sci. U.S.A.* 70:2687–2691, 1973.
21. Elzinga, M., Maron, B. J., Adelstein, R. S. Human heart and platelet actins are products of different genes. *Science* 191:94–95, 1976.
22. Vanderkerckhove, J., and Weber, K. At least six different actins are expressed in a higher mammal: An analysis based on the amino acid sequence of the amino terminal peptide. *J. Mol. Biol.* 126:783–802, 1978.
23. Straub, F. B., and Feuer, G. Adenosine triphosphate: The functional group of actin. *Biochim. Biophys. Acta* 4:455–470, 1950.
24. Martonosi, A., Gouvea, M. A., and Gergely, J. Studies on actin. III. G–F transformation of actin and muscular contraction (experiments in vivo). *J. Biol. Chem.* 235:1707–1710, 1960.
25. Lowey, S., et al. Substructure of the myosin molecule. I. Subfragments of myosin by enzymatic degradation. *J. Mol. Biol.* 42:1–29, 1969.
26. Trayer, I. P., Harris, C. I., and Perry, S. V. 3-Methylhistidine and adult and fetal forms of skeletal muscle myosin. *Nature* 217:452–453, 1968.
27. Huszar, G., and Elzinga, M. ε-N-methyllysine in myosin. *Nature* 223:834–835, 1969.

28. Kuehl, W. M., and Adelstein, R. S. The absence of 3-methylhistidine in red, cardiac, and fetal myosin. *Biochem. Biophys. Res. Commun.* 39: 956–964, 1970.

29. Watkins, C. A., and Morgan, H. E. Relationship between rates of methylation and synthesis of heart protein. *J. Biol. Chem.* 254:693–701, 1979.

30. Haverberg, L. M., et al. Myofibrillar protein turnover and urinary N-methylhistidine output. Response to dietary supply of protein and energy. *Biochem. J.* 152:503–510, 1975.

31. Sarkar, S., Sreter, F. A., and Gergely, J. Light chains of myosins from fast, slow, and cardiac muscles. *Proc. Natl. Acad. Sci. U.S.A.* 68:946–950, 1971.

32. Frank, G., and Weeds, A. G. The amino acid sequence of some alkali light chains of rabbit skeletal muscle myosin. *Eur. J. Biochem.* 44:317–334, 1974.

33. Sarkar, S. Stoichiometry and sequential removal of light chains of myosin. *Cold Spring Harbor Symp. Quant. Biol.* 37:14–17, 1972.

34. Holt, J. C., and Lowey, S. Distribution of alkali light chains in myosin: Isolation of isozymes. *Biochemistry* 16:4398–4403, 1977.

35. Hoh, J. F. Y., and Yeoh, G. P. S. Rabbit skeletal myosin isoenzymes from fetal, fast-twitch and slow-twitch muscles. *Nature* 280:321–322, 1979.

36. Pires, E. M. V., and Perry, S. V. Purification and properties of myosin light chain kinase from fast skeletal muscle. *Biochem. J.* 167:137–146, 1977.

37. Yagi, K., et al. Identification of an activator protein for myosin light chain kinase as the Ca^{2+}-dependent modulator protein. *J. Biol. Chem.* 253: 1338–1340, 1978.

38. Sherry, J. M. F., et al. Roles of calcium and phosphorylation in the regulation of the activity of gizzard myosin. *Biochemistry* 17, 4411–4418, 1978.

39. Ebashi, S., et al. The regulatory role of calcium in muscle. *Ann. N.Y. Acad. Sci.* 307:451–461, 1978.

40. Malhotra, A., Huang, S., and Bhan, A. Subunit function in cardiac myosin: Effect of removal of LC_2 (18,000 molecular weight) on enzymatic properties. *Biochemistry* 18:461–467, 1979.

41. Barany, K., et al. Phosphorylation-dephosphorylation of the 18,000 dalton light chain of myosin during the contraction-relaxation cycle of frog muscle. *J. Biol. Chem.* 254:3617–3623, 1979.

42. Wagner, P. D., et al. Studies on the actin activation of myosin. Subfragment-1 isozymes and the role of myosin light chains. *Eur. J. Biochem.* 99: 385–412, 1979.

43. Pepe, F. A. The myosin filament: II. Interaction between myosin and actin filaments observed using antibody staining in fluorescent and electron microscopy. *J. Mol. Biol.* 27:227–236, 1967.

44. Huxley, H. E. The mechanism of muscle contraction. *Science* 164:1356–1366, 1969.

45. Huxley, H. E., and Brown, W. The low-angle X-ray diagram of vertebrate striated muscle and its behaviour during contraction and rigor. *J. Mol. Biol.* 30:383–434, 1967.

46. Mendelson, R. A., Morales, M. F., and Botts, J. Segmental flexibility of the S-1 moiety of myosin. *Biochemistry* 12:2250–2255, 1973.

47. Thomas, D. D., Seidel, J. C., Hyde, J. S., and Gergely, J. Motion of subfragment 1 in myosin and its supramolecular complexes: Saturation transfer electron paramagnetic resonance. *Proc. Natl. Acad. Sci. U.S.A.* 72:1729–1733, 1975.

48. Highsmith, S., et al. Flexibility of myosin rod, light meromyosin and myosin subfragment 2 in solution. *Proc. Natl. Acad. Sci. U.S.A.* 74:4986–4990, 1977.

49. Tregear, R. T., and Squire, J. M. Myosin content and filament structure in smooth and striated muscle. *J. Mol. Biol.* 77:279–290, 1978.

50. Morimoto, K., and Harrington, W. F. Substructure of the thick filament of vertebrate striated muscle. *J. Mol. Biol.* 83:83–97, 1974.

51. Engelhardt, W. A., and Ljubimova, M. N. Myosin and adenosine triphosphatase. *Nature* 144: 668–669, 1939.

52. Ebashi, S., Endo, M., and Ohtsuki, I. Control of muscle contraction. *Q. Rev. Biophys.* 4:351–384, 1969.

53. Greaser, M. L., et al. Troponin subunits and their interactions. *Cold Spring Harbor Symp. Quant. Biol.* 37:235–244, 1972.

54. Potter, J. D., and Gergely, J. Troponin, tropomyosin and actin interactions in the Ca^{2+} regulation of muscle contraction. *Biochemistry* 13:2697–2703, 1974.

55. Hitchcock, S. E. Regulation of muscle contraction: Binding of troponin and its components of actin and tropomyosin. *Eur. J. Biochem.* 52:255–263, 1975.

56. Haselgrove, J. C. X-ray evidence for a conformational change in the actin-containing filaments of vertebrate striated muscle. *Cold Spring Harbor Symp. Quant. Biol.* 37:341–352, 1972.

57. Huxley, H. E. Structural changes in the actin- and myosin-containing filaments during contraction. *Cold Spring Harbor Symp. Quant. Biol.* 37:361–376, 1972.

58. Potter, J. D., and Gergely, J. The calcium- and magnesium-binding sites on troponin and their role in the regulation of muscle contraction. *J. Biol. Chem.* 250:4628–4633, 1975.

59. Perry, S. V. The regulation of contractile activity in muscle. *Biochem. Soc. Trans.* 7:593–617, 1979.

60. Mak, A., Smillie, L. B., and Barany, M. Specific phosphorylation at serine-283 of α-tropomyosin from skeletal and rabbit skeletal and cardiac muscle. *Proc. Natl. Acad. Sci. U.S.A.* 75:3588–3592, 1978.

61. MacLennan, D. H. Resolution of the calcium transport system of sarcoplasmic reticulum. *Can. J. Biochem.* 53:251–261, 1975.

62. MacLennan, D. H., et al. Assembly of Sarcoplasmic Reticulum. In S. Fleischer et al. (eds.), *The Molecular Biology of Membranes.* New York: Plenum, 1978. Pp. 309–320.

63. Martonosi, A., et al. The biosynthesis of sarcoplasmic reticulum. *Fed. Proc.* 1981.

64. Hill, A. V. The effect of load on the heat of shortening of muscle. *Proc. Roy. Soc. Lond. (Biol.) Ser. B* 159:297–318, 1964.

65. Hill, A. V. The variation of total heat production in a twitch with velocity of shortening. *Proc. Roy. Soc. Lond. (Biol.) Ser. B* 159:596–605, 1964.

66. Cain, D. F., and Davies, R. E. Breakdown of adenosine triphosphate during a single contraction of working muscle. *Biochem. Biophys. Res. Commun.* 18:361–366, 1962.

67. Gilbert, C., Kretzschmar, K. M., and Wilkie, D. R. Heat, work, and phosphocreatine splitting during muscular contraction. *Cold Spring Harbor Symp. Quant. Biol.* 37:613–618, 1972.

68. Gordon, A. M., Huxley, A. F., and Julian, F. J. The variation in isometric tension with sarcomere lengths in vertebrate muscle fibers. *J. Physiol. (London)* 184:170–192, 1966.

69. Reedy, M. K., Holmes, K. C., and Tregear, R. T. Induced changes in orientation of the cross bridges of glycerinated insect flight muscle. *Nature* 207:1276–1280, 1965.

70. Tonomura, Y., and Inoue, A. Energy Transducing Mechanisms in Muscle. In E. Racker (ed.), *Energy Transducing Mechanisms.* London: Butterworth, 1975. Pp. 121–161.

71. Huxley, A. F. Muscular contraction. *J. Physiol. (London)* 243:1–43, 1974.

72. Eisenberg, E., and Hill, T. L. A cross-bridge model of muscle contraction. *Prog. Biophys. Mol. Biol.* 33:55–82, 1978.

73. Cohen, P. The role of cyclic AMP–dependent protein kinase in the regulation of glycogen metabolism in mammalian skeletal muscle. *Curr. Top. Cell. Regul.* 14:117–196, 1978.

74. Cohen, P., et al. Identification of the Ca^{2+}-dependent modulator protein as the fourth subunit of rabbit skeletal muscle phosphorylase kinase. *FEBS Lett.* 92:287–293, 1978.

75. Mansour, T. E. Phosphofructokinase. *Curr. Top. Cell. Regul.* 5:1–46.

76. Pettigrew, D. W., and Frieden, C. Rabbit muscle phosphofructokinase. A model for regulatory kinase behaviour. *J. Biol. Chem.* 254:1876–1901, 1979.

77. Heywood, S. M., and Rich, A. In vitro synthesis of native myosin, actin, and tropomyosin from embryonic chick polysomes. *Proc. Natl. Acad. Sci. U.S.A.* 59:590–597, 1968.

78. Sarkar, S., and Cooke, P. In vitro synthesis of light and heavy polypeptide chains of myosin. *Biochem. Biophys. Res. Commun.* 41:918–925, 1970.

79. Low, R. B., Vournakis, J. N., and Rich, A. Identification of separate polysomes active in the synthesis of the light and heavy chains of myosin. *Biochemistry* 10:1813–1818, 1971.

80. Mondal, H., et al. Highly purified mRNA for myosin heavy chain:size and polyadenylic acid content. *Biochem. Biophys. Res. Commun.* 56:988–996, 1974.

81. Hunter, T., and Garrels, J. I. Characterization of the mRNAs for α- and β- and γ-actin. *Cell* 12:767–781, 1977.

82. Heywood, S. M., Kennedy, D. S., and Bester, A. J. Stored myosin messenger in embryonic chick muscle. *FEBS Lett.* 53:69–72, 1975.

83. Patterson, B. M., and Bishop, J. O. Changes in the mRNA population of chick myoblasts during myogenesis in vitro. *Cell* 12:751–765, 1977.

84. Dym, H. P., Kennedy, D. S., and Heywood, S. M. Subcellular distribution of the cytoplasmic myosin heavy chain mRNA. *Differentiation* 12:145–155, 1979.

85. Morales, M. F., et al. Creatine and Muscle Protein Synthesis. In A. T. Milhorat (ed.), *International Conference on Exploratory Concepts in Muscular Dystrophy.* II. New York: Elsevier, 1974. Pp. 212–220.

86. Hammond, G. L., Wizben, E., and Markert, C. L. Molecular signals for initiating protein synthesis in organ hypertrophy. *Proc. Natl. Acad. Sci. U.S.A.* 76:2455–2459, 1979.

87. Close, R. I. Specialization among fast-twitch muscles. In A. T. Milhorat (ed.), *International Conference on Exploratory Concepts in Muscular Dystrophy.* II. New York: Elsevier, 1974. Pp. 309–316.

88. Kaplan, N. O., and Goodfriend, J. L. Role of the types of lactic dehydrogenase. *Enzyme Regul.* 2:203–212, 1964.

89. Sreter, F. A., Seidel, J. C., and Gergely, J. Studies on myosin from red and white skeletal muscle of the

rabbit. I. Adenosine triphosphate activity. *J. Biol. Chem.* 241:5772–5776, 1966.

90. Barany, M. Activation of myosin correlated with speed of muscle shortening. *J. Gen. Physiol.* 50:197–216, 1967.

91. Nakamura, A., Sreter, F., and Gergely, J. Comparative studies of light meromyosin paracrystals derived from red, white, and cardiac muscle myosins. *J. Cell Biol.* 49:883–898, 1971.

92. Dhoot, G. K., and Perry, S. V. Distribution of polymorphic forms of troponin components and tropomyosin in skeletal muscle. *Nature* 238:714–718, 1979.

93. Edjtehadi, G. D., and Lewis, D. M. Histochemical reactions of fibres in a fast twitch muscle of the cat. *J. Physiol.* (London) 207:439–453, 1979.

94. Brooke, M. H., and Kaiser, K. K. Muscle fiber type: How many and what kind. *Arch. Neurol.* 23:369–379, 1979.

95. Gauthier, G. F., and Lowey, S. Distribution of myosin isoenzymes among skeletal muscle fiber types. *J. Cell Biol.* 81:10–25, 1979.

96. Arndt, L., and Pepe, F. Antigenic specificity of red and white muscle myosin. *J. Histochem. Cytochem.* 23:159–168, 1975.

97. Weeds, A., Hall, R., and Spurway, N. Characterization of myosin light chains from histochemically identified fibers of rabbit psoas muscle. *FEBS Lett.* 49:320–324, 1975.

98. Buller, A. J., Eccles, J. C., and Eccles, R. M. Interactions between motoneurons and muscles in respect of the characteristic speeds of their responses. *J. Physiol.* 150:417–439, 1960.

99. Buller, A. J., Mommaerts, W. F. H. M., and Seraydarian, K. Enzymatic properties of myosin in fast- and slow-twitch muscles of the cat following cross-innervation. *J. Physiol.* (London) 205:581–597, 1969.

100. Barany, M., and Close, R. I. The transformation of myosin in cross-reinnervated rat muscle. *J. Physiol.* (London) 213:458–474, 1971.

101. Sreter, F. A., Gergely, J., and Luff, A. L. The effect of cross reinnervation on the synthesis of myosin light chains. *Biochem. Biophys. Res. Commun.* 56:84–89, 1974.

102. Weeds, A. G., et al. Myosin from cross-reinnervated cat muscles. *Nature* 247:135–139, 1974.

103. Dubowitz, V. Cross-innervated mammalian skeletal muscle. Histochemical, physiological, and biochemical observations. *J. Physiol.* (London) 193:481–496, 1967.

104. Romanul, F. C. A., and Van Der Meulen, J. P. Slow and fast muscles after cross innervation:

enzymatic and physiological changes. *Arch. Neurol.* 17:387–402, 1967.

105. Guth, L., Watson, P. K., and Brown, W. C. Effects of cross reinnervation on some chemical properties of red and white muscles of rat and cat. *Exp. Neurol.* 20:52–69, 1968.

106. Mommaerts, W. F. H. M., Buller, A. J., and Seraydarian, K. The modification of some biochemical properties of muscle by cross-innervation. *Proc. Natl. Acad. Sci. U.S.A.* 64:128–133, 1969.

107. Guth, L. Trophic influences of nerve on muscle. *Physiol. Rev.* 48:645–687, 1968.

108. Drachman, D. B. Trophic actions of the neuron: An introduction. *Ann. N. Y. Acad. Sci.* 238:3–5, 1974.

109. Salmons, S., and Vrbova, G. The influence of activity on some contractile characteristics of mammalian fast and slow muscle. *J. Physiol.* (London) 201:535–549, 1969.

110. Salmons, S., and Sreter, F. A. Impulse activity in the transformation of skeletal muscle type. *Nature* 263:30–34, 1976.

111. Romanul, F. C. A., et al. The effect of a changed pattern of activity on histochemical characteristics of muscle fibers. In A. T. Milhorat (ed.), *International Conference on Exploratory Concepts in Muscular Dystrophy.* II. New York: Elsevier, 1974. Pp. 344–348.

112. Pette, D., et al. Effects of long-term electrical stimulation on some contractile and metabolic characteristics of fast rabbit muscles. *Pflügers Arch.* 338:257–272, 1973.

113. Heilmann, C., and Pette, D. Molecular transformations in sarcoplasmic reticulum of fast-twitch muscle by electrostimulation. *Eur. J. Biochem.* 93:437–446, 1979.

114. Rubinstein, N., et al. Use of type-specific antimyosins to demonstrate the transformation of individual fibers in chronically stimulated rabbit fast muscles. *J. Cell Biol.* 79:252–261, 1978.

115. Pette, D., and Schnez, U. Coexistence of fast- and slow-type myosin light chains in single muscle fibers during transformation as induced by long-term stimulation. *FEBS Lett.* 83:128–130, 1977.

116. Guth, L., and Wells, J. B. Physiological and histochemical properties of the soleus muscle after denervation of its antagonists. *Exp. Neurol.* 51:310–325, 1976.

117. Samaha, F. J., and Theis, W. H. Actomyosin changes in muscles with altered function. *Exp. Neurol.* 51:310–325, 1976.

118. Walton, J. N. (ed.). *Disorders of Voluntary Muscle* (4th ed.). London: Churchill, 1981.

119. Pennington, R. J. T. Serum Enzymes. In L. P. Rowland (ed.), *Pathogenesis of Human Muscular Dystrophies.* Amsterdam: Excerpta Medica, 1977. Pp. 341–350.

120. Albers, M. C., and Samaha, F. J. Serum pyruvate kinase in muscle disease and carrier states. *Neurology* (Minneapolis) 24:462–464, 1974.

121. Ionasescu, V., et al. Identification of carriers of Duchenne muscular dystrophy by muscle protein synthesis. *Neurology* (Minneapolis) 23:497–502, 1973.

122. Ionasescu, V., et al. Protein synthesis in muscle cultures from patients with Duchenne muscular dystrophy. *Acta Neurol. Scand.* 54:241–247, 1976.

123. Mokri, B., and Engel, A. G. Duchenne dystrophy: Electron microscopic findings pointing to a basic or early abnormality in the plasma membrane of the muscle. *Neurology* (Minneapolis) 25:111–1120, 1975.

124. Schotland, D. L., Bonilla, E., and Wakayama, Y. Application of a freeze-fracture technique to the study of human neuromuscular disease. *Muscle Nerve* 3:21–27, 1980.

125. Mawatari, S., Miranda, A., and Rowland, L. P. Adenyl cyclase abnormality in Duchenne muscular dystrophy: Muscle cells in culture. *Neurology* (Minneapolis) 26:1021–1026, 1976.

126. Susheela, A. K., et al. Adenyl cyclase activity in Duchenne dystrophic muscle. *J. Neurol. Sci.* 24: 361–363, 1975.

127. Mawatari, S., Schonberg, M., and Olarte, M. Biochemical abnormalities of erythrocyte membranes in Duchenne dystrophy. *Arch. Neurol.* 33:489–493, 1976.

128. Roses, A. D., Herbstreith, M. H., and Appel, S. H. Membrane protein kinase alterations in Duchenne muscular dystrophy. *Nature* 254:350–351, 1975.

129. Roses, A. D., et al. Carrier detection in Duchenne muscular dystrophy. *N. Engl. J. Med.* 294:193–198, 1976.

130. Matheson, D. W., and Howland, J. L. Erythrocyte deformation in human muscular dystrophy. *Science* 184:165–166, 1974.

131. Sugita, H., et al. Biochemical Alterations in Progressive Muscular Dystrophy with Special Reference to the Sarcoplasmica Reticulum. In A. T. Milhonat (ed.), *Exploratory Concepts in Muscular Dystrophy and Related Disorders.* Amsterdam: Excerpta Medica, 1967. Pp. 321–326.

132. Samaha, F. J., and Gergely, J. Biochemical abnormalities of the sarcoplasmic reticulum in muscular dystrophy. *N. Engl. J. Med.* 280:184–188, 1969.

133. Peter, J. B., and Worsfold, M. Muscular dystrophy and other myopathies: Sarcotubular vesicles in early disease. *Biochem. Med.* 2:364–371, 1969.

134. Takagi, A., Schotland, D. L., and Rowland, L. P. Sarcoplasmic reticulum in Duchenne muscular dystrophy. *Arch. Neurol.* 28:380–384, 1973.

135. Peter, J. B., and Worsfold, M. Oxidative phosphorylation and calcium transport by sarcotubular vesicles in myotonic dystrophy. *Biochem. Med.* 2:457–460, 1969.

136. Samaha, F. J., and Congedo, C. Z. Abnormalities in Duchenne dystrophic sarcoplasmic reticulum proteins. *Trans. Am. Neurol. Assoc.* 100:25–30, 1975.

137. Samaha, F. J., and Congedo, C. Z. Two biochemical types of Duchenne dystrophy: Sarcoplasmic reticulum membrane proteins. *Ann. Neurol.* 1:125–130, 1977.

138. Buchthal, F., Schmalbruch, H., and Kamieniecka, Z. Contraction times and fiber types in patients with progressive muscular dystrophy. *Neurology* (Minneapolis) 21:131–139, 1971.

139. Furukawa, T., and Peter, J. B. Superprecipitation and adenosine triphosphatase activity in myosin B in Duchenne muscular dystrophy. *Neurology* (Minneapolis) 21:920–924, 1971.

140. Samaha, F. J. Actomyosin alterations in Duchenne muscular dystrophy. *Arch. Neurol.* 28: 405–407, 1973.

141. Penn, A. S., Cloak, R. A., and Rowland, L. P. Myosin from normal and dystrophic human muscle. *Arch. Neurol.* 27:159–173, 1972.

142. Samaha, F. J. Tropomyosin and troponin in normal and dystrophic human muscle. *Arch. Neurol.* 26:547–550, 1972.

143. Weinstock, I. M., and Iodice, A. A. Acid hydrolase activity in muscular dystrophy and denervation atrophy. In J. T. Dingle and W. B. Fell (eds.), *Lysosomes in Biology and Pathology.* Amsterdam: North-Holland, 1969. Pp. 450–468.

144. McGowan, E. B., Schafig, S. A., and Stracher, A. Delayed degeneration of dystrophic and normal muscle cultures treated with pepstatin, leupeptin, and antipain. *Exp. Neurol.* 50:649–657, 1976.

145. Libby, P., and Goldberg, A. L. Leupeptin, a protease inhibitor, decreases protein degradation in normal and diseased muscle. *Science* 199:534–536, 1978.

146. Huff, T. A., Horton, E. S., and Lebovitz, H. E. Abnormal insulin secretion in myotonic dystrophy. *N. Engl. J. Med.* 277:837–841, 1967.

147. Barbosa, J., et al. Plasma insulin in patients with myotonic dystrophy and their relatives. *Medicine* (Baltimore) 53:307–323, 1974.

148. Pollock, M., and Dyck, P. J. Peripheral nerve morphometry in myotonic dystrophy. *Arch. Neurol.* 33:33–39, 1976.

149. Drachman, D. B., and Fambrough, D. M. Are muscle fibers denervated in myotonic dystrophy? *Arch. Neurol.* 33:358–488, 1976.

150. Winer, N., et al. Induced myotonia in man and goat. *J. Lab. Clin. Med.* 66:758–769, 1965.

151. Peter, J. B., et al. Myotonic induced by diazacholesterol: Increased $(Na^+ + K^+)$-ATPase activity of erythrocyte ghosts and development of cataracts. *Exp. Neurol.* 41:738–744, 1973.

152. Roses, A. D., and Appel, S. J. Protein kinase activity in erythrocyte ghosts of patients with myotonic muscular dystrophy. *Proc. Natl. Acad. Sci. U.S.A.* 70:1855–1859, 1973.

153. Appel, S. H., and Roses, A. D. Membranes and Myotonia. In L. P. Roland (ed.), *Pathogenesis of Human Muscular Dystrophies.* Amsterdam: Excerpta Medica, 1977. Pp. 747–758.

154. Hull, K. L., and Roses, A. D. Stoichiometry of sodium and potassium transport in erythrocytes from patients with myotonic muscular dystrophy. *J. Physiol.* (London) 254:169–181, 1976.

155. Butterfield, D. A., Chesnut, D. B., Roses, A. D., and Appel, S. H. Electron spin resonance studies of erythrocytes from patients with myotonic muscular dystrophy. *Proc. Natl. Acad. Sci. U.S.A.* 71:909–913, 1974.

156. Roses, A. D., et al. Phenytoin and membrane fluidity in myotonic dystrophy. *Arch. Neurol.* 32:535–538, 1975.

157. Luft, R., et al. A case of severe hypermetabolism of non-thyroid origin with a defect in the maintenance of mitochondrial respiratory control: A correlated clinical, biochemical, and morphological study. *J. Clin. Invest.* 41:1776–1804, 1962.

158. Haydar, N. A., et al. Severe hypermetabolism with primary abnormalities of skeletal muscle mitochondria. Functional and therapeutic effects of chloramphenicol treatment. *Ann. Intern. Med.* 74:548–558, 1971. DiMauro, S., et al. Biochemical and ultrastructural studies of mitochondria in Luft's disease: Implications for "mitochondrial myopathies." *Trans. Am. Neurol. Assoc.* 97:265–267, 1973.

159. DiMauro, S., et al. Mitochondrial Myopathies: Which and How Many? In A. T. Milhonat (ed.), *Exploratory Concepts in Muscular Dystrophy.* II. Amsterdam: Excerpta Medica, 1973. Pp. 506–515.

160. DiMauro, S., et al. Fatal infantile mitochondrial myopathy and renal dysfunction due to cytochrome-c-oxidase deficiency. *Neurology* 30:795–804, 1980.

161. Bank, W. J., et al. A disorder of muscle lipid metabolism and myoglobinuria. Absence of carnitine palmityltransferase. *N. Engl. J. Med.* 292:443–449, 1975.

162. Engel, A. S., and Siekert, R. S. Lipid storage myopathy responsive to prednisone. *Arch. Neurol.* 27:174–181, 1972.

163. Engel, A. S., and Angelini, C. Carnitine deficiency of human skeletal muscle with associated lipid storage myopathy: A new syndrome. *Science* 179:899–902, 1973.

164. Engel, A. S., Angelini, C., and Nelson, R. A. Identification of Carnitine Deficiency as a Cause of Human Lipid Storage Myopathy. In A. T. Milhorat (ed.), *Exploratory Concepts in Muscular Dystrophy.* II. Amsterdam: Excerpta Medica, 1974. Pp. 601–617.

165. Markesbery, W. R., et al. Muscle carnitine deficiency. *Arch. Neurol.* 31:320–324, 1974.

166. Van Dyke, D. H., et al. Hereditary carnitine deficiency of muscle. *Neurology* (Minneapolis) 25:154–159, 1975.

167. Jerusalem, F., Spiess, H., and Baumgartner, G. Lipid storage myopathy with normal carnitine levels. *J. Neurol. Sci.* 273–282, 1975.

168. Karpati, G., et al. The syndrome of systematic carnitine deficiency: Clinical, morphological, biochemical, and pathophysiological features. *Neurology* (Minneapolis) 25:16–24, 1975.

169. Smyth, D. P. L., et al. Inborn error of carnitine metabolism ("carnitine deficiency") in man. *Lancet* 1:1198–1199, 1975.

170. Angelini, C., Lucke, S., and Cantarutti, F. Carnitine deficiency of skeletal muscle: Report of a treated case. *Neurology* (Minneapolis) 26:633–637, 1976.

171. Blass, J. P., Kark, R. A. P., and Engel, W. K. Clinical studies of a patient with pyruvate decarboxylate deficiency. *Arch. Neurol.* 25:449–460, 1971.

172. Engel, W. K., et al. A skeletal muscle disorder associated with intermittent symptoms and a possible deficit in lipid metabolism. *N. Engl. J. Med.* 282:697–704, 1970.

173. Chanarin, I., et al. Neutral-lipid storage disease: A new disorder of lipid metabolism. *Br. Med. J.* 1:553–555, 1975.

174. Walton, J. N. (ed.). *Disorders of Voluntary Muscle* (4th ed.). London: Churchill, 1981. Pp. 676–678.

175. Stanbury, J. B., Wyngaarden, J. B., and Frederickson, D. S. (eds.). *The Metabolic Basis of Inherited Disease.* New York: McGraw-Hill, 1972. Pp. 1181–1203.

176. Creutzfeldt, O. D., et al. Muscle membrane potentials in episodic adynamia. *Electroencephalogr. Clin. Neurophysiol.* 15:508–519, 1963.

177. Brooks, J. E. Hyperkalemic periodic paralysis. Intracellular electromyographic studies. *Arch. Neurol.* 20:13–18, 1969.

178. Hofmann, W. W., and Smith, R. A. Hypokalaemic periodic paralysis studied in vitro. *Brain* 93:445–474, 1970.

179. Samaha, F. J. Sodium-potassium adenosine triphosphate in diseased muscle. Studies on periodic paralysis, myasthenia gravis, and Eaton-Lambert syndrome. *Neurology* (Minneapolis) 19:551–552, 1969.

180. Engel, A. G., and Lambert, E. H. Calcium activation of electrically inexcitable muscle fibers in primary hypokalemic periodic paralysis. *Neurology* (Minneapolis) 19:851–858, 1969.

181. Au, K. S., and Yeung, R. T. T. Thyrotoxic periodic paralysis. Periodic variation in muscle calcium pump activity. *Arch. Neurol.* 26:543–546, 1972.

182. Takagi, A., et al. Thyrotoxic periodic paralysis. Function of sarcoplasmic reticulum and muscle glycogen. *Neurology* (Minneapolis) 23:1008–1016, 1973.

183. Ionasescu, V., et al. Hypokalemic periodic paralysis. Low activity of sarcoplasmic reticulum and muscle ribosomes during an induced attack. *J. Neurol. Sci.* 21:419–429, 1974.

184. Cori, G. T., and Cori, C. F. Glucose-6-phosphatase of the liver in glycogen storage disease. *J. Biol. Chem.* 199:661–667, 1952.

185. Stanbury, J. B., Wyngaarden, J. B., and Frederickson, D. S. (eds.). *The Metabolic Basis of Inherited Disease.* New York: McGraw-Hill, 1972.

186. Curtecuisse, V., et al. Glycogenose musculaire par deficit d-alpha-1,4-glycosidase simulant une dystrophie musculaire progressive. *Arch. Fr. Pediatr.* 22:1153–1164, 1965.

187. Zellweger, H., et al. A mild form of muscular glycogenosis in two brothers with alpha-1, 4-glucosidase deficiency. *Ann. Paediatr.* 205:413–437, 1965.

188. Roth, J. C., and Williams, H. E. The muscular variant of Pompe's disease. *J. Pediatr.* 71:567–573, 1967.

189. Swaiman, K. F., Kenneth, W. R., and Sauls, H. S. Late infantile acid maltase deficiency. *Arch. Neurol.* 18:642–648, 1968.

190. Hudgson, P., et al. Adult myopathy from glycogen storage disease due to acid maltase deficiency. *Brain* 91:435–462, 1968.

191. Engel, A. G., et al. The spectrum and diagnosis of acid maltase deficiency. *Neurology* (Minneapolis) 23:95–106, 1973.

192. Engel, A. G. Acid maltase deficiency in adults: Studies in four cases of a syndrome which may mimic muscular dystrophy or other myopathies. *Brain* 93:599–616, 1970.

193. Chou, S. M., et al. Adult-type acid maltase deficiency: Pathological features. *Neurology* (Minneapolis) 24:394, 1974.

194. Mehler, M., and DiMauro, S. Late-onset acid maltase deficiency: Detection of patients and heterozygotes by urinary enzyme assay. *Arch. Neurol.* 33:692–695, 1976.

195. Hers, H. G. Alpha-glucosidase deficiency in generalized glycogen storage disease (Pompe's). *Biochem. J.* 86:11–21, 1963.

196. Angelini, C., and Engel, A. G. Subcellular distribution of acid and neutral α-glucosidases in normal, acid maltase–deficient, and myophosphorylase-deficient human skeletal muscle. *Arch. Biochem. Biophys.* 156:350–355, 1973.

197. Angelini, C., and Engel, A. G. Comparative study of acid maltase deficiency. *Arch. Neurol.* 26:344–349, 1972.

198. Dreyfus, J. C., and Alexandre, Y. Electrophoretic characterization of acidic and neutral amylo-1,4-glucosidase (acid maltase) in human tissues and evidence for two electrophoretic variants in acid maltase deficiency. *Biochem. Biophys. Res. Commun.* 48:914–920, 1972.

199. Dreyfus, J. C., Proux, D., and Alexandre, Y. Molecular studies on glycogen storage diseases. *Enzyme* 18:60–72, 1974.

200. Koster, J. F., Slee, R. G., and Hulsmann, W. C. The use of leukocytes as an aid in the diagnosis of glycogen storage disease type II (Pompe's disease). *Clin. Chim. Acta* 51:319–325, 1974.

201. Illingworth-Brown, B., Brown, D. H., and Jeffrey, P. L. Simultaneous absence of α-1,4-glycosidase and α-1,6-glycosidase activities (pH 4) in tissues of children with type II glycogen storage disease. *Biochemistry* 9:1423–1427, 1970.

202. Porte, D., et al. Cardiovascular and metabolic responses to exercise in a patient with McArdle's syndrome. *N. Engl. J. Med.* 275:406–412, 1966.

203. Pernow, B. B., Havel, R. J., and Jennings, D. B. The second-wind phenomenon in McArdle's syndrome. *Acta Med. Scand.* 472:294–307, 1967.

204. Schmid, R., and Mahler, R. Chronic progressive myopathy with myoglobinuria: Demonstration of a glycogenolytic defect in the muscle. *J. Clin. Invest.* 38:2044–2058, 1959.

205. Schmid, R., and Hammaker, L. Hereditary absence of muscle phosphorylase (McArdle's syndrome). *N. Engl. J. Med.* 264:223–225, 1961.

206. Engel, W. K., Eyerman, E. L., and Williams, H. E. Late-onset type of skeletal muscle phosphorylase deficiency. *N. Engl. J. Med.* 268:135–137, 1963.

207. McArdle, B. Myopathy due to a defect in muscle glycogen breakdown. *Clin. Sci.* 10:13–35, 1951.

208. Mommaerts, W. F. H. M., et al. Functional disorder of muscle associated with the absence of phosphorylase. *Proc. Natl. Acad. Sci. U.S.A.* 45:791–797, 1959.

209. Rowland, L. P., Araki, S., and Carmel, P. Contracture in McArdle's disease. *Arch. Neurol.* 13: 541–544, 1965.

210. Brody, I. A., Gerber, C. J., and Sidbury, J. B. Relaxing factor in McArdle's disease. Calcium uptake by sarcoplasmic reticulum. *Neurology* (Minneapolis) 20:555–558, 1970.

211. Chui, L. A., and Munsat, T. L. Dominant inheritance of McArdle's syndrome. *Arch. Neurol.* 33:636–641, 1976.

212. Rowland, L. P., Fahn, S., and Schotland, D. L. McArdle's disease. *Arch. Neurol.* 9:325–342, 1963.

213. Grunfeld, J. P., et al. Acute renal failure in McArdle's disease. *N. Engl. J. Med.* 286:1237–1241, 1972.

214. Dreyfus, J. C., and Alexandre, Y. Immunological studies on glycogen storage diseases type III and V. Demonstration of the presence of an immunoreactive protein in one case of muscle phosphorylase deficiency. *Biochem. Biophys. Res. Commun.* 44:1364–1370, 1971.

215. Feit, H., and Brooke, M. H. Myophosphorylase deficiency: Two different molecular etiologies. *Neurology* (Minneapolis) 26:963–967, 1976.

216. Roelofs, R. I., Engel, W. K., and Chauvin, P. B. Histochemical phosphorylase activity in regenerating muscle fibers from myophosphorylase-deficient patients. *Science* 177:795–797, 1972.

217. Tarui, S., et al. Phosphofructokinase deficiency in skeletal muscle. A new type of glycogenosis. *Biochem. Biophys. Res. Commun.* 19:517–523, 1965.

218. Layzer, R. B., Rowland, L. P., and Ranney, H. M. Muscle phosphofructokinase deficiency. *Arch. Neurol.* 17:512–523, 1967.

219. Serratrice, G. Forme myopathique du deficit en phosphofructokinase. *Rev. Neurol.* (Paris) 120: 271–277, 1969.

220. Tobin, W. E., et al. Muscle phosphofructokinase deficiency. *Arch. Neurol.* 28:128–130, 1973.

Yujen Edward Hsia
Barry Wolf

Chapter 28. Disorders of Amino Acid Metabolism

Inherited single-gene disorders share a common mechanism. A mutant gene causes quantitative or qualitative abnormalities of gene products. When the protein product controlled by the mutant gene is supposed to serve a metabolic function, the mutation will result in an inborn error of metabolism. These functional errors can arise from defective enzyme or membrane functions.

When the gene is on an autosomal chromosone, generally only a double dose of the mutant gene in a homozygous individual will cause metabolic disease (exceptions are found in type II hyperlipidemia and some of the porphyrias, described later in this chapter), single doses of these mutant autosomal genes being asymptomatic. Hence these are inherited as autosomal recessive disorders that affect either sex, with 25 percent risk to brothers and sisters; both parents are obligatory heterozygotes.

When the gene is on an X chromosome, the heterozygous female carrier may be asymptomatic (or less severely affected, as in ornithine transcarbamylase deficiency); the hemizygous male, who has no compensatory normal gene, is affected, as is the homozygous female (a much rarer occurrence). Hence these are inherited as X-linked recessive disorders, affecting males but transmitted through sisters, mothers and daughters, with 50 percent risk to sons of known female carriers.

Much of intermediary metabolism comprises complex pathways. Interruption of one step by an inherited functional defect can have widespread consequences. If any of the intermediate metabolites of the pathway is necessary for brain metabolism or composition, or has neurotransmitter activity, affected individuals may show neurological disturbances. Knowledge about the disturbed

pathways is critical for effective treatment of these inborn errors. Furthermore, these "experiments" of nature offer unique opportunities to investigate the neurochemical roles of affected metabolites. Accumulation of metabolites prior to the interrupted step can cause toxicity, while depletion of a substance distal to the step can produce symptoms, if the substance is critical for normal function.

The inherited disorders of amino acid metabolism and of their organic acid derivatives [1–4] are illustrated in Figs. 28-1 to 28-4 and 28-8. These illustrations contain almost all the aminoacidopathies of neurological significance, except for those of proline metabolism. Together, these illustrations provide an overall perspective of individual biochemical disorders among the major pathways of intermediary metabolism (for those of carbohydrate metabolism see Chap. 29).

Disturbances of Brain Nutrition and Development

Spongy degeneration and decreased myelination have been demonstrated in patients with several aminoacidopathies [5–7]. This may result from the decreased synthesis of myelin protein, caused by the imbalanced amino acid concentrations seen in these disorders. Whenever the concentration of any single plasma amino acid is significantly altered, the active transport of other individual amino acids across the blood-brain barrier may be seriously imbalanced (Chap. 17). Experimentally, the uptake of labeled amino acids across the blood-brain barrier varies with each amino acid and is strongly influenced by the concentrations of other amino acids. The essential amino acids and tyrosine, precursors of the biogenic amines, are most actively taken up by the brain, whereas the nonessential amino acids, notably those with neurotransmitter properties, such as aspartate, glutamate, and glycine, are taken up least actively [5–8].

Abnormalities of Amino Acid Transport

HARTNUP DISEASE

Hartnup disease is a particularly apt example of systemic amino acid imbalance with indirect nutritional consequences on neurological function. The biochemical lesion in this condition is defective transport of neutral amino acids by the intestinal mucosa and renal tubule. Tryptophan malabsorption and tryptophanuria are prominent features of this condition, but the transport defect involves all the aromatic and neutral amino acids to greater or lesser degree. This lesion can be benign, and individuals with the disorder often remain asymptomatic.

A well-recognized complication of Hartnup disease is a pellagralike syndrome. *Pellagra,* characterized by a photosensitive, erythematous skin rash, gastrointestinal upset, ataxia, emotional disturbances, and dementia, is caused classically by nutritional lack of niacin, a precursor of nicotinamide (Chap. 33). In humans, probably half of the body's requirement for nicotinamide is met from dietary tryptophan, so patients with Hartnup disease are prone to nicotinamide deficiency. Therapeutic doses of niacin will reverse the cutaneous and neurological lesions, confirming that in Hartnup disease the pellagralike syndrome is an indirect consequence of the transport defect. In one case, neuropathological examination revealed cortical and cerebellar atrophy with severe generalized loss of neurons and Purkinje cells [9]. Other transport abnormalities are shown in Table 28-1.

Metabolic Acidosis

Severe metabolic acidosis, often together with ketosis and lactic acidosis [10], occurs in many disturbances of carbohydrate metabolism (Chap. 29) and of amino acid metabolism (Table 28-2). These conditions produce vomiting, altered respiration, clouding of consciousness, and extreme acidosis that leads to irreversible brain damage or to coma and death; chronic acidosis may also result in general debility and malnutritional brain damage. It is conceivable that moderately severe, but brief, periods of acidosis do no permanent harm to the brain. For instance, one child, who succumbed to severe acidosis without being retarded in any way, appeared to have a deficiency of 3-ketoacid CoA-transferase (succinyl-CoA → acetoacetyl-CoA CoA-transferase) (Fig. 28-1, reaction 5). The intense recurrent acidosis suffered by this patient and by patients with pyroglutamic aciduria argue against irreversible short-term neurotoxicity of acidosis per se.

Branched-Chain Amino Acids

In disorders of branched-chain amino acid catabolism (Fig. 28-2), the nonspecific symptoms of acute irritability, hypertonicity, and drowsiness are attributable to severe acidosis or to hyperammonemia, but, for the brain damage, the failure of postnatal myelination may be a common mechanism in several of the disorders [3, 4, 6, 7]. Cerebellar ataxia has been reported in some patients, but not consistently in any single disorder.

MAPLE SYRUP URINE DISEASE

Maple syrup urine disease was the first of this group of disorders to be recognized. The basic enzyme defect is of branched-chain-ketoacid decarboxylase, a multienzyme complex (see Fig. 28-2, reaction 3) analogous to pyruvate dehydrogenase. The intermediate steps are similar and depend on the same cofactors: thiamine pyrophosphate, lipoic acid, nicotinamide adenine dinucleotide, flavine adenine dinucleotide, and coenzyme A. A single enzyme complex appears to serve all three branched-chain amino acids. The classical variant of this disease is usually lethal in early infancy unless treated with restricted intake of leucine, isoleucine, and valine. In untreated patients who survive longer, there is defective myelination, which has been mimicked experimentally in rat cerebellum cultures by exposure to α-ketoisocaproic acid in concentrations comparable to those found in the blood of patients (and in the brain of one patient) with maple syrup urine disease [11]. This same

Table 28-1. Inherited Abnormalties of Amino Acid Transport

Condition	Location of Lesion	Amino Acids Involved	Neurological Features	Comments
Hartnup disease	Intestine and kidney	Tryptophan and neutral amino acids	Ataxia, dementia, psychosis	Causes nicotinamide deficiency
Blue diaper syndrome*	Intestine	Tryptophan	Irritability	Hypercalcemia, indolyluria
Oasthouse urine disease*	Intestine and kidney	Methionine	Seizures, retardation, hyperpnea	White hair, odd smell, α-hydroxybutyric aciduria
Cystinuria	Intestine and kidney	Cysteine and dibasic amino acids	Possible liability to mental illness	Renal stones
Isolated cystinuria	Kidney	Cysteine	Probably benign	—
Pancreatitis and cystine-lysinuria	Kidney	Lysine and cysteine	None	Hereditary pancreatitis
Lysinuric protein intolerance	Intestine and kidney	Dibasic amino acids	Abdominal cramps, hyperammonemia	Occasional growth retardation
Iminoglycinuria	Kidney	Proline, hydroxyproline, and glycine	Benign	—
Glycinuria	Kidney	Glycine	Benign	Kidney oxalate stones
β-Aminoisobutyric aciduria	Kidney	β-Aminoisobutyrate	Benign	A common normal variant
Hyperornithinemia and homocitrullinemia*	Mitochondria	Ornithine	Hyperammonemia	—
Folate malabsorption	Intestine	Pteroylglutamates	Retardation, athetosis, seizures	Megaloblastic anemia
Vitamin B$_{12}$ malabsorption	Intestine	Vitamin B$_{12}$	Growth retardation, risk of brain damage	Megaloblastic anemia
Intrinsic factor deficiency	Intestine	Vitamin B$_{12}$	Growth retardation, risk of brain damage	Megaloblastic anemia
Transcobalamin II deficiency	Extracellular	Vitamin B$_{12}$	Growth retardation, risk of brain damage	Megaloblastic anemia

*Disorders described in only one or two families.

Table 28-2. Disorders of Amino Acids and Organic Acids that Cause Metabolic Acidosis and Are Associated with Neurological Lesions[a]

Condition	Location of Defective Enzyme	Neurological Lesions
Maple syrup urine disease	Fig. 28-2, reaction 3	Hypotonia, rigidity, retardation, failure of myelination
Isovaleric acidemia	Fig. 28-2, reaction 4	Drowsiness, cerebellar ataxia, hyperreflexia, psychomotor retardation
Biotin responsive multiple carboxylase deficiencies	Fig. 28-2, reactions 5, 7 Fig. 28-1, reaction 2	Prostration, irritability, lethargy, seizures, retardation, rash, and alopecia. Hyperammonemia, lactic acidosis in some
β-Ketothiolase deficiency[b]	Fig. 28-2, reaction 6	Retardation, hyperammonemia in one; benign in the second
Acetoacetyl-CoA thiolase deficiency		Retardation, ataxia, chorea, hypotonia, in one girl with lactic acidemia
Propionic acidemia	Fig. 28-2, reaction 7	Lethargy, prostration, seizures, retardation; hyperammonemia in some
Methylmalonic acidemia	Fig. 28-2, reactions 8, 9, 10	As for propionic acidemia
Methylmalonic acidemia with homocystinuria	Fig. 28-2, reaction 6	May have cerebellar lesions, severe brain damage, convulsions
Pyroglutamic acidemia	Fig. 28-3, reaction 1	Retardation, athetosis, and tetraplegia in one of three known patients

[a]For disorders of carbohydrate metabolism and the hyperalaninemic lactic acidoses, see Chap. 29.
[b]Disorders described in only one or two families.

Fig. 28-1. Metabolic map of citric acid metabolism and related catabolism of some amino acids, indicating sites of inborn errors causing biochemical disturbances. The conversion of triose phosphates through pyruvate to acetyl CoA (top left) leads to the citric acid cycle. The glutamate cycle, with the important biogenic amine γ-aminobutyric acid is included, as well as β-alanine and its metabolism. The catabolism of phenylalanine and tyrosine are at the top right indicating pathways of pigment and hormone formation from tyrosine; that of tryptophan and lysine are at the bottom, including the relation of serotonin, 5-hydroxytryptamine, to tryptophan. Within the citric acid cycle is diagramed the oxidative pathway of energy metabolism by which protons are transferred from NADH to molecular oxygen. The following abbreviations are used for coenzymes, which are included only when relevant to the cause or treatment of an inborn error. Abbreviations: Ad-B₁₂, 5'-Deoxyadenosyl-cobalamin; CoA, coenzyme A; CoQ, coenzyme Q; FAD, flavine adenine dinucleotide; FADH, reduced FAD; Me-B₁₂, methylcobalamin; NAD, nicotinamide adenine dinucleotide; NAD⁺, oxidized form of NAD; NADH, reduced NAD; OH-B₁₂, hydroxycobalamin; PyrP, pyridoxal phosphate; ThPP, thiamine pyrophosphate. The sites of metabolic blocks causing albinism are labeled A, and defects of thyroid hormone synthesis are labeled T. The symbol F locates the site of action of formiminofolate transferase on histidine catabolism (see Fig. 28-8). Enzymes: (1) pyruvate dehydrogenase complex; (2) pyruvate carboxylase; (3) phosphoenolpyruvate carboxykinase; (4) undetermined; (5) 3-ketoacid CoA-transferase; (6) phenylalanine hydroxylase; (7) cytosol tyrosine aminotransferase; (8) p-hydroxyphenylpyruvate dioxygenase; (9) homogentisate oxygenase; (10) glutamate decarboxylase; (11) ? β-alanine aminotransferase; ? γ-aminobutyrate aminotransferase; (12) histidase; (13) carnosinase; (14) ? glutaryl-CoA dehydrogenase; (15) kynureninase; (16) undetermined; (17) lysine dehydrogenase; (18) undetermined; (19) saccharopine dehydrogenase; (20) undetermined; (21) lysine hydroxylase; (22) ? α-aminoadipate aminotransferase.

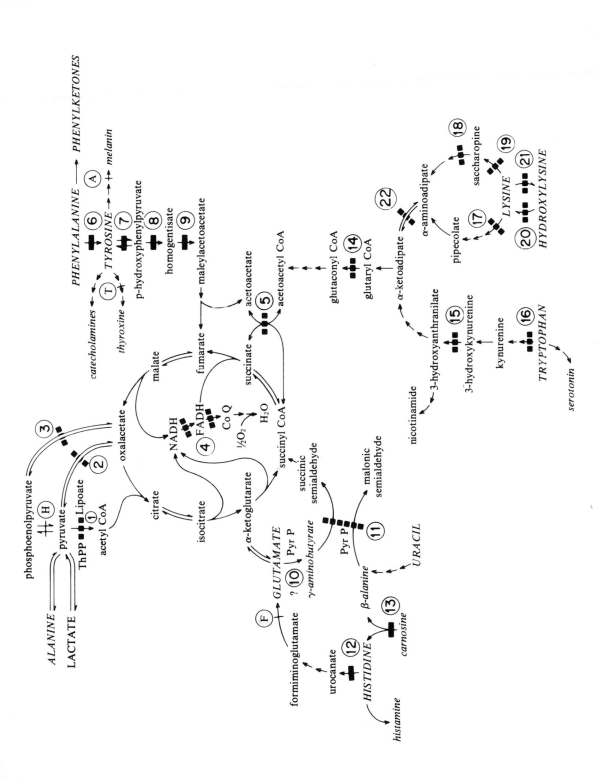

© Y. E. Hsia, 1979

derivative of leucine has been shown experimentally to inhibit oxidation of pyruvate and of α-ketoglutarate [12, 13] suggesting a possible mechanism for lactic acidosis and ketoacidosis in this disease. The odor of maple syrup characteristic of this disease must be from a fragrant ketoacid or ester, the smell being not unlike that of α-ketobutyrate. There are milder, intermittent, and thiamine-responsive variants of maple syrup urine disease.

HYPERVALINEMIA AND HYPERLEUCINE-ISOLEUCINEMIA

Hypervalinemia (Fig. 28-2, reaction 2) and hyper-leucine-isoleucinemia [1] (Fig. 28-2, reaction 1) are shown in Fig. 28-2 and Table 28-4. Perhaps the imbalanced accumulation of valine or of leucine and isoleucine prevents normal metabolism or normal transport of other amino acids into the brain [8]. Rats force-fed a diet low only in valine became very weak but were not weakened by a diet low in both valine and leucine [14]; this confirms that imbalance may be more harmful than combined deficiencies.

ISOVALERIC ACIDEMIA

Isovaleric acidemia [2] (Fig. 28-2, reaction 4) is characterized by severe ketoacidosis associated with an offensive odor, like that of cheese or sweaty feet, from free isovaleric acid. Although acute symptoms were attributable to the recurrent attacks of acidosis, the first reported patients had only mild mental retardation and no other neurological symptoms. Half of the known patients have died in infancy, but a few have survived with normal intelligence. One patient with isovaleric acidemia was intact neurologically despite a series of critical acidotic episodes until aged 40 months [15]. Isovaleric acid itself has been shown to be neurotoxic when given to experimental animals, producing lethargy and coma; and free isovaleric acid levels in the serum of patients have correlated with their symptoms. In fact, Krieger and Tanaka [16] have shown that administration of glycine will enhance formation of the conjugate isovalerylglycine, with improved tolerance to dietary protein. Thus, glycine can be protective in this disorder [17].

The Ketotic Hyperglycinemic Syndromes

A series of organic acidemias in the pathway of isoleucine and valine catabolism (Fig. 28-2, reactions 6–10) produce a common syndrome [2, 18] of protein-induced ketoacidosis with intermittent hyperglycinemia, low counts of white blood cells and blood platelets, hypoglycemia [19] and hyperammonemia [20, 21]. These patients may succumb to acute metabolic imbalance in infancy; they may survive with episodic attacks of ketoacidosis or hyperammonemia; or they may have moderate retardation and seizures without serious metabolic symptoms.

PROPIONIC ACIDEMIA

In propionic acidemia (Fig. 28-2, reaction 7) keto-acidosis, hyperglycinemia and severe hyper-ammonemia occur [2, 3, 20]. The disorder has been associated clinically with serious neurological damage in many of those who survived past early infancy. This neurotoxicity must be due in part to hyperammonemia, but may also be caused by toxic organic-acid by-products (Fig. 28-2). A significant correlation has been shown between the serum propionate and blood ammonia concentrations of two patients [21], but how propionate excess causes hyperammonemia is not clear. One patient with propionic acidemia had abnormal odd-chain and branched-chain fatty acids in the liver [22]; incorporation of these into myelin and other brain lipids could be detrimental (Chap. 32). Many precursors and by-products of propionate that might be neurotoxic have been identified in these patients, ranging from tiglic acid to β-hydroxypropionate and methyl citrate [2, 18]. Some patients with propionic acidemia and intermittent hyperglycinemia have moderate mental retardation and seizures without overt episodes of ketoacidosis. This raises the possibility that glycine is as neurotoxic in these patients as in patients with primary defects of glycine catabolism [23]. Against a neurotoxic role for either propionate or glycine is the finding of two untreated patients with propionic acidemia who were neurologically intact [24]. The sibling of one severely retarded athetotic child has been treated

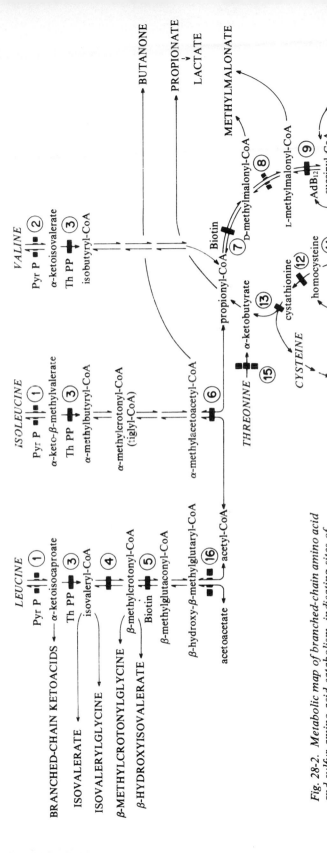

Fig. 28-2. Metabolic map of branched-chain amino acid and sulfur amino acid catabolism, indicating sites of inborn errors of metabolism. The catabolism of leucine, isoleucine and valine descend to common intermediary metabolites from the top. Organic acids and other compounds excreted in these metabolic disorders are indicated on the left or right. The catabolism of threonine and methionine, with the pathways of vitamin B₁₂ coenzyme synthesis, are below. Metabolic blocks at 6, 7, 8, 9, and 10 have all produced the syndrome of ketotic hyperglycinemia (see tables 2-2 and 28-4). Enzymes: (1) ? branched-chain-amino-acid aminotransferase; (2) ? valine-isoleucine aminotransferase; (3) branched-chain-ketoacid decarboxylase complex; (4) isovaleryl-CoA dehydrogenase; (5) β-methylcrotonoyl-CoA carboxylase; (6) β-ketothiolase; (7) propionyl-CoA carboxylase; (8) ? methylmalonyl-CoA racemase; (9) methylmalonyl-CoA mutase; (10) steps in B₁₂ coenzyme synthesis; (11) homocysteine:methionine methyltransferase and steps in folate coenzyme turnover; (12) cystathionine synthase; (13) cystathionase; (14) sulfite oxidase; (15) ? threonine deaminase; (16) β-hydroxy-β-methylglutaryl-CoA lyase.

© Y. E. Hsia, 1979

by restricting toxic precursors from birth and has survived. She displayed superior intelligence at age 10 years [25].

Propionyl-CoA carboxylase, the deficient enzyme in propionic acidemia, is a biotin-dependent enzyme, and there are reports of successful treatment by large doses of this vitamin [26, 27]. Some of these patients have a rare multiple carboxylase deficiency syndrome affecting three or four biotin-carboxylases, due to an abnormality of biotin metabolism [27, 28].

METHYLMALONIC ACIDEMIAS

Methylmalonic acidemias are of special neurochemical interest because the enzyme methylmalonyl-CoA mutase, deficient in primary methylmalonic acidemia (Fig. 28-2, reaction 9), is the only mammalian enzyme known to require the 5'-deoxyadenosyl-cobalamin derivative of vitamin B_{12} as a cofactor [3, 18]. In one of the inherited abnormalities of vitamin B_{12} metabolism (Fig. 28-2, reaction 10), there is also deficient production of methylcobalamin, a cofactor for homocysteine: methionine methyltransferase (Fig. 28-2, reaction 11, and Fig. 28-8, reaction 6). The effects of these inherited metabolic defects can be compared and contrasted with acquired vitamin B_{12} deficiency, pernicious anemia, in which there is degeneration of the long neuronal tracts of the spinal column, peripheral neuropathy, psychological deterioration, and occasionally amblyopia (Chap. 33). In pernicious anemia, there is a metabolic block in both the methylmalonate oxidation and homocysteine:methionine methyl transfer pathways, and patients have elevated urine methylmalonate excretion.

In methylmalonyl-CoA mutase deficiency (Fig. 28-2, reaction 9) and in vitamin B_{12}-responsive methylmalonic acidemias (Fig. 28-2, reaction 10), patients have the syndrome of ketotic hyperglycinemia. Urine methylmalonate excretion is generally elevated many times higher than in pernicious anemia. In one patient with vitamin B_{12}-responsive methylmalonic acidemia, there was impressive clinical improvement, including improved developmental quotient, after treatment with large doses of vitamin B_{12}. His urine methylmalonate output, although lower after B_{12} was administered, was still far higher than in patients with pernicious anemia [29]. Observations on this patient indicated that methylmalonate was not neurotoxic, although sural nerve biopsies of patients with pernicious anemia have shown that [^{14}C]propionate is incorporated into odd-chain fatty acids and branched-chain fatty acids (see Chap. 33). When this patient was ill or exposed to a large oral load of isoleucine, he excreted abnormal branched-chain ketones, including methylethyl ketone (butanone) (Fig. 28-2) and higher analogs. In rats, inhalation of methylbutyl ketone (hexanone) and possibly also methylethyl ketone caused acute muscular weakness and axonal hypertrophy, with beading and degenerative changes in the sural nerve [30]. Therefore, the branched-chain ketones may have specific neurotoxic effects.

METHYLMALONIC ACIDEMIA WITH HOMOCYSTINURIA

Caused by defective formation of both vitamin B_{12} cofactors [3, 18] (Fig. 28-8, reaction 6), methylmalonic acidemia with homocystinuria has been associated with inanition, convulsions, and death at age 2 months in one boy; with very mild mental retardation in 1 of 2 affected brothers; and with severe mental retardation progressing to dementia in 1 girl who died at age 7 years. Postmortem examination of the girl's brain revealed cerebral atrophy and histological changes resembling those observed in pernicious anemia [31]. Chemical analysis of the nervous system lipids in the infant boy showed abnormal branched-chain and odd-chain fatty acids in the phosphatides of his brain, spinal cord, and sciatic nerve [32]. It is curious that, apart from the girl, none of these patients had the severe megaloblastic anemia that is the hallmark of pernicious anemia.

ALPHA-METHYLACETOACETYL-CoA THIOLASE DEFICIENCY

α-Methylacetoacetyl-CoA thiolase deficiency (also referred to as β-ketothiolase deficiency [33], Fig. 28-2, reaction 6) has been associated with two

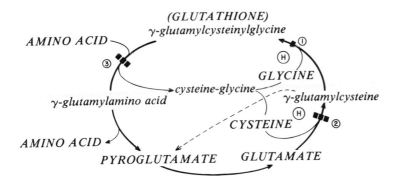

Fig. 28-3. Glutathione metabolism. Enzymes: (1) gluta-thione synthetase; (2) γ-glutamylcysteine synthetase; (3) γ-glutamyltransferase. γ-Glutamylcyclotransferase catalyzes the formation of pyroglutamate from γ-glutamylamino acid and also from γ-glutamylcysteine. The symbol H represents enzyme defects causing hemo-lytic anemia.

clinical syndromes. In one syndrome, ketoacidosis alone occurred in three families; in another syndrome, a single patient had hyperammonemia, hyperglycinemia, and developmental retardation.

Glutathione

Glutathione, a tripeptide, protects red cells from oxidative hemolysis and, in its reduced state, is present in high concentration in the brain, although it is rapidly oxidized after death. The enzyme γ-glutamyltransferase (Fig. 28-3, reaction 3) has high activity in the choroid plexus of the ventricles and the ciliary bodies of the eye; it has been found histochemically on the surface of certain neurons. The functional role of glutathione in the nervous system is unclear, with no proved relationship to amino acid transport. Figure 28-3 illustrates Meister's postulated γ-glutamyl cycle, by which amino acids conjugated with glutamate could be transported across membranes by a membrane-bound enzyme, γ-glutamyltransferase. Release of the amino acid after it traversed the membrane would depend on the action of γ-glutamylcyclotransferase. The pyroglutamate formed by the cyclotransferase is recycled back to glutathione in three steps, each step

dependent on the hydrolysis of ATP to ADP and phosphate.

Glutathione is a potent reducing agent, being reversibly oxidized to a disulfide. In the red blood cells, enzymatic deficiencies of carbohydrate metabolism (that decrease the supply of ATP), of glutathione oxidation, and of glutathione synthesis, all lead to hemolytic anemias [34]. Neurological abnormalities are associated with two abnormalities of glutathione synthesis and one of glutathione degradation. Glutathione synthctase deficiency causes disorders of red-cell integrity and white-cell function, but has no neurological effects [34].

PYROGLUTAMIC ACIDEMIA

This disorder has been recognized in one severely retarded man with athetosis and tetraplegia, and in two neurologically intact infant sisters. Another patient revealed no neurological impairment at 14 months [35]. They all excreted many grams of pyroglutamate (5-oxoproline) in the urine daily and had a severe metabolic acidosis approximately equimolar to the massive accumulation of pyroglutamate in the blood (2 to 5 mM).

The younger patients were found to have low red-cell glutathione and hemolytic anemia, and enzyme studies showed a deficiency not of 5-oxoprolinase, but of glutathione synthetase [35, 36] (Fig. 28-3, reaction 1). In pyroglutamic aciduria, γ-glutamylcysteine seems to be an alternate substrate for the transferase and the cyclotransferase, so that pyroglutamate accumulates beyond the capacity of 5-oxoprolinase to catabolize it.

GAMMA-GLUTAMYLCYSTEINE SYNTHETASE DEFICIENCY (Fig. 28-3, reaction 2)

γ-Glutamylcysteine synthetase deficiency was associated in one adult woman with mild hemolytic anemia, psychotic behavior, and signs of spinocerebellar degeneration [38]. Her brother showed similar symptoms, except for the psychotic behavior, but he had abnormal electromyographic changes. Both patients showed evidence of mental deterioration and exhibited generalized aminoaciduria. Glutathione was reduced in the blood cells and muscles of both patients, and γ-glutamylcysteine synthetase was less than 7 percent of control activity in the red cells of both patients. The aminoaciduria may be secondary to defective glutathione-mediated amino acid transport in the kidney, but the relation between the metabolic disorder and the neurological abnormalities is not clear.

GLUTATHIONEMIA (Fig. 28-3, reaction 3)

Caused by deficiency of γ-glutamyltransferase, this disease has been reported in one moderately retarded man [39]. Again, it was not clear why he was retarded. He had normal renal tubular reabsorption of amino acids [40] despite the absence of this enzyme, which is supposed to be a mediator for the transport of amino acids across cell membranes.

Ammonia, the Urea Cycle, and Dibasic Amino Acids

Ammonia is normally present in relatively constant concentrations in the brain, and its turnover is closely regulated by the active enzymes that shuttle amino groups among glutamine, glutamate, and aspartate [20, 41] (Table 28-3 and Fig. 28-4). These are discussed in Chaps. 12 and 17.

Clinically, severe hyperammonemia in infants produces vomiting, lethargy, alternating hypertonia and hypotonia, sometimes a coarse tremor reminiscent of the asterixis of hepatic coma, and, finally, coma and a decerebrate state with or without seizures. In older children, moderate hyperammonemia has milder manifestations, and often a characteristic aversion to protein-rich foods is seen. The symptoms are episodic and are aggravated by high protein intake, constipation, or intercurrent infection, each of which causes hyperammonemia in susceptible patients.

Ammonia accumulates in liver disease (Chaps. 17 and 35); in the ketotic hyperglycinemia syndromes; in disorders of the urea-cycle enzymes; and in some disorders of the dibasic amino acids. The dibasic amino acids are implicated in hyperammonemia because ornithine and arginine participate in the urea cycle, and lysine loading results in hyperammonemia in patients with hyperlysinemia (Table 28-3).

Synergism between ammonia and other metabolites could also account for neurotoxicity in some inborn errors of metabolism. Subtoxic levels of ammonia in mice interact with mercaptans or with short-chain fatty acids to precipitate lethargy and coma [20], so a combination of metabolites could produce serious neurotoxic effects without markedly elevated concentrations of any single agent. Typical histological changes in astrocytes have been reported in these hyperammonemic patients [20]. Several diamine derivatives of amino acids, such as putrescine (Fig. 28-4), have important neurochemical interactions. These derivatives may increase with hyperammonemia.

The Urea Cycle

As illustrated in Fig. 28-4, detoxification of ammonia is by immediate reversible incorporation into glutamate, glutamine, and aspartate, and by eventual fixation as urea through the Krebs-Henseleit arginine cycle. Both aspartate and carbamoylphosphate feed nitrogen into the cycle, and the cycle synthesizes arginine, urea, and ornithine. Surprisingly, in defects of the urea-cycle enzymes, urea biosynthesis is never totally deficient, perhaps because total blockage of urea biosynthesis is not compatible with fetal survival.

Orotic aciduria occurs in defects of the distal urea-cycle enzymes because intramitochondrial accumulation of carbamoyl phosphate will result in its leakage into the cytoplasm [20], where it is converted to carbamoyl aspartate, the rate-limiting step in pyrimidine biosynthesis, thus accelerating orotate production (Chap. 19). This concept is con-

Table 28-3. Hyperammonemia Caused by Disorders of Amino Acid and Intermediary Metabolism

Condition	Location of Defective Enzyme	Comments
Disorders of arginine-urea cycle		
Carbamoyl-phosphate synthetase deficiency*	Fig. 28-4, reaction 1	Several variants reported, ranging from lethal neonatal syndrome to milder syndromes; each variant was unique to one or two cases
Ornithine transcarbamylase deficiency	Fig. 28-4, reaction 2	X-linked dominant, variable severity in females, lethal in neonatal period in males. Variants are known
Citrullinemia	Fig. 28-4, reaction 3	Variable severity, ranging from lethal neonatal syndrome to milder syndromes
Argininosuccinic aciduria	Fig. 28-4, reaction 4	Hyperammonemia is inconstant and moderate. Neurological toxicity may be due to argininosuccinate, with ataxia. Psychoses may occur
Argininemia*	Fig. 28-4, reaction 5	Variants reported. Hyperammonemia is mild or absent; patients have all been retarded
Disorders of dibasic amino acids		
Hyperornithinemia*	Fig. 28-4, reaction 8	One boy with mild hyperammonemia, myoclonic spasms, and moderate retardation. No hyperammonemia in other forms of hyperornithinemia
Hyperlysinemia*	Fig. 28-1, reaction 17	Moderate hyperammonemia, spasticity, seizures
Hyperlysinuria	? Transport defect	Postprandial hyperammonemia, severe mental retardation
Lysinuric dibasic aminoaciduria	? Transport defect	Variable hyperammonemia; episodic abdominal upset, with pain and distension; inconstant hyperammonemia
Hyperornithinemia and homocitrullinemia	? Mitochondrial transport ? Fig. 28-4, reaction 8	Variable retardation, seizures, and ataxia in one family; severe retardation and stupor in another
Also disorders of branched-chain amino acids, see Table 28-2 and Fig. 28-2.		

*Disorders described in only one or two families.

firmed by the fact that rats on an arginine-free diet have decreased capacity to synthesize urea and develop orotic aciduria [42].

Because the transamination of amino acids is a major source of ammonia and most essential amino acids can be formed by transamination of the corresponding ketoacid carbon skeletons, a synthetic diet that includes these ketoacids could fulfill nutritional needs while drastically curtailing nitrogen intake. This has been tried in patients with urea-cycle enzyme defects with variable success [43–45].

CARBAMOYL-PHOSPHATE SYNTHETASE DEFICIENCY

Carbamoyl-phosphate synthetase deficiency (Fig. 28-4, reaction 1) has been reported in several patients with hyperammonemia. Clinical severity and the degrees of enzyme deficiency have varied considerably [20, 46, 47]. The exclusively hepatic mitochondrial enzyme, carbamoyl-phosphate synthetase I, preferentially accepts ammonia as a substrate and is the primer for urea biosynthesis. In addition, a ubiquitous cytoplasmic enzyme, carbamoyl-phosphate synthetase II, preferentially accepts

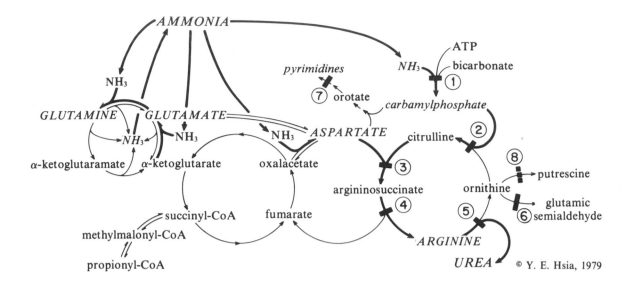

Fig. 28-4. *Metabolic map of ammonia metabolism. The important relationships between ammonia, glutamine, glutamate, and aspartate are emphasized. The purine nucleotide cycle, which releases large amounts of ammonia from muscle, has been omitted. The relationship of the citric acid cycle to the arginine cycle is shown, as is the synthesis of pyrimidines from aspartate and carbamoyl phosphate. How disorders of propionate metabolism produce hyperammonemia is not clear. α-Ketoglutaramate, depicted on the left, has been found in the cerebrospinal fluid of patients with hepatic coma (see Tables 28-3 and 28-4). Enzymes: (1) carbamoyl-phosphate synthetase; (2) ornithine transcarbamylase; (3) argininosuccinate synthetase; (4) argininosuccinase; (5) arginase; (6) ornithine transaminase; (7) orotidine-5'-phosphate pyrophosphorylase and orotidine-5'-phosphate decarboxylase; (8) ornithine decarboxylase. A transport defect of ornithine reentry into the mitochondrion is the probable cause of hyperornithinemia with homocitrullinemia.*

glutamine as a substrate and is the primer for pyrimidine biosynthesis. Unless assays have differentiated carefully between these two enzymes, deficiency of the hepatic mitochondrial enzyme may be missed. Further confusion has arisen because secondary deficiency of the mitochondrial enzyme I may result from low protein diets or from toxic inhibition, as in Reye's syndrome. It also has led to misdiagnosis in one patient with methylmalonic aciduria and in another who was thought to have primary carbamoyl-phosphate synthetase deficiency [48], but who probably had a mitochondrial ornithine transport defect.

ORNITHINE TRANSCARBAMYLASE DEFICIENCY

Ornithine transcarbamylase deficiency (Fig. 28-4, reaction 2) is an excellent example of a systemic metabolic disorder that produces major toxicity in the central nervous system. Some patients have prominent secondary orotic aciduria and, in severely affected patients, amino acid imbalances follow liver-cell damage and hepatic necrosis. In ornithine transcarbamylase deficiency, hyperammonemia appears to be primarily responsible for both the neurotoxicity and the hepatotoxicity.

Its X-linked pattern of inheritance has been confirmed in more than 50 families. It is lethal in affected males and is of variable severity in affected females, who risk transmitting the condition to their offspring. Variants of the disorder have been described that may be related to different mutations of the enzyme molecule [49]. Therapy with low-protein diet and ketoacid analogs of essential amino acids in affected females has been satisfactory [50], but no long-term therapy has yet succeeded in salvaging an affected male [45, 51], except in mild variants.

CITRULLINEMIA
Caused by deficiency of argininosuccinate synthetase (Fig. 28-4, reaction 3 [3, 20, 44]), citrullinemia can be fatal in early infancy as a result of acute liver failure, or it can cause severe neurological dysfunction by late infancy. At least 6 infants with citrullinemia have presented with lethargy, followed by hypertonia, convulsions, and coma in the first few days of life. They had marked elevation of ammonia and citrulline in body fluids, and several also developed acute hepatic necrosis. A similar number of infants showed vomiting, irritability, and seizures beginning a few months after birth, and later displayed severe mental retardation and sometimes ataxia; their electroencephalograms often were abnormal. Pathologically, some of these patients were found to have cerebral atrophy and hepatic-cell damage. Neurotoxicity in this condition may be caused mostly by hyperammonemia, but argininosuccinate synthetase, an enzyme normally found in brain tissue, was defective in these patients, and the subsequent massive elevation of citrulline in brain and cerebrospinal fluid may also have been toxic. The clinical variability of citrullinemia includes a retarded adult and a neurologically intact boy, neither of whom had hyperammonemia. Variants from heterogeneous mutations of this enzyme molecule have been demonstrated [52].

ARGININOSUCCINIC ACIDURIA
Argininosuccinic aciduria is the result of deficiency of argininosuccinase (Fig. 28-4, reaction 4) and is inconstantly associated with hyperammonemia [3, 20]. It can be lethal in early infancy, but the majority of the more than 50 patients reported have survived longer, although almost invariably with retardation and seizures, and usually with intermittent ataxia. One infant's brain had markedly elevated argininosuccinate and altered amino acid concentrations at autopsy [53]. There is suggestive evidence for arginine deficiency in these patients, so the enzyme defect in the condition may cause symptoms because of both a toxic precursor and a deficient product. The best therapy, therefore, may be a combination of restricted protein intake, together with arginine supplements in the diet.

HYPERORNITHINEMIA
Hyperornithinemia has been claimed to be due to ornithine decarboxylase deficiency in one retarded boy with myoclonic seizures and postprandial hyperammonemia [54] (Fig. 28-4, reaction 8). Two other retarded patients with milder hyperornithinemia and similar symptoms had reduced hepatic ornithine transaminase (Fig. 28-4, reaction 6). Another remarkable form of hyperornithinemia has been observed in 22 Scandinavian patients with tapetoretinal degeneration. Patients had gyrate atrophy of the retina and choroid, extinguished electroretinogram, and progressive loss of vision, but no other consistent neurological abnormalities. A defect in ornithine transaminase has been confirmed [55, 56].

Hyperornithinemia and homocitrullinemia, with hyperammonemia, were reported in two families. They were thought to be due to ornithine decarboxylase deficiency, but are from a mitochondrial transport defect. Studies on 6 members of a Canadian family [48], all of whom were afflicted with various degrees of retardation, seizures, and ataxia, reportedly showed decreased carbamoyl-phosphate synthetase I activity in leukocytes. Tissue from a liver biopsy revealed abnormal mitochondria on electron microscopy and contained decreased activity of this enzyme. A severely retarded British woman with episodes of stupor and limited motor ability also had this condition [57]. Both studies [48, 57] reported protein intolerance and increased homocitrullinuria after protein or lysine ingestion. The British patient exhibited lower blood ammonia levels and improved tolerance to protein when her diet was supplemented with either ornithine or arginine, even though the former increased her hyperornithinemia.

Ornithine transcarbamylase, the intramitochondrial enzyme, can also transcarbamylate lysine to homocitrulline. Hence, impaired transport of ornithine into the mitochondrion could result in impeded ammonia detoxification; accumulation of ornithine and homocitrulline; and improved protein tolerance on a diet supplemented with ornithine or arginine [48, 57].

ARGININEMIA
Argininemia is also associated with brain damage [3, 20, 58].

Lysine and Hydroxylysine
Lysine is an essential diamino acid that does not participate in the transamination reactions of the general amino acid pool. It can be carbamylated to form homocitrulline, which, in turn, can form homoarginine in a manner analogous to arginine formation from citrulline (Fig. 28-4). Lysine is catabolized by at least two pathways (Fig. 28-1): one through ε-N-acetyllysine and pipecolate, and the other through saccharopine. Both pathways form α-aminoadipate, which then joins the degradative pathway for tryptophan at α-ketoadipate. Hydroxylysine is formed by hydroxylation of lysyl residues in the polypeptides of collagen. No specific neurochemical action is known for lysine, hydroxylysine, or their derivatives, except that pipecolate is structurally similar to some hypnotic or cerebrotoxic agents such as piperidine.

Various forms of hyperlysinemia are listed in Table 28-4 [1, 3]. The conditions affecting lysine catabolism, together with the hyperornithinemia due to a mitochondrial-membrane transport block, suggest a definite but inconstant relationship between lysine and ammonia metabolism. The mechanism for neurotoxicity of hyperlysinemia is still obscure.

LYSINURIC FAMILIAL PROTEIN INTOLERANCE
Lysinuric protein intolerance is associated with intermittent hyperammonemia [1, 3, 59]. Almost two dozen patients, mostly interrelated, have been reported from Finland and elsewhere. Typically, the patients have an aversion to protein and develop abdominal cramps, diarrhea, and vomiting after protein ingestion, sometimes accompanied by hyperammonemia and obtundation of consciousness. They are thin, short-statured, and may have mild retardation or enlarged livers. Blood urea, lysine, and arginine are low; urine lysine, arginine,

and sometimes cystine are elevated. The defect apparently lies in the transport of dibasic amino acids by renal and intestinal mucosa. Oral loading with lysine has aggravated abdominal symptoms, and intravenous infusion of lysine or arginine, or both, showed a defect in their common renal reabsorptive mechanism. Three of five patients improved clinically on long-term supplementation with arginine, so in this condition, too, there may be a secondary arginine deficiency, which could explain the hyperammonemia.

PIPECOLATEMIA
One patient with pipecolatemia has been described as exhibiting irritability, intention tremor, nystagmus, and hypotonia, progressing to paralysis and death in the third year [60]. He had elevated brain pipecolate but low brain homocarnosine (γ-aminobutyrylhistidine). His brain showed scattered demyelination with gliosis and accumulation of lipid; his muscles were atrophied, and both muscles and liver were fibrotic.

The cerebrohepatorenal syndrome was reported to be associated with pipecolatemia [61]; it has also been related to a block in mitochondrial oxidation between the succinic dehydrogenase flavoprotein and coenzyme Q [62] (Fig. 28-1).

Tryptophan, Xanthurenate, and Glutarate
Tryptophan is an essential amino acid [1, 6] that is hydroxylated and decarboxylated to yield the biogenic amine serotonin [63] (Chap. 11). Its catabolism is through the kynurenines to α-ketoadipate, glutaryl-CoA, and eventually acetoacetyl-CoA (Fig. 28-1).

Kynureninase (Fig. 28-1, reaction 15) is a pyridoxal phosphate–requiring enzyme. Urinary excretion of hydroxykynurenine and of its byproduct, xanthurenic acid increases in vitamin B_6 deficiency. Clinically, vitamin B_6 deficiency causes convulsions and other neurological disturbances in infants (Chap. 33).

Glutaric acidemia I (Fig. 28-1, reaction 14) is a disorder of lysine, hydroxylysine, and tryptophan metabolism characterized by intermittent or chronic metabolic acidosis, choreoathetosis and

Table 28-4. Other Amino Acid Disorders with Neurological Lesions

Condition	Location of Defective Enzyme	Neurological Lesions	Comments
Branched-chain amino acids			
Hypervalinemia*	Fig. 28-2, reaction 2	Lethargy, retardation	
Hyperleucine-isoleucinemia*	Fig. 28-2, reaction 1	Retardation, seizures, retinal degeneration, deafness	Also had prolinemia type II
β-Hydroxy-β-methyl-glutaryl-CoA lyase deficiency	Fig. 28-2, reaction 16	Hypotonia in one, spasticity and stupor in another	Hypoglycemia in one
Glutathione			
Pyroglutamic acidemia	Fig. 28-3, reaction 1	Retardation, athetosis, tetraplegia in one adult	Severe acidosis
γ-Glutamylcysteine synthetase deficiency*	Fig. 28-3, reaction 2	Spinocerebellar degeneration, psychotic behavior in one patient; myopathy in the other	
Glutathionemia*	Fig. 28-3, reaction 3	Moderately retarded adult	
Dibasic amino acids			
Ornithinemia*	Fig. 28-4, reaction 6	Lethargy, ataxia, myoclonic seizures, retardation	
Gyrate atrophy with ornithinemia	? Fig. 28-4, reaction 6	Choroidoretinal degeneration	Hypoammonemia
Persistent hyper-lysinemia*	Fig. 28-1, reaction 19	Two of three sisters were normal	No hyperammonemia
Hyperlysinemia*	?	Severe retardation, hypotonia	No hyperammonemia, lax ligaments
Saccharopinemia and lysinemia*	Fig. 28-1, reaction 18	Severe retardation	No hyperammonemia, cerebrospinal fluid lysine increased
Pipecolatemia*	?	Irritability, tremor, hypotonia, nystagmus, paralysis	Low brain homocarnosine
Cerebrohepatorenal syndrome	? Fig. 28-1, reaction 4	Hypotonia, retardation	Biochemical lesion might be in electron transfer system
Hydroxylysinuria	Fig. 28-1, reaction 2	Retardation, myoclonic seizures	
α-Aminoadipic acidemia*	?	Borderline intelligence in one of two affected brothers	
Tryptophan and metabolites			
Tryptophanemia*	Fig. 28-1, reaction 16	Retardation, cerebellar ataxia	Photosensitive rash

*Disorders described in only one or two families.

(continued)

Table 28-4 (Continued)

Condition	Location of Defective Enzyme	Neurological Lesions	Comments
Xanthurenic aciduria	Fig. 28-1, reaction 15	Some patients had sub-normal intelligence	One variant is responsive to vitamin B_6
Hydroxykynurenic acidemia*	Fig. 24-1, reaction 15	Mildly retarded girl	Unresponsive to vitamin B_6
α-Ketoadipic acidemia*	?	One of two affected brothers was retarded, selfabusive, and without speech	
Glutaric acidemia I	? Fig. 28-1, reaction 14	Dystonia, athetosis, retardation	
Glutaric acidemia II	multiple acyl-CoA carboxylases		
Glutamate and metabolites			
Glutamatemia	Nongenetic	? Neonatal susceptibility to neuronal necrosis and retinal degeneration	Also reported in Menke's syndrome
Pyridoxine-dependent seizures	? Fig. 28-1, reaction 10	Neonatal seizures, retardation	Dramatically responsive to vitamin B_6
β-Alaninemia*	Fig. 28-1, reaction 11	Somnolence, seizures	
Carnosinemia	Fig. 28-1, reaction 13	Retardation, seizures, lethargy, spasticity	
Homocarnosinosis*	?	Spastic tetraparesis, retardation	
Phenylalanine and tyrosine			
Phenylketonuria	Fig. 28-1, reaction 6	Retardation, microcephaly, hyperactivity, occasional seizures, psychoses	Treatable by restricted dietary phenylalanine
Maternal phenyl-ketonuria		Embryopathy and intra-uterine brain damage	
Hyperphenylalaninemia variants	Fig. 28-1, reaction 6	Probably benign	
Dihydrobiopterin reductase deficiency*	Fig. 28-6, reaction 2	Early retardation, myo-clonus, seizures, hypo-tonia, chorea	
Albinisms*: Cross syndrome	Fig. 28-1, reaction A	Microcephaly, retardation, athetosis. Abnormal lateral geniculate bodies	Microphthalmia. Other variants have no consistent neurological lesions
Tyrosine amino-transferase deficiency	Fig. 28-1, reaction 7	Agitation, tics, moderate retardation	Corneal ulcers, keratosis palmoplantaris
Neonatal tyrosinemia	Fig. 28-1, reaction 8	Risk of some retardation	Immature enzyme responsive to ascorbate
Hereditary tyrosinemia	Fig. 28-1, reaction 8	Irritability, mild retardation	Liver and kidney damage

*Disorders described in only one or two families.

Table 28-4 (Continued)

Condition	Location of Defective Enzyme	Neurological Lesions	Comments
Alcaptonuria	Fig. 28-1, reaction 9	None	Urine turns black, arthropathy
Sulfur amino acids and metabolites			
Methioninemia*	Fig. 28-6, reaction 5	One healthy infant	
Homocystinemia	Fig. 28-2, reaction 12	Borderline retardation and mental instability in some patients	Marfanoid habitus, ectopia lentis, thromboembolic complications Vitamin B₆ responsive variant
Cystathioninemia	Fig. 28-3, reaction 13	Benign	Vitamin B₆ responsive variant
Cystinosis	? Lysosomal transport	Photophobia, retinopathy	Progressive nephropathy, aminoaciduria
Taurine deficiency*	?	Depression, insomnia, dysphagia, visual abnormality, parkinsonism, respiratory failure	Three brothers, their mother, and her brother were similarly affected
β-Mercaptolactate cysteine disulfiduria	? β-Mercaptopyruvate sulfurtransferase	One retarded man with seizures, one retarded man without seizures, two sisters who were normal	Second man had ectopia lentis
Sulfite oxidase deficiency*	Fig. 28-2, reaction 14	Severe retardation, multiple abnormalities, decerebrate rigidity	Ectopia lentis
Glycine and sarcosine			
Nonketotic hyperglycinemia	Fig. 28-6, reaction 7	Lethargy, hypotonia, myoclonus, seizures, severe retardation in survivors, hypertonia and decerebrate rigidity	
Other glycinemic syndromes*	?	Extremely variable	
Sarcosinemia	Sarcosine dehydrogenase	Inconsistent association with retardation	May be benign
Proline and hydroxyproline			
Type I hyperprolinemia	Proline oxidase	Possible retardation or seizures	Renal disease may be coincidental
Type II hyperprolinemia	Pyrroline carboxylate dehydrogenase	Retardation, seizures	
Hydroxyprolinemia*	? Hydroxyproline oxidase	Retardation in two of three known cases	

*Disorders described in only one or two families.

(continued)

Table 28-4 (Continued)

Condition	Location of Defective Enzyme	Neurological Lesions	Comments
Iminopeptiduria*	Prolidase	Borderline intelligence	Abnormal collagen
Folate metabolites (and histidine)			
Dihydrofolate reductase deficiency*	Fig. 28-6,	None	Megaloblastic anemia
Cyclohydrolase deficiency*	Fig. 28-6, reaction 3	Retardation	Probably nonexistent entity
Formimino-transferase deficiency	Fig. 28-6, reaction 4	Retardation, cerebral atrophy; another two were very clumsy; one was normal; three had speech problems	Histidine catabolism is blocked
Histidinemia	Fig. 28-1, reaction 12	Perhaps speech problems, mild retardation, and infantile spasms	
Homocysteine-methionine methyl-transferase deficiency	Fig. 28-6, reaction 6	Retardation, cerebral atrophy	
$N^{5,10}$-methylene-tetrahydrofolate reductase deficiency*	Fig. 28-6, reaction 8	Two sisters were retarded; the third patient was hypotonic with seizures; one of the sisters had psychotic episodes	Patients had homocystinemia. The psychotic episodes appeared to respond to folate therapy

*Disorders described in only one or two families.

dystonia, with potentially neurotoxic mono- and dicarboxylic fatty acids, as well as glutaric and β-hydroxyglutaric acids in the urine [3, 64, 65]. Glutaric acidemia II also is characterized by acidosis and hypoglycemia, with increased glutaric and lactic acid in the urine together with a number of organic dicarboxylic acids and their metabolites [66]. The defect in type II perhaps affects several medium-chain acyl-CoA dehydrogenases with a common subunit.

Table 28-4 lists several rare disorders in this group, including tryptophanemia [67], xanthurenic aciduria, hydroxykynurenic acidemia, α-amino-adipic aciduria [68], and α-ketoadipic acidemia [69].

Glutamate, GABA, and Beta-Alanine
The metabolism and functional significance of glutamate and its derivatives are discussed in Chaps. 12 and 17. Metabolic disturbances within this group have been reported in a few cases (Table 28-4).

GLUTAMIC ACIDEMIA
Glutamic acidemia has been reported as an enigmatic finding in Menkes' syndrome, in which the relation of glutamate elevation to the disturbed copper metabolism, profound mental retardation and seizures, is obscure. Excessive ingestion of glutamate as a food additive causes acute symptoms similar to those induced by acetylcholine administration. Experimental, long-term administration of glutamate to young animals produces damage to retinal ganglion cells and results in neuronal necrosis in the hypothalamus, arcuate nucleus, and elsewhere in the developing brain, paradoxically without measurable increase in brain glutamate levels [70].

PYRIDOXINE-RESPONSIVE SEIZURES

This disorder, presumed to be due to impaired interaction of glutamic acid decarboxylase with its cofactor pyridoxal phosphate (Fig. 28-1, reaction 10), is discussed in Chap. 33.

BETA-ALANINEMIA

β-Alaninemia has been reported in an infant who had somnolence from birth and seizures that were unresponsive to anticonvulsants [3, 4]. β-Alanine and GABA were present in high concentrations in the brain, cerebrospinal fluid, blood, and urine of this patient. This is one basis for the postulate that β-alanine and GABA share the same transaminase (Fig. 28-1, reaction 11). Carnosine and β-alanylhistidine also were increased in the brain of this patient.

CARNOSINEMIA

Carnosinemia, which has been described in a few patients [71], is caused by the absence of carnosinase (Fig. 28-1, reaction 13). Carnosine is synthesized in brain and muscle from β-alanine and histidine; the same enzyme will synthesize homocarnosine from GABA and histidine. The compound anserine, β-alanylmethylhistidine, is found in the muscle of many mammals, but is not synthesized in human tissues. The role of these dipeptides in brain and muscle is not known, although anserine and carnosine are both potent activators of muscle ATPase [1]. All but one of the affected patients were retarded and had seizure disorders; some also were lethargic and spastic. Autopsy findings in one affected patient showed demyelination of white matter, loss of Purkinje fibers, cortical atrophy, unidentified "spheroids" in the cerebral gray matter, severe axonal degeneration, and atrophic fibrosis of muscle fibers [72].

HOMOCARNOSINOSIS

Homocarnosinosis has been reported in one adult woman with spastic tetraparesis and mental retardation [73]. Homocarnosine in her cerebrospinal fluid was increased by 10 to 20 times normal. She had normal carnosine levels; as the homocarnosine elevation could not have arisen from carnosinase deficiency, this is circumstantial evidence for a separate homocarnosinase enzyme. It is

intriguing that spasticity occurred both in this condition and in carnosinemia. Homocarnosine, a derivative of GABA, has no known neurochemical function. It is normally present in brain and cerebrospinal fluid, and is reported to raise the electroconvulsive threshold when injected into the cerebrospinal fluid of dog brain. Homocarnosine was reduced in the brain of the original patient with pipecolatemia.

Phenylalanine and Tyrosine

These aromatic amino acids are of major significance neurochemically because they are precursors of the catecholamines [6, 63] (Chap. 10) and of thyroid hormone. Phenylalanine has only one major catabolic reaction, hydroxylation to tyrosine. Tyrosine can be decarboxylated to tyramine, hydroxylated to dihydroxyphenylalanine (dopa), iodinated to the iodotyrosines and thyroid hormone, or catabolized through p-hydroxyphenylpyruvic acid to produce homogentisic acid and maleylacetoacetate (Fig. 28-1).

The hydroxylases for these aromatic amino acids and tryptophan have common properties [74]: cross-specificity for aromatic amino acid derivatives; complex substrate- and product-inhibition behavior; and requirements for a reduced pteridine cofactor and molecular oxygen. Phenylalanine hydroxylase is a microsomal enzyme with high activity in liver, pancreas, and kidney, but not in nervous tissue. Tyrosine hydroxylase is present in noradrenergic and adrenergic neurons of the central and sympathetic nervous systems. It is the rate-limiting enzyme for catecholamine biosynthesis. In the brain, tryptophan hydroxylase has distribution similar to that of serotonin; presumably it is localized in serotoninergic neurons. it is the rate-limiting enzyme for serotonin biosynthesis.

The natural pteridine cofactor for phenylalanine hydroxylase is tetrahydrobiopterine (Fig. 28-5), which is formed from 7,8-dihydrobiopterin in a reaction catalyzed by a dihydrofolate reductase or from pteridine precursors (Fig. 28-6, reaction 2). During the phenylalanine hydroxylase reaction, tetrahydrobiopterin is oxidized to the quinonoid form of dihydrobiopterin. The aromatic amino acid hydroxylases will accept many synthetic cofactors,

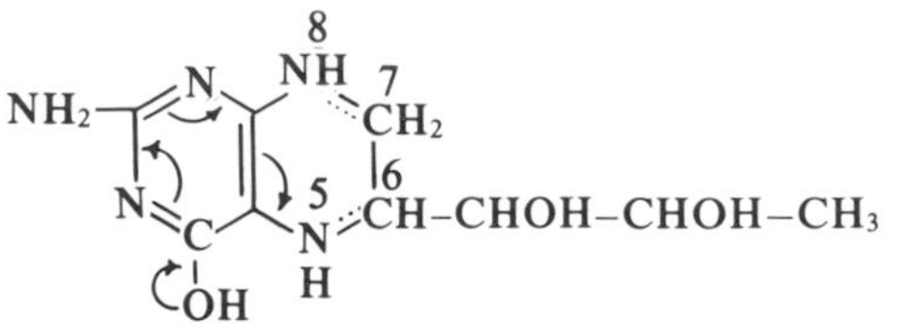

Tetrahydrobiopterin

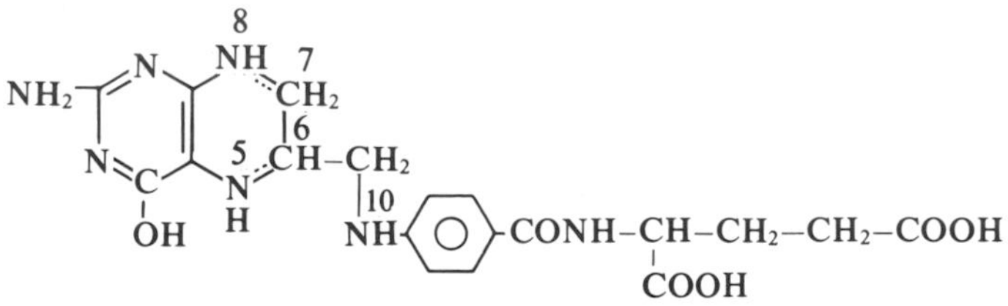

Tetrahydrofolate (monoglutamate form)

but their biochemical activities are considerably modified unless the natural cofactor is used. Tetrahydrobiopterin is presumed to be the natural cofactor for the brain tyrosine and tryptophan hydroxylases, too.

Phenylketonuria

Phenylketonuria (PKU) is the commonest of the inborn errors of metabolism that threaten neurological integrity. In the United States, it affects about 1 in 20,000 of all infants born [1, 7]. The genetic defect in PKU is of hepatic phenylalanine hydroxylase (Fig. 28-1, reaction 6). Patients with PKU have no detectable immunoreactive phenylalanine hydroxylase, but careful assays in one patient's liver showed 0.27 percent of normal enzyme activity, with altered substrate affinities [75, 76]. This confirms that the genetic defect is a structural mutation that seriously compromises the function of this enzyme, which loses its immunoreactive properties but apparently not its cofactor affinity [77]. In this condition, there is microcephaly, hypertonicity, mental retardation, and hyperactive, aggressive behavior. Patients often have seizures, eczema, pigment dilution, and a pungent, mousy odor. Histochemically, there is generalized failure of myelination, but the composition of the myelin, despite conflicting reports, is probably normal (see also Chap. 32).

PKU is the first of the inborn errors of metabolism shown to be treatable by diet restriction [1, 3, 4, 78] and for which large-scale, presymptomatic, screening programs have been effective [79]. Soon after birth, infants with PKU have abnormal elevations of serum phenylalanine that can be detected in a drop of dried blood by one of several efficient techniques. If PKU is confirmed, the patients

Fig. 28-5. Molecular structure of tetrahydrobiopterin and tetrahydrofolate. Biopterin, like folate, has the double bonds within the heterocyclic nucleus indicated by the dotted lines. Dihydrobiopterin and dihydrofolate have reduction of the bond between C^7 and N^8. The quinonoid form of dihydrobiopterin has the rearrangements indicated by the arrows plus a double bond probably between C^7 and N^8. The substitutions on tetrahydrofolate in Fig. 28-8 are at positions N^5 and N^{10}.

should be given a restricted diet that limits their serum phenylalanine to levels between two and five times normal. On this regimen, PKU children are protected from severe brain damage, but only if the diet is started in early infancy [1, 3, 80]. The hyperactive, aggressive behavior of older, retarded, PKU patients may be ameliorated by diet therapy. Inappropriate therapy by overzealous restriction or imbalance of the diet can lead to malnutrition, which can itself cause mental retardation. For instance, in children with PKU, tyrosine becomes an essential amino acid and must be supplied in sufficient quantity to fulfill nutritional needs.

Exceptionally, a few adults have been identified who have had all the metabolic abnormalities of PKU but have escaped with intact intelligence. Some of these individuals have had severely retarded siblings and parents who were chemically heterozygous for PKU [81]. Unrecognized adult PKU has three important implications for the neurochemical understanding of this condition. First, unidentified innate biochemical differences or exceptional environmental factors have somehow protected these individuals during their vulnerable period of brain growth. Second, some of these adults have had major psychotic illnesses, perhaps caused by their biochemical abnormality. Third, adult PKU women, whether brain-damaged or unscathed, offer a hostile intrauterine environment for their offspring [82].

Maternal PKU provides compelling substantiation of the concept that the neurotoxicity of PKU is secondary to changes in the *milieu interieur*. PKU women have a high risk of having spontaneous abortions or children born with congenital malformations. In addition, almost all children born to these mothers have had growth failure, microcephaly, and severe mental retardation [82]. Diet restriction during pregnancy has reportedly protected the human fetus from intrauterine brain damage in some instances, but in other cases has failed to be effective [83].

The neurological consequences of PKU must be produced indirectly, through altered composition of the extracellular fluid, because phenylalanine hydroxylase is not found normally in neural tissue; dietary corrective measures can avert the brain damage in this condition; and maternal PKU is toxic to the fetus.

Possible neurochemical mechanisms for the brain damage, however, are still confusing. Gaull and coworkers have presented a detailed review [7] of many possible neurotoxic mechanisms responsible for the brain damage in PKU, among which are the following:

1. Extreme hyperphenylalaninemia opens several alternate minor pathways for phenylalanine metabolism, and abnormal concentrations of phenylpyruvic acid, phenyllactic acid, phenylacetic acid, *o*-hydroxyphenylacetic acid, and phenylethylamine, among others, all are increased in the body fluids of untreated PKU patients. Some of these compounds may have physiological roles in the nervous system, and some do have neuropharmacological properties. Recent identification of a tetrahydroisoquinoline in PKU indicates another possible neurochemical basis of brain damage, as this compound is taken up actively into the brain and is a noncompetitive inhibitor of dopamine-β-hydroxylase [84]. Aggressive behavior in some violent criminals has been associated with elevated blood phenylacetic acid [85].

2. Relative dietary deficiency of tyrosine in PKU is aggravated by the inhibitory effect of high phenylalanine levels on tyrosine transport [6, 8]. This may deprive the brain of an adequate supply of tyrosine and its derivatives, including tyramine and its hydroxylated product octopamine as well as the catecholamines. This deficiency state might prevent brain growth and impair normal neurotransmission. Relative tyrosine deficiency in late fetal development has seemed to be detrimental to the IQ scores of PKU siblings who were heterozygous, with reduced conversion of phenylalanine to tyrosine [86].

3. Increased concentrations of phenylalanine also inhibit transport of the other neutral amino acids [8], producing an imbalance of amino acids in the brain that could upset regulatory control of neuroactive derivatives and interfere with protein synthesis.

4. Phenylalanine or its by-products may inhibit key metabolic pathways:
   a. Tyrosine hydroxylase will accept phenylalanine as an alternate substrate [6, 74], but elevated phenylalanine inhibits this enzyme [74], blocking catecholamine synthesis. Catecholamine concentrations were found to be much lower in the caudate nucleus, brain stem, and cerebral cortex of four PKU patients than in controls who were mentally retarded from other causes [87].
   b. Tryptophan metabolism is altered in untreated patients with PKU and in experimental hyperphenylalaninemia. Tryptophan hydroxylase is inhibited by excess of phenylalanine. (The concentration of phenylpyruvate required to inhibit this aromatic amino acid decarboxylase exceeds that found in patients with phenylketonuria). Although much of the disturbance of tryptophan metabolism is probably systemic, brain serotonin levels can be reduced experimentally [88] and have been found reduced also in the four PKU brains with reduced catecholamines [87]. Untreated PKU patients had reduced cerebrospinal levels of serotonin

derivatives; these levels rose after dietary restriction of phenylalanine.

c. Energy metabolism is suppressed in PKU, perhaps by inhibition of pyruvate kinase. The utilization of ATP also may be altered as phenylalanine has been reported to stimulate $(Na^+ + K^+)$-ATPase.

5. Protein synthesis in the brain may be impaired seriously by the marked imbalance of amino acid concentrations and by disaggregation of polyribosomes. This disaggregation was shown experimentally to occur in the brains of imma-ture rats [89]. The defect in myelination found in the brains of PKU patients may reflect gen-eralized inhibition of protein synthesis or specific inhibition of proteolipid synthesis.

Experimental models for PKU have been gen-erally unsatisfactory. Simply feeding phenylalanine produces combined elevations of both tyrosine and phenylalanine; specific inhibitors of phenylalanine hydroxylase such as p-chlorophenylalanine may have other pharmacological actions [7]; in vitro tests of phenylalanine on single enzymes or single pathways cannot duplicate the complex metabolic disturbances known to occur in PKU; an identical mutant animal model has not been found; the effects of experimental PKU could never be fully correlated with the intellectual impairment and behavioral changes that are found in humans [90–92]. Perhaps the most convincing animal model is that for maternal PKU. If a pregnant rat is fed large amounts of phenylalanine, with or without a phenylalanine hydroxylase inhibitor, the effects of the maternal hyperphenylalanimenia can be analyzed in her fetuses or, after birth, in her off-spring [89, 90].

ATYPICAL HYPERPHENYLALANINEMIA

Atypical phenylketonuria or benign hyperphenyl-alaninemia variants have been discovered from screening programs which identify infants with high blood phenylalanine. Neonatal hyperphenylalani-nemia can be secondary to any cause of tyro-sinemia, including prematurity; other hyperphenyl-alaninemia variants have been transient or more

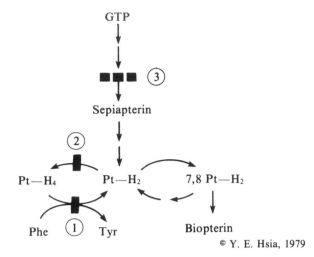

© Y. E. Hsia, 1979

Fig. 28-6. Generation and regeneration of tetrahydro-biopterin (Pt-H_4). The pterin cofactor for the aromatic amino acid is Pt-H_4, which is oxidized to the quinonoid form of dihydrobiopterin, Pt-H_2. Pt-H_2 spontaneously isomerizes to 7.8 Pt-H_2, which is oxidized to biopterin and excreted, or is salvaged by dihydrofolate reductase to yield Pt-H_4. De novo synthesis of Pt-H_2 is from guanosine triphosphate (GTP) through sepiapterin. Enzymes: (1) phenylalanine hydroxylase; (2) dihydro-biopterin reductase; (3) a step in sepiapterin synthesis.

persistent but with lower blood phenylalanine than in classical phenylketonuria [1, 3]. Immuno-reactive hepatic phenylalanine hydroxylase was reduced, but not absent (the enzyme showed altered kinetics), in one patient with atypical hyper-phenylalaninemia [75]. Whether these variants are indeed benign has not yet been resolved. Whatever the neurotoxic mechanism might be in PKU, if it were directly proportional to the degree of hyper-phenylalaninemia, the potential toxicity of the milder variants would be proportional to the blood phenylalanine level found during the vulnerable period of brain growth.

PHENYLKETONURIA VARIANTS

Perhaps one percent of patients diagnosed as hav-ing PKU by newborn blood phenylalanine concen-trations do not respond to diet treatment at all. Some of the patients developed intractable seizures and choreiform movements, and all have had early, progressive mental retardation despite apparently

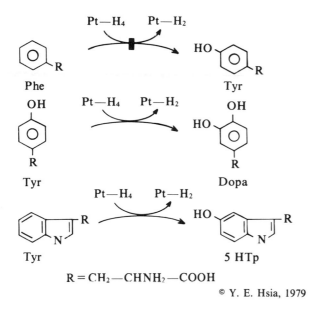

$$R = CH_2 - CHNH_2 - COOH$$

© Y. E. Hsia, 1979

Fig. 28-7. The three aromatic amino acid hydroxylase reactions that require tetrahydrobiopterin as a cofactor. The top reaction is conversion of phenylalanine to tyrosine by phenylalanine hydroxylase, defective in phenylketonuria; the middle reaction is conversion of tyrosine to dihydroxyphenylalanine (Dopa); the bottom reaction is conversion of tryptophan to 5-hydroxy-tryptophan (5HTP), the precursor of serotonin.

satisfactory dietary control of blood phenylalanine levels.

Dihydropteridine reductase deficiency has been demonstrated in some patients [93], associated with reduced tissue concentrations of tetrahydrobiopterin (Fig. 28-6). In another patient, this enzyme activity was present, but nonetheless tetrahydrobiopterin was only 10 percent of normal, suggesting a defect in biosynthesis of biopterin [94].

Since tetrahydrobiopterin is a cofactor for tyrosine hydroxylase and tryptophan hydroxylase as well as for phenylalanine hydroxylase (Fig. 28-7), a block in either its biosynthesis or regeneration (Fig. 28-6) would be expected to interfere with catecholamine and serotonin formation. This has been confirmed in the brain and tissue fluids of these patients. The deficiency of these neurotransmitters provides a rational neurochemical explanation for the refractory neurological disturbances in these patients. Treatment has been attempted with L-dopa and 5-hydroxytryptophan.

TYROSINE AMINOTRANSFERASE DEFICIENCY
Tyrosine aminotransferase deficiency (Fig. 28-1, reaction 7) causes tyrosinemia, with painful dendritic corneal ulcers, keratosis palmoplantaris, agitation, tics, and moderate mental retardation [3, 95–97]. The biochemical defect is in the cytosol enzyme, which accepts the cosubstrate α-ketoglutarate to form p-hydroxyphenylpyruvate and glutamate, requiring pyridoxal phosphate as a cofactor. Because mitochondrial tyrosine aminotransferase (15 percent of tyrosine aminotransferase activity in the liver) remains intact, these patients can still produce p-hydroxyphenylpyruvate and p-hydroxyphenyllactate, which appear in the urine in this syndrome. In the brain, tyrosine aminotransferase is mainly mitochondrial, and its role in tyrosine metabolism appears to be overshadowed by that of tyrosine hydroxylase, so degradation of tyrosine is superseded in the brain by catecholamine biosynthesis. It is not clear how neurotoxicity is produced in this condition, but dietary restriction to control tyrosine levels in blood has improved at least the ocular and cutaneous manifestations of this condition; any observed behavioral improvement could have resulted from symptomatic relief of the distressing eye and skin lesions [96, 97]. p-Hydroxyphenylpyruvate dioxygenase deficiency (Fig. 28-1, reaction 8) produces another hereditary [3, 98] hypertyrosinemia syndrome associated with severe liver damage (Table 28-4).

NEONATAL TYROSINEMIA
Not at all uncommon in premature infants, neonatal tyrosinemia occurs in many full-term infants as well. There is increased urinary p-hydroxyphenylpyruvic, p-hydroxyphenyllactic, and p-hydroxyphenylpyruvate dioxygenase (Fig. 28-1, reaction 8) [1]. This enzyme has low activity in the fetus and is subject to substrate inhibition, so developmental immaturity of the enzyme is worsened by hypertyrosinemia. Administration of ascorbic acid, a reducing substance that stimulates the en-

zyme, will suppress the tyrosinemia. Whether transient neonatal tyrosinemia is benign or neurotoxic has not been fully established, but careful studies have shown that almost 10 percent of affected infants may develop reduced mental capacities [99, 100].

THE ALBINISMS

The albinisms are due to defective melanosome synthesis of melanin, in some variants caused by tyrosinase deficiency (Fig. 28-1, reaction A). Curiously, melanin formation in the central nervous system (e.g., in the substantia nigra) is never affected. Mammals with generalized albinism have been found to have failure of decussation of the optic pathways to the lateral geniculate bodies. In patients with generalized albinism there is physiological evidence for faulty lateralization of visual stimuli [101] and of auditory stimuli [102].

The Sulfur Amino Acids: Methionine, Cysteine, Taurine

Methionine has great biological significance, because S-adenosylmethionine (Fig. 28-8) is the major methyl donor in many biochemical reactions, including the synthesis of such biogenic amines as choline and epinephrine; the inactivation of such neurotransmitters as serotonin and the catecholamines; and the methylation of creatine, of proteins, and of nucleotides [1]. It may also be a precursor of polyamines. S-adenosylhomocysteine, the product of these reactions, can be recycled to methionine through homocysteine by methyltetrahydrofolate methyltransferase (Fig. 28-2, reaction 11 and Fig. 28-8, reaction 6) or by hepatic betaine-homocysteine methyltransferase (see also Chap. 33). By this means, methionine, an essential amino acid, is regenerated using one-carbon fragments from serine and glycine (Fig. 28-8) for its methylation reactions. Methionine deficiency interferes with growth; in excess, it exacerbates the psychotic behavior of chronic schizophrenics. Hypermethioninemia occurs clinically in acute liver failure, and results also from blocked methionine and homocysteine metabolism.

Homocysteine reacts with serine to form cystathionine (Fig. 28-2, reaction 12), a compound with no known biological function. Cystathionine is found in high concentration in the brain, predominantly in white matter. It is also in liver, kidney, and muscle. It is hydrolyzed by cystathionase to cysteine and homoserine (Fig. 28-2, reaction 13). Homoserine, like threonine, is a precursor of α-ketobutyrate and is catabolized through the propionate pathway (Fig. 28-2).

Cysteine is an important component of proteins, glutathione, coenzyme A, and many other biologically active compounds. The further catabolism of cysteine is either by removal and eventual oxidation of the sulfur radical (Fig. 28-2, reaction 14) to sulfate (which accounts for 80 percent of urinary sulfur) or by oxidation to cysteinsulfinate, decarboxylation to hypotaurine, and oxidation to taurine.

Taurine is found in very high concentration in the brain, especially in the cerebellar cortex. It may act as an inhibitory modulator of synaptic transmission or as a transmitter [103]. It is also present in high concentration in the retina, in muscle, and in the liver, where it forms bile salts that participate in fat absorption and are excreted in the stool.

METHIONINEMIA

Caused by hepatic deficiency of methionine adenosyltransferase activity, methioninemia (Fig. 28-8, reaction 5) has been found in one clinically healthy normal infant [104]. S-adenosylmethionine has a vital role in transmethylation reactions, so it is surprising that this condition is compatible with survival, let alone with neurological normality. The biochemical abnormalities were a persistent methioninemia, 30 times normal, which was nevertheless nontoxic; no change in the other sulfur amino acids; and a high serum folate. The only enzyme found to be low was methionine adenosyltransferase, which was about 10 percent of normal in two liver biopsies. Perhaps the partial enzyme block was overcome by the huge excess of methionine.

HOMOCYSTINURIA

Caused by cystathionine synthase deficiency (Fig. 28-2, reaction 12) homocystinuria results in tissue accumulation of homocysteine and methionine,

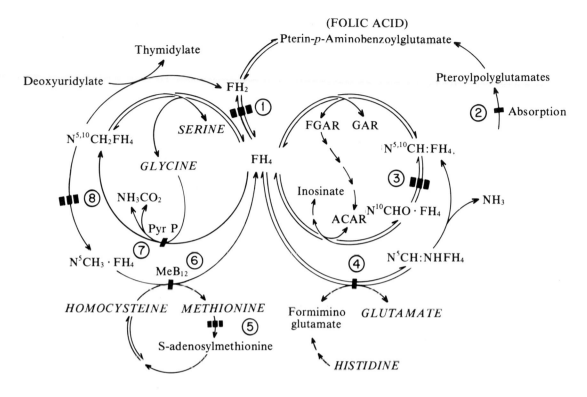

Fig. 28-8. Folate and glycine metabolism. The relationships of derivatives of FH_4 to glycine metabolism are indicated in the circle on the left and to purine biosynthesis in the circle on the right. Acronyms: ACAR, 5-aminoimidazole-4-carboxyamide ribinucleotide; FGAR, N-formylglycinamide ribonucleotide; GAR, glycinamide ribonucleotide. Enzymes: (1) dihydrofolate reductase; (2) folate absorption; (3) cyclohydrolase; (4) formiminotransferase; (5) methionine adenosyltransferase; (6) homocysteine:methionine methyltransferase; (7) glycine cleavage enzyme; (8) $N^{5,10}$-methylene-FH_4 reductase.

and depletion of cystathionine, with the resultant appearance of urinary homocystine and even traces of S-adenosylhomocysteine [1, 3]. Patients with homocystinuria share with Marfan's syndrome patients a characteristic lanky body habitus, long extremities and digits, and abnormal lens capsular ligaments that predispose to dislocation of the lens. Homocystinuric patients often suffer from mental retardation, are liable to psychiatric disturbances, and have a propensity for thromboembolic occlusion of arteries and veins. In homocystinuria it

has been speculated that an abnormality of connective tissue might be the cause for lens dislocation and joint laxity and perhaps for endothelial vulnerability to fibrin deposition, too. The brain damage might then be due to multiple, repeated, small cerebral thromboses.

Vitamin responsiveness to large doses of pyridoxal phosphate has been demonstrated biochemically in some patients, with or without enzymatic evidence of enhanced cystathionine synthase activity, indicating there are variants of this disorder. Some patients have abnormal liver mitochondria [105].

Neurochemically, toxicity from cystathionine deficiency or from other disturbances of homocysteine metabolism has neither been proved nor disproved. Dietary treatment with low methionine intake has resulted in clinical improvement, especially when started in infancy; dietary treatment with serine and cysteine to stimulate reverse synthesis of homocysteine via cystathionase has been recommended. A substantial fraction of plasma homocysteine is claimed to be protein-bound [106].

Hence, clinical studies based on free plasma homo-cysteine may require reevaluation.

Homocystinuria may also be due to abnormalities of vitamin B_{12} metabolism and folate metabolism discussed elsewhere in this chapter.

CYSTATHIONINEMIA
Deficiency of cystathionase (Fig. 28-2, reaction 13) is associated with abnormally elevated concentrations of cystathionine in the brain [1, 3, 7]. Patients are often asymptomatic, but some have had severe mental retardation, and a few have had seizures. The association of this condition with neurological abnormalities has been considered to be coincidental. There are vitamin B_6-responsive and -unresponsive variants [1].

CYSTINOSIS
Cystinosis is not due to deficiency of an enzyme of intermediary metabolism, but almost certainly to an abnormality of lysosomal transport of cysteine or its disulfide, cystine [3, 7]. The severe variant is nephrotoxic, producing generalized aminoaciduria and leading to renal failure by the second decade of life. Apart from patchy depigmentation of the retina and photophobia, possibly related to cystine crystal deposition in the cornea, this condition is neurologically benign. Unlike many of the other lysosomal storage diseases (Chaps. 30 and 31), in this disease there is no brain involvement.

TAURINE DEFICIENCY
Taurine deficiency has been reported in three brothers; their mother, maternal uncle, and maternal grandfather had similar clinical symptoms [103]. Presentation was not until mid-adulthood, with mental depression, insomnia, anorexia and dysphagia, dyspnea, and loss of visual depth perception; they then developed signs of parkinsonism and mental confusion; finally, all the brothers died of respiratory failure. Only one brother had detailed biochemical investigations, and these showed less than half of normal plasma taurine levels and very low cerebrospinal fluid taurine. At autopsy, his brain taurine was reduced in all regions tested, particularly the cerebellum,

compared with controls or patients with Huntington's and Parkinson's diseases. There were no abnormalities of other metabolites of sulfur amino acids or of GABA. Histologically there was distinct depigmentation of the substantia nigra, with extensive loss of neurons and some gliosis in his brain and that of one brother. A younger sister has become depressed and is developing low plasma taurine concentrations, but showed no measurable metabolic abnormality in response to an oral taurine loading test.

Taurine has inhibitory neurotransmitter properties in the central nervous system and retina, so the findings in this patient are tantalizingly suggestive of an inborn error of cysteine conversion to taurine with very specific neurochemical consequences. In immature kittens, dietary taurine deficiency produces a specific retinal degeneration [107], which demonstrates that taurine does have an essential functional role in the nervous system. Because oral taurine in humans has had no untoward effects and can enter the central nervous system, taurine therapy should be tried if other patients are ever found with this disorder.

TAURINE-RELATED DISORDERS
Other rare disorders involving tyrosine (Table 28-4) are β-mercaptolactate cysteine disulfiduria and sulfite oxidase deficiency [108, 109].

Glycine and Sarcosine
Glycine is abundantly present in most tissue fluids and cells. Its general metabolism has been extensively studied, and it participates in innumerable metabolic reactions. In the nervous system, it can be formed from glyoxylate and serine, but it is formed only slowly from glucose (Chap. 17). Glycine degradation in the brain is primarily by the glycine cleavage enzyme system (Fig. 28-8). It is a putative inhibitory neurotransmitter, present in very high concentration in spinal gray matter associated with inhibitory interneurons (Chap. 12).

HYPERGLYCINEMIA
Hyperglycinemia (Fig. 28-8, reaction 7) is caused by deficiency of glycine-cleavage enzyme; it must be

differentiated from a host of genetic and non-genetic causes of hyperglycinemia, including the disorders of branched-chain amino acid catabolism [3, 23, 110]. The patients with defective glycine cleavage have early onset of lethargy, hypotonia, myoclonic jerks, and generalized seizures that are unresponsive to anticonvulsant therapy, but no attacks of ketoacidosis or hyperammonemia. Profound mental retardation appears in those who survive beyond infancy. In the later stages of the condition, hypertonia and decerebrate rigidity may supervene. Tracer studies have shown delayed oxidation of glycine and a defect in liver and brain glycine-cleavage enzyme. The activity of this enzyme was almost equally decreased in one patient with the ketotic hyperglycinemia syndrome due to methylmalonic acidemia [3]. Suppressed enzyme activity in the ketotic hyperglycinemia syndromes would explain the presence of hyperglycinemia in metabolic disorders of branched-chain amino acid and propionate catabolism, but the mechanism of inhibition is not known.

Glycine concentrations in the urine and blood are markedly elevated in all the conditions causing hyperglycinemia. Glycine concentrations in brain and cerebrospinal fluid, however, were found to be very elevated only in patients with nonketotic hyperglycinemia [23]. In two such patients, examined postmortem, glycine cleavage-enzyme activity was undetectable in brain, although the activity in liver was decreased to just a third of normal. The distribution of excess glycine in these patients was in every region of the brain that was analyzed [110]. Strychnine administration to affected infants has produced dramatic improvement in some [111] but not all. The rationale for this treatment is the competitive binding of strychnine to glycine receptors in the central nervous system (see Chap. 12).

HYPERGLYCINURIA

This is a prominent feature of any generalized amino aciduria, ranging from immaturity to drug toxicity, and includes the aminoacidurias secondary to galactosemia (Chap. 29), Wilson's disease (Chap. 36), and cystinosis. Inherited transport defects of glycine alone are rare. Iminoglycinuria, due to defective shared renal transport mechanisms for proline, hydroxyproline, and glycine, is benign. In the other prolinurias, hyperglycinuria is also found [1, 3].

Glycinuria and glycinemia have been reported in individual patients with neurological disorders, such as a family with spinal cord lesions [112] and one patient with an oculocerebral syndrome [113]. These associations may be coincidental.

The Iminoacids: Proline and Hydroxyproline
Proline is a nonessential amino acid synthesized from glutamate through pyrroline-5-carboxylate. It is degraded by the independent catabolic enzymes, mitochondrial proline oxidase and cytosol pyrroline-carboxylate dehydrogenase, back to glutamate. This degradation can occur in the brain. Hydroxyproline is found mostly in collagen, where it is formed by hydroxylation of proline residues during collagen synthesis. Degradation is through oxidation to hydroxypyrroline-carboxylate, hydroxyglutamate and α-hydroxy-γ-ketoglutarate to glyoxylate and pyruvate. Most iminoacid is excreted as oligopeptides; at least one transport system for the free iminoacids is shared with glycine [1, 3].

Type I hyperprolinemia, a proline-oxidase deficiency, has had coincidental association with renal disease and possible mental retardation or seizures. Type II hyperprolinemia, a pyrroline-carboxylate-dehydrogenase deficiency, has been more frequently associated with mental retardation and seizures and causes a greater degree of hyperprolinemia. In both conditions, there is overflow renal prolinuria with competitive saturation of the common reabsorptive mechanism shared with hydroxyproline and glycine.

Hydroxyprolinemia and iminopeptiduria [114] have also been reported (Table 28-4). Iminopeptiduria occurs also in other conditions as a nonspecific expression of disturbed collagen metabolism.

Folate
Folic acid (Fig. 28-8), pteroylglutamic acid, is present in food mainly as polyglutamates. Absorp-

tion of these polyglutamates is preceded by hydrolysis to folate monoglutamate by the enzyme conjugase. Extracellular folic acid is then reduced intracellularly to tetrahydrofolate (FH_4), which serves as a cofactor that transfers one-carbon units in many key regions of intermediary metabolism, including glycine catabolism (the left circle in Fig. 28-8) and purine biosynthesis (the right circle in Fig. 28-8). Folic-acid deficiency, like vitamin B_{12} deficiency, produces megaloblastic anemia, but usually without serious neurological consequences (Chap. 33). Cerebrospinal fluid folates are normally three times the concentration of blood folates. Every cell probably has the capacity to synthesize and recycle the folate intermediates necessary for its own metabolism [115], although nerve cells are supposed to lack dihydrofolate reductase activity and so would be unable to utilize oxidized folic acid.

CONGENITAL MALABSORPTION OF FOLATE

Congenital malabsorption of folate (Fig. 28-8, reaction 2), unlike folic-acid deficiency in older patients, presents in infancy with ataxia or athetosis, seizures and mental retardation, as well as megaloblastic anemia [116, 117]. One older patient was found to have punctate calcification of the basal ganglia. The condition has been reported only four times, in three families. One patient had no neurological abnormality apart from poor school performance, but had been treated with large doses of parenteral folate from the age of 3 months. The severe neurological damage in this disorder may be due to susceptibility of the developing brain to folate deficiency; in one patient, the seizures were aggravated and in another they were reduced by folate treatment.

FORMIMINOTRANSFERASE DEFICIENCY

Formiminotransferase deficiency (Fig. 28-8, reaction 4) blocks the catabolism of histidine and causes a large increase in urinary formiminoglutamate excretion [115, 118, 119]. Four Japanese patients had elevated serum folate, formiminoglutamic aciduria exacerbated by histidine loading, mental retardation, abnormal electroencephalograms, and

cerebral cortical atrophy. One of two Swiss sisters had much worse formiminoglutamic aciduria, normal serum folate, retarded speech, and borderline-normal IQ; her sister had similar chemical findings, but had perfect speech and intelligence. A Canadian brother and sister had persistent formiminoglutamic aciduria, normal serum folate, delayed speech, hypotonia, and clumsiness. Aminoimidazole carboxyimide, the riboside of which is converted to inosinic acid by an enzyme requiring N^{10}formyl-FH_4 as a cofactor (Fig. 28-8), was present in excess in the urine of three of the Japanese patients.

Myelin structure has contained abnormally low cerebroside hydroxy-fatty acids in one patient, who presented in infancy with a megaloblastic anemia that improved with folate or pyridoxine therapy [120].

$N^{5,10}$-METHYLENE-FH_4 REDUCTASE DEFICIENCY

Methylene tetrahydrofolate blocks the synthesis of methyl-FH_4 [115, 121, 122] (Fig. 28-8, reaction 8). It has aroused interest because one patient had psychiatric disturbances that fluctuated with periods on and off folic acid therapy. This condition has been found in two affected sisters and one unrelated boy. The patients had elevated homocysteine in the urine and plasma, marginally low plasma methionine and serum folate, but no measurements were made of amino acids in cerebrospinal fluid. The older of the sisters was retarded mentally, had an abnormal electroencephalogram, and showed features of catatonic schizophrenia at the age of 14. On therapy with pyridoxine and then folate, her mental status improved, but she developed peripheral neuropathy. Off therapy, she relapsed; she improved on reinstitution of pyridoxine and folate or of folate alone, which suppressed her homocysteine production at the same time that her mental derangement improved. Her platelet monoamine oxidase was decreased during a relapse, but it was normal in her younger sister. This sister, also retarded, had no psychotic symptoms. The boy had proximal muscle weakness, abnormal electroencephalogram and seizures, but no reported mental instability.

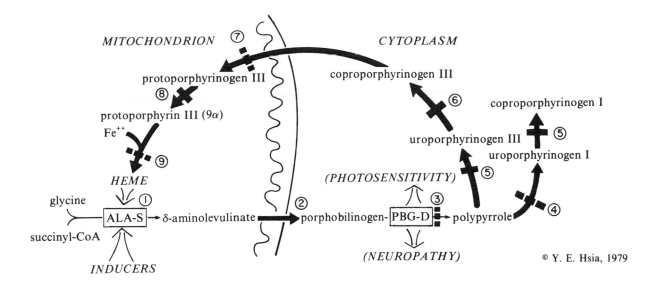

Fig. 28-9. Metabolic map of heme synthesis. The intra-mitochondrial generation of δ-aminolevulinate, shown at the lower left, is the rate-limiting step repressed by the end-product heme and induced by many agents. Two molecules of δ-aminolevulinate condense asymmetrically to form cyclic porphobilinogen; its deamination is thought to be a secondary rate-limiting step, overactivity of which produces excess of photosensitizing porphyrinogen products, and underactivity of which results in accumulation of neurotoxic precursors. Tetracyclic polymerization to the polypyrroles is followed by successive decarboxylations, re-entry into the mitochondrion, oxidation of side-chains, and finally insertion of the ferrous ion to form heme. The compounds on the left are excretion products found in some of the porphyrias (see table 28-5). Abbreviations: ALA-S, δ-aminolevulinate synthetase (1); PBG-D, porphobilinogen deaminase (3); Fe^{2+}, ferrous iron. Enzymes: (1) δ-aminolevulinate synthetase; (2) δ-aminolevulinate dehydratase; (3) ? porphobilinogen deaminase; (4) ? urobilinogen I synthetase; (5) uroporphobilinogen III cosynthetase; (6) uroporphobilinogen decarboxylase; (7) coproporphyrinogen oxidase; (8) ? protoporphyrinogen oxidase; (9) ferrochelatase.

The enzyme activity, demonstrated in liver and cultured skin fibroblasts, was less than 20 percent of normal. FAD coenzyme addition doubled enzyme activity in cells from the sisters and from controls, but stimulated it fivefold in cells from the affected male. Because methyl-FH₄ is a cofactor for the vitamin B₁₂-dependent regeneration of methionine from homocysteine (Fig. 28-8, reaction 6), its decrease in this condition would interrupt the re-supply of S-adenosylmethionine for other methyl transfer reactions. Although degradation of administered methionine to sulfate in these patients was normal, their cultured cells did not grow in a medium when homocysteine was substituted for methionine, confirming that remethylation of homocysteine to methionine was impaired in this condition.

OTHER METHYL-FH₄ DISORDERS

Other disorders in the methyl-FH₄ group (Fig. 28-8) [115] include single reported cases of dihydrofolate reductase (reaction 1), cyclohydrolase (reaction 3), and homocysteine:methionine methyltransferase (reaction 6) deficiencies.

Porphyrins

Heme is a tetrapyrrole ring with a central iron atom that can convert molecular oxygen to its first activated state. It is a prosthetic group for many enzyme reactions involving electron transfer, oxygen transport, activation or breakdown of peroxide, and protein synthesis [123–125]. The porphyrin tetrapyrroles (Fig. 28-9) are synthesized by the union of glycine with succinyl-CoA to form δ-aminolevulinate (δ-ALA), the asymmetrical condensation of two molecules of δ-ALA to form the pyrrole porphobilinogen, deamination and cyclization of four porphobilinogen rings to form urobilinogens, successive decarboxylations of the pyrrole side chains to convert the urobilinogens to coproporphyrins, oxidation to protoporphyrins, and finally incorporation of iron. Only the first enzyme, δ-ALA synthetase (Fig. 28-9, reaction 1), and the last few enzymes are mitochondrial. δ-ALA synthetase, the rate-limiting enzyme, has a very rapid biological turnover with a half-life of just 1 or 2 hours; it is repressed by heme and is induced by steroid hormones, drugs, alcohol, and many other agents.

Porphobilinogen deaminase (Fig. 28-9, reaction 3) is a secondary rate-limiting enzyme, activity of which may determine the relative concentrations of its precursors and its products. Its precursors appear to be neurotoxic; δ-ALA is present in high concentration in the hypothalamus, and has been shown to inhibit human brain $(Na^+ + K^+)$-ATPase; porphobilinogen has inhibited rat presynaptic transmission [123, 124]. Its products, the tetrapyrroles, are potent photosensitizing agents. Heme is an essential component of all mitochondrial electron-transfer systems in every cell, but the major portion of body heme production is in hematopoietic tissue for incorporation into hemoglobin.

Degradation of heme is only partial. Iron is released from reutilization, and the porphyrin ring is broken to form biliverdin and bilirubin. In liver microsomes, this bilirubin conjugates with glucuronic acid, glycine or taurine, and is excreted mainly in the bile.

The Porphyrias

Porphyria is caused by exogenous toxins such as lead and alcohol, metabolic diseases such as tyrosinemia, and several inherited abnormalities of porphyrin synthesis (Table 28-5). Unlike almost all other clinically significant inherited enzyme abnormalities, these are anabolic (also deficient ganglioside G_{M3} biosynthesis, see Chap. 30) and most are autosomal dominant disorders. A few of these have neurological and psychological manifestations, often precipitated by medications or other exogenous factors.

ACUTE INTERMITTENT PORPHYRIA (SWEDISH TYPE)

This is associated with up to 50-fold overproduction of porphyrins, fourfold increase of δ-ALA synthetase activity, half of normal porphobilinogen deaminase or uroporphobilinogen I synthetase activities (Fig. 28-9, reactions 3 or 4) and decreased steroid 5α-reductase activity [123, 124]. Affected individuals may remain asymptomatic, but postpubertally, they are prone to acute attacks that are often precipitated by any drug capable of inducing δ-ALA synthetase, including the barbiturates and alcohol; febrile illnesses; exogenous and endogenous steroid hormones, particularly estrogens (e.g., during the menstrual cycle); and starvation.

A unifying concept of the protean symptoms in this disorder is that most are due to neuropathy [123–125]:

1. Abdominal pain and gastrointestinal upset may be caused by autonomic nervous system disturbances, which would also account for the sweating, labile blood pressure, urinary retention, and skin blanching that occur in the acute attacks or crises.
2. Poly- or mononeuropathy may appear; it may be sensory, with pain and parasthesia, or motor, with weakness and paralysis. If respiratory muscles are weakened, life becomes endangered.
3. Hypothalamic damage and inappropriate secretion of antidiuretic hormone can account for the episodes of water retention and hyponatremia associated with attacks; disturbances of consciousness may also arise from toxicity to the brain stem or hypothalamus.
4. Mental illness occurs in up to one-third of all affected patients. Some of the acute symptoms of irritability and irrationality may be caused by discomfort or by disturbed fluid and electrolyte balance, but other forms of organic brain syndrome, ranging from depression through anxiety states to frank schizophrenia, have been observed.

Unlike the other porphyrias, there are no skin rashes, hemolytic anemia, or liver abnormalities in acute intermittent porphyria.

Table 28-5. The Porphyrias

Type	Postulated Metabolic Block (Fig. 28-9)	Clinical Features					Mode of Inheritance
		Skin Photosensitivity	Hemolytic Anemia	Liver Toxicity	Neurological Involvement		
Acute intermittent porphyria (Swedish type)	3 or 4	None	None	None	Severe acute attacks		Autosomal dominant
Congenital erythro-poietic porphyria (Günther's disease)	5	Bullous scarring	Usual	None	None		Autosomal recessive
Porphyria cutanea tarda	6	Bullous scarring	None	Frequent	None		Autosomal dominant
Hereditary copro-porphyria	7	Mild	None	None	Milder acute attacks		Autosomal dominant
Variegate Porphyria (South African type)	8 or 9	Mild scarring	None	None	Infrequent attacks		Autosomal dominant
Erythropoietic protoporphyria	9	Solar urticaria	Minimal	Present	None		Autosomal dominant

Metabolically, there is increased urinary excretion of δ-ALA and porphobilinogen, especially during attacks; they increase in the cerebrospinal fluid, as well. The neurochemical basis for the toxicity is a mystery, but may be due to toxic effects of precursor accumulation because of rate-limited porphyrin biosynthesis [124]. Although there is no absolute correlation between the degree of metabolic abnormality and the neurological symptoms in a given patient, fluctuating urine excretion of porphyrin precursors tends to correspond with clinical attacks.

Biochemically, δ-ALA synthetase is actively repressed by heme and may be derepressed if heme production is diminished in this condition (Fig. 28-9, reaction 1) [123]. Based on observations in one patient and his two parents, steroid 5α-reductase deficiency has been proposed as an independent genetic mutation, and symptomatic disease would appear only when both abnormalities coincided in a patient [123]. Reduced steroid 5α-reductase activity may explain the vulnerability of affected individuals to estrogen steroids, since degradation to 5β-H derivatives that would induce δ-ALA synthetase could be enhanced if 5α-H derivatives were less readily formed.

Treatment is primarily by avoidance of precipitating factors such as known toxic drugs or starvation; generous carbohydrate intake is protective. Infusions of heme or its ferrihydroxy derivative, hematin, have suppressed red-cell plasma and urine porphyrins in this condition [126, 127]. This approach should suppress excess production of δ-ALA and porphobilinogen while supplying the putatively missing end product, heme. Even if there is systemic biochemical improvement, however, there is no evidence yet that infused heme can penetrate into nerve cells or improve neuronal function.

HEREDITARY COPROPORPHYRIA
Hereditary coproporphyria appears to be the result of a defect of coproporphyrin oxidation (Fig. 28-9, reaction 4), because affected patients excrete an excess of urinary δ-ALA, porphobilinogen, and coproporphyrins but not the more mature porphyrins or heme [123, 124]. Affected individuals (Table 28-5) can have acute neuropathic attacks, as in acute intermittent porphyria, but, as is not the case for that condition, there can be photosensitive skin rashes as well.

Metabolically, coproporphyrin excretion is increased 50-fold, mainly in the stool, with inconstant urinary excretion of δ-ALA, porphobilinogen, and coproporphyrins, which tend to be increased during acute attacks.

VARIEGATE PORPHYRIA (SOUTH AFRICAN TYPE)
Variegate porphyria appears to be due to a partial defect of protoporphyrinogen oxidase (Fig. 28-9, reaction 8) [123–125, 128]. Affected individuals (Table 28-5) have highly variable clinical manifestations, including acute neuropathic attacks and a scarring photosensitivity of the skin.

Metabolically, there is intermittent urinary excretion of δ-ALA, porphobilinogen, and coproporphyrins, with increased fecal coproporphyrins and protoporphyrins. During attacks, urine and fecal uroporphyrins are much increased. These findings are compatible with blocked biosynthesis of heme from protoporphyrin and derepressed δ-ALA synthetase.

Bilirubin
Basal ganglia degeneration can be caused by many diseases, including toxic accumulation of bilirubin and of copper (Chap. 36, [3]). Neonatal hyperbilirubinemia, usually resulting from prematurity or one of the neonatal hemolytic anemias, is characterized by high concentrations of unconjugated bilirubin, which is less efficiently excluded by an immature blood-brain barrier, resulting in bilirubin staining of the brain, particularly of the basal ganglia. Bilirubin appears to be toxic to the central nervous system, producing staining and cystic degeneration of the basal ganglia (*kernicterus*) with disorders of movement, mental retardation, and deafness [3, 130].

CRIGLER-NAJJAR SYNDROME
The Crigler-Najjar syndrome is a genetic deficiency of bilirubin conjugation that generally causes

kernicterus in infancy. Two patients, however, after being neurologically intact for over 15 years, developed disorders of movement, myotonia, intellectual deterioration, and seizures. One was improved by phototherapy [130]. The other eventually lapsed into coma and died; autopsy findings showed neuronal loss and gliosis of the thalamus, and considerable neuronal loss in the basal ganglia and cerebellum [131]. Although there was no staining in the brain, these patients can be considered to have had late onset of bilirubin neurotoxicity equivalent to neonatal kernicterus.

Treatment

Treatment must be a prime consideration for patients with inherited metabolic errors [78]. Specific therapeutic approaches have been discussed in relation to the various disorders, but curative replacement or restoration of a defective protein is seldom possible (see also Chaps. 30 and 31). Better understanding of the neurochemical disturbances in these inborn errors of metabolism may eventually produce rational therapies that will benefit both the common and the rare disorders, and advance our understanding of basic neurochemistry.

Acknowledgment

This work has been supported by a National Foundation–March of Dimes Medical Service Grant C-297.

References

*1. Bondy, P. K., and Rosenberg, L. E. (eds.). *Metabolic Control and Disease* (8th ed.). Philadelphia: Saunders, 1980.

*2. Tanaka, K. Disorders of Organic Acid Metabolism. In G. E. Gaull (ed.), *The Biology of Brain Dysfunction.* New York: Plenum, 1975. Vol. III, pp. 145–214.

*3. Stanbury, J. B., Wyngaarden, J. B., and Frederickson, D. S. (eds.). *The Metabolic Basis of Inherited Disease* (4th ed.). New York: McGraw-Hill, 1978. P. 1862.

4. Hsia, Y. E. Inherited Metabolic Disorders. In G. Avery (ed.), *Neonatology* (2nd ed.). Philadelphia: Lippincott, 1981.

5. Shuman, R. M., Leech, R. W., and Scott, C. R.

*Key reference.

The neuropathology of the nonketotic and ketotic hyperglycinemias: Three cases. *Neurology* 28: 139–146, 1978.

*6. Ciba Foundation Symposium 22 (New Series). *Aromatic Amino Acids in the Brain.* Amsterdam: Associated Scientific Publishers, 1974.

*7. Gaull, G. E., Tallan, H. H., Lajtha, A., and Rassin, D. K. Pathogenesis of Brain Dysfunction in Inborn Errors of Amino Acid Metabolism. In G. E. Gaull (ed.), *The Biology of Brain Dysfunction.* New York: Plenum, 1975. Vol. III, pp. 47–144.

*8. Oldendorf, W. H. Saturation of blood brain barrier transport of amino acids in phenylketonuria. *Arch. Neurol.* 28:45–48, 1973.

9. Tahmoush, A. J., Alpers, D. H., Feigin, R. D., Armbrustmacher, V., and Prensky, A. L. Hartnup disease. *Arch. Neurol.* 33:797–807, 1976.

10. Robinson, B. H., Taylor, J., and Sherwood, W. G. The genetic heterogeneity of lacticacidosis: Occurrence of recognizable inborn errors of metabolism in a pediatric population with lactic acidosis. *Pediatr. Res.* 14:956–962, 1980.

11. Silberberg, D. H. Maple syrup urine disease metabolites studied in cerebellum cultures. *J. Neurochem.* 16:1141–1146, 1969.

12. Bowden, J. A., Brestel, E. P., Cope, W. T., McArthur, C. L., Westfall, D. N., and Fried, M. α-Ketoisocaproic acid inhibition of pyruvate and α-ketoglutarate oxidative decarboxylation in rat liver slices. *Biochem. Med.* 4:69–76, 1970.

13. Bowden, J. A., McArthur, C. L., and Fried, M. Metabolic diseases and mental retardation. I. The chick embryo as a model system in branched-chain ketoaciduria; the effect of α-ketoisocaproic acid. *Int. J. Biochem.* 5:391–396, 1974.

14. Kimura, T., and Tahara, M. Effect of force-feeding diets lacking leucine, valine, isoleucine, threonine or methionine on amino acid catabolism in rats. *J. Nutr.* 101:1647–1656, 1971.

15. Guibaud, P., Divry, P., Dubois, Y., Collombel, C., and Larbre, F. Une observation d'acidemie isovalerique. *Arch. Fr. Pediatr.* 30:633–645, 1973.

16. Krieger, I., and Tanaka, K. Therapeutic effects of glycine in isovaleric acidemia. *Pediatr. Res.* 10:25–29, 1976.

17. Cohn, R. M., Yudkoff, M., Rothman, R., and Segal, S. Isovaleric acidemia: Use of glycine therapy in neonates. *N. Engl. J. Med.* 299:996–999, 1978.

18. Ando, T., and Nyhan, W. L. Propionic Acidemia and the Ketotic Hyperglycinemia Syndrome. In W. L. Nyhan (ed.), *Heritable Disorders of Amino Acid Metabolism.* New York: Wiley, 1974. Pp. 37–60.

19. Schutgens, R. B. H., Heymans, H., Ketel, A., Veder, H. A., Duran, M., Ketting, D., and Wadman, S. K.

Lethal hypoglycemia in a child with a deficiency of 3-hydroxy-3-methylglutarylcoenzyme A lyase. *J. Pediatr.* 94:89–91, 1979.

*20. Hsia, Y. E. Inherited hyperammonemic syndromes. *Gastroenterology* 67:347–374, 1974.

21. Wolf, B., Hsia, Y. E., Tanaka, K., and Rosenberg, L. E. Correlation between serum propionate and blood ammonia concentrations in propionic acidemia. *J. Pediatr.* 93:471–473, 1978.

22. Gompertz, D., Storrs, CN. M., Ban, D. C. K., and Peters, T. J. Localization of enzymatic defect in propionic acidemia. *Lancet* 1:1140–1143, 1970.

23. Perry, T. L., Urquhart, N., McLean, J., Evans, M. E., Hansen, S., Davidson, A. G. F., Applegarth, D. A., MacLeod, P. J., and Lock, J. E. Nonketotic hyperglycemia: Glycine accumulation due to absence of glycine cleavage in brain. *N. Engl. J. Med.* 292:1269–1273, 1975.

24. Wolf, B., Paulsen, E. P., and Hsia, Y. E. Asymptomatic propionyl CoA carboxylase deficiency in a thirteen-year-old girl. *J. Pediatr.* 95:563–565, 1979.

25. Brandt, I. K., Hsia, Y. E., Clement, D. H., and Provence, S. A. Propionic-acidemia (ketotic hyperglycemia): Dietary treatment resulting in normal growth and development. *Pediatrics* 53: 391–395, 1974.

26. Barnes, W. D., Hull, D., Balgobin, L., and Gompertz, D. Biotin responsive propionic-acidemia. *Lancet* 2:244–245, 1970.

27. Weyler, W., Sweetman, L., Maggio, D. C., and Nyhan, W. L. Deficiency of propionyl CoA carboxylase and β-methylcrotonyl CoA carboxylase in a patient with methylcrotonylglycinuria. *Clin. Chim. Acta* 76:321–328, 1977.

28. Saunders, M., Sweetman, L., Robinson, B., Roth, K., Cohn, R., and Gravel, R. A. Biotin-responsive organic-aciduria: Multiple carboxylase defects and complementation studies with propionicacidemia in cultured fibroblasts. *J. Clin. Invest.* 64: 1695–1702, 1979.

29. Hsia, Y. E., Scully, K. J., and Rosenberg, L. E. Vitamin-B_{12} dependent methylmalonicacidemia. *Pediatrics* 46:497–505, 1970.

30. Duckett, S., Williams, N., and Francis, S. Peripheral neuropathy associated with inhalation of methyl-*n*-butyl ketone. *Experientia* 30:1283–1284, 1974.

31. Dillon, M. J., England, J. M., Gompertz, D., Goodey, P. A., Grant, D. B., Hussein, H. A.-A., Linnell, J. C., Matthews, D. M., Mudd, S. H., Newns, G. H., Seakins, J. W. T., Uhlendorf, B. W., and Wise, I. J. Mental retardation, megaloblastic anemia, methylmalonic aciduria and abnormal homocysteine metabolism due to an error in vita-

min B_{12} metabolism. *Clin. Sci. Mol. Med.* 47:43–61, 1974.

32. Kishimoto, Y., Williams, M., Moser, H. W., Hignite, C., and Bieman, K. Branched-chain and odd-numbered fatty acids and aldehydes in the nervous system of a patient with deranged vitamin B_{12} metabolism. *J. Lipid Res.* 14:69–77, 1973.

33. Hillman, R. E., and Keating, J. P. Beta-keto-thiolase deficiency as a cause of the "ketotic hyperglycinemia syndrome." *Pediatrics* 53:221–225, 1973.

34. Boxer, L. A., Oliver, J. M., Spielberg, S. P., Allen, J. M., and Schulman, J. D. Protection of granulocytes by vitamin E in glutathione synthetase deficiency. *N. Engl. J. Med.* 301:901–905, 1979.

35. Larsson, A., Zetterstrom, R., Hagenfeldt, L., Andersson, R., Dreborg, S., and Hornell, H. Pyroglutamic aciduria (5-oxoprolinuria), an inborn error in glutathione metabolism. *Pediatr. Res.* 8:852–856, 1974.

36. Wellner, V. P., Sekura, R., Meister, A., and Larsson, A. Glutathione synthetase deficiency, an inborn error of metabolism involving the γ-glutamyl cycle in patients with 5-oxoprolinuria (pyroglutamic aciduria). *Proc. Natl. Acad. Sci. U.S.A.* 71:2505–2509, 1974.

37. Hagenfeldt, L., Larsson, A., and Andersson, R. The γ-glutamyl cycle and amino acid transport: Studies of free amino acids, γ-glutamyl-cysteine and glutathione in erythrocytes from patients with 5-oxoprolinuria (glutathione synthetase deficiency). *N. Engl. J. Med.* 299:587–590, 1978.

38. Richards, F., Cooper, M. R., Pearce, L. A., Cowan, R. J., and Spurr, C. L. Familial spinocerebellar degeneration, hemolytic anemia, and glutathione deficiency. *Arch. Intern. Med.* 134:534–537, 1974.

39. Goodman, S. I., Mace, J. W., and Pollak, S. Serum gamma-glutamyl transpeptidase deficiency. *Lancet* 1:234–235, 1971.

40. Schulman, J. D., Patrick, A. D., Goodman, S. I., Tietze, F., and Butler, J. Gamma-glutamyl transpeptidase (GGTPase): Investigations in normals and patients with inborn errors of sulfur metabolism. *Pediatr. Res.* 9:355, 1975 (abstract).

41. Krebs, H. A., Hems, R., and Lund, P. Some regulatory mechanisms in the synthesis of urea in the mammalian liver. *Adv. Enzyme Regul.* 11:361–377, 1973.

42. Milner, J. A., and Visek, W. J. Orotate, citrate, and urea excretion in rats fed various levels of arginine. *Proc. Soc. Exp. Biol. Med.* 147:754–759, 1974.

43. Batshaw, M., Brusilow, S., and Walser, M. Keto-acid therapy of carbamyl phosphate synthetase deficiency. *N. Engl. J. Med.* 292:1085–1090, 1975.

44. Thoene, J. T., Batshaw, M., Spector, E., Kulovich, S., Brusilow, S., Walser, M., and Nyhan, W. Neo-

natal citrullinemia: Treatment with ketoanalogues of essential amino acids. *J. Pediatr.* 90:218–224, 1977.

45. McReynolds, J. W., Mantagos, S., Brusilow, S., and Rosenberg, L. E. Treatment of complete ornithine transcarbamylase deficiency with nitrogen free analogues of essential amino acids. *J. Pediatr.* 93: 421–427, 1978.

46. McReynolds, J. W., Crowley, B., Mahoney, M. J., and Rosenberg, L. E. Evidence for autosomal recessive inheritance of mitochondrial carbamyl phosphate synthetase deficiency. *Pediatr. Res.* 12: 453, 1978 (abstract).

47. Mantagos, S., Psagaraki, S., Burgess, E. A., Oberholzer, V., Palmer, T., Sacks, J., Baibas, S., and Valaes, T. Neonatal hyperammonaemia with complete absence of liver carbamyl synthase activity. *Arch. Dis. Child.* 53:230–234, 1978.

48. Gatfield, P. D., Taller, E., Wolfe, D. M., and Haust, M. D. Hyperornithinemia, hyperammonemia and homocitrullinuria associated with decreased carbamyl phosphate synthetase I activity. *Pediatr. Res.* 9:488–497, 1975.

49. Cathelineau, L., Saudubray, J.-M., and Polonovski, C. Heterogenous mutations of the structural gene of human ornithine carbamyltransferase as observed in five personal cases. *Enzyme* 18:103–113, 1974.

50. Glasgow, A. M., Kraegel, J. H., Schulman, J. D. Studies of the cause and treatment of hyperammonemia in females with ornithine transcarbamylase deficiency. *Pediatrics* 62:30–37, 1978.

51. Gelehrter, T. D., and Rosenberg, L. E. Ornithine transcarbamylase deficiency: Unsuccessful therapy of neonatal hyperammonemia with *N*-carbamyl-*l*-glutamate and *l*-arginine. *N. Engl. J. Med.* 292: 351–352, 1975.

52. Kennaway, N. G., Harwood, P. J., Rambert, D. A., Koler, R. D., and Buist, N. R. M. Citrullinemia: Evidence for genetic heterogeneity. *Pediatr. Res.* 9:554–558, 1975.

53. Perry, T. L., Wirtz, M. L. K., Kennaway, N. G., Hsia, Y. E., Atienza, F. C., and Uemura, H. S. Amino acid and enzyme studies of brain and other tissues in an infant with argininosuccinic aciduria. *Clin. Chim. Acta* 105:257–267, 1980.

54. Shih, V. E., and Mandell, R. Metabolic defect in hyperornithinemia. *Lancet* 2:1522–1523, 1974.

55. O'Donnell, J. J., Sandman, R. P., and Martin, S. R. Gyrate atrophy of the retina: Inborn error of *l*-ornithine: 2-oxoacid aminotransferase. *Science* 200:200–201, 1978.

56. Shih, V. E., Berson, E. L., Mandell, R., and Schmidt, S. Y. Ornithine ketoacid transaminase

deficiency in gyrate atrophy of the choroid and retina. *Am. J. Hum. Genet.* 30:174–179, 1978.

57. Fell, V., Pollitt, R. J., Sampson, G. A., and Wright, T. Ornithinemia, hyperammonemia, and homocitrullinemia: A disease associated with mental retardation and possibly caused by defective mitochondrial transport. *Am. J. Dis. Child.* 127:752–756, 1974.

58. Synderman, S. E., Sansaricq, C., Chen, W. J., Norton, P. M., and Phansalkar, S. V. Argininemia. *J. Pediatr.* 90:563–568, 1977.

59. Simell, O., and Perheentupa, J. Renal handling of diamino acids in lysinuric protein intolerance. *J. Clin. Invest.* 54:9–17, 1974.

60. Gatfield, P. D., Taller, E., Hinton, G. G., Wallace, A. C., Abdelnour, G. M., and Haust, M. D. Hyperpipecolatemia: A new metabolic disorder associated with neuropathy and hepatomegaly. *Can. Med. Assoc. J.* 99:1215–1233, 1968.

61. Danks, D. M., Tippett, P., Adams, C., and Campbell, P. Cerebro-hepatorenal syndrome of Zellweger: A report of eight cases with comments upon the incidence, the liver lesion, and a fault in pipecolic acid metabolism. *J. Pediatr.* 86:382–387, 1975.

62. Goldfischer, S., Moore, C. L., Johnson, A. B., Spiro, A. J., Valsamis, M. P., Wisniewski, H. K., Ritch, R. H., Norton, W. T., Rapin, I., and Gartner, L. M. Peroxisomal and mitochondrial defects in the cerebro-hepato-renal syndrome. *Science* 182: 62–64, 1973.

*63. Cooper, J. R., Bloom, F. E., and Roth, R. H. *The Biochemical Basis of Neuropharmacology* (2nd ed.). New York: Oxford University Press, 1977. P. 272.

64. Brandt, N. J., Gregersen, N., Christensen, E., Grøn, I. H., and Rasmussen, K. Treatment of glutaryl-CoA dehydrogenase deficiency (glutaric aciduria). *J. Pediatr.* 94:669–673, 1979.

65. Gregersen, N., and Brandt, N. J. Ketotic episodes in glutaryl-CoA dehydrogenase deficiency (glutaric aciduria). *Pediatr. Res.* 13:977–981, 1979.

66. Sweetman, L., Nyhan, W. L., Trauner, D. A., Merritt, T. A., and Singh, M. Glutaric aciduria type II. *J. Pediatr.* 96:1020–1026, 1980.

67. Wong, P. W. K., Forman, P., and Justice, P. A new inborn error of tryptophan metabolism. *Pediatr. Res.* 9:358, 1975 (abstract).

68. Fischer, M. H., Gerritsen, T., and Opitz, J. M. α-Aminoadipic aciduria, a non-deleterious inborn metabolic defect. *Hum. Genet.* 24:265–270, 1974.

69. Wilson, R. W., Wilson, C. M., Gates, S. C., and Higgins, J. V. α-Ketoadipic aciduria: A description of a new metabolic error in lysine-tryptophan degradation. *Pediatr. Res.* 9:522–526, 1975.

70. Olney, J. W. Toxic Effects of Glutamate and Related Amino Acids on the Developing Central

Nervous System. In W. L. Nyhan (ed.), *Heritable Disorders of Amino Acid Metabolism.* New York: Wiley, 1974. Pp. 501–512.

71. Murphey, W. H., Lindmark, D. G., Patchen, L. I., Housler, M. E., Harrod, E. K., and Mosovich, L. Serum carnosinase deficiency concomitant with mental retardation. *Pediatr. Res.* 7:601–606, 1973.

72. Terplan, K. L., and Cares, H. L. Histopathology of the nervous system in carnosinase enzyme deficiency with mental retardation. *Neurology* 22:644–654, 1972.

73. Gjessing, L. R., and Sjaastad, O. Homocarnosinosis: A new metabolic disorder associated with spasticity and mental retardation. *Lancet* 2:1028, 1974.

74. Kaufman, S., and Fisher, D. B. Pterin Requiring Aromatic Amino Acid Hydroxylases. In O. Hayaishi (ed.), *Molecular Mechanism of Oxygen Activation.* New York: Academic, 1974. Pp. 285–369.

75. Friedman, P. A., Kaufman, S., and Kang, E. S. Nature of the molecular defect in phenylketonuria and hyperphenylalaninemia. *Nature* 240:157–159, 1972.

76. Friedman, P. A., Fisher, D. B., Kang, E. S., and Kaufman, S. Detection of hepatic phenylalanine 4-hydroxylase in classical phenylketonuria. *Proc. Natl. Acad. Sci. U.S.A.* 70:552–556, 1973.

77. Cotton, R. G. H., and Danks, D. M. Purification of inactive phenylalanine hydroxylase protein from liver in classical phenylketonuria. *Nature* 260:63–64, 1976.

*78. Hsia, Y. E. Treatment in Genetic Diseases. In A. Milunsky (ed.), *The Prevention of Genetic Disease and Mental Retardation.* Philadelphia: Saunders, 1975. Pp. 277–305.

79. Bush, J. W., Chen, M. M., and Patrick, D. L. Health Status Index in Cost Effectiveness: Analysis of PKU program. In R. L. Berg (ed.), *Health Status Indexes.* Chicago: Hospital Research and Educational Trust, 1973. Pp. 174–208.

80. Smith, I., and Wolff, O. H. Natural history of phenylketonuria and influence of early treatment. *Lancet* 1:540–544, 1974.

81. Perry, T. L., Hansen, S., Tischler, B., Richards, F. M., and Sokol, M. Unrecognized adult phenylketonuria: Implications for obstetrics and psychiatry. *N. Engl. J. Med.* 289:395–398, 1973.

82. Howell, R. R., and Stevenson, R. E. The offspring of phenylketonuric women. *Soc. Biol.* 18:519–527, 1971 (Suppl.).

83. Smith, I., Erdohaz, M., Macartney, F. J., Pincott, J. R., Wolff, O. H., Brenton, D. P., Biddle, S. A., Fairweather, D. V. I., and Dobbing, J. Fetal damage despite low-phenylalanine diet after conception in a phenylketonuric woman. *Lancet* 1:17–19, 1979.

84. Lasala, J. M., and Coscia, C. J. Accumulation of a tetrahydroisoquinoline in phenylketonuria. *Science* 203:283–284, 1979.

85. Sandler, M., Ruthven, C. R. J., Goodwin, B. L., Field, H., and Matthews, R. Phenylethylamine overproduction in aggressive psychopaths. *Lancet* 2:1269–1270, 1978.

86. Bessman, S. P., Williamson, M. L., and Koch, R. Diet, genetics, and mental retardation interaction between phenylketonuric heterozygous mother and fetus to produce nonspecific diminution of IQ: Evidence in support of the justification hypothesis. *Proc. Natl. Acad. Sci. U.S.A.* 75:1562–1566, 1978.

87. McKean, C. M. The effects of high phenylalanine concentrations on serotonin and catecholamine metabolism in human brain. *Brain Res.* 47:469–476, 1972.

88. Loo, Y. H. Serotonin deficiency in experimental hyperphenylalaninemia. *J. Neurochem.* 28:139–147, 1974.

89. Copenhaver, J. H., Vacanti, J. P., and Carver, M. J. Experimental maternal hyperphenylalaninemia: Disaggregation of fetal brain ribosomes. *J. Neurochem.* 21:273–280, 1973.

90. Andersen, A. E., Rowe, V., and Guroff, G. The enduring behavioral changes in rats with experimental phenylketonuria. *Proc. Natl. Acad. Sci. U.S.A.* 71:21–25, 1974.

91. Beckner, A. S., Centerwall, L. R., and Holt, L. Effects of rapid increase of phenylalanine intake in older PKU children. *J. Am. Diet. Assoc.* 69:148–151, 1976.

92. Marholin, D., Pohl, R. E., Stewart, R. M., Touchette, P. E., Townsend, N. M., and Kolodny, E. H. Effects of diet and behavior therapy on social and motor behavior of retarded phenylketonuric adults: An experimental analysis. *Pediatr. Res.* 12:179–187, 1978.

93. Brewster, T. G., Moskowitz, M. A., Kaufman, S., Breslow, J. L., Milstien, S., and Abroms, I. F. Dihydropteridine reductase deficiency associated with severe neurologic disease and mild hyperphenylalaninemia. *Pediatrics* 63:94–99, 1979.

94. Kaufman, S., Berlow, S., Summer, G. K., Milstien, S., Schulman, J. D., Orloff, S., Spielberg, S., and Pueschel, S. Hyperphenylalaninemia due to lack of biopterine: A variant form of phenylketonuria. *N. Engl. J. Med.* 299:673–679, 1978.

95. Goldsmith, L. A., Kang, E., Bienfang, D. C., Jimbow, K., Gerald, P., and Baden, H. P. Tyrosinemia with plantar and palmar keratosis and keratitis. *J. Pediatr.* 82:798–805, 1973.

96. Zaleski, W. A., and Hill, A.   Tyrosinosis: A new variant. *Can. Med. Assoc. J.* 108:477–484, 1973.

97. Lemonnier, F., Charpentier, C., Odievre, M., Larreque, M., and Lemonnier, A.   Tyrosine aminotransferase isoenzyme deficiency. *J. Pediatr.* 94:931–932, 1979.

98. Lindlad, B., Lindstedt, S., and Steen, G.   On the enzymic defects in hereditary tyrosinemia. *Proc. Natl. Acad. Sci. U.S.A.* 74:4641–4646, 1977.

99. Menkes, J. H., Welcher, D. W., Levi, H. S., Dallas, J., and Gretsky, N. E.   Relationship of elevated blood tyrosine to the ultimate intellectual performance of premature infants. *Pediatrics* 49: 218–224, 1972.

100. Mamunes, P., Prince, P. E., Thornton, N. H., Hunt, P. A., and Hitchcock, E. S.   Intellectual deficits after transient tyrosinemia in the term neonate. *Pediatrics* 57:675–680, 1976.

101. Creel, D., O'Donnell, F. E., and Witkop, C. J.   Visual system anomalies in human ocular albinos. *Science* 201:931–933, 1978.

102. Creel, D., Garber, S. R., King, R. A., and Witkop, C. J.   Auditory brainstem anomalies in human albinos. *Science* 209:1253–1255, 1980.

103. Perry, T. L., Bratly, P. J. A., Hansen, S., Kennedy, J., Urquhart, N., and Dolman, C. L.   Hereditary mental depression and parkinsonism with taurine deficiency. *Arch. Neurol.* 32:108–113, 1975.

104. Gaull, G. E., and Tallan, H. H.   Methionine adenosyltransferase deficiency: New enzymatic defect associated with hypermethioninemia. *Science* 186:59–60, 1974.

105. Gaull, G., Sturman, J. A., and Schaffuer, F.   Homocystinuria due to cystathionine synthase deficiency: Enzymatic and ultrastructural studies. *J. Pediatr.* 84:381–390, 1974.

106. Kang, S. S., Wong, P. W. K., and Becker, N.   Protein-bound homoocyst(e)ine in normal subjects and in patients with homocystinuria. *Pediatr. Res.* 13:1141–1143, 1979.

107. Hayes, K. C., Carey, R. E., and Schmidt, S. Y.   Retinal degeneration associated with taurine deficiency in the cat. *Science* 188:949–951, 1975.

108. Shih, V. E., Abroms, I. F., Johnson, J. L., Carney, M., Mandell, R., Robb, R. M., Cloherty, J. P., and Rajagopalan, K. V.   Sulfite oxidase deficiency: Biochemical and clinical investigations of a hereditary metabolic disorder in sulfur metabolism. *N. Engl. J. Med.* 297:1022–1028, 1977.

109. Crawhall, J. C.   The Unknown Disorders of Sulfur Amino Acid Metabolism: β-Mercapto-lactate-Cysteine Disulfiduria, Sulfite Oxidase Deficiency, the Methionine Malabsorption Syndrome, and Hypermethionemia. In W. L. Nyhan (ed.), *Heritable Disorders of Amino Acid Metabolism.* New York: Wiley, 1974. Pp. 467–476.

110. Tada, K., Corbeel, L. M., Eeckels, R., and Eggermont, E.   A block in glycine cleavage reaction as a common mechanism in ketotic and nonketotic hyperglycinemia. *Pediatr. Res.* 8:721–723, 1974.

111. Gitzelmann, R., Steinmann, B., Otten, A., Dumermuth, G., Herdan, M., Reubi, J. C., and Cuénod, M.   Nonketotic hyperglycinemia treated with strychnine, a glycine receptor antagonist. *Helv. Paediatr. Acta.* 32:517–525, 1977.

112. Bank, W. J., and Morrow, G.   A familial spinal cord disorder with hyperglycinemia. *Arch. Neurol.* 27:136–144, 1972.

113. Balci, S., Say, B., and Firat, T.   Corneal opacity, microphthalmia, mental retardation, microcephaly and generalized muscular spasticity associated with hyperglycinemia. *Clin. Genet.* 5:36–39, 1974.

114. Powell, G. F., Rasco, M. A., and Maniscalco, R. M.   A prolidase deficiency in man with iminopeptiduria. *Metabolism* 23:505–513, 1974.

115. Erbe, R. W.   Inborn errors of folate metabolism. *N. Engl. J. Med.* 293:753–757, 807–812, 1975.

116. Lanzkowsky, P.   Congenital malabsorption of folate. *Am. J. Med.* 48:580–583, 1970.

117. Santiago-Borrero, P. J., Santini, R., Perez-Santiago, E., and Maldonado, N.   Congenital isolated defect of folic acid absorption. *J. Pediatr.* 82:450–455, 1973.

118. Niederwieser, A., Giliberti, P., Tatasouvic, A., Pluznik, S., Steinmann, B., and Baerlocher, K.   Folic acid non-dependent formiminoglutamic aciduria in two siblings. *Clin. Chim. Acta* 54:293–316, 1974.

119. Perry, T. L., Applegarth, D. A., Evans, M. E., Hansen, S., and Jellum, E.   Metabolic studies of a family with massive formiminoglutamic aciduria. *Pediatr. Res.* 9:117–122, 1975.

120. Chida, N., and Arakawa, T.   Decrease in long-chain hydroxy fatty acids of myelin cerebroside in formiminotransferase deficiency. *Tohoku J. Exp. Med.* 108:279–381, 1972.

121. Mudd, S. H., Uhlendorf, B., Freeman, J. M., Finkelstein, J. D., and Shih, V. E.   Homocystinuria associated with decreased methylenetetrahydrofolate reductase activity. *Biochem. Biophys. Res. Comm.* 46:905–915, 1972.

122. Freeman, J. M., Finkelstein, J. D., and Mudd, S. H.   Folate-responsive homocystinuria and "schizophrenia," a defect in methylation due to deficient 5,10-methylenetetrahydrofolate reductase activity. *N. Engl. J. Med.* 292:491–496, 1975.

123. Tschudy, D. P., and Lamon, J. M.   Porphyrin Metabolism and the Porphyrias. In P. K. Bondy and

L. E. Rosenberg (eds.), *Metabolic Control and Disease* (8th ed.). Philadelphia: Saunders, 1980. Pp. 939–1007.

124. Brodie, M. J., Moore, M. R., and Goldberg, A. Enzyme abnormalities in the porphyrias. *Lancet* 2:699–701, 1977.

125. Bloomer, J. R. The hepatic porphyrias: Pathogenesis, manifestations, and management. *Gastroenterology* 71:689–701, 1976.

126. Watson, C. J., Dhar, G. J., Bossenmaire, I., Cardinal, R., and Petryka, Z. J. Effect of hematin in acute porphyric relapse. *Ann. Intern. Med.* 79: 80–83, 1973.

127. Lamon, J. M., Frykholm, B. C., Bennett, M., and Tschudy, D. P. Prevention of acute porphyric attacks by intravenous hematin. *Lancet* 2:492–494, 1978.

128. Brenner, D. A., and Bloomer, J. R. The enzymatic defect in variegate porphyria: Studies with human cultured skin fibroblasts. *N. Engl. J. Med.* 302: 765–769, 1980.

129. MacAlpine, I., Hunter, R., and Rimington, C. Porphyria in the royal houses of Stuart, Hanover and Prussia: A follow-up study of George III's illness. *Br. Med. J.* 1:7–17, 1968.

130. Berk, P. D., Jones, E. A., Howe, R. B., and Berlin, N. I. Disorders of Bilirubin Metabolism. In P. K. Bondy and L. E. Rosenberg (eds.), *Metabolic Control and Disease* (8th ed.). Philadelphia: Saunders, 1980. Pp. 1009–1088.

131. Blashke, T., Berk, P. D., Scharschmidt, B. F., Guyther, J. R., Vergalla, J. M., and Waggoner, J. G. Crigler-Najjar syndrome: An unusual course with development of neurologic damage at age eighteen. *Pediatr. Res.* 8:573–590, 1974.

132. Gardner, W. A., and Konigsmark, B. W. Familial nonhemolytic jaundice: Bilirubinosis and encephalopathy. *Pediatrics* 43:365–376, 1969.

David B. McDougal, Jr.

Chapter 29. Defects in Carbohydrate Metabolism

It is surprising that, although glucose has long been established as the primary source of energy for brain (Chap. 24), the mechanisms by which disorders of carbohydrate metabolism produce their effects on neural function are still essentially unknown. Because these disorders may afford opportunities that cannot be duplicated in the laboratory, their study in human beings can be expected to make unique contributions to the understanding of carbohydrate metabolism and its role in the function of the nervous system.

The commonest disorders of carbohydrate metabolism affect the use or storage of glucose. Diabetes mellitus is discussed in detail below. Others, such as galactosemia and several disorders of hepatic glycogen metabolism, appear to act on the nervous system by depriving it of glucose.

A handful of rare diseases are characterized by the accumulation of pyruvic or lactic acids, or both, in blood or urine. In some of these the nervous system is permanently affected; in others it appears to be normal once the metabolic acidosis is controlled. The reader should consult Chap. 17 for a general review of carbohydrate metabolism.

Diabetes Mellitus

Certainly, the commonest disease of carbohydrate metabolism is diabetes mellitus, which is characterized by elevated blood glucose levels and inappropriately low plasma insulin. The term *diabetes mellitus* designates a group of similar disorders, in which heritable factors may play a role in the response of the subject to such external insults as environmental chemicals or viruses [1]. The peripheral, autonomic, and central nervous systems may be affected.

ENCEPHALOPATHY

An untreated or inadequately treated diabetic may go, more or less suddenly, into a state of metabolic acidosis and then into coma. The clinical chemistry includes marked elevation of the blood and urine glucose levels, ketone bodies in the urine, and depressed plasma PCO_2 and pH. Occasionally, coma is seen with very high blood glucose levels without acidosis. This has been attributed to hyperosmolarity.

Some patients who have had diabetes for many years suffer central nervous system effects that are considered by some to constitute a true diabetic encephalopathy [2]. These patients often lose tendon reflexes, and many have mental disturbances, sometimes severe. Neurological symptoms and signs include attacks of vertigo, transitory hemiparesis, intellectual impairment, dyspraxia, incoordination, and orthostatic hypotension.

A relatively constant pattern of pathological changes is observed in diabetic encephalopathy: diffuse degenerative abnormalities, often with severe pseudocalcinosis of the cerebellum, demyelination of cranial nerves, leptomeningeal fibrosis, and angiopathy.

Experimentally, the effect of diabetic acidosis (produced by alloxan) on cerebral metabolites in mice has been studied in animals in a state of relative immobility before coma or loss of righting reflexes supervened [3]. Cerebral phosphocreatine levels were elevated 70 percent, glucose-6-P was elevated, and fructose diphosphate was depressed, suggesting depressed cerebral and glycolytic activity. Glycogen levels were decreased in most animals, despite a tenfold increase in brain glucose. Lactate levels were decreased, but pyruvate levels were unchanged.

Table 29-1. The Effect of Various Experimentally Produced Alterations
of Glucose Metabolism upon Cerebral Levels of ATP and P-Creatine[a]

	ATP	P-Creatine (mmol per kg)	Glucose
Diabetes[b]	2.98 ± 0.05	4.86 ± 0.015	10.6 ± 1.1
Control[b]	2.80 ± 0.02	2.86 ± 0.05	1.01 ± 0.07
Hypoglycemia[c]			
Stupor	3.02 ± 0.03	4.50 ± 0.08	0.07 ± 0.01
Convulsions	2.98 ± 0.12	4.08 ± 0.30	0.07 ± 0.01
Control[c]	2.90 ± 0.04	4.08 ± 0.07	1.66 ± 0.08
Galactosemia[d]	1.67 ± 0.06	1.70 ± 0.07	0.07 ± 0.05
Control[d]	1.95 ± 0.12	1.92 ± 0.17	1.2 ± 0.4

[a]In none of these conditions does there appear to be serious interference with energy supply. The rise in P-creatine in diabetes suggests a reduction in energy use.
[b]Whole mouse brain [3].
[c]Frontal cerebral cortex of mouse brain [32].
[d]Whole chick brain [20].

In an effort to ascertain to what extent these changes could be attributed to the dehydration that accompanies diabetic acidosis, mannitol loading combined with water deprivation was used to dehydrate animals. The changes were similar to those found in alloxan diabetes, except that the decrease in lactate was accompanied by a decrease in pyruvate. The brain glucose level was not increased.

In another type of experiment, acute diabetes was produced by the injection of antiinsulin serum, which promptly resulted in hyperglycemia. During the first day, cerebral glycogen rose 50 percent and pyruvate rose 40 percent.

It may be concluded that, as far as these studies go, changes observed in experimental diabetes are those expected of depressed neuronal activity, dehydration, and hyperglucosemia. The only apparent exception is the elevation of brain pyruvate soon after the administration of antiinsulin serum and its maintenance at control levels after alloxan treatment. This suggests an increase in the $NAD^+/NADH$ ratio, but the change has not been explained. Despite considerable interference with glucose (and other) metabolism, both in the brain and elsewhere, the brain clearly has no difficulty in maintaining its energy supply (Table 29-1).

NEUROPATHY

Symptoms and signs of peripheral nerve involvement may occur early in the development of diabetes in some individuals, or may be a late manifestation [4]. Any nerve may be involved, and symptoms and signs may be sensory, motor, or autonomic. Tendon jerks may disappear, and neurotropic arthropathy and perforating ulcers of the skin are not uncommon. There is some correlation between these effects and control of the diabetic state, so that the symptoms and signs tend to improve with better diabetic control, and even to disappear. This is not always the case, unfortunately, and signs may persist despite apparently good control.

Physiological studies of nerve and muscle in patients with diabetic neuropathy have shown reduced conduction velocity in motor and sensory nerves [5]. It is said that stimulation of nerve trunks in diabetic patients of long standing requires higher voltages [4]. The data supporting this statement have not been published. It is also said, without support, that the elevated threshold is indicative of "poor axoplasmic flow" [4].

Experimentally, a 25 to 30 percent reduction of conduction velocity in nerve has been observed in rats made diabetic by subtotal pancreatectomy or by injection of alloxan [6]. In this experiment, insulin treatment of diabetic animals was unsuccessful in restoring the conduction velocity to normal. The nerves were found to have reduced levels of myoinositol in animals made diabetic by injections of alloxan or streptozotocin. When myoinositol was added to the diet of diabetic animals, conduction velocity in nerve returned to normal, although the severity of the diabetes was not otherwise reduced [7]. In an earlier study, myoinositol levels in the sciatic nerves of rats treated with alloxan were reduced by 40 percent, whether the animals became diabetic or not [8]. The nerves of the diabetic animals had greatly elevated fructose and sorbitol levels, 10 and 20 times higher, respectively, than the levels in the alloxan-treated, non-diabetic controls. Brain-level elevations of these substances were less dramatic (about fourfold).

A 20 percent reduction in axoplasmic transport of AChE activity has, in fact, been observed in the sciatic nerves of rats made diabetic by treatment with streptozotocin [9]. Whether this was the result of a reduction in rate of transport or in the amount of enzyme activity transported was not determined.

A crucial question for understanding the pathogenesis of neural and cerebral dysfunction in diabetes is whether insulin affects neural metabolism directly. Several studies have been performed in an attempt to answer this question. The results of a careful clinical study suggest that insulin enhances glucose transport into brain [10]. In mice, too, increased blood-to-brain glucose transport is suggested because insulin produces an increase in the ratio of brain glucose to blood glucose [11]. It has been suggested that insulin has a direct effect on both K^+ and Na^+ uptake into cerebral cells [12, 13], but no evidence supporting this suggestion has been obtained [14]. Experiments on the isolated, perfused rat brain showed no direct effects of insulin on the cerebral metabolism of either glucose or K^+ [15]. Whether any portion of the disordered function of brain and nerve in diabetes is the direct result of insulin lack cannot be answered at present.

Both insulin receptors and insulin have been found in brain. These insulin levels were said not to respond to large changes in insulin levels in blood, so it appears that the insulin is of endogenous origin [16].

Galactosemia

Galactosemia is an inherited defect of galactose metabolism in which galactose-1-P uridylyltransferase activity is deficient (Table 29-2, Fig. 29-1) [17]. Whether the enzyme protein is entirely lacking has not been determined.

Vomiting or diarrhea occurs within a few days after the patient first ingests milk. Jaundice or hepatomegaly occurs early. There may be ascites. Cataracts have been seen soon after birth. After a few months, if the disease is not recognized, mental retardation occurs. Chemically, liver-function tests give evidence of derangement, blood galactose is elevated, and galactosuria, albuminuria, and amino aciduria are present. Rarely, blood glucose levels may be depressed. Red-cell galactose-1-P content is elevated in these patients, and the demonstration that the red cells lack galactose-1-P uridylyltransferase activity is diagnostic.

The mechanism by which the derangement of neural function is brought about has been the subject of considerable experimental work. There are no known specific inhibitors of galactose-1-P uridylyltransferase that might be used to produce an experimental model. It is possible, however, to elevate cerebral galactose levels in experimental animals enormously by giving them large amounts of galactose in the diet. In one experiment with rats [8], for example, feeding galactose for 5 weeks produced a serum galactose level of 10 mM and a brain level of 5 mmol per kilogram. The galactitol level in brain was 9 mmol per kilogram (in control animals, the level was less than 0.04 mmol per kilogram). In nerve, galactitol levels reached 17 mmol per kilogram. Despite these changes, the animals appeared to be in good health, except that they developed cataracts.

Table 29-2. Enzyme Deficits in Carbohydrate Metabolism, Most with Neurological Consequences

Disorder	References	Enzyme Affected and Number in Fig. 29-1	Principal Organ Affected	Neurological Involvement
Aglycogenosis	[24, 27]	1. Glycogen synthetase	Liver, muscle	Hypoglycemia
Glycogenoses				
I. Von Gierke's	[24, 25]	8. Glucose 6-phosphatase	Liver, kidney	Severe hypoglycemia, convulsions
II. Pompe's	[24]	Lysosomal acid maltase	General	Hypotonia, loss of motor skills
III. Cori's	[24, 25]	3, 4. Debranching enzymes	General, liver (leukocytes)	Mild hypoglycemia
IV. Andersen's	[24, 25]	2. Branching enzyme	General	
V. McArdle's	[24, 25]	5. Phosphorylase	Muscle	
VI. Hers'	[24, 27]	5. Phosphorylase	Liver, leukocytes	Mild hypoglycemia
VII.	[24, 25]	11. Phosphofructokinase	Muscle, erythrocytes	
VIII.	[24, 27]	9. Phosphohexose isomerase	Muscle	
VIII or IX.	[24, 27]	6. Phosphorylase b kinase	Liver, leukocytes	Mild hypoglycemia
Ketotic hypoglycemia	[28]	10. Fructose 1,6-diphosphatase	Liver, intestine	Severe hypoglycemia
Galactosemia	[17]	7. Galactose-1-P uridylyl-transferase	Liver, lens (erythrocytes)	Severe hypoglycemia, retardation, seizures
Hereditary fructose intolerance	[26]	12. Fructose-1-P aldolase	Liver	Hypoglycemia, vomiting
Familial lactic acidosis	[35, 47, 48]	14. Pyruvate carboxylase?	Liver	Acidosis, hypotonia, tachypnea, convulsions
Subacute necrotizing encephalomyelopathy (Leigh's)	[37, 40]	Inhibitor of thiamine triphosphate formation? Pyruvate carboxylase?	Brain	Retardation, weakness, ataxia, cranial nerve palsies
Lactic acidosis	[42–46]	13. Pyruvate decarboxylase	Liver, brain	Ataxia, confusion, choreoathetosis

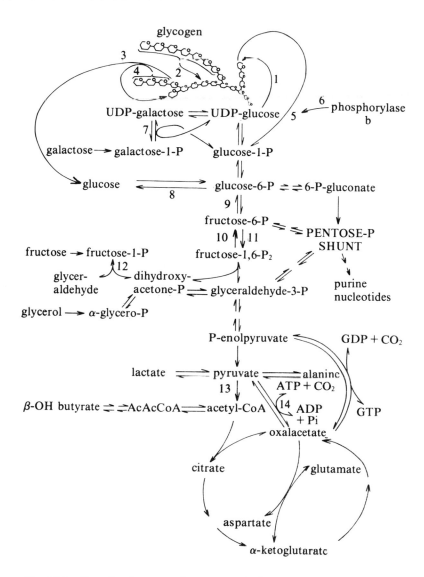

Fig. 29-1. Overall scheme of glucose metabolism.
Some aspects of galactose and fructose metabolism are
also shown. Numbers refer to reactions catalyzed by
enzymes, absence of which leads to one of the glycogenoses (Table 29-2, Chap. 27, and [24, 25]), and
reactions catalyzed by other enzymes mentioned in the
text or in Table 29-2. The reader is reminded that the
activities of some of the enzymes shown are significant
only in extracerebral tissues and that reactions of the
same name may, in different tissues, be catalyzed by very
different proteins. Two arrows in sequence indicate multiple steps. Adapted from Y. E. Hsia.

In young chickens, however, galactose feeding soon produces signs of cerebral dysfunction. They have high cerebral levels of galactose and galactitol (as much as 15 to 20 mmol per kilogram) and relatively high levels of galactose-1-P (0.2 to 1 mmol per kilogram) [18]. After 50 hours on the diet and after allowing for the blood content of the brain (1.75 percent), the brain glucose level was 0.07 mmol per kilogram, only 6 percent of control, despite normal blood glucose levels. As might have been expected, concentrations of glycolytic metabolites were also reduced, and brain glycogen was one-third of control [19]. Studies with radioactive glucose showed that penetration of glucose from blood to brain was reduced by at least 90 percent. Relatively rapid phosphorylation of galactose occurs under these conditions in vivo, and yet the galactose-1-P concentration, after an initial rise in the first few hours of feeding, falls gradually during the next two days. The existence of a "futile cycle" that uses ATP to phosphorylate galactose was postulated, and has been further supported by the discovery of a brain enzyme that hydrolyzes galactose-1-P [18]. No evidence was found for the participation of the cycle when the cerebral metabolic rate was measured, late in the course of the intoxication (after 2 days). However, early in the disease there is a small drop in cerebral ATP and a small rise in AMP at the time when cerebral galactose-1-P levels are highest and before the levels of glycolytic intermediates or glucose have started to fall. This tends to substantiate the notion of an energy-wasting process. Whether the galactose-1-P phosphatase in brain is sufficiently active to account for the observed turnover of galactose-1-P has not been reported. In any event, the disturbance of energy metabolism does not appear to be severe, even when the cerebral glucose levels are exceedingly low (Table 29-1).

Because there is good evidence that glucose penetration into the brain is severely inhibited by the high plasma galactose levels, the effects of a large dose of intraperitoneal glucose were examined in chicks [20]. The animals showed at least a partial reversal of symptoms, concomitant with an increase toward control levels of intracerebral glu-

cose, lactate, and fructose 1,6-P_2, and an increase in intracerebral ATP and P-creatine. Cerebral galactose, galactitol, and galactose-1-P levels were unchanged.

Plasma hyperosmolality, equivalent to that seen in galactose-fed chicks, induced by NaCl or xylose in the drinking water, produced no apparent change in cerebral energy status [20]. Although xylose feeding (but not NaCl) produced a decrease in cerebral glucose to one-fifth of control levels and an increase in xylose and xylitol, lactate and fructose-1,6-P_2 levels were unchanged and cerebral glycogen was nearly 80 percent of control. The chicks showed no sign of neurotoxicity.

Whether the galactose-fed chick is a good model for the galactosemic child has been debated [21, 22]. One criticism has been that the chick recovers promptly when galactose feeding is discontinued, whereas the galactosemic child does not. However, psychological and neuropathological studies of chicks treated with galactose and reared to adulthood have not been reported.

Hypoglycemia

The principal symptoms of hypoglycemia are referable to the nervous system (Chap. 17). The causes may originate almost anywhere in the body [23]. For example, a variety of tumors produce insulin and, consequently, hypoglycemia. In addition, large malignant tumors are sometimes associated with hypoglycemia. It is thought that a tumor of this kind may use large amounts of glucose and, at the same time, may be the source of such substances as tryptophan and its metabolites, which inhibit hepatic gluconeogenesis at the level of phosphoenolpyruvate formation. Some of the tumors have been found to contain increased levels of insulinlike activity, although circulating insulinlike activity is almost never elevated.

Diffuse liver disease, such as acute viral or toxic necrosis or the severe chronic passive congestion associated with heart failure, may give rise to hypoglycemia. In such cases, hepatic output of glucose is reduced because of impaired gluconeogenesis, glycogenesis, and glycogenolysis.

Hypopituitarism is occasionally associated with hypoglycemia as a consequence of increased sensitivity to insulin. Adrenocortical failure is commonly marked by hypoglycemia because the glucocorticoids stimulate some of the key enzymes for gluconeogenesis in the liver. Furthermore, the glucocorticoids play a permissive role in the action of glucagon and epinephrine in producing gluconeogenesis and glycogenolysis.

Hypoglycemia is also a feature of a variety of specific hepatic enzyme deficiencies. In three glycogen-storage diseases (types I, III, and VI, Table 29-2) the capacity to convert glycogen to glucose, and hence to elevate blood glucose levels, is impaired [24, 25]. Although the hypoglycemia produced is severe in glucose 6-phosphatase deficiency, often accompanied by convulsions, permanent cerebral damage appears to be rare. Hypoglycemia is less severe in the type III glycogenosis and least severe in phosphorylase deficiency (see also Chap. 17).

Hepatic fructose-1-P aldolase deficiency [26] (Table 29-2), galactose-1-P uridylyl transferase deficiency (see above), glycogen synthetase deficiency [27] (Table 29-2), fructose 1,6-diphosphatase deficiency [28] (Table 29-2), and maple syrup urine disease (deficiency of branched chain α-keto acid decarboxylases, see Chap. 28) are also characterized by hypoglycemia.

Finally, there is a miscellaneous group of conditions of which hypoglycemia is a more or less constant accompaniment: alcohol ingestion, hyperinsulinism after gastrectomy, reactive hypoglycemia in early diabetes mellitus, and leucine hypersensitivity in children. The list may be extended almost indefinitely by reference to any medical textbook.

PATHOPHYSIOLOGY
A rapidly falling blood glucose level will evoke epinephrine secretion. The chain of events probably involves activation of the adrenal medulla by way of the sympathetic outflow from the central nervous system, perhaps by means of glucose-sensitive neurons in the hypothalamus. The elevated epinephrine level in blood produces symptoms of sweating, weakness, tachycardia, hunger, and "inward trembling." If hypoglycemia persists, symptoms of brain involvement will be added: headache, blurred vision, diplopia, confusion, coma, and convulsions. When hypoglycemia develops slowly, epinephrine secretion and its attendant symptoms may not be evoked but the signs of brain involvement develop in any event. Chronic or repeated hypoglycemia may lead to permanent brain damage [29].

EXPERIMENTAL
It seems evident that if an organ derives most of its energy from glucose it will show signs of malfunction when glucose is withheld. It would appear to follow that the malfunction is the result of energy lack. In brain, at least, this does not appear to be so.

In rats, electroencephalographic evidence of cerebral malfunction occurs at about the time that the calculated intracellular glucose concentration falls to zero [30, 31]. Citric acid cycle intermediates are reduced about 20 percent and pyruvate, glucose-6-P, and glycogen are somewhat lower. But there is no depression of ATP or P-creatine levels, and AMP, a more sensitive indicator of difficulty with the maintenance of ATP levels, does not rise. Even when the animals start to convulse, adenine nucleotide and P-creatine levels remain unchanged, although there is marked depletion of metabolites all along the glycolytic path and around the citric acid cycle, and glycogen has fallen to 30 percent. When electrical activity finally disappears from the EEG, the energy levels in brain fall precipitously. A regional study of the brain in hypoglycemic, unanesthetized mice suggests that symptoms probably develop before the intracellular glucose has completely disappeared [32]. Otherwise, the results of this regional study were similar to those obtained with rats, with no changes in cerebral energy levels at times when cerebral function is severely impaired (Table 29-1).

During hypoglycemia in man and, presumably, in mouse, cerebral glucose and oxygen consumption are reduced (Chap. 24). But there is a parallel reduction in the rate of energy utilization [32] with a consequent preservation of steady-state cerebral ATP and P-creatine levels (in mouse and, presumably, in man). Therefore hypoglycemia appears to reduce the rate of cerebral function (hence the confusion and, finally, coma), but, unless there is a very local energy deficit, as, for example, in synaptic terminals, some metabolic defect other than that of energy supply is the basis of the functional derangement.

To date, the evidence favoring a pivotal role for any of the possible metabolic defects studied is inconclusive. For example, it has been known for many years that in hypoglycemia cerebral aspartate levels rise, and glutamate levels fall. But the changes lag behind the expression of EEG signs of cerebral involvement [30, 31]. Other amino acids also change: Alanine rises, glutamine falls, but the timing of the chemical changes, with respect to that of the EEG signs, does not suggest a precursor-product relationship. When all electrical activity disappears from the EEG, cerebral ammonia levels rise tenfold. Intracellular pH, as indicated by the creatine kinase equilibrium and by the bicarbonate-to-carbonic acid ratio, remains constant throughout the course of the hypoglycemia. The lactate-to-pyruvate ratio falls relatively early in the course of the experiment. It is conceivable that the depression in free cytoplasmic NADH which this suggests could have functional repercussions. What they might be is unknown.

Obviously, if insulin has a direct effect on nervous tissue, the hypoglycemia produced by insulin may be different from that occurring as the result of other causes.

The production of hypoglycemia in hereditary fructose intolerance has been approached experimentally using fructose loading in normal animals. The apparent explanation is based upon the multiplicity of events that occur in the liver after injection of fructose, including increased fructose-1-P and IMP levels, decreased P_i, inhibition of fructose-1-P aldolase by IMP, inactivation of liver phosphorylase, and inhibition of fructokinase, and fructose diphosphate aldolase and phosphorylase by fructose-1-P (for reviews, see [26, 33, 34]).

Disorders of Pyruvate and Lactate Metabolism

Lactic acidosis has been seen in a variety of clinical conditions. Some instances are obvious, as when oxygenation of the patient is impaired because of pulmonary or cardiac disease. Lactic acidosis is also seen in some disorders of amino acid and glycogen metabolism. Of the several causes of hypoglycemia mentioned above, glucose 6-phosphatase deficiency and fructose diphosphatase deficiency are both characterized by lactic acidosis. In a small group of patients, however, the causes of the acidosis are far from clear. Only now is some order being brought to a group of patients who are characterized by metabolic acidosis and sometimes physical retardation and signs of central nervous system disorder. Schärer [35] believes that congenital lactic acidosis can be divided into four types: (1) transitory, seen in full-term newborn infants who recover spontaneously in a few months; (2) early fatal, exemplified by one infant who died a week after birth; (3) slowly progressive, with death in one to four years; and (4) late onset, beginning in the second year of life and usually having a fatal outcome. In all of these types, the most frequent clinical manifestations are periodic attacks of dyspnea, tachypnea and hyperpnea, lethargy, hypotonia, and often obesity. Twitching, convulsions, and psychomotor retardation are not uncommon. Biochemically, there is a metabolic acidosis with elevated blood lactate from 5 to 10 times normal. The rise in pyruvate is often less striking. Lactate levels are elevated in the urine and, less frequently, urinary α-ketoglutarate and amino acids are elevated. Israels and coworkers [36] provide an extensive review of lactic acidosis, including a summary of 23 cases in which the cause was not established. Sixteen of these patients were mentally retarded.

LEIGH'S DISEASE: SUBACUTE NECROTIZING ENCEPHALOMYELOPATHY
Leigh's disease, a disease of children, is characterized pathologically by symmetrical lesions of the mesencephalic tegmentum, pons, medulla, and sometimes the spinal cord (see also Chap. 33). The distribution of lesions is reminiscent of that seen

in Wernicke's encephalopathy (see Chap. 33). Clinically, the patients often show failure of nervous and mental development, with difficulty in standing, sitting, and swallowing. Motor weakness is frequent. Ataxia and abnormalities of the pupillary reflexes are reported less frequently. Cranial nerve palsies are common [37].

Chemically, lactic acidosis is seen frequently, but it tends to be relatively mild and episodic [35]. Subnormal levels of thiamine triphosphate are reported from postmortem specimens of brain, but not of liver [38], and an inhibitor of cerebral thiamine pyrophosphate:ATP phosphotransferase has been found in the blood and urine of children thought to be suffering from this disease and in that of their relatives [39], but rarely in patients with other diseases.

At present, the status of this disorder is not clear. In some, the phosphotransferase inhibitor has been found; in others, an apparent defect in pyruvate carboxylase (Fig. 29-1; also see below) has been reported [40]. In one of the latter patients, the pyruvate carboxylase activity of a liver biopsy sample was within normal limits early in the disease, but nearly absent from a sample obtained at autopsy [41]. Therefore, the loss of the enzyme, at least in this case, cannot have been the cause of the disease.

PYRUVATE DECARBOXYLASE DEFICIENCY

Two children have been described whose clinical histories were marked by repeated episodes of cerebellar ataxia combined with choreoathetosis or confusion which usually followed nonspecific febrile illnesses or other stresses [42–45]. One of these patients is mildly retarded, but the other appears to be above average in intelligence, although even between attacks he is somewhat clumsy.

Biochemically, the blood pyruvate and urine alanine levels were elevated. Blood alanine and lactate were also somewhat increased. Blood glucose levels were within the normal range, and intravenous glucose tolerance tests were also normal. No change was seen in blood glucose levels after an oral glucose load, however, suggesting a defect in in-

testinal glucose absorption. The rate of decarboxylation of pyruvate by whole white cells and fibroblasts and by cell-free preparations of fibroblasts was 25 percent or less than that of the lowest of several preparations from normal subjects (Table 29-2, Fig. 29-1). When glutamate, palmitate, or acetate decarboxylation was studied, the patients' rates were not different from those of controls. Each patient had one parent whose cells showed pyruvate decarboxylation rates intermediate between those of the patient and those of the control. The other parent's cells gave rates equal to the lowest control rates.

Thiamine deficiency did not appear to be a factor, since addition of thiamine pyrophosphate stimulated pyruvate oxidation in cell-free preparations from 20 to 40 percent in both controls and in one patient, but not in the other.

Quite a different sort of patient was described recently by Farrell et al. [46]. An infant with congenital lactic acidosis failed to thrive and died at six months of age. Biochemical examination of brain and liver showed that pyruvate dehydrogenase activity was completely missing, due to a lack of pyruvate decarboxylase. The activities of both dihydrolipoyl transacetylase and dihydrolipoyl dehydrogenase were present in normal amounts. Perhaps the most remarkable thing about this infant was that he survived so long with a defect of this magnitude.

PYRUVATE CARBOXYLASE DEFICIENCY

Several patients have been described as being deficient in hepatic pyruvate carboxylase activity (Fig. 29-1, Table 29-2). As an example, one had hypoglycemia and convulsions early in life with psychomotor retardation [47]. Acidemia was severe, and pyruvate, lactate, and alanine in blood were all three to ten times normal levels. Blood thiamine levels were adjudged to be normal. (The data as reported do not inspire confidence because the control values for free and total thiamine were identical.) Pyruvate decarboxylation by white blood cells and fibroblasts was normal. The patient's liver was not tested for its capacity to decarboxylate pyruvate. In normal livers, pyruvate carboxylase activity was thought to be the result of at least two enzymes, one with a K_m for pyruvate of 0.2 to 0.4 mM, the other with a K_m ten times as high. The activity of the high K_m enzyme appeared to be normal in the patient's liver, but there was no evidence for the presence of the enzyme with the low K_m. Despite the lack of evidence of thiamine deficiency, the patient was put on massive doses of thiamine. The acidemia improved. (There was actually a phase of alkalosis after initiation of thiamine treatment.) Mental retardation persisted, however.

Another patient, seen at age 9, had normal blood glucose, but also showed mental retardation and motor dysfunction [48]. Blood pyruvate levels were two to three times normal, and lactate and alanine levels were at the upper limits of normal. This patient had deficient hepatic pyruvate carboxylase activity (20 percent of controls). A kinetic study was not performed, but the rate of incorporation of pyruvate-2-^{14}C into glycogen by liver slices was only 5 percent of that of a normal control preparation. The patient's pyruvate decarboxylase activity (in liver) was not different from that of two normal controls.

A careful study of partially purified pyruvate carboxylase from human liver [49] has illuminated its properties and called sharply into question previous measurements of its activity in human liver samples obtained by biopsy or at autopsy. These workers found that the enzyme could be made to act at one-fifth of its maximal activity in the absence of acetyl coenzyme A (acetyl-CoA) by increasing substrate levels greatly. In the presence of acetyl-CoA, however, the affinity of the enzyme for its substrates ($MgATP^{2-}$, HCO_3^-, and pyruvate) is enhanced about 30 times. The affinity of the human enzyme for acetyl-CoA was only one-sixth that of the enzyme from chicken liver (which shows no activity without acetyl-CoA). The enzyme appears to have two binding sites for acetyl-CoA and two or more for pyruvate. Scrutton and White [49] point out that, when the enzyme activity is measured in crude tissue preparations by means of the two-step assay used in the studies of patients already cited, precautions should be taken to assure a constant

level of acetyl-CoA during the first step. In an assay of crude tissue, acetyl-CoA would be produced by the action of pyruvate dehydrogenase and destroyed by hydrolysis and by reaction through citrate synthetase with oxalacetate, a product of the pyruvate carboxylase reaction. Therefore, the apparent pyruvate carboxylase activity found in the tissue would be determined both by the balance of influences acting on the acetyl-CoA level during the assay and by the amount of pyruvate carboxylase present.

The questions raised by this study have not yet been examined in a patient in whom the conventional pyruvate carboxylase assay suggests a deficit. The patient reported by Yoshida and coworkers [48] was said to have hepatic pyruvate decarboxylase activity within normal limits. Willems and coworkers [50] report the case of a baby with mental and motor retardation, microcephaly, and hypotonia, who had metabolic acidosis, blood pyruvate levels three to four times higher than normal, and somewhat elevated blood lactate. There was some improvement after massive doses of thiamine were administered. At autopsy, the pyruvate decarboxylase activity was found to be greatly reduced in the liver (it was normal in white blood cells and fibroblasts), and pyruvate carboxylase activity was reduced to 20 percent of normal. Although the data might suggest a double enzyme deficiency, other factors seem likely to account for the low pyruvate carboxylase activity in this patient [49].

Since then, two more cases of pyruvate carboxylase deficiency have been reported [51, 52]. Both children exhibited psychomotor retardation and hypotonia. Both appeared to be well nourished, with ample deposits of subcutaneous fat. One became hypoglycemic, with convulsions, after an extended fast [51], as one would expect. Pyruvate dehydrogenase activities were normal, and there seems to be no reason to doubt the enzyme deficit, although the precautions prescribed by Scrutton and White [49] were not taken. On the basis of a detailed analysis of the patient's hepatic metabolites, one group postulated that although pyruvate carboxylase has a role in gluconeogenesis, its role as a modulator of acetyl-CoA distribution among several pathways and as a governor of citric acid cycle activity may be more important [52]. These functions presumably result from the enzyme's role in oxalacetate production, and hence the rate of the citrate synthetase reaction (Fig. 29-1), a major consumer of acetyl-CoA.

References

1. Craighead, J. E. Current views on the etiology of insulin-dependent diabetes mellitus. *N. Engl. J. Med.* 299:1439–1445, 1978.

*2. Reske-Nielsen, E., and Lundbaek, K. Diabetic Encephalopathy. In E. F. Pfeiffer (ed.), *Handbook of Diabetes Mellitus.* Munich: Lehman, 1971. Vol. II, pp. 719–725.

3. Thurston, J. H., Hauhart, R. E., Jones, E. M., and Ater, J. L. Effects of alloxan diabetes, anti-insulin serum diabetes, and non-diabetic dehydration on brain carbohydrate and energy metabolism in young mice. *J. Biol. Chem.* 250:1751–1758, 1975.

*4. Schneider, T. Diabetic Neuropathy. In E. F. Pfeiffer (ed.), *Handbook of Diabetes Mellitus.* Munich: Lehmann, 1971. Vol. II, pp. 607–630.

5. Mulder, D. W., Lambert, E., Bastron, J. A., and Sprague, K. G. The neuropathies associated with diabetes mellitus. *Neurology* 11:275–284, 1961.

6. Eliasson, S. G. Nerve conduction changes in experimental diabetes. *J. Clin. Invest.* 43:2353–2358, 1964.

7. Greene, D. A., DeJesus, P. V., Jr., and Winegrad, A. I. Effects of insulin and dietary myoinositol on impaired peripheral motor nerve conduction velocity in acute streptozotocin diabetes. *J. Clin. Invest.* 55:1326–1336, 1975.

8. Stewart, M. A., Sherman, W. R., Kurien, M. M., Moonsammy, G. I., and Wisgerhof, M. Polyol accumulations in nervous tissue of rats with experimental diabetes and galactosemia. *J. Neurochem.* 14:1057–1066, 1967.

9. Schmidt, R. E., Matschinsky, F. M., Godfrey, D. A., Williams, A. D., and McDougal, D. B., Jr. Fast and slow axoplasmic flow in sciatic nerve of diabetic rats. *Diabetes* 24:1081–1085, 1975.

10. Goffstein, U., Held, K., Sebening, H., and Walpurger, G. Glucose verbrauch des Gehirns nach intravenösen Infusionen von Glucose, Glucagon und Glucose-Insulin. *Klin. Wochenschr.* 43:965–975, 1965.

11. Nelson, S. R., Schulz, D. W., Passonneau, J. V., and Lowry, O. H. Control of glycogen levels in brain. *J. Neurochem.* 15:1271–1279, 1968.

12. Arieff, A. I., Doerner, T., Zelig, H., and Massry, S. G. Evidence for a direct effect of insulin on electrolyte transport in brain. *J. Clin. Invest.* 54:654–663, 1974.

13. Arieff, A. J., and Kleeman, C. R. Studies on mechanisms of cerebral edema in diabetic comas: Effects of hyperglycemia and rapid lowering of plasma glucose in normal rabbits. *J. Clin. Invest.* 52:571–583, 1973.

14. Thurston, J. H., Hauhart, R. E., Dirgo, J. A., and McDougal, D. B., Jr. Insulin and brain metabolism. Absence of direct action of insulin on K^+ and Na^+ transport in normal rabbit brain. *Diabetes* 26:1117–1119, 1977.

15. Sloviter, H. A., and Yamada, H. Absence of a direct effect of insulin on metabolism of the isolated perfused rat brain. *J. Neurochem.* 18:1269–1274, 1971.

16. Havrankova, J., Schmechel, D., Roth, J., and Brownstein, M. Identification of insulin in rat brain. *Proc. Natl. Acad. Sci. U.S.A.* 75:5737–5741, 1978.

*17. Segal, S. Disorders of Galactose Metabolism. In J. B. Stanbury, J. B. Wyngaarden, and D. S. Fredrickson (eds.), *The Metabolic Basis of Inherited Disease* (4th ed.). New York: McGraw-Hill, 1978. Pp. 160–181.

18. Kozak, L. P., and Wells, W. W. Studies on the metabolic determinants of D-galactose-induced neurotoxicity in the chick. *J. Neurochem.* 18:2217–2228, 1971.

19. Granett, S. E., Kozak, L. P., McIntyre, J. P., and Wells, W. W. Studies on cerebral energy metabolism during the course of galactose neurotoxicity in chicks. *J. Neurochem.* 19:1659–1670, 1972.

20. Knull, H. R., and Wells, W. W. Recovery from galactose-induced neurotoxicity in the chick by the administration of glucose. *J. Neurochem.* 20:415–422, 1973.

21. Knull, H. R., Wells, W. W., and Kozak, L. P. Galactose toxicity in the chick: Hyperosmolality or depressed brain energy reserves. *Science* 176:815–816, 1972.

22. Malone, J. I., Wells, H. J., and Segal, S. Galactose toxicity in the chick: Hyperosmolality or depressed brain energy reserves. *Science* 176:816–817, 1972.

*23. Conn, J. W., and Pek, S. Current Concepts on Spontaneous Hypoglycemia. *Scope Monograph.* Kalamazoo: Upjohn, 1970.

*24. Howell, R. R. The Glycogen Storage Diseases. In J. B. Stanbury, J. B. Wyngaarden, and D. W. Fredrickson (eds.), *The Metabolic Basis of Inherited Disease* (4th ed.). New York: McGraw-Hill, 1978. Pp. 137–159.

*25. Brown, B. I., and Brown, D. H. Glycogen-

*Key reference.

Storage Diseases: Types I, III, IV, V, VII and Un-classified Glycogenoses. In F. Dickens, P. J. Randle, and W. J. Whelan (eds.), *Carbohydrate Metabolism and Its Disorders.* London: Academic, 1968. Vol. 2, pp. 124–150.

*26. Froesch, E. R. Essential Fructosuria, Hereditary Fructose Intolerance and Fructose-1,6-Diphosphatase Deficiency. In J. B. Stanbury, J. B. Wyngaarden, and D. S. Fredrickson (eds.), *The Metabolic Basis of Inherited Disease* (4th ed.). New York: McGraw-Hill, 1978. Pp. 121–136.

27. Sidbury, J. B., Jr. The Glycogenoses. In L. I. Gardiner (ed.), *Endocrine and Genetic Diseases of Childhood.* Philadelphia: Saunders, 1975. Pp. 1002–1018.

28. Baker, K., and Winegrad, A. I. Fasting hypoglycemia and metabolic acidosis associated with deficiency of hepatic fructose-1,6-diphosphatase activity. *Lancet* 2:13–16, 1970.

29. Blau, A., Reider, N., and Bender, M. B. B. Extrapyramidal syndrome and encephalographic pictures of progressive internal hydrocephalus in chronic hypoglycemia. *Ann. Intern. Med.* 10: 910–920, 1936.

30. Lewis, L. D., Ljunggren, B., Ratcheson, R. A., Siesjö, B. K. Cerebral energy state in insulin induced hypoglycemia, related to blood glucose and to EEG. *J. Neurochem.* 23:673–679, 1974.

31. Lewis, L. D., Ljunggren, B., Norberg, K., and Siesjö, P. K. Changes in carbohydrate substrates, amino acids, and ammonia in the brain during hypoglycemia. *J. Neurochem.* 23:659–671, 1974.

32. Ferrendelli, J. A., and Chang, M.-M. Brain metabolism during hypoglycemia. *Arch. Neurol.* 28:173–177, 1973.

33. Thurston, J. H., Jones, E. M., and Hauhart, R. E. Decrease and inhibition of liver glycogen phosphorylase after fructose: An experimental model for the study of hereditary fructose intolerance. *Diabetes* 23:597–604, 1974.

34. Thurston, J. H., Jones, E. M., and Hauhart, R. E. Failure of adrenaline to induce hyperglycemia after fructose injection in young mice. *Biochem. J.* 148: 149–151, 1975.

*35. Schärer, K. Congenital Lactic Acidosis. In J. Stern, and C. Toothill (eds.), *Organic Acidurias.* Edinburgh: Churchill-Livingstone, 1972. Pp. 46–51.

*36. Israels, S., Haworth, J. C., Dunn, H. G., and Applegarth, D. A. Lactic acidosis in childhood. *Adv. Pediatr.* 22:267–303, 1976.

*37. Cooper, J. R., and Pincus, J. H. Thiamine Triphosphate Deficiency in Leigh's Disease (Subacute Necrotizing Encephalomyelopathy). In F. A.

Hommes, and C. J. van den Berg (eds.), *In' orn Errors of Metabolism.* London: Academic, 1973. Pp. 119–127.

38. Cooper, J. R., Itokawa, Y., and Pincus, J. H. Thiamine triphosphate deficiency in subacute necrotizing encephalomyelopathy. *Science* 164:74–75, 1969.

39. Pincus, J. H., Cooper, J. R., Piros, K., and Turner, V. Specificity of the urine inhibitor test for Leigh's disease. *Neurology* 24:885–890, 1974.

40. de Groot, C. J., Jouxis, J. H. P., and Hommes, F. A. Further Studies on Leigh's Encephalomyelopathy. In J. Stern, and C. Toothill (eds.), *Organic Acidurias.* Edinburgh: Churchill-Livingstone, 1972. Pp. 40–45.

41. Grover, W. D., Auerbach, V. H., and Patel, M. J. Biochemical studies and therapy in subacute necrotizing encephalomyelopathy (Leigh's disease). *J. Pediatr.* 81:39–44, 1972.

42. Blass, J. P., Avigan, J., and Uhlendorf, B. W. A defect in pyruvate decarboxylase in a child with an intermittent movement disorder. *J. Clin. Invest.* 49:423–432, 1970.

43. Blass, J. P., Kark, A. P., and Engel, W. P. Clinical studies of a patient with pyruvate decarboxylase deficiency. *Arch. Neurol.* 25:449–460, 1971.

44. Lonsdale, D., Faulkner, W. R., Price, J. W., and Smeby, R. R. Intermittent cerebellar ataxia associated with hyperpyruvic acidemia, hyperalaninemia and hyperalaninuria. *Pediatrics* 43:1025–1034, 1969.

45. Blass, J. P., Lonsdale, D., Uhlendorf, B. W., and Horn, H. Intermittent ataxia with pyruvate-decarboxylase deficiency. *Lancet* 1:1302, 1971.

46. Farrell, D. F., Clark, A. F., Scott, C. R., and Wennberg, R. P. Absence of pyruvate decarboxylase activity in man: A cause of congenital lactic acidosis. *Science* 187:1082–1084, 1975.

47. Brunette, M. G., Delvin, E., Hazel, B., and Scriver, C. R. Thiamine responsive lactic acidosis in a patient with deficient low K_m pyruvate carboxylase activity in liver. *Pediatrics* 50:702–711, 1972.

48. Yoshida, T., Tada, K., Konno, T., and Arakawa, T. Hyperalaninemia with pyruvicemia due to pyruvate carboxylase deficiency of the liver. *Tohoku J. Exp. Med.* 99:121–128, 1969.

49. Scrutton, M. C., and White, M. D. Purification and properties of human liver pyruvate carboxylase. *Biochem. Med.* 9:271–292, 1974.

50. Willems, J. L., Monnens, L. A. H., Trijbels, J. M. F., Sengers, R. C. A., and Veerkamp, J. H. Pyruvate decarboxylase deficiency in liver. *N. Engl. J. Med.* 290:406–407, 1974.

51. Van Biervliet, J. P. G. M., Bruinvis, L., van der Heiden, C., Ketting, D., Wadman, S. K., Willemse,

J. L., and Monnens, L. A. H.   Report of a patient with severe, chronic lactic acidaemia and pyruvate carboxylase deficiency. *Devel. Med.* 19:392–401, 1977.

52. DeVivo, D. C., Haymond, M. W., Leckie, M. P., Bussmann, Y. L., McDougal, D. B., Jr., and Pagliara, A. S.   The clinical and biochemical implications of pyruvate carboxylase deficiency. *J. Clin. Endocrinol. Metab.* 45:1281–1296, 1977.

Roscoe O. Brady

A major group of inherited metabolic disorders characterized by profound deleterious effects on the CNS is distinguished by the accumulation of excessive quantities of lipids in various organs and tissues of the afflicted individuals. There are a dozen conditions of this type whose abnormal biochemistry and mode of inheritance are now known. Each of these diseases is caused by an inherited deficiency of a particular enzyme required for the catabolism of a specific lipid. Most of these disorders are inherited as autosomal recessive traits; therefore both parents, who may be perfectly healthy, must be heterozygotes to produce an affected offspring. When two carriers mate, there is one chance in four that the fetus will be affected; two will be heterozygotes like the parents, and one will be spared the defective gene. This distribution of the harmful genes occurs with each pregnancy. On the other hand, one of the lipid-storage diseases, known as Fabry's disease, is transmitted as an X-linked recessive condition. Here, only the female need be a heterozygote to produce an affected (hemizygote) male child. Half of her sons will have the disorder; half of her daughters will be carriers; the others will not be affected.

Pathways of Sphingolipid Catabolism

Most of the disorders considered in this chapter are caused by defects in catabolism of one of a specific group of lipids in which one portion of the molecule is ceramide (Cer). *Ceramide* $[CH_3 - (CH_2)_{12} - CH = CH - CH(OH) - CH(NH - CO - R) - CH_2OH]$ is a long-chain fatty-acyl derivative of the amino alcohol sphingosine. Various oligosaccharides or a molecule of phosphorylcholine may be joined to C_1 of ceramide. The nomenclature for this group of substances is described in Chap. 18.

On a weight basis, the major lipid of myelin is galactocerebroside (Cer-Gal), which consists of one molecule each of sphingosine, fatty acid, and galactose. The ceramide tetrasaccharide called *globoside* is the major neutral glycolipid of erythrocyte membranes (Fig. 30-1). Acidic glycolipids known as gangliosides have from 1 to 4 molecules of N-acetylneuraminic acid in addition to ceramide and an oligosaccharide portion. Gangliosides that contain a tetrahexosyl oligosaccharide moiety are highly concentrated in brain and appear to play a major role in the development of the CNS and, in particular, may be related to proper synaptic function. Gangliosides are sequentially degraded by a group of catabolic enzymes, indicated in schematic form in Fig. 30-2. The individual disorders of lipid catabolism are described below.

Gaucher's Disease

Gaucher's disease, like many other lipid-storage diseases, bears the name of the clinician who first described the clinical manifestations. The disease is an autosomal recessive disorder, and patients exhibiting it have been divided into three clinical categories. The first, type I, is the "adult" form and is manifested by hepatosplenomegaly, a hemorrhagic diathesis, and extreme pain and pathological fractures of the long bones, vertebrae, and pelvis, caused by the osteoporosis that attends the infiltration of glycolipid-storing cells in the marrow. Patients with type II, the infantile form, have an early onset of the systemic manifestations that occur in patients with type I. Those with type II also have severe mental retardation because of CNS involvement. Patients with type III, the juvenile form, have the systemic signs and symptoms of

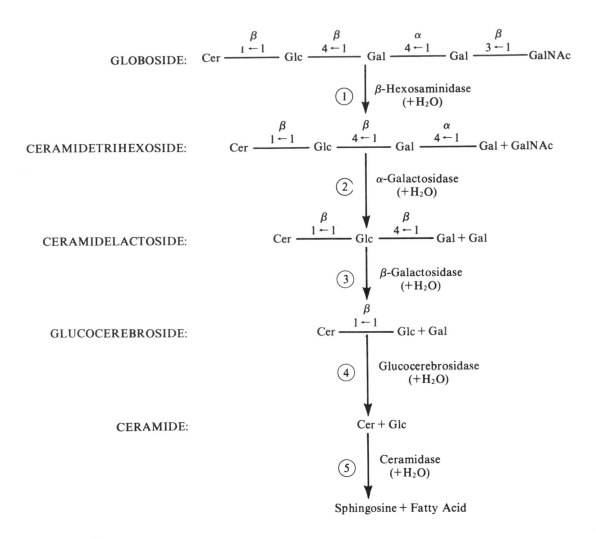

Fig. 30-1. Pathway of catabolism of globoside, the major neutral glycolipid of erythrocyte stroma. Cer = ceramide; Glc = glucose; Gal = galactose; GalNAc = N-acetyl-galactosamine.

type I; they develop seizures and show gradual CNS deterioration, usually beginning in their teens.

An excessive quantity of the glucocerebroside (Cer-Glc) is found in the organs and tissues of patients with this disease. The accumulation is caused by a deficiency of the β-glucosidase, which catalyzes step 4, as shown in Fig. 30-1 [1]. Patients with the infantile form of the disease have virtually no detectable glucocerebrosidase activity in their tissues [2]. Patients with the adult form always have some residual glucocerebrosidase; in this type it is usually greater than 25 percent and may be as high as 44 percent of that in normal individuals. Patients with type III Gaucher's disease can have up to 20

percent of normal glucocerebrosidase activity, although it is generally somewhat less than this but higher than in type II patients.

Most of the glucocerebroside that accumulates in the reticuloendothelial cells of the liver, spleen, and bone marrow appears to be derived primarily from senescent leukocytes and erythrocytes. The principal neutral glycolipid in leukocytes is ceramidelactoside, and its catabolism (through

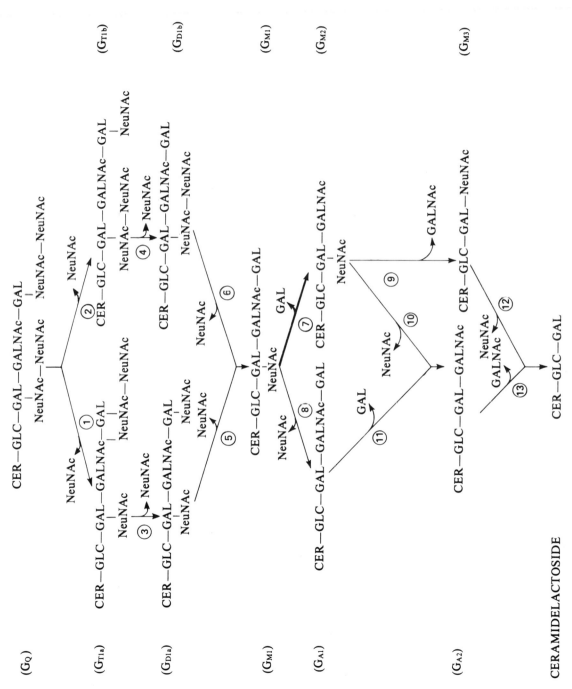

CERAMIDELACTOSIDE

Fig. 30-2. Pathways of catabolism of gangliosides. The major gangliosides of brain are G_Q, G_{T1a}, G_{T1b}, G_{D1a}, G_{D1b}, and G_{M1}. Abbreviations as in Fig. 30-1. NeuNAc = N-acetylneuraminic acid.

steps 3, 4, and 5 in Fig. 30-1) is impaired by the deficiency of glucocerebrosidase (step 4). In like fashion, the catabolism of erythrocyte globoside proceeds through reactions 1 through 3, but cannot be further metabolized at a normal rate by patients with Gaucher's disease. In addition, erythrocytes contain hematoside (G_{M3}, Fig. 30-2), which also contributes to the quantity of glycolipid that must be removed. Actually, erythrocytes have some ceramidetrihexoside (see Fig. 30-1) and glucocerebroside itself in association with their membranes. Leukocytes also normally contain a small quantity of glucocerebroside.

The cause of CNS damage in patients with type II and type III Gaucher's disease is believed to be an impairment of the catabolism of glucocerebroside derived from the metabolism of gangliosides (Fig. 30-2 and Fig. 30-1, steps 3 to 5). Ganglioside turnover is very rapid in the neonatal period and thereafter slows considerably. It is assumed that the residual glucocerebrosidase activity in the brain of patients with the adult form of Gaucher's disease is sufficient to catabolize the glucocerebroside derived from gangliosides, since nerve cells in type I patients do not have a pathological accumulation of this lipid.

The diagnosis of homozygotes and the detection of heterozygotes can be carried out easily through determinations of glucocerebrosidase activity by using washed leukocytes or by enzyme assays in extracts of cultured skin fibroblasts [3]. Glucocerebroside labeled with ^{14}C in the D-glucose portion of the molecule is the preferred substrate; however, a fluorescent agent, 4-methylumbelliferyl-β-D-glycopyranoside, has also been employed for diagnosis [4, 5].

The possible therapy of Gaucher's disease has recently been investigated. When glucocerebrosidase isolated from human placental tissue was injected into 2 patients with Gaucher's disease, there was a 26 percent reduction in the amount of stored glucocerebroside in their livers [6]. The elevated level of erythrocyte glucocerebroside in these patients returned to normal after glucocerebrosidase had been administered. This effect persisted over a period of many months [7]. These findings provide much hope for the amelioration of the adult form of Gaucher's disease by enzyme-replacement therapy [8]. For prenatal diagnosis, glucocerebrosidase assays can be performed on extracts of cultured amniotic cells [9], and, if indicated, genetic counseling is available for type II and type III patients.

Niemann-Pick Disease

Niemann-Pick disease also is transmitted as an autosomal recessive trait. Patients with this disorder have been subdivided into four categories on the basis of the clinical findings. Type A is the severe infantile form, with extensive neurological involvement, emaciation, hepatosplenomegaly, and foam cells in the bone marrow. Patients with type B have organomegaly but are generally without CNS involvement. Patients with type C have both organomegaly and neurological abnormalities, the latter appearing in late childhood or in the teens. Patients with type D disease have organomegaly and CNS damage resembling that in type C; the ancestry of these individuals is confined to the Nova Scotia area.

The enzymatic defect in Niemann-Pick disease is a deficiency of sphingomyelinase that causes the accumulation of sphingomyelin throughout the body [10]:

$$\text{Cer-phosphorylcholine} + H_2O \xrightarrow{\text{sphingomyelinase}} \text{Cer} + \text{phosphorylcholine}$$

Sphingomyelin is a ubiquitous component of the membranes of cells. Therefore its accumulation is assumed to be a consequence of normal cellular turnover.

Homozygotes and heterozygotes may be diagnosed by using radioactive sphingomyelin labeled in the choline portion of the molecule with sonicated leukocyte preparations or extracts of cultured skin fibroblasts [3]. A chromogenic substrate proposed several years ago [3] has recently been synthesized (Fig. 30-3). Gal and coworkers have found this substance reliable also for the diagnosis of Niemann-Pick patients and for the detection of heterozygotes [11].

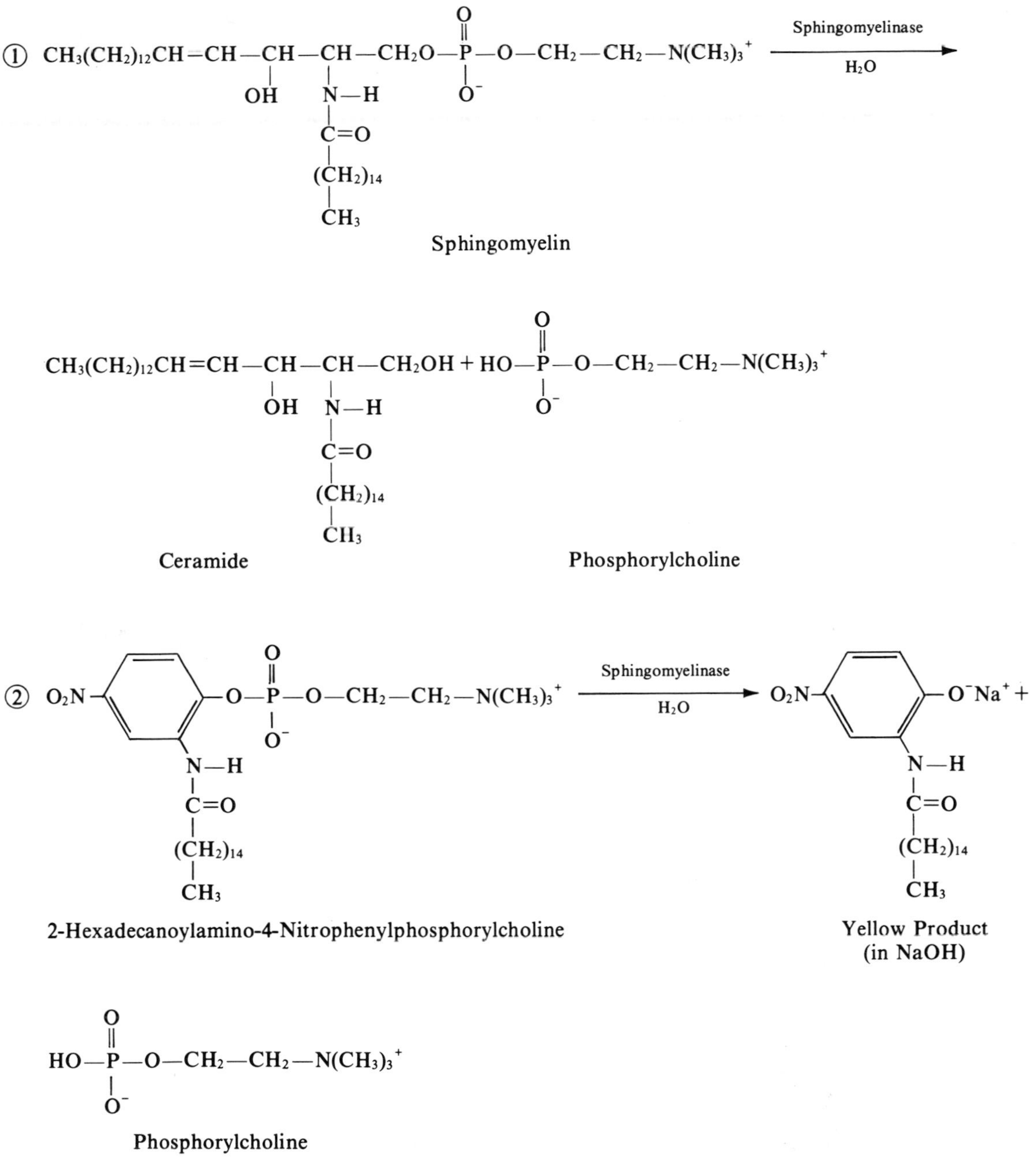

① $CH_3(CH_2)_{12}CH—CH—CH—CH—CH_2O—P—O—CH_2—CH_2—N(CH_3)_3^+$

Sphingomyelin

Sphingomyelinase
H_2O

$CH_3(CH_2)_{12}CH=CH—CH—CH—CH_2OH + HO—P—O—CH_2—CH_2—N(CH_3)_3^+$

Ceramide   Phosphorylcholine

② $O_2N—$ ... $—O—P—O—CH_2—CH_2—N(CH_3)_3^+$

Sphingomyelinase
H_2O

$O_2N—$ ... $—O^-Na^+ +$

2-Hexadecanoylamino-4-Nitrophenylphosphorylcholine

Yellow Product
(in NaOH)

$HO—P—O—CH_2—CH_2—N(CH_3)_3^+$

Phosphorylcholine

Fig. 30-3. *The enzymatic hydrolysis of sphingomyelin (1) and the chromogenic analog of sphingomyelin (2). Reproduced by permission from ref. 16.*

Sphingomyelinase has recently been isolated from human placental tissue [12]. So far, however, no enzyme replacement trials have been carried out. Because of the wide distribution of sphingomyelin, extensive investigations in experimental animals will have to be carried out before sphingomyelinase can be administered to humans. Fortunately, a potentially useful animal model of Niemann-Pick disease has recently been developed [13]. It is anticipated that a number of important problems concerning enzyme replacement in this disorder may be resolved with the pharmacologically produced analog of the human disease.

The prenatal diagnosis of Niemann-Pick disease by amniocentesis has been helped by the availability of the radioactive substrate [14]. The chromogenic substrate was found to be equally reliable for monitoring pregnancies at risk for Niemann-Pick disease [15, 16].

Globoid Leukodystrophy (Krabbe's Disease)

Krabbe's disease, an autosomal recessive disorder, is characterized by hyperirritability, hyperesthesia, and an episodic fever that begins about the fourth or fifth month of age. These symptoms are followed by convulsions, mental retardation, hyperactivity, blindness, and deafness. There is no organomegaly or net accumulation of a specific lipid in the brain. The metabolic defect is a deficiency of a β-galactosidase, which catalyzes the hydrolysis of galactocerebroside [17]:

$$\text{Cer-Gal} + H_2O \xrightarrow{\text{galactocerebroside-}\beta\text{-galactosidase}} \text{Cer} + \text{Gal}$$

A diagnostic test is available that employs galactocerebroside labeled with ^3H in the hexose moiety. Washed leukocytes, cultured skin fibroblasts, and even serum samples may be used for this test [18]. Prenatal detection of Krabbe's disease is feasible through enzyme assays on cultured amniotic cells [19], and a chromogenic analog of galactocerebroside has been developed for the diagnosis of this disorder [20, 21]. There is no specific therapy at this time, although allosteric activation of the mutated galactocerebrosidase has been proposed [22].

Metachromatic Leukodystrophy

Patients with the most common form of this autosomal recessive disorder show progressive flaccidity and weakness of the arms and legs between 12 and 18 months of age. These signs are followed by loss of ability to stand plus mental retardation, which is manifested initially by a loss of speech. The clinical aspects of the disorder progress to blindness and complete mental retardation. In other patients, many of the same signs and symptoms appear in the early teens, and a slower clinical course is followed.

The underlying pathological chemistry in this disorder is the accumulation of large quantities of sulfatide, the 3-O-sulfate ester of galactocerebroside. Sections of peripheral nerves show brownish yellow, metachromatic deposits when stained with cresyl violet dye. The cause of the accumulation is a deficiency of a sulfatase, which catalyzes the conversion of cerebroside sulfate to cerebroside [23]:

$$\text{Cer-Gal-SO}_3\text{H}_2\text{O} \longrightarrow \text{Cer-Gal} + H_2SO_4.$$

Sulfatidase was partially purified from hog kidney, and evidence was obtained for the requirement of a heat-stable factor for the hydrolysis of the sulfated glycolipid in buffers (ionic strength ≥ 0.2) with osmolarity in the physiological range [8].

The diagnosis of homozygotes and heterozygous carriers can be carried out easily on washed leukocytes [24] or on cultured skin fibroblasts, and by assaying the hydrolysis of nitrocatechol sulfate, as described by Austin and coworkers [25].

The therapy of patients with metachromatic leukodystrophy has been undertaken by intravenous and intrathecal injection of crude preparations of a sulfatase, *arylsulfatase A*. There was no improvement in the patients' conditions, and in several instances, there were severe pyrogenic reactions. Genetic counseling is available, based on the determination of arylsulfatase activity in cultured amniotic cells.

Austin's laboratory presented convincing evidence for the presence of a novel protein in tissues from patients with metachromatic leukodystrophy. Although catalytically inactive, this protein cross-reacted with antibody against normal human arylsulfatase A [26]. This was the first evidence of a catalytically inactive protein in patients with a lipid-storage disease, and it provided strong support for the occurrence of structural mutations in the enzymes of patients with such disorders [8].

Ceramidelactoside Lipidosis

A few years ago, Dawson and Stein described a patient [27] in the early teens with progressive mental retardation, hepatosplenomegaly, and lipid-storage cells in the bone marrow. The principal accumulating lipid was reported to be ceramidelactoside (see Fig. 30-1). At first, the disorder was attributed to a deficiency of the β-galactosidase that catalyzes steps 3 in Fig. 30-1. Although this type of enzymatic defect would appear to be logical, subsequent reexamination of enzyme activities in this patient's cultured skin fibroblasts showed, instead, a partial deficiency in sphingomyelinase activity [28]. However, a deficiency of a "neutral" β-galactosidase has been cited as a possible site of defective glycolipid metabolism in the propositus [8].

Fabry's Disease

Fabry's disease is inherited as an X-linked recessive characteristic, and the major clinical manifestations occur primarily in males. Those afflicted have reddish-purple maculopapular lesions in the skin over the buttocks, inguinal region, and scrotum. Fabry patients experience excruciating attacks of peripheral neuralgia in the hands and feet. They are also unable to sweat. Ceramidetrihexoside accumulates progressively (cf. Fig. 30-1) in the walls of the blood vessels and in the glomeruli of the kidneys. Males with the disorder usually experience complete renal failure in their late 40s or early 50s. Some have myocardial infarctions or cerebrovascular thromboses caused by the extensive arteriosclerosis that attends the deposition of lipid in the blood vessels. Heterozygous females may exhibit some of the manifestations of the disease, including corneal opacification and signs of renal impairment. The symptoms are usually milder in females, although recently, several women have been reported with severe manifestations of the disease.

The metabolic defect is a deficiency of the α-galactosidase that catalyzes step 2 in Fig. 30-1 [29]. The principal source of the accumulating lipid are globoside and ceramidetrihexoside, derived from the stroma of senescent erythrocytes (Fig. 30-1). A diagnosis can be made by using artificial chromogenic or fluorogenic galactopyranosides as substrates to determine α-galactosidase activity in leukocytes or cultured skin fibroblasts [30]. Heterozygotes also may be detected by enzyme assays with these substrates, and a reliable procedure has been developed for the prenatal diagnosis of Fabry's disease [31].

Possible therapies for Fabry's disease have come under investigation in several laboratories. A primary consideration is the amelioration of renal failure; for this purpose, kidney transplantation has been used with some degree of success. Reports of the efficacy or lack of benefit from this procedure are cited [32]. A more direct approach to the correction of the enzymatic deficiency was undertaken by using intravenous infusion of purified ceramidetrihexosidase isolated from human placental tissue [32]. Two males with the disorder received a highly purified preparation of the enzyme. They tolerated the procedure without untoward effects. The ceramidetrihexosidase cleared from the circulation rapidly, and much of it appeared in the liver. The elevated level of ceramidetrihexoside in the blood was dramatically lowered after the enzyme had been administered. Several observations make it seem likely that the placental enzyme exerted its catabolic effect outside the circulation: (1) the enzyme is catalytically active at moderately acid pHs and is virtually inactive at the pH of blood; (2) the enzyme had almost completely disappeared from the circulation before the plasma ceramidetrihexoside decreased; (3) there was no elevation of plasma ceramidelactoside, the immediate product of the reaction at a time when ceramidetrihexoside was falling. Another potentially important observation was made in the course of these investigations. There appeared to be three or four times more α-galactosidase activity in the postinfusion liver biopsy sample from a patient than actually was administered. This finding suggests that the placental enzyme may have activated the patient's mutated catalytically inactive protein.

Tay-Sachs Disease

Tay-Sachs disease, a lipid-storage disorder, is transmitted as an autosomal recessive trait. There are several clinical and biochemically distinct forms of Tay-Sachs disease. The signs and symptoms of the classic infantile form of the disorder are restricted to the CNS. These patients appear normal for the first 5 or 6 months of life and then fail to develop motor and mental capacities properly. Convulsions, apathy, and blindness follow. Death usually occurs about the third year. A cherry-red spot is present in the macular region of the eye. Other patients may have delayed onset of these manifestations until 12 to 18 months of age. Here, the progression is slower, with death occurring at 5 or 6 years of age. Occasionally, a patient may experience a very early onset and rapid progression of the signs and symptoms, along with some hepatomegaly. This is the so-called Sandhoff-Jatzkewitz form of Tay-Sachs disease.

The metabolic defect in all of the different clinical forms of Tay-Sachs disease is a deficiency of the hexosaminidase that catalyzes step 9 in Fig. 30-2 [33, 34]. The enzyme is normally found in brain lysosomes. Its absence in patients with Tay-Sachs disease causes lipids and protein to accumulate in the form of membranous cytoplasmic bodies. The catabolism of ganglioside G_{M2} by purified enzymes requires the presence of a suitable detergent or heat-stable factor [8].

The diagnosis of *most* homozygotes and heterozygotes for Tay-Sachs disease can be made through the use of the fluorogenic substrate 4-methyl-umbelliferyl-β-D-N-acetylglucosaminide [35]. Patients with the most frequently seen form of the disease lack hexosaminidase A—one of two normally occurring hexosaminidase "isozymes." Hexosaminidase B activity in these patients is higher than normal. Patients with the Sandhoff-Jatzkewitz form have no detectable hexosaminidase activity in their tissues. Patients with still another mutation show good activity with the fluorogenic substrate but cannot catabolize G_{M2}.

Because of these variations, much caution must be exercised in detecting heterozygotes and homozygotes via artificial substrates. It has recently been shown, furthermore, that there are perfectly normal, but rare, individuals who lack any detectable hexosaminidase A activity in their tissues, as ascertained by using the fluorogenic substrate, but who nevertheless can catabolize G_{M2} [36]. If one were to use the fluorogenic substrate for prenatal detection, as commonly practiced today, such a fetus could be classified mistakenly as a Tay-Sachs homozygote.

The therapy of Tay-Sachs disease has been investigated via the intravenous administration of purified hexosaminidase A, isolated from human urine, to an infant with this disorder [37]. A normal level of hexosaminidase A was quickly reached in the bloodstream after the infusion. None of the hexosaminidase A appeared to cross the blood-brain barrier, however, since there was no detectable increase of hexosaminidase activity in brain biopsy specimens or in the cerebrospinal fluid. Thus, replacement therapy by intravenous administration of exogenous enzyme, which appears promising for patients with Gaucher's [6] or Fabry's disease [32], does not seem likely to be of benefit for Tay-Sachs disease unless the blood-brain barrier or the enzyme is altered. Recent experiments with rodents and primates have revealed that the blood-brain barrier can be altered temporarily so that such enzymes as mannosidase and horseradish peroxidase can enter the substance of the brain [38]. It has further been found that rat brain synaptosomes contain a high-affinity, saturable system that is capable of binding purified human β-hexosaminidase A [39]. Together, these results provide a strong impetus for further studies of the feasibility of enzyme-replacement therapy for inherited disorders that involve the central nervous system.

Generalized Gangliosidosis

This inherited disorder is also transmitted as an autosomal recessive trait. Patients with generalized (G_{M1}) gangliosidoses exhibit severe mental deterioration and frequently have a cherry-red spot in the retina. They also have hepatosplenomegaly, bony abnormalities, and foam cells in the marrow and viscera. At least two clinical forms—the classic infantile type and the juvenile form—have been described on the basis of the age of onset and rapidity of progression of the disease.

Generalized gangliosidosis is the result of a deficiency of the β-galactosidase that catalyzes step 7 in Fig. 30-2 [40]. In some patients, acid mucopolysaccharides also accumulate because of the drastic diminution of total β-galactosidase activity. The generalized reduction of β-galactosidase makes the diagnosis of homozygotes and heterozygotes readily available through the use of such chromogenic or fluorogenic substrates as p-nitrophenyl-β-D-galactopyranoside or 4-methylumbelliferyl-β-D-galactopyranoside.

An interesting feature of generalized gangliosidosis is that the activities of such other neutral lipid β-galacto-sidases as galactocerebrosidase and ceramidelactosidase must be accommodated within the residual 7 to 9 percent of total normal β-galactosidase activity in the tissues of patients. In fact, the activity of these enzymes, as well as that of glucocerebrosidase and ceramidetrihexosidase, may be increased as much as sixfold over that in braintissue samples from human controls. These observations have at least two implications. First, there is a compensatory increase in lysosomal hydrolases in the brains of patients with generalized gangliosidosis (and other lipid-storage disease, as well), and second, the major portion of tissue β-galactosidase activity is involved in ganglioside turnover. The latter point suggests that there are aspects of ganglioside turnover, particularly in parenchymal organs, the metabolic relevance of which is still unrecognized.

There is no known therapy for G_{M1}-gangliosidosis. However, genetic counseling may be indicated, because cultured normal amniotic cells have readily demonstrable β-galactosidase activity with artificial substrates.

Farber's Disease

The signs and symptoms of Farber's disease begin about the third or fourth month after birth, with the onset of hoarseness and a brownish, desquamating dermatitis. Later, foam cells infiltrate the bones and joints, and a granulomatous reaction takes place in the lymph nodes, subcutaneous tissues, heart, and lungs. CNS damage causes psychomotor retardation. The disorder is assumed to be transmitted as an autosomal recessive characteristic, because it has been reported in both male and female infants.

The metabolic lesion in this disease appears to be a deficiency of ceramidase (Fig. 30-1, step 5) [41]. The conditions for the assay of maximal ceramidase activity are stringent, and an important lesson can be derived from investigations of this disorder. Whenever a metabolic defect is suspected, great care should be taken to establish, in tissue samples from both animal and human controls, the optimal conditions for the assay of the enzyme in question. It is mandatory that the precise parameters for maximal catalytic activity in lipid storage diseases be determined, especially with regard to the type and concentration of detergents used to solubilize the natural substrates.

Wolman's Disease

Wolman's disease is probably an autosomal recessive condition, since both males and females may be afflicted. The symptoms, which appear a few weeks after birth, include vomiting, diarrhea, and abdominal distention. Hepatosplenomegaly and, usually, enlargement and calcification of the adrenals are also present. There are no signs of nervous system dysfunction. The course of the disease progresses through cachexia, and death usually occurs by the age of 6 months. Triglycerides and cholesterol esters accumulate in many tissues, particularly the liver, spleen, and adrenals. The enzymatic defect is a deficiency of an acid lipase; the hydrolysis of triglycerides and cholesteryl esters is normal at neutral or alkaline pH [42]. Long-chain fatty esters of p-nitrophenol appear to be useful for the diagnosis of homozygotes and may provide a convenient procedure for the identification of heterozygotes. So far there has been no reported attempt at enzyme-replacement therapy for this disorder, and treatment has been directed primarily toward amelioration of symptoms.

Refsum's Syndrome

Refsum's syndrome is an autosomal recessive condition characterized by retinitis pigmentosa, peripheral polyneuropathy with both motor and sensory deficiencies, elevated cerebrospinal fluid protein, deafness, anosmia, pupillary abnormalities, ichthyosislike alterations of the skin, and epiphyseal dysplasia. Phytanic acid, a 20-carbon branched-chain fatty acid, accumulates in most tissues; especially large quantities of it are present in the liver and kidneys of the afflicted individuals. The major source of the accumulating substance is dietary phytanic acid and phytol; the latter compound is converted to phytanic acid in the body. The metabolic defect is an inability to oxidize phytanic acid to α-hydroxyphytanate [43]. The hydroxylase catalyzing this reaction is present in cultured skin fibroblasts. Homozygotes and heterozygotes can be detected by assaying the activity of the enzyme in extracts of these cells. Patients with the syndrome seem to benefit from restriction of phytol and phytanic acid in their diet.

Batten's Disease

Batten's disease is a heritable, cerebrodegenerative disorder characterized by progressive mental deterioration, cerebellar dysfunction, grand mal seizures, and changes in the retina that eventually result in blindness. The onset of the disease may vary; it can begin in infancy or early childhood, with initial symptoms of visual impairment. The neuronal cells in the brains of patients with Batten's disease accumulate a brown, autofluorescent, pigmented mixture in the form of small, crescentic stacks of lamellae called *curvilinear bodies*. Most of the material in these inclusions is soluble in organic solvents. Much of the accumulated substance appears to consist of phospholipids that are common to the brain, except for an acidic, lipid polymer of uncertain composition. A number of reports have implicated a deficiency of peroxidase activity, especially in leukocyte preparations, from patients with this disorder; however, there is considerable disagreement on this point. More recently, Wolfe and his associates reported the occurrence of retinoyl complexes in the stored material [44]. The

complete identification of the autofluorescent substance has not yet been accomplished.

In spite of these uncertainties, the consistent appearance of "fingerprint bodies" in a sizeable proportion of lymphocytes in patients with this disorder lends support to the notion of an impaired catabolic reaction, and the search for the metabolic lesion continues.

Disorder of Ganglioside Biosynthesis

An entirely new type of sphingolipodystrophy may be represented in a patient whose primary neurological manifestation is severe mental retardation associated with extreme hypomyelination in the CNS. In this patient, there was failure to synthesize ganglioside G_{M2} from G_{M3} [16]. There was a fourfold accumulation of G_{M3}, and a total absence of all higher ganglioside homologs in the brain. This defect is not simply the reverse of step 9 in Fig. 30-2, but is caused by a deficiency of the enzyme that catalyzes the transfer of a molecule of N-acetylgalactosamine from UDP-N-acetylgalactosamine to ganglioside G_{M3}. However, the significance of this metabolic lesion in the pathogenesis of the clinical syndrome recently has been brought into question. Subsequent to the birth of the proband, a male sibling with many of the same clinical features was born. The latter infant died at 6 months of age. In contrast to the subject, there was no lack of higher ganglioside homologs in the brain of the second child [45]. Thus, the relevance of the altered ganglioside pattern in the initial subject remains to be determined, as does the primary metabolic error in both infants with this unusual disease.

References

1. Brady, R. O., Kanfer, J. N., and Shapiro, D. Metabolism of glucocerebrosides. II. Evidence of an enzymatic deficiency in Gaucher's disease. *Biochem. Biophys. Res. Commun.* 18:221–225, 1965.
2. Brady, R. O., et al. Demonstration of a deficiency of glucocerebroside-cleaving enzyme in Gaucher's disease. *J. Clin. Invest.* 45:1112–1115, 1966.
3. Brady, R. O., Johnson, W. G., and Uhlendorf, B. W. Identification of heterozygous carriers of lipid storage disease. *Am. J. Med.* 51:423–431, 1971.
4. Beutler, E., and Kuhl, W. Diagnosis of the adult

type of Gaucher's disease and its carrier state by demonstration of a deficiency of β-glucosidase activity in peripheral blood leukocytes. *J. Lab. Clin. Med.* 76:747–755, 1970.

5. Ho, M. W., et al. Adult Gaucher's disease: Kindred studies and demonstration of a deficiency of acid β-glucosidase in cultured fibroblasts. *Am. J. Hum. Genet.* 24:37–45, 1972.

6. Brady, R. O., et al. Replacement therapy for inherited enzyme deficiency: Use of purified glucocerebrosidase in Gaucher's disease. *N. Engl. J. Med.* 291:989–993, 1974.

7. Pentchev, P. G., et al. Replacement therapy for inherited enzyme deficiency: Sustained clearance of accumulated glucocerebroside in Gaucher's disease following infusion of purified glucocerebrosidase. *J. Mol. Med.* 1:73–78, 1975.

*8. Brady, R. O. Sphingolipidoses. *Annu. Rev. Biochem.* 47:687–713, 1978.

9. Schneider, E. L., et al. Infantile (type II) Gaucher's disease: In utero diagnosis and fetal pathology. *J. Pediatr.* 81:1134–1139, 1972.

10. Brady, R. O., et al. The metabolism of sphingomyelin. II. Evidence of an enzymatic deficiency in Niemann-Pick disease. *Proc. Natl. Acad. Sci. U.S.A.* 55:366–369, 1966.

11. Gal, A. E., et al. A practical chromogenic procedure for the detection of homozygotes and heterozygous carriers of Niemann-Pick disease. *N. Engl. J. Med.* 293:632–636, 1975.

12. Pentchev, P. G., et al. The isolation and characterization of sphingomyelinase from human placental tissue. *Biochim. Biophys. Acta* 488:312–321, 1977.

13. Sakuragawa, N., et al. Niemann-Pick disease experimental model: Sphingomyelinase reduction induced by AY-9944. *Science* 196: 317–319, 1977.

14. Epstein, C. J., et al. In utero diagnosis of Niemann-Pick disease. *Am. J. Hum. Genet.* 23: 533–535, 1971.

15. Patrick, A. D., et al. Prenatal diagnosis of Niemann-Pick disease type A using chromogenic substrate. *Lancet* 2:144, 1977.

*16. Brady, R. O. Heritable catabolic and anabolic disorders of lipid metabolism. *Metabolism* 26:329–345, 1977.

17. Suzuki, K., and Suzuki, Y. Globoid cell leukodystrophy (Krabbe'd disease): Deficiency of galactocerebroside beta-galactosidase. *Proc. Natl. Acad. Sci. U.S.A.* 66:302–309, 1970.

18. Suzuki, Y., and Suzuki, K. Krabbe's globoid leukodystrophy: Deficiency of galactocerebro-

sidase in serum, leukocytes, and fibroblasts. *Science* 171:73–75, 1971.

19. Suzuki, K., Schneider, E. L., and Epstein, C. J. In utero diagnosis of globoid cell leukodystrophy (Krabbe's disease). *Biochem. Biophys. Res. Commun.* 45:1363–1366, 1971.

20. Gal, A. E., et al. A practical chromogenic procedure for the diagnosis of Krabbe's disease. *Clin. Chim. Acta* 77:53–59, 1977.

21. Besley, G. T. N., and Bain, A. D. Use of a chromogenic substrate for the diagnosis of Krabbe's disease with special reference to its application in prenatal diagnosis. *Clin. Chim. Acta* 88:229–236, 1978.

22. Arora, R. C., and Radin, N. S. Stimulation in vitro of galactocerebroside galactosidase by N-decanoyl-2-amino-2-methylpropanol. *Lipids* 7: 56–9, 1972.

23. Mehl, E., and Jatzkewitz, H. Evidence for the genetic block in metachromatic leukodystrophy (ML). *Biochem. Biophys. Res. Commun.* 19: 407–411, 1965.

24. Percy, A. K., and Brady, R. O. Metachromatic leukodystrophy: Diagnosis with samples of venous blood. *Science* 161:594–595, 1968.

25. Austin, J., et al. A controlled study of enzymatic activities in three human disorders of glycolipid metabolism. *J. Neurochem.* 10:805–816, 1963.

26. Stumpf, D., et al. Metachromatic leukodystrophy (MLD). X. Immunological studies of the abnormal sulfatase A. *Arch. Neurol.* 25:427–431, 1971.

27. Dawson, G., and Stein, A. O. Lactosyl ceramidosis: Catabolic defect of glycosphingolipid metabolism. *Science* 170:556–558, 1970.

28. Wenger, D., Sattler, M., Clark, C., Tanaka, H., Suzuki, K., and Dawson, G. Lactosyl ceramidosis: Normal activity for two lactosyl ceramide β-galactosidases. *Science* 188:1310–1312, 1975.

29. Brady, R. O., et al. Enzymatic defect in Fabry's disease: Ceramidetrihexosidase deficiency. *N. Engl. J. Med.* 276:1163–1167, 1967.

30. Kint, J. A. Fabry's disease: Alpha-galactosidase deficiency. *Science* 167:1268–1269, 1970.

31. Brady, R. O., Uhlendorf, B. W., and Jacobson, C. B. Fabry's disease: Antenatal detection. *Science* 172:174–175, 1971.

32. Brady, R. O., et al. Replacement therapy for inherited enzyme deficiency: Use of purified ceramidetrihexosidase in Fabry's disease. *N. Engl. J. Med.* 289:9–14, 1973.

33. Kolodny, E. H., Brady, R. O., and Volk, B. W. Demonstration of an alteration of ganglioside metabolism in Tay-Sachs disease. *Biochem. Biophys. Res. Commun.* 37:526–531, 1969.

*Key reference.

34. Tallman, J. F., Johnson, W. G., and Brady, R. O. The metabolism of Tay-Sachs ganglioside: Catabolic studies with lysosomal enzymes from normal and Tay-Sachs brain tissue. *J. Clin. Invest.* 51: 2339–2345, 1972.

35. Okada, S., and O'Brien, J. S. Tay-Sachs disease: Generalized absence of a beta-hexosaminidase component. *Science* 165:698–700, 1969.

36. Tallman, J. F., et al. Ganglioside catabolism in hexosaminidase A deficient adults. *Nature* 252: 254–255, 1974.

37. Johnson, W. G., et al. Intravenous Injection of Purified Hexosaminidase A into a Patient with Tay-Sachs Disease. In D. Bergsma (ed.), *Enzyme Therapy in Genetic Diseases,* Birth Defects Original Article Series. Baltimore: Williams & Wilkins, 1973. Vol. 9, no. 2, pp. 120–124.

38. Barranger, J. A., et al. Modification of the blood-brain barrier: Increased concentration and fate of enzymes entering the brain. *Proc. Natl. Acad. Sci. U.S.A.* 76:481–485, 1979.

39. Kusiak, L. W., et al. Specific binding of ^{125}I-β-hexosaminidase A to rat brain synaptosomes. *Proc. Natl. Acad. Sci. U.S.A.* 76:982–985, 1979.

*40. O'Brien, J. S. The Gangliosidoses. In J. B. Stanbury, J. B. Wyngaarden, and D. S. Frederickson (eds.), *The Metabolic Basis of Inherited Disease* (3rd ed.). New York: McGraw-Hill, 1972. Pp. 841–865.

41. Sugita, M., Dulaney, J. T., and Moser, H. W. Ceramidase deficiency in Farber's disease (lipogranulomatosis). *Science* 178:1100–1102, 1972.

*42. Patrick, A. D., and Lake, B. D. Wolman's Disease. In H. G. Hers, and F. Van Hoof (eds.), *Lysosomes and Storage Diseases.* New York: Academic, 1973. Pp. 453–473.

*43. Steinberg, D. Phytanic Acid Storage Disease: Refsum's Syndrome. In J. B. Stanbury, J. B. Wyngaarden, and D. S. Fredrickson (eds.), *The Metabolic Basis of Inherited Disease* (4th ed.). New York: McGraw-Hill, 1978. Pp. 688–706.

44. Wolfe, L. S., et al. Identification of retinoyl complexes as the autofluorescent component of the neuronal storage material in Batten disease. *Science* 195:1360–1362, 1977.

*45. Brady, R. O. Inherited metabolic diseases and pathogenesis of mental retardation. *Ann. Biol. Clin.* (Paris) 36:113–119, 1978.

Larry J. Shapiro
Elizabeth F. Neufeld

Chapter 31. Genetic Mucopolysaccharidoses and Mucolipidoses

The *mucopolysaccharidoses* and the *mucolipidoses* are related groups of inherited human diseases caused by abnormal lysosomal function and storage of mucopolysaccharides, sphingolipids, and glycoproteins [1, 2]. These disorders are often considered together because their similar clinical phenotypes frequently necessitate differential diagnosis. They are rare, affecting collectively perhaps only 1 in 20,000 liveborn infants. Although some of these disorders have long been recognized by virtue of their dramatic clinical expression, it is only recently that a biochemical explanation of their pathogenesis has been found. As a result of the demonstration that these conditions are caused by a deficiency of various lysosomal enzyme activities, understanding of normal physiological processes has been enhanced. Practical application of this knowledge has resulted in more accurate diagnosis and counseling, as well as in prenatal diagnosis.

The Biochemical Basis of the Mucopolysaccharidoses

Sulfated mucopolysaccharides (also called *glycosaminoglycans*) are polymeric molecules composed of carbohydrate chains in which amino sugars alternate either with uronic acids (dermatan sulfate, heparan sulfate, chondroitin sulfate) or with hexoses (keratan sulfate). The chains are sulfated in varying degrees and are connected to protein "backbones" by specific linkage regions [3]. These polymers are widely distributed in mammalian tissues and, together with collagen, constitute most of the intercellular matrix. Several of the mucopolysaccharides are major constituents of cartilage, skin, and blood vessels; one, heparan sulfate, is a small, but rapidly turning-over, component of all cell membranes [4]. No doubt such ubiquitous

molecules are involved in the pathogenesis of a number of disease states; however, only inherited disorders of dermatan sulfate, heparan sulfate, and keratan sulfate catabolism will be considered here.

The disorders now known as the mucopolysaccharidoses were described clinically in the first half of this century [1], but were considered derangements of lipid metabolism ("lipochondrodystrophies"). It was only after Brante [5], Brown [6], and Meyer and coworkers [7] identified the stored material as mucopolysaccharide, rather than lipid, that understanding the biochemical basis of these conditions became possible. The discovery by Dorfman and Lorincz [8] of mucopolysacchariduria allowed relatively easy identification of affected patients. From careful comparison of clinical features, mode of inheritance, and chemistry of excreted mucopolysaccharides, McKusick [9] proposed, in 1966, a systematic classification that was adopted widely. This classification was subsequently revised as information about the basic defect in each disorder became available [1, 2]. The revised classification of McKusick and coworkers [2] will be used in this chapter; each mucopolysaccharidosis (MPS) is designated by the eponym and a Roman numeral, followed, where further subdivision is warranted, by a capital letter (e.g., Hurler's syndrome, MPS IH).

MUCOPOLYSACCHARIDOSES AS CATABOLIC DISORDERS

On the basis of pathological findings in *Hurler's syndrome* (the prototype mucopolysaccharidosis), van Hoof and Hers [10] suggested that the disease might be a lysosomal storage disorder. Danes and Bearn [11] found that fibroblasts derived from mucopolysaccharidosis patients stored mucopolysaccharide in culture. The use of radioactive sulfate to measure the fate of mucopolysaccharide in such cultured fibroblasts showed that the storage was a result of faulty degradation, rather than of an increased rate of synthesis, decreased secretion, or abnormal structure of the accumulated polymer [12–14].

Through subsequent work, a specific deficiency of a lysosomal enzyme necessary for the catabolism of mucopolysaccharide has been described for each of the classic phenotypic syndromes [14, 2] (Figs. 31-1 through 31-3). The best interpretation of available data is that the normal degradation of dermatan sulfate, heparan sulfate, and keratan sulfate proceeds unidirectionally from the nonreducing end of the carbohydrate chain by the sequential actions of lysosomal exoglycosidases, exosulfatases, and an acetyltransferase. The absence of any one of these enzymes results in a block in catabolism, although a limited degradation by endoglycosidases may occur in certain tissues. Each of the inherited disorders of mucopolysaccharide metabolism corresponds to the absence of activity of one of these enzymes. The relationship is analogous to that among the disorders of ganglioside catabolism, described in Chap. 30. It should be noted that almost all the linkages known to occur in the three polymers are now associated with a specific enzyme-deficiency disease; however, deficiencies of enzymes that hydrolyze as yet undescribed linkages or that degrade other mucopolysaccharides can reasonably be anticipated.

The spectrum of clinical phenotypes that can be associated with each enzymatic error is great. On the other hand, as might be predicted with a multienzyme pathway, patients with different enzymatic lesions may appear to the clinician phenotypically similar. This complexity requires an integrated biochemical, clinical, and genetic approach if one is to give accurate prognostic information and counseling.

ALPHA-L-IDURONIDASE DEFICIENCY
Patients deficient in the enzyme α-L-iduronidase [15, 16] are variably affected. At one end of the spectrum are those with classic Hurler's syndrome [1, 2]. The disorder has its apparent clinical onset in infancy, although pathological and biochemical manifestations may be recognized earlier. The patients have diminished linear growth after approximately the first year, resulting in significantly shortened stature, and have severe psychomotor retardation. The characteristic facial appearance of these patients and the excretion of dermatan sulfate and heparan sulfate (usually in a 2:1 ratio) in the urine are major criteria for establishing the clinical diagnosis. Hepatosplenomegaly is prominent, as is opacification of the corneas. There is often retinal degeneration as well as optic atrophy, which may be the result of increased intracranial pressure. Characteristic skeletal manifestations are noted clinically and radiographically. These include dysostosis multiplex, kyphosis with a hump deformity, and stiff joints. Deafness and hydrocephalus occur frequently, the latter probably due to meningeal infiltration with mucopolysaccharide. Mucopolysaccharide deposition in walls of blood vessels and heart valves frequently leads to cardiac complications. Congestive heart failure and repeated pulmonary infections are common causes of death, usually before the age of 10.

Patients classified clinically as having a distinct disorder, *Scheie's syndrome* (MPS IS), have also been found to be deficient in α-L-iduronidase activity. Scheie's and Hurler's syndromes represent disorders at opposite ends of the spectrum of clinical variability. Scheie's syndrome is compatible with a normal life-span and normal intelligence. Stature is near normal. Clinical problems include clouding of the cornea and retinitis pigmentosa, aortic valve involvement, and hand deformities associated with median nerve entrapment.

Some patients who are also devoid of α-L-iduronidase activity have a phenotype intermediate between those of the Hurler and Scheie syndromes [17]. These are designated the Hurler-Scheie genetic compound (MPS IH/S). The onset of clinical symptoms occurs later than in Hurler's, and development is less affected. Somatic stigmata are, however, considerably more severe than in Scheie's syndrome, and a number of these patients have developed hydrocephalus with subsequent neuro-

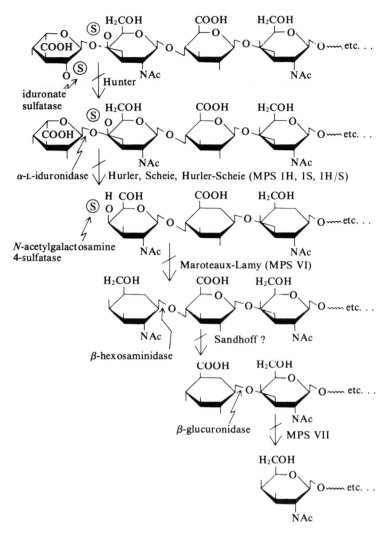

Fig. 31-1. Degradation of dermatan sulfate. Known enzymes and associated deficiency diseases are indicated; a question mark (?) denotes a step about which there is uncertainty [2]. The polymer consists of sulfated N-acetylgalactosamine alternating with uronic acid residues; the latter may be iduronic acid, sulfated iduronic acid, or glucuronic acid, in irregular order.

logical deterioration. The Scheie's patients and those of the intermediate type also have mucopolysacchariduria, the quantity or distribution of which bears no obvious relationship to the severity of the clinical disease.

The relationships among the mutations in these diseases, all of which are inherited in autosomal recessive fashion, is uncertain. All lack iduronidase activity to the same extent (<0.1% of normal) according to in vitro assays that employ artificial substrates. It has been suggested that Hurler's and Scheie's syndromes are due to homozygosity for two different sets of alleles at the same genetic locus, and that the MPS IH/S phenotype carries a Scheie's allele and a Hurler's allele at this locus [2, 17]. This would be analogous to hemoglobinopathies in which one can identify individuals with two different mutant alleles at the same locus (e.g.,

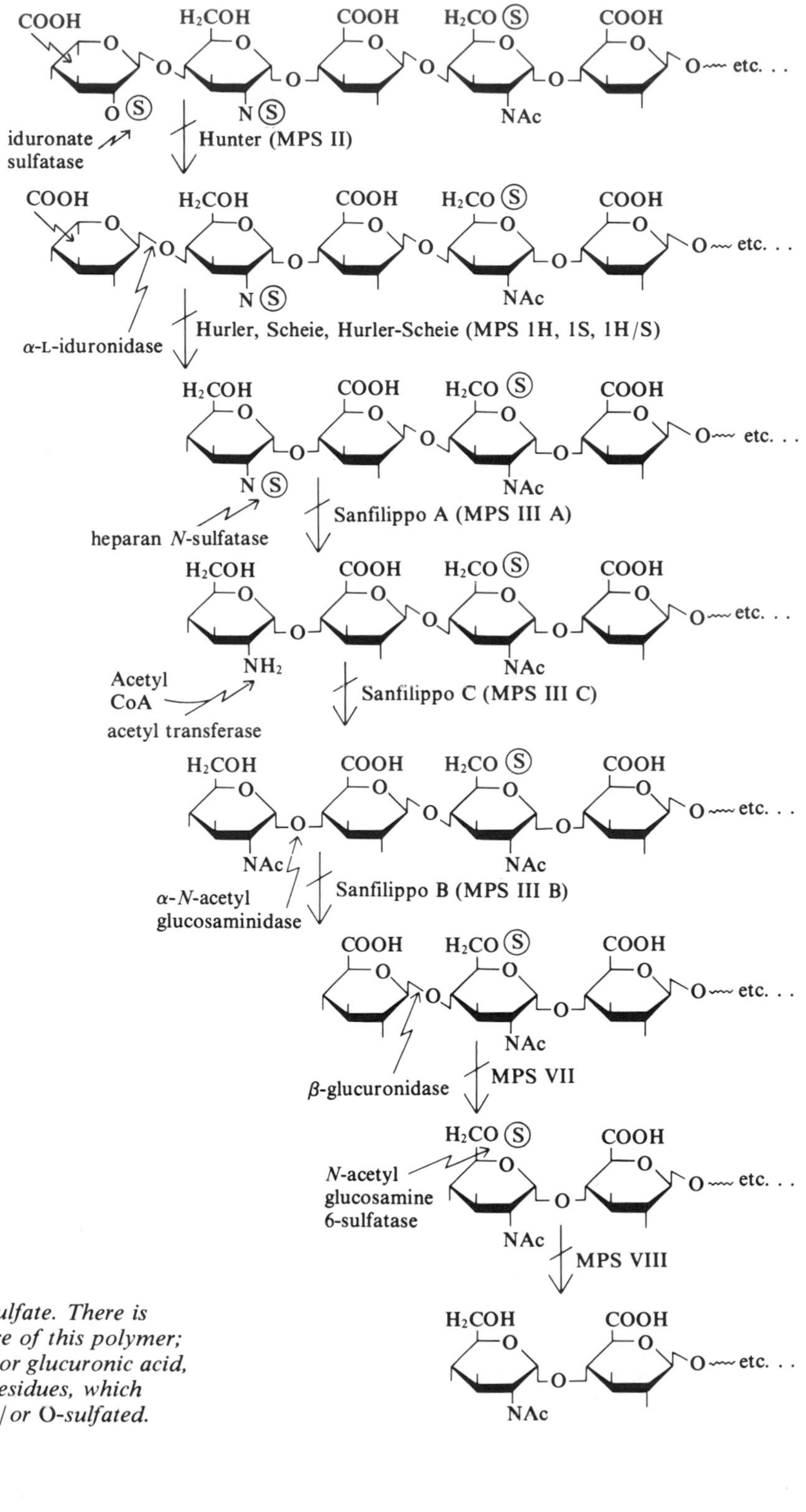

Fig. 31-2. Degradation of heparan sulfate. There is
considerable variation in the structure of this polymer;
sulfated or unsulfated iduronic acid, or glucuronic acid,
alternate with N-acetylglucosamine residues, which
may be N-sulfated, N-acetylated and/or O-sulfated.

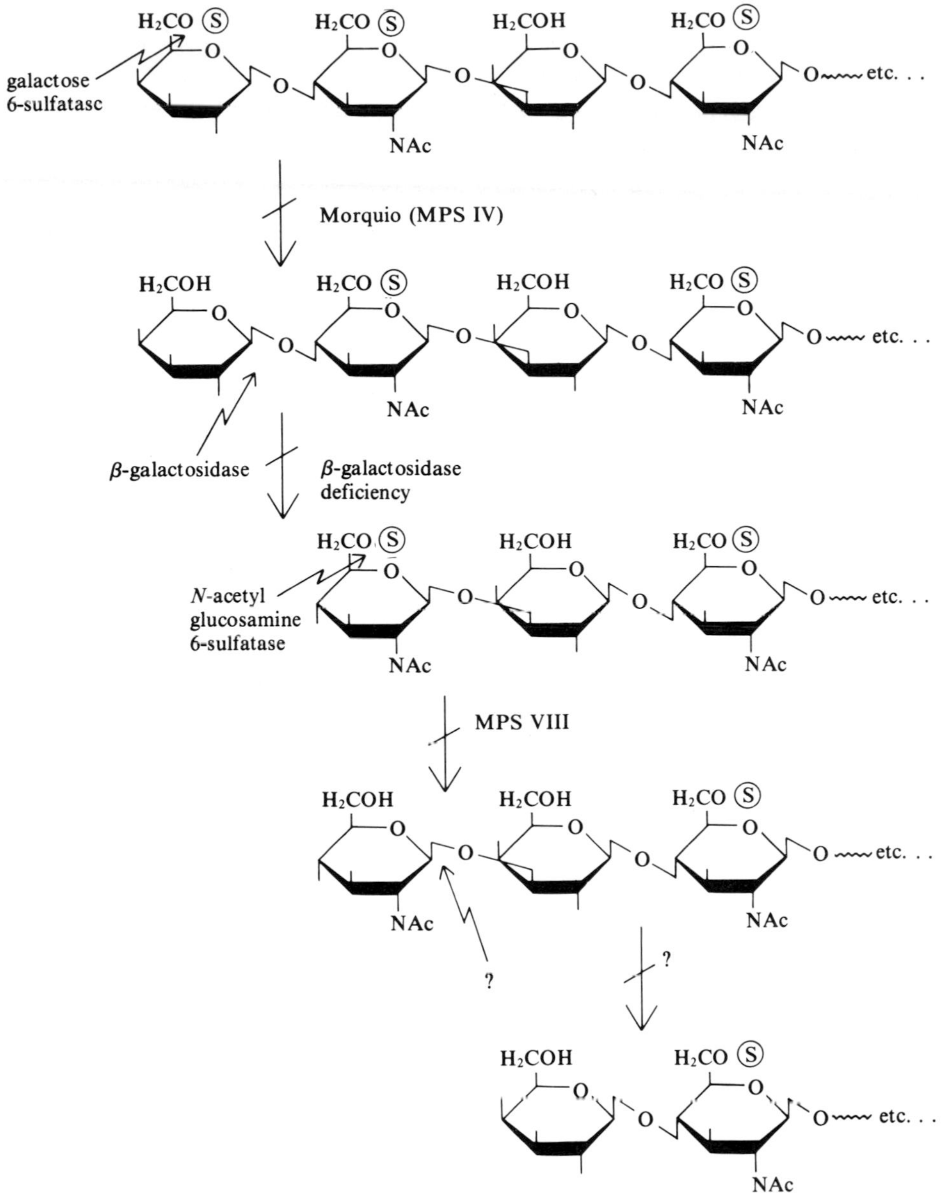

Fig. 31-3. Schematic representation of the degradation of keratan sulfate. A question mark (?) denotes a step about which there is uncertainty.

hemoglobin S-C disease). Alternative explanations are possible, however, and there may well be more than two mutant alleles involved. Resolution of this question must await development of techniques for characterizing the molecular structure of the mutant iduronidase proteins, if such indeed exist, or, alternatively, of sequencing the DNA that encodes the structure of iduronidase.

IDURONATE SULFATASE DEFICIENCY
The gene corresponding to iduronate sulfatase [18], or to some function essential for its expression, resides on the X-chromosome. Deficiency of this enzyme is inherited as a sex-linked recessive trait, the clinical expression of which is *Hunter's syndrome* (MPS II), described below [1, 2]. As might be anticipated, most affected patients have been males. There have been, however, two females identified as having Hunter's syndrome and who lack iduronate sulfatase activity [19]. this is probably due to a defect in an autosomal gene controlling enzyme expression, although an extreme form of "lyonization*" of the typical X-linked genetic defect cannot be ruled out. It has been possible to identify, in fibroblast cultures from clinically normal female carriers, clones of cells deficient in iduronate sulfatase activity, and other clones which have normal enzyme activity as predicted by the Lyon principle* [20]. Owing to the variability of the percentage of cells that may express the mutant X-linked gene in various tissues of heterozygotes, wide ranges of enzyme activity may be observed in carriers. At present, an abnormal result obtained in any of several tests for the carrier state may be taken as good evidence of heterozygosity. However, a normal result in the same tests cannot be used to exclude carrier status [21]. The most prudent course is to advise all female relatives of a Hunter's patient of their calculated risk from their position in the pedigree and to offer them the option of prenatal diagnostic studies.

*The *Lyon principle* states that one X chromosome in each somatic cell of the XX female is randomly inactivated early in embryogenesis. The inactivated X chromosome in each cell may be derived from either parent and the female thus is a mosaic of two classes of cells, those with active maternal X and those with active paternal X.

The clinical spectrum encompassed by iduronate sulfatase deficiency is very broad. Mild and severe variants have been described. Because these occur consistently in families having several affected males, they are thought to constitute distinct genetic entities [22]. Once again, this may be caused by different mutational alterations in the same gene. Severely affected individuals may be similar in appearance to patients with Hurler's syndrome. At times, however, the somatic manifestations may be milder, and CNS dysfunction may predominate to the extent of causing confusion with Sanfilippo's syndrome patients. Hunter's is distinguished from Hurler's syndrome by the absence of corneal clouding, although retinal lesions are usual. Characteristic nodular infiltrations in the skin are frequently seen. The milder variant may have normal or near-normal intelligence, and patients may live well into adulthood; however, only two Hunter's patients are known to have reproduced. Dermatan sulfate and heparan sulfate are excreted in the urine, usually in equal amounts, although an occasional patient will excrete heparan sulfate only.

HEPARAN N-SULFATASE AND ALPHA-N-ACETYLGLUCOSAMINIDASE DEFICIENCIES
Heparan N-sulfatase [23, 24] and α-N-acetylglucosaminidase [25, 26] are two of the enzymes involved in the degradation of heparan sulfate. Deficiency of these activities results in the *Sanfilippo A* (MPS IIIA) or the *Sanfilippo B* (MPS IIIB) syndromes, respectively [1, 2]. Heparan sulfate is the only mucopolysaccharide excreted in these disorders. Heparansulfaturia may be greatly underestimated for methodological reasons, however, and even its absence should not exclude a probable diagnosis in the context of an appropriate clinical situation. The two disorders are essentially indistinguishable clinically and must be differentiated by enzyme assays. In general, somatic manifestations are milder than in the other mucopolysaccharidoses, but again, there is some overlap. The corneas are clear, and organomegaly and cardiac manifestations are variable. Early psychomotor development is often normal, but later in

childhood, progressive loss of intellectual and motor skills results in severe impairment and eventual loss of most cortical functions. Seizures are common. Skeletal and joint involvement is usually much less striking than in the other mucopolysaccharidoses. Both the A and B forms of Sanfilippo's syndrome are inherited as autosomal recessive disorders, with the former considerably more common.

ACETYLTRANSFERASE DEFICIENCY

Quite recently, a novel defect has been described in a third group of patients who clinically have Sanfilippo's syndrome and excrete heparan sulfate (Sanfilippo C) [27]. These patients lack an enzyme that catalyzes the acetylation of glucosamine residues in heparan sulfate. After the removal of N-sulfate groups from heparan sulfate by the N-sulfatase just described, the free amino group generated must be acetylated before the α-N-acetylglucosaminidase can act. Acetyl-CoA functions as cofactor in the reaction. This represents the first documented lysosomal storage disease that is not the result of a defect in a hydrolytic enzyme.

N-ACETYLGALACTOSAMINE 4-SULFATASE DEFICIENCY

N-acetylgalactosamine 4-sulfatase activity is a property of a well-known lysosomal enzyme, arylsulfatase B. The physiological role of this hydrolase is the degradation of appropriate residues of dermatan sulfate [27–31], and the result of its deficiency is the *Maroteaux-Lamy syndrome* (MPS VI) [1, 2]. As in MPS I and MPS II, the manifestations of the Maroteaux-Lamy syndrome are variable. The index case [1] most closely resembles the Hurler-Scheie compound, whereas, in their clinical features, milder variants most closely resemble patients with Scheie's syndrome or those with mucolipidosis III (see below). Characteristic, large, white-cell inclusions are said to be striking in this disease, in contrast to the less impressive bodies seen in cells of patients with other mucopolysaccharidoses. Dermatan sulfate, but not heparan sulfate, appears in the urine of affected individuals, because the chemical linkage involved is unique to

the former. The disease is inherited in an autosomal recessive fashion.

BETA-GLUCURONIDASE DEFICIENCY

β-Glucuronidase is a well-known lysosomal enzyme, but its involvement in the catabolism of mucopolysaccharides came to light only with the description of a patient deficient in this activity [32, 33]. The index case had unusual facies, skeletal deformities, hepatosplenomegaly, and delayed development. A few more patients have been described since then, with widely different manifestations [34].

This disorder (MPS VII) is of some historic interest because it was the first mucopolysaccharidosis to have its enzymatic basis elucidated and its autosomal recessive mode of inheritance established on the basis of enzyme levels in one patient and his close relatives. The mucopolysacchariduria is puzzling: it consists mainly of dermatan sulfate and heparan sulfate, although one would predict from chemical consideration that fragments of chondroitin sulfate and hyaluronic acid should also be excreted. It is likely that the last two polymers are effectively degraded by endoglycosidases (e.g., hyaluronidase).

GALACTOSE 6-SULFATASE DEFICIENCY

Keratan sulfate is an important constituent of cartilage and cornea. Although its total structure is not known, a major portion of the molecule is made up of alternating galactose and N-acetylglucosamine residues, in most of which the primary alcohol is sulfated as indicated in Fig. 31-3. In addition to this characteristic unit, fucose, mannose, and sialic acid also occur in the polymer. A number of patients with urinary excretion and presumptive lysosomal storage of keratan sulfate have been known for some time. These individuals have *Morquio's syndrome* (MPS IV). Corneal clouding, aortic valvular disease, and normal intelligence are usually seen. These patients have a spondyloepiphyseal dysplasia with pronounced short stature. As cartilage and cornea are the only tissues that produce keratan sulfate, it might be expected that these would be the principal sites of pathological involvement as a result of disturbed metabolism of this polymer. Pectus carinatum deformity and marked kyphoscoliosis are prominent. Neurosensory deafness is reported commonly. A major complication is spinal-cord and medullary compression, caused by odontoid hypoplasia and subsequent atlantoaxial subluxation.

Several groups have now documented the deficiency of galactose 6-sulfatase activity in fibroblasts and white blood cells from patients with typical Morquio's syndrome [35–38]. This enzyme also can remove 6-sulfate groups from N-acetylgalactosamine 6-sulfate residues, which probably explains the chondroitin sulfaturia that has been reported to occur in these patients [36]. Morquio's syndrome is inherited as an autosomal recessive trait.

N-ACETYLGLUCOSAMINE 6-SULFATASE DEFICIENCY

Recently, a single patient has been described who manifested some clinical features of both Morquio and Sanfilippo syndromes and who excreted both keratan sulfate and heparan sulfate in his urine [38]. A deficiency of N-acetylglucosamine 6-sulfatase activity was demonstrated [37]. This is interesting, as the linkage involved is found in both of these polymers, which would account for their joint storage and excretion (Figs. 31-2 and 31-3). The disorder has been designated *MPS VIII* [2].

BETA-GALACTOSIDASE DEFICIENCY

Although there are several molecularly and genetically distinct human enzymes capable of removing β-galactosyl residues from different substrates, one of those enzymes appears to have broad substrate specificity and to cleave galactose from ganglioside G_{M1}, keratan sulfate, and a variety of glycoproteins. Most patients who lack this particular β-galactosidase activity have significant neurological abnormalities, due to neuronal storage of G_{M1} ganglioside. Storage of other β-galactosides occurs, as well. However, two patients with β-galactosidase deficiency have been described who lack neurological abnormalities, but have severe skeletal involvement reminiscent of the Morquio

syndrome [39, 40]. The best current explanation for the findings is that the enzyme in these unusual patients is so affected by a mutational event as to have higher residual activity for G_{M1} ganglioside than for keratan sulfate.

The Biochemical Basis of the Mucolipidoses

A number of patients have been described with diseases that clinically or pathologically resemble the mucopolysaccharidoses but lack mucopolysacchariduria. A superficial similarity to diseases of sphingolipid metabolism, as well, has led to their classification as "mucoplipidoses" [41]. These conditions comprise a heterogeneous group of disorders, several of which have turned out to be defects of glycoprotein metabolism.

NEURAMINIDASE DEFICIENCY

Sialic acid is widely distributed in nature, and is present in a variety of glycoproteins and glycolipids. An unknown number of neuraminidases play roles in the degradation of these compounds; it is thought that neuraminidases acting on sialogangliosides are different from those acting on glycoproteins.

Isolated deficiency of glycoprotein neuraminidase has been reported only recently [42]. The spectrum of clinical phenotypes appears to be broad. For instance, children affected with mucolipidosis I have been found to lack that enzyme [43, 44]. They have a mild, Hurlerlike appearance, with hepatosplenomegaly and bony changes, moderate mental retardation, cherry-red spots in the macula, and in some cases, progressive neurological degeneration. Other patients with the so-called cherry-red spot–myoclonus syndrome have also been found to have neuraminidase deficiency [45, 46]. The principal clinical features are late-childhood onset of intention myoclonus without significant intellectual problems, and macular degeneration. In some patients, a deficiency of β-galactosidase, believed to be secondary, accompanies the neuraminidase deficiency [42, 46].

ALPHA-L-FUCOSIDASE DEFICIENCY

As is the case with other lysosomal storage diseases, deficiency of α-L-fucosidase results in a clinical spectrum of disease [47]. Most patients have coarse facies, thickened skin, hepatosplenomegaly, and progressive neurological deterioration. Some have a characteristic rash that resembles the angiokeratoma seen in Fabry's disease. Although the disease is quite rare, there seems to be an increased incidence among individuals of Italian ancestry. It is transmitted in autosomal recessive fashion.

In addition to the enzymatic studies that have established the etiology of this condition, much detailed investigation has been performed characterizing the stored material. Fucose-containing oligosaccharides, glycopeptides, and glycolipids are stored in tissues or excreted in urine [48, 49]. Interestingly, the structure of the glycolipids resembles blood-group substance H. However, no correlation of clinical symptoms with blood type has been observed.

ALPHA-MANNOSIDASE DEFICIENCY

Deficient activity of lysosomal α-mannosidase leads to the autosomal recessive disorder, *mannosidosis* [50]. It is characterized by mental retardation, coarse facial features, dysostosis multiplex, hepatosplenomegaly, hearing loss, and recurrent infections. Clinically, the disease may be confused with Sanfilippo's syndrome or with mucolipidosis I (neuraminidase deficiency). Lack of α-mannosidase activity results in the accumulation of mannose-rich oligosaccharides in brain, liver, and urine. The activity of α-mannosidase may be influenced by certain cations, and the small amount of residual activity in fibroblasts from deficient patients may be stimulated by addition of cobalt or zinc.

MUCOLIPIDOSIS IV

Mucolipidosis IV is a newly recognized condition of unknown pathogenesis that is transmitted as an autosomal recessive trait [51]. So far, the patients have all been of Ashkenazi Jewish descent. The disorder manifests itself as progressive psychomotor retardation without skeletal abnormalities or hepatosplenomegaly. Corneal clouding is present from an early age. Striking inclusions are reported in conjunctival biopsies, cultured fibroblasts, and amniotic fluid cells. The basic defect that causes this condition is as yet unknown, but accumulation of sialogangliosides and mucopolysaccharides has been observed in cultured fibroblasts [52, 53].

MULTIPLE LYSOSOMAL ENZYME DEFICIENCIES

Disorders that are now coming under increasing scrutiny are those associated with multiple lysosomal enzyme deficiencies. Although these conditions are rare, they are very instructive; it is of fundamental biological interest to clarify how a single mendelian genetic defect can lead to the reduction of multiple enzymatic activities.

I-cell disease (inclusion-cell disease, or *mucolipidosis II*) derives its name from the grossly enlarged lysosomes visible as phase-dense inclusions in the fibroblasts of affected patients. The clinical phenotype is similar to that of Hurler's syndrome, although it is even more severe and has more obvious manifestations in the neonatal period [1, 2]. Psychomotor retardation is severe. Most patients die in early childhood.

Mucolipidosis III (pseudo-Hurler's polydystrophy) is milder and evolves more slowly than mucolipidosis II [1, 2]. Corneal clouding and skeletal radiographic changes are milder than in the Hurler syndrome, and intelligence is normal or minimally impaired. Stature is short. Clinically, the disease may be confused with the Maroteaux-Lamy or Hurler-Scheie syndromes. Both mucolipidoses, II and III, are inherited in autosomal recessive manner.

Fibroblasts cultured from skin of patients with either mucolipidosis II or III are deficient in a whole panel of lysosomal hydrolases [reviewed in 54]. Because of this multiple enzyme deficiency, the fibroblasts accumulate a variety of undegraded materials. However, the culture fluid surrounding these fibroblasts, as well as serum, urine, and cerebrospinal fluid from affected individuals, contain markedly elevated levels of some of the enzymes that are deficient intracellularly. Thus, the two disorders appear due to an inappropriate localization of hydrolytic enzymes. It was suggested that the primary biochemical defect is in the synthesis of a recognition marker that would direct the enzymes into lysosomes [55, 56]. This hypothesis recently has been validated. The postulated marker has been identified as 6-phosphomannosyl residues on oligosaccharide chains of the enzymes [57], and this residue is deficient in enzymes produced by fibroblasts from patients with I-cell disease [58].

Multiple sulfatase deficiency is a rare disorder associated with reduced levels of arylsulfatase A, N-acetylgalactosamine 4-sulfatase (arylsulfatase B), heparan N-sulfatase, iduronate sulfatase, steroid sulfatase, and perhaps yet other sulfatases. It is inherited as an autosomal recessive condition, and affected patients have symptomatology reminiscent of both metachromatic leukodystrophy and mucopolysaccharidosis [59]. It is not clear how a single gene defect results in loss of lysosomal and microsomal (steroid sulfatase) enzyme activities, which are thought to be encoded in genes on several autosomal chromosomes as well as on the X chromosome. Because expression of these enzymes is possible in cultured fibroblasts under appropriate conditions [60], it has been suggested that the mutation may be regulatory or may affect enzyme stability.

Clinical Implications

Knowledge of the biochemical defects in the mucopolysaccharidoses and the mucolipidoses permits the dissemination of accurate diagnostic and counseling information. Prenatal diagnosis with selective abortion can be offered to families desiring this option. Total prevention of these disorders by amniocentesis and selective abortion is not possible, however, because the families who are at risk for producing affected offspring can be ascertained only through the production of a previously affected child (except in the case of the X-linked Hunter's syndrome). Heterozygote detection for the autosomal recessive mucopolysaccharidoses and mucolipidoses, analogous to that established for

Tay-Sachs disease [61], does not appear likely. This is because of the large variation of normal values of the relevant lysosomal enzymes and the lack of defined and limited populations suitable for screening.

Hope of replacement therapy for mucopolysaccharidosis patients has been encouraged by the ease with which their fibroblasts can be cured in vitro when the missing enzyme is added to the medium [13, 54]. In the absence of highly purified enzymes for administration to patients, both whole or fractionated plasma and leukocytes have been used. Although early experiments were considered promising [62, 63], further evaluation has resulted in a much less optimistic outlook [64, 65]. The therapeutic failures are attributable in part to the low levels of the relevant enzymes in plasma and other blood fractions used. An additional difficulty lies in the requirement that enzymes have specific recognition markers (see above) in order to enter cells efficiently and lodge in lysosomes [66]. Infusion of purified enzymes that possess the correct marker to insure high uptake in the target tissue, and perhaps modified for greater stability in vivo, will no doubt receive attention in the near future. A further approach to therapy is the use of fibroblast transplantation in the hope that engraftment will result in a continuous supply of enzyme that can be taken up by host tissue [67]; so far, no clinical changes have been observed.

The genetic mucopolysaccharidoses and mucolipidoses are caused by inherited deficiencies of lysosomal enzymes required for mucopolysaccharide and glycoprotein catabolism. Through the study of these disease states, the normal degradative pathways have been elucidated. Further investigation of the defect in certain mucolipidoses should yield information about the processes by which the lysosomal enzymes arrive at their proper intracellular location. From a clinical standpoint, the diversity of phenotypes of individuals who share a common enzymatic deficiency still requires explanation, and patients with as yet undescribed defects of mucopolysaccharide and glycoprotein catabolism must be expected.

References

*1. McKusick, V. A. *Heritable Disorders of Connective Tissue* (4th ed.). St. Louis: Mosby, 1972. Pp. 521–686.

*2. McKusick, V. A., Neufeld, E. F., and Kelly, T. E. Mucopolysaccharide Storage Disorders. In J. B. Stanbury, J. B. Wyngaarden, and D. S. Fredrickson (eds.), *The Metabolic Basis of Inherited Disease* (4th ed.). New York: McGraw-Hill, 1978. Pp. 1282–1307.

*3. Sharon, N. *Complex Carbohydrates. Their Chemistry, Biosynthesis and Function.* Reading, Mass.: Addison Wesley, 1975. Pp. 258–281.

4. Kraemer, P. M. Heparan sulfates of cultured cells. *Biochemistry* 10:1445–1451, 1971.

5. Brante, G. Gargoylism: A mucopolysaccharidosis. *Scand. J. Clin. Lab. Invest.* 4:43–46, 1952.

6. Brown, D. H. Tissue storage of mucopolysaccharides in Hurler-Pfaundler's disease. *Proc. Natl. Acad. Sci. U.S.A.* 43:783–790, 1957.

7. Meyer, K., Hoffman, P., Linker, A., Grumback, M., and Sampson, P. Sulfated mucopolysaccharides of urine and organs in gargoylism (Hurler's syndrome). *Proc. Soc. Exp. Biol. Med.* 102:587–590, 1959.

8. Dorfman, A., and Lorincz, A. E. Occurrence of urinary acid mucopolysaccharide in the Hurler syndrome. *Proc. Natl. Acad. Sci. U.S.A.* 43:443–446, 1957.

9. McKusick, V. A. *Heritable Disorders of Connective Tissue* (3rd ed.). St. Louis: Mosby, 1966. Pp. 325–339.

10. Van Hoof, F., and Hers, H. G. L'ultrastructure des cellules hépatiques dans la maladie de Hurler (Gargoylisme). *C. R. Acad. Sci. [D.]* (Paris) 259: 1281–1283, 1964.

11. Danes, B. S., and Bearn, A. G. Hurler's syndrome; demonstration of an inherited disorder of connective tissue in cell culture. *Science* 149:987–989, 1965.

12. Fratantoni, H. C., Hall, C. W., and Neufeld, E. F. The defect in Hurler's and Hunter's syndromes: Faulty degradation of mucopolysaccharide. *Proc. Natl. Acad. Sci. U.S.A.* 60:699–706, 1968.

*13. Neufeld, E. F., and Cantz, M. The Mucopolysaccharidoses Studied in Cell Culture. In H. G. Hers, and F. Van Hoof (eds.), *Lysosomes and Storage Diseases.* New York: Academic, 1973. Pp. 261–275.

14. Neufeld, E. F. The biochemical basis for mucopolysaccharidoses and mucolipidoses. *Prog. Med. Genet.* 10:81–101, 1974.

*Key reference.

15. Matalon, R., and Dorfman, A. Hurler's syndrome, an α-L-iduronidase deficiency. *Biochem. Biophys. Res. Commun.* 47:959–964, 1972.

16. Bach, G., Friedman, R., Weissmann, B., and Neufeld, E. F. The defect in the Hurler and Scheie syndromes: Deficiency of α-L-iduronidase. *Proc. Natl. Acad. Sci. U.S.A.* 69:2048–2051, 1972.

17. McKusick, V. A., Howell, R. R., Hussels, I. E., Neufeld, E. F., and Stevenson, R. Allelism, nonallelism and genetic compounds among the mucopolysaccharidoses. *Lancet* 1:993–996, 1972.

18. Bach, G., Eisenberg, R., Jr., Cantz, M., and Neufeld, E. F. The defect in the Hunter syndrome: Deficiency of sulfoiduronate sulfatase. *Proc. Natl. Acad. Sci. U.S.A.* 70:2134–2138, 1973.

19. Neufeld, E. F., Liebaers, I., Epstein, C. J., Yatziv, S., Milunsky, A., and Migeon, B. R. The Hunter syndrome in females: Is there an autosomal recessive form of iduronate sulfatase deficiency? *Am. J. Hum. Genet.* 29:455–461, 1977.

20. Migeon, B. R., Sprenkle, J. A., Liebaers, I., Scott, J. F., and Neufeld, E. F. X-linked Hunter syndrome: The heterozygous phenotype in cell culture. *Am. J. Hum. Genet.* 29:448–454, 1977.

21. Nwokoro, N., and Neufeld, E. F. Detection of Hunter heterozygotes by enzymatic analysis of hair roots. *Am. J. Hum. Genet.*, in press, 1981.

22. Spranger, J. W. The systemic mucopolysaccharidoses. *Ergeb. Inn. Med. Kinderherlk.* 32: 165–265, 1972.

23. Kresse, H. Mucopolysaccharidosis III A (Sanfilippo A disease): Deficiency of a heparin sulfamidase in skin fibroblasts and leukocytes. *Biochem. Biophys. Res. Commun.* 54:1111–1118, 1973.

24. Matalon, R., and Dorfman, A. Sanfilippo A syndrome: Sulfamidase deficiency in cultured skin fibroblasts and liver. *J. Clin. Invest.* 54:907–912, 1974.

25. O'Brien, J. S. Sanfilippo syndrome: Profound deficiency of alpha-*N*-acetylglucosaminidase activity in organs and skin fibroblasts from type B patients. *Proc. Natl. Acad. Sci. U.S.A.* 69:1720–1722, 1972.

26. von Figura, K., and Kress, H. The Sanfilippo B corrective factor: An *N*-acetyl-α-glucosaminidase. *Biochem. Biophys. Res. Commun.* 48:262–269, 1972.

27. Klein, U., Kresse, H., and von Figura, K. Sanfilippo syndrome type C: Deficiency of acetyl-CoA: α-glucosaminidine-*N*-acetyltransferase in skin fibroblasts. *Proc. Natl. Acad. Sci. U.S.A.* 75:5185–5189, 1978.

28. Stumpf, D. A., Austin, J. H., Crocker, A. C., and La France, M. Mucopolysaccharidosis type VI (Maroteaux-Lamy syndrome). 1. Sulfatase B deficiency in tissues. *Am. J. Dis. Child.* 126:747–755, 1973.

29. O'Brien, J. F., Cantz, M., and Spranger, J. W. Maroteaux-Lamy disease (mucopolysaccharidosis VI), subtype A: Deficiency of a *N*-acetylgalactosamine-4-sulfatase. *Biochem. Biophys. Res. Commun.* 60:1170–1177, 1974.

30. Matalon, R., Arbogast, B., and Dorfman, A. Deficiency of chondroitin sulfate *N*-acetylgalactosamine-4-sulfatase in Maroteaux-Lamy syndrome. *Biochem. Biophys. Res. Commun.* 61:1450–1457, 1974.

31. Fluharty, A. A., Stevens, R. L., Fung, D., Peak, S., and Kihara, H. Uridine phospho *N*-acetylgalactosamine 4-sulfate sulfohydrolase activity of human arylsulfatase B and its deficiency in the Maroteaux-Lamy syndrome. *Biochem. Biophys. Res. Commun.* 64:955–962, 1975.

32. Sly, W. S., Quinton, B. A., McAllister, W. H., and Rimoin, D. L. β-Glucuronidase-deficiency: Report of clinical, radiologic, and biochemical features of a new mucopolysaccharidosis. *J. Pediatr.* 82:249–257, 1973.

33. Hall, C. W., Cantz, M., and Neufeld, E. F. A β-glucuronidase deficiency mucopolysaccharidosis: Studies in cultured fibroblasts. *Arch. Biochem. Biophys.* 155:32–38, 1973.

34. Beaudet, A. C., DiFerrante, N., Ferry, G., Nichols, B. L., and Mullins, C. E. Variation in the phenotypic expression of β-glucuronidase deficiency. *J. Pediatr.* 86:388–394, 1975.

35. Matalon, R., Arbogast, B., Justice, P., Brandt, I., and Dorfman, A. Morquio's syndrome: Deficiency of a chondroitin sulfate *N*-acetylhexosamine sulfate sulfatase. *Biochem. Biophys. Res. Commun.* 61:759–765, 1974.

36. Horwitz, A. L., and Dorfman, A. The enzymatic defect in Morquio's disease: The specificity of *N*-acetylhexosamine sulfatases. *Biochem. Biophys. Res. Commun.* 80:819–825, 1978.

37. DiFerrante, N., Ginsberg, L. C., Donnelly, P. V., DiFerrante, D. T., and Caskey, C. T. Deficiency of glucosamine-6-sulfate or galactosamine-6-sulfate sulfatases are responsible for different mucopolysaccharidoses. *Science* 199:79–81, 1978.

38. Ginsberg, L., DiFerrante, D. T., Caskey, C. T., and DiFerranti, N. Glucosamine 6-sulfate sulfatase deficiency: A new mucopolysaccharidosis. *Clin. Res.* 25:471A, 1977.

39. Arbisser, A. I., Donnelly, K. A., Scott, C. I., DiFerrante, N., Singh, J., Stevenson, P. E., Ayelsworth, A. S., and Howell, R. R. Morquio-like syndrome with β-galactosidase deficiency and normal hexosamine sulfatase activity. *Am. J. Med. Genet.* 1:195–205, 1977.

40. O'Brien, J. S., Gugler, E., Giedion, A., Wiesmann, U., Herschkowitz, M., Meier, C., and Leroy, J. Spondyloepiphyseal dysplasia, corneal clouding, normal intelligence and β-galactosidase deficiency. *Clin. Genet.* 9:495–504, 1976.

41. Spranger, J. W., and Wiedemann, H. R. The genetic mucolipidoses: Diagnosis and differential diagnosis. *Humangenetik* 9:113–139, 1970.

42. Lowden, J. A., and O'Brien, J. S. Sialidosis: A review of human neuraminidase deficiency. *Am. J. Hum. Genet.* 31:1–18, 1979.

43. Cantz, M., Gehler, J., and Spranger, J. Mucolipidosis I: Increased sialic acid content and deficiency of an α-*N*-acetylneuraminidase in cultured fibroblasts. *Biochem. Biophys. Res. Commun.* 74:732–738, 1977.

44. Kelly, T. E., and Groetz, G. Isolated neuraminidase deficiency: A distinct lysosomal storage disease. *Am. J. Med. Genet.* 1:31–46, 1977.

45. Thomas, G. H., Tipton, R. E., Ch'ien, L. T., Reynolds, L. W., and Miller, L. S. Sialidase deficiency: The enzyme defect in an adult with macular cherry-red spots and myoclonus without dementia. *Clin. Genet.* 13:369–379, 1978.

46. Wenger, D. A., Tarby, T. J., and Wharton, C. Macular cherry-red spots and muoclonus with dementia: Coexistent neuraminidase and β-galactosidase deficiencies. *Biochem. Biophys. Res. Commun.* 82:589–595, 1978.

*47. Van Hoof, F. Fucosidosis. In H. G. Hers and F. von Hoof (eds.), *Lysosomes and Storage Disease.* New York: Academic, 1973. Pp. 277–290.

48. Dawson, G., and Tsay, G. C. Fucosidosis. *Adv. Exp. Med. Biol.* 68:187–203, 1976.

49. Nishigaki, M., Yamashita, K., Matsuda, I., Aroshima, S., Kobata, A. Urinary oligosaccharides of fucosidosis. *J. Biochem.* 84:823–834, 1978.

50. Desnick, R. J., Sharp, H. L., Grabowski, G. A., Brunning, R. D., Quie, P. G., Sung, J. H., Gorlin, R. J., and Ikonne, J. U. Mannosidosis: Clinical, morphologic, immunologic, and biochemical studies. *Pediatr. Res.* 10:985–996, 1976.

51. Berman, E. R., Livni, N., Shapira, E., Merin, S., and Levij, I. S. Congenital corneal clouding with abnormal systemic storage bodies: A new variant of mucolipidosis. *J. Pediatr.* 84:519–526, 1974.

52. Bach, G., Cohen, M., and Kohn, G. Abnormal ganglioside accumulation in cultured fibroblasts from patients with mucolipidosis IV. *Biochem. Biophys. Res. Commun.* 66:1483–1490, 1975.

53. Bach, G., Ziegler, M., Kohn, G., and Cohen, M. M. Mucopolysaccharide accumulation in cultured skin fibroblasts derived from patients with Mucolipidosis IV. *Am. J. Hum. Genet.* 29:610–618, 1977.

*54. Neufeld, E. F., Lim, T. W., and Shapiro, L. J. Inherited disorders of lysosomal metabolism. *Annu. Rev. Biochem.* 44:357–376, 1975.

55. Hickman, S., and Neufeld, E. F. A hypothesis for I-cell disease: Defective hydrolases that do not enter lysosomes. *Biochem. Biophys. Res. Commun.* 49:992–994, 1972.

56. Hickman, S., Shapiro, L. J., and Neufeld, E. F. A recognition marker required for uptake of a lysosomal enzyme by cultured fibroblasts. *Biochem. Biophys. Res. Commun.* 57:55–61, 1974.

57. Kaplan, A., Achord, D. T., and Sly, W. S. Phosphohexosyl components of a lysosomal enzyme are recognized by pinocytosis receptors on human fibroblasts. *Proc. Natl. Acad. Sci. U.S.A.* 74: 2026–2030, 1977.

58. Hasilik, A., Rome, L. H., and Neufeld, E. F. Processing of lysosomal enzymes in skin fibroblasts. *Fed. Proc.* 38:467, 1979.

*59. Moser, H. W., and Dulaney, J. T. Sulfatide Lipidosis: Metachromatic Leukodystrophy. In J. B. Stanbury, J. B. Wyngaarden, and D. S. Fredrickson (eds.), *The Metabolic Basis of Inherited Disease* (4th ed.). New York: McGraw-Hill, 1978. Pp. 770–809.

60. Fluharty, A. L., Stevens, R. L., Davis, L. L., Shapiro, L. J., and Kihara, H. Presence of arylsulfatase A in multiple sulfatase deficiency disorder fibroblasts. *Am. J. Hum. Genet.* 30:249–255, 1978.

61. Kaback, M. M., Zeiger, R. S., Reynolds, L. W., and Sonneborn, M. Approaches to the control and prevention of Tay-Sachs disease. *Prog. Med. Genet.* 10:103–134, 1974.

62. DiFerrante, N., Nichols, B. G., Donnelly, P. V., Neri, G., Hrgovcic, R., and Berglund, R. K. Induced degradation of glycosaminoglycans in Hurler's and Hunter's syndromes by plasma infusion. *Proc. Natl. Acad. Sci. U.S.A.* 68:303–307, 1971.

63. Knudson, A. G., DiFerrante, N., and Curtis, J. E. Effect of leukocyte transfusion in a child with type II mucopolysaccharidosis. *Proc. Natl. Acad. Sci. U.S.A.* 68:1738–1741, 1971.

64. Crocker, A. C. Plasma infusion therapy for Hurler's syndrome. *Pediatrics* 50:683–685, 1972.

65. Moser, H. W., O'Brien, J. S., Atkins, L., Fuller, T. C., Kliman, A., Janowska, S., Russell, P. S., Bartsocas, C. S., Cosimi, B., and Dulaney, J. T. Infusion of normal HL-A identical leukocytes in Sanfilippo disease type B. *Arch. Neurol.* 31: 329–337, 1974.

66. Neufeld, E. F. The Uptake of Enzymes into Lysosomes: An Overview. Second Symposium on Enzyme Therapy in Genetic Disease. New York: National Foundation, 1980.

67. Dean, M. F., Stevens, R. L., Muir, H., Benson, P. F., Button, L. R., Anderson, R. L., Boylston, A., and Mowbray, J. Enzyme replacement therapy by fibroblast transplantation, long-term biochemical study in three cases of Hunter's syndrome. *J. Clin. Invest.* 63:138–146, 1979.

Pierre Morell
Murray B. Bornstein
Cedric S. Raine

Chapter 32. Diseases Involving Myelin

The title of this chapter has been selected to emphasize that myelin cannot in any way be considered an isolated entity. For its maintenance in the peripheral nervous system (PNS), myelin depends on the normal functioning of a Schwann cell, and in the central nervous system (CNS), an oligodendrocyte. The integrity of the myelin sheaths is also dependent upon the viability of the axons that they ensheath and the neuronal cell bodies from which the axons emanate. It is well known, for example, that neuronal death inevitably leads to subsequent degeneration of axons and myelin. Although many conditions are recognized in which preferential loss of myelin occurs, damage to myelin is a common consequence of a multitude of unrelated pathological stigmata (e.g., genetically determined disorders, viral infection, toxic agents, neoplasia, trauma, and anoxia) that happen to affect myelin or myelin-supporting cells either selectively or initially.

General Classification

Many of the diseases involving demyelination can be subdivided into primary and secondary categories on the basis of morphological observations. *Primary demyelination* involves the early destruction of myelin with relative sparing of axons; subsequently, other structures may be affected. *Secondary demyelination* includes those disorders in which myelin is involved after damage to neurons or axons. The classification scheme detailed in this chapter is based on etiology as well as comparative neuropathology, and includes four categories: (1) acquired inflammatory demyelinating disorders, (2) genetically determined metabolic disorders, (3) toxic and nutritional disorders, and (4) disorders with secondary involvement of myelin.

BIOCHEMISTRY OF DEMYELINATING DISEASES—GENERAL COMMENTS

The chemical alterations in whole brain (or white matter, which usually shows more pronounced changes) are similar in demyelinating diseases, regardless of the etiology [1, 2]. The water content of white matter increases markedly because myelin (which is relatively rich in solids) is lost, leaving behind comparatively more hydrated material. Other changes include a decrease of myelin constituents—especially proteolipid protein, cerebroside, ethanolamine phosphatides, and cholesterol—and the appearance of cholesterol esters. Table 32-1 details the results of demyelination caused by genetically determined metabolic disorder, adrenoleukodystrophy [3], and of demyelination secondary to a viral infection, subacute sclerosing panencephalitis (SSPE) [4]. These changes can often be explained by the breakdown and gradual loss of myelin and its replacement by tissue components (e.g., extracellular fluid, astrocytes, inflammatory cells) that are more hydrated, relatively lipid-poor, and free of myelin-specific constituents. The magnitude of these changes varies considerably from specimen to specimen in the same disease. Variations undoubtedly are related to the severity, duration, and activity of the disease process.

Acquired Inflammatory Demyelinating Diseases

Probably the most complete outline of human diseases in this category has been given by Adams and Sidman [5]. In contrast to the metabolic disorders of myelin, nervous system damage in this group of demyelinating diseases is more specifically directed against myelin, and there is relatively little damage to other parenchymal elements. With

Table 32-1. Human White Matter Composition in Two Diseases Compared with Controls

	SSPE[a]		ALD[b]	
	Control	Patient	Control	Patient
Water[c]	72	88.5	72.5	84.3
Proteolipid[d]			8.2	1.4
Total lipid[d]	60	23.4	56.3	34.7
Cholesterol	14	6.1	14.4	9.3
Cholesterol ester	0.2	1.8		9.9
Cerebroside	13	0.8 ⎫	⎧ 10.6	⎧ 0.8
Sulfatide	3.5	3 ⎭	⎩	⎩
Total phospholipid	30	15	25	8.5
Ethanolamine phosphatides	10.2	4.7	7.9	1.3
Lecithin	7.5	4.8	7.3	2.7
Sphingomyelin	5.4	2.9	4.2	1.6
Serine phosphatides	5.9	1.7	5.0	1.6
Phosphatidylinositol	0.8	0.7	0.3	0.7

[a]Subacute sclerosing panencephalitis. Data was recalculated from ref. 3.
[b]Adrenoleukodystrophy. Data was recalculated from ref. 3; originally this case was classified as Schilder's disease, but see ref. 1.
[c]Percentage of wet weight.
[d]Proteolipid, total lipid, and individual lipids as percentages of white matter dry weight.

one exception, lesion formation appears to be related to an immunological response. It is not always clear, however, whether the immunological activity is autoimmune in nature or whether it is related primarily to an antecedent viral infection; nor is the extent of damage directly ascribable to putative viral agents known at the present time.

CLASSIFICATION OF THE ACQUIRED INFLAMMATORY DEMYELINATING DISEASES

Of the many *human demyelinating diseases* encountered, the following are the best-characterized examples:

1. *Multiple sclerosis (MS)* is the paradigm of the demyelinating diseases [6, 7] and the most common, typically showing a chronic relapsing course. Large plaques of primary demyelination, frequently in a periventricular distribution, are typical. Some variants exist by pathological criteria—for example, Devic's disease. The active lesions are inflammatory and are believed to have an immunogenical basis that may be linked to an antecedent viral infection. Genetic factors are considered possible but have not been proved. A distinction is often made between the chronic and acute forms of MS. The so-called acute form is rarer, presents a more fulminant picture, and is of shorter duration. Lesions are more inflammatory than in chronic MS, and a viral infection is also suspected.

2. *Acute disseminated encephalomyelitis,* also called *postinfectious* or *postimmunization encephalitis,* represents a group of disorders of usually mixed viral-immunological etiology. The condition is most commonly related to a spontaneous viral infection (e.g., measles, smallpox, or chickenpox) [6].

3. *Acute hemorrhagic leukoencephalopathy* is a rare condition in which demyelination is accompanied by multiple and focal hemorrhages and inflammation. A viral infection is implicated, and the disease is considered by some [8] to

represent a hyperacute form of acute disseminated encephalomyelitis.

4. *Progressive multifocal leukoencephalopathy (PML)* is a rare demyelinating disease that is usually associated with disorders of the reticuloendothelial system, neoplasias, and immunosuppressive therapy [9]. Lesions are noninflammatory and are believed to be etiologically related to a papovavirus infection.

5. *Landry-Guillain-Barré syndrome* is an inflammatory disease of the peripheral nerves and their roots that is encountered in many forms, ranging from acute-monophasic to chronic-remitting [10].

A number of *spontaneously occurring animal models* (see [11] for a more complete listing and description) are recognized in which inflammatory changes, primarily demyelination and, frequently, a viral infection, are the major components of the disease process.

1. *Canine distemper encephalomyelitis* is a viral-induced CNS demyelinating disease in dogs. Lesions show a strong inflammatory response [11]. Some similarities to acute disseminated encephalomyelitis exist.

2. *Coonhound paralysis* is claimed by some to be the animal counterpart of the Landry-Guillain-Barré syndrome [12].

3. *Marek's disease,* a lymphomatous condition in chickens associated with demyelination in the PNS, is caused by a member of the herpes virus group [11].

4. *Visna,* a viral-induced demyelinating disease of sheep, is claimed by some to be of relevance to the study of MS. Other workers consider visna not specifically demyelinative in type [11].

5. *Mouse hepatitis virus encephalomyelitis* is caused by a neurotropic corona virus strain (JHM virus) and is considered a model for the study of acute disseminated encephalomyelitis [13].

6. *Theiler's virus encephalomyelitis* is a picornavirus-induced disease of the CNS associated with demyelination and other abnormalities related to an autoimmune response [14].

Certain *experimental demyelinating disease models* in animals are of considerable interest to neurochemists. Because the disease process can be initiated when desired and the course of the disease is known, experiments to elucidate the metabolic events associated with the disease process are possible.

1. *Experimental allergic encephalomyelitis (EAE)* is an autoimmune demyelinating disease inducible in most animal species by the inoculation of CNS material. The disease is usually acute and has certain morphological features reminiscent of acute MS and human disseminated encephalomyelitis [15–18].

2. *Experimental allergic neuritis (EAN),* the PNS counterpart of EAE, is caused by sensitization against PNS material. This model is relevant to the study of Landry-Guillain-Barré syndrome [18].

PATHOLOGY OF THE ACQUIRED INFLAMMATORY DEMYELINATING DISEASES

The criteria listed below apply to virtually all the acquired demyelinating diseases with one notable exception, progressive multifocal leukoencephalopathy, in which lesions are noninflammatory. The extent to which criteria (1) through (7) are fulfilled depends on the phase of the disease.

1. Perivenular demyelination
2. Perivenular inflammation
3. Relative sparing of axons
4. Macrophage activity in lesions
5. Disseminated lesions
6. Pia-arachnoid inflammation
7. Sudanophilic deposits, presumably products of myelin degradation

These primary demyelinating disorders (with the exception of progressive multifocal leukoencephalopathy) are characterized pathologically by perivascular cuffs of mononuclear cells that appear early in the disease process. This, coupled with studies that demonstrate blood-brain barrier damage in EAE, implies the participation of hematogenous elements in the destruction of myelin. Locally derived macrophages are also involved, and it is sometimes difficult to quantitate the relative role of the two classes of cells. It has been demonstrated definitely that, during EAE and EAN, hematogenously derived macrophages attack myelin. Among human diseases, a similar phenomenon has been seen only in Landry-Guillain-Barré syndrome and MS. In these two diseases, pieces of myelin are stripped from axons and engulfed by phagocytic cells. Frequently, however, myelin degradation is seen in EAE whereby myelin is lost from axons without the direct participation of invading cells. Once inside macrophages, the myelin presumably is then degraded by lysosomal enzymes. Cholesterol, however, is apparently one myelin constituent that cannot be degraded to smaller units and is esterified, often remaining in phagocytes for some time at the site of the lesion. Cholesterol esters are essentially absent in mature brain so that their presence in myelin disorders is considered indicative of recent demyelination. Such compounds are also responsible for the neutral fat staining, or sudanophilia, demonstrated histochemically in many demyelinating diseases.

The presence of macrophages and cholesterol esters in a particular region of the brain may be a relatively transient phase in the disease process. In demyelinated MS plaques, the center of the plaque might not contain macrophages or cholesterol esters, whereas the margins of the plaque frequently have both. Much of our knowledge of the disease process relating to inflammatory demyelinating disorders comes from work with the experimental model EAE, described in the following section.

Experimental Allergic Encephalomyelitis

The first suggestion of a possible autoallergic cause for multiple sclerosis arose from observations of patients who had been treated with the Pasteur antirabies vaccine. A small minority of these patients developed an acute, severe, sometimes fatal, postinoculation encephalomyelitis. These lesions somewhat resembled those in MS brain, and they were unrelated to the pathological changes observed in an untreated case of rabies.

The laboratory counterpart to the clinical observations was a series of studies demonstrating that animals undergo an immunological response to inoculations of CNS tissue and that a series of such inoculations could lead to neurological symptoms of paralysis, ataxia, and sphincter disturbance. This condition was histologically accompanied by a characteristic lesion consisting of perivascular and diffuse lymphocytic infiltrations, as well as demyelination with sparing of axons. If nerve tissue was emulsified with Freund's adjuvant—a combination of mineral oil, killed mycobacteria, and a binding agent—the allergenic potency of the tissue was increased, and the onset of the disease appeared within 2 to 3 weeks, rather than months, after inoculation. The assumed relation of EAE to MS is based largely on the similarities between the histological lesions in EAE cases and those seen in some acute forms of MS.

Much effort has been spent on isolating the specific CNS components responsible for induction of EAE. This research gained momentum when Kies and Alvord succeeded in establishing a quantitative assay system based on clinical symptoms and histopathological lesions in guinea pigs. Eventually, the major encephalitogenic component was identified as a myelin protein, a basic protein with a molecular weight of about 18,000. As a result of work by Eylar, Hashim, Brostoff, and coworkers, Carnegie and coworkers, and Kibler, Shapira, and coworkers, the complete sequences of bovine and human basic proteins have been elucidated [for review, see 18–22]. It is of interest that the sequence of this protein is highly conserved during evolution: bovine and human proteins differ by only 11 residues. The complete sequences of these proteins are shown in Fig. 32-1. There is some disagreement about certain parts of the sequence, but the discrepancies are relatively minor. The sequence is similar in different species, but different portions of the molecule are antigenic in different species [see 14 for review]. A peptide of 9 amino acids (114–122

```
                                                          His—Gly
NAc—Ala—Ser—Ala—Gln—Lys—Arg—Pro—Ser—Gln—Arg—Ser—Lys—Tyr—Leu—Ala—
                                                            10
Thr
Ser—Ala—Ser—Thr—Met—Asp—His—Ala—Arg—His—Gly—Phe—Leu—Pro—Arg—His—
               20                                                30
                                          Ile                    Gly
Arg—Asp—Thr—Gly—Ile—Leu—Asp—Ser—Leu—Gly—Arg—Phe—Phe—Gly—Ser—Asp—
                              40                         _____
                                                 Ser             Pro
Arg—Gly—Ala—Pro—Lys—Arg—Gly—Ser—Gly—Lys—Asp—Gly—His—His—Ala—Ala—
         ____50_____                    _____60_____
         Ala
Arg—Thr—Thr—His—Tyr—Gly—Ser—Leu—Pro—Gln—Lys— Ala—Gln—Gly—His—Arg—
_____70_____
Thr
Pro—Gln—Asp—Glu—Asn—Pro—Val—Val—His—Phe—Phe—Lys—Asn—Ile—Val—Thr—
_____90
80                                                   Methyl
                                                       |
Pro—Arg—Thr—Pro—Pro—Pro—Ser—Gln—Gly—Lys—Gly—Arg—Gly—Leu—Ser—Leu—
              100                                                110
                                             Arg
Ser—Arg—Phe—Ser—Trp—Gly—Ala—Glu—Gly—Gln—Lys—Pro—Gly—Phe—Gly—Tyr—
         _____
                      120
                                                   Phe
Gly—Gly—Arg—Ala—Ser—Asp—Tyr—Lys— Ser—Ala—His—Lys—Gly—Leu—Lys—Gly—
         130                      _____
                                                   140
Val
His—Asp—Ala—Gln—Gly—Thr—Leu—Ser—Lys—Ile—Phe—Lys—Leu—Gly—Gly—Arg—
_____
                      150
Asp—Ser—Arg—Ser—Gly—Ser—Pro—Met— Ala—Arg—Arg—COOH
_____
160                                      170
```

Fig. 32-1. Amino acid sequence of basic protein of bovine myelin. Substitutions in human basic protein are shown above the appropriate position of the bovine sequence. Between positions 10 and 11, a His-Gly dipeptide occurs in the human protein. (From S. W. Brostoff, in P. Morell (ed.), Myelin. *New York: Plenum, 1977.)*

in Fig. 32-1) has been isolated and shown to produce EAE in guinea pigs. A study using chemically synthesized peptides demonstrated that the minimal sequence requirement for this peptide to induce EAE was Trp-...-...-...-...-Gln-Lys (Arg); various amino acid substitutions for the amino acids between tryptophan and glutamine do not eliminate encephalitogenic activity. Peptides containing this sequence induce EAE in rabbits and guinea pigs but are inactive in monkeys. Another peptide (44–89 in Fig. 32-1) is active in rabbits but inactive in guinea pigs, and has been studied and sequenced. Still a third EAE-inducing peptide, active in monkeys but not in rabbits and guinea pigs, also has been characterized (153–166 in Fig. 32-1). The interest in the chemistry of this protein is closely related to the possibility of developing modified amino acid sequences that might suppress the immune reaction [21].

The obligate participation of the immune system in the disease process of EAE [see 18 and 19 for review] was shown by demonstrating passive transfer of the disease by the use either of viable lymph node cells or circulating cells obtained directly from the peripheral blood of various animals during the deelopment of EAE. The immune system of mammals involves both B cells, which produce humoral antibodies, and T cells, which are responsible for cell-mediated responses. The disease process in EAE is primarily T cell mediated, and in fact, the disease can be induced in normal animals by injection of circulating blood leukocytes from animals with EAE. There is also evidence showing that B cells play a part in EAE, and the participation of circulating antibody must be considered. One test for circulating factors in EAE has been the use of organotypic cultures of CNS tissue. For this, fragments of rat cerebellum are cultured in vitro in such a way that the various cellular elements interact to form myelin [23, 24].

The presence of factors that interfere with myelination can be determined directly by microscopic comparison with control cultures. Serum or lymphocytes obtained from animals immunized with whole CNS tissue or myelin cause demyelination or a block in myelin synthesis, as does serum from MS patients. Demyelination takes place consistently only if the experimental serum is derived from animals immunized against whole CNS tissue or myelin. Serum from animals immunized against purified basic protein, although containing antibodies against basic protein, often does not cause demyelination. In fact, it appears that the demyelination is in part due to antibodies against cerebroside, although other factors are also involved [25]. The block in myelin synthesis is dependent on complement; cultures treated with decomplemented serum continue to make myelin, but it is produced in a disorganized array, rather than in organized lamellae around axons in a normal pattern [26].

As implied by the above discussion, the term *EAE* really describes a class of experimental disorders. The clinical course, the histopathology, and the details of the immune mechanisms involved may vary greatly, depending on the conditions used to induce the disease process [15]. There is great species variability; the disease is usually terminal

in monkeys (and lesions similar to those in human MS cases are found), whereas rats (with less severe lesions) generally recover. There is even considerable strain difference; Lewis rats show a more severe form of the disease than do Wistar rats. It is of importance to note that a chronic form of EAE can be induced that occasionally follows a fluctuating clinical course, thus approaching the relapsing course of MS in humans [16, 17].

No change in the amount of myelin recovered from EAE rats has been observed. Indeed, by histological criteria, only a small amount of the total myelin is involved. There is no marked difference in the composition of CNS myelin between EAE animals and controls.

Proteolytic enzymes have been implicated in the hydrolysis of myelin basic proteins during EAE [27]. The levels of acid proteinase, neutral proteinase, and cathepsin A are increased in the vicinity of lesions in monkeys with EAE. It is likely that some of these enzymes are released from mononuclear cells, including lymphocytes.

Although only a relatively small amount of myelin is involved in EAE, there appear to be some marked changes in CNS metabolism as measured in vitro in spinal-cord slices. Slices from EAE animals show depressed incorporation of radioactive precursors into lipids and increased protein synthesis, relative to slices from control animals [28]. Part of the increased rate of protein synthesis is due to the metabolism of invading mononuclear cells, and part represents increased synthesis of myelin proteins.

Multiple Sclerosis
Extensive biochemical investigations have been carried out on autopsy material from MS brains. In MS, the loss of myelin is more severe than in EAE. White matter in MS shows a decreased yield of myelin, the expected decrease of myelin-specific components, and a buildup of cholesterol esters. Careful studies report no significant compositional differences between myelin from control brains and that from normal-appearing areas of MS brains [29]. This makes it unlikely that the etiology of MS is an underlying defect in myelin composition. The

likelihood that myelin in the periphery of active plaques is abnormal has been reported [30]; the decreased basic protein content of such myelin is relevant to the hypothesis that this is the myelin component most susceptible to damage. The presence in the CSF of material immunologically characterized as myelin basic protein, or a peptide derived from it, correlates with the exacerbation of MS symptoms [31, 32]. Various histochemical and biochemical techniques have been used to demonstrate that the periphery of active plaques is greatly enriched in acid-proteinase activity and that the enzyme levels correlate with the loss of basic protein in these microscopic regions [20].

An interesting observation has been made on the possible role of phagocytes in the breakdown of myelin during EAE and MS. It has been demonstrated that neutral proteases released by stimulated macrophages may serve as a plasminogen activator in vitro [33]. The released plasmin rapidly degrades the basic protein of myelin. This suggests that such an "amplification system" may be involved in various inflammatory demyelinating disorders.

ETIOLOGICAL FACTORS IN MULTIPLE SCLEROSIS

It is now well established that both humorally mediated and cell-mediated factors are involved in producing the observed demyelination in EAE [18, 24]. Evidence is incomplete regarding the role of the immune system in the pathogenesis of MS. Some of the positive evidence is discussed here. MS patients have a significantly elevated level of a particular immunoglobulin, IgG, in the CSF. Furthermore, this IgG often separates into discrete bands on agarose gel electrophoresis (oligoclonal IgG bands) [34]; the immunological implications of this pattern are not clearly understood. There is evidence that some IgG is specifically localized in the region of MS plaques and that IgM, another immunoglobulin, is elevated in the CSF of many MS patients [35]. Increased levels of antibodies to myelin basic protein have also been found in patients with MS [36]. These data suggest involve-

ment of humoral factors, as do results from tissue culture.

There is also evidence suggesting cell-mediated abnormalities. Lymphocytes from MS patients may show hypersensitivity to CNS antigen. It is known that lymphocytes isolated from guinea pigs with EAE produce a soluble factor that inhibits migration of macrophages taken from normal animals. This *migration inhibition factor* (MIF) is assayed by comparing the various rates of migration of macrophages out of a capillary tube into a medium containing cell-free supernatant obtained from the subject's lymphocytes cultured in the presence or absence of myelin basic protein. In a significant number of cases, lymphocytes from patients with MS produce MIF; the lymphocytes from control patients do not [37, 38]. There also appears to be suppression of cellular immunity in MS patients; they have a specific lack of cellular recognition for measles antigen [see 7 and 8]. Recent work has shown that, unlike lymphocytes from normal adults, when lymphocytes from MS patients are exposed to inactivated measles virus, they fail to exert significant suppression of mitogenic (concanavalin A) responses of cryopreserved autochthonous cells. Lymphocytes from MS patients also failed to produce significant amounts of interferons in response to measles challenges in vitro [39]. Despite the positive data presented above and that from other studies, there is still "a paucity of evidence that cell-mediated immune responses directed against neuroantigens have a pathogenic role in MS" [40].

Another immunological result pertinent to a possible slow-virus etiology for MS, is a specific increase in CSF antibodies against measles antigen in MS patients. The abnormal response to measles antigens by soluble and cell-mediated components of the immunological system of MS patients suggests the involvement of measles or a related virus in the initiation of the disease process. Epidemiological studies of the geographical distribution of MS, together with population migration studies, demonstrate that residence in a "high risk" region during the first 15 to 20 years of life sets the pattern for susceptibility to MS, regardless of later geographical relocation [41]. This pattern suggests the involvement of a slow-virus infection. However, despite a great amount of research [see references cited in 42 and 43], an infectious agent specific to MS has not been identified. Presently available evidence contains many inconsistencies; alternate explanations are possible [44]. Claims from several laboratories of finding MS-associated antigens in autopsy material have been challenged vigorously [45].

Studies of genetic factors involved in pathogenesis of MS are based on measurements of the frequency of histocompatibility antigens in populations of MS patients. The HL-A (human leukocyte antigen) system, which determines certain cell-surface immunological specificities, is the major identifiable histocompatibility site in humans. A number of different alleles are present at each of the four regions of the gene in this system. An individual heterozygote at each of the four subloci would express up to eight major HL-A specificities (four maternal and four paternal). Different antigens can be distinguished on the basis of cytotoxicity tests involving interactions with certain standard antisera (prepared from patients who have undergone an immune challenge by virtue of multiple pregnancies, whole-blood transfusion, organ-graft rejection, etc.). The HL-A D series may be identical to a series of immune response–associated antigens expressed on the surface of B lymphocytes. Because the identity is not proved, the nomenclature for the immune response-associated antigen series is HL-A DRw (D-related workshop). The suffix was added by the World Health Organization committee on nomenclature to distinguish Ia-like antigens.

Several studies have shown that, in northern European and North American Caucasian populations, multiple sclerosis is associated with HL-A B7, HL-A Dw2, and HL-A DRw2 [46]. The last two may be the same antigen but are detected by different methods. This association does not hold for all ethnic groups; a population of patients in Florence, Italy, showed an association with HL-A DRw4. The immunogenetic studies demonstrate "weak" relationships (i.e., although they are highly significant statistically, they are not cause-and-

effect relationships, as the control populations also carried a significant percentage of these genes).

The operational hypothesis derived from the above data is that the possession of a certain genotype increases susceptibility to MS. We can only speculate about the molecular basis of the correlation of HL-A antigen distribution with increased susceptibility to MS. Possible explanations are (a) certain HL-A antigens may function more efficiently than others as receptors for a virus that triggers an autoimmune reaction; (b) some HL-A antigens may have a structure that induces immunological tolerance to such a virus; or (c) the HL-A antigen may not be involved at all, but may be genetically linked, and in linkage disequilibrium, with an immunoresponsive gene that plays a part in MS. These investigations may provide a basis for explaining various reports that indicate a weak trend toward familial aggregation of MS.

Demyelination produces impairment of conduction [47, 48]. The relationship of myelin to conduction is described in Chap. 4. However, as is there discussed, the destruction of myelin in a particular disease does not imply that this is the initial lesion or the only cause of malfunction of the nervous system. The CNS tissue culture system offers a model for correlating demyelination with other pathological events. Neurons in the cultured fragments form synaptic interrelationships and develop complex polysynaptic functions that often disappear within a few minutes after the application of EAE or MS serum, whereas axon spikes can still be evoked [23, 24]. The complex polysynaptic functions may return within minutes after removal of the offending serum. Although normal sera may also block the electrical responses of CNS in vitro, special assay conditions [24] or a frog-derived test system [49] may be used to demonstrate differences between normal and EAE or MS sera. The rapid onset of electrical disturbances and the rapid return to the normal state after the offending serum is removed imply that this functional disturbance is independent of the demyelinating response.

Because of the possible implications for treatment of MS, much effort has been devoted to developing methods for suppression of EAE. Various immunosuppressive agents are effective in such treatment, but their action is limited in time, and they may have toxic side effects. In principle, the most effective approach is to counteract the sensitized lymphocytes in situ. This can be done by giving inoculations of the encephalitogen itself [18–21] in either a native or a modified form, and often with incomplete Freund's adjuvant. The mechanism by which the excess of antigen protects the nervous system is not known. There is evidence that pretreatment with basic protein generates suppressor cells that prevent the subsequent development of EAE [50]. It is thought [51] that suppressor cells may influence the course of multiple sclerosis in humans. Clinical trials involving injection of myelin basic protein into MS patients have not been successful, however [52].

OTHER ACQUIRED INFLAMMATORY DEMYELINATING DISORDERS

Experimental allergic neuritis (EAN) is the PNS counterpart of EAE and the experimental analog of the Landry-Guillain-Barré syndrome in humans. EAN is induced by injection of whole peripheral nerve tissue emulsified in an adjuvant. There is evidence that the P2 protein, a protein of PNS myelin that is not present in CNS myelin, is a component of the primary antigenic stimulus [53]. There have been few neurochemical studies of the Landry-Guillain-Barré syndrome; with proper treatment, there usually is almost complete recovery. With regard to PNS disorders, it should be kept in mind that CNS and PNS myelin, although morphologically related, differ significantly in chemical composition, especially in protein composition (see Chap. 4).

Extensive neurochemical studies of the experimentally induced animal virus diseases, targeted primarily against myelin, have not been carried out. Relevant virology and pathology have been reviewed [13, 33, 54].

Genetically Determined Metabolic Disorders of Myelin

A large group of myelin-related diseases consists of genetically determined degenerative disorders of CNS white matter; most of these have their onset in humans before the age of 10 years. The various members of this class of myelin disorders have been outlined [55–57]. These diseases are classified as *inborn errors of metabolism* (presumably due to a genetic insufficiency of a particular enzyme) because they are familial.

CLASSIFICATION OF GENETIC METABOLIC DISORDERS OF MYELIN

A morphological distinction can be made between diseases in which there is apparent accumulation of an abnormal storage product (e.g., metachromatic leukodystrophy) and genetically determined hypomyelinating disorders, in which there is an extreme paucity of myelin formation (e.g., Pelizaeus-Merzbacher disease). Meaningful distinctions within the group of metabolic disorders are possible by biochemical criteria.

The following are examples of genetic disorders of myelin in humans. The examples cited do not represent all the genetic diseases, and each example may well have several variants. It must be emphasized that the pathology observed in the human disorders describes the end results of the disease process.

1. *Metachromatic leukodystrophy (MLD)* is a disorder (Chap. 30) characterized by loss of myelin and the presence of spherical granular masses within oligodendroglial cells, neurons, and macrophages, as well as free in the white matter. These granules and inclusions are metachromatic. In contrast to most leukodystrophies, there is striking involvement of the PNS. An adult variant of this disorder exists.

2. *Krabbe's (globoid) leukodystrophy* shows normal white matter that is deficient owing to widespread diffuse demyelination (Chap. 30). There is astrocytic gliosis and, most striking, characteristic abnormal mononuclear or multinuclear globoid cells scattered in white matter. In some cases, these cells may constitute up to one-half of the total white matter.

3. *Adrenoleukodystrophy (sex-linked Schilder's disease)*, a disease usually of young males, differs from other leukodystrophies by the presence of inflammatory changes in the CNS lesions. Involvement of the adrenals is obligatory. The

morphological picture suggests a lipid-storage disorder [58].

4. *Refsum's disease,* a PNS-myelin disorder, is characterized by swelling of the peripheral nerves, thinning of the myelin sheath, and myelin degradation. CNS lesions are also present (Chap. 30).

5. *Pelizaeus-Merzbacher disease (subanophilic leukodystrophy)* is an early appearing, slowly progressive CNS-degenerative condition resulting in a lack of proper myelination (hypomyelination) [59].

6. *Alexander's disease* is usually apparent in the first year of life, and pursues a variable course thereafter [60].

7. *Canavan's disease (spongy degeneration of the white matter)* is a disease of infants resulting in widespread edema of white matter [57]. Myelin is diminished in certain brain areas, but without the accumulation of sudanophilic myelin products that is characteristic of many metabolic disorders of myelin.

8. *Nonspecific hypomyelination* is a term encompassing a wide variety of chronic metabolic insults, which if present at a particular early developmental stage (the first few years of life), may result in a decrease in the amount of myelin deposited. This grouping is based primarily on chemical data, since quantitation of myelin deficits is difficult by morphological techniques. Histological and ultrastructural data indicate, however, a thinner myelin sheath in certain of these disorders. Genetically determined causes of hypomyelination include disorders of amino acid metabolism (phenylketonuria), familial hypothyroidism, and disorders involving copper metabolism (trichopoliodystrophy).

Genetic disorders involving myelin have been studied in animals, notably several murine mutants:

1. *Myelin defects.* Among the genetically determined hypomyelinating disorders in mice are those exhibited by the quaking mouse and the jimpy mouse [61], which show deficiencies in myelin production. Ultrastructurally, adult quaking animals show an impediment of myelination, thin myelin sheaths, lack of myelin compaction with pockets of oligodendroglial-cell cytoplasm evident, and uneven growth of lateral loops, all of which are typical of the immature (5–10-day-old) mouse. Jimpy mice show severe hypomyelination with sudanophilic deposits. Murine muscular dystrophy is characterized by regional deficiencies in myelin in the PNS.

2. *Globoid leukodystrophy.* Several breeds of dogs and cats are known to carry genetic factors for a disease analogous to human Krabbe's disease [62].

CRITERIA FOR GENETIC METABOLIC DISEASES OF MYELIN
The following criteria are generally characteristic of this group of disorders:

1. Loss of myelin from areas of white matter
2. Concomitant loss of axons
3. Preservation of axotomized neurons
4. Diffuse and symmetrical lesions
5. Lack of inflammatory changes (except adrenoleukodystrophy). Macrophages, however, are present, except in the hypomyelinating disorders

BIOCHEMICAL STUDIES OF GENETIC DISORDERS OF MYELIN
Generally, the demyelination resulting from genetic disorders is often accompanied by abnormal composition of white matter, increase in water, decrease in myelin constituents, and the presence of cholesterol esters. Compositional studies of brain, especially of isolated abnormal myelin from autopsy material, have proved a powerful tool in the study of genetic disorders relating to the myelin sheath. On the basis of such work, we feel justified in subclassifying these disorders largely on the basis of chemical criteria. Chemical analysis indicates that pathological myelin can be divided into two categories, specific and nonspecific [1, 2]. The *specific* category is characterized by an abnormal myelin that contains an accumulation of a particular compound due to a primary genetic lesion that prevents its catabolism. Disorders in the *nonspecific*

Table 32-2. Human Myelin Composition in Three Diseases Compared with Controls[a]

Lipids[b]	Control	Spongy Degeneration	SSPE	MLD
Total lipid, percent of dry weight	70.0	63.8	73.7	63.2
Cholesterol	27.7	58.0	43.7	21.2
Cerebrosides	22.7	8.0	18.8	9.0
Sulfatides	3.8	2.0	2.8	28.4
Total phospholipids	43.1	33.4	36.6	36.1
Ethanolamine phosphatides	15.6	9.8	9.7	8.1
Plasmalogen[c]	12.3		9.1	5.3
Lecithin	11.2	11.3	10.4	10.7
Sphingomyelin	7.9	5.9	8.8	7.1
Serine phosphatides	4.8	5.5	4.6	3.8
Phosphatidylinositol	0.6	0.8	1.4	3.1

[a]The values listed are from the laboratory of W. Norton except for the spongy degeneration data [63].
[b]Individual lipids expressed as weight percentage of total lipid.
[c]Most of the plasmalogen is phosphatidal ethanolamine and is also included in the ethanolamine phosphatides column.

category are characterized by the presence of myelin in which the compositional abnormality is not directly related to the genetic lesion. A third category of genetic disorders, established on the basis of both chemical and morphological observation, is *hypomyelination,* an impediment in normal myelinogenesis.

Diseases in which myelin shows a specific chemical pathology can also be correctly referred to as *dysmyelinating* in accordance with the definition of Poser [55], which states that this category would include those inborn errors of metabolism in which "myelin initially formed is abnormally constituted, thus inherently unstable, vulnerable, and liable to degeneration." The student should be warned that the term *dysmyelinating disorder* is often used rather loosely. According to the original definition, the term has primarily a chemical basis, and the common use of dysmyelination to describe morphological observations has no precise meaning.

Specific Abnormalities
Metachromatic leukodystrophy (MLD) is a sphingolipidosis characterized at the molecular level by inability to catabolize sulfatide (Chap. 30). Mor-

phological observations are consistent with the hypothesis that a certain amount of myelin (normal by morphological criteria, but presumably abnormal chemically) is formed initially. With time, however, the sulfatide which would normally be catabolized (albeit at a very slow rate) continues to accumulate in myelin (Table 32-2) and oligodendroglial cells as its synthesis proceeds. One theory is that the molecular architecture of the myelin is disturbed to such a point that it becomes unstable and breaks down. Sulfatide also accumulates in the oligodendroglial cells and macrophages and presumably gives rise to the metachromatic bodies characteristic of this disorder.

In *Refsum's disease,* a genetic disorder clearly classified as dysmyelinating, the ability to degrade branched-chain fatty acids by oxidation is lacking (Chap. 30). Although the defective enzyme is not essential for degradation of normal fatty acids, it is necessary for degradation of phytanic acid (3,7,11,14-tetramethylhexadecanoic acid). Phytanic acid has been found to accumulate in myelin phospholipids as it does in other tissues of the body. The effects are more serious in the PNS than in the CNS, perhaps because some of this fatty acid is excluded by the blood-brain barrier. The possibility cannot be eliminated that some dysmyelinating disorders have not been classified as such because current analytical methods are not sensitive enough to detect the myelin abnormality.

Globoid-cell leukodystrophy is also a sphingolipidosis, characterized at a genetic level by a β-galactosidase deficit and the consequent inability to catabolize cerebroside (Chap. 30). Curiously, excess amounts of cerebroside are not found upon whole-brain analysis. The ratio of cerebroside to sulfatide is abnormally high, however, indicating a disproportionate preservation of cerebroside, rather than lack of sulfatide. The excess cerebroside accumulates in a specific storage cell, the globoid cell. Poser [55] considered this to be a dysmyelinating disease, and one would expect that the myelin would contain abnormal accumulations of cerebroside (analogous with the findings in MLD; see above). However, this is not the case; the very small amounts of myelin that can be isolated from brains of such patients is normal. The reason for this is not clear, but it is believed that the myelin present is formed during early myelination, before the enzyme deficiency is fully manifested. It has been postulated that the accumulation of cerebroside then elicits the globoid-body response, followed by death of oligodendroglia and little further production of myelin, normal or otherwise. Thus, this disease might better be classified as a hypomyelinating disease.

In the three disorders discussed above, the primary genetic lesion is known. The enzyme deficit is expressed in all cells, so it is possible to utilize fibroblasts or circulating blood elements for diagnosis, detection of heterozygotes, and related studies. Floating cells of fetal origin can be obtained early in pregnancy by amniocentesis and cultured for prenatal diagnosis.

Nonspecific Abnormalities

The genetic disorders characterized by the accumulation of "nonspecific" pathological myelin include *adrenoleukodystrophy* [1, 58], *Canavan's disease* or *spongy degeneration* [63] (Table 32-2), and probably, a number of disorders in which the my-

elin has not yet been analyzed. The primary genetic lesion is not known in these diseases. It is important to note that myelin isolated from these two disorders and myelin isolated from patients with a wide variety of disorders involving secondary demyelination have similar "abnormal" chemical compositions. Certain experimental disorders induced in animals by toxic agents show the same type of abnormality with respect to isolated myelin. In each case, the isolated pathological myelin has a grossly normal ultrastructural appearance. However, it has much more cholesterol, less cerebroside, and less phosphatidal ethanolamine than does normal human myelin. When a considerable accumulation of cholesterol esters is found in whole brain, such compounds are not in the myelin itself. The purification of myelin involves discontinuous sucrose gradients; and a light fraction, containing cholesterol esters, is separated from the denser myelin. The abnormal myelin probably represents a partially degraded form. It is possible that the degradation involves locally derived macrophages.

Hypomyelination

A third category of genetic disorders, hypomyelination, includes the very rare *Pelizaeus-Merzbacher disease* of humans, characterized ultrastructurally by failure of mature myelin to accumulate [59]. It bears some structural resemblances to the disorder of the quaking mouse. Certain disorders of amino acid metabolism result in diminished levels of myelin. Globoid-cell leukodystrophy can also be considered to be in the category of hypomyelinating disorders. In these disorders, there is a great diminution in amounts of myelin constituents, often without the presence of phagocytic cells.

A number of animal models of such disorders are available, most notably the murine mutants [61]. Although oligodendroglial cells appear relatively normal in the adult quaking mouse, myelinated axons have only a few lamellae of myelin. The ultrastructural picture, as well as the composition of isolated myelin, of adult quaking mouse is characteristic of the developing 7- to 10-day-old CNA of normal mice. Enzymatic activity for cerebroside formation (UDP-galactose-ceramide galactosyltransferase) is more than 60 percent depressed in the mutants as compared with control littermates at various points, but the regulatory enzymes that are involved in biosynthesis of sphingolipids in gray matter are completely normal. Two other murine mutants (jimpy and MD), characterized histologically by pathologically low levels of myelin, are defective in enzymatic activity for the biosynthesis of myelin-specific lipids.

Although these observations are certainly relevant to an understanding of the pathology involved, there is no reason to believe that any of the enzymatic deficits are primary. The murine mutants are powerful tools for elucidating details of myelin assembly by contrasting these genetically perturbed animals with controls in various metabolic experiments. A variety of other interesting animal models exist for study of hypomyelinating disorders [61]. *Border disease* (hypomyelinogenesis congenita) of sheep is of interest because, although the amount of myelin in the CNS is decreased, in vitro assay indicates an increased role of cerebroside synthesis. This is an acquired congenital disorder, which can be induced experimentally by inoculating pregnant ewes with a suspension of brain from affected lambs. It is mentioned in this section because, with regard to cerebroside synthesis, it contrasts with the genetic hypomyelinating disorder of mice.

Certain disorders of amino acid metabolism cause some hypomyelination. *Phenylketonuria* (see Chap. 28) is quantitatively the most significant condition. On histological examination, the amount of myelin in brains of patients suffering from phenylketonuria appears abnormally low, and the white matter may be up to 40 percent deficient (as compared to controls) in such myelin-specific components as proteolipid protein and cerebroside [2, 64, 65]. One possible explanation of the myelin deficit is that the high phenylalanine levels depress uptake into brain of tyrosine, or another large neutral amino acid, by competing for a common active transport system. Because of the lack of this essential amino acid, protein synthesis is severely depressed, and myelin, which is usually synthesized rapidly early in life, is not formed. It

has also been suggested that the imbalance of amino acids may depress the initiation of protein synthesis (see Chap. 19) by causing competition at the level of aminoacylation of transfer RNA species [66]. Another explanation may be that the alternate pathways used for phenylalanine metabolism (present normally, but of quantitative significance only in this disease state) cause significant accumulation of phenylpyruvic acid and other metabolites that may be toxic. In any case, protein synthesis is depressed during the period of maximal myelin accumulation. The literature suggests, based on work with model systems, that redressing the amino acid imbalance by supplementation with a mix of large neutral amino acids may have therapeutic potential [see 65 for review]. A further complication exists: at autopsy, untreated cases show significant demyelination. This has led to suggestions that phenylketonuria is a dysmyelinating disorder, but (as in MS) consistent evidence of significant abnormalities in myelin from such patients remains to be demonstrated. Finally, it should be emphasized that phenylketonuria is not only a disorder of myelin; levels of tyrosine and tryptophan, amino acids which are neurotransmitter precursors, presumably are perturbed in such patients.

The model system of *experimental hyperphenylalaninemia* (induced by injecting animals with large doses of phenylalanine) is characterized by a deficit in myelin accumulation and a decreased ability, both in vitro and in vivo, to incorporate radioactive precursors into cerebral lipids and proteins [see 2, 28, 65 for review]. This model is not identical with phenylketonuria, because, as phenylalanine hydroxylase is present at normal levels, both phenylalanine and tyrosine levels are elevated.

A related model for phenylketonuria [2, 28, 65] is obtained by injections of parachlorophenylalanine, which inhibits phenylalanine hydroxylase and causes a rise in blood phenylalanine levels. More important, tyrosine levels are not significantly elevated, thus approximating the human disorder more closely. Again, there is both a deficit in myelin accumulation and a decreased uptake of radioactive precursors into brain lipids and proteins. The incorporation into myelin proteolipid protein is depressed more severely than is incorporation into nonmyelin proteins. This inhibition may not be the result of the phenylalanine itself but of the abnormal deaminated metabolites that accumulate.

Toxic and Nutritional Disorders of Myelin

TOXIC DISORDERS

Certain toxic agents to which humans have been accidentally exposed are known to result in primary demyelination. Ultrastructural observations vary with the toxic agents [see 57 for examples].

In humans, diphtheritic neuropathy is a possible complication of *Corynebacterium diphtheriae* infection. Paralysis, often following a terminal course, is induced by bacterial exotoxin. Swelling and vacuolation is followed by fragmentation of myelin sheaths in the peripheral nervous system, leading to segmental demyelination. A similar disorder can be induced in animals by injection of the toxin.

Hexachlorophene is a recent addition to the list of myelinotoxic compounds. Overexposure of infants in hospital nurseries to hexachlorophene causes a spongy change in myelinated areas in both CNS and PNS [57]. In experimental animal studies, as well, these neurotoxins cause a spongy degeneration of myelin and an edema similar to that seen in the metabolic disorder of Canavan's disease [28].

Carbon monoxide poisoning that leads to postanoxic encephalopathy sometimes also leads to massive destruction of myelin with relative sparing of axons [57].

The list of toxic agents known to cause neurological damage in humans or animals is extensive, and a number of animal model systems have been developed so that the extent of myelin involvement in particular disorders may be assessed by biochemical methods [28].

A number of chemical studies have been done on the *triethyltin model,* brought about by the inclusion of this compound in the drinking water of rats. Acute intoxication involves severe myelin edema, specifically in the CNS, where myelin sheaths become highly vacuolated. The splitting in

the myelin is associated with the intraperiod line. Chronic administration of triethyltin may result in a loss of one-fourth to one-half of the total myelin, relative to untreated control animals [28, 66]. The myelin isolated is of the nonspecific pathological type. This massive myelin loss is not accompanied by inflammatory cells, and the levels of various proteinases are not elevated as they are in such disorders of EAE. There is also no buildup of sudanophilic deposits of degraded myelin. The mechanism by which myelin is damaged under these conditions is unknown, but it clearly contrasts with the situation observed in the acquired demyelinating disorders. Interestingly, there may be almost complete recovery of myelin after triethyltin is removed from drinking water. In vitro metabolic studies demonstrated a greatly increased incorporation of leucine into myelin proteins during chronic administration of triethyltin [28]. Incorporation of acetate into lipid was depressed initially; later in the course of the disease it was somewhat elevated. The goal of the increasing number of metabolic experiments of this type is to elucidate the mechanism of myelin destruction and, perhaps even more important, to study the degree of recovery possible and the mechanism involved. For example, might the increased myelin synthesis associated with triethyltin intoxication be, in part, compensation for degradation of myelin?

In neurochemical studies of this type, *loss of myelin* is an operational term; that is, myelin is not recovered by the standard isolation procedures. The myelin need not be degraded to molecular constituents; it may only be broken down to vesicles too small (or too different in density) to be isolated with normal myelin. Indeed, when animals are treated with triethyltin [67] or with hexachlorophene [68, 69], a "floating fraction," somewhat lighter than normal myelin, but containing many myelin constituents, can be recovered.

Lead encephalopathy, an acquired toxic disorder leading to hypomyelination, has been studied in detail. The disorder can be induced in developing rats by adding lead carbonate to the diet of nursing mothers or by intubation of a lead acetate solution to the pups. The hypomyelination observed appears to be related primarily to retarded growth and maturation of the neuron [70]. Axons are reduced in size, but the previously established relationship between axon size and number of myelin lamellae in particular regions is the same in experimental and control animals. Chemical studies indicate that the number of glial cells is not affected, nor is the myelin composition. These results are in contrast to the starvation model, in which glial-cell proliferation is decreased and myelinogenesis retarded.

Certain drugs, although not normally a risk factor for human populations, have been used to perturb myelin synthesis in an attempt to understand normal myelin metabolism. Many inhibitors of cholesterol synthesis have been studied pharmacologically as being of potential utility in treatment of arteriosclerosis. Cholesterol is a major component of myelin, and application of inhibitory drugs during the time of myelin deposition may have relatively specific effects on myelin [28]. The drug AY9944, an inhibitor of Δ7-reductase, causes 7-dehydrocholesterol to accumulate in myelin, taking the place of normal cholesterol. Not only is the isolated myelin abnormal; its yield is also greatly reduced; this implies that a deficiency of a particular lipid will limit the assembly of myelin. In vitro experiments show a decreased uptake of radioactive glucose into myelin lipids and proteins.

NUTRITIONAL DISORDERS

As was discussed in Chaps. 4 and 23, much of the CNS myelin in mammals is formed during a relatively restricted time period, corresponding to the first few years of life in humans and days 15 to 30 in rats. Just before this rapid deposition of myelin, there is a burst of oligodendroglial cell proliferation. During these restricted periods of time, a major part of the metabolic activity of brain and, even more important, possibly most of the brain's protein and lipid synthetic capacity are involved in myelinogenesis. This developmental phenomenon has practical input for the understanding of hypomyelinations. Any metabolic insult during this "vulnerable period" may lead to a preferential reduction in myelin formation (Chap. 23). A model system for such studies is obtained by restricting access of rat pups to the mother and thus inducing undernourishment. Starvation of rats from birth onward leads to a deficit in myelin lipids and a reduced amount of isolatable myelin compared with normally fed littermate controls. The size of whole brain is also somewhat reduced, but it is clear that the depression of myelin-specific lipids and proteins is greater than that of other brain components [see 27 for review]. The implication is that, during starvation, there is preferential depression in synthesis of myelin-specific components. This has been directly demonstrated by the use of in vivo isotope experiments [71]. Possibly there is not only depression in the amount of myelin deposited (in part due to a lessened number of oligodendroglial cells), but also the developmental program with regard to myelinogenesis is somewhat delayed.

An experimental dietary copper-deficiency model has been used with developing animals. A highly significant decrease in myelinogenesis is observed [72], possibly secondary to the generalized metabolic insult caused by decreased activity of the copper-requiring cytochrome oxidase. This system may be an experimental analog of the sex-linked disorder called trichopoliodystrophy (Menkes' kinky hair disease), in which there appears to be a disorder of copper metabolism.

Disorders with Secondary Involvement of Myelin

A large number of disorders of the human nervous system that preferentially cause lesions in gray matter, in particular neurons, and that are associated with "accidental" brain damage (infarcts, trauma, tumors, etc.) eventually result in regions of demyelination. Such diseases can be of viral (e.g., subacute sclerosing panencephalitis), genetic (Tay-Sachs disease), or of unknown etiology (amyotrophic lateral sclerosis).

SUBACUTE SCLEROSING PANENCEPHALITIS

The first human disease to be studied with respect to myelin composition during secondary demyelination was *subacute sclerosing panencephalitis* (SSPE), a CNS disease caused by a defective measles-virus infection [see 1 and 2 for review]. It is probable that this disease involves destruction of both neurons and oligodendroglia. The brain white matter shows the typical changes for severe demyelination. The isolated myelin has a grossly normal ultrastructural appearance and a normal lipid-protein ratio. However, it was found to have much more cholesterol, less cerebroside, and less ethanolamine phosphatides than normal human myelin (Table 32-1). No cholesterol esters were found in the myelin, although they were abundant in the white matter. Such abnormal myelin has also been isolated from such sphingolipidoses as Tay-Sachs disease, generalized gangliosidosis, and Niemann-Pick disease (see Chap. 30).

WALLERIAN DEGENERATION

The archetypical model for secondary demyelination is *Wallerian degeneration* [for review of relevant biochemistry see 2 and 27]. When a nerve (in the PNS) or a myelinated tract (in the CNS) is sectioned surgically, the proximal segment not infrequently survives and regenerates. In the distal segment, Wallerian degeneration occurs, and both axons and myelin degenerate rapidly. Debris is phagocytosed by the myelinating cell and by macrophages. Eventually, the denervated region is replaced by scar tissue. From such experiments, it is clear that the integrity of the myelin sheath depends on continued contact with a viable axon. The nature of this interrelationship is not known. Any disease that results in a general impairment of neuronal function also will result in axonal degeneration and cause onset of myelin breakdown secondary to the neuronal damage. Most biochemical studies on Wallerian degeneration have been done on whole sciatic nerve, because isolation of myelin from PNS tissue is difficult. There is a rapid loss of myelin-specific lipids within a period of a week or two. Loss of myelin-specific proteins proceeds even more rapidly, and the disappearance of the major PNS myelin protein may precede slightly the loss of the slower-moving basic protein [73]. There is also a concomitant increase in many lysosomal enzymes.

Paradoxically, there is also an increase in certain enzymes implicated in myelinogenesis; for example, NADP$^+$-dependent isocitrate dehydrogenase in-

creases greatly during Wallerian degeneration. This may be related to the Schwann cell proliferation that takes place as these cells phagocytose the myelin they originally synthesized. Cholesterol esters accumulate and cholesterol esterase activity decreases during the degenerative phase that follows the lesion [74]. It is not clear whether the decrease in cholesterol esterase activity reflects decreased synthesis of myelin (developmentally, this enzyme is implicated in myelinogenesis in the CNS), or whether the decrease reflects only the loss of myelin, since a considerable portion of this enzyme (as studied in the CNS) may be localized in myelin [75].

As indicated earlier, analytical studies of the chemical composition of tissue during a disease process may be difficult to interpret because the analysis is indicative of the entire past history of the tissue with regard to total accumulation of any compound, no matter at what time point it is studied. Metabolic studies, in vitro, with incorporation of labeled precursors into the myelin isolated from degenerating rat sciatic nerve, make possible investigations in which various stages of tissue injury and consequent block in the synthesis of new myelin can be separated from a recovery stage, when new myelin sheath is being formed.

Wallerian degeneration has been studied in the CNS by enucleating eyes in rats and examining the optic nerve at different times [76]. The degeneration of CNS myelin is a much slower process than is PNS myelin degeneration and takes place within macrophages (not within the myelin-synthesizing cells, as in the PNS). By using this system, it has been demonstrated that the myelin isolated after enucleation, although present in decreasing amounts as degeneration progresses, does not differ significantly in composition from control myelin. It is not of the nonspecific pathological type encountered in other disease processes that lead to secondary demyelination. This may indicate a real difference in the degenerative processes during surgically induced Wallerian degeneration and the secondary demyelination that follows naturally occurring disease processes (also generally referred to as "Wallerian" degeneration by neuropathological criteria). Another explanation might be that, because of the morphological uniformity of the optic nerve, the existence of the degraded myelin (nonspecific pathological myelin) might be a transitory process and so might not have been detected.

Acknowledgments

During the course of writing this review, P. Morell was partially supported by USPHS grants HD-03110 and NS-11615; C. S. Raine by USPHS grant NS-08952; and M. B. Bornstein by USPHS grant NS-11920 and National Multiple Sclerosis Society grant 433. M. B. Bornstein is a Kennedy Scholar of the Rose F. Kennedy Center for Research in Mental Retardation and Human Development.

References

*1. Suzuki, K. Biochemistry of Myelin Disorders. In S. D. Waxman (ed.), *Physiology and Pathobiology of Axons.* New York: Raven, 1978. Pp. 337–348.

*2. Norton, W. T. Chemical Pathology of Diseases Involving Myelin. In P. Morell (ed.), *Myelin.* New York: Plenum, 1977. Pp. 383–407.

3. Suzuki, Y., Tucker, S. H., Rorke, L. B., and Suzuki, K. Ultrastructural and biochemical studies of Schilder's disease. II. Biochemistry. *J. Neuropathol. Exp. Neurol.* 29:405–419, 1970.

4. Svennerholm, L., Haltia, M., and Sourander, P. Chronic sclerosing panencephalitis. II. A neurochemical study. *Acta Neuropathol.* 14:292–303, 1970.

*5. Adams, R. D., and Sidman, R. L. *Introduction to Neuropathology.* New York: McGraw-Hill, 1968.

6. Adams, R. D., and Kubick, C. S. The morbid anatomy of the demyelinative diseases. *Am. J. Med.* 12:510–546, 1952.

*7. Raine, C. S. The etiology and pathogenesis of multiple sclerosis: Recent developments. *Pathobiol. Annu.* 7:347–384, 1977.

8. Johnson, R. T., and Weiner, L. P. The Role of Viral Infections in Demyelinating Diseases. In F. Wolfgram, G. W. Ellison, J. G. Stevens, and J. M. Andrews (eds.), *Multiple Sclerosis: Immunology, Virology and Ultrastructure.* New York: Academic, 1972. Pp. 245–264.

9. Richardson, E. P., Jr. Progressive Multifocal Leukoencephalopathy. In R. J. Vinken and G. W. Bruyn (eds.), *Handbook of Clinical Neurology: Multiple Sclerosis and Demyelinating Disorders.* Amsterdam: North-Holland, 1970. Vol. 9, pp. 485–499.

10. Asbury, A. K., Arnason, B. W. G., and Adams, R. D. The inflammatory lesion in idiopathic polyneuritis. *Medicine* 48:173–215, 1969.

11. *Animal Models of Human Disease.* Washington, D.C.: Armed Forces Institute of Pathology Registry of Comparative Pathology, 1972.

12. Cummings, J. F., and Haas, D. C. Coonhound paralysis: An acute idiopathic polyradiculoneuritis in dogs resembling the Landry-Guillain-Barré syndrome. *J. Neurol. Sci.* 4:51–81, 1967.

13. Weiner, L. P., and Stohlman, S. A. Viral models of demyelination. *Neurology* 28:111–114, 1978.

14. Dal Canto, M., and Lipton, H. Primary demyelination in Theiler's virus infection: An ultrastructural study. *Lab. Invest.* 33:626–637, 1975.

*15. Raine, C. S. Experimental allergic encephalomyelitis and related conditions. *Prog. Neuropathol.* 3:225–251, 1976.

16. Raine, C. S., and Stone, S. H. Animal model for multiple sclerosis: Chronic experimental allergic encephalomyelitis in inbred guinea pigs. *N.Y. State J. Med.* 77:1693–1696, 1977.

17. Raine, C. S., Snyder, D. H., Valsamis, M. P., and Stone, S. H. Chronic experimental allergic encephalomyelitis in inbred guinea pigs. *Lab. Invest.* 31:369–380, 1974.

*18. Brostoff, S. W. Immunological Responses to Myelin and Myelin Components. In P. Morell (ed.), *Myelin.* New York: Plenum, 1977. Pp. 415–440.

*19. Kies, M. W. Experimental Allergic Encephalomyelitis. In G. E. Gaull (ed.), *Biology of Brain Dysfunction.* New York: Plenum, 1973. Vol. 2, pp. 185–224.

*20. Rauch, H. C., and Einstein, E. R. Specific brain proteins: A biochemical and immunological review. *Rev. Neurosci.* 1:283–343, 1974.

21. Raine, C. S., Traugott, U., and Stone, S. H. Suppression of chronic allergic encephalomyelitis: Relevance to multiple sclerosis. *Science* 201:445–448, 1978.

22. Carnegie, P. R., and Dunkley, P. R. Basic proteins of central and peripheral nervous system myelin. *Adv. Neurochem.* 1:95–135, 1975.

*23. Bornstein, M. B. Immunopathology of demyelinating disorders examined in organotypic cultures of mammalian central nervous tissue. *Prog. Neuropathol.* 0:69–90, 1972.

*24. Bornstein, M. B. Immunobiology of Demyelination. In S. D. Waxman (ed.), *Physiology and Pathobiology of Axons.* New York: Raven, 1978. Pp. 313–336.

*Key reference.

25. Dorfman, S. H., Fry, J. M., Silberberg, D. H., Grose, C., and Manning, M. C. Cerebroside antibody titers in antisera capable of myelination inhibition and demyelination. *Brain Res.* 147: 410–415, 1978.

26. Diaz, M., Bornstein, M. B., and Raine, C. R. Disorganization of myelinogenesis in tissue culture by anti-CNS antiserum. *Brain Res.* 154:231–239, 1978.

*27. Smith, M. E. The role of proteolytic enzymes in demyelination in experimental allergic encephalomyelitis. *Neurochem. Res.* 2:233–246, 1977.

*28. Smith, M. E., and Benjamins, J. A. Model Systems for Study of Perturbations of Myelin Metabolism. In P. Morell (ed.), *Myelin.* New York: Plenum, 1977. Pp. 447–480.

29. Suzuki, K., Kamoshita, S., Eto, Y., Tourtellotte, W. W., and Gonatas, J. O. Myelin in multiple sclerosis: Composition of myelin from normal-appearing white matter. *Arch. Neurol.* 28:293–297, 1973.

30. Althaus, H. H., Pilz, H., and Muller, D. The protein composition of myelin in multiple sclerosis (MS) and orthochromatic leukodystrophy (OLD). *Z. Neurol.* 205:229–241, 1973.

31. Cohen, S. R., Herndon, R. M., McKhann, G. M. Radioimmunoassay of myelin basic protein in spinal fluid. *N. Engl. J. Med.* 295:1455–1457, 1976.

32. Whitaker, J. N. Myelin encephalitogenic protein fragments in cerebrospinal fluid of persons with multiple sclerosis. *Neurology* 27:911–920, 1977.

33. Cammer, W., Bloom, B. R., Norton, W. T., and Gordon, S. Degradation of basic protein in myelin by neutral proteinases secreted by stimulated macrophages. A possible mechanism of inflammatory demyelination. *Proc. Natl. Acad. Sci. U.S.A.* 75: 1554–1558, 1978.

*34. Johnson, K. P., and Nelson, B. J. Multiple sclerosis: Diagnostic usefulness of cerebrospinal fluid. *Ann. Neurol.* 2:425–431, 1972.

35. Williams, A. C., Mingioli, E. S., McFarland, H. F., Tourtellotte, W. W., and McFarlin, D. E. Increased CSF IgM in multiple sclerosis. *Neurology* 28:996–998, 1978.

36. Panitch, H. S., Hafler, D. A., and Johnson, K. P. Antibodies to myelin basic protein in multiple sclerosis: Clinical correlation. *Neurology* 28:394 (Abstract), 1978.

37. Colby, S. P., Sheremata, W., Bain, B., and Eylar, E. H. Cellular hypersensitivity in attacks of multiple sclerosis. *Neurology* 27:132–139, 1977.

38. Johnson, R. T. Current knowledge of multiple sclerosis. *South. Med. J.* 71:2–3, 1978.

39. Neighbour, P. A., and Bloom, B. R. Absence of virus-induced lymphocyte suppression and interferon production in multiple sclerosis. *Proc. Natl. Acad. Sci. U.S.A.* 76:476–480, 1979.

40. Paterson, P. Y. Multiple sclerosis: An immunologic reassessment. *J. Chronic Dis.* 26:119–126, 1973.

41. Kurtzke, J. G., and Kurland, L. T. Multiple Sclerosis in the Epidemiology of Neurologic Disease. In A. B. Baker, and L. H. Baker (eds.), *Clinical Neurology.* Hagerstown, Md.: Harper & Row, 1973. Vol. 3, pp. 22–30.

*42. Wolfgram, F., Ellison, G. W., Stevens, J. G., and Andrews, J. M. *Multiple Sclerosis: Immunology, Virology, and Ultrastructure.* New York: Academic, 1972.

*43. Palo, J. *Myelination and Demyelination.* New York: Plenum, 1978.

44. Nathanson, N., and Miller, A. Epidemiology of multiple sclerosis: Critique of the evidence for a viral etiology. *Am. J. Epidemiol.* 107:451–461, 1978.

45. Gravell, M., Hamilton, R. S., Kiefer, R. H., Madden, D. L., Sever, J. L., and Tourtellotte, W. W. PAM cell assay as a test for multiple sclerosis associated agent. *Neurology* 18:1050–1052, 1978.

*46. Compston, A. HL-A and neurologic disease. *Neurology* 28:413–414, 1978.

47. Rogart, R. B., and Ritchie, J. M. Pathophysiology of Conduction in Demyelinated Nerve Fibers. In P. Morell (ed.), *Myelin.* New York: Plenum, 1977. Pp. 353–379.

48. Rasminsky, M. Physiology of Conduction in Demyelinated Axons. In S. D. Waxman (ed.), *Physiology and Pathobiology of Axons.* New York: Raven Press, 1978. Pp. 361–376.

*49. Schauf, C. L., and Davis, F. A. The occurrence, specificity, and role of neuroelectric blocking factors in multiple sclerosis. *Neurology* 28:34–39, 1978.

50. Swierhosz, J. E., and Swanborg, R. H. Immunoregulation of experimental allergic encephalomyelitis: Conditions for induction of suppressor cells and analysis of mechanism. *J. Immunol.* 119: 1501–1506, 1977.

51. Antel, J. P., Arnason, B. G. W., and Medot, M. E. Suppressor cell function in multiple sclerosis: Correlation with clinical disease activity. *Ann. Neurol.* 5:338–342, 1979.

52. Campbell, B., Vogel, P. J., Fisher, E., and Lorenz, R. Myelin basic protein administration in multiple sclerosis. *Arch. Neurol.* 29:10–15, 1973.

53. Brostoff, S. W., Levit, S., and Powers, J. M. Induction of experimental allergic neuritis with a peptide from myelin P_2 basic protein. *Nature* 268: 752–753, 1977.

*54. ter Meulen, V., and Wege, H. Virus Infection in Demyelinating Diseases. In J. Palo (ed.), *Myelina-*

tion and Demyelination. New York: Plenum, 1978. Pp. 383–394.

55. Poser, C. M. Diseases of the Myelin Sheath. In J. Minckler (ed.), *Pathology of the Nervous System.* New York: McGraw-Hill, 1968. Vol. 1, pp. 767–820.

56. Vinken, P. J., and Bruyn, G. W. *Handbook of Clinical Neurology: Leucodystrophies and Polio-dystrophies.* Amsterdam: North-Holland, 1970. Vol. 10.

*57. Raine, C. S., and Schaumburg, H. H. The Neuro-pathology of Myelin Diseases. In P. Morell (ed.), *Myelin.* New York: Plenum, 1977. Pp. 271–319.

58. Schaumburg, H. H., Powers, J. M., Raine, C. S., Suzuki, K., and Richardson, E. P., Jr. Adreno-leukodystrophy. *Arch. Neurol.* 32:577–591, 1975.

59. Watanabe, I., Patel, V., Goebel, H. H., Siakotos, A. N., Zeman, W., DeMyer, W., and Dyer, J. S. Early lesion of Pelizeus-Merzbacher disease: Electron microscopic and biochemical study. *J. Neuropathol. Exp. Neurol.* 32:313–333, 1972.

60. Herndon, R. M., Rubinstein, L. J., Freedman, J. M., and Mathieson, G. Light and electron microscopic observations on Rosenthal fibers in Alexander's disease and in multiple sclerosis. *J. Neuropathol. Exp. Neurol.* 29:524–551, 1970.

*61. Hogan, E. L. Animal Models of Genetic Disorders of Myelin. In P. Morell (ed.), *Myelin.* New York: Plenum, 1977. Pp. 489–515.

62. Fletcher, T. F., Suzuki, K., and Martin, F. B. Galactocerebrosidase activity in canine globoid leukodystrophy. *Neurology* 27:758–766, 1977.

63. Kamoshita, S., Rapin, I., Suzuki, K., and Suzuki, K. Spongy degeneration of the brain. A chemical study of two cases including isolation and characterization of myelin. *Neurology* 18:975–985, 1968.

64. Shah, S. N., Peterson, N. A., and McKean, C. M. Lipid composition of human cerebral white matter and myelin in phenylketonuria. *J. Neurochem.* 19:2369–2376, 1972.

*65. Hughes, J. V., and Johnson, T. C. Abnormal amino acid metabolism and brain protein synthesis during neural development. *Neurochem. Res.* 3: 381–399, 1978.

66. Eto, Y., Suzuki, K., and Suzuki, K. Lipid composition of rat brain myelin triethyl tin-induced edema. *J. Lipid Res.* 12:570–579, 1971.

67. Smith, M. E. Studies on the mechanism of demyelination: Triethyl tin-induced demyelination. *J. Neurochem.* 21:357–372, 1973.

68. Matthieu, J. M., Zimmerman, A. W., Webster, H. deF., Ulsamer, A. G., Brady, R. O., and Quarles, R. H. Hexachlorophene intoxication: Characterization of myelin and myelin related fractions in the rat during early postnatal development. *Exp. Neurol.* 45:558–575, 1974.

69. Cammer, W., Rose, A. T., Norton, W. T. Biochemistry and pathological studies of myelin in hexachlorophene intoxication. *Brain Res.* 98: 547–559, 1975.

70. Krigman, M. R., Druse, M. J., Traylor, T. D., Wilson, M. H., Newell, L. R., and Hogan, E. L. Lead encephalopathy in the developing rat: Effect upon myelination. *J. Neuropathol. Exp. Neurol.* 33:58–73, 1974.

71. Wiggins, R. C., Miller, S. L., Benjamins, J. A., Krigman, M. R., and Morell, P. Myelin synthesis during postnatal nutritional deprivation and subsequent rehabilitation. *Brain Res.* 107:257–273, 1976.

72. Prohaska, J. R., and Wells, W. W. Copper deficiency in the developing rat brain: A possible model for Menkes- steely-hair disease. *J. Neurochem.* 23:91–98, 1974.

73. Wood, J. G., and Dawson, R. M. C. Lipid and protein changes in sciatic nerve during Wallerian degeneration. *J. Neurochem.* 22:631–635, 1974.

74. Mezei, C. Cholesterol esters and hydrolytic cholesterol esterase during Wallerian degeneration. *J. Neurochem.* 17:1163–1170, 1970.

75. Eto, Y., and Suzuki, K. Cholesterol ester metabolism in rat brain: A cholesterol ester hydrolase specifically localized in the myelin sheath. *J. Biol. Chem.* 248:1986–1991, 1973.

76. Bignami, A., and Eng, K. F. Biochemical studies of myelin in Wallerian degeneration of rat optic nerve. *J. Neurochem.* 20:165–173, 1973.

Pierre M. Dreyfus
Stanley E. Geel

Chapter 33. Vitamin and Nutritional Deficiencies

Vitamins are indispensable to the normal metabolic activity of the nervous system. A severe deficiency of these fundamental nutrients results in the improper functioning of a number of enzyme systems that are essential to the synthesis of basic constituents or to the removal of potentially toxic metabolites; such deficiencies interfere with normal development, growth, and function of the nervous system.

The most obvious cause for depletion of vitamins and other nutrients is an inadequate or improper diet. Vitamin deficiency can occur, however, even in the presence of an adequate diet, when the absorption of nutrients is limited. Vitamins, to be metabolically useful, must first be absorbed in the gastrointestinal tract and transported by the plasma. Then they must gain entry into cells, be converted into their active cofactor forms, and interact with specific apoenzyme proteins.

It has been demonstrated that, under normal circumstances, homeostatic mechanisms in the brain insure normal concentrations of vitamins, nutrients that are not synthesized by that organ [1]. Most, if not all, of the water-soluble vitamins (thiamine, ascorbic acid, pyridoxine, niacin, and folate) reach the extracellular space of the brain directly from blood by way of cerebral capillaries (blood-brain barrier) and indirectly from CSF by way of the choroid plexus [1–5]. To date, three different transport systems for vitamins have been identified: (1) an active, carrier-mediated, energy-dependent system in the choroid plexus that transports the unchanged vitamin against a concentration gradient from blood into CSF (ascorbic acid, methyletrahydrofolate); (2) a facilitated diffusion transport system between blood and CSF (niacin and niacinamide); and (3) a complex system

that may involve phosphorylation-dephosphorylation after facilitated diffusion of nonphosphorylated vitamins through various membranes (thiamine and pyridoxine). It has been postulated that malfunction of these transport systems may be responsible for unexplained neuropsychiatric disorders in humans.

A number of genetically determined diseases—referred to as vitamin-responsive or vitamin-dependent states—have been identified. In these, at least one of the steps involved either in vitamin utilization or in the conversion of vitamins to active forms is faulty or incomplete [6].

Of the various vitamins, some appear to be more essential to the well-being of the nervous system than do others. Despite increasing knowledge about the role of vitamins in general metabolism, the specific mechanisms by which a deficiency state affects the development and function of the nervous system remain essentially unknown.

Vitamin deprivation leads to several readily identifiable biochemical lesions that invariably antedate clinical manifestations and histopathological alterations. In most instances, the correlation between the duration or the severity of these biochemical lesions and the irreversibility of symptoms or tissue changes has not been established; nor has it been possible to elucidate which of the various biochemical lesions are responsible for the neurological manifestations.

Knowledge about the neurochemical changes that attend nutritional disorders of the nervous system has been gleaned mainly from the experimentally induced deficiency of single vitamins, without other associated variables, or by the use of specific antivitamins. The results of these studies, for the most part, bear little or no resemblance to the naturally occurring disorders, which are usually the result of combined multiple deficiencies. Any discussion of the neurochemistry of vitamin and other nutritional deficiencies therefore relies mainly on information derived from studies on experimental animals; speculations about human disease states are based on fragmentary clinical and biochemical observations.

An attempt will be made to summarize, rather than to review in detail, current knowledge of the effects of vitamin and nutritional deprivation on the nervous system.

Thiamine

Thiamine (vitamin B_1), in its phosphorylated form (thiamine diphosphate, also known as thiamine pyrophosphate or cocarboxylase), acts as cofactor in two major enzyme systems that are present in all mammalian tissues, including the nervous system. The first relates to glycolysis and involves the oxidative decarboxylation of pyruvic and α-ketoglutaric acid. The second concerns two transketolation steps of the phosphoglyconate pathway (hexose monophosphate shunt), an alternate route of carbohydrate metabolism of importance in biosynthetic mechanisms (see Chap. 17):

ribose 5-phosphate + xylulose 5-phosphate $\rightleftharpoons$
  sedoheptulose 7-phosphate + glyceraldehyde
           3-phosphate

xylulose 5-phosphate + erythrose 4-phosphate
 $\rightleftharpoons$ fructose 6-phosphate + glyceraldehyde
           3-phosphate.

In addition to its function as a coenzyme, thiamine has been shown to play a unique role in the function of excitable membranes [7]. Experimentally induced thiamine deficiency in animals bears certain clinical and pathological similarities to naturally occurring thiamine deficiency in humans, as exemplified by the Wernicke-Korsakoff syndrome, an affliction of the CNS, and by beriberi, a disease of the peripheral nervous system. The histopathological changes observed in animals and humans assume a fairly constant topography. Although the afflicted regions or parts of the nervous

system differ from species to species, the lesions appear to have a definite predilection for bilaterally symmetrical parts of the CNS and distal parts of the peripheral nerves. Neurochemical data gathered to date have elucidated only partially some of the pathophysiological mechanisms that underlie this apparently selective vulnerability [8].

Much of the current knowledge concerning thiamine, its role in intermediary carbohydrate metabolism, and some of the metabolic consequences brought about by its deficiency in diets was first elucidated by the classic studies of Peters and coworkers [9]. The concept of the *biochemical lesion,* first articulated in relation to thiamine deficiency and the nervous system by Peters's group, has formed the basis for more recent biochemical investigations.

EXPERIMENTAL THIAMINE DEPLETION

Brain thiamine in normal rat and human brain tends to be fairly evenly distributed, the content being higher in cerebral cortex and cerebellum than in white matter [10]. In human brain, the mammillary bodies, structures that are invariably afflicted in Wernicke's disease, appear to have particularly high concentrations of the vitamin. The monophosphate and diphosphate esters make up about 80 percent of the total thiamine in brain; the triphosphate ester and free thiamine each constitute approximately 10 percent of the total thiamine in that organ. Observations made on rat brain during progressive depletion have shown that brain thiamine begins to fall during the second week of deprivation, experiencing its greatest drop during that week. Total brain thiamine has to be reduced to less than 20 percent of normal before severe neurological signs of deficiency (ataxia, loss of equilibrium, opisthotonus, loss of righting reflexes) and irreversible tissue changes (pannecrosis in the lateral pontine tegmentum) become manifest. Reversal of neurological manifestations is noted when brain thiamine returns to 30 percent of normal. These observations suggest that normal cerebral tissue has a substantial reserve of this vitamin. It has been demonstrated that, during progressive depletion, it is predominantly brain thiamine diphosphate that is decreased; whereas free thiamine and thiamine monophosphate remain fairly constant, and thiamine triphosphate tends to increase. It is of interest that the loss of thiamine diphosphate is greater in the pons, the site of major pathological changes, than it is in any other part of rat brain [11].

THIAMINE-DEPENDENT ENZYME SYSTEMS

Studies of thiamine-dependent enzyme systems both in normal and in deficient rat nervous systems suggest that selective vulnerability and the character of histopathological changes may be attributed to the enzymatic topography of the normal nervous system and to the effect of vitamin deprivation on these enzyme systems. In normal adult rat brain, the activity of pyruvate dehydrogenase (the enzyme responsible for the decarboxylation of pyruvate) is highest in areas richly endowed with neurons, such as the cerebellum and the cerebral cortex, and is considerably lower in the spinal cord white matter. During progressive vitamin depletion, no appreciable decreases in activity can be measured in the brain when the animals are vitamin-deficient, yet asymptomatic. Even at the most advanced stage of deficiency, when the animals exhibit severe neurological impairment, only the brain stem shows a 25 percent reduction in enzymatic activity. By contrast, even at the stage when animals are asymptomatic neurologically, the ability to decarboxylate pyruvate is sharply decreased in such other organs as the heart, liver, and kidney. Lactate and pyruvate levels, measured in various parts of the rat nervous system during progressive depletion, generally tend to mirror the enzymatic defect [12]. Normal brain transketolase activity is highest in the spinal cord white matter and pons, whereas gray matter, such as the cerebral cortex and the caudate nucleus, have the lowest enzymatic activity. The lateral pontine tegmentum, where the histological changes are most pronounced, exhibits a significant decrease in transketolase activity during progressive vitamin depletion when compared with other parts of the brain. Severe signs and symptoms of deficiency and irreversible pathological changes become manifest when brain transketolase activity has been reduced by 58 percent. It appears that the defect in transketolation tends to reverse more slowly than does the abnormality of pyruvate metabolism.

THIAMINE DEFICIENCY IN DEVELOPING BRAIN

Studies performed on immature thiamine-deficient rats during a period when the brain develops rapidly and is most susceptible to nutritional insults have failed to demonstrate changes in myelin lipids or other lipid components that could be separated from the effects of simple undernutrition in either the whole brain or the areas most vulnerable to the lack of thiamine. Thiamine deficiency induced during pregnancy has resulted in offspring with reduced body and brain growth. Brain DNA concentration tended to be higher and protein-DNA ratio lower, suggesting smaller cell size. RNA levels expressed per unit DNA were significantly reduced. Ganglioside concentrations tended to be elevated, cholesterol levels were normal, and cerebroside and total sphingolipid (minus gangliosides) concentrations were markedly reduced. Total phospholipid concentration and the distribution of individual phospholipids were normal. Similar results were noted in pair-fed animals that were undernourished but adequately supplied with thiamine [13]. These studies support the notion that thiamine is not related to myelin or its formation in the nervous system. Barchi and Braun [14] could not find any correlation between the content of thiamine and the state of myelination of the nervous system of developing animals, nor did they detect reduced levels of the vitamin in demyelinated areas of human brain afflicted with multiple sclerosis.

Experimental evidence suggests that thiamine-dependent metabolism differs in the nervous systems of the developing and the mature rat. During fetal development, transketolase activity is half of that measured in adult brain. Within the first 10 days of life, the activity rises sharply to about twice the fetal level, reaching a plateau (adult level) thereafter (Fig. 33-1). When the results are expressed in terms of the DNA or cellular content of the samples, a similar curve is obtained. The rise in brain transketolase activity during the first 10 days of life correlates with the rise of enzymes involved in oxidative phosphorylation and glycolysis. Transketolase activity may reflect an increase in glial cell duplication, proliferation, and migration. Animals born to thiamine-deprived mothers tend to be smaller, and their growth rate is retarded. The cerebral transketolase activity of suckling rats is considerably more depressed than is that of their deficient mothers. This may be a reflection of enzyme immaturity or of a difference in coenzyme binding in newborn rat brain, rather than of a selective reduction of the vitamin in neonatal brain.

BIOCHEMICAL PATHOLOGY

The extensive investigations carried out by Peters and coworkers on abnormal pyruvate metabolism in thiamine deficiency and its consequences on brain metabolism as a whole [9] seemed to provide a logical explanation for the neurological symptoms and signs, as well as for the observed histopathological changes. More detailed scrutiny of this biochemical lesion, however, has failed to substantiate the previously postulated theories. One would expect severe thiamine deficiency, by virtue of faulty pyruvate and α-ketoglutaric acid metabolism, to impair ACh synthesis and to bring about a change in ATP levels, particularly in the most severely involved parts of the brain (e.g., the brain stem). Some investigators have shown normal regional ACh levels accompanied by significantly reduced acetylcholine utilization [15]; others have found markedly reduced ACh and acetyl-CoA levels in the face of normal pyruvate dehydrogenase, choline acetyltransferase, and AChE activities [16].

It is generally accepted that the pentose phosphate pathway plays an important role in synthetic mechanisms by virtue of NADPH production for lipid synthesis and ribose production for nucleic acid synthesis. Whereas this metabolic pathway is operative in the CNS, some controversy remains about its importance. In the adult brain, it probably plays a relatively minor role, although it may assume greater importance in the developing nervous system and chronically thiamine-depleted nervous system. In severe thiamine deficiency, the

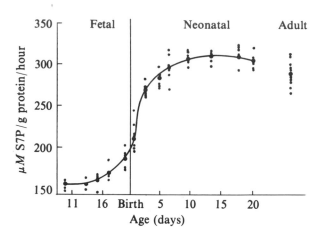

Fig. 33-1. *Whole-brain transketolase activity as a function of age.*

conversion of oxidized glutathione to its reduced form (GSH) is decreased in the brain stem of symptomatic thiamine-deficient animals [12], but no reduction in overall shunt activity has been demonstrated [17]. Cerebral DNA and protein synthesis are significantly decreased in experimental animals with neurological dysfunction. These metabolic abnormalities may be due in part to a vitamin deficiency and in part to the hypothermia and decreased food assimilation and utilization that occur as consequences of thiamine deficiency [18]. It has been shown that cultured glial [C 6] and neuroblastoma cells grown in thiamine-deficient medium exhibit impaired fatty acid synthesis by virtue of decreased activity of two key lipogenic enzymes, acetyl-CoA carboxylase and fatty acid synthetase. The lowered enzyme activity appears to be due to reduced enzyme synthesis. Impaired fatty acid synthesis is readily reversed by the addition of small concentrations of thiamine. Thiamine deficiency has also been shown to affect cholesterol biosynthesis, apparently because of a significant reduction in the activity of the key regulatory enzyme—3-hydroxy-3-methylglutaryl-CoA (HMG-CoA) reductase. The effect of thiamine deficiency on lipid synthesis appears to be more marked in cultured glial cells than in cultured neuroblastoma cells. Since fatty acid and cholesterol are major constituents of cell membranes, any abnormality in their synthesis would have severe effects on membrane function and integrity within the nervous system [19].

There is a significant decrease in the uptake of serotonin by synaptosomal preparations of cerebellum obtained from animals rendered deficient in thiamine by dietary means or by the administration of the vitamin analog pyrithiamine. These observations suggest that some of the neurological manifestations of thiamine deficiency may be due to the failure of serotoninergic neurons in the cerebellum [20].

NEUROCHEMICAL STUDIES IN HUMANS

The neurochemical observations that have been made on the human nervous system are limited. Estimation of transketolase activity in normal brain obtained 6 hr after sudden death has shown high transketolase activity in the mammillary body, a structure invariably affected in cases of Wernicke's disease, and in other structures of the brain stem and diencephalon that are not involved in this disease entity [8]. To date, it has not been possible to define the biochemical lesion in patients suffering from thiamine deficiency. Elevation of pyruvate levels in blood before, and a marked increase in pyruvate after, the administration of glucose was for many years the standard method of estimating thiamine deficiency; this has proved to lack specificity because other metabolic disorders can cause an elevation of pyruvate levels in blood.

Evidence of a severe impairment of tissue transketolase activity has been obtained, however, by simple biochemical measurements of blood. Determinations of such transketolase levels reflect, in a highly sensitive and specific manner, the state of thiamine nutrition in humans [21]. Transketolase assays reveal the levels of available coenzyme and also differentiate an acute from a chronic state of deficiency by reflecting the levels of available apoenzyme. Blood transketolase assays provide clinical and biochemical evidence that at least some of the signs and symptoms of Wernicke's disease, particularly ophthalmoplegia, result from a specific

lack of thiamine and that their prompt reversibility must be attributed to the presence of a biochemical lesion that antedates irreversible histopathological alterations [22]. It has been demonstrated that a magnesium deficiency interferes with the restoration of transketolase activity usually produced by the in vitro addition of thiamine diphosphate to thiamine-deficient red blood cells [23].

Fibroblast transketolase from patients afflicted with the Wernicke-Korsakoff syndrome appears to bind thiamine diphosphate less avidly than does enzyme extracted from control cells. Furthermore, the aberration in coenzyme binding persists after serial passages in tissue culture, suggesting a genetically determined, rather than an acquired, enzymatic defect. The aberration of transketolase presumably constitutes a predisposition to the development of the Wernicke-Korsakoff syndrome only when the individual diet is marginal in thiamine [24].

ROLE OF THIAMINE IN MEMBRANE FUNCTION

Since von Muralt [7] first demonstrated that thiamine, in addition to its function as a coenzyme, plays a unique role in nerve excitation, a number of important observations have been made that have immediate relevance to neurological disease in humans. Experimental evidence has shown that electrical stimulation of peripheral nerves and spinal cord promotes the release of thiamine [25]. Physiological concentrations of such drugs as ouabain and tetrodotoxin have a similar effect [25]. The release appears to involve thiamine triphosphate predominantly, and it is observed in a subcellular fraction rich in axonal membranes [25]. Pyrithiamine produces neurological symptoms of deficiency in experimental animals and has a profound and irreversible effect on the electrical activity of nerve preparations. This appears to be due to a displacement of the vitamin, rather than to inhibition of thiamine-dependent enzyme systems.

Studies have suggested that either thiamine diphosphate or thiamine triphosphate, both of which occupy sites on the nerve membrane, is involved in the sodium-gating mechanisms of excitable membranes, and that agents such as pyrithiamine and other analogs interfere with membrane sites cata-lyzing the voltage-dependent changes in membrane permeability to sodium [26]. There appears to be general agreement that the phosphatases and phos-photransferases that regulate the tissue levels of thiamine and its phosphoesters are localized in axonal membranes [25]. The effects of thiamine deficiency on membrane function could readily explain the dramatic evolution of the clinical events and some of the subtle early ultrastructural changes—despite the lack of demonstrable changes noted by conventional histological methods in most severely affected animals. It is conceivable that the thiamine-deficient membrane is unable to maintain osmotic gradients, and that a failure of the energy-dependent component of glial electrolyte and water transport is the result of relatively acute thiamine deficiency.

THIAMINE-RELATED GENETIC DISEASES

At least three thiamine-related genetic diseases that affect the nervous system have been identified. In many cases of *subacute necrotizing encephalo-myelopathy* (Leigh's disease), a genetically deter-mined disease of infants that resembles Wernicke's disease, there appears to be a total lack of triphos-phothiamine in the brain [27]. Furthermore, patients afflicted with the disease—and some normal carriers—seem to elaborate a factor found in blood, urine, and CSF that inhibits thiamine pyrophosphate-ATP phosphoryltransferase, the enzyme responsible for the synthesis of thiamine triphosphate in brain. In some cases of Leigh's disease, the inborn error of metabolism consists of a deficiency of pyruvate carboxylase [28]; this sug-gests that variants of the disease exist. An in-herited defect in pyruvate oxidation associated with intermittent ataxia has been reported by Blass and coworkers [29]. In these patients, a defect in the thiamine-dependent first enzyme of the pyruvate dehydrogenase complex has been found. Finally, it has been demonstrated that thiamine diphosphate increases the activity of the branched-chain α-keto acid dehydrogenase complex of hepatic tissue and fibroblasts cultured from the skin of individuals

afflicted with *maple syrup urine disease,* an in-herited disorder characterized by mental retarda-tion and neurological deterioration [30] (see also Chap. 28). The oral administration of thiamine and the dietary restriction of branched-chain amino acids, begun soon after birth, have proved bene-ficial. α-Ketoisocaproic acid, the derivative of leucine, one of the three branched-chain amino acids that accumulate in the plasma of affected children, inhibits the decarboxylation of pyruvate in rat brain [31].

Although thiamine deficiency has been the sub-ject of extensive investigation, large gaps exist in our knowledge concerning the sequence of events that ultimately leads to severe neurological dys-function and irreversible histopathological changes.

Vitamin B$_6$ (Pyridoxine)

Several forms of vitamin B$_6$ and its active phos-phorylated coenzymes have been identified in mam-malian tissue, including brain. The vitamin B$_6$ group bears the collective name of *pyridoxine,* and consists of *pyridoxal, pyridoxol,* and *pyridox-amine.* The predominant coenzyme forms of the vitamin in animal tissue are the phosphates of pyridoxal and pyridoxamine. The relative content and the rate of disappearance of these coenzymes during states of deficiency vary from species to species. Pyridoxal 5-phosphotransferase is re-sponsible for the phosphorylation of the vitamin in brain and other organs. Isonicotinic acid hydrazide (the drug used in the treatment of tuberculosis) and 4-deoxypyridoxine (a vitamin B$_6$ antagonist) inter-fere with the phosphorylating enzyme and cause a decrease in the tissue levels of pyridoxal phosphate.

The dietary deprivation of pyridoxine has been shown to lower the seizure threshold in a variety of mammalian species, including humans; the young appear to be more susceptible to convulsions than do the older and more mature. Pyridoxine de-ficiency in pigs is said to result in both convulsions and ataxia, the latter being caused by pathological changes in peripheral nerves, posterior root ganglia, and the posterior funiculi of the spinal cord.

Table 33-1. Distribution of Glutamic Decarboxylase Activity in the Nervous System of Normal and Pyridoxine-Deficient Rats

Area Sampled	Micromoles Glutamic Acid Decarboxylated/Gram Protein/Hour	
	Normal*	Deficient*
Caudate nucleus	73.0	32.2
Cerebral cortex	74.3	34.0
Thalamus	96.7	33.8
Hypothalamus	101.2	47.2
Cerebellar hemisphere	65.8	42.2
Midbrain	100.7	42.8
Spinal cord	31.8	15.2

*Means of 7 animals. All determinations carried out in triplicate. Data of P. M. Dreyfus, F. Meier, and C. York, 1967.

PYRIDOXINE-DEPENDENT ENZYMES

The coenzyme forms of vitamin B_6 act as catalysts in a number of important enzymatic reactions related to the synthesis, catabolism, and transport of amino acids and the metabolism of glycogen and unsaturated fatty acids [32]. Many pyridoxine-dependent enzyme systems have been identified in the nervous system, yet knowledge of the biochemical pathology of vitamin B_6 deficiency remains limited.

Pyridoxine-dependent enzymes in the nervous system fall into two major categories: transaminases and L-amino acid decarboxylases (see Chap. 17). Some of these enzymes are involved in the γ-aminobutyric acid (GABA) shunt, an alternate oxidative pathway restricted to nervous tissue, in which α-ketoglutaric acid is metabolized to succinate by way of glutamate and GABA. Vitamin B_6 deprivation leads to significant enzymatic depression in all tissues. The affinity of the coenzyme for its apoenzyme varies from enzyme to enzyme. Decarboxylases tend to have a lower affinity for coenzyme than do other enzymes; thus, the de-

carboxylases tend to be more readily affected than are the transaminases. Severe vitamin deprivation also results in a decrease in enzyme protein. The addition of excess pyridoxal phosphate to a vitamin-deficient enzyme preparation in vitro fails to restore complete activity; apoenzyme production stimulated by the addition of excess vitamin B_6 to a normal tissue extract can be inhibited by puromycin. Thus it would appear that pyridoxal phosphate regulates intracellular enzyme synthesis. It is generally believed that organs or cells with a high rate of protein turnover are most sensitive to pyridoxine depletion. Finally, pyridoxine is required for cellular proliferation and for the synthesis of specific proteins involved in immunological reactions [33].

Of the various pyridoxine-dependent enzymes, two decarboxylases appear to be of particular importance to the integrity of neuronal function. The first, glutamate decarboxylase, is responsible for the production of the neuroinhibitor GABA from glutamic acid (see Chap. 12). Although generally believed to be restricted to neurons, this enzyme may also be active in other mammalian tissue. In rat CNS, enzymatic activity is highest in the hypothalamus and midbrain and lowest in the spinal cord (see Table 33-1). Although significant enzymatic activity can be demonstrated in human cerebral cortex (32 μmol of glutamic acid decarboxylated per gram of protein per hour), none can be measured in white matter.

The second enzyme, 5-hydroxytryptophan decarboxylase, is localized in nerve terminals and is involved in the synthesis of serotonin (5-hydroxytryptamine, 5-HT). The same enzyme may be involved in the decarboxylation of L-dopa to dopamine (see also Chap. 10). Exogenous pyridoxine reduces the effectiveness of L-dopa in treating Parkinson's disease, presumably because of increased peripheral decarboxylation of L-dopa. In the rat, the activity of this enzyme appears to be highest in the caudate nucleus, the hypothalamus, and the midbrain, which may be rich in serotoninergic terminals. The activity is low in cerebral and cerebellar cortex (see Table 33-2).

EXPERIMENTAL PYRIDOXINE DEFICIENCY

When weanling rats are fed a diet dificient in vitamin B_6 for several weeks, severe depression of growth and acrodynia of paws, nose, ears, and tail ensue. The animals demonstrate unusual irritability; however, they rarely suffer convulsive seizures or motor weakness. This is in sharp contrast to the frequent seizures observed in pyridoxine-deficient newborn rats. When SGOT activity reaches 50 percent of normal, glutamate decarboxylase and 5-HTP decarboxylase activities are sharply reduced. The loss of glutamate decarboxylase activity is 36 to 65 percent, while that of 5-HTP decarboxylase is 46 to 84 percent, depending on the area of the nervous system (see Tables 33-1 and 33-2). Decreased enzymatic activity is even greater in pyridoxine-deficient neonatal animals that convulse; this suggests that there is a correlation between the seizure threshold and the level of activity of these two brain enzymes that are dependent on vitamin B_6 [34]. The DNA, RNA, and protein content of the brain of immature, pyridoxine-deficient rats is reduced significantly, although it remains normal in deficient adult animals [35].

Vitamin B_6 deficiency induced in the maternal rat results in significant cytoarchitectural changes and hypomyelination in the brains of the progeny [36, 37]. The latter is reflected by a reduction in the activity of 2′,3′-cyclic nucleotide 3′-phosphohydrolase, a marker enzyme for myelin, in the brains of the offspring [38].

Vitamin B_6 deficiency produced in immature animals during a period of rapid myelination results in decreased incorporation of labeled acetate into total lipid extracts of brain and into the cholesterol, glycolipid, and phospholipid fractions of brain. Cerebroside and sulphatide levels are markedly decreased [39]. The deficiency state causes a decrease in the polyunsaturated fatty acid content of myelin phosphatides. It seems that vitamin B_6 is essential to the activity of the enzyme serine palmitoyltransferase (3-ketohydrosphingosine synthetase), which is reduced in deficient brain. Vitamin B_6 deficiency also affects the biosynthesis of long-chain polyunsaturated fatty acids

Table 33-2. Distribution of 5-Hydroxytryptophan Decarboxylase Activity in the Nervous System of Normal and Pyridoxine-Deficient Rats

Area Sampled	Nanomoles [14C]Serotonin Formed/Gram Protein/Hour	
	Normal*	Deficient*
Caudate nucleus	4,417.9	2,390.1
Cerebral cortex	621.6	99.5
Thalamus	1,319.3	428.0
Hypothalamus	4,332.0	1,767.2
Cerebellar hemisphere	474.7	165.2
Midbrain	4,204.1	805.3
Spinal cord	1,150.1	226.1
Liver	13,494.6	1,722.2

*Means of 7 animals. All determinations carried out in triplicate. Data of P. M. Dreyfus, F. Meier, and C. York, 1967.

[40]. Thus, the deficiency causes a delay or reduced rate of myelin formation in the CNS.

VITAMIN B_6 DEFICIENCY IN HUMANS

Evidence of vitamin B_6 deficiency in humans can be obtained from a number of biochemical determinations on blood and urine. None is thought specifically to reflect involvement of the nervous system. Pyridoxal estimations in blood and CSF are of limited usefulness. Under normal circumstances, vitamin B_6 and its derivatives can be measured in the urine; none can be found during severe depletion, regardless of the patient's protein intake. Pyridoxine deficiency causes increased urinary excretion of the tryptophan metabolites, xanthurenic and kynurenic acids, after a high dose of tryptophan. Decreased activity of 5-HTP decarboxylase results in decreased excretion of 5-HIAA in the urine, and faulty activity of cysteine sulfinic acid or cysteic acid decarboxylase causes decreased taurine levels in urine. Vitamin B_6 deficiency affects cystathione cleavage, with resultant cystathioninuria (see Chap. 28). Occasionally, reduced activity of SGOT and glutamic-pyruvic transaminase can be demonstrated along with oxaluria.

In recent years, pyridoxine dependency has been the subject of a number of investigations (see also Chap. 28). This is a familial disorder of infants, characterized by seizures and a high daily requirement of vitamin B_6 (10 mg per day). The seizures respond promptly to the administration of pyridoxine, and possibly to GABA. Biochemical evidence of vitamin deficiency is lacking.

Observations made in a child who died as a consequence of vitamin B_6-dependent seizures revealed an abnormally sparse quantity of myelinated fibers in the cerebral hemispheres. Glutamic acid concentrations were elevated and GABA levels reduced in the frontal and occipital cortices, but not in the spinal cord. All other amino acid concentrations were normal, except for increased cystathionine in the occipital cortex. Pyridoxal 5-phosphate was reduced in the frontal cortex. Glutamic acid decarboxylase activity, comparable to that of controls, was detected when the tissue pyridoxal 5-phosphate concentration was greater than 0.05 mM. These findings suggest that pyridoxine-dependent seizures in humans are associated with reduced GABA concentrations in the brain caused by an abnormality of glutamic acid decarboxylase and with hypoplasia of central myelin [41].

Other pyridoxine-responsive genetic diseases affecting the nervous system have been identified [42]. *Homocystinuria, cystathioninuria,* and *xanthurenic aciduria,* associated with mental retardation and occasionally with seizures, may be amenable to effective treatment with large doses of vitamin B_6, which have been shown to enhance the residual activity of the affected enzymes [6].

Vitamin B_{12}

Although a great deal is known about the role of vitamin B_{12} (cyanocobalamin) in biochemical reactions, virtually nothing is known about its function in the nervous system. However, biochemical studies on nervous tissue of animals suffering from experimentally induced vitamin B_{12} deficiency may assume greater importance in view of the recent discovery that rhesus monkeys maintained on a deficient diet for 4 years develop neurological manifestations and demyelinating lesions in the CNS [43].

HISTOPATHOLOGY IN VITAMIN B_{12} DEFICIENCY

In humans, the insufficient absorption of vitamin B_{12} may result in definite histopathological changes, that is, those seen in subacute degeneration of the spinal cord, optic nerves, cerebral white matter, and peripheral nerves. This failure of absorption may be caused by the absence of intrinsic factor, disease of the gastrointestinal tract (postgastrectomy, sprue, fish tapeworm infestation), or vegetarianism. The earliest visible change in the affected parts consists of swelling of individual myelinated nerve fibers in small foci. This is followed by coalescence of the lesions into large, irregular, spongy, honeycomblike zones of demyelination. Fibers with the largest diameter seem to be predominantly affected, and axon cylinders tend to be spared. Although demyelination appears to be the primary lesion, the possibility of initial involvement of axonal metabolism and axoplasmic flow has not been entirely excluded.

B_{12}-DEPENDENT ENZYMES

Only microorganisms that inhabit the mammalian gastrointestinal tract have the capacity to synthesize vitamin B_{12}. Although large amounts of the vitamin are manufactured in the rumens of some herbivorous animals, humans depend on a dietary source, largely meat. The natural vitamin cyanocobalamin must be metabolized by the body to its active coenzyme form, 5-deoxyadenosylcobalamin. Two reactions dependent on vitamin B_{12} have been demonstrated in human and other mammalian tissue (Table 33-3) [44]. The isomerization of L-methylmalonyl-CoA to succinyl-CoA requires the active coenzyme form of the vitamin, whereas the transmethylation of homocysteine to methionine probably depends on another coenzyme form of the vitamin, methyl-B_{12}. The enzymes catalyzing these two reactions are L-methylmalonyl-CoA mutase and N^5-methyltetrahydrofolate homocysteine methyltransferase. Ribonucleotide reductase, an enzyme of great importance in the synthesis of DNA in microorganisms, has not as yet been measured in mammalian tissue, and virtually nothing is known about B_{12}-dependent enzyme systems involved in sulfhydryl reduction.

VITAMIN B_{12} DEFICIENCY AND METHYLMALONYL-CoA METABOLISM

Vitamin B_{12} deficiency in humans and experimental animals results in decreased conversion of methylmalonyl-CoA to succinyl-CoA in the tissues, and the urinary excretion of methylmalonic acid ensues (see also Chap. 28). It is not known to what extent reduced levels of vitamin B_{12} coenzyme and consequent reduction in methylmalonyl-CoA mutase activity are responsible for the neurological complications of vitamin B_{12} deficiency. The dietary restriction of vitamin B_{12} results in decreased coenzyme levels in the liver, kidney, and brain of rats and immature pigs [45]; the percentage decrease is approximately the same in each organ. When rats or miniature pigs are fed a diet free of vitamin B_{12}, methylmalonic aciduria is detectable after 4 to 6 weeks. The presence of this organic acid in the urine of animals and humans has been found to be both a specific and a sensitive index of vitamin B_{12} deficiency; it is, in fact, a more reliable indicator than is the level of B_{12} in serum. Levels of methylmalonic acid in CSF exceed those in plasma; this suggests that the acid may be elaborated by cerebral tissue as a consequence of faulty proprionate metabolism in the brain [46].

Although rats kept on a deficient diet for 8 to 12 months appear clinically to be intact, miniature pigs show a significant reduction in food consumption and body weight, generalized weakness, and intermittent lethargy after 3 months of deprivation. Brain, spinal cord, and peripheral nerves examined by standard light microscope methods reveal no histopathological alterations.

It has been shown that, in deficient liver, kidney, and brain, methylmalonyl-CoA mutase activity is reduced; methylmalonyl-CoA is hydrolyzed to methylmalonic acid rather than to succinyl-CoA.

Table 33-3. Vitamin B_{12}-Dependent Reactions in Mammalian Tissue

Reaction	Active Cofactor
Methylmalonyl-CoA mutase	B_{12} coenzyme
Ribonucleotide reductase (?)	B_{12} coenzyme
Methionine synthetase	Vitamin B_{12}
Sulfhydryl reduction	B_{12} coenzyme (?)

The rate of disappearance of methylmalonyl-CoA, however, is essentially the same in normal and deficient tissue [31]. These observations suggest that, in the deficient state, adaptive mechanisms exist that rid the organism of high levels of methylmalonyl-CoA.

Recent investigations into fatty acids and their metabolism in sural nerve samples obtained from patients afflicted with pernicious anemia have revealed the presence of branched-chain (C_{15}) and odd-chain (C_{17}) fatty acids. In addition, the mean content of total lipids and fatty acids, as well as the in vitro rate of synthesis of fatty acids, was significantly reduced in nerve samples from pernicious anemia patients [47]. It has been shown that methylmalonyl-CoA inhibits both acetyl-CoA carboxylase and fatty acid synthetase activity [48]. These findings may explain, in part, the structural changes observed in central and peripheral myelin.

VITAMIN B_{12} DEFICIENCY AND METHIONINE METABOLISM

The enzyme N^5-methyltetrahydrofolate homocysteine methyltransferase is involved in the synthesis of methionine from homocysteine. The remethylation of homocysteine to methionine is accomplished together with the regeneration of tetrahydrofolate from N^5-methyltetrahydrofolate. The reaction requires trace amounts of S-adenosylmethionine and a vitamin form of B_{12}, most likely methyl-B_{12}. The activity of the enzyme has been estimated in liver and brain of both humans and rats [35]. In deficient rat liver and brain, enzymatic activity is drastically reduced (Table 33-4). The addition in vitro of excess vitamin B_{12} par-

Table 33-4. Activity of N^5-Methyltetrahydrofolate Homocysteine Methyl Transferase in Normal and Vitamin B_{12}-Deficient Rat Liver and Brain[a]

	Controls (6)		Deficient (6)	
	Plain	$+B_{12}$[b]	Plain	$+B_{12}$[b]
Liver	246.8 ± 8	248.2 ± 10	36.8 ± 5	48.8 ± 7
Brain	212.0 ± 10	341 ± 35	47.0 ± 3	97.3 ± 10

[a]Animals on deficient diet for 8 months. Results expressed as CPM/mg protein/hr $\pm$ SEM. Numbers in parentheses represent number of animals. All determinations were carried out in triplicate.
[b]Cyanocobalamin (0.3 μmol) was added to the incubation mixture.
Data of P. M. Dreyfus and C. Gross, 1968.

tially restores the activity of the enzyme in brain but has no significant effect on liver enzyme activity.

The stimulation in vitro of enzymatic activity in normal and deficient brains suggests that this tissue contains excessive amounts of apoprotein. This may represent a protective mechanism against vitamin B_{12} deficiency. A substantial decrease in enzymatic activity may result in a critical reduction of methionine synthesis in neural tissue, which in humans could lead to neurological manifestations and histopathological changes in the nervous system.

Even though methionine is considered an essential dietary amino acid, metabolic pathways exist for its synthesis at the cellular level. Methionine is an important constituent of neural protein and may also be a constituent of proteolipids. The rate of its incorporation into protein is rapid; it is greatest in regions of the nervous system that contain the highest density of cells, and it is more active in microsomes than in either nuclei or mitochondria. Profound changes in concentrations of amino acid in brain affect the incorporation of amino acid into protein and influence protein synthesis and degradation. It can be postulated that, in the nervous system, prolonged and severe vitamin B_{12} deprivation results in a critical reduction of methionine levels in tissue, which in turn, may alter protein synthesis and turnover and, conceivably, structure and function. In support of this contention, it has been demonstrated that when 1-aminocyclopentane carboxylic acid (a powerful inhibitor of the transmethylation reaction that converts homocysteine to methionine) is administered to adult mice, ataxia and paralysis, as well as spongiform demyelination of the spinal cord, result [50].

OTHER DISORDERS RELATED TO
VITAMIN B_{12}

Vitamin B_{12} deficiency has been shown to cause hydrocephalus in newborn rats. It is believed that the anatomical defect is caused by stenosis of the aqueduct of Sylvius, associated with aplasia of the subcommissural organ, a special group of columnar ependymal cells in the roof of the aqueduct and the posterior part of the third ventricle [51]. It has been postulated that the congenital abnormality may be the result of faulty ribonucleic acid metabolism in the newborn brain. Levels of RNA per cell are decreased, whereas the amount of DNA remains normal.

Two distinct types of genetically determined vitamin B_{12}-dependent methylmalonic acidurias associated with developmental arrest, ataxia, and coma have been identified [52] (see also Chap. 28). Examination of the brain, spinal cord, and sciatic nerve obtained from an infant who died of methylmalonic aciduria in which vitamin B_{12} was not converted to deoxyadenosyl-B_{12} revealed an accumulation of branched-chain and odd-numbered fatty acids. The former were identified as a mixture of methylhexadecanoic acids. The phosphatides separated from the spinal cord were shown to contain methyl-substituted palmitic acid, with the highest concentration occurring on the beta position of the phosphatidylcholine [53].

Folic Acid Deficiency

Folic acid depletion occurs as a consequence of dietary deficiency, which is sometimes caused by unmet increased needs during pregnancy or by gastrointestinal defects in absorption. The neurological manifestations engendered in some patients by folic acid depletion alone are thought to be similar to those caused by the lack of vitamin B_{12} (see Chap. 28). In general, however, most folate-deficient patients are neurologically intact.

It is now well established that patients receiving anticonvulsant medications, particularly diphenylhydantoin, may develop folate deficiency. Conversely, the administration of folic acid significantly reduces the levels of these drugs in blood [54]. Presumably the vitamin and the drug compete for intestinal absorption.

Folic acid and its derivatives are involved in the formation of methionine from homocysteine and in the synthesis of purines and pyrimidines and, hence, of RNA and DNA. Folate is therefore fundamental to normal cell division and growth. The active coenzyme form of folate contains four additional hydrogen atoms (tetrahydrofolate). Folic acid reductase permits the reduction of folate to tetrahydrofolate. Various derivatives of tetrahydrofolate have been identified, including methyl-, methenyl-, methylene-, hydroxymethyl-, formyl-, and formiminotetrahydrofolate. In general, the various forms of folate are instrumental in the transfer of single-carbon units. As yet, the specific role of folic acid in cerebral metabolism has not been elucidated, although it is interesting to note that folate levels in CSF are two to three times those in serum, even in states of folate deficiency [46]. Clinical studies have shown that anticonvulsant therapy does not alter the relationship between serum and CSF folate levels.

The neurological complications of pernicious anemia may be precipitated when folic acid without adequate levels of B_{12} is administered to treat the anemia. This phenomenon remains essentially unexplained.

Niacin, Pantothenic Acid, and Vitamin E

NIACIN

In the nervous system, as in other tissues, niacin (nicotinic acid) is a constituent of the two coenzymes that transfer hydrogen or electrons. These coenzymes are *nicotinamide adenine dinucleotide (NAD)* and *nicotinamide adenine dinucleotide phosphate (NADP)*. Both of these nucleotides are essential to a number of important enzymatic reactions involved in carbohydrate, fatty acid, and glutathione metabolism. The significance of these biochemical reactions has been covered in other chapters (see Chaps. 17 and 18).

Most mammalian cells synthesize nicotinic acid from tryptophan. It is not known whether this synthesis can also take place in the cells of the nervous system. In humans, a deficiency of niacin is responsible for the neurological and psychological manifestations of *pellagra:* encephalopathy associated with signs of spinal cord and peripheral nerve involvement. The pathological changes observed in this disorder are known as *central chromatolysis,* or *central neuritis,* and consist of a characteristic degeneration of the large pyramidal cells (*Betz cells*) of the motor cortex.

A deficiency of niacin brings about visible alterations of neuronal Nissl substance, but the mechanism involved is not yet known. It has been demonstrated that niacin deficiency causes a reduction of cerebral NAD and NADP levels and decreased activity of the enzymes that depend upon these nucleotides. No specific neurochemical lesion, however, has been identified. It is well recognized that, in patients afflicted with pellagra, NAD levels in red blood cells are reduced and the urinary excretion product of niacin (*N*-methylnicotinamide) is diminished. The administration of niacin to pellagrins and to niacin-deficient animals causes the nucleotide content of the blood and the tissues to rise temporarily above normal levels. An experimental myelopathy (*rigid paraplegia*) has been produced in rats by the administration of 6-aminonicotinamide, an analog of nicotinamide that results in 6-amino-NADP. This agent inhibits the activity of 6-phosphogluconate dehydrogenase and a 1,000-fold increase in 6-phosphogluconate levels ensues. 6-Aminonicotinamide, which induces structural changes in glial cells, interferes with the activity of the pentose phosphate pathway. This is believed to result in abnormalities of lipid, nucleic acid, and protein metabolism within glial cells and neurons [55].

PANTOTHENIC ACID

Pantothenic acid, a constituent of CoA, is widely distributed in mammalian tissue. In addition to pantothenic acid, CoA contains ribose, adenine, phosphoric acid, and β-mercaptoethylamine. The sulfhydryl group of the latter is the site that links acid and acetyl groups.

As part of CoA, pantothenic acid participates in a variety of biochemical reactions involved in fatty acid synthesis and oxidation as well as in the metabolism of steroids and ACh. Generally speaking, the reactions mediated by CoA fall into two categories: acetokinases and transacetylases [56]. The vitamin is also essential to the formation of certain amide and peptide linkages.

Relatively high concentrations of pantothenic acid exist in the brain, which does not readily yield its stores. Experimentally induced pantothenic acid deficiency in animals results in lesions of the peripheral nerves. In humans, pantothenic acid deficiency causes numbness and tingling of hands and feet and occasionally a "burning-foot" syndrome. Biochemical changes that have been noted in such patients are characterized by the impaired ability to acetylate p-aminobenzoic acid and by a decline in blood levels of cholesterol and its esters. In addition, evidence of adrenocortical hypofunction has been described [57]. It has been noted that a deficiency of the vitamin in experimental animals results in deranged synthesis of ACh, cholesterol, glucosamine, and galactosamine, in faulty fatty acid oxidation, and in reduced energy production. More specific information concerning the neurochemistry of pantothenic acid deficiency is lacking.

VITAMIN E

α-Tocopherol, the major component of vitamin E, is generously distributed in nature. Investigations aimed at delineating the metabolic role of tocopherols strongly suggest that the vitamin acts as a nonspecific antioxidant and, as such, prevents the peroxidation of polyunsaturated fatty acids, a nonenzymatic reaction that occurs normally in the course of intracellular metabolism. The resultant products of peroxidation are highly damaging to the cell (see also Chap. 34). It is of interest that human infant brain, which is relatively abundant in highly unsaturated fatty acids, contains less tocopherol than does any other tissue, including adipose tissue. It is therefore conceivable that the requirements for vitamin E are higher in infants than in adults. There is evidence that the antioxidant effect of tocopherol preserves reduced glutathione stability through the maintenance of sulfhydryl bonds. It also may play a role in the stabilization of biological membranes.

Experimentally induced vitamin E deficiency in animals has resulted in a number of interesting observations. Myocardial degeneration, a dystrophic process of voluntary muscles, encephalomalacia, axonal dystrophy (particularly pronounced in the dorsal funiculi of the spinal cord), and ceroid (a form of lipochrome pigment) deposits in muscles and neurons have all been described. The persistent inability to absorb fats is the most likely mechanism by which human subjects become deficient in this fat-soluble vitamin. In children, the most common underlying causes of deficiency are celiac disease, cystic fibrosis, and biliary atresia. In the adult, sprue and chronic pancreatitis have been the most frequent offenders. On occasion, a progressive myelopathy, ceroid deposition in smooth muscles, and skeletal muscle lesions that resemble muscular dystrophy have been reported.

It has been postulated that, in the course of *Batten's disease,* the massive peroxidation of essential fatty acids leads to the neuronal accumulation of cross-linked polymers in the form of lipopigments, and ceroid [44, 58]. Normal levels of blood and tissue α-tocopherol have been found in patients afflicted with this disorder (see also Chap. 30).

Protein-Calorie Malnutrition

According to current estimates, approximately one-fourth of the world population may be suffering from varying forms of undernutrition. Although the problem in general is cause for concern, particular significance is attached to the proportion of this population represented by children. The possibility that undernutrition during a period of functional development of the brain may seriously impair subsequent intellectual function has provided a considerable impetus to the study of a causal relationship at the molecular level. Two extreme forms of clinical malnutrition exist that differ in etiology, symptomatology, age of onset, and duration: (1) *marasmus* is a chronic condition that develops in infants between the ages of 6 and 18 months as a result of a deprivation of both calories and proteins; (2) *kwashiorkor* commonly occurs in the second year of life and is due to a deficiency of protein. In practice, intermediate forms of these two syndromes affect the greatest percentage of the undernourished population.

A unifying concept that has emerged is that the brain is markedly susceptible to environmental insults during a period of intense functional differentiation [59, 60] (see also Chap. 23). In the rat, this corresponds to a period of ontogenesis between birth and about 21 days of age, when the growth of neuronal processes and the proliferation of glial cells and myelinogenesis is most rapid. A comparable period in the human is from approximately 30 weeks of gestation to 18 to 24 months of age. Most of our knowledge about neurochemical changes accompanying undernutrition during early life has been derived from animal experimentation. Often, however, too little regard has been given to the timing and duration of experimental undernutrition to make it comparable to that occurring in humans [61]. In addition, the variety of procedures employed to produce nutrient deficiency in animals—restricting periods of suckling, increasing litter size, and decreasing protein alone or protein and calories—makes comparison and interpretation of results difficult. A further complicating factor often lost sight of is the heterogeneous nature of the brain, which is reflected in differences in regional rates of development. However, animal models have provided valuable information, much of which may be extrapolated to the human condition.

Recent reviews have catalogued the structural and biochemical changes in the brain produced by a dietary deficiency of either protein or calories or combination thereof during the prenatal or postnatal period, or both [62–64]. Whole brain and regional cellular proliferation is impaired in both animals and humans exposed to undernutrition, and the severity of the deficit and its persistence is closely related to the timing of the nutritional insult [65]. The decrease in brain DNA content is a reflection of the marked suppression of the synthesis rate observed in rats undernourished during gestation and lactation [66]. Furthermore, it has been suggested that the alteration of DNA levels in undernourished suckling rats results from a delayed glial cell proliferation and migration [67], which has obvious repercussions on myelin formation. Indeed, several lines of evidence have demonstrated the adverse affects of undernutrition on myelinogenesis. The decreased myelin recovery in undernourished infant rats [68–70] is consistent with the reduced whole-brain and regional concentration [66, 71] and synthesis [72] of myelin-associated lipids. An analysis of myelin fractions of protein-calorie malnourished rats during infancy suggests an immaturity of myelin composition [73]. In rats undernourished during lactation, qualitative differences in the composition of myelin proteins exist [73] and their rate of synthesis is markedly reduced [69]. A comparison of general undernutrition and protein deficiency during the suckling period in the rat indicates that the latter has a more severe effect on myelin concentration and composition [74]. The myelin deficit produced in the rat by a deprivation of food from birth was not apparent when undernutrition was initiated at a later age [70]; this confirms the notion that an abnormal myelin synthesis may be secondary to an impairment in glial cell proliferation. Malnourished infants have also been reported to possess a deficiency of myelin [75].

The modification of certain key brain constituents by undernutrition conceivably may mediate changes in behavior. Neonatal undernutrition in rats severely retards the conversion of glucose to amino acids [76]; protein malnutrition in immature pigs [77] and rats [64, 78, 79] alters the levels and metabolism of amino acids. Postnatal protein malnutrition [80, 81] and protein deprivation during gestation and lactation [64] in the rat produces alterations in the levels of neurotransmitters. General undernutrition, as well as severe protein malnutrition, in developing rats specifically decreases the activity of enzymes associated with nerve endings [64, 80, 82, 83, 84]. The incorporation of precursors into brain RNA of perinatally malnourished mice [85] and postnatally undernourished rats [86] is diminished, whereas the rate of cerebral protein synthesis is impaired in young rats malnourished both in utero and during suckling [79].

An important consideration is the extent of reversibility of changes induced by nutritional deficiency: a distinction must be made between biochemical alterations that represent a temporary adaptive response and those due to pathological change that are not reversible by nutritional rehabilitation. Most evidence favors the view that undernutrition during a critical phase of brain development induces biochemical changes that are not reversible by subsequent reinstitution of an adequate diet, even for a prolonged period.

A fundamental question is whether learning capacity is altered by nutritional inadequacy in early life. The subject is covered in several recent reviews [87–89]. It has been suggested that tests designed to increase intellectual performance may be compounded by emotional and maturational defects and other variables arising from non-nutritional causes [90, 91]. In human studies in particular, a multitude of coexisting variables, including disease, cultural differences, and psychological factors, interact with malnutrition and make the interpretation of results difficult. Furthermore, data frequently are obtained from a limited population whose clinical history often is both unknown and compared to an inadequate control population. Nevertheless, studies on severely protein-calorie–deficient children [87–89] and on experimental rats [92, 93] have suggested that intellectual function is drastically altered.

A frequently overlooked consideration is the endocrine status of nutritionally deprived populations [94]: a diminished thyroid function [95], for example, can be expected to contribute to the modification of brain development and mental capacity.

In conclusion, many important findings have recently emerged from animal and human studies. There appears to be a marked correlation between the extent and persistence of neurochemical changes and the age of onset and duration of malnutrition. It seems well established that certain molecular indices of CNS structure and function are irreversibly altered by protein-calorie malnutrition. In the future, controlled studies will be necessary to establish whether specific biochemical changes attributable to nutritional deprivation are reflected in defective learning ability and diminished intellectual development.

References

1. Spector, R. Vitamin homeostasis in the central nervous system. *N. Engl. J. Med.* 296:1393–1398, 1977.
2. Spector, R. Vitamin B$_6$ transport in the central nervous system: In vivo studies. *J. Neurochem.* 30:881–887, 1978.
3. Spector, R., and Greenwald, L. L. Transport and metabolism of vitamin B$_6$ in rabbit brain. *J. Biol. Chem.* 253:2373–2379, 1978.
4. Spector, R. Folic Acid. In M. I. Botez and E. H. Reynolds (eds.), *Neurology, Psychiatry and Internal Medicine.* New York: Raven, 1979. Pp. 187–194.
5. Spector, R. Niacin and niacinamide transport in the central nervous system: In vivo studies. *J. Neurochem.* 33:895–904, 1979.
*6. Rosenberg, L. E. Vitamin-Responsive Inherited Diseases Affecting the Nervous System. In F. Plum (ed.), *Brain Dysfunction in Metabolic Disorders.* New York: Raven, 1974. Pp. 263–271.
*7. von Muralt, A. The role of thiamine in neurophysiology. *Ann. N.Y. Acad. Sci.* 98:499–507, 1962.
*8. Dreyfus, P. M. Transketolase Activity in the Nervous System. In G. E. W. Wohlstenholme, (ed.), *Thiamine Deficiency: Biochemical Lesions and Their Clinical Significance.* Boston: Little, Brown, 1967.

*Key reference.

*9. Peters, R. A. *Biochemical Lesions and Lethal Synthesis.* London: Pergamon, 1963.

10. Dreyfus, P. M. The quantitative histochemical distribution of thiamine in normal rat brain. *J. Neurochem.* 4:183–190, 1959.

11. Pincus, J. H., and Grove, I. Distribution of thiamine phosphate esters in normal and thiamine deficient brain. *Exp. Neurol.* 28:477–483, 1970.

12. McCandless, D. W., and Schenker, S. Encephalopathy of thiamine deficiency: Studies of intracerebral mechanisms. *J. Clin. Invest.* 47:2268–2280, 1968.

13. Geel, S. E., and Dreyfus, P. M. Brain lipid composition of immature thiamine-deficient and undernourished rats. *J. Neurochem.* 24:353–360, 1975.

14. Barchi, R. L., and Braun, P. E. Thiamine in neural membranes. A developmental approach. *Brain Res.* 35:622–624, 1971.

15. Voorhees, C. V., Schmidt, D. E., Barrett, R. J., and Schenker, S. Effects of thiamine deficiency on acetylcholine levels and utilization in vivo in rat brain. *J. Nutr.* 107:1902–1908, 1977.

16. Heinrich, C. P., Stadler, H., and Weiser, H. The effect of thiamine deficiency on the acetylcoenzyme A and acetylcholine levels in the rat brain. *J. Neurochem.* 21:1273–1281, 1973.

17. McCandless, D. W., Curley, A. D., and Cassidy, C. E. Thiamine deficiency and pentose phosphate pathway: Intracerebral mechanisms. *J. Nutr.* 106:1144–1151, 1976.

18. Henderson, G. I., Hoyumpa, A. M., Jr., and Schenker, S. Effects of thiamine deficiency on cerebral and visceral protein synthesis. *Biochem. Pharmacol.* 1677–1683, 1978.

19. Volpe, J. J., and Marasa, J. C. A role for thiamine in the regulation of fatty acid and cholesterol biosynthesis in cultured cells of neural origin. *J. Neurochem.* 30:975–981, 1978.

20. Plaitakis, A., Nicklas, W. J., and Berl, S. Thiamine deficiency: Selective impairment of cerebellar serotonergic system. *Neurology* 28:691–698, 1978.

21. Brin, M. Erythrocyte transketolase in early thiamine deficiency. *Ann. N.Y. Acad. Sci.* 98:528–541, 1962.

22. Dreyfus, P. M. Clinical application of blood transketolase determinations. *N. Engl. J. Med.* 267:596–598, 1962.

23. Zieve, L. Influence of magnesium deficiency on the utilization of thiamine. *Ann. N.Y. Acad. Sci.* 162:732–743, 1969.

24. Blass, J. P., and Gibson, G. E. Deleterious aberrations of a thiamine-requiring enzyme in four patients with Wernicke-Korsakoff syndrome. *N. Engl. J. Med.* 297:1367–1370, 1977.

25. Itokawa, Y., Schulz, R. A., and Cooper, J. R. Thiamine in nerve membranes. *Biochim. Biophys. Acta* 266:293–299, 1972.

*26. Barchi, R. L. The Nonmetabolic Role of Thiamine in Excitable Membrane Function. In C. J. Gubler, M. Fujiwara, and P. M. Dreyfus (eds.), *Thiamine.* New York: Wiley, 1976. Pp. 283–305.

*27. Pincus, J. H. Subacute necrotizing encephalomyelopathy (Leigh's disease): A consideration of clinical features and etiology. *Dev. Med. Child Neurol.* 14:87–101, 1972.

28. Tang, T. T., Good, T. A., Dyken, P. R., Johnsen, S. D., McCreadie, S. R., Sy, S. T., Lardy, H. A., and Rudolph, F. B. Pathogenesis of Leigh's encephalomyelopathy. *J. Pediatr.* 81:189–190, 1972.

29. Blass, J. P., Avigan, J., and Uhlendorf, B. W. A defect in pyruvate decarboxylase in a child with an intermittent movement disorder. *J. Clin. Invest.* 49:423–432, 1970.

*30. Elsas, L. J., Danner, D. J., and Rogers, B. L. Effect of Thiamine on Normal and Mutant Human Branched-chain α-ketoacid Dehydrogenase. In C. J. Gubler, M. Fujiwara, and P. M. Dreyfus (eds.), *Thiamine.* New York: Wiley, 1976. Pp. 335–349.

31. Bowden, J. A., McArthur, C. L., and Fried, M. The inhibition of pyruvate decarboxylation in rat brain by α-ketoisocaproic acid. *Biochem. Med.* 5:101–108, 1971.

*32. Williams, M. A. Vitamin B$_6$ and amino acids: Recent research in animals. *Vitam. Horm.* 22:561–579, 1964.

*33. Axelrod, A. E., and Trakatellis, A. C. Relationship of pyridoxine to immunological phenomena. *Vitam. Horm.* 22:591–607, 1964.

34. Wiss, O., and Weber, F. Biochemical pathology of vitamin B$_6$ deficiency. *Vitam. Horm.* 22:495–501, 1964.

35. Bhagavan, H. N., and Coursin, D. B. Effects of pyridoxine on nucleic acid and protein contents of brain and liver in rats. *Int. J. Vitam. Nutr. Res.* 41:419–423, 1971.

36. Morré, D. M., Kirksey, A., and Das, G. D. Effects of vitamin B$_6$ deficiency on the developing central nervous system of the rat. Gross measurements and cytoarchitectural alterations. *J. Nutr.* 108:1250–1259, 1978.

37. Morré, D. M., Kirksey, A., and Das, G. D. Effects of vitamin B$_6$ deficiency on the developing central nervous system of the rat. Myelination. *J. Nutr.* 108:1260–1265, 1978.

38. Morré, D. M., and Kirksey, A. The effect of a deficiency of vitamin B$_6$ on the specific activity of 2′,3′-cyclic nucleotide 3′-phosphohydrolase of neonatal rat brain. *Brain Res.* 146:200–204, 1978.

39. Stephens, M. C., and Dakshinamurti, K. Brain lipids in pyridoxine-deficient young rats. *Neurobiology (Copenh)* 5:262–269, 1975.

40. Kurtz, D. J., and Kanfer, J. N. Composition of myelin lipids and synthesis of 3-keto-dihydrosphinosine in the vitamin B_6-deficient developing rat. *J. Neurochem.* 20:963–968, 1973.

41. Lott, I. T., Coulombe, T., Di Paolo, R. V., Richardson, E. P., and Levy, H. L. Vitamin B_6-dependent seizures: Pathology and chemical findings in brain. *Neurology (Copenh)* 28:47–54, 1978.

42. Mudd, S. H. Pyridoxine-responsive genetic disease. *Fed. Proc.* 30:970–976, 1971.

43. Agamanolis, D. P., Victor, M., Chester, E. M., Kark, J. A., Hines, J. D., and Harris, J. W. Neuropathology of experimental vitamin B_{12} deficiency in monkeys. *Neurology (Copenh)* 26:905–914, 1976.

44. Stadtman, T. C. Vitamin B_{12}. *Science* 171:859–867, 1971.

45. Cardinale, G. J., Dreyfus, P. M., Auld, P., and Abeles, R. H. Experimental vitamin B_{12} deficiency. *Arch. Biochem. Biophys.* 131:92–99, 1969.

46. Girdwood, R. H. Abnormalities of vitamin B_{12} and folic acid metabolism: Their influence on the nervous system. *Proc. Nutr. Soc.* 27:101–107, 1968.

47. Frenkel, E. P. Abnormal fatty acid metabolism in peripheral nerves of patients with pernicious anemia. *J. Clin. Invest.* 52:1237–1245, 1973.

48. Frenkel, E. P., Kitchens, R. L., and Johnston, J. M. The effect of vitamin B_{12} deprivation on the enzymes of fatty acid synthesis. *J. Biol. Chem.* 248:7540–7546, 1973.

49. Levy, H. L., Mudd, S. H., Schulman, J. D., Dreyfus, P. M., and Abeles, R. H. A derangement in B_{12} metabolism associated with homocystinemia, cystathioninemia, hypomethioninemia and methylmalonic aciduria. *Am. J. Med.* 48:390–397, 1970.

50. Gandy, G., Jacobson, W., and Sidman, R. Inhibition of transmethylation reaction in the central nervous system: An experimental model for subacute combined degeneration of the cord. *J. Pathol.* 109:13–14, 1973.

51. Woodard, J. C., and Newberne, P. M. The pathogenesis of hydrocephalus in newborn rats deficient in vitamin B_{12}. *J. Embryol. Exp. Morphol.* 17:177–187, 1967.

*52. Mahoney, M. J., and Rosenberg, L. E. Inherited defects of B_{12} metabolism. *Am. J. Med.* 48:584–593, 1970.

53. Kishimoto, Y., Williams, M., Moser, H. W., Hignite, C., and Biemann, K. Branched-chain and odd-numbered fatty acids and aldehyde in the nervous system of a patient with deranged vitamin B_{12} metabolism. *J. Lipid Res.* 14:69–77, 1973.

54. Bayliss, E. M., Crowley, J. M., Preece, J. M., Sylvester, P. E., and Marks, V. Influence of folic acid on blood-phenytoin levels. *Lancet* 1:62–64, 1971.

55. Herken, H., Lange, K., Kolbe, H., and Keller, K. Antimetabolic Action on the Pentose Phosphate Pathway in the Central Nervous System Induced by 6-Aminonicotinamide. In E. Genazzani and H. Herken (eds.), *Central Nervous System—Studies on Metabolic Regulation and Function.* Berlin: Springer-Verlag, 1974. Pp. 41–54.

56. Novelli, G. D. Metabolic functions of pantothenic acid. *Physiol. Rev.* 33:525–543, 1953.

57. Bean, W. B., and Hodges, R. E. Pantothenic acid deficiency induced in human subjects. *Proc. Soc. Exp. Biol. Med.* 86:693–698, 1954.

58. Zeeman, W. Studies in the neuronal ceroid-lipofuscinoses. *J. Neuropathol. Exp. Neurol.* 33:1–12, 1974.

*59. Dobbing, J. Undernutrition and the Developing Brain. In A. Lajtha (ed.), *Handbook of Neurochemistry.* New York: Plenum, 1971. Vol. 6, pp. 255–264.

60. Dobbing, J., and Smart, J. L. Vulnerability of developing brain and behavior. *Br. Med. Bull.* 30:164–168, 1974.

61. Dobbing, J. Prenatal Development and Neurological Development. In J. Cravioto, L. Hambraeus, and B. Vahlquist (eds.), *Early Malnutrition and Mental Development.* Vol. XII. Uppsala: Almquist and Wiksell, 1974. Pp. 96–110.

*62. Shoemaker, W. J., and Bloom, F. E. Effect of Undernutrition on Brain Morphology. In R. J. Wurtman and J. J. Wurtman (eds.), *Nutrition and the Brain.* New York: Raven, 1977. Vol. 2, pp. 147–192.

*63. Nowak, T. S., and Munro, H. N. Effects of Protein-Calorie Malnutrition on Biochemical Aspects of Brain Development. In R. J. Wurtman and J. J. Wurtman (eds.), *Nutrition and the Brain.* New York: Raven, 1977. Vol. 2, pp. 193–260.

64. Morgane, P. J., Miller, M., Kemper, T., Stern, W., Forbes, W., Hall, R., Bronzino, J., Kissane, J., Hawrylewicz, E., and Resnick, O. The effect of protein malnutrition on the developing CNS in the rat. *Neurosci. Biobehav. Rev.* 2:137–145, 1978.

65. Winick, M. *Malnutrition and Brain Development.* London: Oxford University Press, 1976.

66. Lewis, P. D., Balazs, R., Patel, A. J., and Johnson, A. L. The effect of undernutrition in early life on cell generation in the rat brain. *Brain Res.* 83:235–247, 1975.

67. Bass, N. H., Netsky, M. G., and Young, E. Effect of neonatal malnutrition on developing cerebrum. I. Microchemical and histologic study of cellular

differentiation in the rat. *Arch. Neurol.* 23:289–302, 1970.

68. Fishman, M. A., Madyastha, P., and Prensky, A. L. The effect of undernutrition on the development of myelin in the rat CNS. *Lipids* 6:458–465, 1971.

69. Wiggins, R. C., Miller, S. L., Benjamins, J. A., Krigman, M. R., and Morell, P. Myelin synthesis during postnatal nutritional deprivation and subsequent rehabilitation. *Brain Res.* 107:257–273, 1976.

70. Wiggins, R. C., and Fuller, G. N. Early postnatal starvation causes lasting brain hypomyelination. *J. Neurochem.* 30:1231–1237, 1978.

71. Geison, R. L., and Waisman, H. A. Effects of nutritional states on rat brain maturation as measured by lipid composition. *J. Nutr.* 100:315–324, 1970.

72. Chase, H. P., Dorsey, J., and McKhann, G. M. The effect of malnutrition on the synthesis of a myelin lipid. *Pediatrics* 40:551–559, 1967.

73. Figlewiez, D. A., Hofteig, J. H., and Druse, M. J. Maternal deficiency of protein and calories during lactation in effect upon CNS myelin subfraction formation in rat offspring. *Life Sci.* 23:2163–2172, 1978.

74. Reddy, P. V., Das, A., and Sastry, P. S. Quantitative and compositional changes in myelin of undernourished and protein malnourished rat brains. *Brain Res.* 161:227–235, 1979.

75. Fox, J. H., Fishman, M. A., Dodge, P. R., and Prensky, A. L. The effect of malnutrition on human central nervous myelin. *Neurology* 22:1213–1216, 1972.

76. Balazs, R., and Patel, A. J. Factors affecting the biochemical maturation of the brain: Effect of undernutrition during early life. *Prog. Brain Res.* 40:115–128, 1973.

77. Badger, T. M., and Tumbleson, M. E. Protein-caloric malnutrition in young miniature swine: Brain free amino acids. *J. Nutr.* 104:1329–1338, 1974.

78. Roach, M. K., Corbin, J., and Pennington, W. Effect of undernutrition on amino acid compartmentation in the developing rat brain. *J. Neurochem.* 22:521–528, 1974.

79. Patel, A. J., Atkinson, D. J., and Balazs, R. Effect of undernutrition on metabolic compartmentation of glutamate and on the incorporation of ^{14}C leucine into protein in developing rat brain. *Dev. Psychobiol.* 8:453–465, 1975.

80. Sobotka, T. J., Cook, M. P., and Bhodie, R. E. Neonatal malnutrition: Neurochemical, hormonal and behavioral manifestations. *Brain Res.* 65:443–457, 1974.

81. Shoemaker, W. J., and Wurtmann, R. J. Effect of perinatal undernutrition on the metabolism of catecholamines in the rat brain. *J. Nutr.* 103:1537–1546, 1973.

*82. Adlard, P. P., and Dobbing, J. Vulnerability of developing brain. V. Effects of total and postnatal undernutrition on regional brain enzyme activities in three-week-old rats. *Pediatr. Res.* 6:38–42, 1972.

83. Rajalashmi, R., Parameswaran, M., Telang, S. D., and Ramakrishnan, C. V. Effects of undernutrition and protein deficiency on glutamate dehydrogenase and decarboxylase in rat brain. *J. Neurochem.* 23:129–133, 1974.

84. Eckhert, C., Barnes, R. H., and Levitsky, D. A. The effect of protein-energy undernutrition induced during a period of suckling on cholinergic enzyme activity in the rat brain stem. *Brain Res.* 101:372–377, 1976.

85. Lee, C. J. Biosynthesis and characteristics of brain protein and ribonucleic acid in mice subjected to neonatal infection or undernutrition. *J. Biol. Chem.* 245:1998–2004, 1970.

86. De Guglielmone, A. E. R., Soto, A. M., and Duvilanksi, B. H. Neonatal undernutrition and RNA synthesis in developing rat brain. *J. Neurochem.* 22:529–533, 1974.

*87. Tizard, J. Early malnutrition, growth and mental development in man. *Br. Med. Bull.* 30:169–174, 1974.

*88. Cravioto, J., Hambraeus, L., and Vahlquist, B. (eds.). *Early Malnutrition and Mental Development.* Vol. XII. Uppsala: Almquist and Wiksell, 1974.

*89. Pollitt, E., and Thomson, C. Protein-Calorie Malnutrition and Behavior: A View from Psychology. In R. J. Wurtman and J. J. Wurtman (eds.), *Nutrition and the Brain.* New York: Raven, 1977. Vol. 2, pp. 261–307.

90. Levitsky, D. A. Early malnutrition and behavior. *N.Y. State J. Med.* 71:350–353, 1971.

91. Levine, S., and Wiener, S. G. Malnutrition and early environmental experience: Possible interactive effects on later behavior. *Behav. Biol.* 17:51–70, 1976.

92. Baird, A., Widdowson, E. M., and Cowley, J. J. Effects of caloric and protein deficiencies early in life on the subsequent learning ability of rats. *Br. J. Nutr.* 25:391–403, 1971.

93. Wells, A. M., Geist, C. R., and Zimmermann, R. R. Influence of environmental and nutritional factors on problem solving in the rat. *Percept. Mot. Skills* 35:235–241, 1972.

94. Pimstone, B. Endocrine function in protein-calorie malnutrition. *Clin. Endocrinol.* 5:79–95, 1976.

95. Shambaugh, G. E., and Wilbur, J. F. The effect of caloric deprivation upon thyroid function in the neonatal rat. *Endocrinology* 94:1145–1149, 1974.

Robert A. Fishman

Chapter 34. Brain Edema

Cerebral edema accompanies a wide variety of pathological processes in brain, and it contributes to the morbidity and mortality of many neurological diseases. It plays a major role in head injury, stroke, and brain tumor. Edema also has a part in cerebral infections, including brain abscess, encephalitis and meningitis, lead encephalopathy, hypoxia, hypoosmolality, the disequilibrium syndromes associated with dialysis and diabetic keto-acidosis, and in the various forms of obstructive hydrocephalus. Clinical investigation and laboratory studies of brain edema using neurochemical, physiological, and ultrastructural techniques have clarified many pathological and clinical uncertainties. It is known that cerebral edema may occur in several different forms and that it is inappropriate to view it as a single pathological or clinical entity. The reader is referred to several monographs and symposia that deal with various aspects of the problem [1–5].

DEFINITIONS

In the early literature, brain edema and brain swelling were considered to be different processes, but these terms are now used synonymously. *Brain edema* is defined as an increase in brain volume caused by an increase in water and sodium content generally associated with a fall in the brain potassium content. When brain edema is well localized or mild in degree, it is associated with little or no clinical evidence of brain dysfunction; when severe, it causes major focal or generalized signs of dysfunction (or both), including various types of cerebral herniation and medullary failure of respiration and circulation.

Brain engorgement is an increase in the blood volume of the brain caused by obstruction of the cerebral veins and venous sinuses, or by arterial vasodilatation, as occurs with hypercapnia. Brain engorgement may result in a major increase in brain volume during craniotomy because of the absence of the rigid restriction of the bony skull, and such vasodilatation may coexist with brain edema. Intracranial hypertension is commonly due to brain edema, but may be due to brain engorgement without edema, as seen with the inhalation of 5% carbon dioxide in normal subjects.

MEASUREMENT OF EDEMA

The usual procedure for the definition of edema in vivo involves sampling the edematous area of brain (or spinal cord) and a control area (preferably the homologous contralateral area) and determining the respective dry-weight percentages. This is most conveniently done by weighing each fresh tissue sample (wet weight) in a tared container, drying the sample at approximately $100°C$ to constant weight (usually within 12–24 hr), and reweighing to obtain the weight of the residue (dry weight). The percentage dry weight (P) is simply calculated as

$$P = (\text{dry weight/wet weight}) \times 100$$

The percentage of swelling (edema) or of shrinkage can then be calculated by the formula of Elliott and Jasper [6]:

$$[(P_{cont} - P_{exptl})/P_{exptl}] \times 100 = \text{Percent swelling (or shrinkage)}$$

The same techniques are suitable for measuring edema in vitro.

Biochemistry of Brain Edema

The chemical basis of brain edema was first established by Stewart-Wallace [7] in terms of the changes in water and electrolyte content of the edematous tissue surrounding brain tumors. He showed that the cortex surrounding tumors showed only a minor increase in swelling (less than 5%) compared to the white matter, where the swelling was increased greatly (77%). These data verified in chemical terms the neuropathological observations that white matter is far more vulnerable to edema formation than is the gray matter. The clinical observations were later confirmed in various experimental models, including freezing lesions, stab wounds, implanted tumors, compressive lesions due to intracranial balloons, and such foreign materials as psillium seeds [3]. With these various disruptive lesions, the edema fluid was shown to have the features of a plasma exudate, that is, a high content of sodium and plasma protein with an increase in the volume of the extracellular fluid space. The most commonly studied lesion has been a freezing lesion of the hemisphere, but the data obtained with the entire gamut of disruptive lesions have been similar.

Laboratory models of hypoxia and water intoxication were shown to have an increase in brain water and sodium, but the extracellular fluid space was decreased in volume, in contradistinction to the findings in the models discussed above. These changes were the basis for the delineation by Klatzo [8] of the vasogenic and cytotoxic brain edemas.

There has also been special interest in the ability of various toxins, most notably triethyl tin and lead, to induce brain edema. Triethyl tin induces a severe degree of brain edema that affects both the white and gray matter in humans and animals [9, 10]. The major accumulation of water and sodium is intracellular, with astrocytic swelling more marked than neuronal swelling. There is a striking abnormality of the white matter, with accumulation of fluid within the myelin sheath; the myelin lamellae split at the interperiod line to form large blebs. Thus, triethyl tin appears to have special effects on the integrity of the oligodendroglia, from whose cellular membranes myelin is derived. The water and sodium content of the white matter is increased, but the integrity of the blood-brain barrier is preserved, as measured with radio-iodinated albumin or vital dyes. Thus, unlike the findings in lead encephalopathy, the integrity of cerebral capillary endothelial cells is preserved in triethyl tin poisoning. The biochemical basis for the toxic effects of triethyl tin is not known specifically. The activity of $(Na^+ + K^+)$-ATPase, the enzyme that functions as the sodium-ion pump in cellular membranes (Chap. 6), has not been shown to be affected. Morphological changes in brain mitochondria have been described, as has inhibition of oxidative phosphorylation, but the significance of these observations in edema formation is not clear. It is of interest that a surgical biopsy obtained in a patient with the brain edema of Reye's syndrome revealed a splitting of the myelin lamellae reminiscent of triethyl tin intoxication, so such changes are not unique to that toxin [11].

By using an animal model of lead encephalopathy, Goldstein and coworkers [12] demonstrated that the capillary endothelial cell is selectively poisoned by lead; this gives rise to massive vasogenic edema, particularly in infants. The special vulnerability of the immature brain to lead intoxication has not been explained.

IN VITRO STUDIES OF BRAIN EDEMA

An extensive literature on factors influencing the swelling of brain slices in vitro has been summarized by Katzman and Pappius [3]. These studies are relevant chiefly to the occurrence of cellular (cytotoxic) edema as opposed to vasogenic edema, because the blood-brain barrier is absent in such preparations. Hypoxic conditions or addition of chemical inhibitors of glycolysis to the incubating medium cause cellular swelling, in each case attributable to a failure of the energy-dependent active transport of sodium and water from the cell, with a fall in brain ATP levels. Increases in the water and sodium content of rat cortex associated with decreased inulin space have been used as an in vitro bioassay for the analysis of factors responsible for tissue swelling [13, 14].

The cardioactive glycoside ouabain has been identified as a specific inhibitor of sodium and potassium transport (see Chap. 6), the effect of which is mediated by its binding to and inhibition of the enzyme $(Na^+ + K^+)$-ATPase. Ouabain causes cellular edema when used in studies either in vitro with brain slices or in vivo. Local application of ouabain to the cortex results in convulsions and in morphological and biochemical changes of edema [15]. Status spongiosus was observed with light microscopy, and evidence of cellular swelling was revealed with electron microscopy. Both neuronal and glial elements probably are affected by the topical application of ouabain in both in vivo and in vitro studies, but there is uncertainty about possible differences in the vulnerability of the two cell types to ouabain and to other edema-producing agents.

FREE RADICALS

An experimental literature supports a role for free radicals in the genesis of the permeability changes that underlie brain edema [16, 17]. *Free radicals* are defined as molecules or atoms with an unpaired electron. Free radicals possess unusual chemical reactivity, including an ability to react with unsaturated bonds (for example, in membrane lipids) to produce fragmentation of the chain. Free radicals are short-lived because they are inactivated rapidly by either direct chemical transmutation or specific enzymes. Three free radicals studied in various biological systems are *superoxide ions* $(O_2^{\cdot})$, *hydroxyl radicals* $(OH^{\cdot})$, and *singlet oxygen* $(O^{\cdot})$. Specific enzymes, including superoxide dismutase and catalase [18], rapidly convert the free radicals to less reactive metabolites. Many publications suggest that free radicals are involved in the peroxidation of membrane lipids [19]. In such peroxidation, two oxygen atoms are added across the $C=C$ bond to form a peroxide; this ultimately leads to disruption of the double bond and formation of aldehydes. The role of free radicals in the pathogenesis of the various types of brain edema is under active study. Experimentally, protective effects of barbiturates on the development of hypoxic edema may be related to the drug's pro-tective action against the effects of free radicals (apart from the protective effects of depressing brain metabolism) [20]. Free radicals have a role in the process of phagocytosis by polymorphonuclear granulocytes that is of special interest because granulocytes and their products are the purulent exudate associated with *granulocytic brain edema*, observed in purulent meningitis and brain abscess. The presence in pus of such polyunsaturated fatty acids as arachidonic and linoleic acids has been considered to contribute to the induction of edema [21]. Data indicate that polyunsaturated fatty acid–induced brain edema is associated with the presence of increased superoxide formation in the cortex [22].

POLYUNSATURATED FATTY ACIDS

The ability of the membranes of polymorphonuclear leukocytes to induce cortical swelling has served as an in vitro model of granulocytic brain edema [14, 21]. Analysis of the granulocytic membranes reveals that only lipid-soluble components are responsible for edema formation. Further analysis of the membrane lipids has demonstrated that several polyunsaturated fatty acids (PUFAs) including arachidonic acid ($C_{20:4}$) and linoleic acid ($C_{18:2}$), produce edema, whereas such saturated fatty acids as palmitic acid ($C_{16:0}$) has no effects. Arachidonic acid is of special interest because it is a major constituent of the cellular and subcellular membranes of normal brain tissue and brain tumors, as well as of granulocytic leukocytes. That arachidonic acid is a precursor of the postaglandins is not considered relevant to edema production. First, other PUFAs were equal to arachidonic acid in their edema-producing effects. Second, the prostaglandins were shown to lack edema-producing effects in the bioassay system [21]. Probably only free PUFAs produce edema, that is, protein-bound PUFAs are inactive in this regard. The special vulnerability of the brain to develop swelling with heterogenous injuries and with malignant tumors may depend on the local release of intrinsic arachidonic acid and other polyunsaturated lipids from a bound to a free form. As noted above, the superoxide free radical may mediate this effect, which is shown by the increased formation of lipid peroxides. Furthermore, adrenal glucocorticoids inhibit the release of arachidonic acid from cell membranes; this may be an important factor in the antiedema effects of such steroids [23]. This hypothesis requires substantiation in various models of brain edema.

NEUROTRANSMITTER EFFECTS

Reports indicate that dopamine, norepinephrine, and the excitatory neurotransmitter amino acids, glutamate and aspartate, and their structural analogs and isomers each may induce brain edema in vitro [22]. However, ACh, choline, 5-HT, and the inhibitory neurotransmitter acids had no such effect. Whether these in vitro effects of the excitatory neurotransmitters on brain permeability and water content contribute to brain edema formation in such disease states as concussion or the convulsive disorders requires further elucidation.

Pathophysiology of Brain Edema

Klatzo [8] separated brain edema into two major categories, vasogenic edema and cytotoxic edema, based on neuropathological and experimental observations. *Vasogenic edema* appropriately indicates the importance of the capillary endothelial cell in the pathogenesis of this type of edema. The term *cellular edema* is preferable to *cytotoxic,* because it focuses on the importance of increased cellular volume as the basis for the edema and avoids assuming that toxic states are necessarily the cause; that is, cellular edema may arise from energy depletion per se. To these has been added a third general category, termed *interstitial* or *hydrocephalic edema* [24, 25], which refers to the increase in brain water that characterizes hydrocephalus. The features of the three forms of cerebral edema are summarized in Table 34-1 in terms of pathogenesis, location, and composition of the edema fluid and changes in capillary permeability. Two additional forms of brain edema, *ischemic* and *granulocytic,* share features of these major categories.

VASOGENIC EDEMA

Vasogenic edema is the most common form of brain edema observed in clinical practice. It is characterized by increased permeability of brain capillary endothelial cells to macromolecules such as albumin and various others, the entry of which is limited by the capillary endothelial cells. The special anatomical features and permeability characteristics of brain capillaries and the blood-brain barrier are described in Chap. 25. In the vasogenic edemas, the functional integrity of the endothelial cells is altered. Increased endothelial permeability has been established in various experimental models already mentioned, including freezing lesions, stab wounds, brain compression, anoxia, experimental brain tumors, and allergic encephalomyelitis [2, 26]. The increase in permeability has been shown to vary inversely with the molecular weight of various markers, with a greater increase in the entry of inulin (molecular weight 5,000) than that of albumin (molecular weight 69,000). There is ultrastructural evidence for defects in the tight endothelial cell junctions characteristic of the blood-brain barrier as well as evidence for an increase in the number of pinocytotic vesicles in the endothelial cells which appear responsible for the transport of macromolecules. Growing evidence indicates that increased vesicular transport is characteristic of the vasogenic edemas [27, 28]. The quantitative importance of each of these changes is not known. The cerebral white matter is far more vulnerable than is the gray matter to vasogenic edema, but this vulnerability is not well understood; it may be related to the low capillary density and blood flow in normal white matter, compared to the cortical and subcortical gray matter. The extracellular fluid volume is increased by the edema fluid, which is a plasma filtrate containing some plasma protein.

Vasogenic edema is associated with clinical disorders in which a positive brain scan is frequently noted, including brain tumor, abscess, hemorrhage, infarction, and contusion. It also occurs with lead encephalopathy and with purulent meningitis. An increase in endothelial-cell permeability is responsible for the characteristic increase in CSF

Table 34-1. Classification of Brain Edema

	Vasogenic	Cellular (Cytotoxic)	Interstitial (Hydrocephalic)
Pathogenesis	Increased capillary permeability	Cellular swelling: glial, neuronal, endothelial	Increased brain fluid due to block of CSF absorption
Location of Edema	Chiefly white matter	Gray and white matter	Chiefly periventricular white matter in hydrocephalus
Edema Fluid Composition	Plasma filtrate, including plasma proteins	Increased intracellular water and sodium	Cerebrospinal fluid
Extracellular Fluid Volume	Increased	Decreased	Increased
Capillary Permeability to Large Molecules (RISA, Inulin)	Increased	Normal	Normal
CLINICAL DISORDERS			
Syndromes	Brain tumor, abscess, infarction, trauma, hemorrhage, lead encephalopathy	Hypoxia, hypoosmolality (water intoxication, etc.); disequilibrium syndromes; ischemia; purulent meningitis (granulocytic edema): Reye's syndrome	Obstructive hydrocephalus; pseudotumor (?)
	Ischemia; purulent meningitis (granulocytic edema)		Purulent meningitis (granulocytic edema)
EEG Changes	Focal slowing common	Generalized slowing	EEG often normal
THERAPEUTIC EFFECTS			
Steroids	Beneficial in brain tumor, abscess	Not effective (? Reye's syndrome)	Uncertain effectiveness (? pseudotumor, ? meningitis)
Osmotherapy	Reduces volume of normal brain tissue only, *acutely*	Reduces brain volume *acutely* in hypoosmolality	Rarely useful
Acetazolamide	? Effect	No effect	Minor usefulness
Furosemide	? Effect	No effect	Minor usefulness

Source: Adapted from Klatzo (*J. Neuropathol. Exp. Neurol.* 26:1–14, 1967), Manz (*Hum. Pathol.* 5:291–313, 1974), and Fishman (In *Cerebrospinal Diseases of the Nervous System.* Philadelphia: Saunders, 1980).

protein observed in these disorders. Vasogenic edema can act as a mass displacing brain and can be responsible for the various types of cerebral herniation. The functional manifestations of vasogenic edema include focal neurological deficits, focal EEG slowing, disturbances of consciousness, and severe intracranial hypertension. In patients with primary or metastatic brain tumor, the clinical deficits are often caused more by the peritumoral edema than by the tumor mass itself.

CELLULAR (CYTOTOXIC) EDEMA

Cellular edema is characterized by swelling of all the cellular elements of the brain (neurons, glia, and endothelial cells), with a concomitant reduction in the volume of the brain's extracellular fluid space.

The occurrence of such changes in acute ischemia was described by van Haarveld [29], who used a rapid increase in electrical impedance as an index. Hossmann [30] studied such changes in cats subjected to clamping of the middle cerebral artery for 30 minutes. This resulted in a rapid increase in electrical resistance of the tissue, which indicated an acute reduction in the volume of the extracellular fluid space from a control value of 19 percent to about 11 percent. Brain cells swell within seconds of hypoxia because the ATP-dependent sodium pump within cells fails; sodium rapidly accumulates within cells, and water follows, to maintain osmotic equilibrium [31]. Capillary permeability usually is not affected in the various cellular edemas; patients have a normal brain scan and normal CSF protein.

The causes of cellular edema include

1. Cerebral energy depletion due to hypoxia, as seen after cardiac arrest or asphyxia. The cellular swelling is osmotically determined by the appearance of increased intracellular osmoles (largely sodium, lactate, and hydrogen ions) which induce the rapid entry of water into cells [32].
2. Acute hypoosmolality of the plasma and extracellular fluid is due to acute dilutional hyponatremia, inappropriate secretion of antidiuretic hormone, or acute sodium depletion [33–35].
3. Osmotic disequilibrium syndromes with hemodialysis or diabetic ketoacidosis, wherein excessive intracellular solutes result in excessive hydration when the plasma osmolality is rapidly reduced with therapy [36]. The precise composition of the osmotically active intracellular solutes responsible for cellular swelling in the disequilibrium syndromes associated with hemodialysis and diabetic ketoacidosis is not known.

In uremia, the intracellular solutes presumably include a number of organic acids that have been recovered in the dialysis bath. In diabetic ketoacidosis, the intracellular solutes include glucose and ketone bodies. However, some osmotically active intracellular solutes have not been identified.

These are called *idiogenic osmoles*. Increased intracellular osmolality in excess of the plasma level causes cellular swelling and also is responsible for complex changes in brain metabolism that affect the concentration of the neurotransmitter amino acids, ammonia, and other metabolites [37]. There is no evidence of cerebral edema in uremic encephalopathy [38] in terms of an increase in brain water content. However, impedance studies have not been conducted in uremic encephalopathy. These might provide evidence of cellular edema, despite lack of evidence of a change in the total water content in brain.

An extensive literature also exists on experimental cellular brain edema induced by toxic metabolic inhibitors, such as dinitrophenol, 3-acetylpyridine, 6-aminonicotinamide, and triethyl tin, which cause variable degrees of cellular swelling [3]. The biochemical basis is not known.

Major changes in cerebral function (stupor, coma, decreased seizure threshold, and diffuse electroencephalographic slowing) occur with the cellular edemas. The encephalopathy in acute hypoosmolality is often severe, but in sustained states of hypoosmolality of the same severity, neurological function may be spared. The brain adapts to hyponatremia by losing intracellular osmoles, chiefly potassium, thereby preserving cellular volume [39].

Reye's Syndrome

Reye's syndrome is an acute, noninflammatory encephalopathy of childhood accompanied by fatty degeneration of the liver. It is associated with hyperammonemia, hypoglycemia, organic acidemia, increased serum amino acids, and severe brain edema [11, 40, 41]. Liver dysfunction, usually present at the onset of the encephalopathy, is characterized by hyperammonemia, but there is usually little or no icterus. Elevation of plasma and urine tyramine and tyrosine has also been reported [42], and it is possible that tyramine or its metabolite, octopamine, may adversely affect the brain as a "false neurotransmitter." A decrease in the plasma ratio of branch-chain to aromatic amino acids also has been reported [43]. Liver biopsy shows aromatic microvesicular fat and prominent mitochondrial swelling. The pathogenesis of the severe brain edema is unknown. Aflatoxins, products of certain strains of *Aspergillus flavus,* have been suggested as toxic agents responsible for the liver injury and brain edema [44]. Elevation of circulating short-chain fatty acids has been suggested as responsible for coma in Reye's syndrome [45]. However, these short-chain fatty acids, unlike the several polyunsaturated fatty acids, have not been shown to cause cellular edema. The brain shows cellular edema with myelin bleb formation, astrocyte and glial swelling, and altered mitochondria with pleomorphism and matrix expansion [11]. The brain edema of Reye's syndrome is not usually seen in other forms of liver failure, except when there is acute and massive hepatic insufficiency.

ISCHEMIC BRAIN EDEMA
Acute hypoxia causes cellular edema, which is followed by the development of vasogenic edema as infarction develops. The onset of vasogenic edema, as reflected by a positive radionuclide scan, usually occurs several days after an acute arterial occlusion. The delay is obtaining a positive radionuclide brain scan after an ischemic stroke illustrates that the passage of time is needed for the defects in endothelial cell function to develop and mature. The delay in abnormal uptake may depend on the appearance of newly formed capillaries, which are more permeable than mature blood vessels [26]. Verhas and coworkers [46] found that the maximal intensity of abnormal technitium-99 uptake in radionuclide brain scans of 84 patients with cerebral infarction took place between 10 and 30 days after onset of symptoms. Most patients with arterial occlusion have a combination of cellular edema, developing first, and then vasogenic edema; together these are termed *ischemic brain edema.* The two phases overlap. The cellular phase takes place over minutes to hours and may be reversible. The vasogenic phase takes place over hours to days and results in infarction, which is an irreversible process. The factors that determine the different

outcomes of both components of ischemic edema are poorly understood.

INTERSTITIAL (HYDROCEPHALIC) EDEMA
Interstitial edema is the third type, best characterized in obstructive hydrocephalus, in which there is an increase in the water and sodium content of the periventricular white matter, due to the movement of CSF across the ventricular walls [47, 48]. Obstruction of the circulation of the CSF within the ventricular system (or of CSF absorption in the subarachnoidal space) results in the transependymal movement of CSF and, thereby, an absolute increase in the volume of the brain's extracellular fluid. The chemical change are those of edema, with one exception: the periventricular white matter is rapidly reduced, rather than increased, in volume, because of the rapid disappearance of myelin lipids as the hydrostatic pressures within the white matter increase. The physiological, biochemical, and temporal factors that determine restoration of the cerebral mantle after shunting require elucidation. There are usually relatively minor functional manifestations of interstitial edema in chronic hydrocephalus unless the changes are advanced, when dementia and gait disorder become prominent. The EEG is often normal. This indicates that the accumulation of CSF in the periventricular extracellular fluid space is much better tolerated than is the presence of plasma in the extracellular fluid space in vasogenic edema, which is characterized by focal neurological signs and EEG slowing. The differences in the ionic and protein composition of plasma and CSF may be a factor in explaining the disparate functional responses.

GRANULOCYTIC BRAIN EDEMA
Severe brain edema occurs with brain abscess and purulent meningitis, the result of collections of pus that often are sterile as a result of antibiotic treatment. Such edema, associated with membranous products of granulocytes (pus), has been termed *granulocytic brain edema.* The features of cellular and vasogenic edema occur concurrently in purulent meningitis, and in severe cases, interstitial (hydrocephalic) edema also develops; that is, granu-

locytic brain edema may include the features of all three types. The vasogenic edema in purulent meningitis is associated with a marked increase in endothelial-cell permeability (as evidenced by the increased CSF protein) and in positive scans using radioisotopes or contrast-enhanced computerized tomography. Graded changes in membrane permeability affecting capillary and arachnoid villus function were found in a canine model of pneumococcal meningitis [49]. In purulent meningitis, the membranes of capillaries, brain cells, and the arachnoid villi are adversely affected. Possibly the presence of free radicals may underlie the membrane damage in each case.

The pharmacological treatment of brain edema is based on the use of (1) glucocorticoids, (2) osmotherapy, and (3) drugs that reduce CSF formation. Hypothermia and barbiturate therapy have also been tested experimentally and in clinical practice. Discussion will be limited to a brief consideration of the mechanisms of action only.

Treatment of Brain Edema

GLUCOCORTICOIDS

The adrenal glucocorticoids were introduced in the treatment of peritumoral brain edema by Galicich and French [50] and by Rasmussen and Gulati [51]. The rationale for the use of steroids was largely empirical in origin. Prompted by Menkin's [52] earlier work, Prados and coworkers [53] showed that crude adrenocortical extract protected capillary integrity in physiological studies of the cat cerebral cortex. Since 1961, various high-potency glucocorticoids, chiefly dexamethasone, have been used widely in the management of intracranial hypertension and brain edema. Widespread conviction exists among neurologists and neurosurgeons that these steroids may dramatically and rapidly (in hours) begin to reduce the focal and general signs of brain tumor. The mechanism of such beneficial effects is poorly understood [54]. There has been much interest in the antiinflammatory, immunosuppressive and antiedema activities of glucocorticoids [4, 5, 55, 56]. The major

mechanism suggested to explain its usefulness in vasogenic brain edema is its direct effect on endothelial cell function that restores normal permeability.

The mechanism of action of adrenal steroids on inflammation and immune mechanisms is a fundamental issue in biology. It is difficult to relate much of the basic information in the literature to the beneficial effects of steroids in brain edema. Of special interest is that glucocorticoids were shown to inhibit the release of arachidonic acid from cellular membranes [23]. In view of the ability of arachidonic acid to induce both vasogenic and cellular edema, it is possible that one of the beneficial effects of steroids may be related to inhibition of release of edema-producing PUFAs from cellular membranes. A specific effect of glucocorticoids on free-radical metabolism has not been shown.

Although published data indicate that dexamethasone has therapeutic value in the treatment of vasogenic edema associated with brain tumor, brain abscess, and head injury, its effectiveness in acute cerebral infarction has not been established [57]. The literature recommending its use in stroke has, in general, been poorly documented and is controversial [2]. Steroids may be useful in the treatment of intracerebral hematoma with extensive vasogenic edema due to the mass effect of the clot. Steroid therapy has been used extensively in head injury. Its effectiveness has been documented [5, 56], but the decrease in morbidity and mortality attributable to steroids is not great. Although existing reports are difficult to assess, there are no convincing data, clinical or experimental, that glucocorticoids have beneficial effects in the cellular edema associated with hypoosmolality, asphyxia, or hypoxia in the absence of infarction with mass effects. There is little basis for recommending steroids in the treatment of the cerebral edema associated with cardiac arrest or asphyxia. Mulley and coworkers [57] have recently provided a double-blind study of the effects of dexamethasome in acute stroke. Results led them to conclude that there is no indication for the routine administration of dexamethasone to a heterogenous group of stroke patients.

OSMOTHERAPY

The effects of a variety of hypertonic solutions, including urea, mannitol, and glycerol, on CSF formation and intracranial pressure have been discussed above. The various solutes have been difficult to compare because a large variety of laboratory models, dosages, time intervals, pathological processes, and other variables have been used. Few data are available regarding the levels of plasma osmolality achieved with the use of various solutions and dosage schedules [58, 59].

A few principles seem certain [39]. First, the brain volume will fall only as long as an osmotic gradient exists between blood and brain that allows the water shift that results in the decrease in brain volume and intracranial pressure. Second, osmotic gradients obtained with hypertonic parenteral fluids are short-lived because each of the solutes in use reaches an equilibrium concentration in the brain after a delay of only a few hours. Third, the parts of the brain most likely to "shrink" are those that have normal endothelial cell permeability; thus, in instances of focal vasogenic edema, the normal regions of the hemisphere shrink, but the edematous regions with increased capillary permeability do not. Fourth, a rebound in the severity of the edema may follow any of the suggested hypertonic solutions, because the solute is not excluded from the edematous tissue; if tissue osmolality rises, the tissue water is increased. Finally, there is a poor rationale for the chronic use of hypertonic fluids, either orally or parenterally, because the brain adapts to sustained hyperosmolality of the plasma with an increase in intracellular osmolality due to entry of the added solute.

ACETAZOLAMIDE AND FUROSEMIDE

As an inhibitor of carbonic anhydrase (the enzyme that catalyzes the formation of carbonic acid from carbon dioxide and water), acetazolamide causes about 50 percent reduction in the rate of CSF formation within the ventricles, presumably by reducing the availability of hydrogen ions to exchange with sodium ions within the cells of the choroid plexus. Bulk formation of CSF, normally about 500 ml per day, is directly dependent upon the rate of sodium transport, with rapid diffusion of water to maintain isoosmolality with the plasma. Acetazolamide may have a limited role in the treatment of the interstitial edema of obstructive hydrocephalus and pseudotumor, because it reduces the bulk formation of CSF and thereby would reduce the transependymal movement of CSF into the adjacent hemisphere [60, 61]. Preliminary data indicate that acetazolamide and furosemide may be useful in the treatment of vasogenic edema, because the induction of reduced CSF formation might facilitate the drainage of edema fluid from the edematous cerebrum to the ventricular system [62, 63]. Furosemide also inhibits the formation of CSF by about 25 percent by a mechanism independent of carbonic anhydrase [64]. When the drugs were used together experimentally in rabbits, CSF formation was reduced by about 75 percent.

HYPOTHERMIA AND BARBITURATES

Hypothermia has been used to treat brain injury and brain edema in both the operating room and critical care units. Its use is based on the reduction in cerebral metabolism, cerebral blood flow, and brain volume obtained with experimental hyperthermia, which has been shown to protect animals from a variety of acute cerebral injuries. Its role in clinical practice is not well defined [65]. Experimentally, barbiturates have been shown partially to protect animals from ischemic infarction [66]. Several preliminary reports suggest that barbiturates may be useful clinically. It is not clear whether the protective effects require anesthetic doses to suppress brain metabolism or whether lesser doses may prove effective, by interfering with the ability of free radicals to induce lipid peroxidation. Whether use of barbiturates will be validated in the therapy of brain edema awaits further study [67, 68].

References

*1. Beks, J. W. F., Bosch, D. A., and Brock, M. (eds.). *Intracranial Pressure*. III. New York: Springer-Verlag, 1976.

*Key reference.

*2. Katzman, R., et al. *Brain Edema in Stroke. Stroke* 8:509–540, 1977.

*3. Katzman, R., and Pappius, H. M. *Brain Electrolytes and Fluid Metabolism.* Baltimore: Williams & Wilkins, 1973.

*4. Pappius, H. M., and Feindel, W. (eds.). *Dynamics of Brain Edema.* New York: Springer-Verlag, 1976.

*5. Reulen, H. J., and Schurmann, K. (eds.). *Steroids and Brain Edema.* Berlin: Springer-Verlag, 1972.

6. Elliott, K. A. C., and Jasper, H. Measurement of experimentally induced brain swelling and shrinkage. *Am. J. Physiol.* 157:122–129, 1949.

7. Stewart-Wallace, A. M. A biochemical study of cerebral tissue and of changes in cerebral edema. *Brain* 62:426–438, 1939.

8. Klatzo, I. Neuropathological aspects of brain edema. *J. Neuropathol. Exp. Neurol.* 26:1–14, 1967.

9. Hirano, A., Zimmerman, H. M., and Levine, S. Intramyelinic and extracellular spaces in tri-ethyl tin intoxication. *J. Neuropathol. Exp. Neurol.* 27:571–580, 1968.

10. Katzman, R., Aleu, F., and Wilson, C. Further observations on tri-ethyl tin edema. *Arch. Neurol.* 9:178–187, 1963.

11. Partin, J. C., Partin, J. S., Schubert, W., and McLaurin, R. L. Brain ultrastructure in Reye's syndrome. *J. Neuropathol. Exp. Neurol.* 34:425–444, 1975.

12. Goldstein, G. W., Wolinsky, J. S., and Csejtey, J. Isolated brain capillaries: A model for the study of lead encephalopathy. *Ann. Neurol.* 1:235–239, 1977.

13. Fishman, R. A., Reiner, M., and Chan, P. H. Metabolic changes associated with iso-osmotic regulation in brain cortex slices. *J. Neurochem.* 28:1061–1067, 1977.

14. Fishman, R. A., Sligar, K., and Hake, R. B. Effects of leukocytes on brain metabolism in granulocytic brain edema. *Ann. Neurol.* 2:89–94, 1977.

15. Lewin, E. Epileptogenic cortical foci induced with ouabain. *Exp. Neurol.* 30:172–177, 1971.

16. Demopoulous, H. B., et al. Antioxidant effects of barbiturates in model membranes undergoing free radical damage. *Acta Neurol. Scand.* (Suppl. 64) 56:152–153, 1977.

17. Demopoulous, H. B., et al. Molecular Aspects of Membrane Structure in Cerebral Edema. In H. J. Reulen (ed.), *Steroids and Brain Edema.* Berlin: Springer-Verlag, 1972. Pp. 29–39.

*18. Fridovich, I. Superoxide dismutases. *Annu. Rev. Biochem.* 44:147–159, 1975.

19. Michaelson, A. M., McCord, J. M., and Fridovich, I. (eds.). *Superoxide and Superoxide Dismutases.* New York: Academic, 1977.

20. Flamm, E. S., et al. Free radicals in cerebral ischemia. *Stroke* 9:445–447, 1978.

21. Chan, P. H., and Fishman, R. A. Brain edema: Induction in cortical slices by polyunsaturated fatty acids. *Science* 201:358–360, 1978.

22. Chan, P. H., et al. Effects of excitatory neurotransmitter amino acids on edema induction in rat brain cortical slices. *J. Neurochem.* 33:1309–1315, 1979.

23. Hong, S. L., and Levine, L. Inhibition of arachidonic acid release from cells as the biochemical action of anti-inflammatory corticosteroids. *Proc. Natl. Acad. Sci. U.S.A.* 73:1730–1734, 1976.

24. Fishman, R. A. Brain Edema. In *Cerebrospinal Fluid in Diseases of the Nervous System.* Philadelphia: Saunders, 1980. Pp. 107–128.

25. Manz, H. J. The pathology of cerebral edema. *Hum. Pathol.* 5:291–313, 1974.

*26. Rapoport, S. I. *Blood-brain Barrier in Physiology and Medicine.* New York: Raven, 1976.

27. Petito, C. K. Early and late mechanism of increased vascular permeability following experimental cerebral infarction. *J. Neuropathol. Exp. Neurol.* 38:222–234, 1979.

28. Westergaard, E., Hertz, M. M., and Bolwig, T. G. Increased permeability to horseradish peroxidase across the cerebral vessels, evoked by electrically induced seizres in the rat. *Acta Neuropathol.* (Berlin) 41:73–80, 1978.

29. Van Harreveld, A. *Brain Tissue Electrolytes.* Washington, D.C.: Butterworth, 1966.

*30. Hossmann, K. A. Development and Resolution of Ischemic Brain Swelling. In H. M. Pappius and W. Feindel (eds.), *Dynamics of Brain Edema.* New York: Springer-Verlag, 1976. Pp. 219–227.

*31. MacKnight, A. D. C., and Leaf, A. Regulation of cellular volume. *Physiol. Rev.* 57:510–573, 1977.

32. Siesjo, B. K. *Brain Energy Metabolism.* New York: Wiley, 1978.

33. Andreoli, T. E., Grantham, J. J., and Rector, F. C., Jr. (eds.). *Disturbances in Body Fluid Osmolality.* Bethesda: American Physiological Society, 1977.

34. Dila, C. F., and Pappius, H. M. Cerebral water and electrolytes: An experimental model of inappropriate secretion of antidiuretic hormone. *Arch. Neurol.* 26:85–90, 1972.

35. Rymer, M. M., and Fishman, R. A. Protective adaptation of brain to water intoxication. *Arch. Neurol.* 28:49–54, 1973.

36. Arieff, A. I., and Kleeman, C. R. Studies on mechanisms of cerebral edema in the diabetic comas. *J. Clin. Invest.* 52:571–583, 1973.

37. Chan, P. H., and Fishman, R. A. Elevation of rat brain amino acids, ammonia and idiogenic osmoles

induced by hyperosmolality. *Brain Res.* 161:293–302, 1979.

38. Fishman, R. A., and Raskin, N. H. Experimental uremic encephalopathy: Permeability and electrolyte metabolism of brain and other tissues. *Arch. Neurol.* 17:10–21, 1967.

39. Fishman, R. A. Cell volume, pumps and neurologic function: Brain's adaptation to osmotic stress. In F. Plum (ed.), *Brain Dysfunction in Metabolic Disorders. Assoc. Res. Nerv. Ment. Dis.* 53:159–171, 1974.

40. De Vivo, D. Reye's syndrome: A metabolic response to an acute mitochondrial insult? *Neurology* 28:105–108, 1978.

41. De Vivo, D., and Keating, J. P. Reye's syndrome. *Adv. Pediatr.* 22:175–229, 1976.

42. Faraj, B. A., et al. Evidence for hypertyraminemia in Reye's syndrome. *Pediatrics* 64:76–80, 1979.

43. Rittenhouse, J. W., Mason, M., and Baublis, J. V. Amino acid ratios in Reye's syndrome. *Lancet* 2:105–106, 1979.

44. Ryan, N. J., et al. Aflatoxin B1: Its role in the etiology of Reye's syndrome. *Pediatrics* 64:71–75, 1979.

45. Trauner, D., et al. Treatment of elevated intracranial pressure in Reye's syndrome. *Ann. Neurol.* 4:275–278, 1978.

46. Verhas, M., et al. Study in cerebrovascular disease: Brain scanning with technetium 99 m pertechnetate; clinical correlations. *Neurology* 25:553–558, 1975.

47. Fishman, R. A., and Greer, M. Changes in the cerebrum associated with experimental obstructive hydrocephalus. *Arch. Neurol.* 8:156–161, 1963.

48. Milhorat, T. H. *Hydrocephalus and the Cerebrospinal Fluid.* Baltimore: Williams & Wilkins, 1972.

49. Prockop, L. D., and Fishman, R. A. Experimental pneumococcal meningitis. Permeability changes influencing the concentration of sugars and macromolecules in cerebrospinal fluid. *Arch. Neurol.* 19:449–463, 1968.

50. Galicich, J. H., and French, L. A. Use of dexamethasone in the treatment of cerebral edema resulting from brain tumors and brain surgery. *Am. Pract. Dig. Treat.* 12:169–174, 1961.

51. Rasmussen, T., and Gulati, D. R. Cortisone in the treatment of post-operative cerebral edema. *J. Neurosurg.* 19:535–544, 1962.

52. Menkin, V. Effect of adrenal cortical extract on capillary permeability. *Am. J. Physiol.* 129:691–697, 1940.

53. Prados, M., Strowger, B., and Feindel, W. Studies on cerebral edema II: Reaction of the brain to the exposure of air; physiologic changes. *Arch. Neurol. Psychiatry* 54:290–300, 1945.

54. Fauci, A. S. Glucocorticosteroid therapy: Mechanism of action and clinical considerations. *Ann. Intern. Med.* 84:304–315, 1976.

55. Axelrod, L. Glucocorticoid therapy. *Medicine* 55:39–65, 1976.

56. Faupel, G., et al. Double Blind Study on the Effects of Steroids on Severe Closed Head Injury. In H. M. Pappius, and W. Feindel (eds.), *Dynamics of Brain Edema.* New York: Springer-Verlag, 1976. Pp. 337–343.

57. Mulley, G., Wikok, R. G., and Mitchell, J. R. A. Dexamethasone in acute stroke. *Br. Med. J.* 2:994–996, 1978.

58. McGraw, C. P., Alexander, E., Jr., and Howard, G. Effect of dose and dose schedule on the response of intracranial pressure to mannitol. *Surg. Neurol.* 10:127–130, 1978.

59. Rottenberg, D. A., Hurwitz, B. J., and Posner, J. B. The effect of oral glycerol on intraventricular pressure in man. *Neurology* 27:600–608, 1977.

60. Huttenlocher, P. R. Treatment of hydrocephalus with acetazolamide. *J. Pediatr.* 66:1023–1030, 1965.

61. Rubin, R. C., et al. The production of cerebrospinal fluid in man and its modification by acetazolamide. *J. Neurosurg.* 25:430–436, 1966.

62. Long, D. M., Maxwell, R., and Choi, K. S. A New Therapy Regimen for Brain Edema. In H. M. Pappius, and W. Feindel (eds.), *Dynamics of Brain Edema.* New York: Springer-Verlag, 1976. Pp. 293–300.

63. Meinig, G., et al. The Effect of Dexamethasone and Diuretics on Peritumor Brain Edema: Comparative Study of Tissue Water Content and CT. In H. M. Pappius, and W. Feindel (eds.), *Dynamics of Brain Edema.* New York: Springer-Verlag, 1976. Pp. 301–305.

64. Sahar, A., and Tsipstein, E. Effects of mannitol and furosemide on the rate of formation of cerebrospinal fluid. *Exp. Neurol.* 60:584–591, 1978.

65. James, H. E., et al. Treatment of intracranial hypertension. Analysis of 105 consecutive recordings of intracranial pressure. *Acta Neurochir.* 36:189–200, 1977.

66. Hoff, J. T., and Marshall, L. F. Barbiturates in neurosurgery. *Clin. Neurosurg.* 26:658–668, 1979.

67. Flamm, E. S., et al. Barbiturates and Free Radicals. In A. J. Popp et al. (eds.), *Neural Trauma.* New York: Raven, 1979. Pp. 289–296.

68. Marshall, L. F., Shapiro, H. M., and Smith, R. W. Barbiturate Treatment of Intracranial Hypertensive States. In A. J. Popp et al. (eds.), *Neural Trauma.* New York: Raven, 1979. Pp. 347–351.

Thomas E. Duffy
Fred Plum

Chapter 35. Seizures, Coma, and Major Metabolic Encephalopathies

Generalized seizures and coma represent extremes in the functional activity of the brain and its requirement for energy. Energy consumption in brain is tightly coupled to the work done. This is principally the electrochemical work associated with neuronal excitation and conduction, the uphill translocation of cations necessary to maintain cell membrane polarization, and the synthesis, release, and reuptake of synaptic transmitters. During seizures, cerebral energy consumption, as reflected either by the uptake of glucose (the major fuel of brain) and oxygen or by the breakdown of endogenous high-energy phosphate compounds, may increase as much as three- to fourfold whereas, during surgical anesthesia or coma, cerebral energy demands may fall by more than 50 percent (Chap. 24). Despite such a wide range in metabolic requirements, the cellular homeostatic mechanisms that regulate cerebral energy production tend to maintain remarkably constant the tissue concentration of the energy transducer molecule, ATP. If this constancy fails, however, irreversible brain damage is likely to ensue.

The control of energy balance is exerted both on the supply of energy precursors and on the work done by the brain, that is, on both the input and the output. Intrinsic mechanisms appropriately increase or decrease the rate of brain metabolism during periods of increased or decreased functional activity. During hypoxia or hypoglycemia, cerebral metabolic activity becomes depressed prior to any measurable depletion of ATP stores in tissue [1, 2], suggesting that adaptive responses can lower energy expenditure when the supply of energy precursors is threatened (see also Hypoglycemia in Chap. 29). As part of this process, the brain exerts homeostatic control over its blood supply. When cerebral functional activity increases, as during physiological stimulation or generalized seizures, the cerebral blood flow increases commensurately, thereby increasing the delivery of substrates and oxygen to the actively metabolizing tissue. The interdependence of function, metabolism, and blood flow must somehow be coupled at the cellular-molecular level. Although no single "coupling" factor has been identified, much evidence suggests that ATP expenditure or, more specifically, the $[ATP]/[ADP][P_i]$ ratio (the "phosphate potential"), is an important intracellular regulator of cerebral carbohydrate and energy metabolism. A change in the phosphate potential, furthermore, may generate the signal that modifies the blood supply.

Seizures

A seizure is the sudden onset of an intense, rapidly repetitive focal or generalized electrical discharge in the brain. Generalized cerebral seizures usually are accompanied by motor convulsions. Although epilepsy is the prototypical disease causing such paroxysmal brain dysfunction, seizures are also a common symptom of many other neurological and systemic abnormalities, including brain tumors, disorders of carbohydrate, amino acid, and lipid metabolism, high fever (in the child), or CNS infections. Experimentally, seizures can be induced by several mechanisms. These include (1) repetitive electrical depolarization of cerebral neurons (electroshock); (2) interference with the supply or processing of substrates for brain energy metabolism (hypoxia, hypoglycemia, fluoroacetate poisoning); (3) pharmacologic agents that directly stimulate the nervous system (pentylenetetrazole, flurothyl, ammonium salts); (4) agents that inhibit the uptake or metabolism of certain amino acids

Table 35-1. Indices of Cerebral Metabolism During Generalized Seizures

Metabolic Index	Relative Increase	References
Glycolytic flux	2- to 8-fold	[3–7, 9]
Oxygen consumption ($CMRO_2$)	0.6- to 2.5-fold	[3, 8, 10, 11]
High-energy phosphate ($\sim$P) utilization	2- to 4-fold	[4, 6, 12]
Cerebral blood flow	1.5- to 9-fold	[3, 8, 10, 11]
Glucose transport into brain	Approximately 3-fold	[13]
Respiratory quotient (RQ)	Rises above 1.0	[3, 8]

(methionine sulfoximine, pyridoxal phosphate antagonists); or (5) agents that antagonize the normal physiological inhibition of specific neurotransmitter molecules (picrotoxin, strychnine, bicuculline). Just as there is no single factor that serves as a common denominator for eliciting all types of seizures, so too it is unlikely that a single chemical agent triggers the abnormal electrical discharge in all cases, and none has been proposed. Consequently, the neurochemistry of seizures relates mainly to those events that accompany or follow secondarily from the abnormal electrical discharges; the chemical pathogenesis of the epileptic attack is still unknown.

OXIDATIVE METABOLISM AND BLOOD FLOW
Generalized seizures place on brain its greatest known metabolic load. Measurements in both animals and man indicate that during a single seizure the overall rate of cerebral metabolism increases from 1.5 to 5 times normal, depending upon the intensity and duration of the cerebral stimulus and upon which particular substrate is taken as an index of metabolic activity (Table 35-1). Schmidt and coworkers [10] gave monkeys pentylenetetrazole and, by multiplying arteriovenous differences across the brain by the blood flow, calculated that during the convulsions the cerebral metabolic rate for oxygen ($CMRO_2$) doubled. In paralyzed, nonanesthetized dogs and monkeys that were ventilated artificially, Plum and colleagues [8] recorded a 60 percent increase in $CMRO_2$ during pentylenetetrazole-induced seizures as well as a twofold to fourfold rise in cerebral blood flow. They noted that, at least during the early stages of the seizure,

CO_2 production by the brain exceeded oxygen consumption so that the apparent respiratory quotient (RQ) rose to 1.45. These observations were subsequently confirmed in studies performed on pentobarbital-anesthetized patients who were undergoing electroconvulsive therapy for the treatment of depression [3]. In those subjects, cerebral blood flow and the cerebral metabolic rates for oxygen and glucose doubled during the seizures, whereas the calculated RQ rose from a resting value of 0.95 to 1.29. The hypermetabolism appears to persist for the duration of the abnormal electrical activity; thus, when Meldrum and Nilsson [11] induced sustained seizures in rats by the injection of bicuculline, they found that $CMRO_2$ increased 2.5-fold during the first minute of seizure activity and remained at this elevated rate during the ensuing 2 hours of status epilepticus. Direct measurements of energy consumption in whole brain, cerebral cortex, or major anatomical subdivisions of the CNS in mice and rats indicate that during electroshock-induced seizures, the turnover of high energy phosphates increases to at least two to four times the resting rate [4, 6, 12], a figure that generally corroborates the observed increase in oxygen consumption. The question remains, however, whether the increased metabolism keeps pace with cellular demands. Indeed, one of the tacit questions concerning the metabolism of epilepsy has been whether the seizures stop because the brain becomes energetically exhausted (see also Chap. 24).

Despite the enormous increase in cerebral oxidative metabolism caused by seizures, blood flow to the brain usually increases proportionately with or exceeds the rate of metabolism so that oxygen tension in the cerebral venous blood can actually rise [5, 8, 14, 15]. This homeostatic response of the blood flow can be attributed to two mechanisms: One is a substantial increase in the systemic blood pressure, mediated over descending sympathetic autonomic pathways from the brain, and the other is a marked reduction in resistance of the cerebral vascular bed [8, 11]. Ordinarily, the rate of blood flow through the normally metabolizing brain remains nearly constant in the face of wide fluctuations in blood pressure, presumably owing to the remarkable ability of cerebral arterioles to constrict or dilate appropriately whenever the pressure rises or falls (vascular autoregulation). During seizures, these vessels dilate and the cerebral vasculature becomes pressure passive, giving rise to the increased blood flow. The mechanism of this loss of autoregulation is still uncertain, but it clearly is linked to the greatly increased metabolism of the tissue (Chap. 24). There is evidence to suggest that increased tissue hydrogen ion concentration, secondary to the accumulation of lactic acid, is at least partially responsible [3, 5, 11]; other vasodilators (e.g., adenosine, cyclic 3′,5′-AMP) which are elevated in brain by seizures [16–18] may also play a role.

CEREBRAL ENERGY BALANCE IN EXPERIMENTAL SEIZURES

Most convulsants that cause major tonic-clonic seizures produce similar disturbances in the energy balance of the brain. Data obtained in convulsing mice, whose brains can be frozen rapidly enough to minimize postmortem artifacts, indicate that within 10 to 20 seconds after the initiation of a seizure by electroshock or the inhalation of flurothyl the concentrations of phosphocreatine and ATP in brain decrease by as much as 50 percent whereas the ADP, AMP, and inorganic phosphate levels increase correspondingly [4, 6, 7, 15]. Simultaneously, there is an increased glycolytic flux as indicated by increased glucose consumption, decreased tissue concentrations of glucose and glycogen, and increase lactic acid [4, 6, 7, 15, 19]. King and colleagues [6] noted that, during electroshock-induced convulsions, lactic acid in brain increased much more than could be accounted for by de-

creases in the endogenous tissue glucose and glycogen stores and concluded that the rate of glucose transport into brain from blood must have been greatly facilitated, exceeding the normal rate by as much as fourfold [5, 6; see also 13]. The initial acceleration of glycolysis undoubtedly results from activation and deinhibition of phosphofructokinase, presumably as a consequence of the changes in ATP, ADP, AMP, and inorganic phosphate. Thus, seizures induced by a variety of agents are associated with decreases in brain glucose 6-phosphate and fructose 6-phosphate, and with substantial increases in fructose 1,6-diphosphate and in all other glycolytic intermediates further "downstream" to lactic acid [7, 19–21]. Changes in lactate, however, are consistently greater than the increases in pyruvate [5, 14, 19, 21]; this results in an increased lactate/pyruvate ratio. A moderate fall in ATP and the accumulation of lactic acid are neurochemical changes that appear to be intrinsic to seizures and are not unique to models of generalized convulsions. Thus, when Collins [22] induced focal motor seizures in rats by application of penicillin to the exposed cerebral cortex, he found that, whereas ATP declined and lactate rose in cortical samples taken from the seizure focus, the concentrations of these metabolites in samples obtained from contralateral, homotypic cortex were not different from control. Moreover, local glucose consumption, assessed by the 2-[^{14}C]deoxyglucose method, was increased twofold at the cortical site of the primary electrical discharge [23].

When assessing the neurochemistry of seizures, a distinction must be made between the primary chemical changes in brain that follow directly from the abnormal electrical discharge and those that are partly, or perhaps entirely, secondary to the motor convulsions. Tonic-clonic convulsions prevent adequate pulmonary ventilation and give rise to intense muscular activity, both of which may deplete the oxygen content of blood. Meyer and coworkers [24] observed in patients undergoing electroshock therapy that, during the convulsions, oxygen tensions and pH in arterial blood both decline sharply, and similar changes in blood gases and pH have been reproduced in animals that were allowed to convulse freely [25, 26].

Table 35-2. Effect of Seizures on Metabolite Concentrations, Lactate/Pyruvate Ratios and Tissue pH in the Cerebral Cortex of Paralyzed-Respirated Rats and Cats[a]

Animal and Convulsant	P-creatine	ATP	Lactate	Lactate/ Pyruvate	pH (tissue)
		(mmol/kg wet weight)			
Rat (electroshock)					
Control	4.90	2.76	0.80	11.8	7.04
Seizure	4.10[b]	2.63[b]	3.62[b]	29.9[b]	6.95[b]
Rat (bicuculline)					
Control	4.59	2.95	1.53	11.1	7.04
Seizure	2.46[b]	2.80[b]	2.95[b]	16.6[b]	6.82[c], 7.06[d]
Cat (flurothyl)					
Control	4.40	2.28	1.26	17.7	7.16
Seizure	3.79[b]	2.00[b]	4.98[b]	37.6[b]	7.07[b]

[a]The cortices were frozen in situ by irrigation with liquid nitrogen 10 sec after the initiation of a generalized seizure by supramaximal electroshock [5], intravenous administration of bicuculline [19], or inhalation of flurothyl [14].
[b]Different from the control value with $p < 0.05$.
[c]Calculated from the concentrations of the components of the creatine kinase reaction.
[d]Calculated from estimations of "buffer base."

Contamination from chemical changes produced by convulsing muscles during experimental seizures can be largely overcome by paralysis and artificial ventilation [26]. As indicated in Table 35-2, however, seizures induced in ventilated, well-oxygenated animals given paralytic drugs are still accompanied by clear-cut changes in the glycolytic and energy metabolism of the brain. During the peak of the EEG-recorded seizure in paralyzed rats or cats, cortical concentrations of ATP and phosphocreatine fell by approximately 5 to 10 percent and 15 to 45 percent, respectively. In both species, seizures caused a lactic acidosis in the cerebral cortex that always was associated with an elevated lactate/pyruvate ratio and in two studies [5, 14], with a lower intracellular pH. These changes were calculated to have resulted in an abrupt shift of the cytoplasmic redox potential (i.e., the NAD^+/NADH ratio) toward a more reduced state. Lack of oxygen in tissue cannot explain these metabolic alterations because cerebral venous oxygen tensions actually rose *above* control during the seizures [5, 14], implying that oxygen supply to the brain was in excess of what was necessary to support oxidative metabolism. There is additional evidence pointing to this same conclusion. When Caspers and Speckmann [27] measured the oxygen tension of the cortical surface in rats given pentylenetrazole, they found that, as long as the cortical blood flow remained high during the seizures, tissue PO_2 increased above control. Furthermore, Jöbsis et al. [28], using the technique of reflectance fluorometry, showed that the fluorescence of the exposed cat cortex decreases during pentylenetetrazole- or strychnine-induced seizures, suggesting that the mitochondrial pool of pyridine nucleotides becomes more oxidized. Similar redox changes have been observed in the region of focal hippocampal seizures [29]. Thus a mild to moderate decline in the cerebral energy balance and the development of a "nonhypoxic" lactic acidosis in the tissue seem to be biochemical responses that are intrinsic to the seizures themselves. The question is: How does this nonhypoxic lactic acidosis come about?

PHOSPHATE POTENTIAL AND METABOLIC REGULATION
In brain, as in other organs, glycolysis (discussed in Chap. 17) is primarily a cytoplasmic process

whose end products are pyruvate and lactate (Fig. 17-2). The activity of lactic dehydrogenase in brain is high, localized to the cytosol, and the reaction catalyzed by the enzyme is maintained close to equilibrium in vivo. Thus the lactate/pyruvate ratio at constant pH is determined by the redox state of the pyridine nucleotide couple, NAD^+-NADH, as expressed in the equation:

$$K_{LDH} = ([Lactate]/[pyruvate]) \cdot ([NAD^+]/[NADH][H^+]) \quad (35\text{-}1)$$

Krebs and Veech [30] showed that under a variety of nutritional influences the redox state of the cytoplasmic NAD^+-NADH couple in liver was determined by the phosphorylation state of the adenine nucleotide system, i.e., the value of the phosphate potential, $[ATP]/[ADP][HPO_4^{2-}]$. The link between the phosphate potential and the pyridine nucleotide couple was provided by the demonstration that two of the intermediate reactions of glycolysis were maintained in equilibrium. These reactions involve the conversion of glyceraldehyde 3-phosphate to 3-phosphoglycerate, catalyzed by the enzymes glyceraldehyde 3-phosphate dehydrogenase and 3-phosphoglycerate kinase, given in the equation:

$$K_{app} = ([3\text{-}P\text{-}glycerate]/[glyceraldehyde\ 3\text{-}P]) \cdot ([ATP]/[ADP][HPO_4^{2-}]) \cdot ([NADH][H^+]/[NAD^+]) \quad (35\text{-}2)$$

Because these reactions are in equilibrium with the same pool of NAD [30], combining equations (35-1) and (35-2) yields an expression that shows the relationship between the lactate/pyruvate ratio and the phosphate potential, given in the equation:

$$K_{app} = ([3\text{-}P\text{-}glycerate]/[glyceraldehyde\ 3\text{-}P]) \cdot ([ATP]/[ADP][HPO_4^{2-}]) \cdot ([lactate]/[pyruvate]) \quad (35\text{-}3)$$

Recent measurements have demonstrated that the apparent equilibrium constant of equation (35-3) is strongly influenced by the ionic strength and the Mg^{2+} concentration in the medium and that a portion of the measured "free" cytosolic ADP may, in fact, be bound in vivo [31]. Nevertheless, with appropriate correction for these variables, measurements of the concentrations of the components of equation 35-3 in whole rat brain [31] or cerebral cortex [32] indicate that K_{app} is near its predicted equilibrium value both in control tissue and during the greatly increased glycolytic flux that accompanies an electroshock-induced seizure [32]. Furthermore, during seizures, the ratio of 3-phosphoglycerate to glyceraldehyde 3-phosphate remains constant although the concentrations of both intermediates increases [32]. It follows, therefore, that, if equilibrium is to be maintained, a fall in the phosphate potential will be accompanied by an elevated lactate/pyruvate ratio. Since equation 35-3 represents an equilibrium situation, the validity of the converse argument, i.e., that increased cytoplasmic reduction raises the lactate/pyruvate ratio causing a fall in the phosphate potential, cannot be ruled out. For example, transport of reduced equivalents from cytoplasm to mitochondria for subsequent oxidation occurs through a carrier system (the malate-aspartate shuttle, Fig. 35-7), the capacity of which could be exceeded during the increased glycolytic flux accompanying seizures. If this took place, NADH would be expected to accumulate in the cytoplasm, causing an increased lactate/pyruvate ratio. It seems more likely, however, that a change in the phosphate potential owing to the increased energy demand imposed by the seizure discharge, is the primary metabolic event.

The homeostatic consequences of a decreased phosphate potential with cerebral lactic acidosis during seizures are summarized in Fig. 35-1. The intense neural activity of the seizure discharge leads to Na^+ and K^+ shifts which stimulate the membrane $(Na^+ + K^+)$-activated ATPase and bring about the breakdown of ATP to ADP and inorganic phosphate. This sequence has several important effects. There will be activation and deinhibition of phosphofructokinase, resulting in increased glycolytic flux [34]. Simultaneously, the rise in tissue ADP and P_i will stimulate mitochondrial oxidative phosphorylation, thereby increasing the rate of oxygen consumption and CO_2 production. In addition, the decreased phosphate potential will

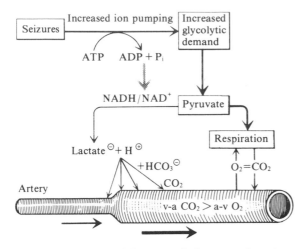

Fig. 35-1. *The blood flow–metabolism couple in brain,*
a hypothesis. From Plum et al. [33], used by permission
of Raven Press.

shift the cytoplasmic redox state toward reduction, promoting the conversion of pyruvate into lactate and causing a nonhypoxic lactic acidosis in the tissue. The increased acidosis, in turn, will titrate tissue bicarbonate to yield CO_2 production in excess of oxygen consumption, accounting for the experimental observations of an apparently increased RQ during seizures [3, 8, 14]. The released CO_2 or, more likely, the increased periarteriolar $[H^+]$ may then act on vessel walls to reduce vascular resistance and thereby increase blood flow to the actively metabolizing tissue. Howse and coworkers [14] showed that in curarized, well-oxygenated cats maximal cerebral vasodilatation during flurothyl-induced seizures coincides precisely with the greatest reduction in the cortical-tissue pH. It seems likely that a similar kind of metabolic control of blood flow also operates during increased physiological stimulation of the brain [35–37], although this has not been directly verified.

STATUS EPILEPTICUS

Status epilepticus is potentially a much more serious clinical problem than the single seizure. Repeated or sustained seizures, particularly in children, are associated with a high incidence of permanent residual brain damage. This limiting effect on growth and development of the brain can be reproduced experimentally in animals [38, 39]. Wasterlain and Plum [38] applied either single daily electroshock seizures or a two-hour episode of status epilepticus to immature rats at different stages of postnatal development and examined the effects of the seizures on subsequent brain growth and chemical content. Animals undergoing convulsive seizures during the immediate 10-day postnatal period, when brain-cell mitosis in the rat is high, had a permanent reduction in brain weight and brain-cell number, as estimated from contents of DNA, RNA, protein, and cholesterol. Such animals were delayed in their achievement of behavioral developmental milestones. Animals undergoing seizures during the second 10 days of life also had permanently smaller brains but with a normal complement of DNA, suggesting a reduction of cell size without change in cell number. After 20 days of life, when cerebral mitotic activity has nearly ceased, neither daily seizures nor status epilepticus caused any permanent alteration in brain weight, cell number, or cell size. Pretreatment of immature, but not adult, rats with glucose reduced mortality during chemically induced status epilepticus and largely reversed the adverse effects of seizures on brain weight, DNA, RNA, and protein content [40]. Because brain ATP concentrations, measured in 4-day-old rats, were not depleted even after as many as 50 seizures, it was concluded that the protection afforded by glucose was more likely related to its role as carbon source in the growing brain, rather than to its role as energy source [40].

In adult animals, at least, many of the acute changes of status epilepticus can be attenuated or reversed by supporting the respiration and circulation during the epileptic attack [26]. This implies that systemic effects of the convulsions (i.e., acidosis, hypotension, hypoxia) are at least partly responsible for the neurological consequences of status epilepticus, although the metabolic effects of the intense abnormal electrical discharges must also contribute to the eventual deterioration of the brain [5, 15, 19].

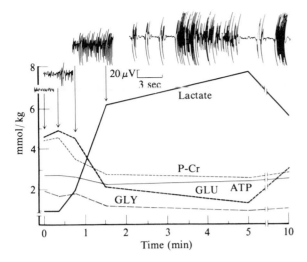

Fig. 35-2. Changes in metabolite concentrations of the mouse forebrain during status epilepticus. Animals were paralyzed and artificially ventilated with oxygen. Seizures were induced with pentylenetetrazole (150 mg/kg, I.P.), and the mice were frozen after periods of continuous epileptiform activity in the EEG lasting up to 10 minutes. EEG tracings from control and treated animals at the time of freezing are shown at the top of the figure. Abbreviations: P-Cr, phosphocreatine; GLU, glucose; GLY, glycogen. Data of Duffy et al. [5]; reproduced in [33]; used by permission of Raven Press.

The complexity of the interactions of intrinsic cerebral metabolic and systemic factors in producing permanent brain damage is illustrated in the study of Blennow and coworkers [41]. These investigators systematically examined the effects of hypoxia, hypoglycemia, hypotension, and hyperthermia on the severity of brain damage produced in paralyzed-ventilated rats during 2 hours of bicuculline-induced status epilepticus. Perhaps surprisingly, there was no correlation between cerebral energy status or lactic acid content and the degree of ischemic neuron damage in cerebral cortex, hippocampus, and striatum; moreover, seizures induced in control animals were associated with a higher incidence of neuronal pathology than in any of the experimental groups, except the hyperthermic animals. This observation emphasizes the particular danger of seizures in a setting of fever, a common clinical presentation in children.

Brain-tissue analyses made after the experimental induction of repeated seizures in both large and small animals indicate that the organ possesses a considerable capacity to maintain its energy balance during at least the early stages of status epilepticus [5, 7]. The experiment illustrated in Fig. 35-2 is typical. Within 30 seconds after the first burst of EEG-recorded seizure activity in paralyzed, well-oxygenated mice treated with pentylenetetrazole, phosphocreatine levels in brain decreased and lactate began to rise. By 90 seconds after injection of the convulsant, there was a second major seizure burst, during which phosphocreatine decreased by 40 percent and ATP by 16 percent, while lactate increased by 500 percent. During the remaining 8.5 minutes of continuous epileptiform activity, only minor further changes were noted in these metabolites, suggesting that a new steady state had been achieved. Animals subjected to as much as 2 hours of continuous pentylenetetrazole-induced [15] or bicuculline-induced [19] seizure activity exhibited a similar stability of high-energy phosphate compounds in the cerebral cortex. However, when mice were given pentylenetetrazole and allowed to convulse freely for 2 hours in an oxygen environment [15], they underwent a progressive deterioration of the cerebral energy state and a depletion of brain glucose, pyruvate, and lactate contents. The implication of these observations is that status epilepticus in freely convulsing animals may lead to failure of cerebral glucose metabolism, possibly as a result of impaired transport of glucose across the blood-brain barrier [40].

A progressive reduction of brain glycogen seems to be a common feature of many types of repeated seizures [5, 7, 19, 42]; this probably reflects both activation of brain glycogen phosphorylase and inhibition of glycogen synthase owing to the seizure-induced rise in cyclic 3',5'-AMP and fall in glucose 6-phosphate, respectively. The physiological significance of the loss of glycogen during status epilepticus is difficult to assess in terms of tissue energy metabolism because the total glycogen stores of brain are low (3 mmol/kg, Fig. 35-2) and could provide glucose 6-phosphate at the normal glycolytic flux rate (approximately 0.7 mmol/kg/min in mice) for only a few minutes at best. However, most cerebral glycogen is confined to the cytoplasm and end feet of astrocytes, implying an intracellular concentration much greater than that of whole brain. Intracellular glycogen exerts little osmotic activity; accordingly, degradation of glycogen to lactic acid and other small molecules could lead to hyperosmolarity within the astrocytes, causing them to take up water from the extracellular space. Swelling of astrocytic end feet around capillaries and neurons has been demonstrated in rat cortex after five minutes of pentylenetetrazole-induced convulsions [43], and has been implicated as the probable cause of abnormalities in the hippocampus after bicuculline-induced status epilepticus in paralyzed, well-oxygenated baboons [44]. Glial cells normally function to buffer the microenvironment of neurons [45], and will take up K^+, NH_4^+, and other ions from the extracellular space. The importance of extracellular K^+ in the *initiation* of seizures is uncertain [46]; however, much evidence suggests that the accumulation of K^+ in the extracellular space (perhaps secondary to failure of the glia to take up the ion) may sustain seizures and predispose the brain to the development of status epilepticus [47].

Coma

Coma represents a great reduction or absence of psychological functions of the brain. Both the neurochemistry and neurophysiology of coma can involve abnormalities that either diffusely affect the cerebral hemispheres, selectively affect the reticular formation, or involve both areas together [48]. This point is well illustrated in a patient studied by Ingvar and colleagues [49, 50]: The subject was in coma due to a destructive lesion confined to the midbrain reticular formation. Despite near-normal morphology of the cerebral hemispheres, cerebral blood flow and oxygen consumption were reduced to 25 percent of normal. Purely focal metabolic abnormalities may produce focal neurological dysfunction, but do not cause coma, except when the reticular activating system of the upper brain stem and diencephalon is involved.

Metabolic studies of the brain of wakeful man during various psychological and physiological activities indicate that, although local changes in metabolism accompany local increases or decreases in cerebral function [29], the metabolically more demanding integrative action of the whole brain hides these variations so that net oxygen consumption normally remains remarkably constant (Chap. 24). Earlier in this chapter, we presented the concept that homeostasis normally maintains energy levels in the brain within very narrow limits and that any deviation from the normal level represents a major threat to the brain. Available evidence in comatose conditions suggests that this is so: Comatose states that are fully reversible are associated with a normal or even supranormal level of ATP and phosphocreatine in brain, whereas states accompanied by a fall in these high-energy phosphates appear to evolve consistently into severe brain damage. As will be seen, with some forms of metabolic encephalopathy, comatose states that are associated with a normal cerebral energy balance, if untreated, tend to deteriorate into states of energy depletion, at which point permanent brain damage may occur. The sequence suggests that coma in such circumstances represents an initial "switching down" of synaptic activity, possibly as a protective adaptive response. Whether such a concept could extend to the effects of anesthetic agents or other nonstructural causes of coma, such as the postictal or postconcussive states, remains to be seen.

ANESTHETIC COMA

General anesthetics produce profound, but fully reversible, depression of nervous system function. The agents vary widely in their chemical structures, so that the molecular basis of their action ordinarily cannot be predicted from their structural configuration alone. Most anesthetics are lipid soluble. Indeed, lipid solubility has been proposed as a mechanism of their actions since this almost inevitably implies an effect on cell membranes [51]. Because equally lipid-soluble agents possess no anesthetic effect, however, the explanation is insufficient, although lipid solubility seems to be essential for these drugs to penetrate cerebral cell membranes.

Drugs that produce general anesthesia affect the cerebral circulation variably, presumably because they differ in the degree to which they affect vascular smooth muscle. Nearly all of them, with the exception of ketamine [52], reduce cerebral oxygen consumption, and most evidence indicates that this reduction occurs as much by a direct and diffuse effect on brain tissue as by any selective depression of the brainstem reticular formation. Physiologically, the anesthetic drugs vary in whether they depress reticular or somatocortical projections more [53–55]. Pentobarbital has been shown selectively to depress excitatory postsynaptic potentials in invertebrates [56], possibly by decreasing the time that postsynaptic ionic channels remain open [57]. However, it is not known to what extent these findings can be extrapolated to the mammalian nervous system.

At present, no satisfactory chemical explanation has been found for the action of any central anesthetic drug. Several physicochemical theories have been tried to relate anesthetic potency to molecular rearrangement within the cell. Perhaps the most attractive hypothesis is that anesthetics occupy hydrophobic sites on nerve cell membranes, causing expansion and disorder of the lipid bilayer [58], and thereby alter membrane permeability, receptor characteristics, or enzyme activities necessary for normal neural function. Virtually all anesthetics increase membrane fluidity, and the application of high hydrostatic pressures can reverse both the anesthetic-induced expansion of lipid membranes and the behavioral depression caused by anesthetics in living organisms [59, 60]. However, the "membrane-expansion" theory does not explain the selectivity of anesthetics, and this has prompted Roth [61] to suggest that the interaction of anesthetic agents with membrane phosphoproteins confers specificity and selectivity on their pharmacological actions.

Barbiturates and other general anesthetics inhibit mitochondrial respiration in vitro when glucose or glutamate (but not succinate) are used as substrates, indicating that the drugs interfere with electron transport at the NADH-dehydrogenase step [62]. At high, nonphysiological concentrations, barbiturates can uncouple oxidative phosphorylation. However, it seems unlikely that anesthesia results from a generalized depression of cellular respiration for several reasons:

1. Not all agents that inhibit cellular respiration cause anesthesia, and some induce convulsions [63].
2. Inhibition of mitochondrial oxidation of NADH would be expected to lead eventually to
   a. A depletion of cerebral energy reserves.
   b. A shift in the tissue redox potential toward a more reduced state.
   c. An acceleration of glycolysis with the accumulation of lactic acid owing to reversal of the Pasteur effect.

In fact, measurements of these variables in the brains of anesthetized animals indicate that just the opposite occurs in almost every instance. Thus, whole brain and cortical concentrations of ATP, phosphocreatine, glucose, and glycogen in anesthetized rodents are either normal or higher than normal, whereas lactate levels, if at all changed, are lower than those in conscious animals [64, 65]. Moreover, cerebral glucose utilization declines during anesthesia in a dose-dependent manner, although neither linearly [66] nor uniformly in all neuroanatomical structures [67]. The cytoplasmic $NADH/NAD^+$ ratio either remains the same or falls [68]. These several observations indicate that the reduced oxygen consumption imposed by most anesthetics is the result, not the cause of the lowered cerebral metabolic activity. During anesthesia, the brain remains in a state of energized readiness.

HYPOXIC COMA

The effects of reduced oxygen supply on the brain must be separated carefully from those of ischemia (see below) because failure of the circulation not only results in absolute oxygen and substrate lack but also fails to rinse the tissue of its metabolic products. Anoxia, also, and perhaps initially, affects the heart and rapidly produces systemic hypotension and cardiac arrhythmias. Accordingly, pure cerebral hypoxia causing coma is relatively uncommon in the clinical setting. Exceptions are provided by the delirium produced at high altitude, and the coma or stupor that may follow carbon-monoxide poisoning, in which high concentrations of carboxyhemoglobin block much of the oxygen transport to brain and other organs.

Chemical changes in the brains of hypoxic animals are dependent on the severity and duration of the hypoxic insult. Perhaps the earliest consistently demonstrable changes, detectable when the arterial PO_2 (PaO_2) falls below about 50 mm Hg, are increases in tissue lactic acid and in the lactate-pyruvate ratio, and a fall in phosphocreatine [13, 69]. Because both the lactic dehydrogenase and the creatine kinase equilibria are pH dependent, a fall in tissue pH (secondary to the accumulation of lactic acid) is thought to be responsible for the changes in phosphocreatine and in the lactate/pyruvate ratio. The initial acceleration of glycolysis during hypoxia, which the rise in lactic acid reflects, is thought to be mediated at the phosphofructokinase step [1, 13]. Exactly how this mediation occurs is uncertain because virtually all of the known activators and inhibitors of brain phosphofructokinase, including ATP, ADP, AMP, cyclic $3',5'$-AMP, inorganic phosphate, NH_4^+, and citrate [34], are normal or near normal when increased glycolysis starts [13]. Although most human beings suffer impaired consciousness if the PaO_2 is reduced acutely below about 30 mm Hg, even at this low level brain tissue concentrations of ATP, ADP, and AMP need not be markedly altered [1, 69, 70] (Table 35-3). With more severe systemic hypoxia (PaO_2 of 21 mm Hg) and as long as cerebral blood pressure is maintained, ATP levels remain normal, but phosphocreatine falls substantially, and a decrease in the phosphate potential also occurs, the latter due to an increase in P_i and ADP. Any further reduction of the oxygen supply—as, for example, by interference with the physiological compensatory hyperemia that normally occurs in the brain during hypoxia—induces a fall in the citric acid cycle intermediates, citrate and α-ketoglutarate, and a substantial drop in cerebral energy reserves. The changes indicate that despite high rates of glycolysis during hypoxia, oxygen availability finally falls sufficiently to inhibit the oxidation of pyruvate and normal mitochondrial oxidative metabolism. In keeping with the chemical observations, morphological studies indicate that the mitochondria undergo the first permanent abnormality during profound cerebral hypoxia-ischemia [71]. With prolonged less severe hypoxia, such as occurs in carbon monoxide poisoning, increased glycolysis from muscle and other systemic tissues results in a pronounced systemic lactic acidosis [72], possibly contributing to the cerebral demyelination that often occurs with severe examples of this disorder.

The exact neurochemical basis for coma in hypoxia is unclear, but it may represent an adaptive response to reduced oxygen supply. Cerebral blood flow increases markedly in hypoxia, conferring a strong homeostatic protection on the brain. Body metabolism and, perhaps, cerebral metabolism also drop. Thus, Duffy et al. [1] found evidence in mice that cerebral energy consumption declined during hypoxia before any effect on tissue concentrations of adenine nucleotides could be observed. Moreover, Fein and coworkers [73] made direct polarographic measurements of cerebral oxygen extraction (utilization) in tranquilized, hypoxemic cats and found that oxygen extraction decreased in cerebral cortex and basal ganglia, but not in white matter, when the PaO_2 was reduced below 50 mm Hg. These findings imply that moderately severe hypoxia may initially exert an anesthetic-like action on the cerebrum, which partially protects the organ against energy failure. On the other hand, the global cerebral metabolic rate for oxygen ($CMRO_2$) in humans does not fall significantly even at a degree of hypoxemia ($PaO_2 = 30$ mm Hg) sufficient to induce EEG slowing and altered consciousness; and measurements in paralyzed, lightly anesthetized rats indicate that $CMRO_2$ may even increase during hypoxia in that species [74]. Thus, whether depression of cerebral energy metabolism contributes to homeostasis in hypoxia is debatable.

Global measurements of cerebral metabolic activity are unlikely to reflect accurately, and may

Table 35-3. Changes in Concentrations of High-Energy Phosphate Compounds of Rat Brain During Severe Hypoxia and Hypoxia-Oligemia[a]

Treatment	PaO$_2$ (mm Hg)	ATP	ADP	AMP	P-creatine	Total ~P
		(mmol/kg wet weight)				
Control	>100	3.06	0.272	0.031	4.98	11.37
Hypoxia (moderate)	28	3.07	0.342[b]	0.039	4.31[b]	10.79
Hypoxia (severe)	21	3.00	0.384	0.046[c]	3.11[b]	9.49
Hypoxia-oligemia	21	2.38[b]	0.576[b]	0.314[c]	1.76[b]	7.10

[a]Data obtained in normotensive, normothermic animals that were paralyzed and artificially ventilated with appropriate oxygen-nitrogen mixtures. Experimental animals had a clamp on one carotid artery ("Levine preparation") and different levels of oxygenation for 30 min, after which the brains were frozen in situ. Oligemia denotes the cerebral hemisphere in which ipsilateral carotid artery occlusion prevented compensatory hyperemia during hypoxic exposure. Data of Salford et al. [70].
[b]$p < 0.001$.
[c]$p < 0.05$.

even mask, the responses of individual structural and functional components of the brain to hypoxia. This point is emphasized by ^{14}C-autoradiographs obtained in hypoxic "Levine" rats in which local cerebral glucose utilization was assessed by the [^{14}C]deoxyglucose method [75] (Fig. 35-3). Hypoxia gave rise to alternating columns of high and low glucose metabolism in the cerebral cortex, increased metabolism in caudate nucleus and hippocampus, and substantially higher metabolism in white matter compared to adjacent gray matter structures. The cortical columns of highest glucose consumption lie between penetrating cortical arteries, and this implies that those areas had become the most hypoxic. In a model of cerebral oligemia in cats, Welsh and coworkers [76, 77] observed cortical columns of high and low NADH fluorescence, indicative of differences in tissue redox state, and a greater accumulation of lactic acid in white matter compared to gray matter. Whether such differences in local cerebral metabolism contribute to the selective vulnerability of the brain to hypoxic-ischemic damage is unknown.

Oxygen lack also exerts profound effects on the metabolism of potential neurotransmitter substances in brain that probably contribute to the early symptoms of neurological impairment. The rate-limiting steps in the synthesis of indole and catechol neurotransmitters depend on molecular oxygen (Chap. 10); Davis and Carlsson [78] observed impaired monoamine metabolism in brain at PaO$_2$ values below about 50 mm Hg. It is unlikely that this produces an altered consciousness, however, because pharmacological measures that produce a similar impairment of monoamine synthesis have little effect on behavior [79]. Hypoxia leads to the accumulation of the inhibitory amino acid GABA, a rise in alanine, and a fall in the excitatory amino acid aspartate [1, 13]. Hypoxia also interferes with ACh synthesis in brain [80, 81], possibly by interfering with the oxidation of pyruvate in the citric acid cycle. The potential significance of cholinergic dysfunction is emphasized by the fact that pretreatment of animals with the cholinesterase inhibitor physostigmine will prolong their survival under a variety of hypoxic conditions [80].

ISCHEMIC COMA
Coma results from total cerebral ischemia or when vascular occlusions involve the blood supply to the reticular formation.

The neurochemistry of carbohydrate and energy metabolism during total cerebral ischemia has been studied in considerable detail [13]. Consciousness is lost within 6 to 9 sec after onset of total cerebral

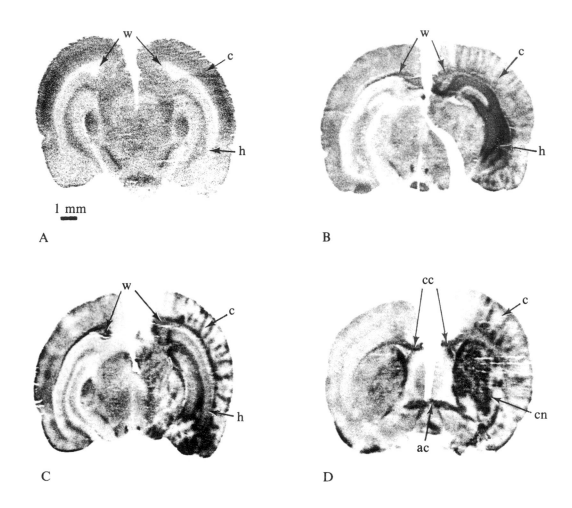

Fig. 35-3. ^{14}C-Autoradiographs of coronal brain sections
from rats subjected to right common carotid artery
ligation, paralysis, and artificial ventilation with either a
normoxic (PaO$_2$ > 90 mm Hg, A) or an hypoxic
(PaO$_2$ = 30 mm Hg, B-D) gas mixture. Animals were
injected IV with a tracer dose of 2–[^{14}C]deoxyglucose
and were decapitated 30 minutes later. The right cerebral
hemisphere is shown on the right side of each photograph.
Labeled anatomical structures include cerebral cortex (c),
hippocampus (h), subcortical white matter (w), corpus
callosum (cc), anterior commissure (ac), and caudate
nucleus (cn). From Pulsinelli and Duffy [75].

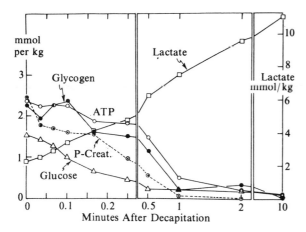

Fig. 35-4. Changes in high-energy compounds and glycolytic intermediates in mouse brain during total ischemia produced by decapitation. Abbreviation: P-Creat., phosphocreatine. From Lowry et al. [82].

ischemia, and the EEG disappears within 15 to 20 sec. The phosphocreatine of brain drops to unmeasurable levels within a minute, and ATP falls by 50 percent within the first minute and to near zero by 2 min (Fig. 35-4). Lactate increases to near maximal values of about 10 mmol/kg by 2 min, paralleling the rapid exhaustion of glucose and glycogen stores during the same period [82]. Ischemia also leads to the accumulation of free fatty acids and ammonium ion in brain, changes in the concentrations of cyclic nucleotides and other putative neurotransmitters, disruption of brain polysomes, and the virtual arrest of protein synthesis [13, 83]. At one time it was believed that permanent brain damage began simultaneously with, or a very short time after, ischemic depletion of cerebral energy reserves. Biochemical studies by several laboratories [84, 85], however, indicate that the brain can regain, for at least brief periods, a considerable proportion of its energy-generating capacity and of other chemical functions after ischemic periods lasting from 15 minutes to as much as an hour. The pressing questions are, therefore: (1) Which, if any, of the observed chemical changes causes irreversible brain damage? (2) Do other neurochemical abnormalities occur during post-ischemic reperfusion of brain that exacerbate the injury and contribute to the development of cerebral edema?

Undoubtedly, failure of cerebral energy metabolism is the precipitating cause of ischemic neuronal damage, but other factors may also be involved. In this connection, lactic acidosis is a leading candidate. Swanson [86] showed that brain cortex slices incubated at pH 6.5 responded normally to electrical stimulation by gaining Na^+ and losing K^+, utilizing high-energy phosphates, and increasing respiration. However, once the stimulation was terminated, the restitution of Na^+ and K^+ gradients and of the concentrations of high-energy phosphates was less complete than in comparably stimulated slices that were incubated at pH 7.5. There is also indirect evidence that lactic acidosis is harmful to the ischemic brain. When monkeys were pretreated with glucose and then subjected to 10 minutes of circulatory arrest, they developed higher lactate concentrations in brain and more extensive cerebral infarction than comparably ischemic monkeys that were not given glucose [87].

The level of cerebral metabolic activity during the reperfusion period following a stroke may also play a role in the development of ischemic brain injury. In several animal models of reversible cerebral ischemia, the insult has been followed by a hypermetabolic phase in which cerebral glucose and oxygen consumption [88] and ATP turnover [89] are all increased. The increased energy demands may reflect enhanced energy requirements for cellular repair superimposed on those for recovering neurological function. If this interpretation is correct, giving metabolic depressants such as barbiturates, even if one initiates them after the ischemic event [90], should protect the brain by suppressing neurological function and thereby channeling more of the available energy toward repair of tissue damage.

HYPOGLYCEMIC COMA

Glucose is the principal substrate for cerebral oxidative metabolism. Normal blood glucose in man is about 5 mM. Levels of approximately 1.5 to 2 mM are associated with confusion or delirium, and levels of 1 mM or less result in deep stupor, coma, or convulsions. Transient hypoglycemic coma that lasts up to an hour usually is fully reversible in man and has been used therapeutically to treat psychosis. More prolonged coma, particularly if accompanied by convulsions, often is followed by irreversible brain damage, with the cerebral cortex suffering pathological changes similar to those incurred during severe sustained anoxia.

Early biochemical studies of hypoglycemia in humans demonstrated a reduction in cerebral glucose consumption accompanied by a disproportionately smaller decrease in cerebral oxygen consumption [91]. The implication that the brain utilizes endogenous substances for oxidative metabolism during hypoglycemia has been borne out by animal experiments that show hypoglycemia-induced decreases in the cerebral concentrations of glutamate, glutamine, and alanine [92, 93]. Alternative, noncarbohydrate fuels, notably ketone bodies, may also be taken up from the plasma. Under conditions of prolonged fasting, which deplete total body carbohydrate stores and mobilize lipid, the cerebral metabolism of acetoacetate and β-hydroxybutyrate can exceed that of glucose [94]. However, though they may supplement cerebral glucose metabolism, ketone bodies alone cannot reverse the metabolic or functional changes caused by hypoglycemia, possibly because their permeability into brain is low and nonuniform [95] and their intermediary metabolism may ultimately inhibit oxidation in the citric acid cycle by depleting the tissue of succinyl-CoA [96].

For a long time it was assumed that coma and slowing of brain metabolism during hypoglycemia were the straightforward results of substrate lack, leading to a failure of oxidative phosphorylation to generate sufficient energy to maintain brain function. More recent studies, however, indicate that whole-brain concentrations of ATP, ADP, AMP, and phosphocreatine remain at normal levels during the early stages of insulin coma, including the stage at which intermittent polyspikes or intermittent isoelectric activity develop in the EEG [2]. With glucose concentrations in blood below 2 mM, the calculated intracellular concentration of glucose in the brains of experimental animals approaches zero and tissue concentrations of glycogen, glucose 6-phosphate, pyruvate, lactate, and citric acid cycle intermediates decline. Roughly concurrent with the development of convulsions, the concentration of the inhibitory agent GABA falls and the stimulants aspartate and ammonia increase.

Although the onset of EEG changes and stupor in animals and, presumably, insulin coma in man occur without changes in the energy state of the cerebral cortex, high-energy phosphate compounds drop rapidly, once glycogen and pyruvate fall to very low levels in the tissue [92]. This stage correlates in animals with the appearance of sustained convulsions and prolonged isoelectricity in the EEG. It is not certain to what degree this stage of energy depletion can be reversed or whether it always presages permanent tissue damage. Agardh and coworkers [97] subjected normothermic, lightly anesthetized rats to insulin hypoglycemia sufficient to deplete brain cortical ATP and phosphocreatine to approximately 15 percent and 8 percent of normal, respectively, and to produce electrical silence in the EEG for 30 min. When glucose was administered to such animals, there was extensive recovery of cortical energy metabolism, and spontaneous activity reappeared in the EEG. Even after 3 hours of normoglycemia, however, the tissue ATP content remained subnormal, and slow waves persisted in the EEG; this implies that some irreversible cell damage had occurred. Hypothermia nearly always accompanies clinical hypoglycemia and undoubtedly partly protects the brain by reducing its rate of metabolism.

The decline in glycolytic and citric acid cycle intermediates, along with the changes in amino acids in brain, is now a well-established sequence in prolonged and severe hypoglycemic coma, but the cause of the initial functional depression is still unknown (Chap. 29). Furthermore, clinical recovery after hypoglycemia occurs in animals before full restoration of all glycolytic and citric acid cycle intermediates takes place [98]. The problem in deducing the functional effects of hypoglycemia from its neurochemistry may be partly methodological: Overall chemical analyses of brain tissue may not disclose local changes in concentration of such critical agents as transmitters. In this respect, it has been shown that hypoglycemia decreases the turnover of ACh in brain [80]; it may also lead to a decrease in the availability of carbon precursors for the synthesis of other, as yet unidentified, neurotransmitter agents.

Encephalopathies

HEPATIC ENCEPHALOPATHY

Impaired brain function is a consistent feature of severe liver disease and occurs with two forms of liver disorder. *Fulminant acute hepatic failure* causes a rapidly developing delirium, progressing to stupor, coma, and even death. *Chronic cirrhosis,* usually secondary to alcoholism, produces a more insidiously developing, relapsing encephalopathy, characterized by episodic stupor, disturbances in mentation, and abnormalities in motor systems indicative of dysfunction of the cerebral hemispheres. It is not known whether these two forms of hepatic encephalopathy share a common pathogenesis, but two major neurochemical theories have been advanced to explain the neurological disorder. One focuses on amino acid and neurotransmitter changes; the other centers around derangements in cerebral ammonia and glutamine metabolism.

Fischer has most actively advanced the hypothesis that a "false neurotransmitter" may explain the neurological changes of hepatic coma [99]. So far, at least, the evidence is inferential. False neurotransmitters are conceived of as structural analogs of naturally occurring biogenic amines that can inappropriately occupy transmitter receptor sites, thereby blocking the effects of normal neurotransmitter action. Amino acids are likely candidates for such a role and a number of amino acids, including phenylalanine, tyrosine and methionine, are elevated in the blood of patients with hepatic coma. In addition, diets rich in the amino acids tyrosine, tryptophan, and phenylalanine are preferentially toxic to animals with portacaval shunts. Monoamine oxidase inhibitors

are reported to accentuate hepatic stupor in man, and L-dopa, the precursor of cerebral dopamine, lightens the coma of some patients with severe liver disease [100]. In the brain of animals with acute hepatic coma, induced by decreasing the blood supply to the liver, norepinephrine falls and octopamine and serotonin increase substantially [99]. These several observations have led to the speculation that the decrease in norepinephrine, or an interference with its normal cerebral action, may account for some or all of the neurological symptoms of acute hepatic failure.

There is other evidence to support a role for abnormal aromatic amino acid concentrations in brain in the production of hepatic encephalopathy. In rats with a portacaval shunt (as a model of chronic liver disease), the transport of phenylalanine, tyrosine, and other neutral amino acids is markedly and specifically enhanced [101]. Moreover, plasma concentrations of the branched-chain neutral amino acids tend to be below normal in patients with liver disease; and Fischer and coworkers [102] observed, in a group of 11 patients with hepatic encephalopathy, that changes in the plasma concentration ratio (valine + leucine + isoleucine)/(phenylalanine + tyrosine) correlated inversely with the severity of the patients' neurological impairment. The branched-chain neutral amino acids compete for the same saturable carrier system at the blood-brain barrier as do the aromatic neutral amino acids, so raising the plasma (valine + leucine + isoleucine) / (phenylalanine + tyrosine) ratio would be expected to inhibit the transport of the aromatic amino acids into brain. In fact, Fischer and coworkers [102] found that parenteral administration of an amino acid mixture rich in branched-chain neutral amino acids and deficient in aromatic neutral amino acids into patients with hepatic encephalopathy improved the neurological status of some of the subjects, perhaps by normalizing the balance of neurotransmitters in their brains. However, other neurochemical mechanisms must contribute to the beneficial effects of such treatment since Morgan and coworkers [103] observed in a much larger series of patients with liver disease of varying etiology and severity that a lowering of the plasma (valine + leucine + isoleucine)/(phenylalanine + tyrosine) ratio was secondary to liver disease but independent of the presence of hepatic encephalopathy.

Abnormal ammonia metabolism has been featured in explanations of hepatic coma ever since the nineteenth century, when investigators were able to induce cerebral symptoms in animals with portacaval shunts by feeding them meat. Soon after, it was learned that orally ingested ammonium salts would do the same thing.

Ammonia is elevated in blood and brain in severe liver disease. Ammonia is generated from the degradation of amines, amino acids, and purines in the body and from the action on the intestinal contents of urea-splitting organisms. Normally ammonia is promptly converted into urea in the liver by the Krebs-Henseleit cycle (see Fig. 28-4). Liver disease interferes with this cycle by (a) impairing venous drainage from the intestine so that ammonia-carrying portal blood bypasses the liver to enter the systemic circulation (portal-systemic shunting) and (b) reducing the tissue capacity for urea synthesis.

Ammonia is constantly formed in brain by deamination of glutamate and aspartate, probably mediated through the enzymes of the purine nucleotide cycle [104], and by the deamidation of glutamine. Ammonia concentrations in brain are always 50 to 100 percent higher than in blood [105–107]. Ammonia leaves brain by diffusion as well as by conversion into glutamate and glutamine (Fig. 35-5). The latter is an energy-requiring process, catalyzed by the enzyme glutamine synthetase. Glutamine can diffuse from brain into blood, and cerebral arteriovenous concentration differences for glutamine in the resting state are moderately negative [108]. Normally, glutamine levels are about 5 mM in brain and 0.6 mM in CSF. With elevated blood ammonia levels, brain ammonia levels rise proportionately, and glutamine promptly increases so that, in severe liver disease, glutamine levels in CSF may reach 4 to 5 mM [109] (see Fig. 35-6). Moreover, an additional metabolite, α-ketoglutaramate, appears in CSF in significant quantities in chronic hepatic encephalopathy

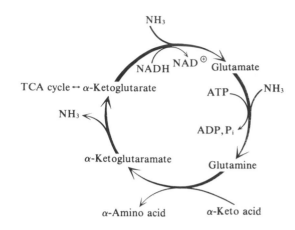

Fig. 35-5. *The pathway of ammonia metabolism in brain. Modified from [109]; used by permission of Raven Press.*

[109]. The mechanism of the rise of α-ketoglutaramate is unknown but it is believed to be formed from glutamine by transamination with an appropriate α-keto acid, possibly phenylpyruvate, glyoxylate, or 4-methyl/thio-2-oxobutyrate [111]. The compound can be broken down subsequently in the presence of the enzyme ω-amidase to yield α-ketoglutarate and ammonia. The entire cycling of one molecule of α-ketoglutarate through glutamate, glutamine, α-ketoglutaramate, and back to α-ketoglutarate removes one molecule of ammonia from the system. Sparing of α-keto acids may be the main normal function of the glutamine transaminase reaction [111].

Considerable physiological evidence indicates that ammonia is toxic to brain. Hyperammonemia accompanies the comas produced by inherited defects in urea synthesis and Reye's syndrome, as well as the coma of liver disease (Chap. 28). Increased ammonia levels in brain have been observed in experimental animals in association with a variety of metabolic disturbances, including cerebral hypoxia-ischemia, hypoglycemia, hypercapnic acidosis, and generalized seizures; this has prompted several investigators to suggest that the accumulation of ammonia in brain may contribute to the pathogenesis of these disorders [13, 93]. Acute hyperammonemia produces both convulsions and coma in experimental animals. Subacute

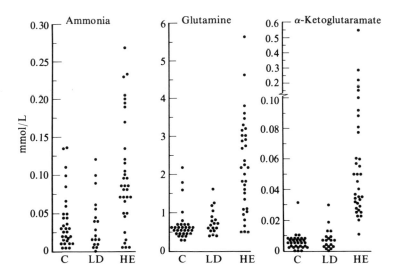

Fig. 35-6. Concentrations of ammonia, glutamine, and α-ketoglutaramate in human CSF. Samples were obtained by routine diagnostic lumbar puncture from control subjects (C), patients with neurologically uncomplicated liver disease (LD), and patients with moderate-to-severe hepatic encephalopathy (HE). Control subjects had a variety of neurological disorders, but normal liver function. The figure includes values reported previously [110], together with more recent, unpublished data from the authors' laboratory.

or chronic hyperammonemia induces dilatation and proliferation of protoplasmic astrocytes in brain; these cells appear to contain large amounts of glutamic dehydrogenase [112] as well as most, if not all, of the brain's glutamine synthetase [113]. Glutamine metabolism is known to be compartmented in brain (Chap. 17), and it has been postulated that the compartment that involves the detoxification of ammonia lies in the protoplasmic astrocytes, which provide a biochemical defense against rising concentrations of ammonia in the adjacent extracellular fluid and neurons [114–116].

The exact mechanism by which elevated ammonia concentrations in brain cause coma is unknown. Bessman and Bessman's [117] earlier theory that α-ketoglutarate is depleted by combining with ammonia to form glutamate was not borne out by experiment: α-ketoglutarate rises, rather than

declines, in brain during hyperammonemia [106, 107, 109]. Present theories center (1) on ammonia's effect on synaptic transmission (it reduces IPSPs and interferes with the chloride pump [118]); (2) on its possible substitution for K^+ in activating the membrane $(Na^+ + K^+)$-ATPase [119]; and (3) on its possible interference with cerebral energy supply.

Marked hyperammonemia produces a significant change in energy metabolism in brain. Hepatic stupor and coma in man and animals are associated with a lowered cerebral oxygen consumption [115]. Also, high concentrations of ammonia inhibit the oxidation of pyruvate in cerebral cortex slices [120]. Schenker and coworkers [106] first noted that coma-producing acute ammonia intoxication in rats lowered phosphocreatine and ATP contents in the brain stem. Hindfelt and Siesjö [105] obtained somewhat similar results, observing significant declines in phosphocreatine and ATP in rat brain 30 minutes after a coma-producing injection of ammonium acetate. In the latter experiments, the fall in high-energy phosphates was maximal in brain stem and cerebellum.

Ammonia-induced stupor and coma in rats with chronic portacaval shunts are associated also with a decline in energy reserves in the brain [107]. When such animals are given moderate amounts of am-

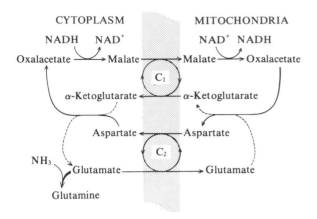

CYTOPLASM   MITOCHONDRIA

Fig. 35-7. Transport of reduced equivalents from cytoplasm to mitochondria through the malate-aspartate shuttle. C_1 and C_2 denote membrane carrier systems for malate–α-ketoglutarate and glutamate-aspartate transport, respectively. Ammonia is represented as interfering with the shuttle by reacting with glutamate in the cytoplasm because glutamine synthetase of brain is predominantly extramitochondrial. From Hindfelt et al. [107].

monium salts, lactate and pyruvate accumulate and the cytoplasmic $NADH/NAD^+$ ratio rises in brain tissue, cerebral oxygen consumption declines, and cerebral concentrations of phosphocreatine and ATP fall. Concentrations of glutamate and aspartate in brain also fall, and glutamine and alanine levels rise. The changes suggest a defect or block in the oxidation of pyruvate and are consistent with an interference by ammonia with the malate-aspartate shuttle that normally transfers reducing equivalents from cytoplasm to mitochondria for oxidation (Fig. 35-7). Studies by Williamson and coworkers [121] with heart mitochondria indicate that the rate of entry of glutamate into mitochondria is an important regulator of the malate-aspartate shuttle but that the affinity of the carrier system for glutamate is low. The accumulation of ammonia in brain could inhibit the shuttle by combining with cytoplasmic glutamate to form glutamine and could ultimately lead to cerebral energy failure by depleting the mitochondria of substrate (NADH) for oxidative phosphorylation. Because most of the glutamine

synthetase of brain is in astrocytes, such an ammonia-mediated inhibition of intracellular hydrogen transport may occur mainly within the glia, perhaps accounting for the astrocytic pathology that is a hallmark of hepatic encephalopathy in humans [114, 115]. Thus, both in vitro and in vivo studies support the view that severe hyperammonemia interferes with the regulation of energy metabolism in the brain, an effect that would explain many clinical aspects of the disorder.

UREMIC ENCEPHALOPATHY

Failure of kidney function leads to the disorder called *uremia*. Measures aimed at the treatment or prevention of uremia, in turn, can cause two additional disorders of cerebral function, namely, the *dialysis-disequilibrium syndrome,* and *progressive dialysis encephalopathy.*

Uremia

Clinically, the patient with severe renal failure suffers from a neurological illness characterized by clouding of consciousness, motor hyperactivity, and overbreathing; the last is a response to the chronic metabolic acidosis of the disease. Rapidly developing renal failure results in a restless delirium; chronic decompensation of kidney function leads to an apathetic, confusional state and eventually to stupor or coma. About one-quarter of the patients suffer transient hemiparesis and other focal neurological weaknesses.

Although a number of biochemical abnormalities are known to occur in uremics, the cause of the encephalopathy has not been identified. Uremia is characterized by retention in the blood of urea, phosphates, hydrogen ions, potentially toxic organic acids and amines, and a number of incompletely identified substances that can be dialyzed from the blood by artificial membranes [122]. Hemodialysis corrects the encephalopathy, so that small, water-soluble molecules are generally thought to be at fault. Urea itself is not the cause of the disorder, because hemodialysis will clear the encephalopathy even when it does not lower the blood urea concentration [123]. Homeostatic physiological and chemical mechanisms protect the brain and spinal fluid against systemic acidosis, and this cannot be incriminated as causing the neurological symptoms [124]. Several neurochemical abnormalities have been identified in animals with experimentally induced uremia. They include decreased rates of glycolysis and energy utilization [125], increased calcium ion content [126], and increased permeability of the bloodbrain barrier [127]. Cerebral blood flow is reduced in renal failure, as is the cerebral metabolic rate for oxygen [128]. Because high-energy phosphate concentrations in the brains of uremic animals remain normal [125], the metabolic changes appear to be a result and not a cause of the disorder. At autopsy, uremic brains do not exhibit cerebral edema, nor do they contain specific neuropathological abnormalities that can be related to the uremic state.

Uremia also produces a chronic, periphral neuropathy, which, unlike the encephalopathy, is not improved by hemodialysis. Clinically, the disorder progresses slowly as a symmetrical, sensorimotor abnormality that affects mainly the lower extremities. The peripheral nerve changes cannot be attributed to any nutritional or vitamin deficiency, to diabetes, or to any other nonspecific complicating factor. Babb and coworkers [129] have suggested that endogenous molecules in the 500 to 2,000 dalton range are responsible, because particles of this size are removed imperfectly by the usual methods of dialysis. No direct evidence supports this hypothesis. However, parathyroid hormone (PTH), a somewhat larger molecule, has been implicated in both the peripheral and central neurological manifestations of uremia [130]. Infusion of PTH into normal dogs induces EEG slowing comparable to that found in uremic animals, whereas parathyroidectomy prior to the induction of uremia prevents the EEG abnormalities [131]. Plasma PTH levels are often elevated in uremic patients, and Avram and coworkers [132] have demonstrated that uremic patients with high serum concentrations of PTH have significantly lower motor-nerve conduction velocities than do uremic patients with normal or moderately elevated levels. The changes in nerve conduction velocity in the subjects studied by Avram and

coworkers [132] could not be correlated with alterations of serum calcium or creatinine; this implies that PTH itself, and not the influence of the hormone on serum calcium levels or the severity of the patients' renal disease, was the causative factor.

Dialysis Dysequilibrium
During the past 20 years, recurrent hemodialysis has become the standard treatment for many patients with chronic renal failure. Hemodialysis is repeated at least weekly, the object being to remove potential toxins from the circulating blood and thereby prevent CNS symptoms of uremia. Perhaps as many as one-half of all patients undergoing dialysis transiently develop uncomfortable neurological symptoms during the procedure. A smaller fraction experience more alarming changes, including impaired consciousness, delirium, or even coma. The condition occurs more commonly during rapid hemodialysis of patients with high blood urea levels.

Symptoms of dialysis dysequilibrium are related to osmolal differences that develop between blood and brain during hemodialysis. The brain responds to uremic hyperosmolality in the blood by slowly increasing its osmolality through the production of molecules (see Chap. 34) that do not readily cross the brain-blood barrier [122]. During hemodialysis, serum osmolality drops rapidly, whereas the osmotically active molecules that have accumulated in brain are cleared more slowly, so the osmolality of the brain and its extracellular water may transiently exceed that of the blood. As a consequence water shifts from the plasma to the brain, causing brain swelling and the symptoms of water intoxication. Dialysis dysequilibrium can be minimized by frequent, slow dialysis.

Progressive Dialysis Encephalopathy
In a small proportion of patients undergoing hemodialysis therapy, a progressively severe, and eventually fatal, encephalopathy has been found to develop. This encephalopathy (*dementia dialytica*) usually occurs in patients receiving chronic dialysis for several years prior to the onset of neurological symptoms. Alfrey and coworkers

[133] first suggested that progressive dialysis encephalopathy is due to chronic aluminum intoxication. Patients with chronic renal failure ingest large quantities of phosphate-binding $Al(OH)_3$ gels to control serum phosphate levels; and body tissues, including the brains of patients dying of dialysis encephalopathy, have been found to contain abnormally high concentrations of aluminum [133, 134]. Recent reports have strongly implicated the aluminum present in untreated or softened tap water used to prepare the dialysis fluid for patients receiving maintenance hemodialysis at home as a major cause of dialysis encephalopathy [134, 135]. Aluminum is highly neurotoxic, and when placed on the brains of experimental animals, will cause focal and generalized seizures [136]. Of possible relevance, elevated levels of aluminum are sometimes found in the brain in association with neurofibrillary degenerative changes characteristic of Alzheimer's dementia [137].

HYPERCAPNIC ENCEPHALOPATHY

Acute pulmonary or ventilatory insufficiency in humans, if untreated, rapidly leads to alterations resembling those of acute hypoxia-ischemia. Chronic pulmonary insufficiency is characterized by mild-to-moderate hypoxemia accompanied by varying degrees of carbon dioxide retention. In the steady state, renal conservation of bicarbonate usually buffers the hypercapnia, and blood pH is normal. The superimposition of infection, the ingestion of a sedative, or fatigue can further compromise pulmonary function, resulting in unbuffered hypercapnia with arterial pH values falling to 7.25 or lower. In metabolic acidosis, physiological buffering mechanisms maintain normal brain pH despite a fall in serum pH. Respiratory acidosis (i.e., CO_2 retention) causes an almost equal accumulation of hydrogen ion in systemic tissues and the CNS [138] because the ventilatory mechanism for excreting carbon dioxide is lost. Patients with chronic pulmonary insufficiency may exhibit lethargy, mental confusion, and stupor. The combination of hypoxia and hypercapnia leads to cerebral vasodilatation, increased cerebral blood flow and, sometimes, to increased intracranial pressure.

Neurological symptoms of chronic pulmonary insufficiency correlate best with the degree of carbon dioxide retention [48]. The associated hypoxemia contributes to, but probably does not cause, the encephalopathy. Moderate, acute hypercapnia (5–10% CO_2 in the inspired air) produces increased arousal and excitability; carbon dioxide concentrations in excess of 35 to 40 percent are anesthetic. Moderate hypercapnia decreases the CMRGlu [13, 139, 140], presumably owing to the inhibitory effect of acidosis on brain phosphofructokinase [34]. Most investigators have observed an unchanged $CMRO_2$ during acute hypercapnia in humans [141] and animals [142, 143]; this implies that the consumption of nonglucose fuels increases to support the continuous high cerebral oxidative rate [13]. Others report that moderate hypercapnia decreases the $CMRO_2$ roughly in proportion to its depression of CMRGlu [140, 144]. This latter view is supported by studies of Kogure and coworkers [145], who used Lowry's closed system technique [82] and found that moderate hypercapnia in rats decreased overall cerebral energy utilization by as much as 17 percent. However, even extreme hypercapnia (20–30% CO_2 in the inspired air) does not deplete brain ATP concentrations [139, 146]. It seems likely, therefore, that the depression of cerebral metabolism during hypercapnia is secondary to decreased neuronal activity and is not the cause of the encephalopathy.

References

1. Duffy, T. E., Nelson, S. R., and Lowry, O. H. Cerebral carbohydrate metabolism during acute hypoxia and recovery. *J. Neurochem.* 19:959–977, 1972.
2. Ferrendelli, J. A., and Chang, M.-M. Brain metabolism during hypoglycemia. *Arch. Neurol.* 28:173–177, 1973.
3. Brodersen, P., Paulson, O. B., Bolwig, T. G., Rogon, Z. E., Rafaelsen, O. J., and Lassen, N. A. Cerebral hyperemia in electrically induced epileptic seizures. *Arch. Neurol.* 28:334–338, 1973.
4. Collins, R. C., Posner, J. B., and Plum, F. Cerebral energy metabolism during electroshock

seizures in mice. *Am. J. Physiol.* 218:943–950, 1970.

5. Duffy, T. E., Howse, D. C., and Plum, F. Cerebral energy metabolism during experimental status epilepticus. *J. Neurochem.* 24:925–934, 1975.

6. King, L. J., Lowry, O. H., Passonneau, J. V., and Venson, V. Effects of convulsants on energy reserves in the cerebral cortex. *J. Neurochem.* 14:599–611, 1967.

7. Sacktor, B., Wilson, J. E., and Tiekert, C. G. Regulation of glycolysis in brain, *in situ,* during convulsions. *J. Biol. Chem.* 241:5071–5075, 1966.

8. Plum, F., Posner, J. B., and Troy, B. Cerebral metabolic and circulatory responses to induced convulsions in animals. *Arch. Neurol.* 18:1–13, 1968.

9. Borgström, L., Chapman, A. G., and Siesjö, B. K. Glucose consumption in the cerebral cortex of rat during bicuculline-induced status epilepticus. *J. Neurochem.* 27:971–973, 1976.

10. Schmidt, C. F., Kety, S. S., and Pennes, H. H. Gaseous metabolism of the brain of the monkey. *Am. J. Physiol.* 143:33–52, 1945.

11. Meldrum, B. S., and Nilsson, B. Cerebral blood flow and metabolic rate early and late in prolonged epileptic seizures induced in rats by bicuculline. *Brain* 99:523–542, 1976.

12. Ferrendelli, J. A., and McDougal, D. B., Jr. The effect of electroshock on regional CNS energy reserves in mice. *J. Neurochem.* 18:1197–1205, 1971.

*13. Siesjö, B. K. *Brain Energy Metabolism.* New York: Wiley, 1978.

14. Howse, D. C., Caronna, J. J., Duffy, T. E., and Plum, F. Cerebral energy metabolism, pH, and blood flow during seizures in the cat. *Am. J. Physiol.* 227:1444–1451, 1974.

15. Howse, D. C. Metabolic responses to status epilepticus in the rat, cat, and mouse. *Can. J. Physiol. Pharmacol.* 57:205–212, 1979.

16. Peterson, E. W., Searle, R., Mandy, F. F., and Leblanc, R. The reversal of experimental vasospasm by dibutyryl-3′,5′-adenosine monophosphate. *J. Neurosurg.* 39:730–734, 1973.

17. Rubio, R., Berne, R. M., Bockman, E. L., and Curnish, R. R. Relationship between adenosine concentration and oxygen supply in rat brain. *Am. J. Physiol.* 228:1896–1902, 1975.

18. Sattin, A. Increase in the content of adenosine-3′,5′-monophosphate in mouse forebrain during seizures and prevention of the increase by methylxanthines. *J. Neurochem.* 18:1087–1096, 1971.

19. Chapman, A. G., Meldrum, B. S., and Siesjö, B. K. Cerebral metabolic changes during prolonged epileptic seizures in rats. *J. Neurochem.* 28:1025–1035, 1977.

20. Carl, J. L., and King, L. J. Hexose and pentose phosphates in brain during convulsions. *J. Neurochem.* 17:293–295, 1970.

21. King, L. J., Carl, J. L., and Lao, L. Carbohydrate metabolism in brain during convulsions and its modification by phenobartitone. *J. Neurochem.* 20:477–485, 1973.

22. Collins, R. C. Metabolic response to focal penicillin seizures in rat: Spike discharge vs. afterdischarge. *J. Neurochem.* 27:1473–1482, 1976.

23. Collins, R. C., Kennedy, C., Sokoloff, L., and Plum, F. Metabolic anatomy of focal motor seizures. *Arch. Neurol.* 33:536–542, 1976.

24. Meyer, J. S., Gotoh, F., and Favale, E. Cerebral metabolism during epileptic seizures in man. *Electroencephalogr. Clin. Neurophysiol.* 21:10–22, 1966.

25. Meldrum, B. S., and Horton, R. W. Physiology of status epilepticus in primates. *Arch. Neurol.* 28:1–9, 1973.

26. Wasterlain, C. G. Mortality and morbidity from serial seizures. *Epilepsia* 15:155–176, 1974.

27. Caspers, H., and Speckmann, E.-J. Cerebral PO_2, PCO_2 and pH: Changes during convulsive activity and their significance for spontaneous arrest of seizures. *Epilepsia* 13:699–725, 1972.

28. Jöbsis, F. F., O'Connor, M., Vitale, A., and Vreman, H. Intracellular redox changes in functioning cerebral cortex. Metabolic effects of epileptiform activity. *J. Neurophysiol.* 34:735–749, 1971.

29. Lewis, D. V., O'Connor, M. J., and Schuette, W. K. Oxidative metabolism during recurrent seizures in the penicillin treated hippocampus. *Electroencephalogr. Clin. Neurophysiol.* 36:347–356, 1974.

*30. Krebs, H. A., and Veech, R. L. Regulation of the Redox State of the Pyridine Nucleotides in Rat Liver. In H. Sund (ed.), *Pyridine Nucleotide-Dependent Dehydrogenases.* New York: Springer-Verlag, 1970. Pp. 413–434.

31. Veech, R. L., Lawson, J. W. R., Cornell, N. W., and Krebs, H. A. Cytosolic phosphorylation potential. *J. Biol. Chem.* 254:6538–6547, 1979.

32. Howse, D. C., and Duffy, T. E. Control of the redox state of the pyridine nucleotides in the rat cerebral cortex. Effect of electroshock-induced seizures. *J. Neurochem.* 24:935–940, 1975.

*33. Plum, F., Howse, D. C., and Duffy, T. E. Meta-

*Key reference.

bolic effects of seizures. *Res. Publ. Assoc. Nerv. Ment. Dis.* 53:141–157, 1974.

34. Lowry, O. H., and Passonneau, J. V. Kinetic evidence for multiple binding sites on phosphofructokinase. *J. Biol. Chem.* 241:2268–2279, 1966.

35. Kennedy, C., Des Rosiers, M. H., Jehle, J. W., Reivich, M., Sharpe, F., and Sokoloff, L. Mapping of functional neural pathways by autoradiographic survey of local metabolic rate with [^{14}C]-deoxyglucose. *Science* 187:850–853, 1975.

36. Raichle, M. E., Grubb, R. L., Jr., Gado, M. H., Eichling, J. O., and Ter-Pogossian, M. M. Correlation between regional cerebral blood flow and oxidative metabolism. *Arch. Neurol.* 33:523–526, 1976.

37. Salford, L. G., Duffy, T. E., and Plum, F. Association of Blood Flow and Acid-Base Change in Brain During Afferent Stimulation. In T. W. Langfitt, L. C. McHenry, Jr., M. Reivich, and H. Wollman (eds.), *Cerebral Circulation and Metabolism.* New York: Springer-Verlag, 1975. Pp. 380–382.

38. Wasterlain, C. G., and Plum, F. Vulnerability of developing rat brain to electroconvulsive seizures. *Arch. Neurol.* 29:38–45, 1973.

39. Meldrum, B. S., and Brierley, J. B. Prolonged epileptic seizures in primates. *Arch. Neurol.* 28:10–17, 1973.

40. Wasterlain, C. G., and Duffy, T. E. Status epilepticus in immature rats. Protective effects of glucose on survival and brain development. *Arch. Neurol.* 33:821–827, 1976.

41. Blennow, G., Brierley, J. B., Meldrum, B. S., and Siesjö, B. K. Epileptic brain damage. The role of systemic factors that modify cerebral energy metabolism. *Brain* 101:687–700, 1978.

42. Minard, F. N., Kang, C. H., and Mushahwar, I. K. The effect of periodic convulsions induced by 1,1-dimethylhydrazine on the glycogen of rat brain. *J. Neurochem.* 12:279–286, 1965.

43. DeRobertis, E., Alberici, M., and Rodriguez de Lores Arnaiz, G. Astroglial swelling and phosphohydrolases in cerebral cortex of metrazol convulsant rats. *Brain Res.* 12:461–466, 1969.

44. Meldrum, B. S., Vigouroux, R. A., and Brierley, J. B. Systemic factors and epileptic brain damage. *Arch. Neurol.* 29:82–87, 1973.

*45. Kuffler, S. W., and Nicholls, J. G. *From Neuron to Brain. A Cellular Approach to the Function of the Nervous System.* Sunderland: Sinauer Associates, 1976.

46. Prince, D. A., Pedley, T. A., and Ransom, B. R. Fluctuations in Ion Concentrations During Excitation and Seizures. In E. Schoffeniels, G. Franck, L. Hertz, and D. B. Tower (eds.), *Dynamic Properties of Glia Cells.* Oxford: Pergamon, 1978. Pp. 281–303.

47. Ward, A. W., Jr. Glia and Epilepsy. In E. Schoffeniels, G. Franck, L. Hertz, and D. B. Tower (eds.), *Dynamic Properties of Glia Cells.* Oxford: Pergamon, 1978. Pp. 413–427.

*48. Plum, F., and Posner, J. B. *Diagnosis of Stupor and Coma* (3rd ed.). Philadelphia: Davis, 1980.

49. Ingvar, D. H., Haggendal, E., Nilsson, N. J., Sourander, P., Wickbom, I., and Lassen, N. A. Cerebral circulation and metabolism in a comatose patient. *Arch. Neurol.* 11:13–21, 1964.

50. Ingvar, D. H., and Sourander, P. Destruction of the reticular core of the brain stem. A pathoanatomical follow-up of a case of coma of three years' duration. *Arch. Neurol.* 23:1–8, 1970.

*51. Meyer, H., and Overton, E. Cited by Andersen, N. B., and Amaranath, L. Anesthetic effects on transport across cell membranes. *Anesthesiology* 39:126–152, 1973.

52. Dawson, B., Michenfelder, J. D., and Theye, R. A. Effects of ketamine on canine cerebral blood flow and metabolism. *Anesth. Analg.* 50:443–447, 1971.

53. Clark, D. L., Hosick, E. C., and Rosner, B. S. Neurophysiological effects of different anesthetics in unconscious man. *J. Appl. Physiol.* 31:884–891, 1971.

54. French, J. D., Verzeano, M., and Magoun, H. W. A neural basis of the anesthetic state. *Arch. Neurol. Psychiatr.* 69:519–529, 1953.

55. Hosick, E. C., Clark, D. L., Adam, N., and Rosner, B. S. Neurophysiological effects of different anesthetics in conscious man. *J. Appl. Physiol.* 31:892–898, 1971.

56. Barker, J. L. Selective Depression of Postsynaptic Excitation by General Anesthetics. In B. R. Fink (ed.), *Molecular Mechanisms of Anesthesia.* New York: Raven, 1975. Vol. 1, pp. 135–153.

57. Torda, T. A., and Gage, P. W. Postsynaptic effect of i.v. anesthetic agents at the neuromuscular junction. *Br. J. Anaesth.* 49:771–776, 1977.

58. Seeman, P., and Roth, S. General anesthetics expand cell membranes at surgical concentrations. *Biochim. Biophys. Acta* 255:171–177, 1972.

59. Trudell, J. R., Hubbel, W. L., and Cohen, E. N. Pressure reversal of inhalation anesthetic-induced disorder in spin-labeled phospholipid vesicles. *Biochim. Biophys. Acta* 291:328–334, 1973.

60. Halsey, M. J., and Wardley-Smith, B. Pressure reversal of narcosis produced by anaesthetics, narcotics and tranquilizers. *Nature* 257:811–813, 1975.

*61. Roth, S. H. Physical mechanisms of anesthesia. *Annu. Rev. Pharmacol. Toxicol.* 19:159–178, 1979.

62. Nahrwold, M. L., and Cohen, P. J. Anesthetics and Mitochondrial Function. In P. J. Cohen (ed.), *Metabolic Aspects of Anesthesia.* Clinical Anesthesia Series. Philadelphia: Davis, 1975. Vol. 1, pp. 25–44.

63. Nahrwold, M. L., Clark, C. R., and Cohen, P. J. Is depression of mitochondrial respiration a predictor of *in-vivo* anesthetic activity? *Anesthesiology* 40:566–570, 1974.

64. Goldberg, N. D., Passonneau, J. V., and Lowry, O. H. Effects of changes in brain metabolism on the levels of citric acid cycle intermediates. *J. Biol. Chem.* 241:3997–4003, 1966.

65. Nilsson, L., and Siesjö, B. K. The effect of anesthetics upon labile phosphates and upon extra- and intracellular lactate, pyruvate and bicarbonate concentrations in rat brain. *Acta Physiol. Scand.* 80:235–248, 1970.

66. Crane, P. D., Braun, L. D., Cornford, E. M., Cremer, J. E., Glass, J. M., and Oldendorf, W. H. Dose dependent reduction of glucose utilization by pentobarbital in rat brain. *Stroke* 9:12–17, 1978.

67. Shapiro, H. M., Greenberg, J. H., Reivich, M., Ashmead, G., and Sokoloff, L. Local cerebral glucose uptake in awake and halothane-anesthetized primates. *Anesthesiology* 48:97–103, 1978.

68. Chapman, A. G., Nordström, C.-H., and Siesjö, B. K. Influence of phenobarbital anesthesia on carbohydrate and amino acid metabolism in rat brain. *Anesthesiology* 48:175–182, 1978.

69. Kogure, K., Scheinberg, P., Utsunomiya, Y., Kishikawa, H., and Busto, R. Sequential cerebral biochemical and physiological events in controlled hypoxemia. *Ann. Neurol.* 2:304–310, 1977.

70. Salford, L. G., Plum, F., and Siesjö, B. K. Graded hypoxia-oligemia in rat brain. Biochemical alterations and their implications. *Arch. Neurol.* 29:227–238, 1973.

*71. Brown, A. W., and Brierley, J. B. The earliest alterations in rat neurones and astrocytes after anoxia. *Acta Neuropathol.* 23:9–22, 1973.

72. Ginsberg, M. D., and Myers, R. E. Experimental carbon monoxide encephalopathy in the primate. I. Physiologic and metabolic aspects. *Arch. Neurol.* 30:202–208, 1974.

73. Fein, J. M., Eastman, R., and Moore, C. Oxidative metabolism in cerebral ischemia. Part 1. Measurement of oxygen extraction slopes of grey and white matter *in vivo. Stroke* 8:472–479, 1977.

74. Berntman, L., Carlsson, C., and Siesjö, B. K. Cerebral oxygen consumption and blood flow in hypoxia: Influence of sympathoadrenal activation. *Stroke* 10:20–25, 1979.

75. Pulsinelli, W. A., and Duffy, T. E. Local cerebral glucose metabolism during controlled hypoxemia in rats. *Science* 204:626–629, 1979.

76. Welsh, F. A., O'Connor, M. J., and Langfitt, T. W. Regions of cerebral ischemia located by pyridine nucleotide fluorescence. *Science* 198:951–953, 1977.

77. Welsh, F. A., O'Connor, M. J., and Marcy, V. R. Effect of oligemia on regional metabolite levels in cat brain. *J. Neurochem.* 31:311–319, 1978.

78. Davis, J. N., and Carlsson, A. Effect of hypoxia on tyrosine and tryptophan hydroxylation in unanesthetized rat brain. *J. Neurochem.* 20:913–915, 1973.

79. Breese, G. R., and Traylor, T. D. Effect of 6-hydroxydopamine on brain catecholamine neurons. *J. Pharmacol. Exp. Ther.* 174:413–420, 1970.

80. Gibson, G. E., and Blass, J. P. Impaired synthesis of acetylcholine in brain accompanying mild hypoxia and hypoglycemia. *J. Neurochem.* 27:37–42, 1976.

81. Gibson, G. E., and Duffy, T. E. Impaired synthesis of acetylcholine by mild hypoxic hypoxia or nitrous oxide. *J. Neurochem.* 36:28–33, 1981.

*82. Lowry, O. H., Passonneau, J. V., Hasselberger, F. X., and Schulz, D. W. Effect of ischemia on known substrates and cofactors of the glycolytic pathway in brain. *J. Biol. Chem.* 239:18–30, 1964.

83. Kleihues, P., and Hossmann, K.-A. Protein synthesis in the cat brain after prolonged cerebral ischemia. *Brain Res.* 35:409–418, 1971.

84. Hossman, K.-A., and Kleihues, P. Reversibility of ischemic brain damage. *Arch. Neurol.* 29:375–384, 1973.

85. Hinzen, D. H., Müller, U., Sobotka, P., Gebert, E., Land, R., and Hirsch, H. Metabolism and function of dog's brain recovering from longtime ischemia. *Am. J. Physiol.* 223:1158–1164, 1972.

86. Swanson, P. D. Acidosis and some metabolic properties of isolated cerebral tissues. *Arch. Neurol.* 20:653–663, 1969.

87. Myers, R. E. Lactic Acid Accumulation as Cause of Brain Edema and Cerebral Necrosis Resulting from Oxygen Deprivation. In R. Korobkin, and C. Guilleminault (eds.), *Advances in Perinatal Neurology.* New York: Spectrum, 1979. Vol. 1, pp. 85–114.

88. Hossmann, K.-A., Sakaki, S., and Kimoto, K. Cerebral uptake of glucose and oxygen in the cat brain after prolonged ischemia. *Stroke* 7:301–305, 1976.

89. Levy, D. E., and Duffy, T. E.   Cerebral energy metabolism during transient ischemia and recovery in the gerbil. *J. Neurochem.* 28:63–70, 1977.

90. Levy, D. E., and Brierley, J. B.   Delayed pentobarbital administration limits ischemic brain damage in gerbils. *Ann. Neurol.* 5:59–64, 1979.

91. Kety, S. S., Woodford, R. B., Harmel, M. H., Freyhan, F. A., Appel, K. E., and Schmidt, C. F. Cerebral blood flow and metabolism in schizophrenia: The effects of barbiturate semi-narcosis, insulin coma and electroshock. *Am. J. Psychiatry* 104:765–770, 1948.

92. Lewis, L. D., Ljunggren, B., Norberg, K., and Siesjö, B. K.   Changes in carbohydrate substrates, amino acids and ammonia in the brain during insulin-induced hypoglycemia. *J. Neurochem.* 23:659–671, 1974.

93. Tews, J. K., Carter, S. H., and Stone, W. E. Chemical changes in the brain during insulin hypoglycaemia and recovery. *J. Neurochem.* 12:679–693, 1965.

94. Owen, O. E., Morgan, A. P., Kemp, H. G., Sullivan, J. M., Herrera, M. G., and Cahill, G. F. Brain metabolism during fasting. *J. Clin. Invest.* 46:1589–1595, 1967.

95. Hawkins, R. A., and Biebuyck, J. F.   Ketone bodies are selectively used by individual brain regions. *Science* 205:325–327, 1979.

*96. Sokoloff, L., Fitzgerald, G. G., and Kaufman, E. E.   Cerebral Nutrition and Energy Metabolism. In R. J. Wurtman, and J. J. Wurtman (eds.), *Nutrition and the Brain.* New York: Raven, 1977. Vol. 1, pp. 87–139.

97. Agardh, C.-D., Folbergrová, J., and Siesjö, B. K. Cerebral metabolic changes in profound, insulin-induced hypoglycemia, and in the recovery period following glucose administration. *J. Neurochem.* 31:1135–1142, 1978.

98. Gorell, J. M., Law, M. M., Lowry, O. H., and Ferrendelli, J. A.   Levels of cerebral cortical glycolytic and citric acid cycle metabolites during hypoglycemic stupor and its reversal. *J. Neurochem.* 29:187–191, 1977.

*99. Fischer, J. E.   False neurotransmitters and hepatic coma. *Res. Publ. Assoc. Nerv. Ment. Dis.* 53:53–73, 1974.

100. Lunzer, M., James, I. M., Weinman, J., and Sherlock, S.   Treatment of chronic hepatic encephalopathy with levodopa. *Gut* 15:555–561, 1974.

101. James, J. H., Escourrou, J., and Fischer, J. E. Blood-brain neutral amino acid transport activity is increased after portacaval anastomosis. *Science* 200:1395–1397, 1978.

102. Fischer, J. E., Rosen, H. M., Ebeid, A. M., James, J. H., Keane, J. M., and Soeters, P. B.   The effect of normalization of plasma amino acids on hepatic encephalopathy in man. *Surgery* 80:77–91, 1976.

103. Morgan, M. Y., Milsom, J. P., and Sherlock, S. Plasma ratio of valine, leucine and isoleucine to phenylalanine and tyrosine in liver disease. *Gut* 19:1068–1073, 1978.

104. Schultz, V., and Lowenstein, J. M.   The purine nucleotide cycle. Studies of ammonia production and interconversions of adenine and hypoxanthine nucleotides and nucleosides by rat brain *in situ. J. Biol. Chem.* 253:1938–1943, 1978.

105. Hindfelt, B., and Siesjö, B. K.   Cerebral effects of acute ammonia intoxication. The effect upon energy metabolism. *Scand. J. Clin. Lab. Invest.* 28:365–374, 1971.

106. Schenker, S., McCandless, D. W., Brophy, E., and Lewis, M.   Studies on the intracerebral toxicity of ammonia. *J. Clin. Invest.* 46:838–848, 1967.

*107. Hindfelt, B., Plum, F., and Duffy, T. E.   Effect of acute ammonia intoxication on cerebral metabolism in rats with portacaval shunts. *J. Clin. Invest.* 59:386–396, 1977.

108. Gjedde, A., Lockwood, A. H., Duffy, T. E., and Plum, F.   Cerebral blood flow and metabolism in chronically hyperammonemic rats: Effect of an acute ammonia challenge. *Ann. Neurol.* 3:325–330, 1978.

*109. Duffy, T. E., Vergara, F., and Plum, F.   α-Ketoglutaramate in hepatic encephalopathy. *Res. Publ. Assoc. Nerv. Ment. Dis.* 53:39–52, 1974.

110. Duffy, T. E., and Plum, F.   α-Ketoglutaramate in the CSF: Clinical Implications in Hepatic Encephalopathy. In D. H. Ingvar, and N. A. Lassen (eds.), *Brain Work. The Coupling of Function, Metabolism and Blood Flow in the Brain.* Copenhagen: Munksgaard, 1975. Pp. 280–292.

111. Cooper, A. J. L., and Gross, M.   The glutamine transaminase-ω-amidase system in rat and human brain. *J. Neurochem.* 28:771–778, 1977.

112. Norenberg, M. D.   Histochemical studies in experimental portal-systemic encephalopathy. Glutamic dehydrogenase. *Arch. Neurol.* 33:265–269, 1976.

113. Norenberg, M. D., and Martinez-Hernandez, A. Fine structural localization of glutamine synthetase in astrocytes of rat brain. *Brain Res.* 161:303–310, 1979.

*114. Cavanagh, J. B.   Liver bypass and the glia. *Res. Publ. Assoc. Nerv. Ment. Dis.* 53:13–38, 1974.

*115. Plum, F., and Hindfelt, B.   The Neurological Complications of Liver Disease. In P. J. Vinken, and G. W. Bruyn (eds.), *Handbook of Clinical Neurology: Metabolic and Deficiency Diseases of* *the Nervous System.* Amsterdam: North-Holland, 1976. Vol. 27, pp. 349–377.

116. Cooper, A. J. L., McDonald, J. M., Gelbard, A. S., Gledhill, R. F., and Duffy, T. E. The metabolic fate of ^{13}N-labeled ammonia in rat brain. *J. Biol. Chem.* 254:4982–4992, 1979.

117. Bessman, S. P., and Bessman, A. N. The cerebral and peripheral uptake of ammonia in liver disease with an hypothesis for the mechanism of hepatic coma. *J. Clin. Invest.* 34:622–628, 1955.

118. Meyer, H., and Lux, H. D. Action of ammonium on a chloride pump: Removal of hyperpolarizing inhibition in an isolated neuron. *Pflüegers Arch.* 350:185–195, 1974.

119. Skou, J. C. Further investigations on a $Mg^{++}+$ Na^{+}-activated adenosintriphosphatase, possibly related to the active, linked transport of Na^+ and K^+ across the nerve membrane. *Biochim. Biophys. Acta* 42:6–23, 1960.

120. McKhann, G. M., and Tower, D. B. Ammonia toxicity and cerebral oxidative metabolism. *Am. J. Physiol.* 200:420–424, 1961.

*121. Williamson, J. R., Safer, B., LaNoue, K. F., Smith, C. M., and Walajtys, E. Mitochondrial-Cytosolic Interactions in Cardiac Tissue: Role of the Malate-Aspartate Cycle in the Removal of Glycolytic NADH from the Cytosol. In D. D. Davies (ed.), *Rate Control of Biological Processes.* New York: Cambridge University Press, 1973. Pp. 241–281.

*122. Raskin, N. H., and Fishman, R. A. Neurologic disorders in renal failure. *N. Engl. J. Med.* 294:143–148, 204–210, 1976.

123. Merrill, J. P., Legrain, M., and Hoigne, R. Observations on the role of urea in uremia. *Am. J. Med.* 14:519–520, 1953.

124. Posner, J. B., Swanson, A. G., and Plum, F. Acid-base balance in cerebrospinal fluid. *Arch. Neurol.* 12:479–496, 1965.

125. van den Noort, S., Eckel, R. E., Brine, K. L., and Hrdlicka, J. Brain metabolism in experimental uremia. *Arch. Intern. Med.* 126:831–834, 1970.

126. Arieff, A. I., and Massry, S. G. Calcium metabolism of brain in acute renal failure. Effects of uremia, hemodialysis, and parathyroid hormone. *J. Clin. Invest.* 53:387–392, 1974.

127. Fishman, R. A., and Raskin, N. H. Experimental uremic encephalopathy. Permeability and electrolyte metabolism of brain and other tissues. *Arch. Neurol.* 17:10–21, 1967.

128. Scheinberg, P. Effects of uremia on cerebral blood flow and metabolism. *Neurology* 4:101–105, 1954.

129. Babb, A. L., Popovich, R. P., Christopher, T. G., and Scribner, B. H. The genesis of the square

meter-hour hypothesis. *Trans. Am. Soc. Artif. Intern. Organs* 17:81–91, 1971.

*130. Massry, S. G. Is parathyroid hormone a uremic toxin? *Nephron* 19:125–130, 1977.

131. Guisado, R., Arieff, A. I., and Massry, S. G. Changes in the electroencephalogram in acute uremia. Effects of parathyroid hormone and brain electrolytes. *J. Clin. Invest.* 55:738–745, 1975.

132. Avram, M. M., Feinfeld, D. A., and Huatuco, A. H. Search for the uremic toxin. Decreased motor-nerve conduction velocity and elevated parathyroid hormone in uremia. *N. Engl. J. Med.* 298:1000–1003, 1978.

*133. Alfrey, A. C., LeGendre, G. R., and Kaehny, W. D. The dialysis encephalopathy syndrome: Possible aluminum intoxication. *N. Engl. J. Med.* 294:184–188, 1976.

134. McDermott, J. R., Smith, A. I., Ward, M. K., Parkinson, I. S., and Kerr, D. N. S. Brain-aluminium concentration in dialysis encephalopathy. *Lancet* 1:901–904, 1978.

135. Elliott, H. L., Dryburgh, F., Fell, G. S., Sabet, S., and MacDougall, A. I. Aluminium toxicity during regular haemodialysis. *Br. Med. J.* 1:1101–1103, 1978.

136. Moseley, J. I., Ojemann, G. A., and Ward, A. A., Jr. Unit activity in experimental epileptic foci during focal cortical hypothermia. *Exp. Neurol.* 37:164–178, 1972.

137. Goetz, C. G., and Klawans, H. L. Neurologic Aspects of Other Metals. In P. J. Vinken, and G. W. Bruyn (eds.), *Handbook of Clinical Neurology: Intoxications of the Nervous System.* Amsterdam: North-Holland, 1979. Vol. 36, pp. 319–345.

*138. Plum, F., and Siesjö, B. K. Recent advances in CSF physiology. *Anesthesiology* 42:708–730, 1975.

*139. Miller, A. L., Hawkins, R. A., and Veech, R. L. Decreased rate of glucose utilization by rat brain *in vivo* after exposure to atmospheres containing high concentrations of CO_2. *J. Neurochem.* 25:553–558, 1975.

140. DesRosiers, M. H., Kennedy, C., Sakurada, O., Shinohara, M., and Sokoloff, L. Effects of hypercapnia on cerebral oxygen and glucose consumption in the conscious rat. *Stroke* 9:98, 1978.

141. Kety, S. S., and Schmidt, C. F. The effects of altered arterial tensions of carbon dioxide and oxygen on cerebral blood flow and cerebral oxygen consumption of normal young men. *J. Clin. Invest.* 27:484–492, 1948.

142. Nilsson, B., and Siesjö, B. K. A method for determining blood flow and oxygen consumption in the rat brain. *Acta Physiol. Scand.* 96:72–82, 1976.

143. Gjedde, A., Caronna, J. J., Hindfelt, B., and Plum, F. Whole-brain blood flow and oxygen metabolism in the rat during nitrous oxide anesthesia. *Am. J. Physiol.* 229:113–118, 1975.

144. Kliefoth, A. B., Grubb, R. L., Jr., and Raichle, M. E. Depression of cerebral oxygen utilization by hypercapnia in the rhesus monkey. *J. Neurochem.* 32:661–663, 1979.

*145. Kogure, K., Busto, R., Scheinberg, P., and Reinmuth, O. Dynamics of cerebral metabolism during moderate hypercapnia. *J. Neurochem.* 24: 471–478, 1975.

146. Folbergrová, J., MacMillan, V., and Siesjö, B. K. The effect of moderate and marked hypercapnia upon the energy state and upon the cytoplasmic NADH/NAD$^+$ ratio of the rat brain. *J. Neurochem.* 19:2497–2505, 1972.

Chapter 36. Parkinson's Disease and Other Disorders of the Basal Ganglia

Some large, anatomically distinct masses of gray matter lie at the base of the brain, and certain of these, namely the caudate nucleus, the putamen, and the globus pallidus, are collectively termed *basal ganglia*. The first two of these constitute the *striatum,* or *neostriatum;* the internal and external parts of the globus pallidus, or pallidum, are known as the *paleostriatum*. This striopallidal system is an integrative unit, the constituent parts of which have many connections between one another and to and from other regions of the brain. Some of the interconnections of the basal ganglia and related structures are shown in Fig. 36-1. The subcortical structures shown in this figure are equivalent to the extrapyramidal system, i.e., the structures of the brain, apart from the cerebral cortex, which send efferent fibers to the spinal cord. Among the body functions regulated by the extrapyramidal system are the tone and posture of the limbs.

Regulatory functions of this type have been recognized since 1911, when S. A. K. Wilson demonstrated in a series of patients the relationship between lesions of the lenticular nucleus (putamen and globus pallidus, considered as a unit), on the one hand, and rigidity, tremor, and postural defects, on the other. At postmortem examination, he discovered previously unsuspected, extensive hepatic cirrhosis. *Wilson's disease* was regarded as the prototype of disorders of the basal ganglia, as well as a prime example of combined liver and brain disease.

The most prevalent disorder of the extrapyramidal system is *Parkinson's disease,* the "shaking palsy," first described in 1817 by the London physician James Parkinson. This disorder is now recognized to stem from degenerative changes in the substantia nigra, a portion of the brain that has extensive connections with the striatum. Besides the shaking, or tremor, of the limbs, patients with Parkinson's disease may also exhibit muscular rigidity, which leads to difficulties in walking, writing, and speaking, masking of facial expression, and flexed posture. Some also suffer loss of volitional movement that may progress to akinesia.

Huntington's disease is a third important disorder of basal ganglia, with the most prominent pathology in the caudate nucleus. This is a familial disorder leading to chorea and to behavioral and cognitive dysfunction.

Biochemical Characteristics of Basal Ganglia and Associated Structures

The basal ganglia are especially sensitive to carbon monoxide and to manganese. This sensitivity probably plays a role in the neurological complications that accompany intoxication with these chemicals. In infants, the predilection of bilirubin for the cells of the basal ganglia may result in *kernicterus* (jaundice of the nuclei of the brain). Historically, kernicterus was the first basal ganglial disease described, and Wilson made use of the parallel in his classic study.

The globus pallidus contains much iron, a property it shares with other nuclei of the extrapyramidal system: the subthalamic nucleus of Luys, the substantia nigra, the red nucleus (nucleus ruber), the dentate nucleus, and the inferior olive. It has been suggested that the metal is present in ferritinlike molecular form.

The basal ganglia are richly innervated with cholinergic fibers. This is particularly evident in the caudate nucleus. Other types of fiber, characterized by their content of substance P or of GABA have now been described.

719

The substantia nigra, the red nucleus, and the locus ceruleus each contain a distinctive pigment. The precursor of the pigmented material is thought to be dopa (3,4-dihydroxyphenylalanine) or a catecholamine, but the specific pathways of pigment formation are not completely known.

Dopamine and Basal Ganglia

Biochemical characteristics that have thrown much light on the functions of the basal ganglia and certain associated structures in humans and animals are the distribution of dopamine and of tyrosine hydroxylase, an enzyme found in catecholamine-containing neurons and cells. The biosynthetic relationships of dopamine are illustrated in Fig. 36-2 (see also Chap. 10). The starting point for its biosynthesis is tyrosine, which is present in the whole brain at a level of about 1.2 mg per 100 g fresh weight of tissue, or 70 μmol per kilogram. The first step is catalyzed by tyrosine hydroxylase; it requires iron and a pteridine cofactor, tetrahydrobiopterin. The latter is oxidized along with tyrosine during the reaction. A system consisting of NADPH and dihydropteridine reductase is also required to regenerate the coenzyme. The product of this oxidation is dopa, an amino acid that is normally present only in the most minute concentrations in the body because it is so readily decarboxylated to dopamine (3,4-dihydroxyphenylethylamine). This is achieved through the action of the widely distributed enzyme AADC (aromatic L-amino-acid decarboxylase). Important physiological substrates for it are dopa and 5-HTP (5-hydroxytryptophan).

Like other amino acid decarboxylases, AADC requires pyridoxal phosphate as its coenzyme. It is inhibited by many compounds, some of which are effective in vivo and have even been used therapeutically in certain diseases. A few decarboxylase inhibitors are illustrated in Fig. 36-3. The first of these, methyldopa, is used as an antihypertensive drug in humans, but it is the only decarboxylase inhibitor with such properties. Its action in essential hypertension is mediated through metabolites, either α-methyldopamine or α-methylnorepineph-

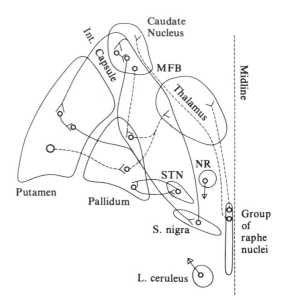

Fig. 36-1. *Major subcortical connections of the basal ganglia and some associated structures. Nigral dopaminergic fibers pass upward in the medial forebrain bundle (MFB) to the caudate nucleus and putamen. These constitute the nigrostriatal tract. GABA-containing fibers pass from the striatum and pallidum to the substantia nigra, where they exert inhibitory actions. Cholinergic neurons (and perhaps others) that are intrinsic to the striatum serve as intermediaries between these two tracts. The major output of the basal ganglia is by way of the globus pallidus, to the lateral and anterior parts of the thalamus and other structures, by presumed cholinergic fibers. The thalamus, in turn, has direct connections with the motor cortex, so that the existence of a striato-pallido-thalamo-cortical circuit, as well as connections to the thalamus from the motor cortex and the cerebellum, emphasize the fact that the basal ganglia are prominently involved in the regulation of motor phenomena. Fibers pass from the pallidum to the subthalamic nucleus (STN, corpus Luysii). The pallidum is reciprocally innervated by fibers originating in the STN. Noradrenergic neurons from locus ceruleus innervate these and other regions of the brain. Serotonergic fibers from certain of the midline raphe nuclei reach the thalamus, striatum (by way of the MFB), and elsewhere. Nucleus ruber (NR, red nucleus) is important as an upper brain stem nucleus from which descending motor pathways, including the rubrotegmentospinal system, originate.*

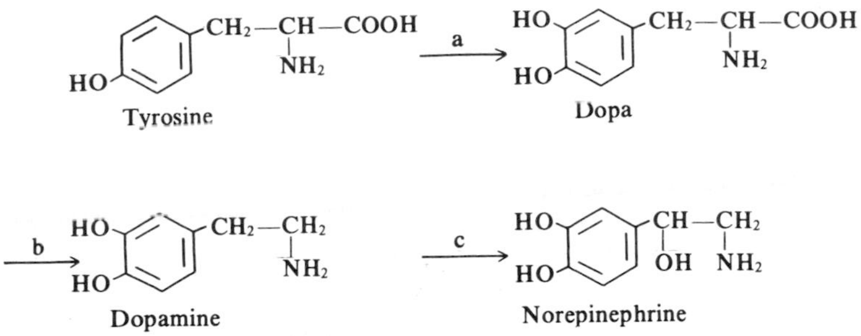

Fig. 36-2. Pathway of biosynthesis of catecholamines. The enzymes catalyzing each step are: (a) tyrosine hydroxylase; (b) aromatic amino acid decarboxylase; and (c) dopamine β-hydroxylase.

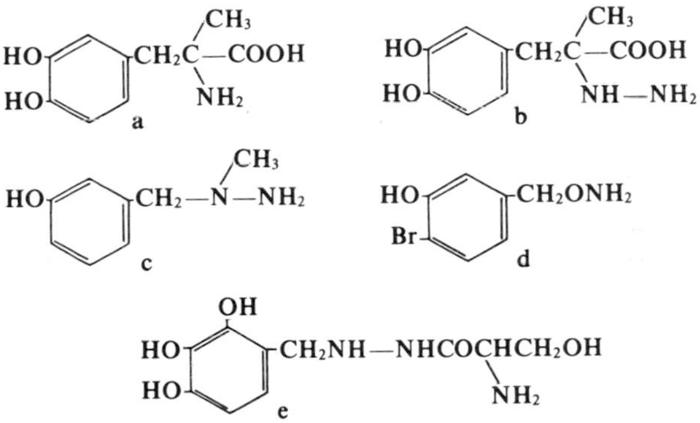

Fig. 36-3. Some frequently used inhibitors of aromatic amino acid decarboxylase: (a) methyldopa (L-alpha-methyldopa); (b) carbidopa, the hydrazino analog of methyldopa; (c) N-m-hydroxybenzyl-N-methylhydrazine; (d) brocresine; (e) benserazide.

rine, formed (among other locations in the body) in the region of the vasomotor centers in the medulla oblongata, where these metabolites initiate their hypotensive action. Methyldopa has been widely used in biochemical and pharmacological studies because of important effects on monoamine metabolism. The other compounds in Fig. 36-3 have also been employed extensively in research when blockade of decarboxylation is required. Carbidopa and benserazide are used in Parkinson's disease.

The formation of dopamine is the terminal step in biosynthesis in certain neurons of the brain. These neurons have been identified by use of the specific fluorescence of derivatives of dopamine and other monoamines developed in situ by histochemical means. By pharmacological pretreatment of animals in a manner that specifically depletes the brain of one amine or another, areas rich in a particular monoamine can be differentiated by ultraviolet histofluorescence. The fiber connections passing from the substantia nigra to the caudate nucleus belong to this group of neurons. They store dopamine in vesicles within the varicosities of the nerve terminations; the intravesicular concentration of the amine may rise to as high as 1 to 10 mg per gram fresh weight, that is, in the range of amine concentration of chromaffin tissue. Other neurons of the brain contain not only tyrosine hydroxylase and AADC but also dopamine β-hydroxylase which is found in the membrane of the storage vesicles. These are the norepinephrine-containing fibers. They can be detected immunohistochemically by preparing an antibody to purified dopamine β-hydroxylase and derivatizing it to produce a fluorescent reagent for use with histologically prepared tissue sections.

Under many circumstances, the biosynthesis of these monoamines is limited by the slow flux through the stage of tyrosine hydroxylase because of the low turnover rate of that enzyme.

The regional distribution of these compounds in the CNS is shown in Table 36-1. Dopamine and norepinephrine are irregularly distributed in the brain and spinal cord. Thus dopamine is found in certain regions along with norepinephrine, but unlike norepinephrine, it is present in unusually

Table 36-1. Regional Distribution of Catecholamines and Related Substances in Human Brain

Brain Region	DA[a]	NE[a]	TH[c]	AADC[b]	DBH[f]
Cerebral cortex	0.13	0–0.06	3–6	0–42	5–10
Caudate nucleus	4.1	0.06	16–121	366	nd[e]
Putamen	5.65		15–198	432	
Globus pallidus	0.4		4–15	22	
Thalamus	0.30–0.46	0.05	8	22	60
Hypothalamus	1.12	1.11	10	149	265
Substantia nigra	0.42	nd[e]	17–38[d]	21	57
Cerebellum			5	28	7
Medulla	0.17	0.14		24	

[a]Micrograms per gram fresh weight of tissue. Data from [1] and [2].
[b]Nanomoles of CO_2 per 100 mg protein in 2 hours [3].
[c]Nanomoles per gram wet weight of tissue per hour [4, 5].
[d]Mackay et al. [5] observed a value for TH in substantia nigra of the same order as for the caudate nucleus.
[e]Not detectable.
[f]Nanomoles per gram wet weight of tissue per hour [5].

high concentrations in some of the basal ganglia. On the other hand, norepinephrine is readily detected in the spinal cord, but dopamine only with difficulty.

For a long time dopamine was regarded as merely the precursor of norepinephrine. This view was upset by the results of neurochemical and histofluorescent mapping of the brain, which revealed the highly uneven distribution of the two compounds. The striking discrepancies in their regional distribution (Table 36-1) suggested a specific neural role for dopamine. The concept of dopamine as a neurohumor acting at certain synapses within the neostriatum and thus assisting in their function has drawn effectively upon our present knowledge of the function of norepinephrine as a transmitter at peripheral synapses served by postganglionic sympathetic fibers. Although conclusive proof is still required, many investigators have tacitly accepted dopamine into the family of neurotransmitters and speak of "dopaminergic" neurons (see Chap. 10).

The major metabolites of dopamine in the body are 3-O-methyldopamine (3-methoxytyramine) and HVA (homovanillic acid, 4-hydroxy-3-methoxyphenylacetic acid). These are depicted in Fig. 36-4, which also shows the various alternative

pathways of metabolism (in addition to the formation of norepinephrine). A sulfate conjugate of dopamine has recently been detected in cerebrospinal fluid. The amine and its O-methyl derivative are both subject to the action of monoamine oxidase (MAO), a flavoprotein that is present in the outer membrane of the mitochondria and one that declines in concentration in iron-deficient animals. Products of this oxidation include the aldehyde that corresponds to the amine substrate, along with hydrogen peroxide and ammonia. Monoamines represent only a minor source of brain ammonia. Most of the aldehyde undergoes further dehydrogenation to form DOPAC (3,4-dihydroxyphenylacetic acid) or HVA. DOPAC, like dopamine, is a substrate for catechol-O-methyl transferase (COMT), an enzyme that catalyzes the transfer of the methyl group from S-adenosylmethionine to an appropriate acceptor. This process appears to be very efficient in the brain because substantial amounts of HVA are normally present in the striatum, whereas only very small quantities of DOPAC are there. A portion of the aldehyde undergoes reduction, catalyzed by alcohol dehydrogenase or a similar enzyme, with participation of a reduced nicotinamide coenzyme. The alcoholic products

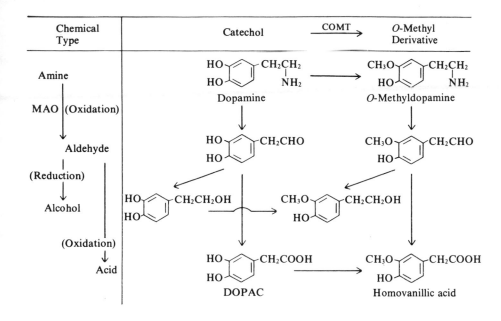

Chemical Type	Catechol	COMT →	O-Methyl Derivative

Fig. 36-4. Alternative pathways of dopamine metabolism. COMT, catechol O-methyltransferase; MAO, monoamine oxidase; DOPAC, 3,4-dihydroxyphenylacetic acid.

that are formed are shown in Fig. 36-4; they are far less abundant as products of dopamine than are the acidic metabolites.

Biological activities have been sought for some of these metabolites of dopamine, so far with little success. There is some interest in the possibility that the aldehyde derivatives of monoamines subserve a significant function.

As the dopamine-rich regions of the brain are preeminently the basal ganglia and some associated structures (apart from the thalamus and hypothalamus) it is natural to investigate diseases of the basal ganglia for evidence of deranged metabolism of catecholamines, in general, and dopamine, in particular. The search for such a faulty metabolism has been especially successful in Parkinson's disease, which now stands as the paradigm of cerebral diseases that involve dysfunction of monoamine-containing fibers. In that respect it may serve as a model for the investigation of monoamine function in nervous and mental diseases.

Chemical Pathology of Parkinson's Disease

The evidence for disturbed metabolism of monoamines comes from the direct measurement of these substances in the brains of patients dying with Parkinson's disease [2, 6–8]. The regional concentrations of catecholamines are shown in Table 36-2. The monoamines that have been measured are all present in lower concentrations than those observed in normal conditions, and the decrease of dopamine is greater than that of norepinephrine (or serotonin). One of the first attempts to restore normal levels of brain monoamines was through administration of MAO inhibitors to patients with Parkinson's disease. MAO inhibitors prevent the oxidative deamination of the amine (see Fig. 36-4); hence, if its biosynthesis is proceeding normally, an excess of the compound could be expected to accumulate. Patients who were treated in the terminal stages of their illness with these inhibitors (some of which are used therapeutically in the treatment of mental depression) showed a significant increase in the brain concentrations of norepinephrine and serotonin, but not of striatal dopamine. These results point clearly to some type of dysmetabolism of monoamines, particularly dopamine, in an important disease of the brain [1, 9].

Table 36-2. Catecholamines and Homovanillic Acid (HVA) in Brain in Parkinson's Disease

Brain Region	Dopamine		HVA		Norepinephrine	
	Normal[a]	P.D.	Normal	P.D.	Normal	P.D.
Caudate nucleus	3.50[b]	0.32	1.87	0.34	0.07	0.03
Putamen	3.57	0.23	2.92	0.69	0.11	0.03
Globus pallidus	0.30	0.14	1.73	0.56	0.09	0.11
Substantia nigra	0.46	0.07	1.79	0.52	0.04	0.02
Thalamus	—	—	0.35	0.21	—	—
Internal capsule (anterior limb)	—	—	1.67	0.42	—	—

[a]Normal = nonneurological cases; P.D. = Parkinson's disease.
[b]Micrograms per gram wet weight of tissue.

Neuropathological and necropsy findings by themselves cannot establish the precise biochemical defect that causes the loss of brain dopamine. Fortunately, one can prepare models in experimental animals for comparison with the clinical state in humans. This has been especially successful with monkeys, in which a small lesion is placed stereotaxically in the ventromedial tegmental area of the upper brain stem. In this way, it has been possible to induce in the animals dyskinesias such as tremor and hypokinesia of the limbs contralateral to the side of the lesion [6, 10–14]. Histological study of the brains of these monkeys indicates that fibers from the substantia nigra to the striatum are interrupted and undergo degenerative changes. Retrograde degeneration entails loss of staining characteristics of the nigra (i.e., loss of cell bodies) accompanied by significant decreases in the concentration of catecholamines in the striatum, without involving its serotonin content. The loss of striatal monoamines is attributed, then, to anterograde degeneration of the nigrostriatal fibers, leading to the disappearance not only of the neuronal structure but also of enzymes and metabolites.

Cats, rabbits, and rats also have been used effectively in the identification of neurochemical events that accompany specific morphological changes. The primates, however, show the motor disturbances that permit neurological and neuropharmacological investigations that have a direct significance for the understanding of human diseases.

Examples of the loss of enzymes and metabolites from the striatum, that is, from the nigrostriatal terminations there, are given in Tables 36-3 and 36-4. Table 36-4 illustrates the progressive neurochemical changes accompanying the nigral degeneration as a result of experimental lesions: the greater the loss of nigral cell bodies and fibers, the greater the loss of AADC and dopamine.

The decreased ability of the diseased nigra to produce dopamine in Parkinson's disease is also reflected in lower concentrations of HVA in the caudate nucleus and putamen (Table 36-2). This can be reproduced experimentally by introducing lesions of the nigrostriatal fibers in monkeys. The concentrations of the acidic metabolites of dopamine—HVA and DOPAC—then decline. Some HVA diffuses into the CSF, particularly from the caudate nucleus, and samples of this fluid have readily detectable amounts of the acid. In patients undergoing brain surgery for the treatment of Parkinson's disease, the concentration of HVA is reduced far below the level in patients who are being operated on for reasons other than a disorder of the basal ganglia. This is clear from the data in Table 36-5. Because of the difficulty in obtaining

Table 36-3. Monoamine Functions of Striatum of Animals with Unilateral Lesions of the Nigrostriatal Tract

Function	Species	No.	Intact Side	Operated Side
Concentration of				
Dopamine[a]	Monkey	5	5.30	0.29
Homovanillic acid[a]	Monkey	4	12.50	6.10
Norepinephrine[a]	Monkey	5	0.30	0.15
Dopamine following injection of DL-DOPA (70 mg/kg)[a]	Cat	10	17.4	6.5
Homovanillic acid in cisternal fluid[b]	Cat	4	16.7[c]	6.8[d]
Dopamine following intraventricular injection of radioactive tyrosine[e]	Monkey	3	6500	750
Activity[f] of				
Succinic dehydrogenase	Cat	6	100	87–110
Tyrosine hydroxylase	Cat	6	100	1–34
Dopa decarboxylase	Monkey	4	100	44
Monoamine oxidase	Monkey	4	100	89

[a]Micrograms per gram fresh weight.
[b]Nanograms per milliliter.
[c]Intact animals.
[d]Bilaterally operated cats.
[e]Counts per minute (as dopamine) per gram of caudate nucleus tissue.
[f]Relative activity.

Table 36-4. Relation of Neurochemical Changes in the Striatum to Histological Changes in the Substantia Nigra After Lesioning of the Nigrostriatal Tract

Cellularity of Substantia Nigra on the Side of the Lesion	Dopa Decarboxylase Activity[a]			Dopamine Concentration[b]		
	No.	Intact Side	Lesion Side	No.	Intact Side	Lesion Side
No cell loss (or nearly none)	6	75	63	16	4.79	4.12
Partial loss of cells	4	113	31	5	2.47	1.07
Complete or nearly complete loss of cells	6	99	0	13	3.35	0.27

[a]Nanomoles of dopamine formed per hour per 100 mg tissue.
[b]Micrograms per gram fresh weight of tissue.

Table 36-5. Concentrations of HVA and 5-HIAA in CSF (ng/ml)

	HVA		5-HIAA		
	No. of Cases	Mean ± SE	No. of Cases	Mean ± SE	References
Lateral ventricles					
Nonextrapyramidal disorders					
Various	15	447 ± 40	17	111 ± 12	[15]
Brain atrophy	3	62 ± 33			[16]
Spasmodic torticollis	4	213 ± 60			[16]
Extrapyramidal disorders					
Parkinson's disease	53	157 ± 17	17	46 ± 7	[16]
Akinesia present	6	52 ± 24			[16]
Akinesia absent	41	169 ± 19			[16]
Attitudinal tremor	21	230 ± 19	5	77 ± 9	[16]
Lumbar space					
Various neurological disorders	20	40 ± 5	20	26 ± 2	[17, 18]
Parkinson's disease	5	15 ± 7	4	24 ± 9	[16]
Progressive supranuclear palsy	6	26 ± 9	6	20 ± 7	[16]
Epilepsy partial complex seizures	7	27 ± 5	7	20 ± 3	[17]
Huntington's chorea	15	23 ± 4	15	28 ± 3	[18]
Spasmodic torticollis*	8	15 ± 6	8	14 ± 2	[19]

*In this study, CSF was drawn from patients who had been recumbent overnight. Less of the metabolites are found under these conditions: the control group gave a mean (± SE) of 18 ± 1.9 ng/ml for HVA (n = 10) and 23 ± 2.6 ng/ml for 5-HIAA (n = 21).

"normal" CSF, the concentration of HVA in ventricular CSF obtained from Parkinson's disease patients must be compared with that from the other groups of patients who show no evidence of extrapyramidal disease or degenerative changes, either focal or general. Within the category of Parkinson's syndrome, the values are much lower in patients who present evidence of akinesia before death than in those without akinesia. This is also true for the dopamine in the caudate nucleus.

It has already been mentioned that serotonin concentrations are abnormally low in the caudate nucleus of patients who have died of Parkinson's disease. Moreover, glutamate decarboxylase activity and the concentrations of GABA in the substantia nigra are lower in Parkinson's disease than in control cases.

CSF taken at the suboccipital and lumbar levels has a much lower concentration of HVA than has the ventricular fluid. Thus the ratio of mean concentrations of this substance in the CSF at ventricular, cisternal, and lumbar levels is approximately 9:4:1 [20–22]. The steep gradient is based on two important facts: (1) All the HVA originates in the brain, much of it in that portion of the caudate nucleus immediately adjacent to the lateral ventricles, that is, the parts lining the floor of the body and anterior horn, and the roof of the inferior horn [23, 24]; the remainder probably comes from dopamine-rich regions contributing HVA to the third and fourth ventricles. Although the cerebral cortex also contains some dopamine, HVA formed there and passing into the fluid bathing that region of the brain would probably not reach lower compartments of the CSF. (2) Once HVA enters the CSF, an active transport mechanism works to remove such metabolic acids as HVA, as well as 5-HIAA.

The compartmental ratio for 5-HIAA corresponding to that given above for HVA is 4:3:1. The lower gradient in this case arises from the fact that 5-HIAA enters the CSF at many levels; serotonin-containing fibers of the spinal cord make a substantial contribution to the 5-HIAA detected in the lumbar CSF, although some of this compound originates from higher compartments of the CSF [20, 22].

The concentration gradient of HVA in the CSF applies in Parkinson's disease as well (Table 36-5). The generally lowered HVA concentration, however, is not specific to Parkinson's disease. It is observed also in patients with inflammatory and other disorders of the CNS. Differentiation may be made by using probenecid (p-dipropylsulfamyl-benzoic acid), a drug that inhibits the transport mechanism operating to remove HVA and similar acids from CSF to blood. While probenecid is present, the concentrations of HVA and 5-HIAA normally increase in the spinal fluid because their efflux is blocked. Parkinsonians tested with this drug show less increase in HVA than do non-parkinsonian patients. There are several types of "probenecid test," but whichever is used, it is important to remember that under certain conditions the accumulation of the acidic metabolites may be determined simply by the level of probenecid attained in the CSF, regardless of other factors.

If an enzymic defect in the brain were accompanied by a comparable one in the liver, the kidneys, or both, the abnormality might be more readily detectable and so could be studied conveniently during the life of the patient. This has motivated clinicochemical studies of Parkinson's disease, including measurement of the urinary excretion of monoamines and some of their metabolites. Such studies have shown that the excretion of epinephrine and norepinephrine is normal, but the excretion of dopamine after a loading dose is subnormal and may be especially low in those patients with the greatest degree of akinesia [8, 25, 26]. The low values cannot be attributed to the use of antiparkinsonian drugs, for these results are found in untreated Parkinson's disease as well [26].

Levodopa Treatment of Parkinson's Disease

An important outgrowth of catecholamine studies has been the use of levodopa (L-dopa) in the treatment of Parkinson's disease. In 1961, neuropharmacological studies in patients with the disease revealed that this amino acid exerts antirigidity and antiakinesic actions; that is, it influences the two most incapacitating symptoms of Parkinson's disease. Today it is said that levodopa produces about 60 percent improvement in the majority of patients with Parkinson's disease; the treatment is considered the best one available.

It is generally assumed that the therapeutic role of levodopa lies in the ease with which it crosses the blood-brain barrier (in contrast to the exclusion from the brain of intravenously infused dopamine) and in its ability to replenish the supply of dopamine at appropriate sites. The passage of levodopa into the parenchymal tissue of the brain entails its transfer from blood through the endothelial cells lining the capillaries (see Chap. 25). These cells, like many other peripheral cells, contain considerable amounts of AADC, so that only a portion of a given amount of levodopa will eventually pass into the brain. Hence, large doses (up to 8 g per day) have been used. By giving the patient such AADC inhibitors as carbidopa and benserazide in doses that affect only the peripherally located enzyme (including that of the brain capillaries) it is possible to reduce the daily dose of levodopa to 2 to 3 g per day while retaining the same therapeutic response [27, 28].

According to the commonly accepted hypothesis of its mode of action, when levodopa has crossed the blood-brain barrier, it must be converted to dopamine. This is an apparent paradox; for if pathological processes have partially eliminated dopaminergic neurons, including their content of AADC, how can the levodopa be effective? An important consideration is that studies with postmortem material have not yet revealed any cases with a total deficiency of AADC in the striatum: there has always been at least a small residue of enzymic activity [29]. Thus, dopamine could be formed in the neighborhood of striatal receptors. Cells of the striatum receive connections from many fibers, including some that contain serotonin. Hence, levodopa could be acted on by the decarboxylase within those neurons, for example, by the enzyme that normally has 5-HTP as substrate. The dopamine formed would then be available in the presynaptic space, although its path of diffusion to sensitive neurons might be longer than usual. Current developments in receptor theory suggest that the diminution in dopamine-releasing fibers results in an increase of the number of dopamine-responsive receptors in the striatum. This structure would become more sensitive to dopamine, so that even small amounts of the amine, as provided by levodopa, could be effective [30, 31].

There are other hypotheses concerning the action of levodopa in Parkinson's disease, but the choice among them must await further research. Whatever the outcome, the use of the amino acid in this disorder represents a successful biochemical treatment of an important neurological disease [32].

The actions of levodopa in Parkinson's disease or of dopamine at receptor sites in the CNS are mimicked by certain compounds, some of which have useful therapeutic actions [33]. Amantadine is used in the treatment of Parkinson's disease as an adjunctive therapy; its action favors the release of dopamine from residual intact neurons in much the same way as does amphetamine. Apomorphine has a brief, levodopalike activity. Its best-recognized action is at the dopamine receptor sites making up the trigger zone of the emetic center; this lies in the area postrema (as has been shown in the cat). Apomorphine also is effective in certain neuroendocrine systems; for example, in humans, subemetic doses provoke a great increase in the concentration of growth hormone in the plasma, presumably by an action on cells producing the appropriate releasing factor. Other dopamine agonists include some ergot alkaloids, such as bromocriptine. Antagonists acting at dopamine receptors include the

major tranquilizers (Chaps. 10 and 38). Reserpine behaves differently from other neuroleptics. It causes depletion of stored monoamines, including dopamine; this depletion is achieved through blockade of the vesicular uptake mechanism for storage of monoamines.

Among the most commonly used drugs in the treatment of parkinsonism are anticholinergic agents. Their use has been rationalized in this way: In the striatum, dopamine has an inhibitory action at postsynaptic sites; if this influence is removed, as in Parkinson's disease (or by treatment with excessive amounts of neuroleptics), the cholinergic neurons in the striatum become overactive, and this hyperactivity can then be regulated by anticholinergic drugs at those postsynaptic sites.

Huntington's Disease

Huntington's disease has been of special interest to the neurochemist because it is genetically transmitted via an autosomal dominant gene and involves the loss of many neurons in the striatum [34]. It is characterized by choreiform movements and progressive dementia. These features usually appear well into adulthood. It presents certain biochemical mirror-image features of Parkinson's disease. One of the newest animal models of extrapyramidal disorder is provided by the use of kainic acid [35, 36]. This rigid analog of glutamate, when injected into the striatum, causes destruction of intrinsic GABA-containing and cholinergic neurons, and spares fibers of passage.

Postmortem studies of Huntington's patients have revealed a small, but significant, decrease in the dopamine and HVA of the caudate nucleus ([7] and Table 36-6). Tyrosine hydroxylase activity is not seriously affected. There is a significant reduction of the glutamate decarboxylase activity in substantia nigra and globus pallidus, and of the concentration of GABA in the same regions, as well as striatum [37–41]. Receptor sites for GABA are also reduced in the caudate nucleus (Table 36-6). Other recent findings in Huntington's disease point to diminished cholinergic function in the basal ganglia. This is characterized by decreases in the

Table 36-6. Analysis of Huntington's-Disease Brains Postmortem

Substance Measured (unit)[a]	Brain Region	Huntington's Disease	Control	Reference
GAD (μmol $^{14}CO_2$/g per hr)	Globus pallidus	1.9	7.1	[37]
	Substantia nigra	2.2	6.5	
	Caudate nucleus	1.5	5.1	
	Putamen	0.9	4.4	
	Hypothalamus	4.4	3.2[b]	
	Frontal cortex	2.7	3.0[b]	
GABA (μmol/g)	Lenticular nucleus	1.8	4.4	[38]
	Caudate nucleus	1.6	2.9	
	Frontal cortex	1.6	1.8[b]	
GABA-receptor sites (pmole/mg protein)	Caudate nucleus	0.11	0.15[b]	[39]
CAT (μmol/g per hr)	Globus pallidus	1.5	0.9[b]	[37]
	Substantia nigra	1.0	1.2[b]	
	Caudate nucleus	5.4	11.9	
	Putamen	9.1	21.8	
	Hypothalamus	0.2	0.2[b]	
	Frontal cortex	1.4	1.2[b]	
ACh-receptor sites, muscarinic (pmole/mg protein)	Caudate nucleus	0.65	1.36	[39]
Tyrosine hydroxylase (nmol/g per hr)	Caudate nucleus	4.1	4.9	[37]
Dopamine (μg/g)	Caudate nucleus	2.6	1.3	[7, 40]

[a]Wet weight of tissue.
[b]Difference is not statistically significant.

activity of choline acetyltransferase in the striatum and in the number of receptor sites for ACh in the caudate nucleus ([32, 33] and Table 36-6).

If GABA normally exerts an inhibitory action over nigrostriatal function (see Fig. 36-1) then this deficiency in Huntington's disease could contribute to an overproduction of dopamine at striatal synapses. Reduced cholinergic function at the output from the basal ganglia could also favor dopaminergic dominance. Both these findings are consistent with the exacerbation of abnormal movements in Huntington's disease caused by the administration of levodopa. Useful drugs in the treatment of this disease have been those that deplete dopamine (among other monoamines), prevent its storage in nerve terminals, or block its synaptic actions. These agents are the *neuroleptics,* and they include reserpine, methyldopa, and others. More recently, inhibitors of GABA-transaminase have been sought, as drugs that might protect GABA from metabolic conversion. Among these are γ-acetylenic GABA, isoniazid, and dipropylacetate (valproate).

Various blood lipids, serum enzymes, and urinary constituents, including trace metals and phenolic and indolic compounds, have been examined in Huntington's disease. None of these is characteristically altered. A number of laboratories are currently studying peripheral cells, such as fibroblasts and erythrocytes, seeking clues for the genetically determined biochemical defect that underlies this disorder.

Wilson's Disease (Hepatolenticular Degeneration)

Much of our knowledge of the metabolism of copper comes from studies of experimental and farm animals [42, 43]. The interest in Wilson's disease, a disorder in which copper accumulates in a number of organs, has helped to stimulate research into the metabolism of this metal in humans. *Wilson's disease* is a combined brain-liver disorder characterized by progressive rigidity, intention tremor, hepatic cirrhosis of the coarse type, and recurrent hepatitis. Renamed *hepatolenticular degeneration* in 1921, it is recognized as a familial disorder inherited in an autosomal recessive fashion. The frequency rate of the gene is estimated to be 1 in 500. Biochemically, hepatolenticular degeneration is characterized by low concentrations of copper and ceruloplasmin in the serum, elevated excretion of the metal in the urine, and deposition of excess copper in the brain (especially in the basal ganglia) and in the liver and kidneys. In some cases, copper is deposited in the cornea, where it is reduced, forming the "Kayser-Fleischer ring." This ring is virtually pathognomonic of the disease but appears also in occasional cases of primary biliary cirrhosis. In addition, there is a constant aminoaciduria, including excretion of some dipeptides and, sometimes, abnormal excretion of monoamines and their metabolites. The amino acid levels in the plasma are normal, so the urinary findings simply may signify a renal defect caused by histotoxicity of copper [8, 43, 44].

Some metal-chelating agents have been tested therapeutically in Wilson's disease. The most effective in treatment has been D-penicillamine (3,3-dimethylcysteine). It is given in doses up to about 3 g per day. Its effectiveness indicates that the cytotoxicity caused by copper can be reversed, even to the extent of bringing about a remission of neurological and other symptoms.

Normal Metabolism of Copper

About 1 to 2 mg of copper suffices daily for adult humans, but most diets supply more than this. The normal infant is born with a large store of the metal in the liver, and this provides temporary protection against the deficiency of the metal in milk (just as with iron). Copper is needed for the utilization of iron in hemoglobin synthesis as well as other functions. In some laboratory species, copper deficiency causes a microcytic hypochromic anemia. Farm animals maintained in regions where the soil (and therefore the pasturage) is deficient in copper may suffer from specific clinical disorders. In the sheep and goat, the primary symptom is anemia, but in other animals there is a neurological disturbance, such as swayback in cattle and posterior paralysis in swine. Myelination of nerve is delayed in lambs born of copper-deficient ewes (see Chap. 32).

The regulation of copper metabolism is attuned to the very small requirement of the metal in adult animals, so most of the copper ingested in the diet is excreted in the feces. A minute fraction of the dietary copper appears in the urine. Balance studies, however, disguise the fact that much copper is absorbed from the intestinal tract and reaches the liver in the portal circulation; a portion of it is utilized there, but most of it is excreted in the bile. Thus, there is an enterohepatic cycle for copper. The mechanism can be overwhelmed in experimental animals by repeated parenteral administration of copper, for example, by daily intraperitoneal injection of solutions of copper sulfate. The metal then accumulates in the liver, kidneys, and other organs, and excess copper is found in all subcellular fractions and in many proteins. The association with proteins is by no means random. Initially, the copper increases in the low molecular weight fraction of cytoplasmic proteins of rat liver. Only later, as the concentration of the metal rises greatly, does it appear in the largest proteins; those of intermediate size are the last to take up the copper [45]. In the rat, under conditions of copper loading, decreases of activity of certain hepatic enzymes can be detected. The toxic action of copper is selective, even among sulfhydryl enzymes; the present evidence runs contrary to the concept of a generalized toxic action on metabolic or respiratory processes [46].

Regulation of the entry of copper into the brain is very strict, even under the aggravated conditions of chronic copper loading, so that the net increase of copper in that organ is significant, but small, and not of the proportions seen in hepatolenticular degeneration in humans [46].

Cuproproteins

Copper is an essential constituent of several important proteins, including cytochrome *c* oxidase, dopamine β-hydroxylase, uricase (present below the level of the primates), ceruloplasmin, superoxide dismutase, diamine oxidase, and lysine oxidase. Copper is found in tyrosinase as the prosthetic group, and in the melanocytes of the skin and certain pigmented regions of the brain. Indeed, there may be as much as 0.4 mg of copper per gram of dry weight in the subthalamic nucleus, with somewhat smaller amounts in the substantia nigra and dentate nucleus. However, all these cuproproteins do not account for the total amount of copper in the body (100 to 150 mg in the human adult), and many other cuproproteins probably will be discovered.

Ceruloplasmin is a blue serum glycoprotein. Its molecular weight is about 155,000, and it contains 6 atoms of copper, not all of which are equivalent in function. The divalent atoms of copper endow the protein with its blue color. The molecule displays some oxidase activity toward polyamines and polyphenols; phenylenediamine is often used as a substrate. Ceruloplasmin has a half-life in the serum of 54 hours. Its sialic acid residues protect it from metabolic degradation because asialoceruloplasmin disappears from the circulation after its injection far more rapidly than does ceruloplasmin.

Normally, the serum contains about 100 μg of copper per 100 ml. Most of this (95%) is present as ceruloplasmin. The concentration of this protein amounts to 20 to 40 mg per 100 ml. In hepatolenticular degeneration, serum copper may fall to one-half this value or less. Ceruloplasmin does not seem to be involved in transport of the metal in the serum; this function is served by serum albumin, which loosely binds most of the nonceruloplasmin copper. It has been demonstrated recently that, when ceruloplasmin is perfused through the isolated liver, there is a specific and rapid shift of transferrin from liver to the perfusate. This result is pertinent to the problem of the copper-iron interaction in metabolism.

A vexing question is that of the relationship between ceruloplasmin and hepatolenticular degeneration. The many investigations in this field have not yet provided a decisive answer, so we do not know what role, if any, the depressed level of ceruloplasmin plays in the pathogenesis of the disorder.

Copper Deficiency and Other Clinical States

Copper deficiency has been demonstrated in a number of mammalian species under laboratory or range conditions. For humans, the metal is so infrequently limiting in the diet that a true dietary deficiency state has been recognized only recently. It has been detected in infants and children on low copper intakes, with peak incidence at about 7 to 9 months of age, that is, at the time that the hepatic stores of the metal have become exhausted [47, 48]. Plasma ceruloplasmin activity, which responds rapidly and sensitively to experimental copper deficiency in animals, is decreased below normal levels. There are changes in bone structure and elastin of the blood vessel walls attributable to diminished lysine oxidase of the connective tissues, and consequently, there is reduced formation of desmosine for cross-linking of the collagen fibers. Altered pigmentation of the hair and skin probably stems from changes in copper-catalyzed melanin formation. Other characteristics are hypotonia, psychomotor retardation, and visual problems. In the genetic disorder *trichopoliodystrophy* (Menkes' kinky hair syndrome) somewhat similar changes have been noted.

From time to time, a relationship between copper metabolism and schizophrenia has been claimed. For example, soon after the oxidase property of serum ceruloplasmin became widely recognized, numerous people studied its activity in the psychosis. There is no valid evidence of a relationship.

Chronic Manganese Poisoning

A small portion of miners exposed to manganese dust develops *manganism*. The disease is ushered in by self-limited psychiatric symptoms, followed by permanent neurological changes. The manifestations are those of extrapyramidal disease. Because the disorder responds to treatment with levodopa, it is thought that dopaminergic neurons of the brain are affected.

Acknowledgment

Research on the title subjects in the author's laboratory is supported by grants from the Medical Research Council of Canada.

References

*1. Hornykiewicz, O. Dopamine (3-hydroxytyramine) and brain function. *Pharmacol. Rev.* 18: 925–964, 1966.

2. Riederer, P., Birkmayer, W., Seemann, D., and Wuketich, S. Brain noradrenaline and 3-methoxy-4-hydroxyphenylglycol in Parkinson's syndrome. *J. Neural. Transm.* 41:241–251, 1977.

3. Lloyd, K. G., and Hornykiewicz, O. Occurrence and distribution of aromatic L-amino acid (L-DOPA) decarboxylase in the human brain. *J. Neurochem.* 19:1549–1559, 1972.

4. McGeer, E. G., McGeer, P. L., and Wada, J. A. Distribution of tyrosine hydroxylase in human and animal brain. *J. Neurochem.* 18:1647–1658, 1971.

5. Mackay, A. V. P., Davies, P., Dewar, A. J., and Yates, C. M. Regional distribution of enzymes associated with neurotransmission by monoamines, acetylcholine and GABA in the human brain. *J. Neurochem.* 30:827–839, 1978.

6. Kopin, I. J. (ed.). *Neurotransmitters.* Vol. 50. Research Publications of the Association for Research in Nervous and Mental Diseases. New York: A.R.N.M.D., 1972.

7. Bernheimer, H., Birkmayer, W., Hornykiewicz, O., Jellinger, K., and Seitelberger, F. Brain dopamine and the syndromes of Parkinson and Huntington. *J. Neurol. Sci.* 20:415–455, 1973.

*8. Sourkes, T. L., Poirier, L. J., and Lal, S. Diseases of the Basal Ganglia. In R. A. Good, S. B. Day, and J. J. Yunis (eds.), *Molecular Pathology.* Springfield, Ill.: Thomas, 1975. Pp. 689–743.

9. Lamprecht, F. Dopaminerge Neurotransmission beim Parkinson-Syndrom. *Fortschr. Neurol. Psychiatr.* 45:459–471, 1977.

10. De Ajuriaguerra, J., and Gauthier, G. (eds.). *Monoamines, Noyaux Gris Centraux, et Syndrome de Parkinson.* Geneva: Georg, and Paris: Masson, 1971.

11. Sourkes, T. L., and Poirier, L. J. Neurochemical bases of tremor and other disorders of movement. *Can. Med. Assoc. J.* 94:53–60, 1966.

*12. Poirier, L. J., Sourkes, T. L., Bouvier, G., Boucher, R., and Carabin, S. Striatal amines, experimental tremor and the effect of harmaline in the monkey. *Brain* 89:37–52, 1966.

13. Goldstein, M., Anagnoste, B., Battista, A. F., Owen, W. S., and Nakatani, S. Studies of amines in the striatum in monkeys with nigral lesions. *J. Neurochem.* 16:645–653, 1969.

14. Gillingham, F. J., and Donaldson, I. M. L. (eds.). *Third Symposium on Parkinson's Disease.* Edinburgh: Livingstone, 1969. (The basic scientific aspects cover a substantial portion of these proceedings).

*15. Moir, A. T. B., Ashcroft, G. W., Crawford, T. B. B., Eccleston, D., and Guldberg, H. C. Cerebral metabolites in cerebrospinal fluid as a biochemical approach to the brain. *Brain* 93:357–368, 1970.

16. Papeschi, R., Molina-Negro, P., Sourkes, T. L., and Erba, G. The concentration of homovanillic and 5-hydroxyindoleacetic acids in ventricular and lumbar CSF. *Neurology* (Minneapolis) 22:1151–1159, 1972.

17. Laxer, K. D., Sourkes, T. L., Fang, T. Y., Young, S. N., Gauthier, S., and Missala, K. Monoamine metabolites in epileptic patients. *Neurology* 29: 1157–1161, 1979.

18. Curzon, G., Gumpert, J., and Sharpe, D. Amine metabolites in the cerebrospinal fluid in Huntington's chorea. *J. Neurol. Neurosurg. Psychiatry* 35:514–519, 1972.

19. Lal, S., Hoyte, K. M., Kiely, M. E., Sourkes, T. L., Baxter, D. W., Missala, K., and Andermann, F. Neuropharmacological investigation and treatment of spasmodic torticollis. *Adv. Neurol.* 24:335–351, 1979.

*20. Garelis, E., Young, S. N., Lal, S., and Sourkes, T. L. Origin of monoamine metabolites in CSF. *Brain Res.* 79:1–8, 1974.

21. Garelis, E., and Sourkes, T. L. Use of cerebrospinal fluid drawn at pneumoencephalography in the study of monoamine metabolism in man. *J. Neurol. Neurosurg. Psychiatry* 37:704–710, 1974.

*22. Ebert, M. H., and Perlow, M. J. Utility of cerebrospinal fluid measurements in studies of brain monoamines. In E. Usdin, N. Weiner, and M. B. H. Youdim (eds.), *Structure and Function of Monoamine Enzymes.* New York: Dekker, 1977. Pp. 963–984.

*Key reference.

23. Sourkes, T. L. On the origin of homovanillic acid (HVA) in the cerebrospinal fluid. *J. Neural Transm.* 34:153–157, 1973.

24. Garelis, E., and Sourkes, T. L. Sites of origin in the central nervous system of monoamine metabolites measured in human cerebrospinal fluid. *J. Neurol. Neurosurg. Psychiatry* 36:625–629, 1973.

25. Sourkes, T. L. Metabolism of monoamines in extrapyramidal disorders. In J. De Ajuriaguerra and G. Gauthier (eds.), *Monoamines, Noyaux Gris Centraux, et Syndrome de Parkinson.* Geneva: Georg, and Paris: Masson, 1971. Pp. 129–141.

26. Hoehn, M. J., Crowley, T. J., and Rutledge, C. O. Dopamine correlates of neurologic and psychologic status in untreated parkinsonism. *J. Neurol. Neurosurg. Psychiatr.* 39:941–951, 1976.

*27. Yahr, M. D. (ed.). *The Treatment of Parkinson's Disease—the Role of DOPA Decarboxylase Inhibitors. Advances in Neurology.* New York: Raven, 1973. Vol. 2.

*28. Poirier, L. J., Sourkes, T. L., and Bédard, P. J. (eds.). *The Extrapyramidal System and Its Disorders. Advances in Neurology.* New York: Raven, 1979. Vol. 24.

29. Lloyd, K., and Hornykiewicz, O. Parkinson's disease: Activity of L-Dopa decarboxylase in discrete brain regions. *Science* 170:1212–1213, 1970.

*30. Melnechuk, T. *Cell Receptor Disorders.* La Jolla, Calif.: Western Behavioral Sciences Institute, 1978.

31. Lloyd, K. G., and Davidson, L. Involvement of gaba neurons and receptors in Parkinson's disease and Huntington's chorea: A compensatory mechanism? *Adv. Neurol.* 24:293–301, 1979.

32. Hornykiewicz, O. Compensatory biochemical changes at the striatal dopamine synapse in Parkinson's disease—limitations of L-DOPA therapy. *Adv. Neurol.* 24:275–281, 1979.

33. Goldstein, M., Lew, J. Y., Nakamura, S., and Battista, A. F. Dopamine agonists: Anti-parkinsonian efficacy in experimental animal models and binding to putative dopamine (DA) receptors. *Adv. Neurol.* 24:247–252, 1979.

*34. Barbeau, A., Chase, T. N., and Paulson, G. W. (eds.). *Huntington's Chorea, 1872–1972. Advances in Neurology.* New York: Raven, 1973. Vol. 1.

35. Coyle, J. T., and Schwarcz, R. Lesion of striatal neurons with kainic acid provides a model for Huntington's chorea. *Nature* 263:244–246, 1976.

36. McGeer, E. G., and McGeer, P. L. Duplication of biochemical changes in Huntington's chorea by intrastriatal injections of glutamic and kainic acids. *Nature* 263:517–519, 1976.

37. Bird, E. D., and Iversen, L. L. Neurochemical findings in Huntington's chorea. In M. B. H. Youdim et al. (eds.), *Essays in Neurochemistry and Neuropharmacology.* New York: Wiley, 1977. Vol. 1, pp. 177–195.

*38. Urquhart, N., Perry, T. L., Hansen, S., and Kennedy, J. GABA content and glutamic acid decarboxylase activity in brain of Huntington's chorea patiens and control subjects. *J. Neurochem.* 24:1071–1075, 1975.

39. Enna, S. J., Bird, E. D., Bennett, J. P., Bylund, D. B., Yamamura, H. I., Iversen, L. L., and Snyder, S. H. Huntington's chorea: Changes in neurotransmitter receptors in the brain. *N. Engl. J. Med.* 294:1305–1309, 1976.

*40. Bird, E. D., and Iversen, L. L. Huntington's chorea: Post-mortem measurement of glutamic-acid-decarboxylase, choline acetyltransferase and dopamine in basal ganglia. *Brain* 97:457–472, 1974.

41. McGeer, P. L., McGeer, E. G., and Fibiger, H. C. Choline acetylase and glutamic acid decarboxylase in Huntington's chorea. *Neurology* (Minneapolis) 23:912–917, 1973.

42. Scheinberg, I. H., and Sternlieb, I. Copper metabolism. *Pharmacol. Rev.* 12:355–381, 1960.

43. Walshe, J. M. The physiology of copper in man and its relation to Wilson's disease. *Brain* 90:149–176, 1967.

44. Cumings, J. N. Trace metals in the brain and Wilson's disease. *J. Clin. Pathol.* 21:1–7, 1968.

45. Bloomer, L. C., and Sourkes, T. L. The effect of copper-loading on the distribution of copper in rat liver cytosol. *Biochem. Med.* 8:78–91, 1973.

46. Lal, S., Papeschi, R., Duncan, R. J. S., and Sourkes, T. L. Effect of copper loading on various tissue enzymes and brain monoamines in the rat. *Toxicol. Appl. Pharmacol.* 28:395–405, 1974.

47. Graham, G. G., and Cordano, A. Copper depletion and deficiency in the malnourished infant. *Johns Hopkins Med. J.* 124:139–150, 1969.

48. Ashkenazi, A., Levin, S., Djaldetti, M., Fishel, E., and Benevisti, D. The syndrome of neonatal copper deficiency. *Pediatrics* 52:525–533, 1973.

Part Three. Behavioral Neurochemistry

Psychopharmacology is concerned with drugs that are active in the CNS and that influence behavior, perception, thought, and affect. In its earliest usage, the Greek word *psychopharmaka* was applied to drugs or measures that had a healing action upon the psyche. Today the term *Psychopharmacology* refers to the selection and use of drugs that have specific actions in the treatment of mental diseases; it embraces the experimental study of such drugs at the biochemical, neural, and behavioral levels. The information obtained in these ways is essential to an understanding of the action of drugs on human thought and action.

The study of the biochemical effects of drugs made little progress until the discovery of the antibacterial effects of the sulfonamides. This was contemporaneous with the replacement of galenic pharmaceuticals by synthetic medicinal chemicals. The structural resemblance of sulfanilamide to *p*-aminobenzoic acid, a bacterial vitamin, led to the recognition of other comparable pairs of presumed antagonists. Antecedents can be found in Emil Fischer's concept of the precise fit of enzyme and substrate; in Ehrlich's work on the relation of drug and cell receptor; and in the concept of "competitive inhibition," as first described by Quastel and Wooldridge. These concepts were then applied to chemotherapy, biochemical pharmacology, and even psychiatric theory, especially through the "antimetabolite hypothesis." For example, the resemblance between the structures of the hallucinogen mescaline and the catecholamine neurotransmitters has played a significant role in biochemical psychiatry by raising the question of whether mescaline and similar drugs act by antagonizing the normal functions of catecholamines in the brain. Although the psychological effects of the so-called phantastica had been known for many years, their special meaning for psychiatric research was largely unrecognized until the accidental discovery in 1943 of the remarkable actions of LSD-25. Because the ingestion of minute amounts of this compound causes acute and protean changes in the subjective experience, one could question whether, in an analogous way, an endogenous chemical resulting from some metabolic derangement might conceivably be responsible for the development of psychoses (see Chap. 38).

In psychiatry, drugs affecting the concentration, synthesis, binding, or release of known and putative neurotransmitters in the brain are of the utmost interest because of the important role that some of these drugs have played in pharmacotherapy. Chlorpromazine's peripheral adrenolytic effects are thought to lie in preventing the attachment of the sympathetic transmitter to a specific receptor site. Reserpine causes the release of amines from the special vesicles in which most of the intracellular content of these substances is stored; it also prevents their being taken up into the vesicles from the external medium. Monoamines are subject to the action of monoamine oxidase (MAO), an enzyme that is inhibited by many compounds, some of which are valuable in the treatment of mental depression. This very brief statement may help to explain why so many neurobiologists have focused their attention on the role of the brain amines in mental diseases.

The neurochemist who is oriented toward pharmacology seeks another type of information that is important in understanding the mode of action of drugs and their clinical uses. This has to do with the metabolism of the drugs themselves—their length of residence in the body, the blood levels attained, the chemical changes they undergo, and their mode and routes of excretion. Knowledge of drug metabolism and kinetics may aid in understanding and even in helping to prevent toxic and side actions of drugs.

An area of pharmacology to which neurochemistry aims to contribute is the classification of CNS-active drugs according to their modes of action. The present classification is necessarily based on analysis by pharmacological and physiological techniques. Although the anatomical, biochemical, and physiological sites of action of many drugs in this category are being clarified, much of the terminology of psychopharmacology currently in use is subjective, and admittedly a compromise.

The general pharmacological and clinical effects of psychopharmacological agents are outlined in Table 37-1. Detailed information can be found in a number of useful monographs and symposia, some of which are described in the references [1–6]. In one reference, valuable chemical and dosage data are given [7]. Pertinent biochemical actions of some psychopharmacological agents are summarized in Table 37-2 and are discussed in more detail below.

Neuroleptics, or Major Tranquilizers

RESERPINE

Reserpine (Fig. 37-1) was the first of the neuroleptics. It is no longer used in psychiatry because of such side effects as mental depression and iatrogenic parkinsonism. However, its biochemical and pharmacological actions, now so well correlated by the results of a vast amount of experimentation, make it a worthwhile—indeed, an essential—topic for discussion in a basic text. Its primary action is on the storage and uptake of monoamines by nerve endings and synaptic vesicles. An interesting experiment has been carried out by injecting labeled reserpine into animals and then isolating the blood platelets. These organelles are rich in serotonin (5-HT), among other constituents, and serve as a model for the study of the release and uptake of monoamines by vesicles of the nervous system. In this experiment, when the membrane of the platelet is separated from the soluble contents, most of the labeled material of the platelets is found to be associated with the membrane. Similar results are obtained even if the platelets are incubated in vitro with the labeled drug. This experiment and others suggest that reserpine acts at the membrane level of the storage organelle by regulating movement of amines through it. Reserpine inhibits the ability of adrenal chromaffin granules to take up catecholamines by a process that is dependent on Mg^{2+} and ATP. When an animal is given a large dose of reserpine, the immediate effect on neurons is the loss of their monoamine content. Much of the amine is released intraneuronally under the influence of reserpine; in this case, it becomes subject to the action of mitochondrial MAO, and ultimately it is lost from the brain as acidic compounds.

The action of reserpine and certain other rauwolfia alkaloids on brain monoamines is indiscriminate. Hence, this effect cannot by itself specify the amine whose loss from the brain is to be correlated with the sedative effect of the drug. A great many experiments have been carried out to establish which cerebral amine is affected by reserpine to bring about the tranquilizing action of the drug. If the amines could pass the blood-brain barrier readily, they could be injected singly to determine which one is effective; but peripherally administered amines do not get into the parenchyma of the brain in appreciable amounts. Their amino acid precursors cross the blood-brain barrier much more easily, although the action of aromatic amino acid decarboxylase in the endothelial wall of the brain capillaries limits the amount that gets into the neurons. Within the brain, an amino acid such as L-dopa or 5-hydroxytryptophan (5-HTP) is readily decarboxylated (Chaps. 10 and 36), and the corresponding amine will be found both in regions of the brain where it is an endogenous constituent, and in others—for instance, in regions that normally do not contain that amine but do have the decarboxylase. Experiments of this kind show that L-dopa temporarily reverses the sedation caused by reserpine. 5-HTP does not do this. It has therefore been deduced that a catecholamine, but not serotonin, is the immediately effective arousal agent. Furthermore, under these experimental conditions,

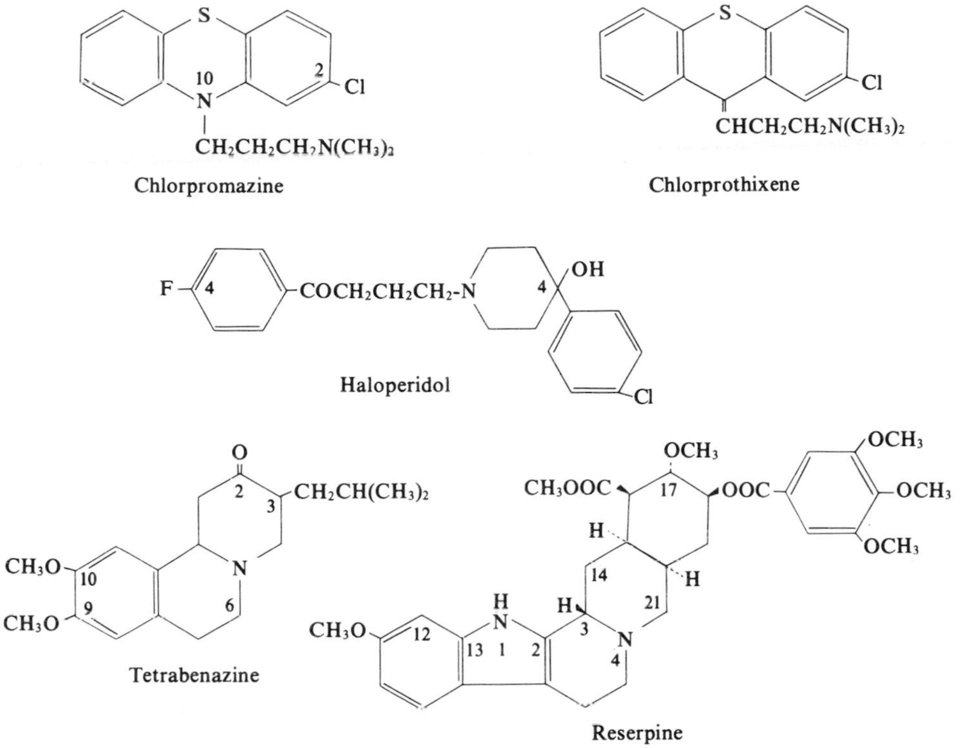

Chlorpromazine

Chlorprothixene

Haloperidol

Tetrabenazine

Reserpine

Fig. 37-1. Some examples of neuroleptics.

the β-oxidation of dopamine (DA) to norepinephrine (NE) is rate-limiting, so the injection of L-dopa brings about large increases in the concentration of DA in many parts of the brain, with little increase of the concentration of NE. This points to DA as the amine with the antireserpine activity.

Some benzoquinolizines have a reserpinelike action both pharmacologically and on the storage of monoamines. One of them, tetrabenazine (Fig. 37-1), has a much shorter-lasting action than does reserpine but has the same type of activity qualitatively.

When reserpine is administered, it is distributed to many organs of the body without any preferential uptake by the brain. Initially, the viscera contain relatively high concentrations, but later the drug moves into adipose tissue. Careful experiments with radiolabeled reserpine have demonstrated the presence of the drug in the brain during

the long period over which it exerts its central depressive action. Reserpine contains two esterified groups, and both of these may be hydrolyzed in the course of metabolism. Among the products are methyl reserpate, reserpic acid, 3,4,5-trimethoxybenzoic acid, and other compounds.

Chlorpromazine

Pharmacologists have shown that chlorpromazine (see Fig. 37-1) acts at the postsynaptic receptor site, thereby blocking the action of transmitter substance released into the synapse. The blockade is long-lasting and not reversed by excessive amounts of the transmitter. Chlorpromazine and haloperidol, for example, block the DA-sensitive receptors of the caudate nucleus (Table 10-1). This results in increased activity within the nigrostriatal dopaminergic system, causing an accelerated rate of turnover of brain DA. Some of this effect is due to the blocking of presynaptic receptors of the DA-releasing fibers themselves, that is, receptors that

Table 37-1. Pharmacological Actions of Psychotropic Compounds

Category	Typical Examples	Broad Pharmacological Effects	Broad Effects in Humans	
			Clinical	Subjective
Neuroleptics, or major tranquilizers	Phenothiazines Butyrophenones Thioxanthenes Reserpine Benzoquinolizines	Decreased autonomic activity, especially of sympathetic branch; hence, antiadrenergic. Decreased motor activity. Decreased conditioned avoidance reflex. No anesthesia.	Tranquilization of overactive psychotic syndromes. Indifference to environment. In high doses, extrapyramidal symptoms produced. Calming action. Antipsychotic effect.	Drowsiness, apathy, indifference to environment, but no effect on intellect. In high doses, extrapyramidal symptoms produced (tardive dyskinesia).
Anxiolytic sedatives, or minor tranquilizers	Meprobamate Benzodiazepines	Actions similar to those of the neuroleptics, but less potent. No anesthesia. Meprobamate in large doses causes paralysis. Benzodiazepines exert anticonvulsant action.	Tranquilization, but without any antipsychotic effect. Sedation of anxious patients.	Muscular and mental relaxation. Less interest in environmental stimuli. Euphoria may occur.
	Barbiturates	As for other minor tranquilizers. Also, there is some blockade of parasympathetic functions. Reduced ability to undergo conditioning. In higher doses, ataxia and then anesthesia.	Tranquilization; hypnotic effect.	Sedation, sleepiness.
Antidepressants Tricyclic types	Imipramine Desipramine Chlorimipramine Amitriptyline Nortriptyline Doxepin	Reduced autonomic activity, especially of cholinergic systems. Sedation especially with the tertiary amines.	Antidepressant action; stimulation; decreased fatigue. Anxiety already present may be increased. If psychotic symptoms are already present, they may be increased.	Reduced motor activity; feeling of relaxation. Increased mental energy; decreased feelings of fatigue; euphoria but less of this with pipradrol. Greater awareness of the surroundings.

Others				
	MAO Inhibitors	Central sympathetic activation. Increased motor activity, with alerting behavior. Reduction of appetite and sleeping time.		In appropriate patients feeling of well-being.
	Lithium salts		In manic-depressive psychosis there is control of the manic attack. On chronic use, there may be prophylaxis against the clinical depression.	
Psychodysleptics or hallucinogenic agents	Lysergide Mescaline Psilocybin Tetrahydrocannabinol	Increased motor activity. Variable autonomic effects. Catatonia.	Marked action on affect, perception, thought processes. Psychotic disturbance may be aggravated.	Autonomic phenomena (e.g., salivation, nausea), followed by psychotic reactions, with distortion of sensory perceptions, color visions, hallucinations.

Source: Based primarily on Tables 8 and 12 in E. Jacobson, *Bull. W.H.O.*, 21:411–493, 1959; and tables in F. T. Von Brücke and O. Hornykiewicz, *The Pharmacology of Psychotherapeutic Drugs*, New York: Springer-Verlag, 1969.

Table 37-2. Biochemical Effects of Psychopharmacological Agents

Haloperidol
Long-lasting blockade of receptors sensitive to NE and DA. Increased concentration of striatal HVA, by feedback-regulated overactivity of nigrostriatal fibers. May cause temporary decrease in brain catecholamines.

Chlorpromazine
Same as for haloperidol. Chlorpromazine causes an increased rate of synthesis of dopamine in brain from tyrosine. Inhibition of some flavin (yellow) enzymes.

Reserpine
Interference with ATP-dependent and Mg^{2+}-dependent reuptake of released monoamines across the vesicular membrane. This results in depletion of monoamines from peripheral sympathetic nerve endings and from central sites. Effects are long lasting. Effects of reserpinization are reversed temporarily by administration of dopa, but not of 5-HTP.

Imipramine
Interference with reuptake of norepinephrine from synaptic cleft. Chlorimipramine has a similar action on reuptake, but it is more potently expressed toward 5-HT. Potentiates depressant action of serotonin on hippocampal neurons.

MAO Inhibitors
Hydrazide type, tranylcypromine, and pargyline cause long-lasting, irreversible inhibition of mitochondrial MAO; monoamines are protected, and increase in concentration (more pronounced for 5-HT in brain than for catecholamines); some of conserved catecholamines may be diverted in increasing amounts into pathway of O-methylation. Harmaline and harmine are reversible, short-acting inhibitors of MAO. Clorgyline yields a double-sigmoid curve of inhibition, corresponding to MAO-A (low range of concentrations) and MAO-B (high range). Deprenyl inhibits MAO-B preferentially.

Amphetamine
Weak inhibitor of MAO; inhibits NE reuptake in peripheral nerve (perhaps also in CNS neurons); effective in releasing monoamines from storage vesicles into synaptic space. Stereotypies caused by amphetamine are mediated by striatal dopaminergic mechanisms.

Lithium salts
Stimulate the rate of turnover of NE and 5-HT in the brain; effect is greater for 5-HT than for NE in chronic experiments. Inhibit the evoked release of monoamines from brain slices. Cause increase in total body water and extracellular water.

monitor the level of synaptic DA and provide retrograde signals to the transmitter-synthesizing apparatus of the neuron. At the same time, there is an increased output of ACh from the caudate nucleus (determined by the "push-pull" technique in cat), which is consistent with the known regulatory action of dopaminergic fibers over the striatal cholinergic system. The increased impulse flow under the influence of neuroleptics is characteristic of dopaminergic fibers.

The concentration of monoamines in the brain reflects the steady state balance of production and utilization. The action of neuroleptics on the rates of these two processes is assessed by kinetic studies with labeled precursors. For example, if radioactive tyrosine is infused into animals, some of it reaches the brain and is synthesized into catecholamines. In animals given chlorpromazine or thioproperazine, a substantial increase in the amount of radioactivity derived from tyrosine can be accounted for as DA (Table 37-3). There is less increase of NE. Moreover, a DA agonist like apomorphine causes ex vivo a drastic reduction in DA synthesis by cerebral cortex, although NE formation is unaffected (Table 37-3).

Chlorpromazine, like many other tranquilizers and anesthetics, blocks excitability of the nerve membrane without affecting the resting membrane potential; at the same time, the membrane expands so that its components assume a somewhat disordered association [11]. CNS depressants, including neuroleptics, have sometimes been reported to

Table 37-3. Effects of Drugs on Rates of Formation of Catecholamines in Brain in Vivo and ex Vivo

Species	Treatment	Precursor	Products Dopamine	Products Norepinephrine
Rat[a]	Control	[^{14}C]Tyrosine	615 cpm $\cdot$ g^{-1}	183 cpm $\cdot$ g^{-1}
	CPZ	[^{14}C]Tyrosine	1262	217
Guinea pig[b]	Control	[^{14}C]Tyrosine		400
	MAOI	[^{14}C]Tyrosine		180
	Control	[^{3}H]Dopa		876
	MAOI	[^{3}H]Dopa		1826
Rat[c]	Control	[^{3}H]Tyrosine	0.36 μCi $\cdot$ g^{-1} $\cdot$ hr^{-1}	0.52 μCi $\cdot$ g^{-1} $\cdot$ hr^{-1}
	TPZ	[^{3}H]Tyrosine	0.70	0.74
	AMP	[^{3}H]Tyrosine	0.14	0.48

[a]Rats were injected IP with chlorpromazine (CPZ), 15 mg/kg, 2 hr before being killed for brain measurements. Labeled tyrosine was infused IV for 25 min immediately preceding death [8].
[b]Guinea pigs were injected with labeled tyrosine or dopa 24 or 7 hr, respectively, after pargyline (MAOI) was given, and were killed 1 hr later. The compounds were then measured in the brain stem [9].
[c]Rats were injected SC with either saline, thioproperazine (TPZ), 10 mg/kg, or apomorphine (APM), 2 mg/kg, and were killed 2 hr (TPZ) or 0.5 hr (APM) later. Cortical slices were incubated in a physiological medium for 15 min in the presence of the precursor. Rates are calculated to 1 hr. Dopamine measurements were made in rats treated earlier with 6-hydroxydopamine, injected bilaterally into the peduncular cerebellaris superior, in order to eliminate noradrenergic fibers from the cortex [10].

cause an increase in the levels of ATP and phosphocreatine in the brain, but when precautions are taken to avoid degradation of these labile esters in the course of their extraction from the brain, there proves to be no effect. Many of these drugs inhibit (Na$^+$ + K$^+$)-ATPase but only at concentrations many times greater than needed to disturb the nerve membrane [12].

Chlorpromazine inhibits the secretion of certain hypothalamic neurohormones that act on the anterior pituitary gland, probably by blocking monoaminergic fibers that innervate the neuroendocrine cells (Chap. 14). One of these hypothalamic factors causes release of growth hormone; in subjects receiving chlorpromazine, the plasma level of growth hormone declines. Another neurohormone inhibits the release of prolactin, and chlorpromazine treatment relieves this inhibition. Accordingly, neuroleptic administration results in raised concentrations of plasma prolactin (see Chap. 38).

The phenothiazine nucleus is a strong electron donor, and charge-transfer properties have been suggested as playing a role in the cellular actions of these compounds. It has also been suggested that they act as chelators of certain trace metals. Chlorpromazine inhibits D-amino acid oxidase and some other flavoproteins, perhaps through its action as a flavin analog.

Chlorpromazine is readily absorbed from the gut, tissues (into which it may be injected), and blood. An oral dose yields a peak plasma concentration of the drug in 2 to 4 hours. In patients receiving chronic treatment with chlorpromazine, the plasma level of the drug shows extremely wide variation, from 10 to 1300 ng per milliliter. There also seems to be some accumulation in the tissues, because cessation of treatment with chlorpromazine is followed by a period of many months during which small amounts of the compound or its metabolites are found in the urine. The brain is easily penetrated by chlorpromazine, and the drug is found in higher concentrations in the cerebral cortex and the basal ganglia than in other parts of the CNS. There is still insufficient information about the factors regulating steady state plasma levels of the antipsychotic drugs. The great variability in these levels has thus far precluded using the values as a guide to adjustment of dosage for the optimal clinical response [13].

In the course of tissue metabolism, chlorpromazine is extensively altered. Its reactions include demethylation of the side chain, oxidation of the ring to yield a phenolic group, conjugation of this hydroxyl with glucuronic acid, oxidation to the sulfoxide and to the N-oxide, and others. Nonenzymic reactions that take place in the gut, skin, and elsewhere contribute further products that have been catalogued for this drug. The result is that very little chlorpromazine itself is excreted unchanged. After long-continued use of the drug, as in the treatment of schizophrenia, a photosensitive metabolite may accumulate in the skin; exposure to sunlight converts this substance to a purple derivative, which then lends a grayish or grayish-purple cast to the patient's complexion. Chlorpromazine-derived pigment may also be deposited in the cornea.

Chlorprothixene (Fig. 37-1) is a member of the thioxanthene family, and is oxidized to the sulfoxide, its major metabolite.

A comprehensive bibliography on the chemistry, metabolism, and pharmacology of phenothiazines and thioxanthenes exists [14].

Anxiolytics, or Minor Tranquilizers

BENZODIAZEPINES

The sedative, anticonvulsant, and taming activity of such benzodiazepines as chlordiazepoxide (Fig. 37-2), along with their relaxing effect on skeletal muscle, has given these drugs a prominent role as minor tranquilizers. They seem to reduce the turnover of monoamines in the brain; this effect is more significant with respect to 5-HT than to NE [15], at least when oxazepam is tested. However, there is growing evidence that a principal action is the production of GABA-like effects. This is achieved by facilitation of GABA transmission; by protecting animals against seizures that are caused by reduced GABA levels; by increasing presynaptic inhibition in the spinal cord; and by decreasing cyclic GMP levels in the cerebellum [16].

A dose of 15 mg of chlordiazepoxide administered orally provides a peak plasma concentration of about 1 μg per milliliter in 1 to 2 hours. The half-life of the radioactivity of the labeled compound in plasma is about 24 hours. Half of the radioactivity of chlordiazepoxide is excreted in the urine in 3 to 3.5 days. In the case of diazepam, 20 mg taken orally provides a peak level in the plasma of 0.5 μg per milliliter in 30 minutes.

The benzodiazepines all undergo similar patterns of metabolism. As exemplified by diazepam (Fig. 37-2) the principal metabolic reactions include N-demethylation and hydroxylation of the heterocyclic ring. Oxazepam results from these two successive changes. Eventually, these metabolites are conjugated with glucuronic acid and are excreted in the urine [17].

BARBITURATES

The barbiturates depress the metabolism of brain tissue to some extent in vitro; their effect is greater on electrically stimulated brain slices than on "silent" tissue. Moreover, some of them inhibit the respiration of brain mitochondria whose metabolism has been stimulated by the uncoupling agent 2,4-dinitrophenol. Thiobarbiturates inhibit oxidative phosphorylation of the liver and brain mitochondria that metabolize pyruvate, and these drugs display some action in uncoupling oxidative phosphorylation; the oxybarbiturates affect only the former process. The site of action of the oxybarbiturates appears to be in the respiratory chain between NAD and cytochrome c; this includes a flavoprotein which, it has been postulated, is inhibited by barbiturates (see also Chap. 35).

Barbiturates effect the neurolemma in the same manner as already described for chlorpromazine, with resulting nerve blockade. Many of them also inhibit $(Na^+ + K^+)$-ATPase [11].

One of the important characteristics that pharmacologists use to classify the barbiturates is their duration of action. This is influenced, of course, by the molecular structure. Thus, the thiobarbiturates undergo metabolism more rapidly

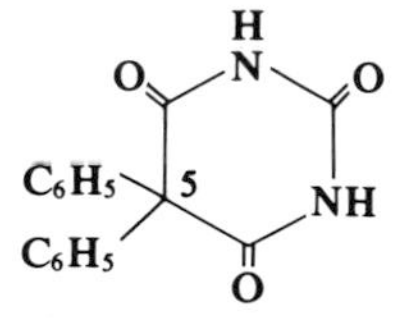

Phenobarbital

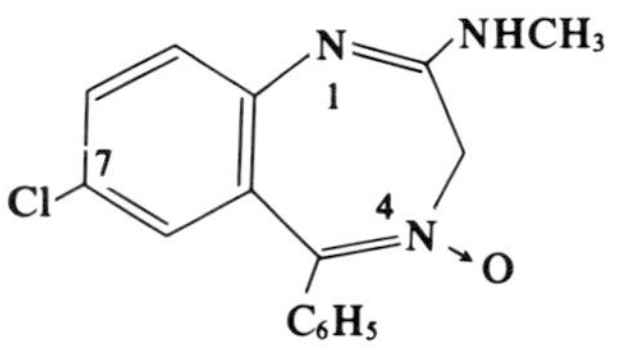

Chlordiazepoxide 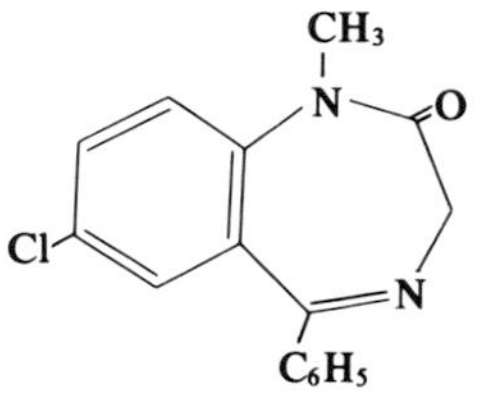   Diazepam

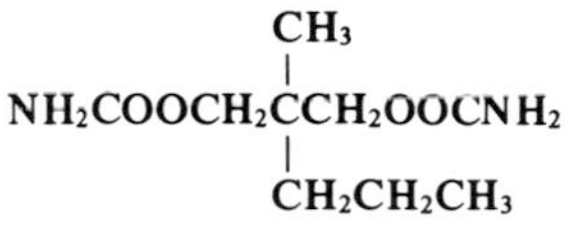

$$CH_3$$
$$NH_2COOCH_2CCH_2OOCNH_2$$
$$CH_2CH_2CH_3$$

Meprobamate

Fig. 37-2. Examples of minor tranquilizers and anxiolytics.

than do the oxybarbiturates; and those with longer aliphatic side chains or an aromatic substituent are metabolized more slowly, presumably because of greater lipid solubility and longer residence in adipose tissue. These substituents are rendered more polar during metabolism through oxidations catalyzed by microsomal enzymes. In phenobarbital (Fig. 37-2), a phenolic group is inserted; in pentobarbital, the alkyl side chain of the compound undergoes hydroxylation.

The administration of phenobarbital to rats causes increased activity of the microsomal oxidizing enzymes of the liver. One of the components of these induced enzymes is hemoprotein.

Antidepressants

MONOAMINE OXIDASE INHIBITORS

MAO inhibitors as a class of antidepressant drugs have had great significance for biochemical pharmacology and for biochemical theory of mental disease (Fig. 37-3; [18]). This significance remains, despite dangers inherent in the clinical use of these drugs. The first member of this class was iproniazid (*N*-isonicotinyl-*N'*-isopropylhydrazide), which was tested originally as an antitubercular drug along with isoniazid (*N*-isonicotinylhydrazide). The elation observed in patients receiving iproniazid was later put to use in the treatment of mental depression. The reversal of depression was then related to the ability of the compound powerfully to inhibit MAO and thereby increase the concentration of monoamines in the brain. Subsequently, chemists synthesized scores of compounds on the model of iproniazid in the search for new MAO inhibitors that might also be useful therapeutically. Other structural models have yielded additional inhibitors. Representative examples are illustrated in Fig. 37-3.

For many years, Zeller's classification of oxidase enzymes into MAO (acting on tyramine, isoamylamine, epinephrine, and similar amines) and

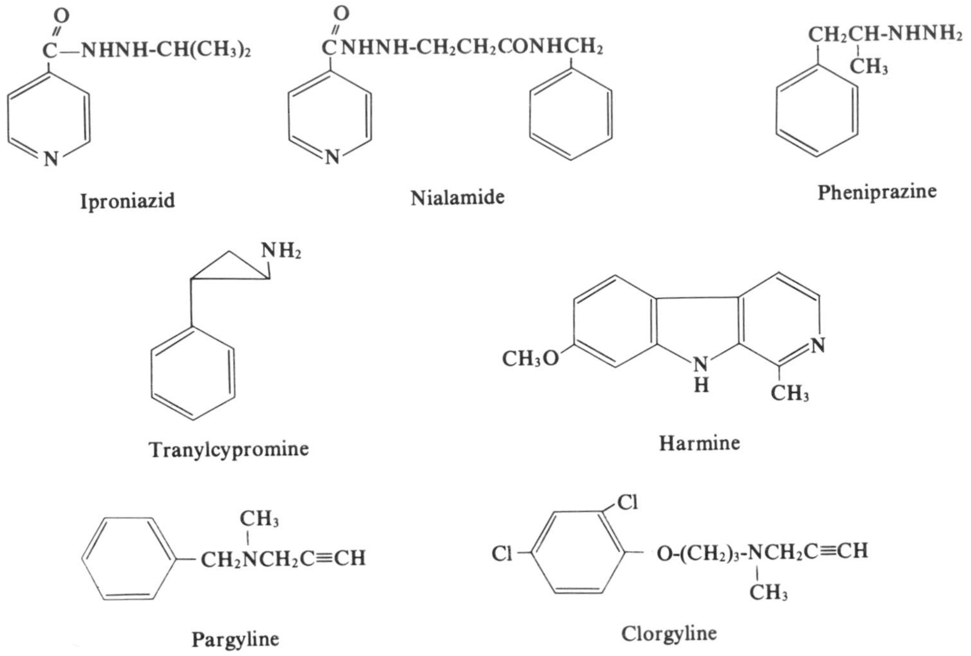

Fig. 37-3. Monoamine oxidase inhibitors.

diamine oxidase (DAO, acting on histamine and putrescine) has been used. As new types of amine oxidase have been discovered and as the physical and chemical properties of these enzymes are elucidated, it is becoming possible to classify them also on the basis of their respective prosthetic groups [19, 20]. For example, classic MAO is a yellow enzyme present in the outer membrane of mitochondria. In the case of the well-studied beef liver enzyme, it bears flavin adenine dinucleotide (FAD) covalently linked through its 8-methyl group to a cysteinyl residue of the peptide chain. DAO employs copper. The pink amine oxidase in the plasma of pig and some other species has similar requirements; its function is unknown. A copper-containing amine oxidase, acting upon the ε-amino group of lysine, has been detected in the connective tissue of birds and other species; it is needed for the formation of desmosine, which serves to cross-link elastin and collagen fibers.

MAO has been purified from the liver of several species and from bovine kidney and pig brain. The molecular weight of the mitochondrial enzyme in rat liver is approximately 150,000 (by ultracentri-

fugation measurements). The enzyme is especially sensitive to certain hydrazine derivatives, although not to hydrazine itself. Many propargylamines ($RR'NCH_2CCH$) like pargyline inhibit MAO irreversibly by forming an adduct at the N^5 position. Two of these, clorgyline (Fig. 37-3) and deprenyl (in which RN represents the amphetamine structure) exhibit some degree of differential inhibition of MAO with respect to substrates. Thus, MAO is especially sensitive to clorgyline with 5-HT or NE as substrate, whereas the enzyme is relatively more sensitive to deprenyl when the substrate is tryptamine, benzylamine, or phenethylamine. Results of this kind have led to the concept of two types of MAO: one, called *MAO-A,* is characterized by great sensitivity to clorgyline, N-cyclopropyl-N-o-chlorophenoxyethylamine (Lilly 51641), and harmaline and another type, called *MAO-B,* has low sensitivity to clorgyline. The proportions of these enzymic activities vary among organs and among species. Brain is said to have a preponderance of MAO-B. Although different investigators have succeeded in physically separating up to five MAO isoenzymes from a given mitochondrial source, the properties of these moieties do not conform clearly to the A and B categories. Hence, there are still important unanswered questions about the chemistry of MAO, and the reputed multiplicity of the enzyme is undergoing continuing evaluation.

MAO has at least two functions. In the intestinal tract it serves to detoxify certain amines produced by the gut flora. On absorption, these amines could exert pharmacological activity, although the liver MAO represents a second defense in regard to any such amines that reach it in the portal circulation. Other amines produced by the organism itself and arriving at the liver through the systemic circulation are subject to MAO action in the hepatocytes. In the nervous system, the enzyme serves to oxidize some of the 5-HT, DA, and NE after their release into the synaptic space, thus terminating their action. Metabolism of catecholamines may be initiated by the action of catechol-O-methyltransferase (COMT), so that the substrates for MAO are then 3-methoxytyramine and normetanephrine. MAO acts within the nerve fiber itself when monoamines leak from the synaptic vesicles. This occurs on a massive scale if reserpine is used to release the stored amines, for this takes place intraneuronally: the free amine within the nerve ending can then be attacked as it diffuses toward the mitochondria.

MAO catalyzes the following reaction:

$$RCH_2CH_2NH_2 + O_2 + H_2O \longrightarrow$$
$$RCH_2CHO + H_2O_2 + NH_3$$

The aldehyde undergoes oxidation by an aldehyde dehydrogenase to form the corresponding carboxylic acid, but some reduction may also take place through the action of alcohol dehydrogenase (aldehyde reductase). The latter reaction is quantitatively important in the cerebral metabolism of NE, but less so for amines that lack the β-hydroxyl group.

If an animal is treated with a MAO inhibitor, the concentrations of many amines increase in the tissues, including the brain. Thus, the rate of synthesis of 5-HT in the brain is essentially unaffected, but because degradation of the amine is slowed, there is a net increase in the amount of the amine. This phenomenon also occurs with the catecholamines, but the increases are more modest because of two other factors: (1) catecholamine biosynthesis is regulated by the NE feedback inhibition of tyrosine hydroxylase (Chap. 10 and [9, 21, 22]); (2) DA and NE are subject to the action of COMT, and the methylated products have less biological potency than do the parent amines. Despite the increased concentration of NE with a MAO inhibitor, the formation of this amine from labeled tyrosine is reduced; this is not true when labeled dopa is used (Table 37-3).

Animals given a MAO inhibitor become alert, even excited, but not if they have received reserpine previously. On the other hand, if a MAO inhibitor is administered before reserpine, the action of the inhibitor is potentiated. In this case, the released amines exert their pharmacological activity for a protracted period, unmitigated by reuptake into the vesicles of the nerve endings or by the reduced degree of catabolism by MAO. The behavioral stimulation caused by the MAO inhibitor is attributed to the increase in concentration of a cerebral monoamine, but which one is not known. It is not even known if the response is mediated by only one amine or by several acting in concert. There have been clinical attempts to use precursors of specific monoamines, for example, dopa, tryptophan, and 5-HTP, to potentiate the action of MAO inhibitors, but the profound activation of autonomic systems caused by such combinations has precluded their use in the treatment of depression. Cardiovascular and other unwanted effects of therapeutically used MAO inhibitors represent autonomic reactions mediated by endogenous amines.

An important precaution in the clinical use of MAO inhibitors is the avoidance of fermented foods (cheeses, especially aged varieties, red wines) and pickled foods as these contain much tyramine. Ordinarily, tyrosine would be metabolized to *p*-hydroxyphenylacetic acid before it could pass into the general circulation, but protected by the MAO inhibitor, the tyramine reaches sympathetic post-ganglionic nerve endings, where it stoichiometrically displaces stored NE. The excessive release of NE to receptor sites initiates the observed, sometimes lethal, autonomic changes. MAO inhibitors can also potentiate the effects of ethanol.

Paradoxically, MAO inhibitors cause a lowering of blood pressure. Several mechanisms for this have been suggested, based on events that may take place centrally or peripherally. One hypothesis suggests that the inhibitor allows the accumulation of abnormal amounts of amine metabolites that are normally not detectable; an example is octopamine (p-hydroxyphenylethanolamine) formed by β-oxidation of tyramine. At sympathetic nerve endings, this derivative would replace NE and then act as a substitute, or false, transmitter, with little musculotropic action. Pargyline (see Fig. 37-3) is a MAO inhibitor that has been used in the treatment of hypertension.

Although the antidepressant action of MAO inhibitors is thought to reside in their ability to conserve monoamines and to increase the concentrations of these compounds in the brain, the drugs exert inhibitory actions on other enzymes as well. These inhibitions have not received the same thorough attention that has been given to blockade of amine oxidation but nevertheless are important toxicologically. For example, the metabolism of ethanol is inhibited by MAO inhibitors, so the effects of alcoholic beverages are potentiated. MAO inhibitors also act on microsomal liver enzymes that catalyze the metabolic transformation or detoxification of other drugs. Thus, additional precautionary measures must be observed when a MAO inhibitor is used therapeutically. For example, the treatment must be stopped some days before a general anesthetic is to be administered.

The long-lasting action that most MAO inhibitors exert suggests that they form a covalent link with the enzyme, as already demonstrated for pargyline. If so, the activity of the enzyme would be restored only when new enzyme has been synthesized. This has been tested experimentally in rats given an inhibitor to block MAO; their mono-amine-oxidizing ability is restored in 4 to 6 days, approximately the time needed for recovery of rats from the MAO-depressing effects of riboflavin or iron deficiency. Riboflavin is needed for the synthesis of the coenzyme of MAO, and iron for maintaining a normal complement of the enzyme in tissues, for example, liver (rat) and platelets (human). It is probably required in the biosynthesis of the enzyme [18].

Tranylcypromine (see Fig. 37-3), a cyclopropylamine derivative, is thought to resemble the transient intermediate species formed by the substrate at the active site of the enzyme.

Harmine (see Fig. 37-3) and harmaline (dihydroharmine) are unique among MAO inhibitors in that they occur naturally. Their action is short-lasting and reversible. Harmine is considered to have some hallucinogenic activity. The mode of action of these compounds is still being explored. Along with their O-demethylated derivatives, harmol and harmalol, and certain related compounds, they antagonize peripheral actions of 5-HT, although only harmine and harmaline in this group inhibit MAO. Many β-carboline analogs have been synthesized in the search for useful therapeutic agents.

The metabolism of hydrazide inhibitors of MAO involves the loss of one or another of the N-substituents. For example, iproniazid yields isonicotinylhydrazide, isopropylhydrazide, isonicotinic acid, and unchanged drug in urine. There is evidence that iproniazid must undergo one of these reactions, perhaps dealkylation, before it acquires its inhibitory property.

Two hydrazine derivatives, carbidopa and benserazide, inhibit aromatic amino acid decarboxylase of peripheral tissues, without affecting the brain enzyme. They do not inhibit MAO and are devoid of antidepressant action. However, they protect easily degraded substrates such as L-dopa and 5-HTP from the action of decarboxylase in the tissues, with the result that a larger portion of the amino acid is conserved for distribution to the brain, where its amine product is needed (see Chap. 36).

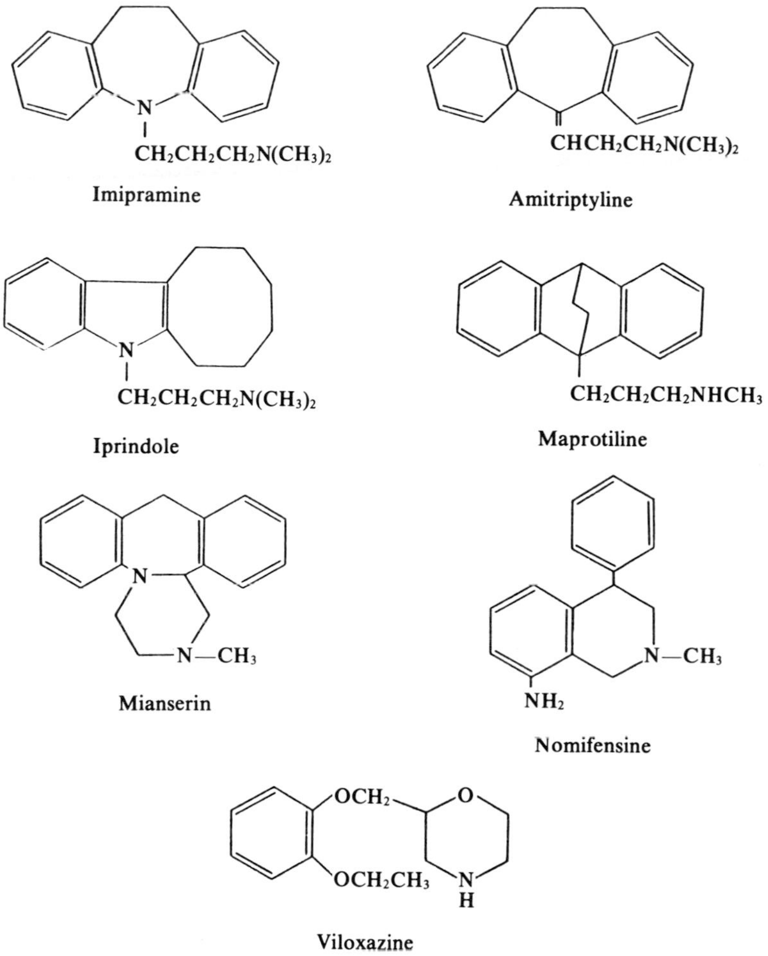

Imipramine

Amitriptyline

Iprindole

Maprotiline

Mianserin

Nomifensine

Viloxazine

Fig. 37-4. Tricyclic and other antidepressant drugs.

TRICYCLIC ANTIDEPRESSANTS

The tricyclic antidepressants (Fig. 37-4), the prototype of which is imipramine, have structures based on those of the phenothiazines. They have been supplemented in recent years by additional polycyclic compounds and by nomifensine and viloxazine. In *imipramine,* the sulfur atom of promazine is replaced by an ethylene bridge, yielding a dibenzazepine or iminodibenzyl; in *amitriptyline,* the further substitution of a carbon atom for the

nitrogen in the middle ring yields a dibenzocycloheptadiene. Doxepin has the same structure as amitriptyline, except for the presence of an oxymethylene bridge instead of ethylene. Despite the resemblance between the structures of imipramine and promazine, the latter molecule is symmetrical, whereas the two benzene rings of imipramine are actually twisted against one another asymmetrically in three-dimensional space.

Originally, some of these drugs were tested unsuccessfully in schizophrenic patients, but ultimately they were applied in the treatment of mental depression. The tricyclic antidepressants have only a weak effect or none at all on MAO, but their therapeutic action has been related in another way to monoamine metabolism. Many of them interfere with the uptake of monoamines from the synaptic cleft back into the nerve ending and its vesicles (see Chap. 10). This inhibition of the membrane pump provides a net increase in the concentration of free amine (i.e., amine not bound in vesicles or to a macromolecule) in the synapse at any one time, and provides increased probabilities of stimulation of sensitive receptors on the postsynaptic neurons [23].

There are some important differences between the tricyclic compounds in this respect; for example, imipramine, chlorimipramine, and amitriptyline strongly inhibit reuptake of 5-HT, whereas desipramine, nortriptyline, protriptyline, maprotiline, and viloxazine are more effective against uptake of NE. The acute administration of imipramine to experimental animals causes a decreased turnover of 5-HT in neurons; this could stem from the reduced rate of reuptake of the amine and its longer residence in the synaptic space. When the drug is given to animals chronically in order to approximate the therapeutic situation, the NE content of the brain decreases and the rate of metabolism of intracisternally injected (labeled) NE increases. The reduced rate of uptake of the amine under the influence of imipramine would render it more accessible to metabolic pathways. According to several hypotheses, the inhibition of monoamine reuptake plays an important role in the antidepressant action of imipramine and its congeners [24] (Chap. 38).

The reuptake of DA is strongly affected by certain anticholinergic and antihistaminic agents, but little by the tricyclic antidepressants. It is interesting that some members of the two classes of drugs inhibiting DA uptake are used in the treatment of Parkinson's disease (see Chap. 36).

There is evidence that mechanisms other than inhibition of uptake play a role in the antidepressive action. For example, iprindole and mianserin are antidepressants without action on uptake. Mianserin acts presynaptically as an α-noradrenergic blocker. Other types of effects are postulated to occur postsynaptically, with mediation by catecholamines or 5-HT. Thus, antidepressant drugs (and also electroshock treatment) given chronically to animals decrease the sensitivity of the adenylate cyclase system of brain tissue to NE [25]. The rate of synthesis of cyclic AMP is regarded in this context as a direct response to the intensity of stimulation of the cerebral noradrenergic receptors (Chap. 15). It has been found that the iontophoretic applications of 5-HT to hippocampal neurons depress their activity. Their sensitivity in this test is increased if the animals have previously received chronic intraperitoneal injections of antidepressant drugs. The interesting point is that the drugs accomplishing this effect are not uniform with respect to their presynaptic action or monoamine uptake [26].

Imipramine is well absorbed on oral administration; a single dose provides gradually increasing concentrations in the plasma for 4 to 8 hours, when a maximum is reached. This compound is metabolized analogously to the phenothiazines: it undergoes dealkylation of the tertiary amine side chain, yielding desipramine, which also has antidepressant properties, as the first product. Microsomal enzymes of the liver catalyze other oxidative reactions, as well, one of them being an aromatic hydroxylation; this represents a major route of metabolism. Glucuronidation of the phenolic group occurs. Metabolism of the drug to the monodemethylated products determines that both parent and derived compound are present in a ratio that varies with time and between subjects. Nevertheless, both will exert pharmacological activity. This is also true in the cases of maprotiline and amitriptyline. Soon after an oral dose of amitriptyline is given, the drug can be detected in the plasma. A few hours later, when its level has attained a peak, nortriptyline is detectable. This compound then increases to its maximal level as the amitriptyline declines in concentration. These facts indicate how difficult it is to predict clinical response from pharmacokinetic data [5]. The therapeutic level of this group of drugs, however, lies in the range of 95 to 120 ng per milliliter of plasma [27].

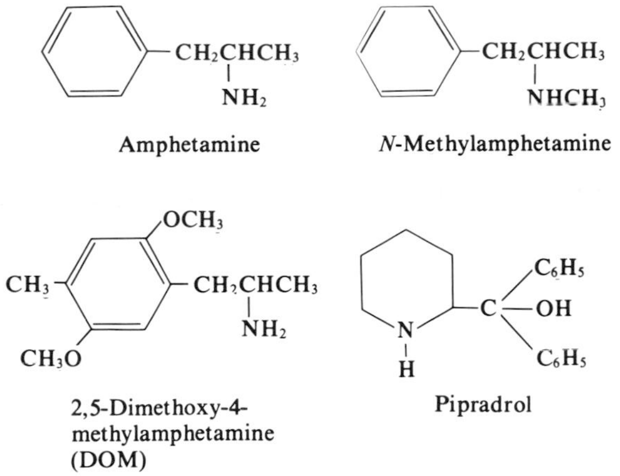

Fig. 37-5. *Amphetamines and pipradrol.*

AMPHETAMINE

Amphetamine (Fig. 37-5) and some other β-phenyl-isopropylamines have been used as therapeutic agents for many years. After World War II, their illicit use as psychological stimulants and hallucinogenic agents expanded greatly. Amphetamine abuse can lead to serious disturbances of mental behavior. The resulting *amphetamine psychosis* may be virtually indistinguishable from paranoid schizophrenia and is often diagnosed correctly only when the patient is discovered to be taking amphetamine (see Chap. 38). Some amphetamine-dependent individuals exhibit peculiar chewing movements, which are related to the stereotypy elicited in laboratory animals by large doses of amphetamine and which entail drug-induced release of newly synthesized (as against long-stored) presynaptic dopamine. This stereotypy is mediated by dopaminergic fibers, with output by way of a cholinergic system, and is also elicited by the dopamine agonist apomorphine. The orolingual activity is related to symptoms seen in tardive dyskinesia, an extrapyramidal disorder that occurs in some individuals who have received phenothiazines, particularly chlorpromazine, over a prolonged period (see Table 37-1). It is difficult to treat.

Amphetamine was recognized early as an inhibitor of MAO. It is not especially potent in this respect in comparison to the newer synthetic derivatives discussed above, but experiments with labeled amines show that it nevertheless exerts some inhibitory action on MAO in vivo. It is not itself a substrate, since MAO acts only on ω-amines.

The stimulant action of amphetamine seems attributable to its ability to inhibit MAO and to two other actions. First, it inhibits reuptake of NE into sympathetic nerve fibers, causing retention of a greater supply of the amine in the synapse for stimulation of the postsynaptic fiber. Second, it penetrates into the amine storage vesicles, and replaces their NE. This resembles the action of tyramine. The amine is released outward, that is, into the synapse. The vector of the releasing mechanism has been shown experimentally: After labeled NE is injected into an animal and time is allowed for the amine to be taken up into sympathetic nerve endings, administration of reserpine leads to a preponderance of *acidic derivatives.* On the other hand, injection of tyramine (or amphetamine) produces a preponderance of labeled *amines,* one fraction of which consists of nor-metanephrine. This indicates that MAO has limited opportunity to act under the influence of amphetamine, but that COMT, an extraneuronal enzyme, serves in the postrelease disposal of the amine.

Despite their CNS-stimulating properties, both amphetamine and pipradrol have found a use in the treatment of hyperkinetic children. For many years it was thought that these drugs exert a paradoxical quieting effect in this condition, but a careful clinical study shows that normal young boys respond to a single dose of *d*-amphetamine in the same way as hyperactive children: by a decrease of motor activity and improvement in the performance of certain cognitive tasks [28].

An interesting derivative of amphetamine is its *p*-chloro analog. This compound inhibits tryptophan hydroxylase, as does *p*-chlorophenylalanine. Both drugs reduce the rate of formation of 5-HT in the brain, with a resulting decrease in its concentration.

The excretion of amphetamine and related compounds is sharply dependent on the urinary pH. For example, an adult taking about 10 mg of *N*-methylamphetamine (methamphetamine) orally, together with ammonium chloride, excretes 55 to 70 percent of the dose unchanged in the urine in 16 hours and an additional 6 to 7 percent as amphetamine. If one takes sodium bicarbonate, which renders the urine alkaline, only 0.6 to 2.0 percent of the total dose appears in the urine in the amine fraction because tubular reabsorption is then favored.

β-Phenylisopropylamines are metabolized along several pathways: *p*-hydroxylation, with or without *O*-glucuronidation; *β*-hydroxylation of the side chain; *N*-dealkylation, if there is a substituent on the amino group; and oxidative deamination, with formation of a ketone, the ketone being either reduced to the corresponding alcohol or further oxidized to an acid after decarboxylation of the *α*-carbon. Considerable species differences exist among these metabolic pathways. In the dog, about one-third of a dose of *d*-amphetamine is excreted unchanged in the urine; another large portion appears as *p*-hydroxyamphetamine, some of which is conjugated. In human and rabbit, deamination is the predominant route. Some of the phenylacetone formed is converted to phenylisopropanol; another portion is oxidized to benzoic acid, most of which appears in the urine as hippuric acid. In the rat and cat, *d*-amphetamine is hydroxylated on both the ring and the side chain, forming *p*-hydroxynorephedrine. A small amount of this metabolite is formed in humans through *p*-hydroxyamphetamine.

The oxidative metabolism of amphetamine is initiated by microsomal enzymes of the liver. These enzymes increase in amount under the influence of certain drugs, so that the rate of catabolism of amphetamine is directly affected. Another pertinent type of drug interaction is simply a matter of competition between amphetamine and another drug that is acted on by the same hepatic enzymes [29]. The first type of interaction leads to a reduction of amphetamine content of the tissues, compared with controls dosed similarly with the compound; the second leads to increased levels.

A comprehensive review of amphetamine exists [30], as well as additional material [31].

LITHIUM SALTS

Lithium salts are the drug of choice in *hypomania* and *mania*. They also are used successfully on a prophylactic basis in the treatment of recurrent, endogenous, affective disorders of both the bipolar and unipolar types, protecting the patient against the depressive as well as the manic episodes of the phasic illness [32]; (see also Chap. 38).

There is good absorption from the gastrointestinal tract, with Li^+ passing from the blood into the tissues. Equilibration takes place quickly in liver, kidneys, and skin, and less rapidly in muscle and brain. The lithium level in serum corresponds to that in tissue. Its determination by flame photometry in the clinical laboratory facilitates therapeutic control. Measurements should be made on blood drawn about 12 hours after the last dose of lithium. Dosage is adjusted to maintain a serum level of 0.5 to 1.2 mEq per liter; this requires 25 to 50 mEq of lithium per day. Side effects in the lower range are rare, but their incidence increases as the serum Li^+ concentration rises. Serum levels above 1.3 mEq per liter should be avoided. The concentration of Li^+ in CSF reaches only about one-half the serum level. Almost all the ingested Li^+ is excreted in urine.

Lithium salts appear to have some influence over the movements of NE at nerve endings and in synapses. There is evidence of a reduced availability of the amine at receptor sites as a result of Li^+ action. This may stem from increased CNS release of NE at a rate that outstrips biosynthesis. However, the dynamics of monoamine metabolism during Li^+ treatment are still being worked out, especially in chronic administration. In acute experiments, DA and 5-HT are not affected.

Li^+ alters somewhat the distribution of Na^+, K^+, and water, but with good therapeutic control of dosage, these changes are not serious. Success with lithium salts has led to research on the actions of rubidium and cesium in manic-depressive psychosis, but as yet there are no therapeutic indications for use of these ions.

TRYPTOPHAN

Tryptophan has been tested for the treatment of mentally depressed patients on many occasions, over a wide dosage range, and with varying results. An important consideration in the use of this amino acid is its induction of hepatic pyrrolase, the increased activity of which results in degradation of proffered tryptophan at a faster rate; it thereby reduces the availability of the amino acid to the brain [33]. Some of the observed variations in response may arise from a nondirect relation of dosage and response. Thus, tryptophan may serve therapeutically in only a limited range of dosage ("therapeutic window"). Attempts to control these sources of variability have enhanced its usefulness [34]. The mode of action of this amino acid in depression is not completely understood, but two possibilities have been proposed. The first is the provision of extra 5-HT, to make up for any relative deficiency that may arise in depression [24, 33]. The other is the direct neurophysiological action of tryptophan in depressing the activity of certain raphe neurons in a dose-dependent fashion [35, 36].

Psychodysleptics, or Hallucinogenic Agents

The psychodysleptics represent a motley group of plant and laboratory products (Fig. 37-6). The remarkably potent D-*LSD-25* is a synthetic derivative of a plant alkaloid, lysergic acid. The hallucinogens can be classified roughly into three major categories: (1) indole derivatives, (2) phenylalkylamine derivatives, and (3) nonnitrogenous compounds. The first two have lent themselves readily to biochemical theories of hallucinogenic actions based on the concept of antagonism to cerebral 5-HT and catecholamines, respectively. This antagonism is thought to interfere in some way with the function of monoamines in mental processes. Molecular orbital calculations also have been used to assess hallucinogenic potency in relation to chemical reactivity. However, our under-

standing of the action of these compounds at the cellular or molecular level remains very limited.

INDOLIC HALLUCINOGENS

The simplest members of this category are the *dialkyltryptamines,* for example, diethyltryptamine (see Fig. 37-6). Others are psilocybin, the *O*-phosphoryl ester of *N*-dimethyl-4-hydroxytryptamine, and D-LSD-25. Bufotenine (*N*-dimethyl-5-hydroxytryptamine) also is reputed to be hallucinogenic; it is found in both plants and the poison gland of the toad. D-LSD-25, now known as *lysergide,* is one of four diastereoisomers of lysergic acid diethylamide, all four of which have been tested for hallucinogenic activity. Only lysergide is active to any extent, and it is exceedingly potent. It is estimated to be present in brain to the extent of only a few picograms per gram of tissue while exerting its psychodysleptic action.

In 1953 and 1954, investigators drew attention to the possible interaction of indole alkaloids with 5-HT receptors; drugs such as lysergide were proposed to act in the brain by opposing the normal action of 5-HT. This application of the antimetabolite hypothesis to psychodysleptics was soon recognized to be inadequate. For example, if lysergide is brominated to 2-bromolysergide, hallucinogenic activity is lost, but antagonism toward musculotropic actions of 5-HT is retained. Thus, presence of an anti-5-HT action in one context does not necessarily insure that it will be manifest in another.

In other experiments, it has been shown that lysergide affects the metabolism of 5-HT in the brain in several ways: it decreases its rate of synthesis from tryptophan; it increases brain 5-HT slightly; and it decreases 5-HIAA correspondingly. This pattern of effects can be explained by assuming that the drug reduces the turnover rate of cerebral 5-HT. There is also evidence that lysergide and other indoleamines specifically inhibit the firing of 5-HT–containing neurons in the median and dorsal raphe nuclei. Hallucinogenic activity in this group is associated with a greater inhibitory

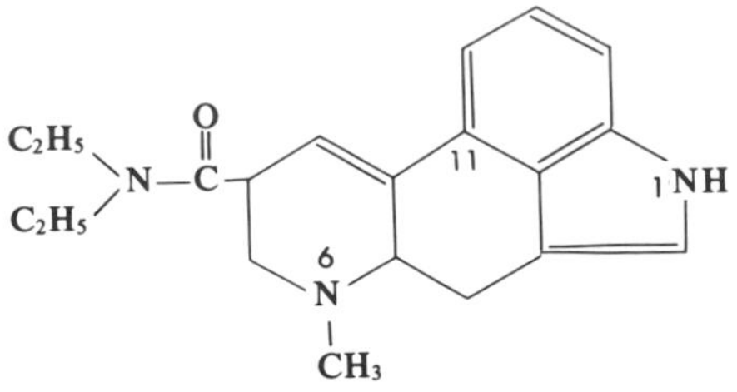

Lysergide

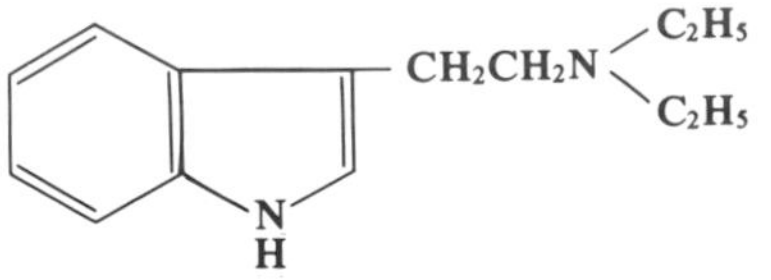

Diethyltryptamine

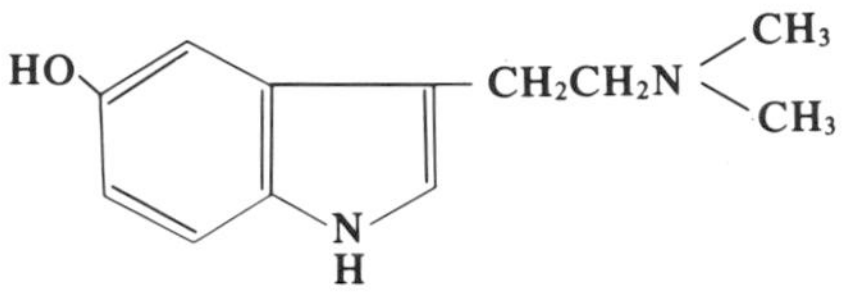

Bufotenine

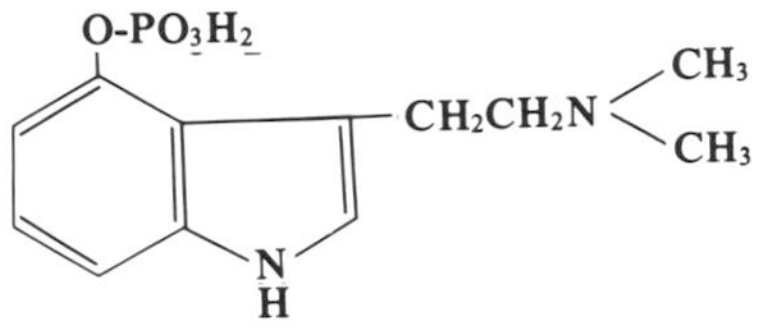

Psilocybin

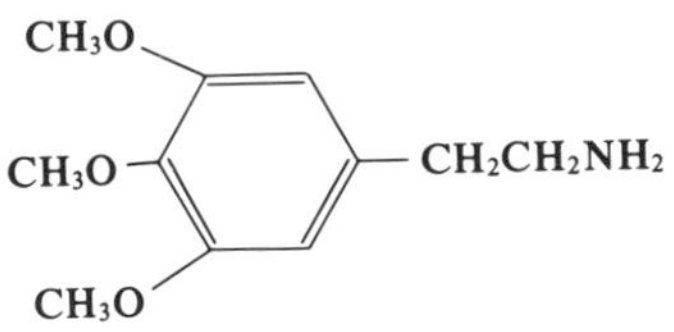

Mescaline

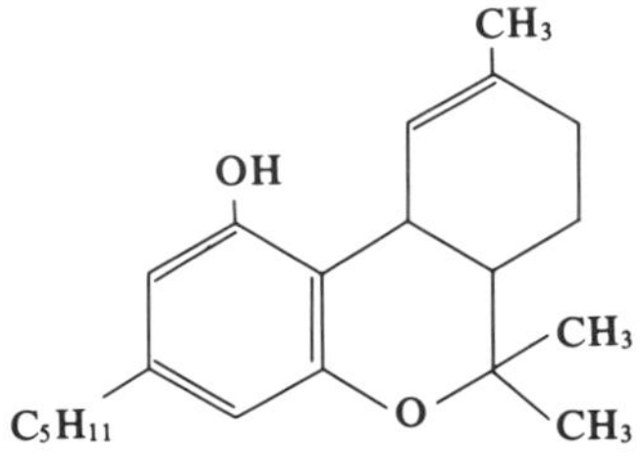

Δ^9-Tetrahydrocannabinol

Fig. 37-6. Some known and putative hallucinogens. Dimethoxyphenylethylamine (DMPEA, referred to in Chap. 38) has the structure of mescaline minus one of the meta methoxy groups.

action on presynaptic than on postsynaptic neurons [35].

Studies of the distribution of 5-HT in the subcellular fractions suggest that the biochemical changes noted above probably take place within the neuron, that is, without its release into the synaptic space. In fact, if the drug is applied in very low doses iontophoretically, it has a direct inhibitory effect on raphe cells in rats and specifically antagonizes the excitatory action of 5-HT on certain cells of the brain stem in cats. In recent years, mixed agonistic and antagonistic actions of some ergot alkaloids, such as bromocriptine and lergotrile, have been described with respect to presynaptic DA receptors [37].

Lysergide is absorbed rapidly from the gastrointestinal tract, but there are large differences in its metabolism among species. The biological half-life of the compound in the blood of rodents is 7 minutes, but in the monkey and cat it is 1.5 to 2 hours. When transported in the blood, it is bound to plasma proteins, but it is readily released into the brain and other organs. Its highest concentration is attained in these organs soon after injection, and it declines over the next few hours. The concentration of lysergide in the brain is always less than in the blood. Highest amounts are found in the liver. Microsomal enzymes in the liver (but not in the brain) oxidize lysergide to its biologically inactive 2-oxy derivative. Other products, more polar than lysergide itself, are formed. The bile serves as one route of excretion of the hallucinogen, but some of it is probably then reabsorbed from the intestine.

Some investigators claim that bufotenine is a constituent of the urine of schizophrenic patients, normal subjects, or both. However, these claims have never received adequate verification. *Psilocybin*, the active principle of certain mushrooms found in the southern highlands of Mexico, is unusual in being an ester of phosphoric acid. Its hydrolytic product is psilocin, the 4-hydroxy analog of bufotenine, and it is also hallucinogenic. An interesting and novel pathway of metabolism of some indolic compounds (including melatonin) is by way of 6-hydroxylation. This route accounts for two-fifths of a dose of N,N'-diethyltryptamine, but for only about one-fifth of the dose of the dimethyl and dipropyl homologs.

MESCALINE
Mescaline, like lysergide, has been investigated for possible inhibitory actions in many enzyme and respiratory systems in the search for specific effects that might be related to its psychodysleptic action. Its structure (Fig. 37-6) suggests that it acts through some catecholamine system in the brain. In fact, when mescaline is given to monkeys, it causes the oral (licking) syndrome [38] seen with amphetamine and with centrally acting DA agonists generally. One suggestion has been that in schizophrenia DA is doubly methylated to 3,4-dimethoxyphenylethylamine (see Chap. 38). The resemblance of this hypothetical metabolite to *mescaline* (3,4,5-trimethoxyphenethylamine) is clear enough (see Chap. 38; Fig. 37-6). The synthetic compound has no hallucinogenic action, however, and on the few occasions when it has been identified in body fluids there has been no evidence of relation to schizophrenia.

The dose of mescaline required to elicit hallucinations is much larger than that needed for many of the other psychodysleptics. It is quite possible that some quantitatively minor metabolite of the drug is responsible for its effects. Oral administration of labeled mescaline to humans shows that the compound is readily absorbed and rapidly metabolized. Among the metabolites detected are the carboxylic acid corresponding to mescaline, N-acetylmescaline, 3,4-dimethoxy-5-hydroxyphenylethylamine, and the N-acetyl derivative of the last compound. Demethylation of the 4-methoxy group can also occur. The deamination of mescaline is catalyzed by DAO, not by MAO.

2,5-Dimethoxy-4-methylamphetamine (Fig. 37-5) resembles both mescaline and amphetamine in structure. It is a hallucinogen.

TETRAHYDROCANNABINOL
Research on the mechanisms of action of hallucinogens is difficult enough when chemically pure agents are available, but it is much more difficult in the case of a galenical agent, such as *marijuana*. The chemistry of cannabis has now been clarified, with the identification of its most important psychodysleptic constituent as $(-)$-trans-Δ^9-tetrahydrocannabinol (THC) [39]. It is effective in humans in oral administration in a dose of 50 to 200 μg per kilogram of body weight and, by smoking, in a dose of 25 to 50 μg per kilogram. This compound (Fig. 37-6) is now used as a standard for biological testing of other cannabinoids, that is, C_{21} compounds characteristically found in the cannabis plant and in preparations made from it, as well as related synthetic compounds and metabolites. Marijuana contains about one percent of Δ^9-THC; *hashish*, the resinous product of cannabis, is much richer. Research in this area is currently directed toward finding synthetic THC-like compounds devoid of hallucinogenic activity but with autonomic actions that are useful in treating hypertension and glaucoma, as has been reported for marijuana.

THC is rapidly accumulated in the liver and then metabolized to more polar products. Its half-life is about 30 min in humans and rats, and even less in rabbits. If smoked, it is temporarily detectable in the lungs. It is carried in the plasma in association with lipoproteins. THC is an effective in vitro inhibitor of the mitochondrial NADH oxidation system of brain and heart, probably acting near the amytal-sensitive site of the electron-transport chain [40].

Hepatic microsomes act quickly on THC to convert it to the 11-hydroxy derivative; this substance is even more potent than the parent compound. Further transformation leads to 8,11-dihydroxy-THC, 11-hydroxycannabinol (in which the cyclohexene ring is aromatized), and other products; side-chain oxidation also occurs. The route of excretion varies from species to species. In humans, fecal excretion of radioactive $\triangle^9$-THC exceeds urinary output after the first day, during which most of the eliminated radioactivity is in the urine. In the rabbit, urinary excretion predominates; but in the rat, the major path of excretion is by way of the bile.

Acknowledgment

Research in the author's laboratory in this field is supported by grants from the Medical Research Council of Canada.

References

1. Jacobson, E.   The comparative pharmacology of some psychotropic drugs. *Bull. W.H.O.* 21:411–493, 1959.
2. Von Brücke, F. T., and Hornykiewicz, O.   *The Pharmacology of Psychotherapeutic Drugs.* New York: Springer-Verlag, 1969.
*3. Efron, D. (ed.).   *Psychopharmacology, a Review of Progress,* 1957–1967. Washington, D.C.: Public Health Service Publication No. 1836, 1968.
*4. Clark, W. G., and Del Giuduce, J. (eds.).   *Principles of Psychopharmacology* (2nd ed.). New York: Academic, 1978.
5. Garattini, S., and Morselli, P. L.   Metabolism and pharmacokinetics of psychotropic drugs. In Ref. 4, pp. 169–182.
*6. Lipton, M. A., DiMascio, A., and Killam, K. F. (eds.).   *Psychopharmacology: A Generation of Progress.* New York: Raven, 1978.
7. Usdin, E., and Efron, D. H.   *Psychotropic Drugs and Related Compounds* (2nd ed.). Washington, D. C.: Department of Health, Education and Welfare, Publication No. (HSM) 72-9074, 1974.
8. Nybäck, H., Sedvall, G., and Kopin, I. J.   Accelerated synthesis of dopamine-C^{14} from tyrosine-C^{14} in rat brain after chlorpromazine. *Life Sci.* 6:2307–2312, 1967.

9. Spector, S.   Regulation of norepinephrine synthesis. In reference 3, pp. 13–16.
10. Scatton, B., Thierry, A. M., Glowinski, J., and Julou, L.   Effects of thioproperazine and apomorphine on dopamine synthesis in the mesocortical dopaminergic systems. *Brain Res.* 88:389–393, 1975.
11. Seeman, P.   The membrane actions of anesthetics and tranquilizers. *Pharmacol. Rev.* 24:583–653, 1972.
12. Landmark, K., and Øye, I.   The action of thioridazine and promazine on biological membranes: Relationship between ATPase inhibition and membrane stabilization. *Acta Pharmacol. Toxicol.* 29:1–8, 1971.
13. Cooper, T. B., Simpson, G. M., and Lee, J. H.   Thymoleptic and neuroleptic drug plasma levels in psychiatry: Current status. *Int. Rev. Neurobiol.* 19:269–309, 1976.
14. Forrest, I. S., Carr, C. J., and Usdin, E. (eds.).   *Advances in Biochemical Psychopharmacology.* New York: Raven, 1974. Vol. 9.
15. Wise, C. D., Berger, B. D., and Stein, L.   Benzodiazepines: Anxiety-reducing activity by reduction of serotonin turnover in the brain. *Science* 177: 180–183, 1972.
16. Iversen, L. L.   Biochemical psychopharmacology of GABA. In ref. 6, pp. 25–38.
17. Shader, R. I., and Greenblatt, D. J.   Clinical implications of benzodiazepine pharmacokinetics. *Am. J. Psychiatry* 134:652–656, 1977.
18. Wolstenholme, G., and Fitzsimmons, D. W. (eds.).   *Monoamine Oxidase and its Inhibition.* New York: American Elsevier, 1976.
19. Blaschko, H.   The natural history of amine oxidases. *Rev. Physiol. Biochem. Pharmacol.* 70: 83–148, 1974.
20. Sourkes, T. L.   Copper, biogenic amines, and amine oxidases. In D. Evered and G. Lawrenson (eds.), *Biological Roles of Copper.* Ciba Foundation Symposium 79. Amsterdam: Associated Scientific Publishers, 1980.
21. Cotten, M. de V. (ed.).   *Regulation of Catecholamine Metabolism in the Sympathetic Nervous System.* Baltimore: Williams & Wilkins, 1972.
*22. Usdin, E., Kopin, I. J., and Barchas, J. (eds.).   *Catecholamines: Basic and Clinical Frontiers* (2 vols.). New York: Pergamon, 1979.
23. Sulser, F., and Sanders-Bush, E.   Effect of drugs on amines in the CNS. *Annu. Rev. Pharmacol.* 11:209–230, 1971.
24. Sourkes, T. L.   Biochemistry of mental depression. *Can. Psychiat. Assoc. J.* 22:467–481, 1977.

*Key reference.

25. Sulser, F., Vetulani, J., and Mobley, P. L.   Mode of action of antidepressant drugs. *Biochem. Pharmacol.* 27:257–261, 1978.

26. De Montigny, C., and Aghajanian, G. K.   Tricyclic antidepressants: Long-term treatment increases responsivity of rat forebrain neurons to serotonin. *Science* 202:1303–1306, 1978.

27. Hollister, L. E.   Tricyclic antidepressants. *N. Engl. J. Med.* 299:1106–1109, and 1172–1186, 1978.

28. Rapoport, J. L., Buchsbaum, M. S., Zahn, T. P., Weingartner, H., Ludlow, C., and Mikkelsen, E. J. Dextroamphetamine: Cognitive and behavioral effects in normal prepubertal boys. *Science* 199: 560–563, 1978.

29. Lal, S., Sourkes, T. L., and Missala, K.   The effect of certain tranquilisers, chlorpromazine metabolites and diethyldithiocarbamate on tissue amphetamine levels in the rat. *Arch. Int. Pharmacodyn. Ther.* 207:122–130, 1974.

*30. Lewander, T.   Effects of Amphetamine in Animals. In W. R. Martin (ed.), *Handbook of Experimental Pharmacology.* Berlin: Springer-Verlag, 1977.

31. Costa, E., and Garattini, S. (eds.).   *International Symposium on Amphetamines and Related Compounds.* New York: Raven, 1970.

*32. Schou, M.   Clinical use of lithium. In ref. 4, pp. 553–560.

33. Young, S. N., and Sourkes, T. L.   Tryptophan in the central nervous system: Regulation and significance. *Adv. Neurochem.* 2:133–191, 1977.

34. Chouinard, G., Young, S. N., Annable, L., and Sourkes, T. L.   Tryptophan-nicotinamide, imipramine and their combination in depression. *Acta Psychiatr. Scand.* 59:395–414, 1979.

35. Haigler, H. J., and Aghajanian, G. K.   Serotonin receptors in the brain. *Fed. Proc.* 36:2159–2164, 1977.

36. Trulson, M. E., and Jacobs, B. L.   Dose-response relationships between systemically administered L-tryptophan or L-5-hydroxytryptophan and raphe unit activity in the rat. *Neuropharmacology* 15: 339–344, 1976.

37. Goldstein, M., Lew, J. Y., Nakamura, S., Battista, A. F., Lieberman, A., and Fuxe, K.   Dopaminephilic properties of ergot alkaloids. *Fed. Proc.* 37: 2202–2206, 1978.

38. Klüver, H.   *Mescal and Mechanisms of Hallucinations.* Chicago: University of Chicago Press, 1966.

*39. Cotten, M. de V. (ed.).   Marihuana and its surrogates. *Pharmacol. Rev.* 23:259–380, 1971.

40. Bartova, A., and Birmingham, M. K.   Effect of Δ^9-tetrahydrocannabinol on mitochondrial NADH-oxidase activity. *J. Biol. Chem.* 251: 5002–5006, 1976.

Philip A. Berger
Jack D. Barchas

Chapter 38. Biochemical Hypotheses of Mental Disorders

Useful pharmacological treatments for mental disorders, which appeared only during the last quarter century, have been of great benefit to psychiatric patients. Perhaps as important, effective drug treatments for mental disorders have stimulated the development of multiple links between psychiatry and biological sciences. Such links should allow the development of rational pharmacological treatments based on attempts to correct or compensate for the presently unknown biochemical abnormalities that are the basis of mental disorders [1].

The purpose of this chapter is to review critically the biochemical hypotheses of the two major mental disorders, *schizophrenia* and *affective illness,* and to suggest directions for future research. A number of practical and conceptual problems make research in biological psychiatry challenging. Despite a number of useful animal models for studying behavior, there is no convincing evidence that schizophrenia or affective disorders occur in any nonhuman species. Studies in human patients are therefore essential, despite the relative inaccessibility of the living human brain. Because indirect approaches must be used, an important task of researchers who study metabolic processes in mental illness is to diminish potential sources of artifactual variability [2], not the least of which arises from assay methodology.

The recent history of research in biological psychiatry has been characterized by the attempt to develop more sensitive and specific assays for measuring metabolic variables in biological tissues and fluids. Because metabolic variables often change according to a circadian rhythm, the time of collection of biological samples can also lead to differences among groups. Patient variability is also important. A difference between two groups of subjects may reflect age or sex distribution, differences in diet, activity level, or physical health. Medication status and the phase of the illness can also modify results. Differences between patients and control subjects may primarily reflect the patients' physiological response to a drug.

Schizophrenia

Schizophrenia is a disease of unknown cause that commonly begins in young adulthood. Symptoms include disturbed thinking, perceptual distortions, altered mood, unpredictable motor activity, and unusual interpersonal behavior. Disturbances in thinking cause distorted concept formation, bizarre speech, and illogical thought patterns. These disturbances are often expressed as *delusions,* ideas that are improbable or erroneous but that cannot be modified by contradictory evidence or persuasion. *Paranoid delusions* often lead schizophrenic patients to believe that they have a special mission or extraordinary powers, or that they are the object of a complex plot against them. (For example, they might be convinced that anything they write will be destroyed by an unscrupulous publisher.) Some schizophrenics believe that unseen forces are controlling their thoughts or behavior, or reading their minds.

Delusional beliefs are often reinforced by misinterpretations of reality. *Perceptual distortions* include hallucinations, which can arise in any sensory modality, although auditory hallucinations (usually "voices") are the most common schizophrenic hallucination. The mood of schizophrenic patients is frequently disturbed. Expressions of emotion are often absent, diminished, or entirely inappropriate to the context in which they occur. Schizophrenics are sometimes overwhelmed by deep rage or intense anxiety for no apparent reason. The motor activity of schizophrenic patients ranges from frenetic, purposeless overactivity to total immobilization. Schizophrenics often adopt unusual postures or have peculiar mannerisms [1, 3, 4].

The most fundamental defect in schizophrenia may be disturbed interpersonal behavior. The profound defects in thinking, perception, mood, and motor activity make it difficult for patients to carry out everyday tasks or to maintain relationships with family and friends. Those close to the patient have increasing difficulty understanding his or her unusual thoughts, beliefs, feelings, and behavior. These two factors increasingly isolate the patients, who often withdraw into themselves to focus on internal experiences. Thus, schizophrenia often leads to almost total disability of the patient and to suffering for both the patient and those around him or her.

How common is this disabling condition? At present there are about 180,000 hospitalized schizophrenics in the United States (occupying about one-quarter of all hospital beds); another 800,000 to 1 million are being treated as outpatients or have active symptoms but are not receiving treatment. The number of individuals who develop schizophrenic symptoms each year is about 150 per 100,000. The chances that a person will develop schizophrenia in his lifetime are approximately 1 in 100. The incidence of schizophrenia appears to be similar in every nation and culture that has been investigated [5].

Research on a possible biochemical basis for schizophrenia has been influenced by two major hypotheses: The *transmethylation hypothesis* proposes that the symptoms of schizophrenia result from an endogenous psychotogen produced by the abnormal methylation of a neurotransmitter amine; the *dopamine hypothesis* proposes that schizophrenia is related to an overactivity of dopaminergic neurons in certain areas of the CNS.

THE TRANSMETHYLATION HYPOTHESIS OF SCHIZOPHRENIA

The transmethylation hypothesis postulates an autointoxicating substance or endogenous psychotogen formed by the abnormal methylation of a neurotransmitter amine. This hypothesis was originally based on the observation of Osmond and Smythies [6] that the hallucinogen mescaline can be considered a methoxylated derivative of the catecholamines (see Fig. 37-6). They suggested that enzymes could methylate hydroxyl positions of catecholamines in vivo to form a mescalinelike substance, such as 3,4-dimethoxyphenylethylamine (DMPEA), and lead to schizophrenic symptoms. The discovery of serotonin (5-hydroxytryptamine,5-HT) in the brain led to a transmethylation hypothesis of schizophrenia, based on the methylation of indoleamines: N,N-dimethyltryptamine (DMT) is a potent hallucinogen that also has been reported to exacerbate the symptoms of schizophrenia [2]. Bufotenine, the N,N-dimethyl derivative of 5-HT, may also have hallucinogenic properties (see Fig. 37-6) [3, 4]. Both of these substances have been proposed to act as endogenous psychotogens [7].

Investigations of the transmethylation hypothesis include three major types of studies: (1) attempts to identify methylated derivatives of neurotransmitters in biological fluids; (2) attempts to increase or decrease the production of these methylated derivatives by pharmacological manipulations; and (3) efforts to identify and characterize enzymes that might lead to the production of methylated catecholamines or indoleamines and could thus form endogenous psychotogens [7].

The original hypothesis of an endogenous psychotogen suggested that DMPEA might play this role in schizophrenia. In 1962, a compound that behaved like DMPEA was reported in the urine of 15 of 19 schizophrenics, but not in 14 controls [8]. DMPEA became known as the "pink spot" because of its color in stained chromatograms. This original report has since been disputed. Today, it is still not certain whether DMPEA plays a role in schizophrenia or even whether it is frequently found in the urine of patients with this diagnosis [9]. DMPEA is probably not a hallucinogen, despite its structural similarity to mescaline [10]. The search for methylated derivatives of indoleamines has also met with mixed results. Bufotenine and DMT have been demonstrated in the urine of both schizophrenics and normal controls [9]. In addition, a possible O-methylated indoleamine derivative, 5-methoxytryptamine, has been reported in the CSF of some psychotic patients [11]. In these studies, it might be fruitful to investigate the excretion pattern of methylated neurotransmitters in individual schizophrenic patients over time, as their disease improves or worsens.

Another method for evaluating the transmethylation hypothesis has been an attempt to alter schizophrenic sysmptoms by administration of an amino acid that could act as precursor for an endogenous psychotogen. In 1961, Kety and associates reported that schizophrenic patients receiving the monoamine oxidase (MAO) inhibitor iproniazid had an increase in schizophrenic symptoms when methionine, a methyl donor, was also given [12]. There have since been at least 15 other studies on the effects of methionine loading in schizophrenia [9]. Despite a wide variety of patient populations, drug regimens, and experimental designs, all studies report an increase in psychotic symptoms in patients given methionine, although the question has been raised whether this worsening is a true increase in schizophrenic symptoms or is the result of a superimposed toxic delirium. Even if schizophrenia is truly exacerbated by the combined actions of methionine and an MAO inhibitor, it is not clear that increased methylation is the cause of this worsening. Methionine ingestion increases the concentration of the methyl donor S-adenosylmethionine (SAM) in rat brain and liver, but not in rat or human blood [10]. Thus, studies with methionine have produced some interesting results, but they neither confirm nor disprove the transmethylation hypothesis of schizophrenia.

Since the methyl donor methionine may worsen schizophrenia, would a decrease in methylation cause improvement? The use of nicotinamide in schizophrenia was based in part on its ability to serve as an acceptor of methyl groups. Despite the continued use of this treatment by some physicians, often as part of megavitamin therapy, careful studies have not found significant improvement in schizophrenia after nicotinamide administration [13]. It has also been reported that a low methionine diet failed to cause significant improvement in schizophrenia [10].

Another strategy for investigating the transmethylation hypothesis is to search for enzymes capable of methylating neurotransmitters. In 1961, Axelrod [14] reported an enzyme capable of transferring a methyl group from SAM to several indoleamine substrates. This SAM enzyme, which was originally isolated from rabbit lung, has also been reported in chicken brain and human lung, blood, and brain. However, to date, no one has shown that schizophrenic patients have greater activity of this enzyme than do normal controls in either the blood or the brain [10].

An enzymatic system has been reported that appeared to use 5-methyltetrahydrofolic acid (5-MTHF), rather than SAM, as a methyl donor for indoleamine substrates. However, this reaction was soon shown to involve a one-carbon-unit transfer from 5-MTHF to the indoleamine substrate, followed by an intramolecular cyclization to form a β-carboline compound (called a tryptoline), and not a methylated indoleamine. Although tryptolines may be formed physiologically, their role remains to be defined [15].

In summary, almost 30 years after the suggestion that schizophrenia may be caused by abnormal methylation, the hypothesis remains neither confirmed nor disproved. As Kety pointed out more than ten years ago, the transmethylation hypothesis transcends consideration of any individual substance [16]. Candidates for the elusive endogenous psychotogen are numerous. Even if their concentrations are shown to be similar in schizophrenics and controls, it is always possible that schizophrenics metabolize the compounds differently, or have receptors that are more sensitive to their actions. Similar considerations apply to methylating enzymes. The SAM enzyme, currently the only enzyme known to *N*-methylate indoleamines, may be regulated or controlled differently in schizophrenics than in controls. Finally, the failure of nictotinamide to improve schizophrenic symptoms does not negate the strategy of testing other pharmacological agents that might alter the formation or metabolism of methylated amines.

THE DOPAMINE HYPOTHESIS OF SCHIZOPHRENIA

Two complementary types of pharmacological data led to the hypothesis that schizophrenic symptoms reflect altered brain dopamine (DA) activity: (1) neuroleptics (used to treat psychoses) that improve schizophrenic symptoms can also be shown to decrease central DA transmission; and (2) drugs that enhance central DA activity can produce psychosislike symptoms in nonpsychotic subjects and worsen symptoms in schizophrenic patients. *α*-Methyl-*p*-tyrosine (AMPT), which reduces DA synthesis, may enhance the activity of neuroleptic antipsychotics. This pharmacological evidence suggesting that DA may be involved in schizophrenia has stimulated the search for direct evidence of dopaminergic hyperactivity in schizophrenic patients.

Neuroleptic Agents and Dopaminergic Transmission

Dopamine is the neurotransmitter in at least three neuronal pathways in the brain: the nigrostriatal, the mesolimbic-mesocortical, and the tuberoinfundibular pathways (Table 38-1). The nigrostriatal pathway (see also Fig. 36-1) has cell bodies in the substantia nigra with axons in the caudateputamen (striatum); the mesolimbic-mesocortical pathway has cell bodies in the substantia nigra and in an area medial to it and has terminals in limbic system and certain cortical regions; the tuberoinfundibular pathway originates in the arcuate nucleus, with terminals in the median eminence (Table 38-1) [17].

Neuroleptic medications are thought to inhibit DA transmission in each of these major DA path-

ways by blocking DA postsynaptic receptors. Nigrostriatal inhibition results in extrapyramidal reactions, including parkinsonian symptoms; tuberoinfundibular inhibition causes prolactin release, while the antipsychotic activity of neuroleptics is thought to result from inhibition of the mesolimbic-mesocortical DA pathway (Table 38-1). There are at least five types of neuropharmacological evidence that suggest that neuroleptics inhibit brain DA transmission:

1. *Neuroleptics and extrapyramidal reactions.* All neuroleptics, except clozapine, can cause extrapyramidal side effects that can be similar to the symptoms of Parkinson's disease. Idiopathic Parkinson's disease is caused by the degeneration of the nigrostriatal DA pathway, leading to a predominance of cholinergic over dopaminergic activity in this area of the brain [18]. The similarity of some neuroleptic-induced extrapyramidal symptoms to Parkinson's disease suggests that neuroleptics inhibit nigrostriatal DA activity. Anticholinergic drugs improve the extrapyramidal symptoms in both situations, so this is further evidence for a common neurochemical basis of these movement disorders. Clozapine may be free of extrapyramidal symptoms because of its potent anticholinergic activity.

Use of the extrapyramidal side effects of neuroleptics as evidence that these drugs inhibit DA neurotransmission can be misleading, because neuroleptics without extrapyramidal side effects might be erroneously excluded by animal-screening procedures.

2. *Neuroleptics and dopamine turnover.* The ability of neuroleptics to increase DA turnover in CNS, first reported by Carlsson and Lindqvist in 1963 [19], was suggested to result from a blockade of DA receptors. The increased turnover might be caused by a feedback mechanism that attempts to overcome the receptor blockade by increasing DA synthesis [19].

Evidence for increased DA turnover during administration of neuroleptics can almost always be found in the spinal fluid of subjects. Clozapine not only fails to cause extrapyramidal reactions,

Table 38-1. Dopamine Tracts in Psychiatric Disorders

Tract	Hypothesized Physiological Role	Pharmacological Involvement	Anatomical Location
Mesolimbic-mesocortical	Emotional tone Schizophrenia	Antipsychotic action of neuroleptics Amphetamine and L-dopa psychoses	Substantia nigra and area medial to substantia nigra (A9, A10) to limbic nuclei and cortical regions
Nigrostriatal	Muscle and movement coordination Parkinson's disease	Animal stereotypy Extrapyramidal symptoms of anti-psychotics Tardive dyskinesia	Substantia nigra (A9) to caudate-putamen (striatum)
Tuberoinfundibular	Modulation of endocrine functions	Antipsychotic drug action on prolactin	Arcuate nucleus to median eminence

but also fails to produce evidence of increased DA turnover in human spinal fluid [20].

3. *Neuroleptics and DA effects on electrical activity.* The electrical response of nigrostriatal neurons to the application of DA is blocked by neuroleptics. When neuroleptics are administered systematically, they cause an increase in the electrical firing rate of dopaminergic neurons in the substantia nigra [21]. This finding parallels the neuroleptic-induced increase in DA turnover.

Amphetamine administration suppresses DA-mediated electrical activity, probably by reversal of the mechanism by which neuroleptics increase neuronal DA turnover. By causing increased DA receptor stimulation, amphetamines may activate a feedback mechanism leading to decreased DA turnover and electrical activity. Neuroleptics reverse amphetamine-induced suppression of dopaminergic neurons; related drugs without antipsychotic activity do not [21]. Clozapine is more effective in reversing amphetamine suppression in mesolimbic DA neurons than in nigrostriatal DA neurons.

4. *Neuroleptics and animal stereotypy.* Amphetamine, apomorphine, and related medications cause stereotyped behaviors in animals. This stereotypy is presumably the result of brain DA activity and is reportedly abolished by destruction of the striatum. Thus, animal stereotypy probably results

from the effect of amphetamine and apomorphine on the nigrostriatal DA neurons [22].

5. *Neuroleptics and dopamine receptors.* The potency of several phenothiazine neuroleptics in inhibiting DA-sensitive adenylate cyclase and in competing with [^{3}H]DA for receptor binding can be correlated with their clinical potency [23–25]. Butyrophenones, however, are not as potent in inhibiting DA-sensitive adenylate cyclase as would be predicted from their clinical potency. This discrepancy might arise because of artifacts of the in vitro enzyme preparations or because butyrophenones act on a class of DA receptors not linked to adenylate cyclase. On the other hand, the clinical potencies of both phenothiazines and butyrophenones can be correlated with their competition for [^{3}H]spiroperidol-binding sites. In addition, there is good correlation, except for clozapine, between the antipsychotic potencies of the various classes of neuroleptics and their stimulation of prolactin release, a useful index of DA antagonists [26, 27]. These topics are discussed with respect to classes of dopamine receptors in Chap. 10 and with respect to adenylate cyclase in Chap. 14.

At the least, one may conclude, first, that there is ample evidence that most neuroleptics act by inhibiting dopaminergic neurotransmission in the brain, probably by blocking DA receptors. Second, one effective neuroleptic, clozapine, has a divergent pharmacological profile and may be unique in having antipsychotic activity that is not entirely attributable to DA inhibition.

Dopaminergic Agents and Schizophrenia

The DA hypothesis of schizophrenia is further supported by studies with drugs that, like the neuroleptics, alter central dopaminergic activity. These drugs include α-methyl-p-tyrosine (AMPT), L-dopa, and amphetamine (see Fig. 37-5). AMPT, which inhibits DA synthesis, has been reported to potentiate the antipsychotic action of phenothiazine neuroleptics (see Fig. 37-1) [28]. In contrast, L-dopa, the immediate precursor of DA, causes psychosis in some patients with Parkinson's disease and increases symptomatology in schizophrenic patients [29]. Such studies may be complicated by the effects of these drugs on other central or peripheral systems.

The behavioral effects of amphetamine or amphetaminelike substances, such as methylphenidate, tend to support the role of DA in producing schizophrenic symptoms. The chemical structure of amphetamine is closely related to DA (see Fig. 37-5). Chronic amphetamine users frequently develop a psychosis that is different from other toxic psychoses: they are usually oriented and have a good memory of the psychotic episode. In many patients, the syndrome is indistinguishable from acute paranoid schizophrenia. Unlike chronic schizophrenics, however, patients with amphetamine psychosis rarely have formal thought disorder or blunted affect [30]. Amphetamines can, however, exacerbate schizophrenic symptoms in some patients with chronic schizophrenia [30].

Although the neurochemical basis of amphetamine psychosis is not known, the actions of amphetamine on catecholamines may be important. Amphetamines increase catecholaminergic activity by increasing catecholamine release and by inhibiting catecholamine reuptake. Whether the major action is on DA or norepinephrine (NE) is less clear. Most investigators believe that the actions of amphetamine that lead to psychotic symptoms are based on its actions on dopaminergic neurons [30].

Physiological Investigations in Schizophrenic Patients

Neuroleptics and amphetamine probably have opposite effects on schizophrenic symptoms because of their opposing actions on dopaminergic symptoms. However, evidence that unmedicated schizophrenic patients have increased DA activity has not been easy to obtain. Neuroleptics inhibit DA and raise prolactin concentrations, but unmediated schizophrenic patients have normal serum prolactin concentrations [10]. Concentrations of the DA metabolite homovanillic acid (HVA) in the spinal fluid of schizophrenic patients (see Fig. 36-4) are within normal limits [31].

Postmortem studies of brains from schizophrenic patients have included examination of the enzymes that aid in the synthesis and breakdown of the catecholamines but have not generally found consistent differences between pathological and normal brains [32].

One group of investigators reports a deficiency in brain dopamine β-hydroxylase (DBH) which they relate to a hypothetical defect in the NE "reward system" in schizophrenics [33]. It is suggested that DBH deficiency leads to DA excess, followed by oxidation of DA to 6-hydroxydopamine, which it is hypothesized, destroys the NE neurons of the system involved in positive reinforcement, or reward, and thus gives rise to schizophrenic symptoms. Investigators have also been studying the concentrations of catecholamines in the nucleus accumbens of brains of schizophrenic patients postmortem. Some find increased NE; others report increased DA levels [34]. A reduction in platelet MAO activity in people with chronic schizophrenia has been reported [35], although there are no significant differences between the MAO activity in their brains compared with that of controls [31].

There are, then, at least three hypotheses that relate DA to psychoses. The hypothesis that neuroleptic antipsychotic activity is based on DA receptor blockade would seem the most compelling. The evidence that amphetamine psychosis is due to the drug's action on DA is less firm but is suggestive. The DA hypothesis of schizophrenia, which proposes that schizophrenic symptoms arise from hyperactive dopaminergic neurons, finds relatively little support by way of direct evidence of altered DA activity or metabolism in schizophrenic patients.

ALTERNATE BIOCHEMICAL HYPOTHESES OF SCHIZOPHRENIA

Phenylethylamine
A possible role for phenylethylamine (PEA) in normal or pathological states is not known. PEA is formed by the decarboxylation of phenylalanine. The proposal that PEA might be involved in schizophrenia [36, 37] is based, in part, on the structural and pharmacological similarities of PEA and amphetamine. Both increase spontaneous motor activity in rats, and both produce stereotypical behavior. Neuroleptics, in doses roughly parallel to their clinical potency, reportedly modify the animal-behavioral actions of PEA and an MAO inhibitor [36]. The MAO inhibitor was used because, unlike amphetamine, PEA is an excellent substrate for MAO. PEA, then, might act as an endogenous amphetaminelike compound to produce a psychosis. Phenylketonuric patients generate increased amounts of PEA and also have autistic behavior. Heterozygotes for phenylketonuria have been evaluated for an increased risk of developing schizophrenia, but evidence is not conclusive [36, 37].

Gamma-Aminobutyric Acid
One hypothesis proposes that the inhibitory influence of GABAergic neurons on dopaminergic pathways in schizophrenic patients is decreased [38]. Because of this decrease, neuronal activities occur that should have been suppressed, and this results in inappropriate behavior. Neuroleptics, according to this hypothesis, do not work by correcting the primary defect, but rather by blocking the secondary increase in dopaminergic activity. GABA concentrations have been reported to be significantly lower in two areas in the autopsied brains of schizophrenic patients. Thus, drugs that alter GABAergic activity may offer a new approach to the treatment of schizophrenia.

Acetylcholine and Neurotransmitter Imbalance
Parkinson's disease is an example of a disorder the symptoms of which are due to a disturbed balance between activity in two neurotransmitter systems, in this case the dopaminergic and cholinergic systems (see Chap. 36). Evidence for a role of the brain's cholinergic systems in schizophrenia comes from suggestive reports that cholinomimetic agents improve schizophrenic symptoms and that anticholinergics may reduce the antipsychotic activity of neuroleptics. Arecoline, a centrally acting cholinomimetic, is reported to produce a brief improvement in schizophrenia [39]. Oral physostigmine (which increases central cholinergic activity) given with neuroleptics to chronic schizophrenics unresponsive to neuroleptics alone [40], reportedly produced a dramatic reduction in symptoms; the reduction was transient, with a rapid return to a baseline pathology.

Anticholinergics have been reported to decrease the efficiency of neuroleptics, but on the other hand, neuroleptics with anticholinergic activity, such as thioridazine, appear to be effective antipsychotic agents. Intravenous physostigmine can prevent the exacerbation of schizophrenic symptoms caused by IV infusion of methylphenidate [41]. This may be the most compelling evidence for the importance of a DA-acetylcholine balance in psychotic behavior.

Endorphins
A massive research effort currently underway attempts to define the role of endorphins in both normal and abnormal physiology [42, 43] (see also Chap. 13). Part of this research focuses on their possible role in schizophrenia. Interestingly, there is controversial evidence for both an excess and a deficiency of endorphin activity in schizophrenia [43, 44]. Rats given β-endorphin exhibit catatoniclike behavior that resembles the postural abnormalities of some schizophrenic patients [45]. In addition, there are reports that some endorphins are elevated in unmedicated schizophrenic patients, and that these increased concentrations return toward normal when the patients are medicated [46]. In contrast, elevated concentrations of β-

endorphin have also been described in schizophrenic patients. Double-blind studies have reportedly shown an improvement in schizophrenic hallucinations or bizarre delusions following IV naloxone administration, although not all investigators have been able to confirm this finding [43, 44]. Finally, an improvement in schizophrenic symptoms has been reported after hemodialysis, a procedure usually performed for patients with kidney failure [43, 44]. The improvement after hemodialysis is proposed to be secondary to the removal of excess leucine-5-β-endorphin [47], but demonstration of elevated concentrations of leucine-5-β-endorphin in either the dialysate or the plasma of schizophrenic patients has not been confirmed [48]. For consideration of possible effects of human dialysis on brain metabolism, see Chap. 35.

Evidence for an endorphin deficiency in schizophrenia is equally controversial [43]. The stiffness produced in rats by β-endorphin has been described as similar to that produced by neuroleptics [49]. Several peptides, including an analog of methionine-enkephalin, FK 33-824 [50], the endorphinlike peptide des-tyrosine-γ-endorphin [51], as well as β-endorphin itself [52], have been reported to have beneficial effects in schizophrenic patients.

Affective Disorders: Depression and Mania

Everyone feels sadness, grief, disappointment, loneliness, or discouragement during the difficult times of life. For the depressed patient, however, such a change in mood is only one of many symptoms. In addition to changes in mood, depressed patients have altered thinking patterns, motor activity, and behavior. They also have somatic or physical symptoms, and commonly have suicidal ideas. Changes in thinking lead to pessimism and low self-esteem. The belief of worthlessness combines with pessimism to rob depressed patients of motivation, making it difficult for them to maintain jobs or interpersonal relationships. Depressed patients often feel guilty about being a burden or not meeting others' expectations. Some severely depressed patients develop psychosis, distorting or

misperceiving reality; they sometimes develop unusual beliefs or behaviors. Many are fearful or anxious. Some are physically hyperactive and agitated; others move slowly, feel weak, tired, and helpless, and have slow or labored thoughts and speech. Both agitated and slowed patients can have trouble concentrating and accomplishing even simple tasks. Physical symptoms are often an important part of the depression syndrome. Weight loss, disturbed sleep, constipation, dry mouth, dizziness, tight feelings in the chest, and aches and pains are all reported by depressed patients. The pattern of physical symptoms is highly varied. Hopelessness, guilt, low self-esteem, and delusional beliefs can all lead to suicidal thinking and behavior.

Most depressed patients have no history of other psychiatric disorders. However, about one-fifth have episodes of both depression and mania, a disorder called bipolar illness. *Unipolar* depressed patients are those who suffer recurrent depressive episodes without episodes of mania. *Mania* is a severe mental disorder that includes changes in mood, thought, motor activity, and behavior. The mood of a manic patient is elated, carefree, overconfident, and sometimes euphoric. Manic patients feel attractive, desirable, clever, alert, and efficient. However, many manic patients become easily irritated if frustrated. The thinking of manic patients is rapid and complex, with one thought leading to another in what is called "flight of ideas." Ideas of special abilities, unique knowledge, or feelings of potency occur in severe mania. Manics have accelerated motor activity, seem to have boundless energy, and often sleep and eat very little. However, they are so restless they frequently move from project to project, unable to complete any. In its most severe form, mania can present with psychosis, usually consisting of delusional beliefs of self-omnipotence [2].

How common are the affective disorders, depression and mania? The incidence of bipolar illness is about 300 per 100,000 per year. Thus, about 600,000 bipolar patients are treated each year in the United States alone. The incidence of unipolar depression is certainly much larger, but epidemiological studies have been hindered by the lack of widely accepted diagnostic criteria. About 1.5 million people are being treated for depression today. Perhaps 3 or even 5 times that number, or 4.5 to 7.5 million individuals, suffer from depression but are not receiving treatment. A National Institute of Mental Health study and a British study both conclude that as many as 15 percent of the population will have at least one depressive episode in their lifetimes [53]. There are at least 26,000 reported deaths by suicide each year, making it the tenth leading cause of death [53].

Research in the affective disorders of mania and depression has been motivated by two major concepts. The first, the *monoamine hypothesis,* proposes that the affective disorders are due to functional changes in the central monoamine neurotransmitters. The second derives from the finding that subgroups of patients with affective disorders may have abnormalities in specific *neuroendocrine systems* [54–56].

THE MONOAMINE HYPOTHESIS OF DEPRESSION AND MANIA

The *biogenic* or *monoamine hypothesis* states that depression is associated with a functional deficit of monoamines at critical synapses, whereas mania is associated with a functional excess of these amines [55, 56]. This hypothesis is based on studies on the mechanism of action of reserpine, of monoamine oxidase (MAO) inhibitors, of tricyclic antidepressants, and of lithium carbonate. Reserpine is an alkaloid of the plant *Rauwolfia serpentina,* which for many centuries was used as a treatment for mental illness in India. It was isolated in the early 1950s and has been used to treat a number of conditions, including schizophrenia and hypertension. After an initial period of stimulation, reserpine produces a syndrome in animals that includes sedation and motor retardation. This syndrome has been proposed as a model for depression, and receives support from the observation that some patients treated for hypertension with this drug may develop a reserpine syndrome similar to endogenous depression. Reserpine is now known to deplete 5-HT, NE, and DA from the CNS [54–56].

The MAO inhibitor iproniazid was synthesized in the early 1950s for the chemotherapy of tuberculosis. The drug was soon reported to produce euphoria and overactive behavior [57, 58], and to increase brain concentrations of NE and 5-HT by inhibiting the enzyme MAO.

The tricyclic antidepressants are thought to counteract depression by potentiating monoamine neurotransmitters at brain receptors through prevention of the reuptake of monoamine neurotransmitters, decreasing monoamine inactivation, and in-theory, increasing their concentration at postsynaptic receptors. Numerous studies have shown that tricyclic antidepressants decrease the uptake by rat brain of intraventricularly administered tritiated NE in vivo [59]. 5-HT reuptake is also blocked by the action of tricyclic antidepressants [60]. The rate of onset of the clinical response is, however, slower than can be explained by these pharmacological effects, as is discussed below.

In controlled clinical trials, lithium salts have been shown to be effective treatments for acute manic episodes. The prophylactic properties of lithium-salt–maintenance treatment against recurrent manic episodes have also been established. The mechanism of action of lithium in mania has not been determined. However, lithium does have effects on monoamine neurotransmitters, including inhibition of the electrically stimulated release of 5-HT and NE from rat-brain slices [61]. These studies, taken together, suggest that tricyclic antidepressants and lithium have opposite effects on monoamine metabolism. In this scheme, lithium would reduce the quantity of monoamine neurotransmitters available at the postsynaptic receptor.

Thus, the monoamine hypothesis of affective disorders finds support in the action of four drugs. Reserpine depletes brain monoamines and may cause depression in some individuals. MAO inhibitors and tricyclic antidepressants increase the quantity of monoamines at the postsynaptic receptor by two different mechanisms, and drugs from both chemical classes are useful treatments for depression. In addition, lithium salts, useful in the treatment of mania, decrease the quantity of monoamines at the postsynaptic receptor.

Several problems with the pharmacological evidence support the monoamine hypothesis. A reevaluation of the incidence of reserpine-induced depression finds it to be only about 6 percent, the approximate percentage of patients with histories of previous depressive episodes. Reserpine may thus precipitate depression only in those individuals who are susceptible to the syndrome. The reserpine animal model of depression is also imperfect. Reserpine-induced motor retardation in animals may be caused by DA depletion and can, in fact, be reversed by administration of L-dopa. Yet L-dopa is not an effective antidepressant in human patients [54].

Furthermore, the suggested mechanism of action of tricyclic antidepressants is hard to reconcile with the pharmacological activity of several other psychoactive compounds. Cocaine, which is not chemically related to the tricyclics, and which does not have significant antidepressant activity, is a potent inhibitor of monoamine reuptake at the synapses [62]. In contrast, iprindole, structurally related to other tricyclic antidepressants, does not inhibit the in vivo reuptake of NE [63]; yet, iprindole is reported to be an effective antidepressant. Wellbatrum, mianserin, and zometapine are all reported to be antidepressants, yet these three drugs have no known effects on DA, NE, or 5-HT.

The delay in the onset of the antidepressant effect of tricyclics is also a problem for the hypothesis that they act by blocking monoamine reuptake. It takes from 1 to 3 weeks for the antidepressant effects of tricyclics to become apparent, but the inhibition of monoamine reuptake occurs after acute administration. The delay in the onset of tricyclic antidepressant action has led to several "receptor-sensitivity" hypotheses of affective disorders. It has been suggested, for example, that depressed patients may have supersensitive catecholamine receptors in limbic or other brain structures and that an excess, rather than a deficit, in monoamine activity occurs [64]—the reverse of

the original monoamine hypothesis. If so, successful treatment would require desensitization, and effective drugs presumably would initiate the receptor's homeostatic response over time to increased monoamine concentrations.

Support for this hypothesis comes from two findings. First, a NE-sensitive adenylate cyclase from limbic forebrain is reported to be inhibited by tricyclic antidepressants, including iprindole, as well as by MAO inhibitor pargyline after a delay of 3 weeks [64]. This decrease in adenylate-cyclase activity may reflect the decrease in activity of NE receptors that occurs in response to increased receptor exposure to NE. The second finding is that NE β-receptors labeled by radioactive isoproterenol decrease in density after a 6-week treatment with the tricyclic antidepressant desipramine [64]. Another group of investigators [65] suggests that a subgroup of patients may have hypersensitive indoleamine receptors, using the same reasoning to explain the delay in onset of tricyclic antidepressants.

The molecular mechanisms of action of lithium and tricyclic antidepressants seem opposite, and they are generally used to treat clinical conditions that also seem opposite. This picture is complicated, however, by the reports that lithium salts are useful in the treatment and prevention of depressive episodes, particularly in patients with a history of both mania and depression. Lithium is reported to alter 5-HT synthesis and tryptophan uptake in such a way as to dampen the acute and chronic effects of stimulant drugs such as amphetamine [66], a finding that could explain the dual clinical action of lithium.

Reserpine, MAO inhibitors, tricyclic antidepressants, and lithium each affects both catecholamines and indoleamines. Thus, one or any of these monoamines may play the prominent role in affective disorders. The tricyclic antidepressants differ in their abilities to alter the metabolism of indoleamines and catecholamines. Tertiary amine tricyclics, such as amitriptyline (see Fig. 37-4), preferentially inhibit 5-HT reuptake; secondary amines, such as desipramine, seem to be more effective inhibitors of catecholamine reuptake [67]. In addition, two of the tertiary amine tricyclics, amitriptyline and imipramine, are metabolized to active secondary amine tricyclics, nortriptyline and desipramine, respectively. This lack of specificity in the actions of antidepressants clouds interpretation of the molecular basis for their pharmacological activity.

The pharmacological evidence supporting the monoamine hypothesis of affective disorders is not definitive. Even if current psychotherapeutic agents act through monoaminergic mechanisms, the etiology of depression may be found in an entirely different physiological system. These problems have led to two additional research strategies. One strategy attempts to manipulate monoamine neurotransmitter activity pharmacologically in patients with affective disorders; the second searches for evidence of their altered monoamine neurotransmitter metabolism.

The "precursor-loading" strategy is an attempt to correct the hypothesized deficit of brain monoamines in depressed patients by providing metabolic precursors of 5-HT, NE, and DA; the monoamines do not cross the blood-brain barrier. L-Tryptophan and 5-hydroxytryptophan have been used in attempts to increase brain 5-HT, and L-dopa has been used to increase brain DA and NE. The use of these neurotransmitter precursors in depressed patients has been largely unsuccessful, either in improving depression or in definitively testing the monoamine hypothesis [54].

Additional attempts to alter monoamine concentrations in patients with mania and depression include the use of enzyme inhibitors and presumed antagonists and agonists of amine receptors. AMPT is a potent competitive inhibitor of tyrosine hydroxylase, the rate-limiting enzyme in DA and NE synthesis. AMPT reduces catecholamine concentrations in the CNS and decreases urinary excretion of the catecholamine metabolite 3-methoxy-4-hydroxymandelic acid (vanillylmandelic acid, or VMA). Some patients with hypertension who receive AMPT may have become depressed, and transient hypomanic reactions have been described when AMPT is discontinued. In a clinical study, some manic patients showed improvement with AMPT [68], whereas others seemed to get worse.

p-Chlorophenylalanine (PCPA) is an inhibitor of tryptophan hydroxylase, the enzyme involved in the rate-limiting step in 5-HT synthesis (see Fig. 11-2). PCPA has been shown to decrease 5-HT synthesis in humans but did not decrease symptoms in manic patients [69].

Methysergide and cinanserin, both 5-HT antagonists, are reported to have antimanic activity, but these findings await confirmation [54].

The DA agonist peribedil and the NE agonist clonidine have both been used in depression and have produced mixed results [70].

Investigations of monoamine transmitter metabolism include measurements of monoamines and their metabolites in body fluids and, when possible, in brain tissue. Enzymes involved in the synthesis and degradation of monoamines have also been measured in patients with affective disorders.

Measurement of Monoamines and Their Metabolites in Biological Fluids

Measurement of the catecholamine precursor tyrosine, the catecholamines DA and NE, and their metabolites homovanillic acid (HVA), VMA, 3-methoxy-4-hydroxyphenylglycol (MHPG) in the blood, urine, and spinal fluid of depressed patients have produced inconsistent results. Similar inconsistencies are found in studies of the indoleamine precursor tryptophan and of the indoleamine metabolite 5-hydroxyindoleacetic acid (5-HIAA). The three most consistent findings are that some depressed patients have decreased concentrations of HVA in spinal fluid after the efflux of this acid dopamine metabolite is blocked; that some depressed patients have lower spinal-fluid concentrations of the 5-HT metabolite 5-HIAA; and that there is a bimodal distribution of the urinary excretion of the NE metabolite MHPG [54].

Urinary MHPG could arise from the peripheral sympathetic nervous system or from the brain. The proportion of urinary MHPG that derives from the CNS is debated. One group of investigators simultaneously injected [^{14}C]NE peripherally, and [^{3}H]NE centrally, into dogs and collected urine for 12 hr. They calculated that 25 to 30 percent of the urinary MHPG came from the brain in the dog, whereas only about 1 percent of the urinary VMA reflected central metabolism [71]. A study in primates given 6-hydroxydopamine, which destroys CNS NE neurons, suggests that at least half of the urinary MHPG reflects brain norepinephrine in these animals [71]. The most novel approach to the origin of urinary MHPG is the measurement of arteriovenous differences in the jugular veins of patients compared to the radial artery. This study suggests that about 60 percent of urinary MHPG in humans comes from the brain [72]. Several studies report decreased urinary excretion of MHPG in depressed patients and increased excretion during manic episodes; other studies do not. Stress and increased motor activity have both been shown to increase MHPG excretion, adding difficulty to the interpretation of these data [54, 71].

Differential responses to antidepressant medications in depressed patients have been correlated with their excretion of urinary MHPG. Depressed patients with low MHPG excretion were reported to respond better to imipramine than did those whose initial MHPG excretion was high [71]. MHPG excretion was reported to be higher in depressed patients who responded to amitriptyline than in those who did not [73]. Depressed patients who respond to imipramine are reported to have lower urinary MHPG excretion than do patients who respond to amitriptyline [74]. To explain these results, one could propose that imipramine is rapidly metabolized to desipramine, yielding more NE reuptake-blocking activity [67]; the tertiary amine amitriptyline is more slowly metabolized; this results in prolonged 5-HT reuptake-blocking activity [71].

Studies of Enzymes Involved in Monoamine Metabolism

The enzyme activities that have been assessed in patients include MAO, DBH, and COMT. Plasma and platelet MAO activities, serum and plasma DBH activities, as well as erythrocyte COMT activities have all been studied in patients with unipolar and bipolar affective disorders. At present, no consistent pattern has emerged [54].

In summary, the data from studies attempting to test the monoamine hypothesis are fragmentary and often contradictory. Some of the inconsistencies must be caused by the multiple actions and different duration of action of drugs. Difficulties in assay reproducibility and sensitivity are compounded by the fact that peripheral measures may poorly reflect CNS activity. A more important problem may be differences among the patients themselves. Nevertheless, affective illness probably can be divided into subtypes based on metabolic measures of monoamine activity. Tests that eventually may prove useful for this purpose are measurement of the concentration of spinal fluid 5-HIAA and HVA, and of the urinary excretion of MHPG, particularly in response to antidepressants.

NEUROENDOCRINE DISTURBANCES IN DEPRESSION

Some patients with depressive illness also have neuroendocrine abnormalities. (Regulatory mechanisms in the brain-pituitary-adrenal axis are discussed in Chaps. 14 and 39.) These abnormalities include hyperactivity of the pituitary-adrenal system, a blunted response of pituitary thyrotropin (thyroid-stimulating hormone, TSH) to stimulation by thyrotropin-releasing hormone (TRH), a blunted growth-hormone (GH) response to stimulation by amphetamine, and hypoglycemia. Elevated plasma cortisol levels, increased cortisol metabolite excretion, increased excretion of urinary free cortisol, and elevated spinal-fluid cortisol have all been reported in depressed patients [75]. This hyperactivity of the pituitary-adrenal system has been further characterized in studies that sample serum cortisol at frequent intervals throughout the day. In these studies, some depressed patients fail to show the usual diurnal pattern of an early sleep-time decrease in cortisol output [75, 76]. After clinical recovery, the pattern returns toward normal. The increase in pituitary-adrenal activity found in some depressed patients has also been reported as resistant to feedback suppression by dexamethasone. Dexamethasone is a potent synthetic steroid that suppresses pituitary-adrenal activity in a standard test of the competence of the negative-feedback system for controlling cortisol levels [77]. This defect in the pituitary-adrenal system of depressed patients may be secondary to the hypothesized deficiencies in monoamine neurotransmitter activity, since both NE and 5-HT can regulate or modulate brain-pituitary-adrenal function.

The TSH response to TRH in depressed patients may be diminished or blunted [78]. Both large, acute elevations of corticosteroids and small, chronic elevations are known to decrease the TSH response to TRH, suggesting a possible interaction.

There is strong evidence that human growth hormone (HGH) secretion is mediated by brain neurotransmitters. Much of the evidence so far points to regulation by NE or by DA, although 5-HT may also play a role. HGH release can be stimulated by L-dopa, by amphetamine, or by hypoglycemia. Insulin-induced [79, 80] and amphetamine-induced HGH stimulation is reduced in some depressed patients. Because of the suggestion that HGH response is controlled by catecholamines, the question arises whether this proposed subgroup of depressed patients with blunted HGH response overlaps with patients who demonstrate abnormalities in catecholamine metabolism.

We may, then, conclude that the development of effective drug treatments for psychiatric disorders has helped to establish connections between psychiatry and the biological sciences and should eventually help elucidate the pathophysiology of schizophrenia and the affective disorders [81].

References

1. Goodwin, F. K., Cowdry, R. W., and Webster, M. H. Predictors of Drug Response in the Affective Disorders: Toward an Integrated Approach. In M. A. Lipton, A. DiMascio, and K. F. Killam (eds.), *Psychopharmacology: A Generation of Progress.* New York: Raven, 1978. Pp. 1277–1288.

2. Berger, P. A. Medical treatment of mental illness. *Science* 200:974–981, 1978.

3. Sack, R. L. Schizophrenia and Manic-Depressive Illness. In A. Freeman, R. Sack, and P. A. Berger (eds.), *Psychiatry for the Primary Care Physician.* Baltimore: Williams & Wilkins, 1979. Pp. 181–197.

4. Lehmann, H. E. Schizophrenia: Clinical Features. In A. Freedman, H. I. Kaplan, and B. J. Sadock (eds.), *Comprehensive Textbook of Psychiatry II.* Baltimore: Williams & Wilkins, 1975. Vol. 1, pp. 890–923.

5. Babigian, H. M. Schizophrenia: Epidemiology. In A. Freedman, H. I. Kaplan, and B. J. Sadock (eds.), *Comprehensive Textbook of Psychiatry II.* Baltimore: Williams & Wilkins, 1975. Vol. 1, pp. 860–866.

6. Osmond, H., and Smythies, J. Schizophrenia: A new approach. *J. Ment. Sci.* 98:309–315, 1952.

7. Elliott, G. R., and Barchas, J. D. The Transmethylation Hypothesis of Schizophrenia: Current Status and Future Prospects. In E. Usdin, R. T. Borchardt, and C. R. Creveling (eds.), *Transmethylation.* New York: Elsevier North-Holland, 1979. Pp. 307–318.

8. Friedhoff, A. J., and Van Winkle, E. The characteristics of an amine found in the urine of schizophrenic patients. *J. Nerv. Ment. Dis.* 135:550–555, 1962.

9. Wyatt, R. J., Termini, B. A., and Davis, J. Biochemical and sleep studies of schizophrenia: A review of the literature—1960–1970. *Schizophr. Bull.* 4:10–66, 1971.

10. Barchas, J. D., Elliott, G. R., and Berger, P. A. Biogenic Amine Hypotheses of Schizophrenia. In J. D. Barchas, P. A. Berger, R. D. Ciaranello, and G. R. Elliott (eds.), *Psychopharmacology: From Theory to Practice.* New York: Oxford University Press, 1977. Pp. 100–120.

11. Koslow, S. Bio-significance of *N*- and *O*-methylated Indoles to Psychiatric Disorders. In E. Usdin, D. A. Hamburg, and J. D. Barchas (eds.), *Neuroregulators and Psychiatric Disorders.* New York: Oxford University Press, 1977. Pp. 210–219.

12. Pollin, W., Cardon, P. V., and Kety, S. S. Effects of amino acid feeding in schizophrenic patients treated with iproniazid. *Science* 133:104–105, 1961.

13. Ban, T. A., and Lehman, H. E. Nicotinic acid in the treatment of schizophrenics. *Can. Psychiatr. Assoc. J.* 15:499–500, 1970.

14. Axelrod, J. Enzymatic formation of psychotomimetic metabolites from normally occurring metabolites. *Science* 134:343–344, 1961.

15. Barchas, J. D., Elliott, G. R., DoAmaral, J., Erdelyi, E., O'Connor, S., Bowden, M., Brodie, H. K. H., Berger, P. A., Renson, J., and Wyatt, R. J. Trypto-

lines: Formation from tryptamine and 5-MTHF by human platelets. *Arch. Gen. Psychiatry* 31:862–867, 1974.

16. Kety, S. S. Summary: The Hypothetical Relationships between Amines and Mental Illness: A Critical Synthesis. In H. E. Himwich, S. S. Kety, and J. R. Smythies (eds.), *Amines and Schizophrenia*. Oxford: Pergamon, 1967. Pp. 271–277.

17. Ungerstedt, U. Stereotaxic mapping of the monoamine pathways in the rat brain. *Acta Physiol. Scand. (Suppl.* 367) 88:1–48, 1971.

18. Hornykiewicz, O. Die topische Lokalisation and das Verhalten von Noradrenalin und Dopamin (3-Hydroxytyramin) in der Substantia Nigra des Normalin und Parkinsonkranken. *Menschen. Wein. Klin. Wschr.* 75:309–312, 1963.

19. Carlsson, A., and Lindqvist, E. Effect of chlorpromazine or haloperidol on the formation of 3-methoxytyramine and normetanephrine in mouse brain. *Acta Pharmacol. Toxicol. (Kovenhavn)* 20:140–144, 1963.

20. Bürki, H. R., Eichenberger, E., Sayers, A. C., and White, T. C. Clozapine and the dopamine hypothesis of schizophrenia: A critical appraisal. *Pharmakopsychiatr. Neuro-Psychopharmakol.* 8:115–121, 1975.

21. Bunney, B. S., and Aghajanian, G. K. Antipsychotic Drugs and Central Dopaminergic Neurons: A Model for Predicting Therapeutic Efficacy and Incidence of Extrapyramidal Side Effects. In A. Sudilovsky, S. Gershon, and B. Beer (eds.), *Predictability in Psychopharmacology: Preclinical and Clinical Correlations*. New York: Raven, 1975. Pp. 225–245.

22. Randrup, A., and Munkvad, J. Pharmacology and physiology of stereotyped behavior. *J. Psychiatr. Res.* 11:1–10, 1975.

23. Kebabian, J. W., Petzold, G. L., and Greengard, P. Dopamine sensitive adenylate cyclase in the caudate nucleus of brain and its similarity to the "dopamine receptor." *Proc. Natl. Acad. Sci. U.S.A.* 69:2145–2149, 1972.

24. Seeman, P., Chau-Wong, J., Tedesco, J., and Wong, K. Brain receptors for antipsychotic drugs and dopamine: Direct binding assays. *Proc. Natl. Acad. Sci. U.S.A.* 72:4376–4380, 1975.

25. Snyder, S. H. The dopamine hypothesis of schizophrenia: Focus on the dopamine receptor. *Am. J. Psychiatry* 133:197–202, 1976.

26. Sachar, E. J., Gruen, P. H., Altman, N., Langer, G., Halpern, F. S., and Liefer, J. Prolactin Responses to Neuroleptic Drugs: An Approach to the Study of Brain Dopamine Blockade in Humans. In E. Usdin, D. Hamburg, and J. Barchas (eds.), *Neuroregulators*

and Psychiatric Disorders. New York: Oxford University Press, 1977. Pp. 242–249.

27. Meltzer, H. Y., Daniels, S., and Fang, V. S. Clozapine increases rat serum prolactin levels. *Life Sci.* 17:339–342, 1975.

28. Carlsson, A. Antipsychotic drugs and catecholamine synapses. *J. Psychiatr. Res.* 11:57–64, 1975.

29. Goodwin, F. K., and Murphy, D. L. Biological Factors in the Affective Disorders and Schizophrenia. In M. Gordon (ed.), *Psychopharmacological Agents*. New York: Academic, 1974. Pp. 19–37.

30. Snyder, S. H. Amphetamine psychosis, a "model" schizophrenia mediated by catecholamines. *Am. J. Psychiatr.* 130:61–67, 1973.

31. Berger, P. A., Elliott, G. R., and Barchas, J. D. Neuroregulators and Schizophrenia. In M. A. Lipton, A. DiMascio, and K. F. Killam (eds.), *Psychopharmacology: A Generation of Progress*. New York: Raven, 1978. Pp. 1071–1095.

32. Barchas, J. D., Berger, P. A., Elliott, G. R., Erdelyi, E., and Wyatt, R. J. Studies of Enzymes Involved in Amine Metabolism in Schizophrenia. In N. Weiner and M. B. H. Youdim (eds.), *Biochemistry and Function of Monoamine Enzymes*. New York: Dekker, 1977. Pp. 868–904.

33. Wise, C. D., Baden, M. M., and Stein, L. Postmortem Measurement of Enzymes in Human Brain: Evidence of a Central Noradrenergic Deficit in Schizophrenia. In S. W. Matthysse and S. S. Kety (eds.), *Catecholamines and Schizophrenia*. Oxford: Pergamon, 1974. Pp. 185–198.

34. Kleinman, J. E., Bridge, P., Karoum, F., Gillan, J. C., and Wyatt, R. J. Postmortem Studies in Chronic Schizophrenia. Presented at the Veterans Administration Conference on Chronic Schizophrenia. Harpers Ferry, West Virginia: Raven, April, 1981, in press.

35. Murphy, D. L., Belmaker, R., and Wyatt, R. J. Monoamine oxidase in schizophrenia and other behavior disorders. *J. Psychiatr. Res.* 11:221–248, 1974.

36. Wyatt, R. J., Gillin, J. C., Stoff, D. M., Moja, E. A., and Tinklenberg, J. R. β-Phenylethylamine and the Neuropsychiatric Disturbances. In E. Usdin, D. Hamburg, and J. D. Barchas (eds.), *Neuroregulators and Psychiatric Disorders*. New York: Oxford University Press, 1977. Pp. 31–45.

37. Sandler, M., and Reynolds, G. P. Does phenylethylamine cause schizophrenia? *Lancet* 1:70–71, 1976.

38. Roberts, E. The γ-Aminobutyric Acid System and Schizophrenia. In E. Usdin, D. Hamburg, and J. Barchas (eds.), *Neuroregulators and Psychiatric Disorders*. New York: Oxford University Press, 1977. Pp. 347–357.

39. Pfeiffer, C. C., and Jenney, E. H. The inhibition of the conditioned response and the counteraction of schizophrenia by muscarinic stimulation of the brain. *Ann. N.Y. Acad. Sci.* 66:753–764, 1957.

40. Rosenthal, R., and Bigelow, L. G. The effects of physostigmine in phenothiazine resistant chronic schizophrenic patients: Preliminary observations. *Compr. Psychiatry* 14:489–495, 1973.

41. Davis, J. M. Janowsky, D., and Casper, R. C. Acetylcholine and Mental Disease. In E. Usdin, D. Hamburg, and J. Barchas (eds.), *Neuroregulators and Psychiatric Disorders.* New York: Oxford University Press, 1977. Pp. 434–441.

42. Hughes, J., Smith, T. W., Kosterlitz, H. W., Fothergill, L., Morgan, B., and Morris, H. Identification of two released pentapeptides from the brain with potent opiate agonist activity. *Nature* 258:577–579, 1975.

43. Watson, S., Akil, H., Berger, P. A., Barchas, J. D. Opiate peptides and schizophrenia. *Arch. Gen. Psychiatry* 36:35–41, 1979.

44. Berger, P. A. Investigating the role of endogenous opioid peptides in psychiatric disorders. *Neurosci. Res. Program Bull.* 16:585–599, 1978.

45. Bloom, F. E., Segal, D., Ling, N., and Guillemin, R. Endorphins: Profound behavioral effects in rats suggest new etiological factors in mental illness. *Science* 194:630–632, 1976.

46. Terenius, L., Wahlström, A., Lindström, L., and Widerlöv, E. Increased levels of endorphins in chronic psychosis. *Neurosci. Lett.* 3:157–162, 1976.

47. Palmour, R., Ervin, F., Wagemaker, H., and Cade, R. Characterization of a Peptide from the Serum of Psychotic Patients. In E. Usdin, W. E. Bunney, Jr., and N. S. Kline (eds.), *Endorphins in Mental Health Research.* New York: Macmillan, 1979. Pp. 581–593.

48. Ross, M., Berger, P. A., and Goldstein, A. Plasma β-endorphin in schizophrenia. *Science* 205:1163–1164, 1979.

49. Jacquet, Y. F., and Marks, N. The C-fragment of β-lipotropin: An endogenous neuroleptic or antipsychotogen. *Science* 194:632–636, 1976.

50. Aage, J., Fog, R., and Veilis, B. Synthetic enkephalin analogue in treatment of schizophrenia. *Lancet* 1:935, 1979.

51. Verhoeven, W. M. A., van Praag, H. M., van Ree, J. M., and de Wied, D. Improvement of schizophrenic patients treated with des-tyr^1-γ-endorphin (DTγE). *Arch. Gen. Psychiatry* 36:294–298, 1979.

52. Kline, N. S., and Lehmann, H. E. β-Endorphin Therapy in Psychiatric Patients. In E. Usdin, W. E. Bunney, Jr., and N. S. Kline (eds.), *Endorphins in Mental Health Research.* New York: Macmillan, 1979. Pp. 500–517.

53. Kline, N. S. Incidence, prevalence and recognition of depressive illness. *Dis. Nerv. Syst.* 37:10–14, 1976.

54. Berger, P. A., and Barchas, J. D. Biochemical Hypothesis of Affective Disorders. In J. D. Barchas, P. A. Berger, R. D. Ciaranelli, and G. R. Elliott (eds.), *Psychopharmacology: From Theory to Practice.* New York: Oxford University Press, 1977. Pp. 151–173.

55. Bunney, W. E., and Davis, J. M. Norepinephrine in depressive reactions. *Arch. Gen. Psychiatry* 13:483–494, 1965.

56. Schildkraut, J. J. The catecholamine hypothesis of affective disorders: A review of supporting evidence. *Am. J. Psychiatry* 122:509–522, 1965.

57. Kline, N. S. Clinical experience with iproniazid (Marsilid). *J. Clin. Exp. Psychopath.* 19 (Suppl. 1): 72–78, 1958.

58. Crane, G. E. Iproniazid (Marsilid) phosphate, a therapeutic agent for mental disorders and debilitating disease. *Psychiatr. Res. Rep.* 8:142–152, 1957.

59. Glowinski, J., and Axelrod, J. Inhibition of uptake of tritiated noradrenaline in intact rat brain by imipramine and related compounds. *Nature* 204: 1313–1319, 1964.

60. Carlsson, A., Corrodi, H., Fuxe, K., and Hokfelt, T. Effect of antidepressant drugs on the depletion of intraneuronal brain 5-hydroxytryptamine stores caused by 5-methyl-α-ethyl-meta-tyramine. *Eur. J. Pharmacol.* 5:357–366, 1969.

61. Katz, R. I., Chase, T. M., and Kopin, I. J. Evoked release of norepinephrine and serotonin from brain slices: Inhibition by lithium. *Science* 162:466–467, 1968.

62. Post, R. M., Kotin, J., and Goodwin, F. K. The effects of cocaine on depressed patients. *Am. J. Psychiatry* 131:511–517, 1974.

63. Gluckman, M. I., and Baum, T. The pharmacology of iprindole, a new antidepressant. *Psychopharmacologia* 15:169–185, 1969.

64. Sulser, F. Functional aspects of the norepinephrine receptor coupled adenylate cyclase system in the limbic forebrain and its modification by drugs which precipitate or alleviate depression: Molecular approaches to an understanding of affective disorders. *Pharmakopsychiatr. Neuro-Psychopharmakologie* 11:43–52, 1978.

65. Shaw, D. M., Riley, G. J., Michalakeas, A. C., Tidmarsh, S. F., and Blazek, R. New direction to the amine hypotheses. *Lancet* 1:1259–1260, 1977.

66. Mandell, J., Knapp, S., and Geyer, M. A. Lithium Decreases and Cocaine Increases the Bilateral Asymmetry of Serotonin in Mesotriatal and Mesolimbic Systems Associated with Changes in the Kinetic Properties of Tryptophan Hydroxylase. In

E. Usdin, I. J. Kopin, and J. Barchas (eds.), *Catecholamines: Basic and Clinical Frontiers*. New York: Pergamon, 1979. Vol. 1, pp. 663–665.

67. Carlsson, A., Jonason, J., and Lindqvist, M. On the mechanism of 5-hydroxytryptamine release by thymoleptics. *J. Pharm. Pharmacol.* 21:769–773, 1969.

68. Brodie, H. K. H., Murphy, D. L., Goodwin, F. K., and Bunney, W. E., Jr. Catecholamines and mania: The effect of alpha-methyl-para-tyrosine on manic behavior and catecholamine metabolism. *Clin. Pharmacol. Ther.* 12:218–224, 1971.

69. Goodwin, F. K., and Murphy, D. L. Biochemical Aspects of Affective Disorders and Schizophrenia. In M. Gordon (ed.), *Psychopharmacological Agents*. New York: Academic, 1974. Pp. 9–37.

70. Post, R. M. Frontiers of Affective Disorder Research: New Pharmacological Agents and New Methodologies. In M. A. Lipton, A. DiMascio, and K. F. Killam (eds.), *Psychopharmacology: A Generation of Progress*. New York: Raven, 1978. Pp. 1323–1335.

71. Maas, J. W. Biogenic amines and depression: Biochemical pharmacological separation of two types of depression. *Arch. Gen. Psychiatry* 32:1357–1361, 1975.

72. Maas, J. W., Greene, N. M., Hattox, S. E., and Landis, H. Neurotransmitter Metabolite Production by Human Brain. In E. Usdin, I. J. Kopin, and J. D. Barchas (eds.), *Catecholamines: Basic and Clinical Frontiers*. Oxford: Pergamon, 1979. Pp. 1878–1880.

73. Schildkraut, J. J. Norepinephrine metabolites as biochemical criteria for classifying depressive disorders and predicting responses to treatment: Preliminary findings. *Am. J. Psychiatry* 130:695–699, 1973.

74. Beckmann, H., and Goodwin, F. K. Antidepressant response to tricyclics and urinary MHPG in unipolar patients: Clinical response to imipramine or amitriptyline. *Arch. Gen. Psychiatry* 32:17–21, 1975.

75. Carroll, B. J., Curtis, G. C., and Mendels, J. Neuroendocrine regulation in depression I and II. *Arch. Gen. Psychiatry* 33:1039–1044; 1051–1057, 1976.

76. Sachar, E. J., Hellman, L., Roffwarg, H. P., Halpern, F. S., Fukushima, D., and Gallagher, T. F. Disrupted 24-hour patterns of cortisol secretion in psychotic depression. *Arch. Gen. Psychiatry* 28:19–24, 1973.

77. Editorial. The dexamethasone test and depression. *Lancet* 1:730, 1980.

78. Maeda, K., Kato, Y., Ohgo, S., Chihara, K., Yoshimoto, Y., Yamaguchi, N., Kuromaru, S., and Imura, H. Growth hormone and prolactin release after injection of thyrotropin releasing hormone in patients with depression. *J. Clin. Endocrinol. Metab.* 40:501–505, 1975.

79. Gruen, P. H., Sachar, E. J., Altman, N., and Sassin, J. Growth hormone responses to hypoglycemia in postmenopausal depressed women. *Arch. Gen. Psychiatry* 32:31–33, 1975.

80. Langer, G., Heinze, G., Reim, B., and Matussek, N. Reduced growth hormone responses to amphetamine in "endogenous" depressive patients. *Arch. Gen. Psychiatry* 33:1471–1475, 1976.

81. Barchas, J. D., Akil, H., Elliott, G. R., Holman, R. B., and Watson, S. J. Behavioral neurochemistry: Neuroregulators and behavioral states. *Science* 200:964–973, 1978.

Bruce S. McEwen

Chapter 39. Endocrine Effects on the Brain and Their Relationship to Behavior

Awareness of endocrine influences on brain function is as old as the field of endocrinology itself. In 1849, Berthold described striking behavioral changes resulting from castration of roosters and the reversal of these changes after testes had been transplanted into the castrated animals [1].

Nearly 100 years later, Dr. Frank Beach published a book entitled *Hormones and Behavior* [2], which has served to instruct and motivate recent generations of investigators to explore in depth the interactions of hormones with the brain. Spectacular growth of the field of neuroendocrinology (i.e., neural control of endocrine function, described in Chap. 14 of this book) offers to the present generation of neurobiologists unparalleled opportunities to explore with great sophistication interrelated problems of the influences of neural activity on endocrine secretion and of endocrine secretion, in turn, on neural activity and behavior.

The relationships among these influences may be summarized as

Endocrine system ⇌ nervous system ⇌ behavior

This emphasizes that associations between behavioral and endocrine events are mediated through the nervous system (Chap. 14). It is the purpose of this chapter to examine chemical and molecular aspects of the influences of hormonal secretion on the nervous system and behavior. But, before doing so, it is necessary to describe briefly the behavioral events and the accompanying neural activity that can trigger hormone secretion.

Behavioral Control of Hormone Secretion

The brain is the producer of master hormones, the hypothalamic releasing factors, which regulate release of the anterior pituitary tropic hormones (see Chap. 14). Neurons in the hypothalamus also produce the hormones oxytocin and vasopressin, which are released by the posterior pituitary into the blood. It is therefore not surprising that behavioral influences are associated with the secretion of these hypothalamic releasing factors and hormones (Fig. 39-1). Consider, for example, the phenomenon of lactation, in which the suckling stimulus to the nipple triggers the release of oxytocin, which facilitates milk ejection, and of prolactin, which helps the mammary gland to replenish the supply of milk [3].

The phenomenon of stress also illustrates the behavioral control of anterior pituitary hormone secretion. Conditions associated with injury and surgical trauma, and the so-called psychic stresses of fear, novelty, and even joy, can activate the release of ACTH, which, in turn, stimulates the secretion of adrenal glucocorticoids. These behavioral stimuli are mediated by complex neural pathways and can be modified readily by learning.

The secretion of the gonadotropins is also subject to behavioral modification. In the female rabbit, the act of copulation activates spinal reflex pathways that stimulate the secretion of luteinizing hormone (LH) and leads to ovulation. In the male rabbit, the act of copulation also activates the secretion of LH and increases plasma testosterone levels [4]. Social stimuli, too, modify gonadotropin secretion. In mice, olfactory cues from other females can interrupt normal estrous cycles and lead to pseudopregnancies or periods of prolonged diestrus (Lee-Boot effect), and olfactory cues from males can shorten the estrous cycle and either cause rapid attainment of estrus (*Whitten effect*) or terminate pregnancy in a newly impregnated mouse (*Bruce effect*) [3]. In male rhesus monkeys, sudden

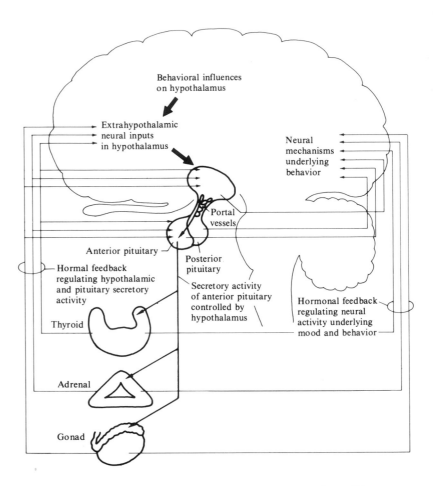

Behavioral influences
on hypothalamus

Extrahypothalamic
neural inputs
in hypothalamus

Neural
mechanisms
underlying
behavior

Portal
vessels

Anterior pituitary

Posterior
pituitary

Hormal feedback
regulating hypothalamic
and pituitary secretory
activity

Secretory activity
of anterior pituitary
controlled by
hypothalamus

Hormonal feedback
regulating neural
activity underlying
mood and behavior

Thyroid

Adrenal

Gonad

Fig. 39-1. Schematic representation of possible reciprocal interactions among hypothalamic, pituitary, thyroid, adrenal, and gonadal hormones.

decisive defeat by other males leads to prolonged reduction in plasma testosterone levels, which can be reversed in the defeated male by the introduction of a female companion [5]. In humans, the anticipation of sexual intercourse has been reported to increase beard growth, a process under control of circulating androgen, although this finding has been disputed [6].

Several points should be stressed concerning such behavioral control by hormone secretion. First, as will become apparent in the next section of this chapter, hormones so secreted act on target tissues, including parts of the CNS, to modify their function. In the brain, this feedback action includes modification of behavior and neuroendocrine function. For example, increased gonadotropin and testosterone levels in the male rabbit that result

from copulation or, in the male rhesus monkey, from exposure to the female, as might be expected facilitate both sexual activity and replenishment of sperm and seminal fluid. This constitutes a form of positive feedback with respect to reproductive function.

A second aspect of behavioral control of neuroendocrine function is that the circumstances under which hypothalamic hormones are released serve to define those behavioral and physiological conditions that, it also might be expected, are subject to feedback actions of target hormones. With such gonadal steroids as testosterone, these conditions are self-evident. With adrenal steroids, analysis of the diverse circumstances leading to ACTH secretion is more difficult but in the end may reveal the role of adrenal steroid interactions with the brain. Each type of stress is a perturbation of the body away from a physiological norm. For example, encounter with a predator may require rapid evasive action, in which neural activity and rapidly mobilized hormones such as epinephrine play a role. Adrenal steroid secretion is slower, reaching a peak minutes after the stressful event, and as such is not expected to play a role in the immediate coping with the situation. If the evasive action is successful and the animal survives, however, it will not only have to reestablish homeostasis; presumably it will learn from its experience in order to minimize the chances of another such encounter. Adrenal steroids might be acting toward such longer adaptations. A special case of this reaction is the extinction of a conditioned avoidance response. Suppose the animal has learned to avoid a certain place where it was previously punished but then discovers that being in that place no longer results in punishment. If, for example, that place also contains a food or water supply, it is in the best interests of the animal to extinguish the avoidance response in order to take advantage of the food or water. Adrenal steroids have, in fact, been found to facilitate such extinction and thus can be said to facilitate a form of behavioral adaptation [7, 8].

We must add to this kind of analysis the fact that, in the absence of external stressors, adrenal steroids are also secreted in varying amounts according to the time of day. In nocturnally active animals such as the rat and in animals such as the human which are active during the day, the peak of this basal secretion always occurs near the end of the sleep period. Thus it is conceivable that adrenal steroid secretion may modulate behavior as a function of the time of day. Indeed it has been reported that adrenal steroids modify the detection and recognition thresholds for a variety of sensory stimuli and influence the occurrence of the so-called rapid eye movement (REM) or paradoxical phase of sleep [8].

Activational and Organizational Effects of Hormones on the Brain

Feedback effects on the brain of hormones that modify behavior and neuroendocrine function may be classified as either activational or organizational. Activational effects are facilitative effects on preexisting neuroendocrine pathways or behavioral patterns that are reversible when the hormone disappears (Fig. 39-1). It is essential to consider activational effects on the behavior as facilitative or permissive because the hormones do not by themselves cause the behavior; rather, they increase its likelihood of occurrence given the proper stimuli. For example, a male rat mounting an estrogen-primed female usually will stimulate her to assume the mating (lordosis) posture, whereas a male mounting a spayed female will only infrequently elicit the lordosis response.

Organizational effects occur during a specific phase of early development and organize aspects of behavior and neuroendocrine function for a period of time beyond the presence of the hormone itself, usually for the remainder of the individual's life. Such effects will be considered below in the last sections.

EXAMPLES OF ACTIVATIONAL EFFECTS
The specific activating or inhibiting effects of the hypothalamic, pituitary, and target gland hormones on neuroendocrine function are considered in Chap. 14. Especially noteworthy among these effects is the positive-feedback action of estrogen on the brain, leading to the surge of LH that triggers ovulation. Concomitant with such hormone effects on neuroendocrine function are effects that modify appropriate behavioral responses of the animal. There are examples of behavioral effects of each class of hormone. Luteinizing hormone-releasing factor (LRF) has been observed to facilitate female mating behavior in estrogen-primed ovariectomized female rats, even in the absence of the normal LRF target gland, the pituitary [9, 10]. One suspects that other hypothalamic releasing hormones may also have behavioral effects. For example, recent reports suggest that both thyrotropin releasing factor (TRF) and melanocyte inhibiting

factor (MIF) may potentiate, respectively, the noradrenergic and dopaminergic systems and exert antidepressant effects [11–13]. The posterior pituitary hormone, vasopressin, has been reported to potentiate conditioned avoidance behavior under extinction conditions in the rat, and the anterior pituitary hormone, ACTH, has been observed to have similar, but less prolonged, effects [14]. Melanocyte-stimulating hormone (MSH), which resembles ACTH in amino acid sequence, has been reported to have behavioral effects similar to those of ACTH [15].

The activational effects of steroid hormones have been studied the most extensively of all hormones. Estradiol facilitates mating activity in female animals of many species. In the female rat, estrogen promotes the lordosis response, increases locomotor activity, decreases food intake [16], and facilitates maternal behavior [17]. Testosterone facilitates male copulatory activity [18] and activates other behaviors, such as intermale aggression in mice [19] and territorial scent-marking activities in gerbils [20]. Progesterone appears to be important in rodents, together with estrogen, in promoting ovulation and facilitating lordosis response [21, 22]. In addition, progesterone antagonizes a variety of androgen effects [23–26] and facilitates food intake and maintenance of body weight in intact and ovariectomized adrenalectomized female rats [27]. Adrenal glucocorticoids have been reported to facilitate extinction of conditioned avoidance behavior, modify thresholds for detection and recognition of sensory stimuli, and influence frequency of occurrence of REM sleep [8].

BIOCHEMICAL ASPECTS OF ACTIVATIONAL HORMONE EFFECTS

Metabolism of Steroid Hormones in Brain Tissue

One important aspect of the interaction of steroid hormones with target tissues is the metabolic transformation of the hormone to more or less active metabolites. Such transformations appear to be of particular importance for the androgen testosterone and lead to the concept that this steroid may be a prehormone. The brain, like the seminal vesicles, is able to convert testosterone to 5α-dihydrotestosterone (DHT) and $3\alpha,5\alpha$-androstanediol (Fig. 39-2, a and b) and also, like the placenta, converts testosterone to estradiol (Fig. 39-2c). Neither conversion occurs equally in all brain regions. Regional distribution of 5α-reductase activity toward testosterone in rat brain is found in midbrain and brain stem; intermediate activity in hypothalamus and thalamus; and lowest activity in cerebral cortex [28]. The pituitary has higher 5α-reductase activity than any region of the brain, and its activity is subject to changes as a result of gonadectomy, hormone replacement, and postnatal age. 5α-Dihydrotestosterone has been implicated in hypothalamus and pituitary as a potent regulator of gonadotropin secretion but is relatively inactive toward male rat sexual behavior [29]. Labeled metabolites with the R_f value of 5α-DHT have been detected in extracts of hypothalamic and pituitary tissue after [^{3}H]testosterone had been administered in vivo to both adult and newborn male rats. It is interesting that progesterone inhibits 5α-reductase activity toward [^{3}H]testosterone and that [^{3}H]progesterone is itself converted to [^{3}H]5α-dihydroprogesterone (Fig. 39-2d). Progesterone competition for the 5α-reductase may explain some of the antiandrogenicity of this steroid [30].

The aromatization of testosterone to form estradiol, and of androstenedione to form estrone (Fig. 39-2c and c', respectively) has been described in brain tissue in vitro and in vivo [31, 32]. Aromatization is higher in hypothalamus and limbic structures than in cerebral cortex or pituitary gland and, in noncastrated animals, is higher in male than in female brains. Aromatization has been found in brains of reptiles and amphibia as well as in mammals [33, 34]. The capacity to aromatize testosterone and related androgens may therefore be a general property of vertebrate brains. The functional role of aromatization has been studied most extensively in the rat: male sexual behavior is facilitated by estradiol [35], and testosterone facilitation of male sexual behavior can be blocked by a steroidal inhibitor of aromatization [36, 37]. There are indications that a similar situation exists

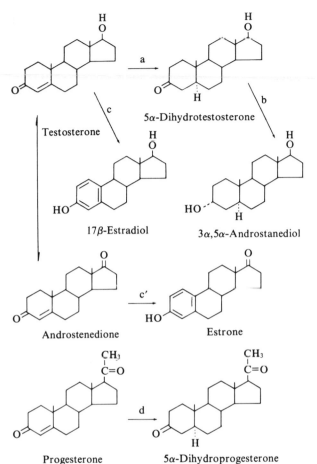

Fig. 39-2. *Some steroid transformations that are carried out by neural tissue.*

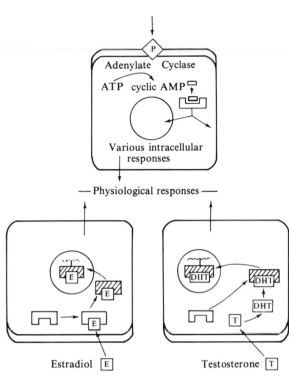

Fig. 39-3. *Schematic representation of interactions of hormones with target cells.* Top: *Certain protein hormones (P) and epinephrine are known to interact with cell surface receptors to stimulate adenyl cyclase.* Bottom: *Steroid hormones interact with intracellular receptors and are transferred into cell nuclear compartment.*

in birds, amphibia, and reptiles; that is, testosterone and estradiol can stimulate heterotypical sexual behavior in males and females. Curiously, not all mammals are like the rat: for example, male sexual behavior of the guinea pig and rhesus monkey is restored by the nonaromatizable androgens androstenedione and dihydrotestosterone [38, 39].

A number of other steroid transformations occur in brain tissue, but this metabolism does not appear to be of importance for interaction of those hormones with the putative receptor sites to be described below: Both [³H]estradiol and [³H]-

corticosterone are recovered from their binding sites in the brain tissue [40].

Cellular Mechanisms of Hormone Action
The study of hormone action has centered around the recognition of putative receptor sites for a variety of hormones and the classification of these receptor sites in terms of two fundamentally different cellular mechanisms of action, which are shown in Fig. 39-3. A number of polypeptide hormones such as glucagon, insulin, ACTH, and possibly the hypothalamic releasing factors are believed to act by way of cell-surface receptors that

are associated with the enzyme adenylate cyclase. Interaction of hormones with such receptors is believed to trigger increased formation from ATP of cyclic 3'5'-AMP, which in turn, is an intracellular second messenger in a variety of cellular events (Fig. 39-3). This mechanism is discussed in Chap. 15. Steroid hormones, on the other hand, interact with intracellular, presumably cytoplasmic, receptor sites and are transferred to the cell nucleus, where they interact with the genome to alter transcription processes (Fig. 39-3). Recent evidence suggests that thyroid hormone also may be able to act through cell nuclear receptor sites [41]. Because of the greater amount of evidence available, the remainder of this section will focus on the cellular mechanism of steroid hormone action on brain and pituitary cells.

Methods for Studying Putative Steroid Hormone Receptor Sites

Before summarizing the evidence for steroid hormone receptor sites in brain and pituitay, let us review the methods that are used to measure such sites. The availability in the early 1960s of tritium-labeled steroids of high specific activity (20 to 25 Ci per mmole at each labeled position) permitted the measurement of specific binding sites of low capacity which had previously escaped detection using ^{14}C-labeled steroids [42]. In the brain, high-resolution autoradiographic methods utilizing ^{3}H-labeled steroids have permitted mapping of steroid-hormone target cells in specific brain regions (Fig. 39-4). It should be noted that tritium permits a high degree of spatial resolution (particle range 1 to 2 μm in light-microscope autoradiography) owing to its low energy of decay [43].

Cell fractionation procedures are basic to the biochemical identification and study of steroid hormone-binding sites. Isolation of highly purified cell nuclei from small amounts of tissue from discrete brain regions is generally accomplished with the aid of a nonionic detergent. Triton X-100, and such methods have been described in detail elsewhere [41]. Cytosol fractions of brain tissue (prepared by centrifugation of homogenates at 105,000 $\times$ g for 60 min) contain the soluble steroid

hormone-binding proteins, and a variety of methods intended to sepaate bound from unbound steroid have been used for measuring their binding activity [42]. The most commonly employed are gel filtration chromatography and sucrose density gradient centrifugation. Dextran-coated charcoal is frequently used because it effectively adsorbs unbound steroid and leaves intact the complexes between steroid and putative receptor. Other methods, such as disc gel electrophoresis and precipitation of putative receptor material by protamine sulfate, have more restricted uses.

Several general comments are in order regarding use of these methods in studies of cytosol hormone receptors. The objective of such studies is to measure the affinity, capacity, and specificity of the hormone-receptor interaction [42; see also Chap. 3]. Measurements of affinity and capacity are accomplished by running concentration-dependence curves of binding and plotting the results in the form of a Scatchard plot or a reciprocal plot (Fig. 39-5). Evaluation of the x and y intercepts yields the association constant (K_a) or its reciprocal, the dissociation constant (K_d), and the capacity of the binding sites at saturation (B_{max}) by an infinite concentration. Problems encountered in measurements of K_d and B_{max} center around the attainment of a true equilibrium: Inasmuch as it may take hours for ligand to equilibrate with receptor, and some kinds of receptors decay measurably during this time of equilibration, there may never be attained more than a quasi equilibrium in which the K_d and B_{max} approach but never reach the true values. Specificity studies are conducted by competing for binding of ^{3}H-ligand by various unlabeled ligands. The relative ability of various unlabeled steroids to compete for binding in increasing molar excesses to ^{3}H-steroid is compared with the effectiveness of the unlabeled homologous steroid in similarly increasing excesses. A large (100- to 1,000-fold) excess of unlabeled homologous steroid is used to estimate nonspecific binding since the techniques for separation of bound from unbound ligand measure total binding. A general criterion for nonspecific binding is that it be linear as a function of ^{3}H-

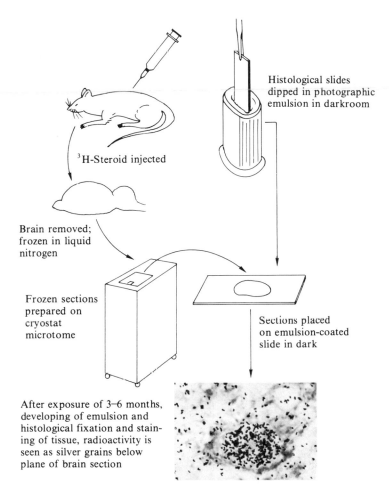

Fig. 39-4. Flow diagram of a frequently used procedure for autoradiographic localization of ^3H steroid hormones in neural tissue.

Histological slides dipped in photographic emulsion in darkroom

^{3}H-Steroid injected

Brain removed; frozen in liquid nitrogen

Frozen sections prepared on cryostat microtome

Sections placed on emulsion-coated slide in dark

After exposure of 3–6 months, developing of emulsion and histological fixation and staining of tissue, radioactivity is seen as silver grains below plane of brain section

ligand in the presence of a large and constant excess of unlabeled ligand, that is, nonsaturable. Subtraction of nonspecific form total binding gives an estimate of the actual limited-capacity binding (saturable).

There are several criteria for calling a steroid hormone-binding site a putative receptor. First, it must be present in hormone-responsive tissues (or brain regions) and absent from nonresponsive ones. Second, it should bind steroids that are either active agonists or effective antagonists of the hormone effect and not bind steroids that are inactive

in either sense. These two criteria will form the basis of the discussion that follows.

Properties and Topography of Putative Steroid Receptor Sites in Brain

Let us now consider the evidence for putative steroid hormone receptor sites in brain and pituitary. In the brain and pituitary, as in other steroid hormone target tissues, there appear to be steroid hormone-binding sites for certain hormones in the cytosol and in cell nuclei. Unlike receptors in many other target tissues, however, putative brain receptors are not distributed uniformly but are concentrated in discrete brain regions.

ESTRADIOL (formula in Fig. 39-2). The first neural steroid hormone-binding sites to be recog-

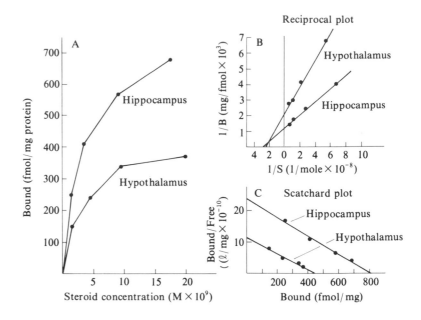

Fig. 39-5. (A) *Concentration-dependence curve for binding of* [3]*H-dexamethasone by cytosis from hippocampus and hypothalamus.* (B) *Expression of data in* (A) *in the form of a reciprocal plot, 1/bound vs. 1/steroid concentration.* (C) *Scatchard plot of same data, bound/free steroid vs. bound (fmol = 10^{-15} mol; 1 = liters).*

nized were those for estradiol [45]. Studies of the in vivo accumulation of ^{3}H]estradiol from the blood revealed extremely high concentrations in pituitary as well as uterus and lower but substantial uptake in the hypothalamic region of the brain. Within brain, ^{3}H]estradiol accumulation is highest in the hypothalamus and preoptic region. A substantial proportion of uptake into these brain regions and into pituitary and uterus can be blocked by concurrent administration of ^{3}H]estradiol and 100- or 1,000-fold excesses of unlabeled 17β-estradiol but not by similar excesses of unlabeled testosterone or 17α-estradiol (an inactive estrogen). Such competition establishes the binding as a phenomenon of limited capacity, with specificity for active estrogens.

Autoradiography has provided more detailed information as to the distribution within the brain of binding sites for ^{3}H]estradiol [46]. Neurons, rather than glial cells, appear to contain the highest concentrations of these putative receptor sites and, in male and female rats, these neurons are concentrated within the hypophyseotropic area (medial preoptic area, anterior and medial-basal hypothalamus) and amygdala and, to a lesser extent, in the midbrain (Fig. 39-6). Not all neurons

within these areas bind estradiol, but many of the cells that do bind the hormone have an intensity of labeling comparable to that found in cells of the uterus and pituitary.

The use of sedimentation rate in sucrose density gradients (approximately 8 S at low ionic strength) and specificity of binding toward active estrogens, such as 17β-estradiol and diethylstilbestrol, cell fractionation studies of the pituitary and hypothalamus, preoptic area, and amygdala demonstrated the existence of soluble (cytosol) binding sites which resemble those found in the uterus. In spite of similarities in sedimentation behavior and hormonal specificity, no one knows for sure if the estrogen-binding proteins are identical in these various estrogen target tissues. In agreement with the autoradiographic results cited above, estrogen-binding proteins are not detectable by sucrose-

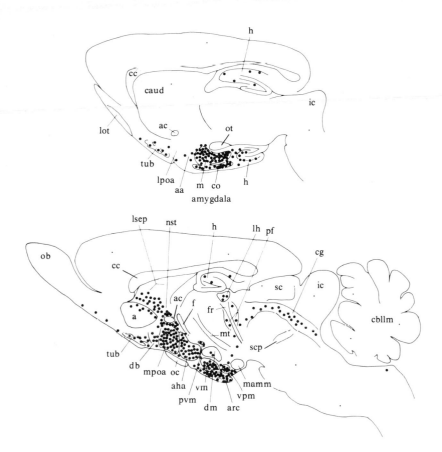

Fig. 39-6. Distribution of estrogen-concentrating neurons in the brain of the female rat represented schematically in two sagittal sections. Most labeled neurons can be represented in a medial plane (bottom). Estradiol-concentrating neurons in the amygdala and hippocampus are represented in a more lateral plane (top). Locations of estradiol-concentrating neurons are represented by black dots (●). Figure reproduced from Pfaff and Keiner [46] by permission of the authors and The Wistar Press, Philadelphia. (Identity of the anatomical abbreviations may be found in [46].)

density gradient centrifugation in cytosols from the cerebral cortex and are demonstrable in cytosols from the pooled preoptic area, hypothalamus, amygdala, and midbrain [16]. Quantitative estimates of estradiol-binding capacity of cytosol based on Scatchard plots (see above) indicate that cerebral cortex has less than one-fourth of the capacity found in amygdala and less than one-

tenth of the capacity found in hypothalamus, whereas the hypothalamus has a capacity around one-thirtieth of that found in either pituitary or uterus [45]. The dissociation constant of the binding (K_d) is between 1 and 5×10^{-10} M, depending on the method used to separate bound from free [^{3}H]estradiol. Based on the DNA content of these tissues, the capacity of uterine and pituitary tissues to bind [^{3}H]estradiol corresponds to 12,000 to 15,000 molecules per cell, whereas the capacity of the whole hypothalamus is around 2,000 to 3,000 molecules per cell. These estimates of binding per cell are, of course, averages which do not take into account the proportion of cells in each tissue that bind with the hormone.

The estradiol which attaches to cytosol estrogen-binding sites is transferred into the cell nuclei, and substantial amounts of the [^{3}H]estradiol in the tissue can be recovered in isolated nuclei from these target tissues [40, 45]. The relative magnitude of binding in cell nuclei closely parallels the relative magnitude of cytosol-receptor content in uterus, pituitary, and various brain regions. Cell nuclear-bound [³H]estradiol can be extracted as a complex with protein using KCl in concentrations of 0.3 M or greater. These complexes from uterine, pituitary, and brain nuclei have lower sedimentation coefficients in sucrose-density gradient centrifugation than those of the corresponding cytosols, when the cytosols are run in low ionic-strength buffers. As reported for calf uterus [45], the 8.6 S estrogen-binding protein in cytosol is believed to be a tetrameric form of a subunit of about 61,000 M_r. Dissociation to a dimeric form (5.3 S) occurs at high ionic strength (0.2 M salt or greater), and further transformation to a monomer (4.5 S) is carried out by a "receptor transforming factor," believed to be an enzyme with limited proteolytic activity that is present in the cytosol. In the calf uterus, the purified cell-nuclear receptor has a sedimentation coefficient of 4.5 S and is believed to be related to the monomeric form of the cytosol receptor. Therefore, the hormone, together with the cytosol monomer, appears to be translocated into the cell nucleus and to interact with the genome.

ANDROGEN (formulas in Fig. 39-2). As noted earlier in this section, testosterone is transformed to 5α-DHT in a number of androgen target tissues, including the brain and pituitary. This transformation was first recognized in the male accessory sex glands, and subsequently receptor sites specific for 5α-DHT were recognized in these tissues [42]. In discussing putative receptor sites in the pituitary and brain, it is necessary to consider both testosterone and 5α-DHT. Measurement of tissues after either [³H]testosterone or [³H]5α-DHT has been administered to castrated male rats has shown the pituitary to have the highest concentration of radioactivity after the prostate and seminal vesicles. Hypothalamus has generally higher concentrations of radioactivity than cerebral cortex, but differences between these two structures are small, in contrast to the concentration difference between hypothalamus and cortex in [³H]estradiol uptake.

Cell nuclear and cytosol androgen receptors, characterized in brain and pituitary tissue [47, 48], resemble those from peripheral tissues such as seminal vesicles. In vivo administration of [³H]-testosterone results in cell nuclear accumulation of both [³H]testosterone and of [³H]5α-DHT, of which are both capable of binding to the androgen receptors. There do not appear to be separate receptors for testosterone and 5α-DHT [49].

Autoradiography has provided more substantial evidence for cellular localization of androgen-binding sites, although this technique does not permit identification of labeled material. ³H-Testosterone uptake has been observed in 10 to 15 percent of the cells of the anterior pituitary and in selected cell groupings within the preoptic area and medial basal hypothalamus as well as in the amygdala [45]. [³H]5α-DHT is also accumulated by cells in anterior pituitary and in the limbic system of the rat [48, 50], and such results are more indicative of true androgen receptors because 5α-DHT, unlike testosterone, cannot be aromatized. Cellular localization of [³H]testosterone has been reported in the hypothalamus, preoptic area, and midbrain of a songbird, the chaffinch *Fringilla coelebs* [45]. The midbrain localization is of particular interest because of androgen effects on bird song, motor control centers for which are located in the area of hormone uptake.

GLUCOCORTICOIDS (formulas in Fig. 39-7). Because of the success achieved in measuring putative estrogen receptors in the brain, attempts were made to find similar receptor molecules for adrenal steroids. Based upon the estrogen studies and on information regarding the importance of the hypothalamus in the control of ACTH secretion, it was anticipated that adrenal steroid receptors would be localized in the hypothalamic region of the brain. Such putative receptors were indeed found in hypothalamus, but the highest concentrations of binding sites for [³H]corticosterone, the predominant adrenal glucocorticoid in the rat, were found in the hippocampus, amygdala, and

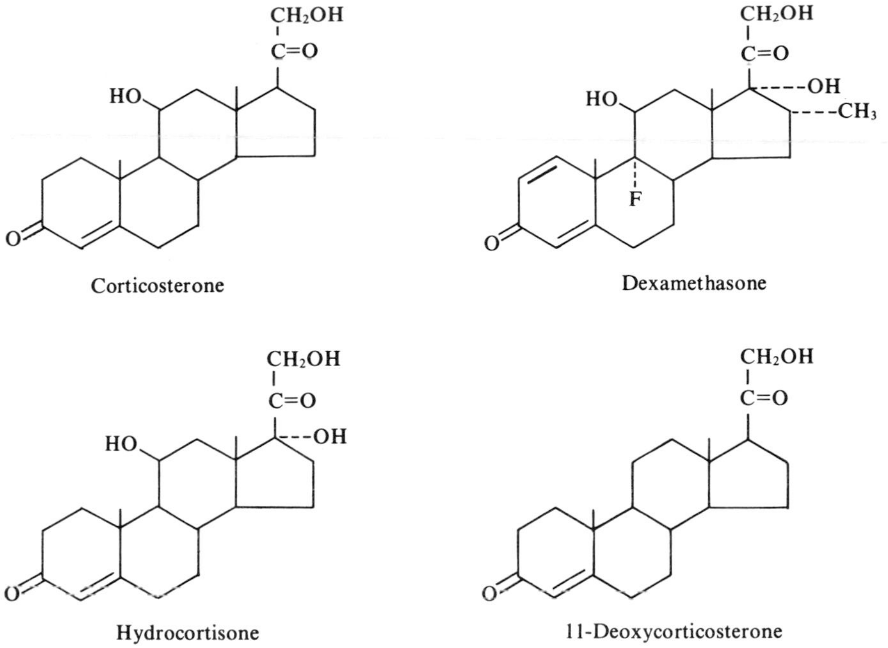

Corticosterone

Dexamethasone

Hydrocortisone

11-Deoxycorticosterone

Fig. 39-7. Formulas of four steroid hormones.

septum [8, 40]. Cell fractionation studies revealed that this binding was due to both cytosol and cell-nucleus binding sites, in the fashion we have seen is typical for many steroid hormones and target tissues. In hippocampus, the capacity of the cytosol corticosterone-binding protein is about 850 fmol (femtomoles per milligram total cytosol protein; Fig. 39-5). This is large compared with the 20 fmoles per mg protein that approximates the capacity of estrogen-binding protein in the hypothalamus. Estimates of binding in cell nuclei in the hippocampus indicate that about 16,000 molecules of corticosterone are bound per cell nucleus. This is also large compared to the figure of 3,000 molecules of estradiol per cell nucleus in the hypothalamus. Differences in the binding capacity for the two steroids are undoubtedly a reflection of two factors: first, that the density of hormone-sensitive cells is different in each brain region; second, that the amount of receptor tends to reflect the amount of hormone in the blood. Physio-

logical estrogen levels in the rat range from 3 to 30 pg per milliliter; corticosterone levels range from 30 to 300 ng per milliliter. As noted in the estrogen section, the presence together of hormone-sensitive and hormone-insensitive cells in a given brain region makes it virtually impossible to estimate the actual hormone capacity in sensitive cells.

The properties of the soluble brain glucocorticoids that bind macromolecules toward [3H]dexamethasone are illustrative of some of the characteristics of steroid hormone-binding proteins in general. These proteins have a high affinity ($K_d = 3$ to 4×10^{-9} M; Fig. 39-5), limited, low capacity ($B_{max} = 810$ fmol per milligram protein; Fig. 39-5), and a high degree of specificity for the glucocorticoids. They do, however, bind progesterone and mineralocorticoids (see below). They may be compared with transcortin, the serum protein. Unlike transcortin, the binding proteins in brain bind dexamethasone, the synthetic glucocorticoid, with high affinity. The steroid–brain receptor complex, unlike the transcortin-steroid complex, can be precipitated by the polycation, protamine sulfate. At low ionic strength, the brain receptor–steroid complex is a macromolecular aggregate of more than 600,000 M_r and has a low mobility in polyacrylamide gel electrophoresis; in contrast, transcortin has a molecular weight of $\approx 60,000$ and a high mobility in polyacrylamide gels, which permits it to be quantitatively separated from the binding proteins in brain.

Autoradiographic examination of the rat brain labeled with [³H]corticosterone reveals that neurons in hippocampus, septum, induseum griseum, and corticomedial amygdala are heavily labeled [8]. Most of the radioactivity appears over the region of the cell nucleus. It should be noted that there is excellent evidence that glial cells also respond to glucocorticoids and contain putative receptor sites. After adrenalectomy, the activity of the enzyme glycerolphosphatedehydrogenase (GPDH) falls in all regions of the brain and can be restored by replacement therapy with glucocorticoids [51]. In tissue culture, a rat glial-cell tumor line, RGC6, shows the glucocorticoid inducibility of GPDH and contains putative receptors for glucocorticoids. In addition, the optic nerve of the rat contains inducible GPDH activity as well as glucocorticoid receptors, and the former has been immunohistochemically localized to oligodendroglial cells in this and other neural tissue [52, 53]. Thus glial cells in the nervous system are a major target for glucocorticoids. It is puzzling that autoradiographic studies of intact nervous tissue labeled with [³H]corticosterone have failed to show specific labeling in cell nuclei associated with nonneural elements. On the other hand, glial cells are very difficult to identify in lightly stained frozen sections, and there is a substantial background of radioactive label in the neuropil surrounding the heavily labeled neurons.

PROGESTERONE (formula in Fig. 39-2). As is true with testosterone, progesterone is likely to undergo one of a number of metabolic transformations in the body [45]. The conversion to 5α-dihydroprogesterone, which has been demonstrated to occur in brain (see p. 778), is one of these. This metabolite can be further reduced to 3α and 3β derivatives. 5α-Dihydroprogesterone and its 3α–OH derivative have been reported to be less active than progesterone itself in inducing lordosis behavior in estrogen-primed, spayed female rats [22]. However, 5α-DHP and not 5β-DHP appears to mimic the effect of progesterone in inhibiting ovulation under rigidly defined experimental conditions in immature rats treated with PMSG, an inducer of precocious ovulation. Another progesterone metabolite, 20α-hydroxyprogesterone, is produced by ovarian tissue and is functionally active in maintaining LH release in the rabbit after mating [45].

Studies of the fate of systemically injected [³H]progesterone and [³H]20α-OH-progesterone have shown that the highest uptake occurs in the midbrain region, somewhat lower uptake in hypothalamus, and still lower uptake in cerebral cortex and hippocampus of rat and guinea pig brains [45]. Midbrain and hypothalamus in guinea pig are both sites at which progesterone implants exert effects on mating that resemble physiological effects of the hormone given systemically. This pattern of uptake is, however, similar to that observed for [³H]corticosterone and [³H]estradiol in guinea pig brains when binding sites are saturated by either endogenous or exogenous hormones. These facts have suggested that an interaction of the steroid with lipids in the brain, and not with specific receptors, determines the pattern of uptake.

Attempts to identify progestin receptor sites in the brain were for a long time unsuccessful owing to the instability of the receptor and of the progesterone-receptor interaction. Recently, successful demonstrations of progestin receptors have utilized a synthetic progestin, 17α,21-dimethyl-19-norpregna-4,9-dione-3,20-dione (R5020), which forms a more stable complex with the receptors than does progesterone [54–57]. Progestin receptors are present throughout the rat brain but only those in hypothalamus and the preoptic area are induced by estrogen treatment [56]. Estrogen inducibility may underlie the synergistic interaction of estradiol and progesterone in activating feminine sexual behavior in the rat. Although the progesterone effect on behavior is rapid (within an hour [58]) there are indications that it involves a cell nuclear action according to the scheme in Fig. 39-3 [57].

The biochemical data on neural progestin receptors is complemented by several autoradiographic studies of the guinea pig and rat brain that show progestin-concentrating neurons in the mediobasal hypothalamus and medial preoptic area [59, 60]. An interesting example of interspecies variability is the observation that, in the monkey, progestin receptors are found only in the mediobasal hypothalamus and immediately adjacent tissue, where they are induced by estradiol [61].

MINERALOCORTICOIDS (formulas in Fig. 39-7). Proteins capable of binding [^{3}H]deoxycorticosterone and [^{3}H]aldosterone have been described in rat brain. Some evidence exists for binding specificity toward mineralocorticoids [62], but a major portion of the binding shows overlap with glucocorticoid binding sites. In fact, the in vivo distribution of [^{3}H]aldosterone in the brains of adrenalectomized rats is virtually identical to that of [^{3}H]corticosterone, with high concentrations of radioactivity in neurons of hippocampus and septum [63]. It will be necessary in the future to devise more selective means of distinguishing between glucocorticoid receptors and bona fide mineralocorticoid binding sites. Physiological and pharmacological evidence indicates that true mineralocorticoid receptors should exist: adrenalectomy increases salt hunger in rats and this behavior is returned to normal levels by replacement therapy with microgram quantities of aldosterone, the naturally occurring mineralocorticoid [62].

Estradiol Action in the Brain and Pituitary: Integration of Behavioral and Neuroendocrine Effects

It is evident from the previous sections that the brain and pituitary gland contain target sites for the action of steroid hormones and that these hormones activate neuroendocrine events and facilitate the occurrence of particular behaviors. Usually the neuroendocrine and behavioral effects of hormone action are coordinated with each other and together contribute to the efficient operation and survival of the individual and the species. Nowhere is this more evident than in reproduction, and this integration is particularly well illustrated by the example of reproduction in the female rat.

The estrous cycle of the female rat is usually of four days' duration (Fig. 39-8). It can be measured by means of vaginal smears, which, when examined under a light microscope, reveal a characteristic pattern of cell types present in the vaginal epithelium [16]. Indeed, the entire reproductive tract undergoes cyclic changes under the direct control of circulating estrogen and progesterone and at about the day of estrus becomes able to receive and maintain a fertilized egg. Plasma levels of circulating estrogen are represented schematically in Fig. 39-8. Basal levels are below 25 pg per milliliter and rise to a peak of around 40 to 80 pg per milliliter on the day of proestrus [64]. Plasma levels of luteinizing hormone, the direct stimulus for ovulation, rise to a sharp peak (the LH surge) on the afternoon of proestrus. That the previous rise in estrogen is required for this surge can be demonstrated by administering antibodies against estrogen on diestrous day 2. In this way, the LH surge is blocked by the effective removal of estrogen from access to target-tissue receptors [65].

In a similar fashion, "antiestrogenic" compounds such as clomiphene or MER-25 (formulas in Fig. 39-9) also block the LH surge when administered on diestrous day 2 [45]. These antiestrogens are known to interact with putative estrogen receptors in the uterus, pituitary, and brain and block access of estradiol to the intracellular receptor sites. It appears, in fact, that the antiestrogens are themselves translocated into the cell nuclei where they remain for long periods of time, unlike estradiol, which comes out of the nucleus after a number of hours [45]. Nuclear retention of antagonist-receptor complexes apparently depletes cytoplasmic receptor levels and prevents newly arriving estrogen from having an effect [66]. A *single* injection of antagonist has been demonstrated to be as effective as estradiol itself in promoting uterine growth; however, the antagonist-loaded tissue is rendered insensitive to further estrogen treatment [66]. The antiestrogenic action thus apparently hinges on the interference with the "amplification" of the initial estrogenic effect that normally occurs through further interaction of target cells with continuing supplies of estrogen. In the uterus, this is seen as an attenuation of the growth and differentiation response to hormone. It remains to be seen what corresponding cellular events are attenuated in brain and pituitary by antiestrogens and what cellular events may actually be induced by antiestrogens as well as by estradiol.

Further indication that events in the cell nucleus are required for the LH surge is provided by experiments in which actinomycin D is able to prevent the LH surge when given systemically to ovariectomized rats before the administration of a dose of estradiol, which otherwise will produce such a surge 30 hours later [45]. It is interesting to note that progesterone is an effective signal for eliciting the LH surge in estrogen-primed rats. In view of the demonstration that progesterone receptors are induced in hypothalamus and pituitary by estradiol, it is attractive to suppose that these receptors may mediate the progesterone effect. Although the latency of progesterone action may be as little as 1 hour [58], compared to a latency of nearly 24 hours for estradiol action, a genomic mode of action is still likely (see discussion above). Genomic effects of steroids have been described with an onset latency of 20 minutes [67].

The site of estrogen action on the LH surge is assumed to lie in the region of the hypothalamus and pituitary, but the exact location of these effects is unclear. As a function of time, estrogen appears first to inhibit and then to facilitate the response of the pituitary to the stimulatory effects of luteinizing hormone releasing factor (LH-RF) [68]. One of the peculiar aspects of estrogen action is that this hormone can have both negative and positive feedback effects on gonadotropin secretion. The negative effects tend to have a short latency and duration. Even these effects appear to involve a receptor mechanism, judging from the fact that antiestrogens can block negative feedback [69].

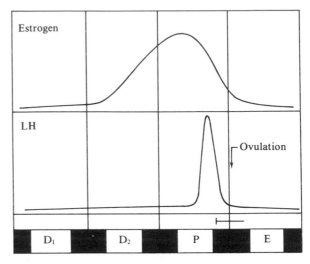

Fig. 39-8. Schematic representation of plasma levels of estrogen and luteinizing hormone (LH) during the 4-day estrous cycle of the female rat. D1, D2 = diestrous days 1 and 2, respectively. P = proestrus; E = estrus. Black panel = night, white panel = day. Bar indicates onset of behavioral estrus.

Concurrently with the neuroendocrine events described above, estrogen acts on target sites in the hypothalamus to prime the sexual behavior of the female rat. The period of behavioral estrus is denoted by the bar in Fig. 39-8, and it is clear that its coordination with ovulation assures a high probability that pregnancy will result from copulation. The estrous female rat shows a number of behavioral changes: increased locomotor activity, characterized by darting motion and dragging the hind quarters to leave a scent; an ear quiver, which may serve as attraction (together with the very important estrous scent) for the sexual motivation of the male; and a decreased food intake, related to the fact that the female in estrus spends less time searching for food and more time searching for a male [16]. Facilitation of lordosis, the mating posture of the female, is also apparent in estrus and is particularly striking because a female not in estrus will run away from or fight off the advances of a male. Implants of estradiol into the ventromedial hypothalamus of the ovariectomized female rat will prime the lordosis response and lead to decreased food intake [68], suggesting that this

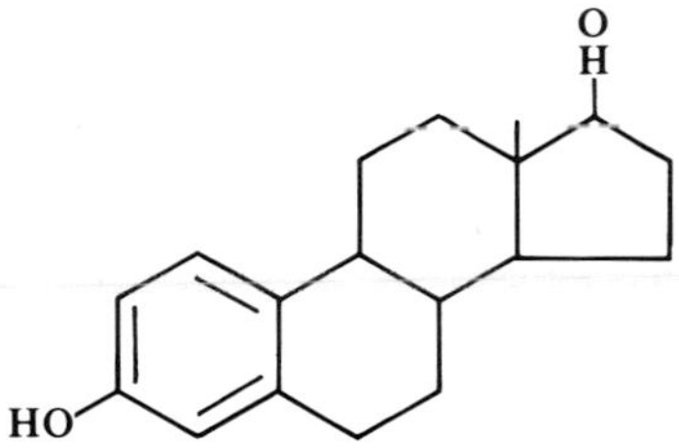

17β-Estradiol

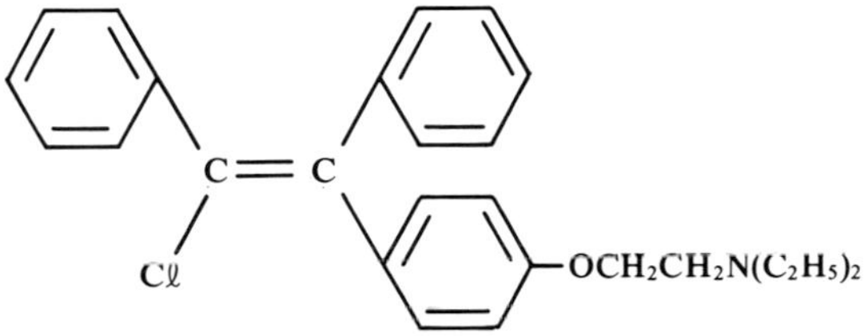

cis-Clomiphene
(MRL-41)

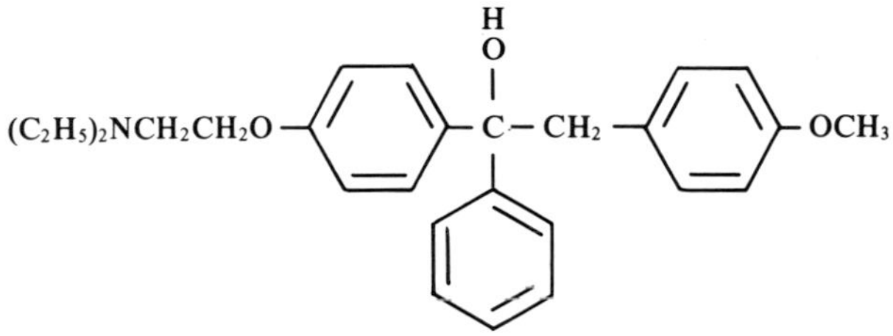

Ethamoxytriphetol
(MER-25)

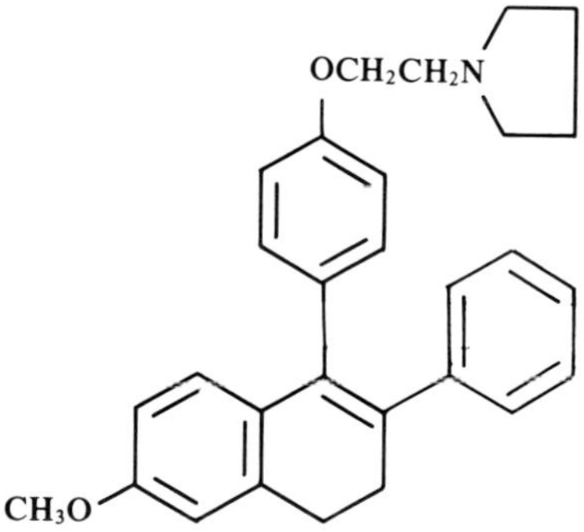

Nafoxidine
(U-11,100)

Fig. 39-9. Formulas of 17β-estradiol and 3 antiestrogens.

part of the hypophysiotropic area of the brain is a target site for the behavioral effects. The role of these receptors is further implicated by experiments using the antiestrogens, MER-25 and *cis*-clomiphene (see Fig. 39-9). These agents, which interfere with estrogen binding to the receptors, block estrogen induction of behavioral receptivity and interfere with behavioral estrus when given during the normal estrous cycle [68]. Actinomycin D, an RNA-synthesis inhibitor, has been reported to block estrogen priming of lordosis. Implantation studies with actinomycin D have delineated the conditions for the action of this drug. It can be given up to 6 hours after estradiol treatment and still have an inhibitory effect over the lordosis response. When the implants are removed, a high percentage of the animals recover their responsiveness to estradiol, indicating that the drug does not simply produce a brain lesion that destroys the capacity to produce the behavior.

Both estrogen induction of the LH surge and estrogen facilitation of lordosis behavior require about 24 hours to be fully manifested. The time course for lordosis is illustrated in Fig. 39-10. The ovariectomized female fails to respond to mounting attempts by the male until more than 16 hours after a single intravenous injection of the steroid. Time-course measurements after a single dose of [^{3}H]-estradiol capable of promoting lordosis behavior reveal that the putative brain and pituitary receptor sites remain occupied for less than 12 hours [68]. The time difference between receptor occupation and the appearance of lordosis behavior, taken together with the actinomycin D effects noted above, suggests that intervening metabolic changes are taking place in the target cells, leading to the change in behavioral responsiveness.

A number of neurochemical markers of gonadal steroid action in brain and pituitary have been uncovered recently. For example, in the pituitary, estradiol treatment induces progestin receptors, increases sensitivity to the LH-releasing effects of LH-RH, and elevates the activity of such oxidative enzymes as glucose 6-phosphate dehydrogenase [68]. In female rat hypothalamus and preoptic area, estradiol induces progestin receptors and

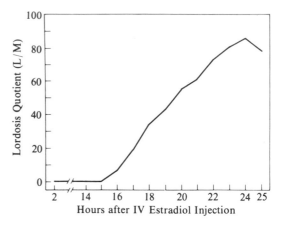

Fig. 39-10. *Time course of lordosis quotient (ratio of lordoses by female to number of times mounted by male) after 100 μg of estradiol was given intravenously. (Redrawn from Green, Luttge, and Whalen, Physiol. Behav. 5:137, 1970. Reprinted with permission of authors and Pergamon Press, copyright 1970.)*

elevates the activity of a number of enzymes, including choline acetyltransferase (ChAT) isocitrate dehydrogenase, and cysteine aminopeptidase. Estrogen treatment depresses the activity of monoamine oxidase in amygdala and hypothalamus. A number of these changes have been shown to be attenuated by the estrogen antagonist MER-25, but MER-25 by itself appears unable to produce similar changes [68]. Another antagonist, CI 628, does mimic estradiol effects on monoamine oxidase and ChAT activities, but it blocks estrogen induction of progestin receptors. It is possible that the effects that are blocked by estrogen antagonists, like progestin-receptor induction, may be related to the behavioral and neuroendocrine effects of estradiol, which are also blocked by these antagonists. The estrogenlike actions of CI 628 may be related to the estrogenlike effects of this drug in mimicking estradiol effects on food intake in the rat [68].

ORGANIZATIONAL EFFECTS OF HORMONES ON DEVELOPING BRAIN

Gonadal Steroids and Sexual Differentiation

During the embryonic development of many vertebrates, the presumptive gonads undergo differen-

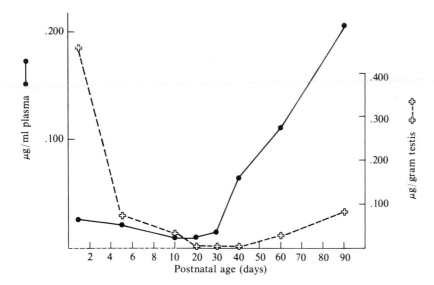

Fig. 39-11. Testosterone levels in plasma (µg per ml) and testis (µg per gram) as a function of postnatal age in days. See [95].

tiation into ovaries or testes as determined by the genetic sex of the animal [70]. In lower vertebrates, especially fish, the gonad retains some of the potentiality to produce gonadal tissue of the opposite sex. As a result, sex reversals can occur under natural conditions or after hormonal administration during adult life. In mammals (and many other vertebrate classes as well), the gonadal tissue is irreversibly determined during early life, and complete sex reversals are not possible.

The secretions of the gonads determine the sex both of the reproductive tract and, apparently, of the brain as well [70, 71]. In mammals and many lower vertebrate classes, the hormonally neutral sex is the female, and testicular secretions determine the differentiation of the male reproductive tract and brain from a basically feminine pattern. In other words, if the testes are removed before this differentiation occurs, the reproductive tract and brain acquire a basically feminine pattern. An important exception to this is found in many species of birds, where the hormonally neutral sex is the male, and ovarian secretion determines feminiza-

tion of brain and body sex from a basically masculine pattern. We shall consider only the mammal, however, and use sexual differentiation of the rat as the principal illustration.

Shortly before the rat is born (and during fetal life in other mammals, including man), the testes secrete substantial amounts of testosterone [71]. This secretion continues for most of the first week of postnatal life (Fig. 39-11). Removal of the testes on the day of birth results in an animal that, as an adult, shows more feminine behavior after estrogen treatment than do animals castrated as adults and that will maintain a cyclic pattern of ovarian secretion when ovaries are implanted. Conversely, if testosterone is administered to female rats on the day of birth or even several days after, the results are animals that, when ovariectomized as adults and treated with gonadal steroids, show more masculine behavior from administration of androgen and less feminine behavior from estrogen than do untreated females ovariectomized as adults. In addition, these androgenized females display anovulatory sterility in the form of persistent vaginal estrus. It should be noted that the reproductive tract of the rat undergoes differentiation during the week preceding birth and is only slightly affected by postnatal manipulations of the type described above.

With respect to brain differentiation, the ability to manipulate neonatally the behavioral responsiveness to gonadal hormones in the adult rat has provided endocrinologists with an excellent experimental system with which to study sexual differentiation of the brain. The two end points usually used to assess such differentiation are, as noted above, the presence or absence of ovulatory cycles and the frequency of occurrence of adult patterns of male or female sexual behavior under gonadal hormone treatment of gonadectomized animals. In this section, we shall consider the neurochemical aspects of sexual differentiation of the brain.

A fundamental problem has been to determine the sites of sexual differentiation within the brain. Several laboratories have shown that ovulation and female sexual behavior are suppressed most effectively by implanting pellets of testosterone in the anterior hypothalamic area and ventromedial hypothalamus; the latter site is perhaps the more effective one [72]. By using implants that can be removed, one laboratory has shown that the minimal exposure time for obtaining anovulatory sterility is at least 48 hours.

Another approach in the localization of neural sites of sexual differentiation has been to measure morphological correlates of the phenomenon. A report by Raisman and Field [73] indicates that neonatal testosterone treatment, as well as the natural secretion of androgen in the neonatal male, results in a decrease in the number of presynaptic endings on dendritic spines within the preoptic area of the rat brain. The origin of these synapses is not known, but it is not the projection of the amygdala via the stria terminalis. Similar morphological differences were not found in the ventromedial hypothalamus, although it is clear from the enormous complexity of synaptic contacts with dendrites and cell bodies that other morphological differences may exist. In fact there is a recent report of a morphological sex difference in the preoptic area of the hamster, involving the shape of the dendritic tree [74]. The region involved turns out to be somewhat different than that studied by Raisman and Field. Another more dramatic sex

difference, again in the preoptic area, was reported for the rat by Gorski and coworkers [75]. This difference is in the size of the medial preoptic nucleus, and it is visible under the light microscope. It appears to be a combination of differences in cell number and in cell size.

A more general conclusion is that, although the preoptic and hypothalamic areas are indeed sites of sexual differentiation, we have no basis for concluding that they are the only sites. For example, recent work has indicated possible effects of treating the neonatal cerebellum with androgen [76].

In view of the long-term organizing effects of neonatal testosterone secretion (or its administration to females) on the sexual differentiation of the brain, it is most attractive to view the primary site of action as the genome of brain cells. There is some evidence for androgen-dependent alterations in the volume of the cell nucleus and incorporation of precursors into RNA in anterior hypothalamus and amygdala during the perinatal period. The most important evidence to date for a genomic role derives, however, from studies of the long-term effects of inhibitors of protein and RNA synthesis on the defeminizing effects of testosterone on ovulatory cycles in female rats [77]. Subcutaneous administration of inhibitors of RNA, protein, and DNA synthesis to 4-day-old female rats, both together with and 6 hours after testosterone propionate in varying doses, blocks or strongly attenuates the development of anovulatory sterility measured on postnatal day 80 [77]. Earlier reports indicated similar effects, although intrahypothalamic administration (in contrast to the subcutaneous route) produced variable results. Thus, while the prognosis for this approach appears to be good, further work is required to delineate the intracranial sites of action of these drugs. One important technical problem is the relatively short period of inhibition produced by the drugs (usually a few hours) in relation to the longer period (at least 48 hours, as noted above) required for the defeminizing effects of testosterone. It is quite likely that a systemic dose of testosterone propionate remains in the body for at least 2 or 3 days. Because of their systemic toxicity, administration of the inhibitory drugs in larger amounts, including repeated administration, risks confounding the experiment.

Testosterone was once assumed to be the active hormone for producing sexual differentiation. This view has been challenged recently, however, on the basis of experiments that compared the potency of various steroids with testosterone. Surprisingly, such estrogens as estradiol and diethylstilbestrol are at least as effective as testosterone in inducing anovulatory sterility and defeminizing behavior [78]. A synthetic estrogen, 11β-methoxy-17α-ethynyl-17β-estradiol (Ru2858), is almost two orders of magnitude more effective than estradiol [79]. 5α-Dihydrotestosterone, the potent androgen, is ineffective in defeminizing behavior or inducing anovulatory sterility in the rat [78].

These findings relate to the discussion of the metabolism of testosterone in the brain and pituitary (see above): Estradiol is formed from testosterone and estrone from androstanedione in hypothalamus and limbic structures but not in pituitary; 5α-DHT is formed from testosterone in pituitary, hypothalamus, and other brain regions. These same transformations are observed to occur in newborn rats. In particular, the aromatization of testosterone to estradiol, which has been observed in vivo as well as in vitro in newborn rats [31, 80], supports the concept that conversion to estrogen may be an obligatory step in sexual differentiation. It should be noted that 5α-DHT cannot be converted to estrogen. Further support for aromatization in sexual differentiation derives from experiments showing that the antiestrogen MER-25 can block testosterone-induced anovulatory sterility in female rats and that another antiestrogen, CI 628, and a competitive inhibitor of aromatization, androst-1,4,6-triene-3,17-dione (ATD), block the defeminizing actions of testosterone on sexual behavior [81]. While there is no doubt that aromatization plays a major role in rat brain sexual differentiation, there may be more to the story, for so-called antiandrogens such as cyproterone acetate and flutamide also interfere with the action of testosterone on brain sexual differentiation [82].

It is conceivable that these drug effects ultimately may be explained by a common mechanism involving aromatization, but it should also be borne in mind that in two other mammalian species, guinea pig and rhesus monkey, there is evidence for a greater role of androgens per se in brain sexual differentiation.

The search for receptors that mediate sexual differentiation must therefore consider both estrogen and androgens. Very little information exists on androgen receptors in the neonatal period, except that receptors resembling those found in adult brain can be found in neonatal mouse brain [83].

The story of estradiol-binding sites in immature brain presents a series of problems. Attempts to measure cytosol estradiol-binding sites led to the discovery of an atypical estradiol-binding protein in fetal and neonatal brains of male and female rats [78]. This protein was found equally in cerebral cortex, hypothalamus, and limbic structures. It bound estradiol but not diethylstilbestrol (which binds to the adult receptor) and disappeared from the brain by the beginning of the fourth postnatal week of life. This protein has a sedimentation coefficient of 4 S, in contrast to the 6 S to 8 S of the adult receptor. By virtue of all of these criteria and the protein's inability to bind columns of DNA cellulose, the protein was judged to be different from the adult receptor and similar to if not identical with a protein found in the blood of fetal and newborn rats. That protein is manufactured in the liver and is the same as the so-called α-fetoprotein [78]. Yet this fetoneonatal estrogen-binding protein (fEBP) remained in the tissue after the brain was perfused to remove blood contamination, and fEBP could be detected in cerebrospinal fluid [78].

The function of such a protein, found in extracellular fluid bathing the brain tissue, as well as in the blood, has been hypothesized to be protective in nature, preventing estrogen present in the maternal blood and estrogen that may be secreted in the neonatal animal from having deleterious, defeminizing effects. Testosterone does not appear to bind to this protein. Thus the hormone secreted by the testes of newborn males is free to enter the brain tissue and produce its effect. Support for the protective role of fEBP has come from studies revealing the ineffectiveness of low doses of estradiol in eliciting sexual differentiation and promoting uterine growth, compared to the potency in comparable doses of a synthetic estrogen that does not bind to the fEBP [78]. Additional support comes from experiments that demonstrate that low doses of [^{3}H]estradiol do not bind in the nuclei of brain cells of female rats until after the fEBP has disappeared from the animal at the beginning of the fourth postnatal week [78].

The detection of estrogen receptor sites in the neonatal rat brain is made possible by a labeled synthetic estrogen, [^{3}H]R2858, which as noted above, does not bind to fEBP and is a highly effective agent for inducing sexual differentiation. R2858 labels cell nuclear sites in vivo at least 30 times more effectively than [^{3}H]estradiol, which binds to EBP. Using [^{3}H]R5828 for in vitro labeling experiments, receptors have been detected in the rat brain as early as the day 21 of gestation (1 day after birth) but not on days 15 or 19. The increase in receptor levels is very rapid from the fetal day 21 (birth on day 22) until the postnatal day 6, after which there is a more gradual rise [84]. Estrogen receptors are found in virtually the same areas of the hypothalamus, preoptic area, and amygdala of the baby and of the adult rat; estrogen receptors are also found in cerebral cortex of the neonate but are absent from the cerebral cortex of the adult [86]. Cortical and hypothalamic estrogen receptors of the neonate resemble each other and resemble receptors of the adult uterus, pituitary, and brain. They translocate estradiol to the cell nucleus. Although they arise at the same time in development, and increase during the same developmental period, cortical but not hypothalamic receptors disappear between postnatal days 12 and 21. The function of cortical estrogen receptors remains obscure.

Due to the presence of fEBP, estrogen receptors are unoccupied in female brains and in the cerebral cortex of male brains for at least the first 8 days of postnatal life [85]. However, in the hypothalamus, preoptic area, and amygdala of the male brain, estrogen receptors are occupied to about 10 percent of their capacity, and this occupation can be detected as early as the receptors themselves can be detected (i.e., around fetal day 21) [84, 85]. Apparently the secretion of testosterone and the enzyme activity that converts testosterone to estradiol appear earlier than the estrogen receptors, which makes it likely that the appearance of the receptors determines the onset of sensitivity of the brain to the effects of testosterone, which are mediated by its conversion to estradiol.

Thyroid Hormone and Brain Development

The euthyroid condition during the first three postnatal weeks of life is essential for normal brain maturation. Both hypothyroidism and hyperthyroid states, induced experimentally, lead to abnormalities in brain structure, chemistry, and behavior. Thyroid hormone deficiency from birth retards myelinization and development of the neuropil, and decreases respiratory activity of brain tissue [87]. Thyroidectomy before day 10 impairs body temperature regulation permanently [87]. Although both RNA and protein content in cerebrum and cerebellum are lower in rats made hypothyroid at birth, total DNA in each structure is normal at day 35, after cell proliferation has ceased, suggesting that absence of thyroid hormones does not reduce total cell numbers but does reduce cell size [88]. In contrast, administration of T$_3$ (triiodothyronine) to euthyroid rats at birth decreases the total number of cells in cerebrum and cerebellum [88].

Synapse formation in the cerebellum has been studied under both hyperthyroid and hypothyroid conditions. The total number of synaptic profiles is decreased in hypothyroid rats after 10 days of age, following chemical thyroidectomy at birth. Hyperthyroidism is associated with an initial increase in synaptic density and number, followed by a reduction in number of synaptic profiles after 21 days of age [89]. Interesting parallels with synapse formation are reported for learning behavior in rats as a result of neonatal hypothyroidism and hyperthyroidism. Learning ability is generally impaired as a result of neonatal hypothyroidism; hyperthyroid rats show an initial acceleration in learning ability but are poorer than euthyroid controls later in life [90].

Attempts to understand the mechanism of thyroid hormone action on the developing brain led one group to the observation that a mitochondrial fraction of neonatal brain (as well as adult and neonatal liver, but not adult brain) responds to thyroid hormone and increases the incorporation of labeled amino acids into protein in vitro [91]. Other evidence for adult pituitary and brain cells points to the existence of possible receptor sites in cell nuclei [41]. Cell nuclear receptor sites that bind iodinated T_3 are found in the late fetal and neonatal rat brain [92]. In whole brain, these sites increase markedly at the time of birth and decrease gradually to reach adult levels during the first month of postnatal life. Receptor sites in cerebellum reach a peak at around 2 weeks of postnatal life, whereas sites in cerebrum are highest immediately after birth [92]. The appearance of T_3-binding sites in neonatal brain cell nuclei precedes by several days of elevation of plasma T_3 levels [92]. Such information is consistent with the above-mentioned effects of T_3 on the structural development of the brain, and the elevated levels of receptors coincides with the critical period of sensitivity to thyroid hormone action. The thyroid state of the animal also affects the sensitivity to gonadal hormones in the perinatal period: the hypothyroid state prolongs the period of sensitivity to the developmental actions of testosterone (see above) [93]; the hyperthyroid state terminates this period of sensitivity prematurely [94]. This latter situation is one of many possible interactions among endocrine factors in the structural and functional maturation of the brain that remain to be elucidated.

Acknowledgments

Research cited in this chapter from the author's laboratory was supported by USPHS Grant NS07080 and by an Institutional Grant RF70095 from the Rockefeller Foundation. The author expresses his appreciation to Mrs. Oksana Wengerchuk for editorial assistance.

References

1. Berthold, A. A. Transplantation der Hoden. *Arch. Anat. Physiol. Wiss. Med.* 16:42–60, 1849.
*2. Beach, F. A. *Hormones and Behavior.* New York: Hoeber, 1948.
*3. Turner, C. D., and Bagnara, J. T. *General Endocrinology* (5th ed.). Philadelphia: Saunders, 1971.
4. Saginor, M., and Horton, R. Reflex release of gonadotrophin and increased plasma testosterone concentration in male rabbits during copulation. *Endocrinology* 82:627–629, 1968.
5. Rose, R. M., Gordon, T. P., and Bernstein, I. S. Plasma testosterone levels in the male rhesus: Influences of sexual and social stimuli. *Science* 178: 643–645, 1972.
6. Anon. Effects of sexual activity on beard growth in man. *Nature* 226:869–870, 1970. See also *Nature* 226:1277, 1970.
7. Bohus, B. Pituitary Adrenal Influences on Avoidance and Approach Behavior of the Rat. In E. Zimmerman, W. H. Gispen, B. Marks, and D. de Wied (eds.), *Progress in Brain Research.* Vol. 39, Drug effects on Neuroendocrine Regulation. Amsterdam: Elsevier, 1973, pp. 407–419.
*8. McEwen, B. S., Gerlach, J. L., and Micco, D. J., Jr. Putative Glucocorticoid Receptors in Hippocampus and Other Regions of the Rat Brain. In R. Isaacson, and K. Pribram (eds.), *The Hippocampus: A Comprehensive Treatise.* New York: Plenum, 1975. Pp. 285–322.
9. Moss, R. L., and McCann, S. M. Induction of mating behavior in rats by luteinizing hormone-releasing factor. *Science* 181:177–179, 1973.
10. Pfaff, D. W. Luteinizing hormone-releasing factor potentiates lordosis behavior in hypophysectomized ovariectomized female rats. *Science* 182:1148–1149, 1973.
*11. Prange, A. J., Jr. *The Thyroid Axis, Drugs, and Behavior.* New York: Raven, 1974.
12. Friedman, E., Friedman, J., and Gershon, S. Dopamine synthesis: Stimulation by a hypothalamic factor. *Science* 182:831–832, 1973.
13. Keller, H. H., Bartholini, G., and Pletscher, A. Enhancement of cerebral noradrenaline turnover by thyrotropin-releasing hormone. *Nature* 248: 528–529, 1974.
14. van Wimersma Greidanus, Tj. B., Bohus, B., and de Wied, D. Differential localization of the in-

*Key reference.

fluence of lysine vasopressin and of ACTH 4-10 on avoidance behavior: A study in rats bearing lesions in the parafascicular nuclei. *Neuroendocrinology* 14:280–288, 1974.

15. Kastin, A. J., Dempsey, G. L., Le Blanc, B., Dyster-Aas, K., and Schally, A. V. Extinction of an appetitive operant response after administration of MSH. *Horm. Behav.* 5:135–140, 1974.

*16. McEwen, B. S., and Pfaff, D. W. Chemical and Physiological Approaches to Neuroendocrine Mechanisms: Attempts at Integration. In L. Martini, and W. F. Ganong (eds.), *Frontiers in Neuroendocrinology*. New York: Oxford University Press, 1973. Pp. 267–335.

17. Rosenblatt, J. S. Views on the Onset and Maintenance of Maternal Behavior in the Rat. In L. R. Aronson, E. Tobach, D. S. Lehrman, and J. S. Rosenblatt (eds.), *Development and Evolution of Behavior: Essays in Memory of T. C. Schneirla.* San Francisco: Freeman, 1970. Pp. 489–515.

18. Johnston, P., and Davidson, J. M. Intracerebral androgens and sexual behavior in the male rat. *Horm. Behav.* 3:345–351, 1972.

19. Owen, K., Peters, P. J., and Bronson, F. H. Effects of intracranial implants of testosterone propionate on intermale aggression in the castrated male mouse. *Horm. Behav.* 5:83–92, 1974.

20. Yahr, P., and Thiessen, D. D. Steroid regulation of territorial scent marking in the Mongolian gerbil (*Meriones unguiculatus*). *Horm. Behav.* 3:359–368, 1972.

21. Mann, D. R., and Barraclough, C. A. Role of estrogen and progesterone in facilitating LH release in 4-day cyclic rats. *Endocrinology* 93:694–699, 1973.

22. Whalen, R. E., and Gorzalka, B. B. The effects of progesterone and its metabolites on the induction of sexual receptivity in rats. *Horm. Behav.* 3:221–226, 1972.

23. Erickson, C. J., Bruder, R. H., Komisaruk, B. R., and Lehrman, D. S. Selective inhibition by progesterone of androgen-induced behavior in male ring doves (*Streptopella risoria*). *Endocrinology* 81:39–44, 1967.

24. Erpino, M. J. Temporary inhibition by progesterone of sexual behavior in intact male mice. *Horm. Behav.* 4:35–339, 1973.

25. Griffo, W., and Lee, C. T. Progesterone antagonism of androgen-dependent marking in gerbils. *Horm. Behav.* 4:351–358, 1973.

26. Luttge, W. G. Activation and inhibition of isolation induced inter-male fighting behavior in castrate male CD-1 mice treated with steroidal hormones. *Horm. Behav.* 3:71–81, 1972.

27. Ross, G. E., and Zucker, I. Progesterone and the ovarian-adrenal modulation of energy balance in rats. *Horm. Behav.* 5:43–62, 1974.

28. Denef, C., Magnus, C., and McEwen, B. S. Sex differences and hormonal control of testosterone metabolism in rat pituitary and brain. *J. Endocrinol.* 59:605–621, 1973.

29. Feder, H. H. The comparative actions of testosterone propionate and 5α androstan 17β ol 3 one propionate on the reproductive behavior, physiology, and morphology of male rats. *J. Endocrinol.* 51:241–252, 1971.

30. Massa, R., and Martini, L. Interference with the 5α Reductase System: A New Approach for Developing Antiandrogens. In P. O. Hubinont, S. M. Hendeles, and P. Preumont (eds.), *Hormones and Antagonists:* Proceedings of the 4th International Seminar on Reproductive Physiology and Sexual Endocrinology, Brussels, May 23–25, 1972. Reprinted from *Gynecol. Invest.* Vol. 2, No. 1–6, 1971/2, and Vol. 3, No. 1–4, 1972.

31. Naftolin, F., Ryan, K. J., Davies, I. J., Reddy, V. V., Flores, F., Petro, Z., and Kuhn, M. The formation of estrogens by central neuroendocrine tissues. *Rec. Prog. Horm. Res.* 31:291–315, 1975.

32. Lieburg, I., and McEwen, B. S. Estradiol-17β: A metabolite of testosterone recovered in cell nuclei from limbic areas of adult male rat brains. *Brain Res.* 91:171–174, 1975b.

33. Callard, G. V., Petro, Z., and Ryan, K. J. Identification of aromatase in the reptilian brain. *Endocrinology* 100:1214–1218, 1977.

34. Kelley, D. B., Lieburg, I., McEwen, B. S., and Pfaff, D. W. Autoradiographic and biochemical studies of steroid hormone-concentrating cells in the brain of *rana pipiens. Brain Res.* 140:287–305, 1978.

35. Davis, P. G., and Barfield, R. J. Activation of masculine behavior by intracranial estradiol benzoate implants in male rats. *Neuroendocrinology* 28:217–227, 1979.

36. Christensen, L. W., and Clemens, L. G. Blockade of testosterone-induced mounting behavior in the male rat with intracranial application of the aromatization inhibitor, androst-1,4,6-triene-3,17-dione. *Endocrinology* 97:1545–1551, 1975.

37. Morali, G., Larsson, K., and Beyer, C. Inhibition of testosterone-induced sexual behavior in the castrated male rat by aromatase blockers. *Horm. Behav.* 9:203–213, 1977.

38. Alsum, P., and Goy, R. W. Actions of esters of testosterone, dihydrotestosterone, or estradiol on sexual behavior in castrated male guinea pigs. *Horm. Behav.* 5:207–217, 1974.

39. Phoenix, C. H.   Effects of dihydrotestosterone on sexual behavior of castrated male rhesus monkeys. *Physiol. Behav.* 12:1045–1055, 1974.

40. McEwen, B. S., Zigmond, R. E., and Gerlach, J. L. Sites of steroid binding and action in the brain. In G. H. Bourne (ed.), *Structure and Function of Nervous Tissue.* New York: Academic, 1972. Vol. 5, pp. 205–291.

41. Oppenheimer, J. H., Schwartz, H. L., and Surks, M. I.   Tissue differences in the concentration of triiodothyronine nuclear binding sites in the rat: Liver, kidney, pituitary, heart, brain, spleen and testis. *Endocrinology* 95:897–903, 1974.

42. King, R. J. B., and Mainwaring, W. I. P.   *Steroid-Cell Interactions.* Baltimore: University Park Press, 1974.

43. Feinendegen, L. E.   *Tritium-Labelled Molecules in Biology and Medicine.* New York: Academic, 1967.

44. McEwen, B. S., and Zigmond, R. E.   Isolation of Brain Cell Nuclei. In N. Marks, and R. Rodnight (eds.), *Research Methods in Neurochemistry.* New York: Plenum, 1972. Vol. 1, pp. 140–161.

45. McEwen, B. S.   Gonadal steroid receptors in neuroendocrine tissues. In B. O'Malley, and L. Birnbaumer (eds.), *Hormone Receptors. Steroid Hormones.* New York: Academic, 1978. Vol. I, pp. 353–400.

46. Pfaff, D. W., and Keiner, M.   Atlas of estradiol-concentrating cells in the central nervous system of the female rat. *J. Comp. Neurol.* 151:121–158, 1973.

47. Barley, J., Ginsburg, M., Greenstein, B. D., Maclusky, N. J., and Thomas, P. J.   An androgen receptor in rat brain and pituitary. *Brain Res.* 100: 383–393, 1975.

48. Lieberburg, I., Maclusky, N. J., and McEwen, B. S.   5α dihydrotestosterone receptors in rat brain and pituitary cell nuclei. *Endocrinology* 100: 598–607, 1977.

49. Ginsburg, M., and Shori, D. K.   Are there distinct dihydrotestosterone and testosterone receptors in brain? *J. Steroid Biochem.* 9:437–441, 1978.

50. Sar, M., and Stumpf, W. E.   Distribution of androgen target cells in rat forebrain and pituitary after ^{3}H-dihydrotestosterone administration. *J. Steroid Biochem.* 8:1131–1135, 1977.

51. deVellis, J., and Inglish, D.   Hormonal control of glycerol phosphate dehydrogenase in the rat brain. *J. Neurochem.* 15:1061–1070, 1968.

52. Leveille, P. J., McGinnis, J. F., Maxwell, D. S., and deVellis, J.   Immunocytochemical localization of glycerol-3-phosphate dehydrogenase in rat oligodendrocytes. *Brain Res.* 196:287–305, 1980.

53. Meyer, J. S., Leveille, P. J., McEwen, B. S., and deVellis, J.   Corticoids and glial cells: Glycerol-phosphate dehydrogenase induction and cytosol binding in normal and degenerated rat optic nerve. Endocrine Society Annual Meeting, Miami, 1978, p. 278. Abstract 406.

54. Kato, J., and Onouchi, T.   Specific progesterone receptors in the hypothalamus and anterior hypophysis of the rat. *Endocrinology* 101:920–928, 1977.

55. Moguilewsky, M., and Raynaud, J-P.   Progestin binding sites in the rat hypothalamus, pituitary and uterus. *Steroids* 30:99–109, 1977.

56. Maclusky, N. J., and McEwen, B. S.   Oestrogen modulates progestin receptor concentrations in some rat brain regions but not in others. *Nature* 274:276–278, 1978.

57. Blaustein, J. D., and Wade, G. N.   Progestin binding by brain and pituitary cell nuclei and female rat sexual behavior. *Brain Res.* 140:360–367, 1978.

58. Kubli-Garfias, C., and Whalen, R. E.   Induction of lordosis behavior in female rats by intravenous administration of progestins. *Horm. Behav.* 9: 380–386, 1977.

59. Sar, M., and Stumpf, W. E.   Neurons of the hypothalamus concentrate ^{3}H-progesterone or its metabolites. *Science* 182:1266–1268, 1973.

60. Warembourg, M.   Uptake of ^{3}H-labeled synthetic progestin by rat brain and pituitary. A radioautographic study. *Neurosci. Lett.* 9:329–332, 1981.

61. Maclusky, N. J., Lieberburg, I., Krey, L. C., and McEwen, B. S.   Progestin receptors in the brain and pituitary of the bonnet monkey (*Macaca radiata*): Differences between the monkey and the rat in the distribution of progestin receptors. *Endocrinology* 106:185–191, 1980.

62. McEwen, B. S.   Influences of adrenocortical hormones on pituitary and brain function. In G. Rousseau and J. Baxter (eds.), *Mechanisms of Glucocorticoid Action.* New York: Springer-Verlag, 1978. Pp. 467–492.

63. Ermisch, A., and Rühle, H-J.   Autoradiographic demonstration of aldosterone-concentrating neuron populations in rat brain. *Brain Res.* 147:154–158, 1978.

64. Butcher, R. L., Collins, W. E., and Fugo, N. W. Plasma concentration of LH, FSH, prolactin, progesterone, and estradiol 17β throughout the 4-day estrous cycle of the rat. *Endocrinology* 94: 1704–1708, 1974.

65. Ferin, M., Tempone, A., Zimmering, P. A., and Van de Wiele, R. I.   Effect of antibodies to 17β estradiol and progesterone on the estrous cycle of the rat. *Endocrinology* 85:1070–1078, 1969.

66. Clark, J. H., Peck, E. J., and Anderson, J. N. Oestrogen receptors and antagonism of steroid hormone action. *Nature* 251:446–448, 1974.

67. Makman, M. H., Dvorkin, D., and White, A.   Evidence for induction by cortisol *in vitro* of a protein inhibitor of transport and phosphorylation processes in rat thymocytes. *Proc. Natl. Acad. Sci. U.S.A.* 68:1269–1273, 1971.

68. McEwen, B. S., Davis, P. G., Parsons, B., and Pfaff, D. W.   The brain as a target for steroid hormone action. In M. Cowan (ed.), *Annual Review of Neuroscience*. Vol. 2. Ann. Rev. Inc., Palo Alto, pp. 65–112, 1979.

69. Krey, L. C., Lieberburg, I., Roy, E., and McEwen, B. S.   Estradiol + receptor complexes in the brain and anterior pituitary gland: Quantitation and neuroendocrine significance. *J. Steroid Biochem.* 11:279–284, 1979.

70. Burns, R. K.   Role of hormones in the differentiation of sex. In W. C. Young (ed.), *Sex and Internal Secretions* (3rd ed.). Baltimore: Williams & Wilkins, 1961. Vol. I, pp. 76–158.

71. Goy, R. W.   Early hormonal influences on the development of sexual and sex-related behavior. In F. O. Schmitt (ed.), *The Neurosciences: Second Study Program*. New York: Rockefeller University Press, 1970. Pp. 196–206.

72. Hayashi, S., and Gorski, R. A.   Critical exposure time for androgenization by intracranial crystals of testosterone proprionate in neonatal female rats. *Endocrinology* 94:1161–1167, 1974.

73. Raisman, G., and Field, P. M.   Sexual dimorphism in the neuropil of the preoptic area of the rat and its dependence on neonatal androgen. *Brain Res.* 54:1–29, 1973.

74. Greenough, W. T., Carter, C. S., Steerman, C., and DeVoogd, T.   Sex differences in dendritic patterns in hamster preoptic area. *Brain Res.* 126:63–72, 1977.

75. Gorski, R. A., Gordon, J. H., Shryne, J. E., and Southam, A. M.   Evidence for a morphological sex difference within the medial preoptic area of the rat brain. *Brain Res.* 148:333–346, 1978.

76. Litteria, M., and Thorner, M. W.   Inhibition of the incorporation of ^{3}H lysine in the Purkinje cells of the adult female rat after neonatal androgenization. *Brain Res.* 69:170–173, 1974.

77. Salaman, D. F., and Birkett, S.   Androgen-induced sexual differentiation of the brain is blocked by inhibitors of DNA and RNA synthesis. *Nature* 247:109–112, 1974.

78. Plapinger, L., and McEwen, B. S.   Gonadal steroid-brain interactions in sexual differentiation. In J. Hutchinson (ed.), *Biological Determinants of Sexual Behavior*. New York: Wiley, 1977. Pp. 193–218.

79. Doughty, C., Booth, J. E., McDonald, P. G., and Parrott, R. F.   Effects of oestradiol 17β, oestradiol benzoate, and the synthetic oestrogen, Ru2858, on sexual differentiation in the neonatal female rat. *J. Endocrinol.* 67:419–424, 1975.

80. Lieberburg, I., Wallach, G., and McEwen, B. S.   The effects of an inhibitor of aromatization (1,4,6-androstatriene-3,17-dione) and an anti-estrogen (CI-628) on *in vivo* formed testosterone metabolites recovered from neonatal rat brain tissues and purified cell nuclei. Implications for sexual differentiation of the rat brain. *Brain Res.* 128:176–181, 1977.

81. McEwen, B. S., Lieberburg, I., Chaptal, C., and Krey, L. C.   Aromatization: Important for sexual differentiation of the neonatal rat brain. *Horm. Behav.* 9:249–263, 1978.

82. Gladue, B. A., and Clemens, L. G.   Androgenic influences on feminine sexual behavior in male and female rats: Defeminization blocked by prenatal antiandrogen treatment. *Endocrinology* 103:1702–1709, 1978.

83. Attardi, B., and Ohno, S.   Androgen and estrogen receptors in the developing mouse brain. *Endocrinology* 99:1279–1290, 1976.

84. Maclusky, N. J., Lieberburg, I., and McEwen, B. S.   The development of estrogen receptor systems in the rat brain: Perinatal development. *Brain Res.* 178:129–142, 1979a,b.

85. Lieberburg, I., Krey, L. C., and McEwen, B. S.   Sex differences in serum testosterone and in exchangeable brain cell nuclear estradiol during the neonatal period in rats. *Brain Res.* 178:207–212, 1979.

86. McEwen, B. S., Plapinger, L., Chaptal, C., Gerlach, J., and Wallach, G.   Role of fetoneonatal estrogen binding proteins in the association of estrogen with neonatal brain cell nucleus receptors. *Brain Res.* 96:400–406, 1975.

87. Hamburgh, M.   An analysis of the action of thyroid hormone on development based on in vivo and in vitro studies. *Gen. Comp. Endocrinol.* 10:198–213, 1968.

88. Balasz, R.   Effects of hormones on the biochemical maturation of the brain. In D. H. Ford (ed.), *Influence of Hormones on the Nervous System*. Proceedings International Society of Psychoneuroendocrinology, Brooklyn, 1970. Basel: Karger, 1971, pp. 150–164.

89. Nicholson, J. L., and Altman, J.   Synaptogenesis in the rat cerebellum: Effects of early hypo and hyperthyroidism. *Science* 176:530–531, 1972.

90. Eayrs, J. T.   Endocrine influence on cerebral development. *Arch. Biol.* (Liege) 75:529–565, 1964.

91. Sokoloff, L., and Roberts, P.   Biochemical mechanisms of the action of the thyroid hormones in nervous and other tissues. In D. H. Ford (ed.), *Influence of Hormones on the Nervous System*.

Proceedings International Society of Psychoneuro-endocrinology, Brooklyn, 1970. Basel: Karger, 1971. Pp. 213–230.

92. Schwartz, H. L., and Oppenheimer, J. H. Ontogenesis of 3,5,3'-Triiodothyronine receptors in neonatal rat brain: Dissociation between receptor concentration and stimulation of oxygen consumption by 3,5,3'-Triiodothyronine. *Endocrinology* 103:943–948, 1978.

93. Kikuyama, S. Alteration by neonatal hypo-thyroidism of the critical period for the induction of persistent estrus in the rat. *Endocrinol. Japon.* 16: 269–273, 1969.

94. Phelps, C. P., and Sawyer, C. H. Postnatal thyroxine modifies effects of early androgen on lordosis. *Horm. Behav.* 7:331–340, 1976.

95. Resko, J. A., Feder, H. H., and Goy, R. W. Androgen concentrations in plasma and testis of developing rats. *J. Endocrinol.* 40:485–491, 1968.

Bernard W. Agranoff

Chapter 40. Learning and Memory: Biochemical Approaches

It is difficult to ask a question more likely to generate conflicting opinions than that of how the brain encodes, stores, and retrieves behavioral information. Little disagreement exists on this puzzle's inherent intellectual challenge or that clinical benefits would likely follow its solution. Conflicts arise from the enormous complexity of the problem, which, together with a rather meager list of experimentally generated constraints, have permitted the continuous generation of hypotheses, often untestable. There is a vast literature on human and animal learning and memory, but experimental results are frequently not comparable. Factors such as the species—and even the strain—of animal used, the details of construction of the experimental apparatus, training sequence, conditions of animal housing, and other factors appear to affect measured behavior drastically. Nevertheless, the various experiments have all been directed at answering the same question: What are the changes that take place in the brain during a few seconds (or less) of experience that will mediate the resulting altered response of an organism for long periods, even for a lifetime? That such changes are permanent and are resistant to subsequently imposed "electrical storms" and "silences" of the brain points to an underlying molecular process leading to covalent structural changes. The various investigations described in this chapter constitute attempts to establish, by chemical and behavioral means, the nature of the physiological changes that lead to the altered performance of an animal measured at various times after a training experience. Experimental approaches can generally be categorized as being either interventive or correlative. That is, we either observe the effects of an extraneous agent, such as a drug, on behavior, or we measure bio-

chemical changes in the brain that accompany behavioral processes. The principal appeal of specific interventive agents is that they permit the block of discrete metabolic processes in the otherwise intact, behaving animal. They have the great disadvantage that one cannot readily distinguish their known actions from possible unknown effects that could lead to altered behavior. Whereas the interventive approach limits us, at best, to inferences about what is going on physiologically, it has the capacity to tell us when and where in the brain a critical process is occurring. In the correlative approach, specific biochemical events are compared and measured in both control and experimental animals. The great potential advantage is that the behavioral process is not perturbed by the experimental probe. Although beset with technical problems, this approach has the attraction that it might eventually identify biochemical processes involved in memory formation.

A number of experimental approaches to the study of brain plasticity are included in this chapter. Additional background is available in previous editions of this book, as well as in a number of relevant reviews, so indicated in the reference list.

Consolidation and Stages of Memory Formation

Our present concept of memory formation and storage began with the observations of the last century that physical trauma to the human brain results in loss of memory [1]. Typically, a blow to the head may lead to a *retrograde amnesia,* that is, loss of memory for events immediately preceding the trauma. The common interpretation of this phenomenon is that memory ordinarily forms after the actual experience, and that "fixation," or *consolidation* of long-term memory (LTM) is blocked by physiological consequences of the blow. A similar conclusion was drawn from animal experiments in which electroconvulsive shock (ECS) administered after training was shown to result in poor subsequent performance, whereas the same treatment given some time after training had no effect. In each instance, the increasing stability of memory following training is thought to reflect a physiological process of consolidation, whereby memory is converted from an unstable, or labile, form to a permanent one. A consolidation process has been observed in innumerable studies, but its reported duration varies from seconds to many hours, depending on the species, the training task, and the disruptive agent employed [2].

Not all psychologists accept the consolidation concept, and alternative explanations for the developing strength of memory with passage of time after training have been offered. It has been argued, for example, that the experimental amnestic treatments, by ECS or some other means, are noxious, and the subject withholds the learned response in order to avoid punishment. The amnestic agent has alternatively been postulated to interfere with performance in some nonspecific way, such as by creating spurious electrical effects in the neuronal networks that mediate the new behavior. Both of these explanations argue that the new memory is not obliterated by the amnestic agent, and that some superimposed process prevents its retrieval. The contraconsolidation arguments might state that after a physical blow to the head, resultant fear or pain has repressed events closely associated in time with the trauma. It can thus be argued that whether there is electrical or behavioral interference with retrieval, learning and formation of memory occur simultaneously during the training session. Although this issue has not been completely resolved, the consolidation hypothesis has gained considerable support from interventive studies like those described in this chapter.

Measurement of Learning and Memory

LEARNING PARADIGMS

Learning could be considered an expression of brain plasticity, and relevant neurochemical in-

sights might be gleaned from biochemical knowledge of such diverse topics as development and regeneration, or of nonassociative behaviors, such as habituation and sensitization, described below. But to the behaviorist, the sine qua non of learning and memory formation is the *conditioned response,* which has served him as the fruitfly long served the geneticist. Commonly, distinction is made between two kinds of associative learning, *classical* and *instrumental* (or *operant*) *conditioning* [3]. In classical, or Pavlovian, conditioning, a stimulus is conditioned by pairing with a subsequent unconditioned stimulus-response sequence. For example, an animal is exposed to a light flash (the conditioned stimulus, CS), followed by a mild electrical shock (the unconditioned stimulus, UCS), which elicits an escape response in the untrained animal. After several pairings, the escape response, or a related one, is seen after presentation of the unpaired CS. In classical conditioning, the UCS presentations do not depend on the animal's response. For example, the animal may be given an inescapable shock. In instrumental conditioning, the response of the subject (such as pressing a bar) determines whether it will receive the UCS. Instead of an aversive stimulus, the UCS may be a reward, such as food, for either type of conditioning.

In most species used, a negative (aversive) UCS results in faster learning and perhaps more lasting memory than does a reward (positive reinforcement). Measured responses may be considered to be either active or passive. In a step-down task, for example, a mouse learns that its natural tendency to step down from a small pedestal results in a mild electrical shock to the foot, and it learns to remain on the pedestal (*passive avoidance*). Alternatively, an animal can be taught that shortly after a light or sound warning signal, it must leave the chamber in which it has been placed (e.g., by jumping over a hurdle) to avoid a punishing foot shock (*active avoidance*).

A further refinement in training techniques is *discrimination learning*. Animals learn to choose, for example, a given limb of an apparatus on the basis of position (right or left), illumination (light or dark), color, geometrical pattern, or other characteristics. An animal may be placed in the

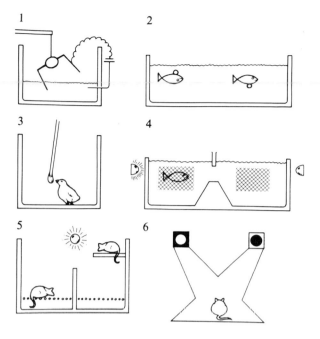

Fig. 40-1. Several training tasks used in the measurement of learning and memory, described in the text.
(1) The headless-insect preparation used to condition a position habit. The suspended experimental leg is shocked when it touches a water reservoir. After several shocks, an elevated position is maintained. The opposite leg does not acquire the new position. (2) Restoration of posture in the goldfish (see text). After a styrofoam float is sutured to the lower jaw (shown on left), fish recover the upright position (shown on right). (3) One-trial avoidance. Newly hatched chicks peck at a glass rod containing a bitter substance, methyl anthranilite. The next day they avoid an uncoated rod. (4) An automated shuttle-box used for goldfish learning an avoidance response to a light stimulus coupled with shock. The light signal is administered to the side of the apparatus which the fish initially occupies. After 15 seconds, if the fish has not escaped to the darkened side, shock is applied to the water through grids. Fish position is determined by photodetectors. (5) A jump-up task for mice. After the CS (a light and buzzer) has been presented, the mouse learns to jump up on a shelf to avoid shock administered through floor grids (right side). On the mouse's escape, the shock to the floor is terminated. The yoked control mouse (left side) receives the same sequence of light and shock, even though it cannot escape. (6) A Y-maze used to teach a discrimination task. Choice of the correct limb results in reward, or avoidance of an aversive stimulus.

starting box (the stem of a Y-maze) and be forced to choose one arm of the maze by application of foot shock in the stem and the other arm of the maze. This is an escape discrimination task in which the subject learns to select the safe arm. In the avoidance variant of this training task, a warning signal is given prior to shock onset, and only those trials in which the animal avoids shock by selecting the safe arm prior to shock onset are scored as correct. Alternatively, food or water reward may be located in one arm. Discrimination tasks have the advantage of minimizing the effects of illness in an experimental subject. If a subject is sick after drug treatment, it is unlikely that the illness will influence the choice in a discrimination task, even though motor performance is impaired. In nondiscriminative avoidance tasks, such as the step-down task, the rate or speed of response might be the index of learning employed, and the animal's state of health could easily affect recorded scores. Thus, it would seem that discrimination tasks are preferable, but timed, nondiscriminative paradigms have several advantages. For example, in the step-down task, a naive animal will step down within 5 sec of being placed on a pedestal, whereas it may take more than 30 seconds after foot shock. By using this response, quick (one-trial) learning is measured rapidly. The score for a single trial in a two-choice discrimination task, on the other hand, is not informative, because on a random basis, an animal will make the correct response 50 percent of the time. Discrimination learning thus requires many trials; and unless an automated apparatus is used, the process limits the number of animals that can be trained by the investigator. Various training procedures are depicted in Fig. 40-1.

METHODS OF QUANTITATION

If we consider *learning* to be a change in performance as a result of training, then *memory* is the demonstration of that new performance at later times. In associative learning experiments, we generally rely on a single characteristic of the animal's response, even though many physiological factors may contribute to the observed overt behavior. One is confronted with a variety of numbers after the experiment. These may include latency (the time between onset of stimulus and response); the tally of correct and incorrect responses for segments of the training session (first five trials, second five trials, etc.); and various other criteria that can be established before, or even after, an experiment (e.g., 9 out of 10 correct responses). From these, the investigator must decide which best measures the "amount" of memory. He might use raw scores (such as number of correct responses), percent of correct responses in trained subjects relative to untrained subjects, or a number of other scoring systems. None of these would a priori seem to be more valid than another, yet opposite conclusions sometimes can be drawn from a given set of data, depending on which scoring method is used. Often, however, the calculated results are not directly comparable to those of another laboratory because of the differences in scoring methods. Given these problems, it is not surprising that conflicting conclusions are often reached.

Loss of memory is variously referred to as *extinction,* forgetting, or amnesia, depending upon the experimental history of the subject [2, 3]. If memory reappears after apparent loss, it is generally proposed that the subject did not lose memory, but was temporarily unable to retrieve it. Dosage-response curves and temporal gradients frequently demonstrate partial impairments of memory. In such instances, we are faced with the dilemma of whether some fraction of the specific components of the learned behavior is lost or whether there is a general impairment of all the components. In experiments in which amnesia has been produced by ECS after training, the "lost" memory can be regained by means of a behavioral "reminder" in some instances [4]. Since performance of the learned response could involve a number of necessary physiological components, the impairment of any one would result in the loss of performance, and its restitution could permit performance of the learned response. The amnesia in this case appears to be for some subset of memories necessary for performance of the measured response.

Experimental Preparations

THE INTACT ANIMAL

For many years, the laboratory rat dominated physiological psychology. Its hardiness under adverse laboratory conditions is somewhat balanced by the disadvantage that much interesting innate behavior may have been bred out of this now-docile beast. For example, it is now recognized that the albino rat has very limited vision. Much variation from experiment to experiment and from laboratory to laboratory can be attributed to diurnal variation and seasonal effects on behavior. Differences in behavior among strains have long been recognized [5]. Inbred strains can vary from supplier to supplier, as can conditions of rearing. Strains of mice that are genetically homogeneous are available, and may reduce this source of variability. For biochemical studies on behavior, mice have the additional advantage, relative to rats, that they are less expensive and require less expenditure in radioisotope costs by virtue of their small size.

Birds also have proved suitable for behavioral studies. The pigeon has long been a standard subject, especially for instrumental conditioning. Although biochemical studies are as yet limited, the songbird has attracted attention because of its lateralization of certain higher functions, a property of the human brain that is largely unknown in other species. The nervous system of the newly hatched chick is myelinated and capable of a repertoire of behavioral responses. Other advantages of the chick are its small size and a relatively undeveloped blood-brain barrier that facilitates the entry of drugs into the brain. Hatcheries dispose of male chicks, so they are usually inexpensive and available. Newly hatched ducklings and chicks also exhibit imprinting phenomena useful in behavioral studies (see below).

Fish have long been studied extensively, from the standpoint of both learning and LTM formation. Because they are cold-blooded, temperature can readily be introduced as an experimental variable. Regeneration occurs in the fish CNS, a property that has made possible studies on specification and regrowth [6, 7]. A gynogenetic strain, *Poecilia formosa,* permits experiments with genetically invariant subjects [8]. Other useful properties include imprinting of the homing response in some teleosts through a highly developed olfactory system and conditioning paradigms that employ the lateral-line system [9]. Fish and birds, unlike land mammals, have highly developed color vision.

Learning has been reported in virtually every readily available species. To say that a species is incapable of demonstrating learning and memory is unwise, because revelation of a new training paradigm can transform a subject from nonlearner to learner status. The search for a useable invertebrate model has met with limited, but increasing, success. Touch and light pairing has been studied extensively in protozoa, and well-documented examples of habituation have been reported in micrometazoa [10, 11]. Coelenterates have an elementary nervous system, and habituation has been reported, as well as learning. "Bait-shyness," the rejection of food previously coupled with an aversive stimulus, has been claimed for a wide variety of species, from sea anemone to human [12, 13]. That planarians can learn is generally accepted, but whether they can retain what they have learned for a long period is less apparent. This uncertainty precludes, for the present, conclusions regarding more complex experiments with this species, such as the chemical transfer of memory. Yerkes, studying a single annelid worm, reported in 1912 that it learned a right-left discrimination task [14]. Behavioral studies of nematodes may be spurred by recent ultrastructural mapping of the brain of *Caenorhabditis elegans* (258 neurons) [15]. Its rapid life cycle and the convenience of storing mutants at low temperatures are attractive experimentally. On the negative side, observable behaviors are limited (swimming appears to be myogenic), and the neurons are too small to penetrate for electrophysiological studies. Larger neurons are seen in *Ascaris*. Echinoderms have been relatively little studied, although learning has been reported in the starfish. Among the mollusks, the octopus can be trained to respond to various visual or tactile stimuli and to retain (for many hours) what it has learned [16]. A number of non-associative behaviors have been observed in

Aplysia, a sea slug, for which there exists an extensive electrophysiological, anatomical, and neurochemical background [17]. Behavioral studies with intact arthropods are dominated by *Drosophila*. While its small size requires special neurochemical methods, *Drosophila* behavioral mutants have been studied extensively by means of various ultrastructural and interventive methods [18]. Considering the size of species in the class Insecta, subjects may yet be discovered that are more ideal for a combined behavioral-genetic study than those that are presently being used. Readers fortunate enough to have seen a flea circus can attest to the potential behavioral skills of insects.

REDUCED SYSTEMS

As a result of ablation studies in the rat, Lashley concluded that all of the brain was involved in learning. His hypothesis of mass action survives in holographic theories of learning and memory [19]. In general, however, that hypothesis has lost ground to connectionist models, which suggest learning and memory reside in specific neuronal ensembles. A number of attempts have been made to demonstrate learned behavior, using only part of the nervous system. For example, the headless insect has been shown to acquire a position habit [20] (see Fig. 40-1,1). Electrodes are connected to a right and left leg of the same segment. When the tip of a leg touches a saline bath beneath it, an electrical contact is made so that leg position (either in or out of the bath) is recorded. Under these conditions, the two legs move independently. During the experiment, a mild shock is administered to the experimental leg whenever it contacts the bath. The paired, or "yoked," leg moves in and out of the bath, but is shocked whenever the experimental leg is extended. It receives as much shock as the experimental leg, but not in relation to a specific position. During a 30 minute trial, the experimental leg develops avoidance of the bath; the paired leg does not. The avoidance seen in the experimental leg appears, then, to be a learned-position habit. Simple neuronal models that could mediate the sensorimotor relationships in acquisition of this habit can be proposed, but even this seemingly simple model appears to be complex and to involve neuronal ensembles [13]. In some species, on the other hand, stimulation of a single cell predictably results in a complex behavior. For example, a withdrawal response can be elicited by stimulation of a single interneuron (a so-called command fiber) in *Tritonia,* a mollusk [21]; the tail flip by the goldfish is mediated by the Mauthner cell [22].

A further reductionist approach is the electrophysiological model, in which brief stimulation of a preparation leads to long-lasting changes in electrical properties. In the past, posttetanic potentiation and heterosynaptic facilitation were proposed as models. At present, there is much interest in hippocampal slice preparations [23], which have been shown to support long-lasting changes after brief stimulation. The involvement of Ca^{2+} and a 40,000 M_r phosphoprotein have been proposed [24].

Interventive Studies

Of various interventive procedures, the simplest and oldest is the selective ablation of brain regions. It has been known for some time that lesion of the hippocampal system in humans results in the inability to form new LTM, whereas memory of events that existed before the injury is unimpaired [25]. While what we usually consider as human memory is primarily verbal (ideational) and cannot be compared directly to animal memory, it is nevertheless interesting that it has not been possible to produce this striking dissociation of learning and memory in animals by means of surgical lesions. However, this dissociation, as well as the demonstration that different brain regions affect memory processes to different extents, has been accomplished (reversibly) in animals by injection of inhibitors of protein synthesis [26, 27] or by electrical disruption [28].

ELECTROCONVULSIVE SHOCK
Retrograde amnesia, the loss of memory of recently learned tasks, can be produced by ECS. Current can be applied transcorneally or through ear or scalp electrodes. The amount of current, frequency

of the pulse, and its duration are important variables. It was once assumed that the resultant convulsion was the amnestic effector, but amnesia has been reported after application of subseizure levels of current [29]. ECS administered before training has been shown to block memory (anterograde amnesia) without measurable effect on acquisition [30], and this suggests that some metabolic sequellae of the treatment produce the amnesia, rather than the electrical effects themselves. It is known that ECS produces long-lasting changes in neurotransmitter metabolism [31], as well as in macromolecular turnover [32].

INHIBITORS OF PROTEIN SYNTHESIS
Parenteral or intracerebral injection of protein synthesis inhibitors have been shown to block the formation of LTM in a number of species, yet such inhibitors do not affect acquisition, or short-term memory (STM) formation. That is, under conditions of a temporary block in protein synthesis, test animals learn as well as uninjected control subjects, but when such test animals are retested some time later, they appear not to have formed stable LTM of the training session, as exemplified in the goldfish studies described below. Examples of these agents are given in Fig. 40-2.

Studies in Goldfish
The behavioral apparatus used in my laboratory is a "shuttle box" (Fig. 40-1,4), which consists of a water-filled plastic tank divided by an opaque barrier with a rectangular opening. The trial starts when a light on the side of the box in which the fish is located goes on; 15 sec later, a repetitive mild electrical shock is administered through the water through grids, unless the fish has swum to the darkened side. The fish shuttles back and forth, receiving 1 trial per minute. During a single, 15 min trial session, the fish learns that by swimming through the opening within 15 sec of light onset, it avoids the shock. This active avoidance is the learned response. The multitrial nature of the task permits one to measure learning and the formation of STM as well as LTM. Figure 40-3 summarizes the effects of the intracranial injection of puro-

Fig. 40-2. Three classes of eukaryotic protein-synthesis inhibitors that block long-term memory formation and do not affect short-term memory formation. Because they bear little structural similarity and block different steps in protein synthesis [33], it is concluded that their common amnestic action is by inhibition of protein synthesis, rather than by side effects. Replacement of the acetoxy group by H of acetoxycycloheximide (AXM) results in the structure of cycloheximide (CXM), while substitution with OH gives the structure of streptovitacin A.

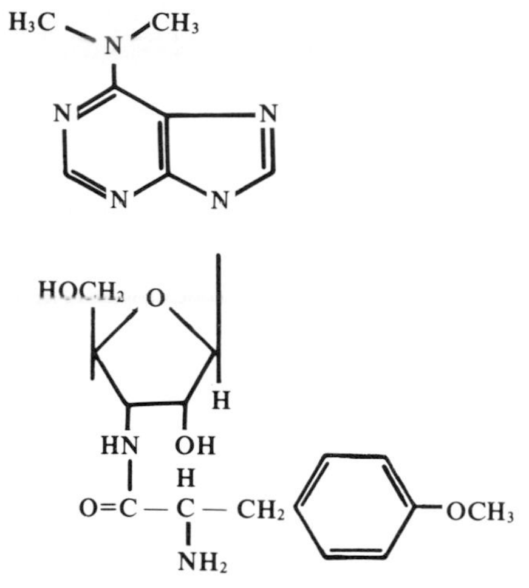

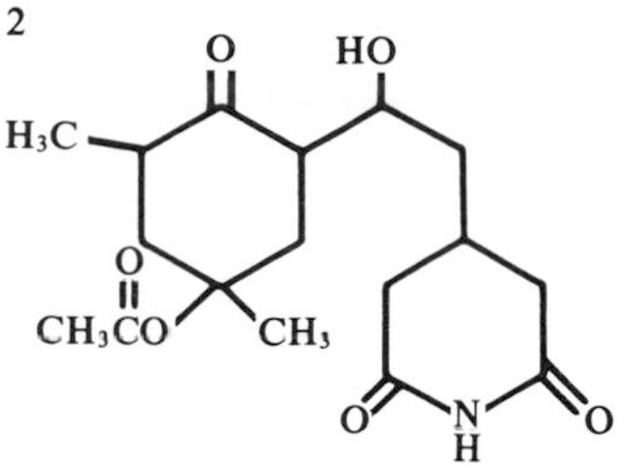

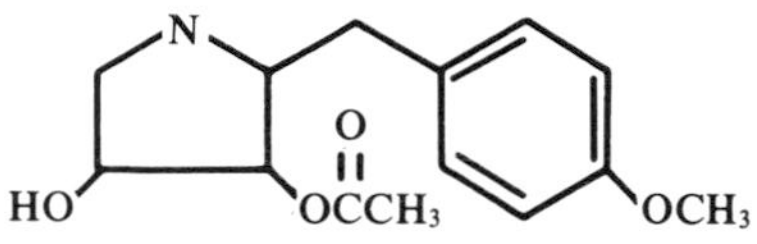

mycin, an inhibitor of protein synthesis. The increased probability of the avoidance response during day 1 training indicates the formation of STM (Fig. 40-3,1). Fish returned immediately to their home tanks and retrained 1 week later show further improvement. When the inhibitor is injected just before the session, normal acquisition is seen, but there is a profound deficit in performance on retraining 1 week later. If the agent is administered sufficiently in advance of the first session, normal retention is seen on retraining, as the inhibitor's effects have worn off before training.

By varying the time of injection before training, the duration of a given agent's amnestic effect can be determined. This is about 24 hours for puromycin and is similar to its known duration of action

as an inhibitor of brain protein synthesis. Treated fish exhibiting a retention decrement in session 2 can be given a third session (not shown) on day 15. In this case, they show the usual improvement in performance seen between sessions 1 and 2. This result indicates that the induced memory block does not permanently damage the fish's ability to learn or to form memory. Similar results have been seen with acetoxycycloheximide (AXM), a glutarimide inhibitor of protein synthesis. These experiments [34] indicate a clear difference between STM and LTM formation: blockers of protein synthesis appear to have no effect on STM but prevent the development of LTM. Memory loss can also be produced by injections administered after training (Fig. 40-3,2). Administration of the amnestic agent immediately after session 1 results in profound deficits on retraining scores 1 week later. The process is time dependent: if fish are returned to their home tanks and not given the injection until a few hours later, no deficit is seen upon retraining on day 8. In fact, fish not treated previously and given the amnestic agent just before retraining on day 8 show the learned response of control fish. This time-dependency of the treatment rules out both chronic (lingering) and acute toxic effects of the amnestic agents as possible explanations for the ob-

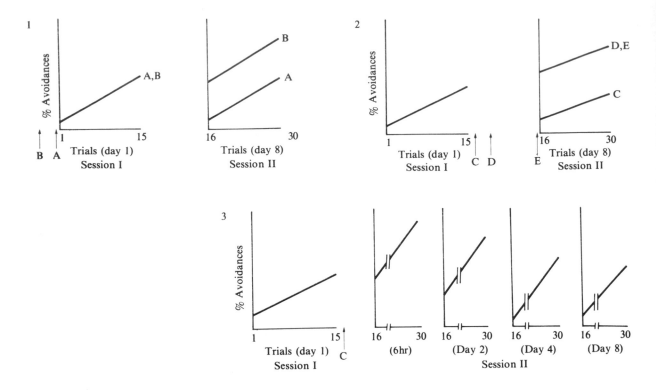

Fig. 40-3. *Effects of agents that block long-term memory of a multi-trial task—the goldfish shuttle box shock avoidance paradigm. Figure 40-3,1 shows that the probability of an avoidance response during 15 trials (session 1) increases, indicating that STM is formed. Fish returned immediately to their home tanks and retrained 1 week later show additional improvement in session 2. If an amnestic agent is injected intracranially just before the session (time A), normal acquisition is seen, but there is a profound deficit in performance on retraining 1 week later. If the agent is administered sufficiently in advance of session 1 (time B), normal retention is seen on day 8, since the effects of the injection will have worn off by the time of the training session. By varying the time of injection before training, the duration of a given agent's amnestic effect can be established. Intracranial injection of puromycin is effective when given 24, but not 72 hours before session 1. Figure 40-3,2 shows the effects of amnestic agents administered after training. An injection immediately after session 1 (C) results in profound deficits on retraining 1 week later.*

The process is time dependent, because fish return to their home tanks and, given the injection a few hours later (D), show no deficit on retraining in session 2, a week later. In fact, fish not treated previously and given the amnestic agent just before retraining on day 8 (E) show a learned response. This time-dependence of the treatment rules out both chronic (lingering) and acute toxic effects of the amnestic agents as possible explanations for the observed reduced responding rates, and indicates that the agent produces a specific memory loss. the decay of STM is shown in Fig. 40-3,3. Injection of a blocking agent just after (or before) session 1 results in failure to form LTM. In this experiment, individual groups of animals so treated and retrained at various times earlier than 8 days (e.g., 6, 48, or 96 hr after session 1) demonstrate the learned response. The experiments thus constitute evidence for the decay of STM (see text). (From B. W. Agranoff, in Y. Tsukada and B. W. Agranoff (eds.), Neurobiological Basis of Learning and Memory, *New York: Wiley, 1980, pp. 135–147).*

served reduced response rates. The decrement in performance is therefore attributed to a specific memory loss. The results suggest that LTM is formed after the training session and is thus analogous to the posttraumatic retrograde amnesia seen clinically.

The decay of STM is seen in Fig. 40-3,3. Groups of animals treated with blocking agents just before or just after training and retrained at various times (6, 48, or 96 hours after session 1) demonstrate progressive loss of the learned response. The experiments constitute evidence for the decay of STM following the training session. They do not, however, tell us whether STM is "hardened" into LTM, or whether STM is a temporary memory that serves the brain while LTM is being formed separately in a slow, protein synthesis–dependent process. In either event, it is clear that STM is not obliterated by such treatments—its presence can be detected behaviorally after the amnestic agent has been administered. Note that the measured consolidation time represents the interaction of an interventive agent and the inferred physiological process of LTM formation. Because fish are poikilothermic, they can be cooled or warmed after a training session, and this property can be used to show that cooling slows LTM formation while warming accelerates it, as is expected of a biochemical process [35].

There are indications that LTM formation is triggered by environmental stimuli. Fish transferred to their home tanks immediately after training lose their susceptibility to amnestic agents in a few minutes, while their detention in the training apparatus prolongs their susceptibility for over an hour [36]. Subsequent studies have shown that this delay in onset of LTM is mediated by visual stimuli. I have postulated elsewhere that these stimuli inform the fish whether it is in the threatening environment of the training apparatus or in the safe environment of the home tank and that the lowering of arousal following a stressful experience triggers the onset of memory formation [37].

Studies in Mice

The application of inhibitors of protein synthesis to learning was introduced by Flexner [38]. Memory of Y-maze training could be obliterated by bilateral temporal injections of puromycin 5 days after training. At later times, amnesia could be produced by injecting puromycin into 6 sites. There was no time limit to the effectiveness in producing amnesia by the latter treatment. While the effects were initially attributed to a block in protein synthesis, a number of other possible explanations were subsequently proposed [39]. Flexner's experiments are difficult to compare to the fish studies or to most studies of other investigators in chicks and mice, because a consolidation curve, which would distinguish illness from effects on memory, was not obtained. Extensive studies in mice from the laboratory of Barondes [40] and, more recently, from that of Squire [41] and Flood [42] have confirmed that the protein synthesis–blocking antibiotics selectively disrupt memory. Consolidation time in mice is much more rapid than in the fish, about 15 to 30 minutes. Possible noxious and amnestic effects of the blockers have been dissociated [43]. The duration of inhibition of protein synthesis necessary to produce retention deficits in mice receiving passive-avoidance training has been examined by means of multiple injections of anisomycin, a short-acting protein-synthesis blocker [42]. Inhibition of protein synthesis immediately after training appears most effective. Most mouse studies involve subcutaneous injections of sufficient amounts of antibiotic to result in profound inhibition in brain. Systemic injections do not permit study of the possible sites in the brain where the block produces the amnestic response. Effects of intracerebral microinjections in mice [26] as well as in rats [27] indicate that hippocampus and amygdala are effective action sites of the protein-synthesis inhibitors. Although the localization studies are not yet precise, they at least confirm that it is inhibition of protein synthesis in the brain, not in other organs, that produces the amnesia!

Studies in Birds

Extensive studies on retention of a one-trial aversive discrimination task (Fig. 40-1,3) have demonstrated that protein synthesis inhibitors block retention of the task. Gibbs has postulated the existence of short-term and intermediate (labile) phases of memory in addition to LTM [44]. Earlier phases of memory are proposed to be mediated by ion transport–dependent processes, whereas LTM formation is blocked by the inhibitors of protein synthesis.

INHIBITION OF DNA AND RNA SYNTHESIS

Experiments in which amnesia is caused by protein-synthesis inhibitors led to the speculation that RNA-synthesis blockers might also block memory. If enzyme induction mediates some aspect of long-term memory formation, a block at the transcriptional level might also be expected to produce a similar effect. If a protein-synthesis blocker simply reduces the level of a rapidly turning-over protein, RNA-synthesis blockers might also cause reduction in a critical protein, if the appropriate messenger RNA is unstable. Earlier studies with agents found to be highly toxic in vivo, such as 8-azaguanine and actinomycin D, as well as more recent studies with less toxic and possibly more selective agents, such as camptothecin and α-amanitin, generally support the proposal that RNA blockers are also effective amnestic agents [45, 46].

Since DNA turnover is linked to cell replication, and since neurons are nondividing end cells, conventional memory theories would preclude DNA synthesis involvement. As anticipated, arabinosyl cytosine, a DNA blocker, does not affect learning or memory in the goldfish [45].

NEUROTRANSMITTERS

The availability of powerful agonists and antagonists of neurotransmitter binding, as well as of enzyme blockers of their metabolism has encouraged investigations on the effects on behavior of neurotransmitter actions. Deutsch has proposed a cholinergic hypothesis, based primarily on studies with the acetylcholinesterase blocker, di-isopropylphosphofluoridate (DFP) [47]. He suggests that optimal levels of ACh are required for memory formation and retrieval. Drachman studied the well-known amnestic action of scopolamine, a muscarinic blocker, on human learning and memory, as well as its reversal by physostigmine [48]. Implications for memory deficits in aging have been proposed. A possible role for catecholamines in learning and memory is inferred from behavioral studies after a block of dopamine β-hydroxylase by diethyldithiocarbamate. Destruction of catecholaminergic sites by 6-OH-dopa has also been reported to produce behavioral impairment. These and other examples are cited in recent reviews [49, 50].

ANTIBODIES

Antibodies to crude extracts of specific brain regions have produced variable behavioral results. As brain-specific proteins have been identified (such as S100, 14-3-2, etc.) effects of their antibodies on behavior have been explored. Antibody to ganglioside G_{M1} has been reported to block a learned avoidance response in rats [51]. The agent also produces epileptiform activity, but this effect appears to be separate from its amnestic action. Identification of other brain-specific proteins, the availability of monoclonal antibodies, and the use of antibody fragments to increase penetrability of injected antibodies should facilitate further progress.

COLCHICINE AND OTHER
TUBULIN-BINDING AGENTS

Tubulin is a major brain protein, and is prominent in neurons in the form of the neurotubules of neuronal processes, where it is believed to provide a rigid endoskeleton upon which contractile proteins provide the mechanism for axonal transport. Intracranial injection of the tubulin-binding drug, colchicine, has been reported to produce behavioral deficits in chicks [52] and goldfish [53]; vinblastine is claimed to block memory formation in mice [54]. Effects of nerve growth [55] and of sensory stimulation on tubulin [56, 57] have also been described.

In adult neurons, protein synthesis is restricted to the cell body, and new protein reaches the synapse through axonal transport. Tubulin-binding agents block axonal transport and other tubulin-mediated processes. Their general toxicity may complicate interpretation of their reported effects on behavior. It should be borne in mind that axonal flow studies are generally performed in neurons with long processes, and it cannot be assumed that cells mediating behavioral plasticity are of this type. In fact, one could argue effectively that small interneurons are the critical participants in the process.

Enhancing Agents

Improvement of memory can be defined experimentally a number of ways, such as better retention scores than those of controls following training associated with drug treatment; protection against the amnestic action of a second substance; increased rate of consolidation; decreased forgetting; or resistance to extinction training. For example, amphetamine is reported to reverse, or protect against, the effects of cycloheximide on memory in mice (see [39] and [46]). Low doses of some conulsants, such as strychnine or pentylenetetrazole, are claimed to accelerate consolidation [58]. Many current investigations are directed at a demonstration that peptides improve memory. They can be traced to the observation that learning defects in hypophysectomized animals can be reversed by injection of pituitary extracts. Both anterior and posterior pituitary hormones have since been reported effective in a number of training paradigms in intact animals, and derivatives of posterior pituitary hormones that no longer possess the parent molecule's hormonal activity are claimed to improve memory [59].

Extensive studies in the laboratory of deWied began with the observation that ACTH fragments block extinction of a pole-jumping task in rats. Many psychologists would claim that the paradigm used, the loss of performance of a task after repeated presentation of the unpaired conditioned stimulus, is actually new learning. According to this interpretation, it would follow that a block of extinction represents the block of new memory formation rather than protection against memory loss (i.e., forgetting). However, a number of ACTH-like peptides have been synthesized and investigated in other training tasks, and have been demonstrated to have behavioral effects that are consistent with enhancement of learning and memory formation. A small, behaviorally effective fragment of ACTH, $ACTH_{4-10}$ (Met-Glu-His-Phe-Arg-Try-Gly), appears to mediate the effect, but is 1,000 times less potent than an analog, Met-Glu-His-Phe-D-Lys-Phe (ORG2766). A somewhat larger peptide possessing 300 times the activity of 2766 has also been reported [59]. The opiate peptides have been found to effect learning, as well as to produce altered behavioral states after intracerebral injection. β-Endorphin injected intraventricularly produces a naloxone-reversible catatonia [60]. A substance derived from the CSF, presumably a peptide, is reported to induce sleep [61]. After injection, a number of peptides evoke intense grooming behavior, the significance of which is not understood. Some of the effects produced by peptides may partially explain previous claims that memory could be transferred by injection into a naive recipient of the extracts of brains from trained "donor" subjects. The isolation of peptides that mediate a light-fear response in rats and color preference in goldfish has been reported [62]. It is likely that many or all of the highly-contested and publicized claims of memory transfer can be attributed to nonspecific effects seen with a variety of natural and synthetic peptides.

From the foregoing interventive studies, it can be concluded that in a number of species and training paradigms, learning and memory have been separated into distinct processes. Most extensive studies have been performed with inhibitors of protein synthesis. A variety of structurally distinct molecules (Fig. 40-2), employed in several experimental species, serve to affirm the conclusion that normally ongoing protein synthesis is not required for the acquisition of a new behavior, but is required for steps related to its encoding into a permanent form. The means by which the biochemical inhibition leads to the behavioral deficit is not known. One could propose two possibilities: that the block leads to a depletion of rapidly turning over proteins required for consolidation of memory; or, after learning, new protein must be synthesized for LTM to form. A number of experiments indicate that inhibiting protein synthesis prior to training has no greater amnestic effect than does a block induced following training [30, 63]. Since presession injections would be expected to have a greater effect on reducing preexisting protein levels than postsession injections, such results indicate that the formation of new protein is required for memory formation. The question then arises: Which protein, and in which cells? Experiments involving local injection of blockers [26, 27] have suggested the hippocampus, amygdala, or both as loci and have also indicated that the critical interval is the period immediately following training. The experiments do not indicate whether the blocked processes are specific to a given learned behavior or whether they are part of a generalized fixation process [34, 37]. The posttraining environment plays a role in initiating the memory-fixation process, as demonstrated in the goldfish, and suggests that arousal and its diminution may be important factors. Block of appetitive learning by the various blockers has also been reported, but the vast majority of interventive studies involve avoidance tasks. It therefore remains possible that they exert their effect by interference with physiological processes that relate fear responses to learning and memory.

A number of studies have been directed at specific actions of the blockers that could mediate the amnestic response. The protein-synthesis blockers have been reported to alter enzyme levels in neurotransmitter synthesis, such as tyrosine hydroxylase. However, elevation of brain tyrosine levels to the same degree as that produced by a protein synthesis inhibitor does not produce amnesia [64]. It may be that the concomitant effects on a number of metabolic steps is necessary for the block of memory formation, and although together they block memory, no one step is of itself critical [39].

Correlative Approaches

Correlative experiments seek a change in structure or in metabolism (usually measured by means of radioisotope incorporation) that accompanies training known to alter behavior. As the term *correlative* indicates, observed changes are not necessarily causally linked to learning or to memory formation. They might, for example, be related to sensorimotor processing, to hormonal or cardiovascular changes associated with stress, or to other possibly unrelated epiphenomena of associative learning. Often, questions can be answered by the use of appropriate controls in the experimental design. Because of the highly complex structure of the brain and the great diversity of possible behavioral repertoires, it seems safe to assume that biochemical alterations causally linked to the associative aspects of new learning will be small, and that one is therefore searching for a biochemical "needle in a haystack." A highly suitable way to search for minor changes within a heterogeneous population of macromolecules, such as RNA or protein, is to use the isotopic double-label technique introduced to behavioral experiments by Glassman [65]. $[^3H]$ or $[^{14}C]$uridine was injected intracerebrally into mice, who were then trained in a "jump-up" task (see Fig. 40-1,5), while the other isotopic precursor was injected into resting or yoked-control mice subjected to the same stimuli and number of shocks, but denied a ledge upon which to escape. Brains were combined and RNA was isolated and separated on gels. Measured radioactivity was normalized to the double-label ratio of the total acid-soluble pool. Rather than one or more specific regions in the RNA profile in which the double-label ratio was altered, a broad increase was seen throughout the RNA, suggesting that the observed alteration is attributable to some aspect of precursor metabolism rather than to de novo RNA synthesis.

The question of precursor-pool sizes is a severe one in whole-animal labeling studies. Even when chemical amounts of such precursors as UMP, UDP, and UTP in brain are recovered and measured accurately, one is not certain of the identity of the relevant precursor pool. In this case, the neuronal nuclear precursor pool presumably should be examined. Although a rather extensive series of experiments was performed involving the use of yoked, overtrained, and quiet control animals, it is still not clear whether the observations were related to learning or to stress of training [39]. A number of other technical questions have been raised regarding the interpretation of these results [46]. Changes in nucleic acid metabolism as a function of training has also been reported by Shashoua [66] in experiments in which goldfish learn to swim upright after a float has been attached to the jaw (see Fig. 40-1,2). In a subsequent session, they swim upright much more rapidly than in the initial session. Although this adaptive response has some properties of associative learning, it is unclear whether possible effects of stress were adequately controlled [46]. Restoration of normal swimming behavior is reportedly accompanied by alterations in nucleic acid and protein labeling. Although an altered double-label ratio is claimed in three protein gel bands, the regions represent the major brain proteins [66], raising again the question of whether some consequence of the behavioral manipulation unrelated to learning is reflected in altered precursor pool sizes. Antibody to one of the proteins is reported to block memory (reacquisition of the normal posture in a second session), and immunohistochemical studies indicate that the material is restricted to the brain ependymal region [67]. The relevance of these experiments to memory and learning is questionable, but they raise the interesting possibility that secretion of a CSF protein might be enhanced during stress. Acquisition of the float task is also reported to be blocked by puromycin [68]. Although extensive interventive studies implicating protein synthesis and memory have been performed on shuttle-box task acquisition of the goldfish, no changes in amino acid incorporation have yet been observed [69].

During the past three decades, Hydèn has developed a number of microtechniques, which have been applied to small numbers of brain cells in an attempt to demonstrate altered structural metabolism related to learning and memory. Recent attention has focused on reversal of "handedness" in the rodent. Rats express a preference for the right or left paw in obtaining food, and once this is established, they are then trained to use the other paw. There are indications that the hippocampus mediates the reversal learning, and overtrained animals can be used to serve as suitable controls for alterations attributable to motor activity. The preparation offers the additional advantage that the two sides of the animal can be compared. Thus, systemic factors, for example, hormonal or cardiovascular responses, are expected to affect both sides equally and should thus be distinguishable from putative changes attributable to learning and memory formation. Altered mRNA [70] as well as protein (notably, S100) labeling is reported, and antibody to S100 is claimed to block the acquisition [71]. This preparation would seem to hold promise, although a number of questions have been raised [72].

An attractive aspect of the handedness experiments—the use of one side of the animal as a control—has also been used in imprinting experiments. Rose and his collaborators have demonstrated that the (surgically) split-brain chick can be imprinted through one eye and remain behaviorally naive when tested with the other [72, 73]. Under these conditions, it was demonstrated that more uracil incorporation is seen in the forebrain roof on the trained side than on the untrained side. In other experiments, with intact chicks, both RNA and protein labeling are selectively increased in the forebrain in imprinted animals compared with overtrained animals [73]. It is not yet clear whether some of the changes seen are simply correlated with light exposure inherent in the task or are true correlates of learning and memory formation. Increased incorporation of $[^{14}C]2$-deoxy-D-glucose (see Chap. 24) suggests increased glucose metabolism in the forebrain as a result of imprinting [74]. Results with the one-trial learning paradigm used by Gibbs [44] indicate increased leucine incorporation into tubulin in the anterior forebrain roof 30 minutes after training, as well as an increase in incorporation of [³H]fucose [73].

In summary, while there appears to be a number of promising biochemical "handles" on learning and memory, none can presently be taken as unequivocal evidence. The history of such claims of biochemical correlates is sobering. Many have been subject to heavy criticism or are somewhat suspect because they were not pursued after the preliminary reports. Current promising approaches await replication and further documentation.

Nonassociative Learning and Other Models of Brain Plasticity

HABITUATION AND SENSITIZATION

Habituation is an adaptive decrease in response to a repeated stimulus. For example, if a puff of air is blown at the eye of a rabbit, it will blink. After repeated stimulation, the reflex is lost. It can be demonstrated in a number of ways that the diminished response is not mediated by sensory or motor fatigue. Spontaneous recovery follows. *Sensitization* is the converse phenomenon, in which application of a UCS results in a response to a previously subthreshold stimulus. Thus, a puff of air that previously had been too mild to elicit an eye blink might become effective after a loud noise. Sensitization can reverse habituation. Since these nonassociative phenomena have been regarded to be of brief duration, they generally have not been considered as valuable for the study of biochemical correlates as those in which LTM is formed. Recently, Kandel and his collaborators, studying the neural basis of habituation and sensitization to gill-withdrawal in *Aplysia* after a waterjet stimulus, have demonstrated that a two-neuron circuit can mediate withdrawal and that the habituated response is mediated by lowered neurotransmitter release from a presynaptic element, which in turn results from a decreased calcium current [17]. After stimulation has been repeated for several days, circuits become completely nonfunctional and remain so for weeks. They can be reactivated centrally by a sensitizing stimulus that appears to involve serotonin. In *Aplysia,* habituation follow-

ing a single session of 10 to 100 stimuli is lost in 2 hr, but after four daily sessions, it can persist for weeks. These weak and persistent effects are referred to as *short-term* and *long-term memory,* respectively [17]. However, these terms have a completely different meaning in this context than they do in interventive studies on learning and memory where they refer to two *stages* of memory resulting from a single training session.

KINDLING

Repeated, mild, electrical stimulation of selected brain regions during a period of days leads to a permanent susceptibility to seizures. There are no indications of scarring or other pathological alterations of the brain as a result of the stimulation, and it has been suggested that the phenomenon is a useful model of synaptic plasticity, because the "trials" lead to permanent alteration [75]. Inhibitors of protein synthesis are reported to block the development of kindling [76, 77], and long-lasting changes in dopaminergic [78] properties, as well as transient alterations in cholinergic receptors [79], have been reported.

DEVELOPMENTAL AND GENETIC MODELS

Tryon first attempted to breed "maze-bright" and "maze-dull" rats [80], and there have been many attempts since to distinguish behavioral properties among related strains of animals [5, 81]. In general, the problem is complicated by the fact that genetic strains are rarely, if ever, single-gene mutants, and even as seemingly simple a response as choosing between two arms of a maze is undoubtedly the result of interactions of multiple physiological mechanisms. It has nevertheless been possible to demonstrate genetically regulated correlations. For example, cross-breeding experiments in mice have been used to correlate ChAT activity with inherited learning traits [82]. Another approach is to vary biochemical and behavioral characteristics by intervention during development, but the relevance of the actions of a toxic substance on development to physiological mechanisms in the intact animal places a severe limitation on this approach. Injection of growth hormone into pregnant rats during the period of rapid brain development reportedly leads to increased brain size and perhaps to increased learning ability of some tasks [83].

It might be reasoned that, since the amount of physical change in brain structure resulting from a single training session probably is beyond detection with present methodology, one should begin by looking for a cumulative effect by comparing brains of animals raised in a complex, stimulating environment (enriched condition, EC), with littermates maintained in an austere, sensory-deprived environment (impoverished condition, IC). An extensive series of experiments over many years has led to the conclusion that environmental stimulation leads to an increase in the size of the occipital cortex, and that increased dendritic branching (about 10%) occurs [84, 85]. More dramatic anatomical changes are seen in comparisons of animals reared in complete darkness compared to those reared in light [85, 86]. Altered rates of labeled amino acid incorporation into protein, as well as levels of a number of enzymes, are reported in the visual cortex. The enzymes include ChAT, AChE, MAO, $(Na^+ + K^+)$-ATPase, and a number of hydrolases [72]. Altered labeling of tubulin [56] and colchicine binding [57] have also been reported.

HYBRIDIZATION STUDIES

DNA and RNA hybridization studies offer the opportunity of examining the degree of heterogeneity, that is, the fraction of the species' genome that is expressed in a cell or organ. Such studies also offer the hope that unique sequences will be identified as the result of a physiological variable. Theoretically, isolation of unique RNA could be followed by translation in vitro to yield the relevant phenotype. As might be anticipated, the brain's heterogeneity is reflected in a greater content of hybridizable RNA (HnRNA) than other organs [87]. In human brain obtained at autopsy, differences in HnRNA are reported in the left (dominant) temporal lobe (compared to the right) [88]. If confirmed, this result would represent a significant advance in our understanding of lateralization in the brain, an important factor in cognition in humans. HnRNA is reportedly altered in

EC compared to IC rats [89]. Since hybridization studies are primarily qualitative, they are not as likely to demonstrate a small increase or decrease in an RNA population as to identify the presence of significant amounts of novel species. Thus, the hope that training in animals will generate measurable alterations in hybridization rests on a purported synthesis of novel RNA sequences. It would seem equally reasonable that we would instead find altered intracellular distribution of preexisting protein species. In this case, we would not expect to find altered hybridization in a tissue extract, although such claims have been made. It is unfortunate, as with memory transfer, that so many such reports go unconfirmed and unrefuted, mingling in the minds of many with a growing body of rigorously conducted research on the neurobiological basis of behavior.

Posttranslational Alteration of Protein: A Possible Role in Behavior

Most proteins are modified after the primary sequence has been synthesized, and there is increasing interest in the effect of such modifications on function [90]. A well-known model is the enzyme phosphorylase, which must be phosphorylated by ATP for activation. CNS-specific phosphoproteins are believed to play a role in synaptic function (see Chap. 19), and a relationship between phosphorylation of brain proteins and behavior has been proposed [91]. The brain contains activity for the tyrosinylation of tubulin, but its functional significance is unknown. Glycosylation of brain proteins has been studied extensively, particularly in synaptic membranes [92].

Specialized structures involved in mediation of plasticity have not been identified, but it is tempting to speculate that the rapid events associated with acquisition are mediated by posttranslational modifications [37], based on the fact that acquisition can occur in a fraction of a second and yet is long-lasting. These temporal considerations favor mediation of acquisition by posttranslational modifications, as stable covalent bond formation can be catalyzed by a single rapid enzyme step.

Protein synthesis, implicated in LTM by the use of interventive agents is undoubtedly too slow to mediate STM formation. Furthermore, the machinery in the cell body that mediates protein synthesis may be at some distance from the synapses mediating the altered behavior, so additional time is necessary for axonal transport.

Clinical Implications

Nowhere in biology is the laboratory animal less appropriate for studying human disease than in the area of higher brain function. Yet, many basic principles established in studies on animal learning and memory have direct implications for practical biomedical problems. For example, the beneficial effects of electroconvulsive shock therapy (ECT) in the treatment of depression has not been explained adequately. We do not yet know whether the amnesia associated with ECT is related to the therapeutic effect. Numerous drugs have been proposed for the aid of defective learning and memory, mainly for the impaired young and for the aged. In the pharmaceutical industry, there is currently much interest in the development of new agents. It is possible, as has occurred in the past in other fields of biomedicine, that a serendipitous discovery will yield drugs that will also serve as valuable tools for understanding basic mechanisms. At present, the effects of most agents purported to improve memory can be attributed to noncognitive actions, such as depression of overactivity, increasing attention span, mild stimulation, and other effects. A number of drugs, such as magnesium pemoline that have been reported to improve memory, have questionable biochemical and behavioral effects [93]. Recent nutritional studies indicate that brain metabolism can be altered by diet [94]. While much is yet to be learned, it is clear from animal experiments that the malnourished fetus and infant may well be destined to a life of restricted usefulness; it is cause for great concern.

Recent technical breakthroughs in positron-emission scanning have made it possible to measure brain metabolism in humans by $[^{11}C]$2-deoxy-D-glucose or $[^{18}F]$2-fluoro-2-deoxy-D-glucose [95].

In addition, positron-emitting derivatives of a number of drugs have been developed, and recently, a quantitative method, which should be adaptable to a human noninvasive technique [96], has been developed for measurement of regional brain protein synthesis. In the next decade, then, we could learn much about memory mechanisms at the molecular level, as well as about specific memory defects in humans.

References

1. Ribot, T. A. *The Diseases of Memory*. New York: Appleton, 1882.
2. McGaugh, J. L., and Herz, M. J. *Memory Consolidation*. San Francisco: Albion, 1972.
*3. Cotman, C. W., and McGaugh, J. L. *Behavioral Neuroscience*. New York: Academic, 1980. Pp. 255–294.
4. Quartermain, D., McEwen, B. S., and Azmitia, E. C. Recovery of memory following amnesia in the rat and mouse. *J. Comp. Physiol. Psychol.* 79: 360–370, 1972.
5. Bovet, D., Bovet-Nitti, F., and Oliverio, A. Genetic aspects of learning and memory in mice. *Science* 163:139–149, 1969.
6. Gaze, R. M. *The Formation of Nerve Connections*. London: Academic, 1970.
7. Jacobson, M. *Developmental Neurobiology*. New York: Plenum, 1978.
8. Agranoff, B. W., Davis, R. E., and Gossington, R. E. Esoteric fish. *Science* 171:230, 1971.
9. Bennett, M. V. L. Neural Control of Electric Organs. In D. Ingle (ed.), *The Central Nervous System and Fish Behavior*. Chicago: University of Chicago Press, 1968. Pp. 147–169.
10. Corning, W. C., Dyal, J. A., and Willows, A. O. D. (eds.). *Invertebrate Learning*. New York: Plenum, 1975.
*11. Krasne, F. B. Invertebrate Systems as a Means of Gaining Insight into the Nature of Learning and Memory. In M. R. Rosenzweig and E. L. Bennett (eds.), *Neural Mechanisms of Learning and Memory*. Cambridge, Mass.: M.I.T. Press, 1974. Pp. 401–429.
12. Garcia, J., and Hankins, W. G. The Evolution of Bitter and the Acquisition of Toxiphobia. In D. Denton and J. P. Coghlin (eds.), *Olfaction and Taste V*. New York: Academic, 1975. Pp. 39–45.
*13. Davis, W. J. Plasticity in the Invertebrates. In M. R. Rosenzweig and E. L. Bennett (eds.), *Neural*

*Key reference.

Mechanisms of Learning and Memory. Cambridge, Mass.: M.I.T. Press, 1974. Pp. 430–462.

14. Yerkes, R. M. The intelligence of earthworms. *J. Anim. Behav.* 2:332–352, 1912.

15. Brenner, S. The genetics of *Caenorhabditis elegans. Genetics* 77:71–94, 1974.

16. Young, J. Z. Short and long memories in *Octopus* and the influence of the vertical lobe system. *J. Exp. Biol.* 52:385–393, 1970.

*17. Kandel, E. R. Cellular Insights into Behavior and Learning. *The Harvey Lectures* 73:19–92, 1979.

18. Quinn, W. G., and Gould, J. L. Nerves and genes. *Nature* 278:19–23, 1979.

19. Arbib, M. A., Kilmer, W. L., and Spinelli, D. N. In M. R. Rosenzweig and E. L. Bennett (eds.), *Neural Mechanisms of Learning and Memory.* Cambridge, Mass.: M.I.T. Press, 1974. Pp. 109–132.

20. Eisenstein, E. M., and Cohen, M. J. Learning in an isolated prothoracic insect ganglion. *Anim. Behav.* 13:104–108, 1965.

21. Willows, A. O. D. Behavioral Acts Elicited by Stimulation of Single Identifiable Nerve Cells. In F. D. Carlson (ed.), *Physiological and Biochemical Aspects of Nervous Integration.* Englewood Cliffs, N.J.: Prentice-Hall, 1968. Pp. 217–243.

22. Diamond, J. The Mauthner Cell. In W. S. Hoar and D. J. Randall (eds.), *Fish Physiology.* New York: Academic, 1971. Vol. V, pp. 265–346.

23. Andersen, P., Sundberg, S. H., Sveen, O., and Wigstrom, H. Specific long-lasting potentiation of synaptic transmission in hippocampal slices. *Nature* 266:736–737, 1977.

24. Lynch, G., Browning, M., and Bennett, W. F. Biochemical and physiological studies of long-term synaptic plasticity. *Fed. Proc.* 38:2117–2122, 1979.

25. Scoville, W. B., and Milner, B. Loss of recent memory after bilateral hippocampal lesions. *J. Neurol. Neurosurg. Psychiatry* 20:11–21, 1957. But see also Woolsey, R. M., and Nelson, J. S. Asymptomatic destruction of the fornix in man. *Arch. Neurol.* 32:566–568, 1975.

26. Eichenbaum, H., Quenon, B. A., Heacock, A. M., and Agranoff, B. W. Differential behavioral and biochemical effects of regional injection of cycloheximide into mouse brain. *Brain Res.* 101:171–176, 1976.

27. Berman, R. F., Kesner, R. P., and Partlow, L. M. Passive avoidance impairments in rats following cycloheximide injection into the amygdala. *Brain Res.* 158:171–188, 1978.

28. Zornetzer, S. F., Chronister, R. B., and Ross, B. The hippocampus and retrograde amnesia: Localization of some positive and negative memory disruptive sites. *Behav. Biol.* 8:507–518, 1973.

29. McGaugh, J. L., and Gold, P. E. Modulation of Memory by Electrical Stimulation of the Brain. In M. R. Rosenzweig and E. L. Bennett (eds.), *Neural Mechanisms of Learning and Memory.* Cambridge, Mass.: M.I.T. Press, 1974. Pp. 549–560.

30. Springer, A. D., Schoel, W. M., Klinger, P. D., and Agranoff, B. W. Anterograde and retrograde effects of electroconvulsive shock and of puromycin on memory formation in the goldfish. *Behav. Biol.* 13:467–481, 1975.

31. Kety, S. S., Javoy, F., Thierry, A.-M., Julou, L., and Glowinski, J. A sustained effect of electroconvulsive shock on the turnover of norepinephrine in the central nervous system of the rat. *Proc. Natl. Acad. Sci. U.S.A.* 58:1249–1254, 1967.

32. Wynter, C. V. A. Persistence of altered RNA synthesis in rat cerebral cortex 12 h after a single electroconvulsive shock. *J. Neurochem.* 32:495–504, 1979.

33. Vazquez, D. Inhibitors of Protein Biosynthesis. In *Molecular Biology, Biochemistry, and Biophysics,* 30. Berlin: Springer-Verlag, 1979.

*34. Agranoff, B. W. Biochemical Events Mediating the Formation of Short- and Long-Term Memory. In Y. Tsukada and B. W. Agranoff (eds.), *Neurobiological Basis of Learning and Memory.* New York: Wiley, 1980. Pp. 135–147.

35. Neale, J. H., Klinger, P. D., and Agranoff, B. W. Temperature-dependent consolidation of puromycin-susceptible memory in the goldfish. *Behav. Biol.* 9:267–278, 1973.

36. Davis, R. E., and Agranoff, B. W. Stages of memory formation in goldfish: Evidence for an environmental trigger. *Proc. Natl. Acad. Sci. U.S.A.* 55:555–559, 1966.

37. Agranoff, B. W., Burrell, H. R., Dokas, L. A., and Springer, A. D. Progress in Biochemical Approaches to Learning and Memory. In M. A. Lipton, A. Demascio, and K. F. Killam (eds.), *Psychopharmacology: A Generation of Progress.* New York: Raven, 1978. Pp. 623–635.

38. Flexner, J. B., Flexner, L. B., and Stellar, E. Memory in mice as affected by intracerebral puromycin. *Science* 141:57–59, 1963.

39. Rainbow, T. C. Role of RNA and protein synthesis in memory formation. *Neurochem. Res.* 4:297–312, 1979.

40. Barondes, S. H. Cerebral protein synthesis inhibitors block long-term memory. *Int. Rev. Neurobiol.* 12:177–205, 1970.

41. Davis, H. P., and Squire, L. Pharmacology of memory. *Annu. Rev. Pharmacol. and Toxicol.* (In preparation, 1981)

*42. Flood, J. F., and Jarvik, M. E. Drug Influences and Learning and Memory. In M. R. Rosenzweig and E. L. Bennett (eds.), *Neural Mechanisms of Learning and Memory.* Cambridge, Mass.: M.I.T. Press, 1974. Pp. 483–507.

*43. Quartermain, D. The Influence of Drugs on Learning and Memory. In M. R. Rosenzweig and E. L. Bennett (eds.), *Neural Mechanisms of Learning and Memory.* Cambridge, Mass.: M.I.T. Press, 1974. Pp. 508–518.

*44. Gibbs, M. E., and Ng, K. T. Psychobiology of memory: Towards a model of memory formation. *Biobehav. Rev.* 1:113–136, 1977.

45. Agranoff, B. W. Biochemical Concomitants of the Storage of Behavioral Information. In L. Jaenicke (ed.), *Biochemistry of Sensory Functions.* 25 Mosbacher Colloquium der Gesellschaft fur Biologische Chemie. Berlin: Springer-Verlag, 1974. Pp. 597–623.

*46. Dunn, A. J. The Chemistry of Learning and the Formation of Memory. In W. H. Gispen (ed.), *Molecular and Functional Neurobiology. Amsterdam: Elsevier, 1976. Pp. 347–387.* See also Dunn, A. J. Neurochemistry of learning and memory: An evaluation of recent data. *Annu. Rev. Psychol.* 31:343–390, 1980.

47. Deutsch, J. A. The cholinergic synapse and the site of memory. *Science* 174:788–794, 1971.

48. Drachman, D. A. Central Cholinergic System and Memory. In M. A. Lipton, A. Dimascio, and K. F. Killam (eds.), *Psychopharmacology: A Generation of Progress.* New York: Raven, 1978. Pp. 651–662.

49. Zornetzer, S. F. Neurotransmitter Modulation and Memory: A New Neuropharmacological Phrenology? In M. A. Lipton, A. DiMascio, and K. F. Killam (eds.), *Psychopharmacology: A Generation of Progress.* New York: Raven, 1978. Pp. 637–649.

50. DeFeudis, F. U. Environment and central neurotransmitters in relation to learning, memory and behavior. *Gen. Pharmacol.* 10:281–286, 1979.

51. Karpiak, S. E., Graf, L., and Rapport, M. M. Antibodies to G_{M1} ganglioside inhibit a learned avoidance response. *Brain Res.* 151:637–640, 1978.

52. Cherfas, J. J., and Bateson, P. Colchicine impairs performance after learning a one-trial passive avoidance task in day-old chicks. *Behav. Biol.* 23:27–37, 1978.

53. Cronly-Dillon, J., Carden, D., and Birks, C. The possible involvement of brain microtubules in memory fixation. *J. Exp. Biol.* 61:443–454, 1974.

54. Murakami, T. H. Microtubules and Memory Effects of Vinblastine on Avoidance Training. In Y. Tsukada and B. W. Agranoff (eds.), *Neurobiological Basis of Learning and Memory.* New York: Wiley, 1980. Pp. 165–178.

55. Heacock, A. M., and Agranoff, B. W. Enhanced labeling of a retinal protein during regeneration of the optic nerve in goldfish. *Proc. Nat. Acad. Sci. U.S.A.* 73:828–832, 1976.

56. Rose, S. P. R., Sinha, A. K., and Jones-Lecointe, A. Synthesis of tubulin enriched fraction in rat visual cortex is modulated by dark rearing and light exposure. *FEBS Lett.* 65:135–139, 1978.

57. Stewart, M., and Rose, S. P. R. Increased binding of [^{3}H]-colchicine to visual cortex proteins of dark-reared rats on first exposure to light. *J. Neurochem.* 30:595–599, 1978.

58. McGaugh, J. L. Drug facilitation of learning and memory. *Ann. Rev. Pharmacol.* 13:229–241, 1973.

*59. deWied, D. Pituitary Neuropeptides and Behavior. In K. Fuxe, T. Hokfelt, and R. Luft (eds.), *Central Regulation of the Endocrine System.* New York: Plenum, 1979. Pp. 297–314.

60. Bloom, F., Segal, D., Ling, N., and Guillemin, R. Endorphins: Profound behavioral effects in rats suggest new etiological factors in mental illness. *Science* 194:630–632, 1976.

61. Pappenheimer, J. R., Fencl, V., Karnovsky, M. L., and Koski, G. Peptides in Cerebrospinal Fluid and Their Relation to Sleep and Activity. In F. Plum (ed.), *Brain Dysfunction in Metabolic Disorders.* New York: Raven, 1974. Pp. 201–210. Vol. 53, A.R.N.M.D.

62. Ungar, G. Evidence for Molecular Coding of Neural Information. In H. P. Zippel (ed.), *Memory and Transfer of Information.* New York: Plenum, 1973. Pp. 317–341.

63. Squire, L. R., and Barondes, S. H. Amnesic effect of cycloheximide not due to depletion of a constitutive brain protein with short half-life. *Brain Res.* 103:183–189, 1976.

64. Spanis, C. W., and Squire, L. R. Elevation of brain tyrosine by inhibitors of brain protein synthesis is not responsible for their amnestic effect. *Brain Res.* 139:384–388, 1978.

65. Glassman, E. The biochemistry of learning: An evaluation of the role of protein and nucleic acids. *Annu. Rev. Biochem.* 38:605–646, 1969.

66. Shashoua, V. E. Brain protein metabolism and the acquisition of new behaviors. I. Evidence for specific changes in the pattern of protein synthesis. *Brain Res.* 111:347–364, 1976.

67. Benowitz, L. I., and Shashoua, V. E. Localization of a brain protein metabolically linked with behavioral plasticity in the goldfish. *Brain Res.* 136:227–242, 1977.

68. Shashoua, V. E.   RNA changes in goldfish brain during learning. *Nature* 217:238–240, 1968.

69. Lim, R., Davis, G. A., and Agranoff, B. W.   Electrophoretic studies on solubilized proteins of goldfish brain. *Brain Res.* 25:121–131, 1971.

70. Cupello, A., and Hydèn, H.   Studies on RNA metabolism in the nerve cells of hippocampus during training in rats. *Exp. Brain Res.* 31:143–152, 1978.

71. Hydèn, H.   Protein changes in neuronal membranes and synapses during learning. *Biosci. Commun.* 4:185–204, 1978.

*72. Rose, S. P. R., and Haywood, J.   Experience, Learning and Brain Metabolism. In A. N. Davison (ed.), *Biochemical Correlates of Brain Structure*. London: Academic, 1977. Pp. 249–292.

*73. Rose, S. P. R.   Neurochemical Correlates of Early Learning in the Chick. In Y. Tsukada and B. W. Agranoff (eds.), *Neurobiological Basis of Learning and Memory*. New York: Wiley, 1980. Pp. 179–191.

74. Kohsaka, S., Takamatsu, K., Aoki, E., and Tsukada, Y.   Metabolic mapping of chick brain imprinting using [^{14}C]2-deoxyglucose technique. *Brain Res.* 172:539–544, 1979.

75. Goddard, G. V., and Douglas, R. M.   Does the engram of kindling model the engram of normal long term memory? *Can. J. Neurol. Sci.* 2:385–394, 1975.

76. Morrell, F., Tsuru, N., Hoeppner, T. J., Morgan, D., and Harrison, W. H.   Secondary epileptogenesis in frog forebrain; effect of inhibition of protein synthesis. *Can. J. Neurol. Sci.* 2:407–416, 1975.

77. Jonec, V., and Wasterlain, C. G.   Effect of inhibitors of protein synthesis on the development of kindled seizures in rats. *Exp. Neurol.* 66:524–532, 1979.

78. Engel, J., Jr., and Sharpless, N. S.   Long-lasting depletion of dopamine in the rat amygdala induced by kindling stimulation. *Brain Res.* 136:381–386, 1977.

79. McNamara, J. O.   Muscarinic cholinergic receptors participate in the kindling model of epilepsy. *Brain Res.* 154:415–420, 1978.

80. Tryon, R. C.   Genetic differences in maze learning abilities on rats. *Yearbook Nat. Soc. Stud. Educ.* 39 (Part 1):111, 1940.

*81. Oliverio, A.   Genetic and Environmental Factors in Relation to Behavioral Rigidity and Plasticity. In Y. Tsukada and B. W. Agranoff (eds.), *Neurobiological Basis of Learning and Memory*. New York: Wiley, 1980. Pp. 193–212.

82. Mandel, P., Ayad, G., Hermetet, J. C., and Ebel, E.   Correlation between choline acetyltransferase activity and learning ability in different mice strains and their offspring. *Brain Res.* 72:65–70, 1974.

83. Zamenhof, S., Mosley, J., and Schuller, E.   Stimulation of the proliferation of cortical neurons by prenatal treatment with growth hormone. *Science* 152:1396–1397, 1966.

*84. Bennett, E. L.   Cerebral Effects of Differential Experience and Training. In M. R. Rosenzweig and E. L. Bennett (eds.), *Neural Mechanisms of Learning and Memory*. Cambridge, Mass.: M.I.T. Press, 1974. Pp. 279–287.

*85. Greenough, W. T.   Enduring Brain Effects of Differential Experience and Training. In M. R. Rosenzweig and E. L. Bennett (eds.), *Neural Mechanisms of Learning and Memory*. Cambridge, Mass.: M.I.T. Press, 1974. Pp. 255–278.

86. Valverde, F.   Rate and extent of recovery from dark rearing in the visual cortex of the mouse. *Brain Res.* 33:1–11, 1971.

87. Brown, I. R., and Church, R. B.   RNA transcription from nonrepetitive DNA in the mouse. *Biochem. Biophys. Res. Commun.* 42:850–856, 1971.

88. Grouse, L., Omenn, G. A., and McCarthy, B. J.   Studies by DNA-RNA hybridization of transcriptional diversity in human brain. *J. Neurochem.* 20:1063–1073, 1973.

89. Grouse, L. D., Schrier, B. K., Bennett, E. L., Rosenzweig, M. R., and Nelson, P. G.   Sequence diversity studies of rat brain RNA effects of environmental complexity on rat brain RNA diversity. *J. Neurochem.* 30:191–203, 1978.

90. Uy, R., and Wold, F.   Post-translational covalent modification of proteins. *Science* 198:890–896, 1977.

91. Routtenberg, A.   Anatomical localization of phosphoprotein and glycoprotein substrates of memory. *Prog. Neurobiol.* 12:85–113, 1979.

92. Mahler, H. R.   Glycoproteins of the Synapse. In R. U. Margolis and R. K. Margolis (eds.), *Complex Carbohydrates of Nervous Tissue*. New York: Plenum, 1979. Pp. 165–184.

93. Agranoff, B. W., Springer, A. D., and Quarton, G. C.   Biochemistry of Memory and Learning. In P. J. Vinken and G. W. Bruyn (eds.), *Handbook of Clinical Neurology*. Amsterdam: North-Holland, 1976. Vol. 2, pp. 459–476.

94. Nowak, T. S., Jr., and Munro, H. N.   Effects of protein-calorie malnutrition on biochemical aspects of brain development. In R. J. Wurtman and J. J. Wurtman (eds.), *Nutrition and the Brain*. New York: Raven, 1977. Pp. 193–260.

95. Reivich, M., Kuhl, D., Wolf, A., Greenberg, J., Phelps, M., Ido, T., Casella, V., Fowler, J., Hoffman, E., Alavi, A., Som, P., and Sokoloff, L.   The

[^{18}]Fluorodeoxyglucose method for the measurement of local cerebral glucose utilization in man. *Circ. Res.* 44:127–137, 1979.

96. Smith, C. B., Davidsen, L., Deibler, G., Patlak, C., Pettigrew, K., and Sokoloff, L. A method for the determination of local rates of protein synthesis in brain. Eleventh Annual Meeting, American Society for Neurochemistry, Houston, Texas, 1980. Abstract, p. 94.

Glossary

Glossary

AADC	aromatic L-amino-acid decarboxylase	CDR	calcium-dependent regulatory protein; calmodulin
ACh	acetylcholine	Cer	ceramide
AChE	acetylcholinesterase (I) specific for ACh; II is unspecific	CG	chorionic gonadotropin
		ChAT	choline acetyltransferase
AChR	acetylcholine receptor	ChE	cholinesterase (II, unspecific)
ACTH	adrenocorticotropic hormone	CMR	cerebral metabolic rate
ADP	adenosine 5′-diphosphate	CMRGlc	cerebral metabolic rate for glucose
ADTN	2-amino-6,7-dihydroxy-1,2,3,4-tetrahydronaphthalene		
		$CMRO_2$	cerebral metabolic rate for O_2
△-ALA	△-aminolevulinic acid	CNS	central nervous system
△-ALA-S	△-aminolevulinic acid synthetase	CoA	coenzyme A
AMP	adenosine 5′-monophosphate (adenylic acid)	COMT	catechol-O-methyltransferase
		CPK	creatine phosphokinase
AMPT	α-methyl-p-tyrosine	CRF	corticotropin releasing factor
APM	apomorphine	CS	conditioned stimulus
APUD	amine precursor uptake and decarboxylation	CSAD	L-cysteinesulfinic acid decarboxylase (side reaction of aspartate 4-decarboxylase)
ATD	androst-1,4,6-triene-3,17-dione		
		CSF	cerebrospinal fluid
ATP	adenosine 5′-triphosphate	cyclic AMP	adenosine 3′,5′-cyclic phosphate
dATP	deoxyadenosine 5′-triphosphate	cyclic GMP	guanosine 3′,5′-cyclic phosphate
ATPase	adenosine triphosphatase	DA	dopamine
AXM	acetoxycycloheximide	DAO	amine oxidase, pyridoxal containing (diamine oxidase, histaminase)
BAL	British antilewisite (2,3-dimercaptopropanol)		
BB	dimer of creatine phosphokinase in brain (see also MB and MM)	DBH	dopamine β-hydroxylase
		DDC	dopa decarboxylase
BCH	2-aminonorbornane-2-carboxylic acid	DEAE	diethylaminoethyl
		DFP	diisopropylphosphofluoridate
α-BTX	α-bungarotoxin	2-DG	2-deoxy-D-glucose
β-BTX	β-bungarotoxin	DHP	dihydroprogesterone
BTX	batrachotoxin	DHT	dihydrotestosterone
BWSV	black widow spider venom	DMPEA	3,4-dimethoxyphenylethylamine
CAM	cell adhesion molecule	DMT	N,N-dimethyltryptamine
CBF	cerebral blood flow	DNA	deoxyribonucleic acid
CDP	cytidine 5′-diphosphate		

DNP	2,4-dinitrophenol	GTP	guanosine 5'-triphosphate
DON	6-diazo-5-oxo-α-norleucine	GTPase	guanosine triphosphatase
DOPAC	3,4-dihydroxyphenylacetic acid	GTT	glucose tolerance test
DPN	diphosphopyridine nucleotide (see NAD)	HC	hemicholinium (HC-1, etc.)
		HGH	human growth hormone
EAE	experimental allergic encephalo-myelitis	HHH	hypothalamic hypophysiotropic hormone
EAN	experimental allergic neuritis	5-HIAA	5-hydroxyindoleacetic acid
EBP	estrogen-binding protein	HIOMT	hydroxyindole-O-methyl-transferase
ECF	extracellular fluid		
ECS	electroconvulsive shock	HMG-CoA	3-hydroxy-3-methylglutaryl coenzyme A
ECT	electroconvulsive shock therapy		
EDTA	ethylene(dinitrilo)tetraacetic acid (ethylenediaminetetraacetic acid)	HMM	heavy meromyosin
		HMM S-1	heavy meromyosin subfragment 1
EEG	electroencephalogram	hnRNA	heterogeneous nuclear RNA
EGTA	ethyleneglycol-bis-(β-aminoethyl ether)-N,N,N',N'-tetraacetic acid	HPLC	high-performance liquid chromatography
EM	electron microscope (or micro-graph)	HPr	histidine-containing protein
		HRP	horseradish peroxidase
EPP	end-plate potential	5-HT	5-hydroxytryptamine (serotonin)
EP	phosphoenzyme (E_1P,E_2P)	5-HTP	5-hydroxytryptophan
EPSP	excitatory postsynaptic potential	HVA	homovanillic acid (4-hydroxy-3-methoxyphenylacetic acid)
ER	endoplasmic reticulum		
FAD	flavin-adenine dinucleotide	IAA	iodoacetic acid
fEBP	fetoneonatal estrogen-binding protein	IF	intermediate filaments
		IMP	inosine 5'-monophosphate
FH$_4$	tetrahydrofolic acid	IP	intraperitoneal
FSH	follicle-stimulating hormone	IPSP	inhibitory postsynaptic potential
GABA	γ-aminobutyric acid	ITT	insulin tolerance test
GABA-T	GABA:α-oxoglutarate trans-aminase	IV	intravenous
		K$^+$-pNPPase	K$^+$-stimulated p-nitrophenyl-phosphatase; phosphatase function of the (Na$^+$ + K$^+$)-ATPase
GAD	glutamic acid decarboxylase		
GAPD	glyceraldehyde 3-phosphate dehydrogenase		
		KA	kainic acid
GDP	guanosine 5'-diphosphate	LH	luteinizing hormone
GFAP	glial fibrillary acidic protein	LHRF	luteinizing hormone-releasing factor
GFP	glial filament protein		
GH	growth hormone	LHRH	luteinizing hormone-releasing hormone (same as LHRF)
GHRF	growth hormone-releasing factor		
Gln synth	glutamine synthetase	LMM	light meromyosin
GMP	guanosine 5'-monophosphate (guanylic acid)	β-LPH	β-lipotropin
		LSD	D-lysergic acid diethylamide, lysergide (also LSD-25)
GPDH	glycerol 3-phosphate dehydro-genase		
		LTM	long-term memory
GSH	growth-stimulating hormone; also, reduced glutathione	MAG	myelin-associated glycoprotein

MAO	monoamine oxidase (MAO-A, MAO-B) amine oxidase, flavin containing	OLDP	β-N-oxalyl-L-α, β-diaminopropionic acid
MAP	microtubule-associated protein	OMP	orotidine 5′-monophosphate
MB	hybrid dimer of creatine phosphokinase (see BB and MM)	PAGE	polyacrylamide gel electrophoresis
MEPP	miniature end-plate potential	2-PAM	pyridine-2-aldoxime methiodide
MER-25	ethamoxytriphelol	PAP	peroxidase-antiperoxidase complex used in an immunocytochemical method
MER-29	tripananol		
MET	metanephrine		
MF	microfilament	PAPS	3′-phosphoadenosine 5′-phosphosulfate
MG	myasthenia gravis		
MHPG	3-methoxy-4-hydroxyphenylglycol	PEA	phenylethylamine
		PFK	phosphofructokinase
MIF	migration inhibition factor; also see MSH-IF	PG	prostaglandin
		P_i	inorganic phosphate
MIF_1	see MSH-IF	PIF	prolactin inhibitory factor
MLD	metachromatic leukodystrophy	PML	progressive multifocal leukoencephalopathy
MM	dimer of creatine phosphokinase found in muscle (see BB and MM)	PMSG	pregnant mare serum gonadotropin
MPS	mucopolysaccharide, glycosoaminoglycan (also mucopolysaccharidosis)	PNMT	phenylethanolamine-N-methyltransferase
		PNS	peripheral nervous system
MS	multiple sclerosis	PSD	postsynaptic density
MSH	melanocyte stimulating hormone	$Pt-H_4$	tetrahydrobiopterin
MSH-IF	melanocyte-stimulating hormone release-inhibiting factor	$Pt-H_2$	dihydrobiopterin
		PTH	parathyroid hormone
MT	microtubule	Q_{10}	ratio of reaction rate at one temperature to the rate of the same reaction at 10°C lower
5-MTHF	5-methyltetrahydrofolic acid		
NAD^+	oxidized nicotinamide-adenine dinucleotide	REM	rapid eye movement [stage of sleep]
NADH	reduced nicotinamide-adenine dinucleotide	RER	rough endoplasmic reticulum
		RIA	radioimmunoassay
$NADP^+$	oxidized nicotinamide-adenine dinucleotide phosphate	RMP	resting membrane potential
		RNA	ribonucleic acid
NADPH	reduced nicotinamide-adenine dinucleotide phosphate	mRNA	messenger RNA
		tRNA	transfer ribonucleic acid
NANA	see Neu-NAc	RQ	respiratory quotient
NE	norepinephrine	SAM	S-adenosylmethionine
NEM	N-ethylmaleimide	SC	slow components [of axonal transport (SCa,SCb)]
Neu-NAc	N-acetylneuraminic acid		
NF	neurofilament	SDS	sodium dodecylsulfate
NFP	neurofilament protein	SDS-PAGE	sodium dodecylsulfate-polyacrylamide gel electrophoresis
NGF	nerve growth factor		
6-OHDA	6-hydroxydopamine	SER	smooth endoplasmic reticulum

SHMT	serine hydroxymethyltransferase	TLCK	N-α-t-tosyl-L-lysinechloromethyl ketone
SR-ATPase	ATPase of the sarcoplasmic reticulum	TnT, TnC, TnI	protein components of troponin
SSADH	succinate-semialdehyde dehydrogenase	TPN	triphosphopyridine nucleotide (see NADP)
SSPE	subacute sclerosing panencephalitis	TPZ	thioproperazine
STM	short-term memory	TRF *or* TRH	thyrotropin-releasing factor (or hormone)
STX	saxitoxin	TSH	thyroid-stimulating hormone
T_3	triiodothyronine	TTX	tetrodotoxin
T_4	thyroxine	UCS	unconditioned stimulus
TBX, TBXA$_1$	thromboxane, thromboxane A$_1$	UDP	uridine 5′-diphosphate
TCA	tricarboxylic acid	UMP	uridine 5′-monophosphate
TEC	triethylcholine	UTP	uridine 5′-triphosphate
TH	tyrosine hydroxylase	VCR	vincristine
THC	l-Δ^9-tetrahydrocannabinol (also referred to as l-Δ^1-THC)	VDS	vindesine
		VIP	vasoactive intestinal polypeptide
Thy-1	[also] theta (ϕ) antigen; alloantigen present on surface of most thymocytes and peripheral T lymphocytes	VLB	vinblastine
		VMA	vanillylmandelic acid

Index

Index